SCHOOL NURSING:
A Comprehensive Text

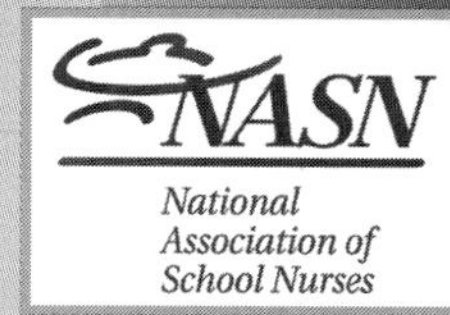

SCHOOL NURSING: A Comprehensive Text

Janice Selekman, DNSc, RN *Editor*

Professor
University of Delaware
Newark, Delaware

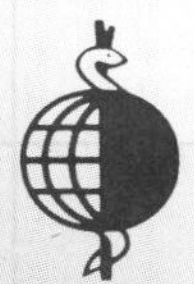

F.A. DAVIS COMPANY • Philadelphia

F. A. Davis Company
1915 Arch Street
Philadelphia, PA 19103
www.fadavis.com

Printed in the United States of America

Last digit indicates print number: 10 9 8 7 6

Acquisitions Editor: Joanne Patzek DaCunha, RN, MSN
Developmental Editor: Kristin L. Kern
Art and Design Manager: Carolyn O'Brien

As new scientific information becomes available through basic and clinical research, recommended treatments and drug therapies undergo changes. The author(s) and publisher have done everything possible to make this book accurate, up to date, and in accord with accepted standards at the time of publication. The author(s), editors, and publisher are not responsible for errors or omissions or for consequences from application of the book, and make no warranty, expressed or implied, in regard to the contents of the book. Any practice described in this book should be applied by the reader in accordance with professional standards of care used in regard to the unique circumstances that may apply in each situation. The reader is advised always to check product information (package inserts) for changes and new information regarding dose and contraindications before administering any drug. Caution is especially urged when using new or infrequently ordered drugs.

Library of Congress Cataloging-in-Publication Data

School nursing : a comprehensive text / edited by Janice Selekman.
p. ; cm.
Includes bibliographical references and index.
ISBN 10: 0-8036-1403-9 ISBN 13: 978-0-8036-1403-1
1. School nursing.
[DNLM: 1. School Nursing. WY 113 S3724 2005] I. Selekman, Janice.
RJ247.S34 2005
371.7'12–dc22 2005053756

TO LINDA, *who restarted this project and was my chief cheerleader;*

TO YETTA AND SONNY, *who gave me life and unconditional love;*

TO AARON, REBECCA, AND DANIEL, *who gave me purpose and give me pride;*

AND TO TRACY *AND* JENNIFER *who love them;*

TO JUSTIN, KATLYN, BRIAN, EMILY, HEATHER, AND EMMA, *who give me joy;*

To all of them, with love

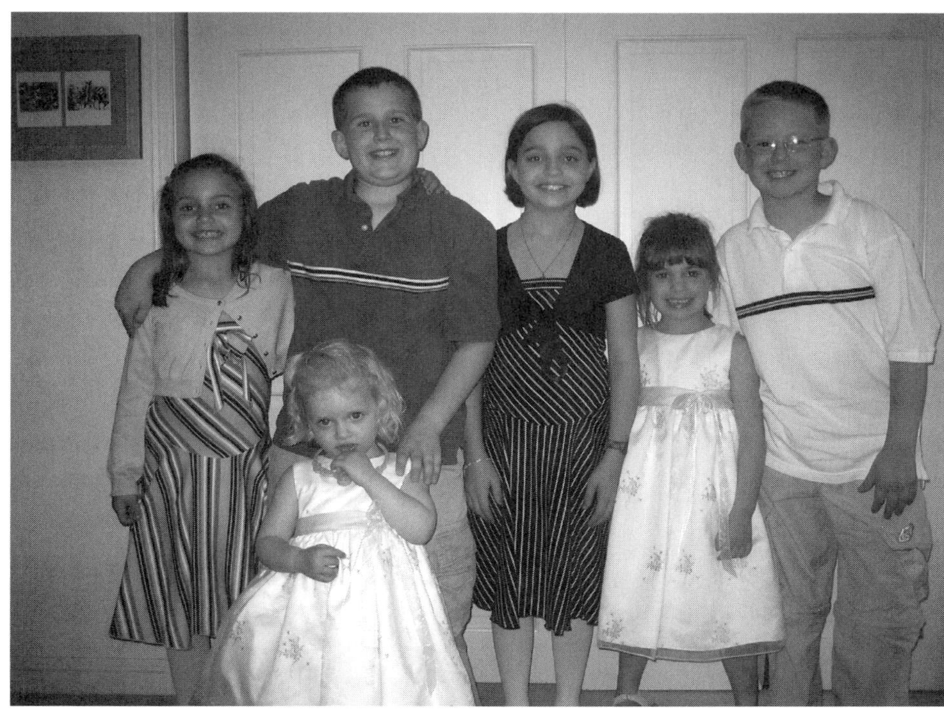

Contributors

Susan Adams, MSN, RN
Former School Nurse
Bennett Community School District, Iowa
Doctoral Student, University of Iowa

Jill Asprey, MA, RN, ARNP
Pediatric Nurse Practitioner
Cedar Rapids Community School District
Cedar Rapids, Iowa

Charlotte D. Barry, PhD, RN, NCSN
Associate Professor
Christine E. Lynn College of Nursing
Florida Atlantic University
Boca Raton, Florida

Janet Sobey Bubert, Esquire
Associate
Bracewell and Patterson LLP
Dallas, Texas

Daryl Canham, EdD, RN, BC
Associate Professor
San Jose State University
San Jose, California

Jayne Chatterton, BSN, RN, CDE
Licensed School Nurse
Certified Diabetes Educator
St. Paul, Minnesota

Mariann Cosby, MPA, MSN, RN, PHN, CEN, LNCC, CCM
Nurse Consultant
California Department of Health Services
Maternal Child Health Branch
Sacramento, California

Carol Costante, MA, RN, NCSN, FNASN
Specialist, Office of Health Services
Baltimore County Public Schools
Baltimore, Maryland
Past President, National Association of School Nurses

Linda Davis-Alldritt, MA, RN, PHN, FNASN
School Nurse Consultant
California Department of Education
Sacramento, California

Janice Denehy, PhD, RN
Associate Professor Emeritus
University of Iowa
College of Nursing
Iowa City, Iowa
Executive Editor, *Journal of School Nursing*

Elizabeth Dietz, EdD, RN, CS-NP
Professor/Nurse Practitioner
San Jose State University
San Jose, California

Michelle Ficca, DNSc, RN
Associate Professor
Bloomsburg University of Pennsylvania
Bloomsburg, Pennsylvania

Betty Fitzpatrick, MS, RN, SNP
Nurse Practitioner
Retired School Nurse
Jefferson County, Colorado
Hospice Nurse
Palm Beach County, Florida

Michael Gamel-McCormick, PhD
Director, Center for Disability Studies
University of Delaware
Newark, Delaware

Gloria Gelmann, PhD, EdD, RN, APN-C
Associate Professor
Director of the Masters of School Nursing Program
Seton Hall University
South Orange, New Jersey

Shirley C. Gordon, PhD, RN, NCSN
Associate Professor
Christine E. Lynn College of Nursing
Florida Atlantic University
Boca Raton, Florida

Margaret Clark Graham, PhD, MSN, CRNP
Professor
Wright State University
Dayton, Ohio

Carol Gray, MSN, CFNP
Nurse Practitioner
Asthma and Allergy Care of Delaware
Newark, Delaware

Elizabeth K. Gregory, PhD, RN, NCSN, FNASN
Retired School Nurse Consultant
Harris County Department of Education
Houston, Texas

Patricia Guilday, MSN, RN, NCSN
School Nurse
Brandywine School District
Wilmington, Delaware

Julie Henderson, MSN, RNC, SN
School Nurse
Camden Board of Education
Camden, New Jersey

Jan Hootman, PhD, RN, NCSN
Supervisor, Multnomah Education Service District
Portland, Oregon
Past President, National Association of School Nurses

Laura Jannone, EdD, RN, CSN
Assistant Professor
Coordinator of the School Nursing Program
Marjorie K. Unterberg School of Nursing
Monmouth University
West Long Branch, New Jersey

Ritamarie John, DrNP, MSN, CPNP
PNP Program Director
Columbia University School of Nursing
New York, New York

Tara Kaup, MSN, RN, CDE
Licensed School Nurse
St. Paul Public Schools
St. Paul, Minnesota

Lynn E. Kelly, PhD, RN, CSN
Associate Professor
Widener University
Chester, Pennsylvania

Jeanne Kiefner, MEd, RNC, FNASN
Adjunct Professor
Rowan University
Glassboro, New Jersey

Barbara Krivda, BSN, RN, SCN
School Nurse
Mercer County Special Services School District
Mercer County, New Jersey

Kathleen Ryan Kuntz, MSN, RN, CRRN, CLCP, Cm
President
Rehab Advantage Inc.
Doylestown, Pennsylvania

Ruth Ellen Luehr, MS, RN, FNASN
School Health/Student Services Specialist
Minnesota Department of Education
Roseville, Minnesota

Marilyn Marcontel-Shattuck, MA, BSN, NCSN, CNA, FNASN
School Nurse Consultant
Former Director of Health Services
Dallas Independent School District
Dallas, Texas

Elizabeth Mattey, MSN, RN, NCSN
School Nurse
Mount Pleasant High School
Brandywine School District
Wilmington, Delaware

Donna J. Mazyck, MS, RN, NCSN, NCC
School Health Services Specialist
Maryland State Department of Education
Baltimore, Maryland
President-Elect, National Association of School Nurses

Ann Marie McCarthy, PhD, RN, FAAN
Professor
Director of Doctoral Program of Nursing
University of Iowa
Iowa City, Iowa

Sandra McHenry, DNSc, RN
Associate Professor
Chair, Department of Special Educational Services/Instruction
Rowan University
Glassboro, New Jersey

Carole E. Moore, BSN, RN, NCSN
School Nurse
Grace School
Houston, Texas
President, Texas School Nurses Organization

Carol Murphy Moore, MSN, RN, CRNP
Assistant Professor
Bloomsburg University of Pennsylvania
Bloomsburg, Pennsylvania

Nancy W. Mosca, PhD, RN
Professor
Coordinator, School Nurse Program
Youngstown State University
Youngstown, Ohio

Berit Peterson, MPH, RN
Health Services Coordinator
Edina Independent School District
Edina, Minnesota

Susan G. Praeger, EdD, APRN, BC, FNASN
Professor of Nursing
Director of School Nurse Program
College of Nursing and Health
Wright State University
Dayton, Ohio

Susan Proctor, DNS, MPH, RN, FNASN
Professor Emeritus
Former Coordinator of School Nursing
California State University
Sacramento, California
Past Executive Editor, *Journal of School Nursing*

Marie Renzi, MSN, RN, CEN
Coordinator, Delaware Division of Public Health
Nemours/A.I. Dupont Hospital for Children
Emergency Medical Services for Children
Wilmington, Delaware

Kathleen Riley-Lawless, PhD, RN, APRN, BC
Assistant Professor
University of Delaware
Advanced Practice Nurse
Nemours/A.I. Dupont Hospital for Children
Wilmington, Delaware

Maria Rivera (Klein)-Matza, MSN, RNC
District School Nurse
West Covina Unified School District
West Covina, California

Leatha Ross, MS, CRNP
Clinical Instructor
Wright State University
Dayton, Ohio

Lynn Rossi-Scott, Esquire
Partner
Bracewell and Patterson LLP
Dallas, Texas

Janice Selekman, DNSc, RN
Professor
University of Delaware
Newark, Delaware

Rebecca Silver, MEd, RN
Adjunct Professor
Rowan University
Glassboro, New Jersey
Executive Director, New Jersey State School Nurse Organization

Mary A. Swanson, MS, RN, LSN
Licensed School Nurse
Robbinsdale Area Schools
Plymouth, Minnesota

Elizabeth L. Thomas, MEd, RN, NCSN
School Health Coordinator
Christina School District
Wilmington, Delaware

Judith Vessey, PhD, MBA, CRNP, FAAN
Lelia Holden Carroll Professor in Nursing
Boston College
Boston, Massachusetts

Linda C. Wolfe, MEd, BSN, RN, NCSN
Education Specialist, Health Services
Delaware Department of Education
Dover, Delaware
Past President, National Association of School Nurses

Donna Zaiger, BSN, RN, NCSN, FNASN
School Nurse
Lee's Summit R-7 School District
Kansas City, Missouri
Past President, National Association of School Nurses

Barbara Zimmerman, DNSc, CNS, RN
Associate Professor
Millersville University
Millersville, Pennsylvania

Reviewers

Margaret Barry, BSN, MEd, NCSN, FNASN
School Nurse
Wuerzburg Elementary School
Wuerzburg, Germany

Martha Dewey Bergren, DNSc, MS, RN
Clinical Assistant Professor
University of Illinois at Chicago
College of Nursing
Chicago, Illinois

Joan Blair, MSN, RN, APRN-BC
Pediatric Nurse Practitioner
Nemours/A.I. Dupont Children's Hospital
Wilmington, Delaware

Nicole Bobo, MSN, RN
Nursing Education Director
National Association of School Nurses
Castle Rock, Colorado

Elizabeth Y. Boone, RN, CSN
Certified School Nurse
Pennridge School System
Perkasie, Pennsylvania

Terry Clark, BS, RN, NCSN
School Nurse
Ironwood Ridge High School
Tucson, Arizona

Carol Gordon Cox, MS, MPH, RN, CS
Professor Emeritus
East Carolina University
Greenville, North Carolina

Sandra Delack, MEd, RN, CSNT
School Nurse Teacher
Health Services Coordinator
Sarah Dyer Barnes Elementary School
Johnston, Rhode Island

Suzey Delger, MSN, RN, FNP-C
Nursing Coordinator
Natrona County School District
Casper, Wyoming

Jacalyn Dougherty, PhD, RN
Project Manager for Asthma Grant
National Association of School Nurses
Castle Rock, Colorado

Janice Doyle, MSN, RN
Nurse Specialist
Bethel School District
Graham, Washington

William Geimeier, MD
Asthma and Allergy Care of Delaware
Newark, Delaware

Margie Golden, BSN, RN
Bureau Director
School Nursing/Public Health Nursing
Utah County Health Department
Provo, Utah

Beverly Hine, MPH, RN, NCSN
Health Services and Medical Director
Las Cruces Public Schools
Las Cruces, New Mexico

Carol Hinton, MS, RN, CSN
Adolescent and School Health
Des Moines, Iowa

Gail Houck, PhD, RN
OHSU School of Nursing
Portland, Oregon

India Husch, PhD, RNC, CDDN
School Nurse
School Health Services
Beckley, West Virginia

Martha Ide, BSN, RN, NCSN
School Nurse
Barre Town Middle and Elementary School
Barre, Vermont

Virginia Incerpi, BA, RN, NCSN
Former School Nurse/Health Educator
Danville School District
Danville, Vermont

Christina Jackson, PhD, APRN, BC, HNC, CSN
Assistant Professor of Nursing
Eastern University
St. David, Pennsylvania

Mitzi Johnson, MSN, RN
Continuing Education Director
National Association of School Nurses
Castle Rock, Colorado

Veronica Kane, PhD, RN, CPNP
Assistant Clinical Professor
MGH Institute of Health Professions
Boston, Massachusetts

Marilyn Kinne, MA, RN, CSNP
Staff
National Association of School Nurses
Castle Rock, Colorado

Kathryn Kolar, PhD, RN, CS-PNP
Professor
Director, Johnson Elementary School Based Health Clinic
University of Mississippi
Jackson, Mississippi

Paul Kravitz, MD
Fairfax, Virginia

Laura Mason, RN
Charge Nurse
Havergal College
Toronto, Ontario

Erin Maughan, PhD(c), RN
Instructor
Brigham Young University
Provo, Utah

Pauline Menger, MHEd, BSN, RN
Adjunct Faculty
Immaculata University
Immaculata, Pennsylvania

Wanda Miller, MA, RN, NCSN, FNASN
Executive Director
National Association of School Nurses
Castle Rock, Colorado

Jean Norris, MSN, RN
School Nurse Administrator
Hoover City School District
Birmingham, Alabama

Katherine Pohlman, JD, MS, RN
Attorney
Minneapolis, Minnesota

Phyllis Powel Pelt, MS, RN
Director of School Nurse Certificate Program
University of Illinois at Chicago
Chicago, Illinois

Kathleen Rose-Grippa, PhD, RN
Professor
Coordinator, School Nurse Program
Ohio University School of Nursing
Athens, Ohio

Janie Sailors, BSN, RN, NCSN
Health Specialist
Bowling Green, Kentucky

Jan Sanderson, MST, BSN, RN
Multnomah Education Service District
Portland, Oregon

Janet Shackelford, BSN, RN, NCSN
Retired School Nurse
Boise, Idaho

Barbara Smith, MPH, MEd, RN
School Nurse Consultant
Oklahoma State Department of Health
Coordinated School Health Program
Oklahoma City, Oklahoma

James Stoycheff
School Psychologist
Waterloo, Iowa

Mary Ann Strawhacker, MPH, BSN, RN
Special Educator
Nurse Consultant
Johnston, Iowa

Jayme Thomson, RN
Supervisor
Multnomah Education Service District
Portland, Oregon

Judith Vessey, PhD, MBA, CRNP, FAAN
Lelia Holden Carroll Professor in Nursing
Boston College
Boston, Massachusetts

Elaine Taboskey Wade, MEd, RN, NCSN, FNASN
Director School Nursing Program
NCH Healthcare System
Naples Community Hospital
Naples, Florida
Past President, National Association of School Nurses

Lynne B. Walsh, EdD, RN, C-FNP
Dean, Professor
College of Nursing and Health Professionals
Marshall University
Huntington, West Virginia

Martha Witt, MEd, RN
School Nurse
Poland, Ohio

Contents

PART I

Foundations of Professional School Nursing

PART II

Roles and Functions of the School Nurse

PART III

Legal Concerns

PART IV

The Well Child: Preschool, School Age, and Adolescent

PART V

Episodic Illnesses of School Children

PART VI

Chronic Conditions of School Children

PART VII

Acting Out and High-Risk Behaviors

PART VIII

Health Services Management

PART I

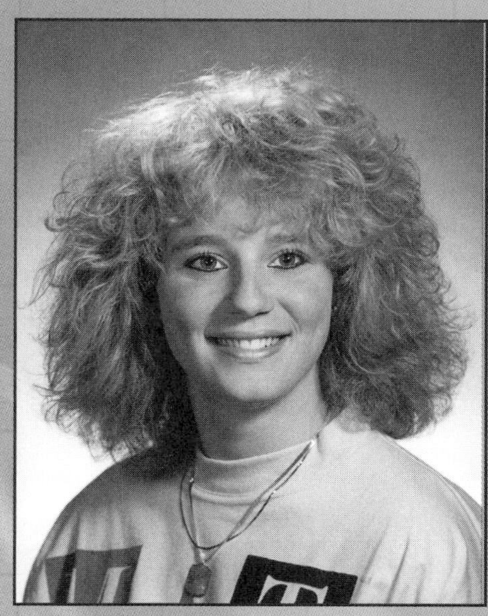

Foundations of Professional School Nursing

Chapter 1

Historical Perspectives of School Nursing

DONNA ZAIGER

Chapter Outline

INTRODUCTION

History tends to make us humble. It often shows us that what we think is original is only repetition of what has been done before. It shows us how our predecessors struggled with problems almost exactly like those that we meet. It lets us see that the conditions under which they worked are often like those of today; that their methods were not wholly unlike ours; and that even their results resembled ours, and were no less conspicuous than those that we laud as remarkable (Goodnow, 1948, p. vii).

The development of school nursing services parallels events and developments in society. Before 1900, most health care was delivered in the home and community. The home was the place where babies were born, old folks died, and the injured and ill were provided care by the family. As society moved from agrarian communities to densely populated industrialized cities, public health issues surfaced. Attempts were made by public officials to address the situations in factories and in the community. With the establishment of compulsory education, concerns about sanitation and disease related to children became prevalent. School health programs were developed. Nurses assisted physicians with inspections and examinations, provided direct care and health education in school and in the home, and made referrals to other community agencies.

The further development of the industrial movement and the establishment of hospitals started moving some aspects of health care from the home to a more physician-oriented environment, with less family and community involvement. Health care focused on identification and treatment of disease and disabilities. During the second quarter of the 20th century, most nurses assisted physicians in caring for patients in hospitals. School nurses assisted physicians with physical examinations and record keeping. This task-oriented practice resulted in less opportunity to promote wellness (Randle, 1944; Wold, 1981; Zaiger, 2000).

Over the decades of the past century, school health services varied widely from state to state and from district to district. Lack of consistency in program expectations promoted role confusion among the nurses, the nursing profession, public health agencies, and educational entities. Each group envisioned the role of the nurse in the school setting from its own perspective. As the programs developed, the confusion over role definition became more evident. Was the nurse a nurse, a teacher, or a nurse-teacher combination? Some states and individual school systems maintained or developed strong school health programs. Students in other districts had no access to a school nurse. In the 1990s, the health care delivery focus moved back to the home and community with an increase in home health agencies providing care. Children returned to school sooner from illnesses and injuries. Children with chronic conditions requiring nursing care were enrolled in public schools. As the 21st century began, the school nurse's role once again included direct services, program planning and management, health education, and integration with the community as the focus of practice (Lordi, 2000).

Those in school nursing practice today share a common bond with the visionary women of action who paved the way to the school door and who have practiced throughout this past century. In a review of school nursing literature, common threads continually reappear: the role of the nurse in an educational setting (public health nurse assigned to schools, nurses employed by an educational agency, nurse-teacher, etc.), the preparation needed to practice school nursing, the need to see the child as an individual, and the importance of the nurse's involvement as a health care provider in the school and in the community at large (Axelson, 1944; Ayling & Johnson, 1949; Brainard, 1922/1985; Hawkins, Hayes, & Cortliss, 1994; Lordi, 2000). School nursing role perception and educational preparation are ongoing dialogues in literature and the workplace. Frustration regarding funding scarcities and challenges in meeting the increasing demands for services continue. However, these are coupled with excitement about ongoing opportunities to participate in shaping the health and educational success of students through delivery of school-, community-, and family-based health systems.

History and the interpretation of history have an impact on today and the future. By examining the evolution of school nursing from early nursing history and especially from its roots in public health, today's practitioner will appreciate the vision and dedication of the early pioneers. Nursing leaders of the past century provided words of wisdom and works of distinction that are worthy of reflection. The lessons learned from history will support leaders today and provide a vision for the future. The historical perspective encourages seasoned practitioners to engage in professional self-renewal to meet the challenging opportunities of providing services to the school community in the 21st century.

PUBLIC HEALTH NURSING EMERGES FROM EARLY NURSING HISTORY

Early nursing in Europe, from the first decade of the 1st century, was heavily influenced by religion and politics. Public health concerns to prevent disease—especially waste disposal, water and food sanitation, and burial of the dead—and segregating the sick have been in place for thousands of years; the practice of visiting the sick to look after the physical, emotional, psychological, and social well-being of others is a commandment from the old testament (Selekman, 2003). School nursing is an outgrowth of public health nursing, which has its roots in the very early Christian deaconesses' work, as well as modern nursing based on special training and educational preparation. The deaconess's movement of 2000 years ago provided visits to the homes of those who were sick or in need of other assistance. Lay deaconesses provided Christian service. Their focus "was to relieve suffering, not to prevent or cure disease" (Woodfill & Beyrer, 1991, p. 1). By the 5th century, care was provided in the early hospitals and in the community by religious nursing orders. The sisters had training in nursing and social work practices. The influence of religion on the care of the sick declined during the Reformation, with the control of hospitals falling into the hands of government officials (Goodnow, 1943). "Graft and mismanagement were rampant, patients were exploited and neglected, living and working conditions were generally deplorable and moral conditions were at a low ebb" (Steward, 1943, p. 24). Both the quality of care and the quality of the caregiver declined.

Fictional European literature and accounts in nursing history describe nursing as an undesirable occupation. The average nurse lacked both skills and morals. Charles Dickens' character, Sairey Gamp, was depicted as a woman given to habitual drunkenness and indifference to her patients, and one who actually enjoyed deathbed scenes (Goodnow, 1943). "The secular nurse was illiterate, heavy-handed, venal, and over-worked. She divided her time between housework, laundry, scrubbing, and a pretense at nursing of the most rough and ready kind.... Strong drink (was) her refuge from the drudgery of her life" (Dock & Stewart, 1938, p. 98).

Nursing began emerging from this dark time in the mid-1800s with the vision, leadership, and determination of Florence Nightingale. "Although Florence Nightingale's accomplishments are many, one of the most important was the establishment in London of the first fully endowed and therefore independent school of nursing in 1860" (Wold & Dagg, 1981, p. 4). Nurses educated nurses. This set the foundation for the independent practice of nursing as an autonomous professional discipline. Trained nurses provided disease prevention information and care for the ill in the community and in schools. Their work gave birth to the specialty of public health nursing.

Early in the 19th century, absenteeism was high in European schools and factories. Officials in government, schools, and businesses looked for ways to curb the conditions that kept children and their parents away from school and work. Illness was quickly identified as the main reason for the absences. Health conditions were recognized as a public issue, not just an individual condition.

Public health is broader than solely nursing services, but nursing emerged as the one discipline that could address health concerns effectively with the family, the school, and the community. "From the standpoint of nursing history, the doctrines of Florence Nightingale mark the turning point from visiting nursing to public health nursing. Nightingale established nursing as a profession with two missions: sick nursing and health nursing" (Woodfill & Beyrer, 1991, p. 2).

By the middle of the 19th century, both religious orders and secular nurses were providing care for the sick in hospitals. After hospital training, those wishing to become district nurses in public health completed additional training in the field under the supervision of a district superintendent, followed by more formalized courses for the purpose of upgrading standards of education and practice. Organized public health agencies sent district nurses into homes of the sick poor. These district nurses provided care for the sick and preventive teaching with a special emphasis on asepsis (Goodnow, 1943; Steward, 1943; Wold & Dagg, 1981; Woodfill & Beyer, 1991).

INITIATION OF SCHOOL HEALTH PROGRAMS IN EUROPE

Medical Inspections

France led the way in school health. By 1837, the French had instituted ordinances that mandated the supervision of schoolchildren's health and mandated that school authorities enforce sanitary conditions. In 1874, Brussels, Belgium, became the first city to establish a citywide system of school inspections conducted by school physicians (Gardner, 1936) (Figure 1.1).

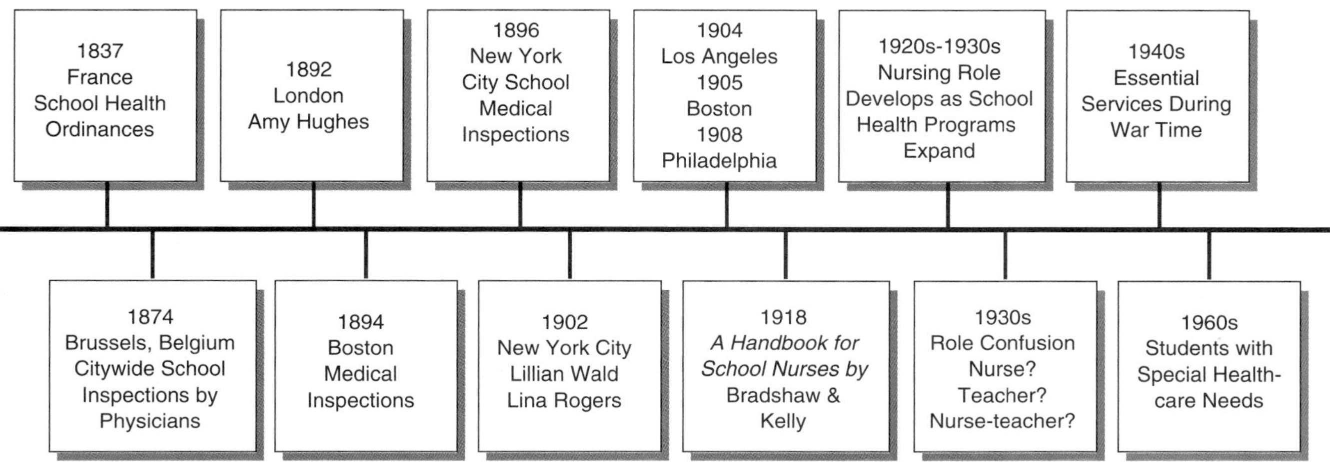

Figure 1.1 ■ Time line for school health programs and nursing services.

Nursing Services

A decade after elementary education became compulsory in England, around 1880, sickness was identified as the chief cause of absenteeism; illness was believed to originate from neglect of care for the children's minor ailments and injuries (Pavey, 1953). Visiting nurses did volunteer work in schools in London and Liverpool. Miss Honnor Morton, a nurse and a London School Board member, urged employment of nurses who would go into schools to provide care and follow-up for children from families they had identified as having some contagious condition (Kelly & Bradshaw, 1918). In 1891, at the International Congress of Hygiene and Demography, Dr. Malcolm Morris gave as his opinion that "a staff of specially educated nurses should visit the elementary school regularly to inspect the children" (Brainard, 1922/1985, p. 263). Amy Hughes, Superintendent of Queen's Nurses in Bloomsbury Square, made daily visits to a school with the poorest and most neglected children in London (see Figure 1.1). The purpose of the visits was to investigate the nutritional status of students, to attend to minor ailments of children in school before they became serious, and to provide follow-up care with home visits. The positive effects of her efforts were recognized. However, the London school officials were reluctant to fund the services.

Within 5 years, the London School Nurse Society was formed as a private charity. The subscriptions (contributions) to the society were not nearly sufficient to meet the requests from schools for school nursing services. The society was able to supply only five nurses to the 500 elementary schools in London. Even in limited numbers, these nurses continued to make such a significant difference and so thoroughly demonstrated their usefulness in decreasing absenteeism that the work was taken over by the London County Council in 1904, allowing the underfunded London School Nurse Society to disband (Brainard, 1922/1985; Pavey, 1953).

INITIATION OF SCHOOL HEALTH SERVICES IN THE UNITED STATES

Medical Inspections

In the United States in 1894, Boston became the first city to utilize physicians to conduct medical inspection of children in school. The goal of these programs was to identify and exclude students with serious communicable diseases such as scarlet fever, diphtheria, pertussis, varicella, and mumps. This service was broadened to include parasitic diseases such as scabies, impetigo, and ringworm (Gardner, 1924; Struthers, 1917) (see Figure 1.1).

In 1896, medical inspections were initiated in New York City. The Department of Health hired 150 doctors to spend 1 hour a day inspecting schoolchildren. Children identified with contagious conditions were sent home. Where the medical inspections were consistent and thorough, classrooms were nearly vacant. Often 15 to 20 children were excluded daily. "In a single school, 300 children were out at one time" (Rogers, 1905, p. 766). Typically, there was no treatment or follow-up care after these school-based physician medical inspections. The focus of these programs was on exclusion (Struthers, 1917). If a child was sent home, it was unlikely that he or she would return.

Education was compulsory in New York City schools by 1900. Children came from homes where parents were often unable to speak or write English, few homes had telephones, and there was a lack of regular medical care. Children coming from tenements exhibited conditions associated with crowded, unsanitary conditions: scabies, ringworm, impetigo, conjunctivitis, and pediculosis. Children were still in the neighborhoods, if not in school. Thus, contagious disease continued to spread (Pavey, 1953). By 1918, twenty-six states had laws requiring medical inspections in school (Kelly & Bradshaw, 1918).

Nursing Services in the Community

In the 1880s, hospital training schools in America were developed to prepare young women in the art of nursing. Lillian Wald was a socially conscious, self-assured woman from a well-to-do Jewish family. In 1891, Miss Wald graduated from the New York Hospital School of Nursing. Shortly after graduation, she experienced an awakening to human needs through an emergency call to the East Side. She decided to become a resident and active participant in the civic and spiritual growth of this community, where 90% of ill patients never entered a hospital (Pennock, 1940).

Miss Wald focused her entire career on relieving the abominable living and working conditions for foreign-born and rural American immigrants living in the tenement sections of New York City's East Side. She established the Henry Street Settlement to address the issues of poverty, homelessness, substandard housing, and lack of primary health care. From the Henry Street Settlement, health care and social services were delivered to those living in the surrounding community. Miss Wald maintained social connections and developed political savvy, necessary components of fund raising for the support of the settlement house work. She is credited with coining the phase "public health nurse." "It was her goal to make it known to the public that the public health nurse was their nurse" (Ohlsom & Wood, 1999, p. 26).

From the opening of the settlement in 1893, she received cooperation from the New York City health officials. The nurses maintained records on the children they encountered who were out of school. They tried to determine the reason for the child's absence. When possible, the nurses provided care or assisted parents in obtaining care. Lillian Wald had read an account of the London experiment that was published in the *American Journal of Nursing* in 1901 (Goodnow, 1948; Hawkins et al., 1994). Miss Wald met with the chairman of the New York Board of Education and the city's health commissioner. The article, along with the documentation collected by the nurses, supported her recommendation that nurses actually treat the children in the schools and make follow-up visits to the homes of those excluded from classes by the medical inspections.

The Month-Long Project in the New York City Schools

Lina Rogers, a young nurse working at the Henry Street Settlement, was chosen to pioneer the New York month-long project that started on October 1, 1902 (see Figure 1.1). The four schools with the greatest number of medical exclusions and highest absenteeism were chosen for the project. They were Public Schools 12, 17, and 147 and a parochial school on Madison Street. The enrollment of these four schools was 8671. During the month, she visited each school for 1 hour each school day. Miss Rogers worked in the space available with only limited supplies and equipment (Hawkins et al., 1994; Rogers, 1905; Struthers, 1917).

In school No. 12, an unused stair closet was the only available space for a dispensary, and, although the nurse could not stand erect here, there was sufficient room to store supplies. In front of an adjacent window, a radiator did duty as a dressing table (Struthers, 1917, p. 19). In another school, the dispensary was in the basement playground, where the nurse used the windowsills as dressing tables (p. 20).

Miss Rogers cleaned and dressed wounds and treated mild cases of conjunctivitis and minor skin infections as directed by the physicians. For those who had to be sent home, Miss Rogers made home visits to instruct parents in care or to assist them as needed in seeking treatment, and to provide follow-up care. The primary objective of her work was to keep children in school or to have them return as soon as possible. Detailed records were kept on each child seen in the school dispensary, including the condition, treatment, and outcome. Careful notes of the home visits described conditions of the home, needs of the family, teaching, treatment, referrals, and follow-up (Struthers, 1917).

"At the end of a month of twenty school days (and six of these were Jewish holidays when sometimes only 30 of 2000 attended school) the result was more than satisfactory" (Rogers, 1905, p. 767). Miss Rogers' careful and complete documentation showed that 893 treatments were given, 137 home visits were made, and 25 children returned to school. Lina Rogers was appointed school nurse by the Board of Health in New York City, the first municipality in the world to take financial responsibility for school nursing. With the nurse's involvement, children could return to the classroom as soon as they received treatment. Miss Rogers emphasized "the saving of school time for the children was of the greatest importance" (p. 766) (FIGURE 1.2).

The project was expanded in December 1902 to include 12 nurses with Miss Rogers as Superintendent of School Nurses. Within 1 year, from October 1902 to September 1903, the number of children excluded for health reasons in the New York Public School system dropped from 10,567 to only 1101. In 1903, more schools were added to the project and were served by a staff of 27 nurses. Documentation showed that 98% of students who had been excluded for medical reasons were now in the classrooms. "It was seen that the work of the nurses connected the efforts of the Department of Health with the homes of the children, this supplying the link needed to complete the chain of medical inspection" (Rogers, 1908, p. 966).

School Health Programs Expand Across the United States

The success of the New York experiment was emulated in Los Angeles in 1904, when a nurse from the Los Angeles City Health Department was sent into the schools (Brainard, 1922/1985). Similar programs were started in Boston in 1905 and Philadelphia in 1908 (see Figure 1.1). Across the nation, steps were taken to provide school health services. Miss Rogers accepted an invitation to initiate a school nurse program in Pueblo, Colorado, in 1909 (Struthers, 1917). In communities where the district nurses from

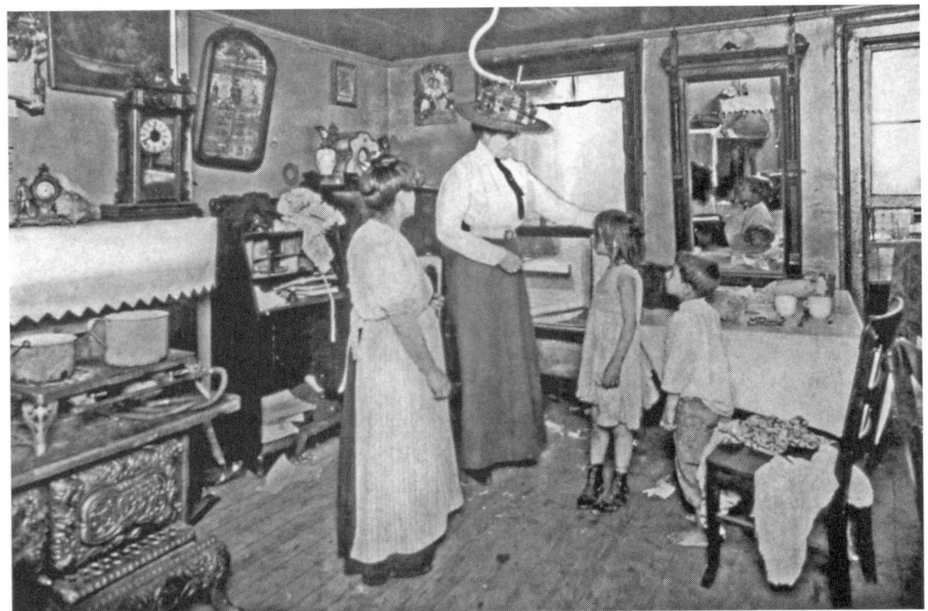

Figure 1.2 ■ The school nurse is the most efficient link between the school and the home. (Courtesy of the National Library of Medicine.)

the health department provided services, children in private and public school received the same care (Kelly & Bradshaw, 1918). Independent school districts also initiated school health programs. The St. Louis (Missouri) Board of Education's Department of Hygiene employed nurses, titling their positions as "Inspector of Hygiene" (Christ, 1957, p. 275). By 1915, all schools ("white, Negro, and schools for exceptional children") were served by 20 nurses and a nursing supervisor (Christ, p. 275).

School programs developed to meet the health needs of children in a particular community were regularly featured in speeches at conferences and in related publications, highlighting the ingenuity of nurses, school personnel, and community leaders in finding funding and implementing programs to address the specific health needs of the children in their care. Throughout the 1920s and 1930s, nurses from municipal, county, and state public health departments in heavily populated areas provided a variety of programs (Table 1.1). Services were also developing in smaller towns of the rural areas across the country. Nursing services in schools were provided under a variety of systems of organization and administration. A private organization or individual often initiated the work. Once the importance of the program was demonstrated, municipal and county authorities were more willing to appropriate funds for the continuance of the programs. Early periodicals such as the *American Journal of Nursing* and *Public Health Nursing,* and later, the *Journal of School Health* routinely published articles describing the programs initiated to meet the needs of the local community.

Early School Nursing in Rural Areas

As early as 1910 or 1915, nurses with the American Red Cross, the Frontier Nursing Service, and other privately funded social or health societies provided services to rural schools. In some cases, nurses were assigned to specific schools and provided ongoing care through regular visits. For most nurses, however, schools were only a part of their public health assignment (Pavey, 1953). Visits to schools were often scheduled for a specific program such as vision screening, or to advise on an outbreak of a contagious disease. These pioneers of rural nursing visited one-room schools, making their rounds by traveling dirt, and sometimes snow-packed, back roads on horseback, by buggy or sled, and later by car. While visiting a school, they learned about health concerns of other family members. The visit to the community often included making home visits, providing health education in the school and home, and making referrals to other resources such as a doctor or welfare agency.

The Red Cross rural nursing program was under the guidance of a local Red Cross committee that was charged with fund raising to support the program and implementing other regulations authorized by the national Red Cross, including local supervision of the nurse. General nursing supervision was directly from the national office of the Red Cross in the form of monthly written reports and occasional visits by the supervisor of rural nursing. The national Red Cross used the

(text continues on page 11)

Table 1.1

WHAT DOES A SCHOOL NURSE DO, ANYWAY? A THREE-DAY SAMPLE FROM 1939

Day 1	
7:50 a.m.	Arrived at school—I like 10 minutes to get my room set up, blanks arranged on my desk, files opened, rest cots and first aid supplies in order before the rush begins.
	Conferred with 3 teachers regarding pupils returning after serious illnesses—worked out postconvalescence modifications of program.
8:10–8:30	Saw students returning from absences caused by illnesses—Quickly disposed of the students with statements from family physician and the one returning from a quarantinable disease for which I already had data from the health department.
	Took temperature of 10 students feeling ill.
	Made appointment with others for later in the day when they had a free period—At that time we will discuss their health problem and plan so they can avoid the condition in the future.
	Two were sent home with instructions to see their physician. They were in no condition to be in school.
8:30–8:45	Interviewed and inspected pupils whom the homeroom teachers had sent to the health office. Three were held over for the school physician to see.
9:00–10:30	Assisted physician with physical examination of high school girls this day. Assisted with removal of clothing, and the donning of "angel robes." Prior to the day of examination, I weighed and measured them, obtained visual acuity by using the Snellen chart and hearing acuity by group audiometer testing. All results were recorded on the pupil's health record, which was provided to the physician for the examination.
	The physician made his own record as he finished each examination. We talked about some of his findings. I made notes on follow-up cards.
10:30	Gave a few instructions to the student assistant and rushed out to catch the 10:35 bus.
11:00	At one of my grade schools until lunchtime. Saw pupils who had been identified by the teachers during the morning inspection with some deviation from normal or with some symptoms of communicable disease.
	The Principal had already sent two that had seemed very ill home. Asked by the Principal to visit one of the children's home where there was no telephone to discuss the child's illness with the parent. I'll do that on my way to lunch.
12:45–1:15 p.m.	At my second grade school. Saw the students that had been identified by the teachers.
	Cared for 2 little boys who had been in a fistfight. It was funny to see them try to take care of each other on the way in. The fight was all out of their systems.

(continued)

Table 1.1 ■ *(Continued)*

Day 1	
1:30	Back to the high school. See the students with whom I made appointments this morning.
	Scheduled work for this afternoon was to finish vision testing, weigh and measure pupils before their scheduled physical examinations.
	Interrupted 13 times, including 3 phone calls. It would be possible to get much more done if one could work in peace for an hour or two.
3:15	School is out.
4:00	Official end of my workday.
	Today I'm in the midst of writing notices to parents of the girls that were seen by the doctor this morning.
	Conferred with 2 teachers who serve with me on the Health Curriculum Committee. It gives me a thrill to see practical health instruction incorporated into social studies and science courses. I would gladly stay later if it would help.

Day 2

School physician is out of town. Scheduled to spend the entire day at the smaller of the two grade schools doing hearing tests with group audiometer (this is minus time spent with interruptions and the regularly scheduled early time at the high school). This year we are trying a quieter location in the general storage area on the third floor. This principal is one after my own heart. Nothing is too much trouble for him if it means better results for his pupils.

Day 3

Started out with the usual office hours at the high school. Completed urgent work at the grade schools. Then on to the community center, where I had three children scheduled for the monthly guidance clinic. I look forward to this opportunity for effective contact with the community public health nurse and the social worker.

Prior to these scheduled conferences in the clinic, I had made home visits and prepared a detailed written history as required by the mental hygiene department.

I had to make a second visit to one of the homes last Sunday because the father is a traveling salesman and only home on that day. He had forbidden his wife to take the daughter to the clinic. He said the only purpose was to take the child from the parents. The father was difficult and so sensitive about the child's backwardness. With the mother's help, he finally understood the value and intent of the clinic and gave his consent.

Adapted from Swanson, M. (1939). What does a school nurse do, anyway? *American Journal of Nursing, 39,* 956–960. The article was written in the form of a letter to two nurses thinking of applying for a school nurse position. The author described the routine of her day and a few of the thoughts about her work.

Visiting Nurses Association (VNA) agencies as training centers for rural nurse preparation. The Red Cross recognized that these nurses needed exposure to various branches of public health and social services in the cities in order to initiate similar work in the rural areas. After the VNA experience, the Red Cross nurses were placed in a rural area with a program for 1 month before being assigned to their own community (Clement, 1913). Red Cross nurses were pioneers in the rural areas they served. The success of the first rural services depended greatly upon the tact of the woman assigned to engage the community. Communication skills were the key to unlocking funds, winning support of old-line physicians not always anxious to share their territory, and establishing programs in the schools and homes (Writers' Program of the Work Projects Administration in the State of Kansas, 1942/1984).

Mary Breckinridge founded the Frontier Nursing Service in 1925 to address health care needs of those families living in the mountains of eastern Kentucky. Routine and preventive care was nonexistent. Most people could not get out of the area to access health care in towns and cities. A "granny woman" (midwife) was called for births and, in the absence of a doctor, was called on for the sickest conditions in children, and for the most serious accidents. Mrs. Breckinridge's cousin documented the work of the nurses on silent film, which has been released as a video recording with narration added (Breckinridge, 1987). As in all communities at the time (the 1920s), childhood communicable diseases swept through the population every few years. On one occasion, the film documented the challenges faced in implementing an immunization program. In preparation, the nurse had to talk with the parents, and gain their confidence and their permission to inoculate their children against diphtheria. The parents met the nurse at the school at the agreed upon time. The teacher did not want to release the children, insisting the needles would be painful. Mrs. Breckinridge used her very best communication skills to convince the teacher, encourage the children, and keep the parents committed to the program. She asked for a volunteer. Who would be first? One little boy said he would be second. Finally a father stepped forward and received the first inoculation, followed by the children (Breckinridge, 1987).

In some areas, public and private agencies teamed with schools and health departments in providing school health services. Such cooperative programs required harmony in philosophy and policies of the varied participants in order for the desired health benefits for the children to be achieved. By the late 1920s in Oregon and in the Territory of Hawaii, the public health concern surrounding tuberculosis gave impetus to expanding school health programming.

In Hawaii, the Department of Public Instruction, the Territorial Board of Health, the Territorial Committee on Sight Conservation, and the Hawaii Tuberculosis Association joined forces to strengthen school health services. At that time in Hawaii, nurses who carried out duties as public health district nurses serving the community at large also served schools. In the school, authorities recognized the public health nurse as a health specialist and health teacher with services focused on education and prevention rather than treatment and first aid. The nurse was a link between school and home. Programs included vision screening, tuberculin testing, x-raying, weight monitoring, and dental screening. Treatment, referral, and follow-up were provided. Health education emphasized basic hygiene and nutrition (Rhea, 1936).

School Health Services in Secondary Schools

From the turn of the century, school health services focused on the younger children. Children going on to secondary school had little, if any, ongoing health screening or health education. At the National Organization for Public Health Nursing (NOPHN) biennial Convention in Los Angeles, California, in June 1936, during a roundtable for school nurses, Foeller (1936) reported that, in Oregon, public health programs were a part of a child's life during the prenatal, infant, preschool, and grade-school periods. There was a gap in health programs and services to address adolescent needs during the 4 years of high school. "Too often a boy or girl goes on to college or into the business world with health handicaps that should have been discovered earlier, when preventive work could have been most effective" (p. 617).

In 1928, the Oregon State Tuberculosis Association financed a demonstration nursing-service partnership with a Portland trade school. The services connected with this project did not specifically relate to tuberculosis but rather to general health education and care. The first role of the nurse was as first aid provider and as teacher of first aid. The program was so successful that the Board of Education took over funding. The program was expanded to other high schools in the Portland system. The nurse was encouraged to provide care, to do individual teaching, and to serve as a resource to science, home economics, and homeroom teachers.

In school nursing programs aimed at younger children, control of communicable diseases was the first consideration. In high school programs, it was a less important component of the nurse's work. Older children were more likely to have acquired immunity to the common "childhood" diseases. The older students had already been exposed to health education and hygiene practices in the lower grades. With continued encouragement to practice these preventive measures, the high school–age student had a decrease in the common respiratory and skin conditions (Foeller, 1936).

Although not compulsory at the time, parents were invited to give permission for school-site physical examinations. The nurse used the information from the examinations to develop a "constructive preventive and corrective program" (Foeller, 1936, p. 617). Follow-up to examinations and programs included contacts "with the home, the family physician, health agencies, and social agencies" (p. 617). The nurse correlated health screenings and programs with the teachers' curriculum. "When the biology classes are studying the eye, the nurse does vision testing in the classroom" (p. 618). Individual health teaching occurred through personal conferences with the students. Cooperative relationships with the dean of boys, the dean of girls, and the nurse assisted students needing extra support in areas of study, attendance, or referral to outside agencies. Mental hygiene was recognized as a significant factor in adolescent health. "Emotional upsets that come in the form of unhappiness in love affairs, anxiety over poor grades, disappointments of various kinds, and sickness used as a means of escape from school difficulties are some of the most outstanding situations" (p. 618).

From the Oregon experience, Foeller (1936) suggested the following were necessary in order for high school health programs to be successful:

- The physical education and health departments should work together under one head.
- A physical examination should be required for all new students, including tuberculosis skin tests, x-ray, and follow-up for reactors.
- The study of anatomy and physiology should be included in the curriculum, taught by persons with an adequate scientific background.
- The nurse for the high school health service must be carefully selected with regard to qualifications for the position. The nurse should be a well-prepared public health nurse, have an understanding of the problems of this age-group, be equipped to teach and to counsel students, and be well informed about the aims, administration, and activities of secondary schools.

THE NURSE'S ROLE DEVELOPS TO MEET THE SCHOOL HEALTH NEEDS OF CHILDREN

Nursing Services

From 1900 to 1950, nursing services provided in the schools took some interesting turns. Wold and Dagg (1981) identified three phases in the developing role of the school nurse during the 1920s and 1930s (Table 1.2). The school health program activities moved from medical inspections (Phase I) to medical examination (Phase II), and then to health education (Phase III). The goal of the programs progressed from control of contagious conditions to assisting students and parents to accept responsibility for their health behavior. The nurse's role expanded from assisting the physician with the inspections to independently inspecting children and making home visits.

Health Education

The nurse's role in health education continued to emerge. The emphasis was changing from a provider being responsible for detection and treatment to having students and parents assume responsibility for health behaviors. Initially, school nurses developed and implemented health education programs without regard to the rest of the curriculum. "The topics of the nurse's 3 to 5 minute talks included cleanliness, food, teeth, and proper rest and sleep for the growing child. These talks were often preceded or followed by inspections for cleanliness" (Wold & Dagg, 1981, p. 9). As health departments and boards of education worked together to improve the health of schoolchildren, the health teaching role of the nurse was valued. However, Brainard (1922-1985) found that didactic teaching of hygiene failed to interest the children. Nurses then "began to tell them stories about the 'Health Fairy' and the 'Old Witch of Finger Nail Care'; kindergarten methods were used, with handkerchief and tooth-brush drills; bright posters illustrated the use of the tooth-brush, the value of good food and fresh air, and the dangers from flies and mosquitoes, and the children were asked to make their own posters, prizes being offered for the best" (Brainard, pp. 270–271). Not only were the presentations unrelated to the students' curriculum, they lacked logical sequencing and were not adjusted to fit the comprehension abilities of the students (Wold & Dagg, 1981).

School nurses then began to develop health education programs that could be incorporated into

Table 1.2 ■
THE DEVELOPING ROLE OF THE SCHOOL NURSE DURING THE 1920s AND 1930s

PHASE	SCHOOL HEALTH PROGRAM ACTIVITY	GOAL	SCHOOL NURSE'S ROLE
I	Medical inspection	Control of contagion	Assist school physician with inspection *or* independently inspect children in the classroom Visit homes for follow-up
II	Medical examination	Identification of: Physical defects Disability limitation through correction of defects	Assist school physician with examination Visit homes for follow-up
III	Medical inspection Medical examination Health education	Same as for Phase II Student attainment of responsible health behavior Student and parental attainment of responsible health behavior	Same as for Phase II Stage one: develop and implement own health education program Stage two: incorporate health education program into teacher's program Stage three: mutual planning of health education program by teacher and nurse

From Wold, S. J., & Dagg, N. (1981). School nursing: A passing experiment. In S. J. Wold (Ed.), *School nursing: A framework for practice* (p. 8). North Branch, MN: Sunrise River Press; used with permission.

the teacher's curriculum. Ultimately, mutual planning of the health education program by teachers and nurses began; this may have resembled the intent of health education described in today's Coordinated School Health Program model (National Association of School Nurses [NASN], 2001a) (see Chapter 3).

Conflicting Expectations of the Nurse's Role

As school health services expanded in school districts across the nation, role confusion swiftly developed. In some cases, nurses were overextended, and in other programs their services were underused. Along the way, state and national organizations and leaders in nursing, medicine, and education attempted to define the role. However, the local nurse, school administrator, or physician did not consistently apply those role descriptions to their situations. Wold (1981) summed up this complicated issue by writing:

> Although school nurses' problems of role confusion and under-use are partially the result of others' misperceptions and inappropriate expectations, school nurses must accept partial responsibility themselves. ...Even among school nurses themselves, there has been no consensus regarding such basic issues as appropriate roles and functions or educational preparation and employment experience needed for school nursing. (p. ix)

School nurses in the 1920s and 1930s continued to expand their role and services until they were overextended. In an effort to meet the demands of the needs they saw and conform to the visions of others, they became confused about their nursing role in the school setting. Efforts to meet the needs of the schoolchildren they served were no longer effective.

A 1934 survey conducted by the National Organization for Public Health Nursing (NOPHN) showed the poorest quality of any phase of public health nursing was that being done in the schools (Gardner, 1936; Wales, 1941, as cited in Wold & Dagg, 1981).

There had been an ongoing discussion about who should administer school nursing programs. "It would seem that health departments consider that school nursing properly belongs there, while boards of education believe the best ends are served if the nurse is a member of the school system" ("Who Shall Administer School Nursing," 1938, p. 134). This debate also led to varying opinions about who is best suited to supervise the school nurse (Chayer, 1945).

While these concerns were administrative in nature, nurses focused on the training and experience needed to serve effectively. "School nursing can be learned only where school children are found. Therefore the school itself is the only available place where the nurse can learn to do school nursing" (Chayer, 1945, p. 468). Nursing educators took up the challenge by recommending that nurses working in public health needed specialized postgraduate preparation and those working full time in the school setting needed to strengthen their public health background.

By the mid-1940s, with the emphasis in the preceding years on the role of health education, many school nurses believed themselves to be more allied with educators and education than with nurses and nursing. Some did not even consider themselves to be public health nurses. Nurses assumed the role of "school nurse teacher" or "teacher-nurse" (Wold & Dagg, 1981, p. 9).

Ayling and Johnson (1949) described the evolving role of the nurse-teacher in the Syracuse, New York schools. They emphasized that the nurse-teacher had to be familiar with both public health nursing and the school health education program. Her role included assisting the physician with physical examinations, tuberculosis testing, and x-raying, and interpreting the results to the students and parents. She assisted with the dental program and was responsible for vision and dental screenings, referral, and follow-up. In addition, the nurse-teacher served as a resource about health concerns to teachers and parents and needed a keen awareness of community resources available in health and social services (FIGURE 1.3).

Dilworth (1937) wrote about the trends in school nursing in the late 1930s: "When good school nursing of today is compared with school nursing as practiced three decades ago, progress is noted in the organization of the service, the preparation of the nurses, the activities selected for major emphasis, and the coordination of school and community efforts" (p. 522). She identified trends in health and social welfare to help determine where the emphasis of school nursing should be. These included

- The acceptance of the family as the unit for all health work.

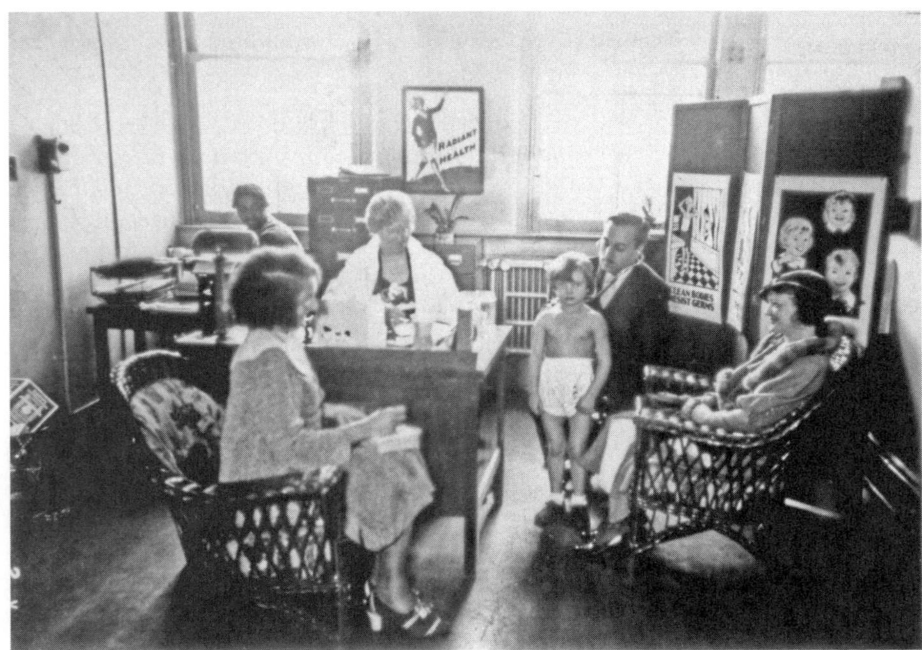

Figure 1.3 ■ Physical examination in the health room. (Courtesy of the National Library of Medicine.)

- Development of a better understanding of human behavior.
- Coordination of all health services in the community.
- An active and intelligent awareness on the part of every nurse in regard to all problems of nursing.
- Close working relationships between the nurse and members of other professional groups with similar aims, such as teachers and social workers.
- A clear-cut conception of our own program, and the ability to state in simple terms its place in the general campaign for human welfare.
- A more comprehensive appreciation of genetics as a factor in public health.
- An increase in lay participation in school nursing.
- More adequate initial preparation for the nurse, followed by sufficient education on the job to keep abreast of the times. (pp. 522, 523, 524)

Many aspects of these trends of the early decades of the 1900s are applicable to the health and social welfare issues addressed by school nurses today.

Evolution and Clarification of the Role of the School Nurse

During the 1930s, two related but external nursing events helped mold the role of school nurses. Some state boards of education set up certification requirements for school nurses. These were generally established on an education system model and did not necessarily relate to the education of nurses or the practice of school nursing (Wold & Dagg, 1981). Additionally, during the 1930s, as nurses grappled with role confusion between identification with nursing or education, they also suffered from overextension of duties (see Figure 1.1). About this same time, the American Medical Association renewed its interest in school health. Physicians took over the leadership of school health programs, formally in some larger school districts and more informally in more rural areas. Physicians provided physical examinations for students in physical education and sports as well as examinations for food handlers and other school employees. In these situations, nurses found that their role was similar to the role of assistant to the physician, as it had been in earlier decades.

In 1944, the School Nursing Section of NOPHN held a conference titled "The Changing School Health Program." Dr. Dorothy B. Nyswandler, health education specialist in the Division of Education of the Office of the Coordinator of Inter-American Affairs, opened the conference by explaining that panel members "represented some of the persons who must work together if a sound plan for the future health programs in the school is to evolve" (Randle, 1944, p. 478). Participants in the panel presentation included a school physician, school nurse, health officer, school administrator, general science teacher, parents, extension service and 4-H agent, school dentist, home economics teacher, classroom teacher, and secondary school teacher. In summarizing the main points of the conference, Randle stated, "It is significant that each participant recognized the necessity for closer cooperation among the school, the community, and the home, and among all the professional groups concerned in the program. The field of school health is so complex that no one person or profession alone can meet its demands, if the program is to fulfill its obligations to the child" (p. 483).

During the 1940s, much of the world was at war, and all national resources were directed toward the war effort. In retrospect, it may seem that school health services would have become less important, but, interestingly, the opposite was the case. Strong young men were needed to supply soldiers for the armed forces. Young women were needed to support the war effort by preparing for jobs at home. Maximizing the health of schoolchildren was viewed as a good investment in the future of the nation. However, the essential elements of school nursing needed to be identified (Dilworth, 1944). NOPHN identified four services that should be maintained by school nurses during the war (Randle, 1944):

- Advisory service to school administrators regarding the school health program and the expanded use of community resources to supplement it.
- Guidance and in-service education for teachers regarding health services they were now expected to perform.
- Interpretation of student health examination data to parents, teachers, and children with referral to community resources for needed follow-up.
- Home visiting to interpret children's health needs to their parents, to discover the family's health needs for interpretation to other school personnel, and to assist the family and school to meet these needs.

Adapting to Change in School Nursing Practice

In order for the school nurse to adequately carry out the activities identified by NOPHN, many of the other duties typically carried out by the nurse but not necessarily requiring nursing skills were delegated to others, including teachers, aides, and volunteers (Palmer, 1944). This was encouraged even after the war as a way to expand and improve school nursing services (Dilworth, 1944). Teachers were expected to take on aspects of care such as first aid for injured children and basic care of ill students, as well as observation for signs of contagious conditions or symptoms of communicable diseases. School administrators had their views on preparation and qualification of the nurse as well as duties to be performed. School administrators acknowledged the school nurse as an important member of the school team. The nurse needed to exhibit superior personal and professional qualifications and a well-balanced personality. Some believed that the school nursing program should focus on health education rather than direct care and treatment. The school nurse's primary objective at that time was to promote healthful living (Nelson, 1944).

Rural school nurses and those in large districts were particularly challenged. Anne Steed (1949), a county school nurse supervisor, was the only nurse in a county program in Indiana. She wondered, "How could one nurse possibly carry out in eleven rural schools, with between 5,000 and 6,000 children, any kind of a good health program?" (p. 609). Recognizing that children learn by doing, she invited teachers and students to actively participate through the development of a student health council in each school. The councils, under faculty sponsorship, took a leadership role in defining the health education and service needs of that school. Students were instructed and supervised in assisting with many aspects of the program, including physical examinations, health screenings, immunization programs, and the milk program for younger children. Through these efforts it was possible to "broaden our total health program in the county" and for "the program itself to become an educational experience to the boys and girls" (p. 611). Through the activities of the student health councils, the students learned lessons in leadership and about health self-care; they also developed an interest in the community. The teachers were pleased that the students learned health education lessons by doing. The health information provided to the teachers assisted them in teaching their students. Steed concluded that "one of the objectives in public health nursing is to have our teachers and students take over the responsibility" (p. 612) for their own health. Steed's innovative rural school health program provided an opportunity for this objective to be implemented.

Following World War II, the nursing staff was nearly depleted in Kershaw County, South Carolina. With a shortage of staff, the school work of the county health nurses had been reduced to the immunization program. In an effort to meet the health needs of schoolchildren, the Kershaw County Tuberculosis Association and the County Department of Health joined into an agreement. The Tuberculosis Association would emphasize case finding and health education (McMaster, 1949). These two agencies agreed to cooperatively promote "a demonstration of a modern school health program" (p. 204). Two schools were selected to begin this demonstration. One was a large consolidated rural elementary and secondary school, and the other was a city elementary school. Many of these children's parents worked in textile factories. A team of people from both agencies gathered and studied materials to determine criteria of successful school health programs. These studies led them to realize that all players in the school and community needed to be welcomed to the group; they needed to be heard and to discuss and participate in the development of the program. It is interesting to note that this concept is very much at the core of today's coordinated school health programs, school health advisory committees, and school-based and school-linked agreements for health services (NASN, 2001a, 2001b, 2001c).

In the South Carolina demonstration project, teachers were trained to teach aspects of general health and hygiene, to conduct daily inspection of children, and to refer children with concerns to the nurse. The nurse's role was that of treating, referral, and follow-up. To be most effective, the nurse needed a collaborative relationship with community physicians and agencies. Immediate health concerns were identified, treated, or referred. The health education component provided information that could be used beyond the school years (McMaster, 1949).

As the United States moved from the war years into the boom years of the 1950s, demands increased on educators and health care providers. Although much of health care was focused on the care of ill patients in hospitals, school nurses realized anew a growing need for collaboration with health agencies in the community. Within the school, nurses collected health education resources for students, parents, and teachers. Flexibility was an important factor in a successful program so that classroom schedules were interrupted as little as possible (Huntsman, 1949).

Meeting the Needs of Students with Special Health Care Conditions

Schools have provided educational opportunities to children with chronic health conditions throughout the history of school nursing. Prior to the enactment of federal law in the mid-1960s, the type of education depended on state laws and local school district policy. Available funding, personnel, and community resources determined the services provided. Children requiring direct nursing care were more likely to be sent to a residential school. Those with conditions that were less involved were enrolled in their local school. Handicapping conditions mentioned in educational and nursing journals included health that was impaired by birth defects, diseases, and infections. These included speech impediments, motor dysfunction, cardiac conditions, hearing and vision impairments, and even enlarged tonsils and adenoids. Chronic enlargement of the tonsils affected the child's speech development as well as general health. The nurse's role in serving children with these physical conditions varied from school to school. Generally, the nurse was the liaison between parent, physician, and the school personnel, monitoring the child's condition, making referrals, providing follow-up as needed, and assisting the family when possible (Rhea, 1936; Struthers, 1917) (see Figure 1.1). The history of the care of children with special needs in the schools is detailed later in this text.

THE MAKING OF A SCHOOL NURSE

"Just to be a 'good nurse' is not enough for the nurse in the school" ("The Nurse in the School," 1949, p. 178). From Lina Rogers to those practicing in private, parochial, and public schools today, the school nurse has defined the roles of effective nursing practice in an educational setting. The effective nurse understands nursing as a discipline set apart and different professionally from medicine and education, while also understanding the roles of the nurse in those settings. During the past century, certain roles of the school nurse may have been more prevalent than another from time to time. However, there are roles that have been consistent in the delivery of quality school nursing services: delivery of direct care; management and leadership of the school health program (planner and coordinator within the school and with the health agencies in the community); case finding and case management (health screenings, referral, and follow-up); communicator/liaison within the school and to the community regarding health concerns; advocate of child and adolescent health and safety needs; provider of health education to individual students, groups of students, the family, and the staff; and finally, mentor and teacher for other nurses (American School Health Association, 1974; Bryan, 1973; NASN, 2002b; Proctor, 1993; Randle, 1944; School Nurses Branch of the Public Health Nurses Section of the American Nurses Association, 1961; Struthers, 1917).

There is timelessness to these roles. The roles seems to become contemporary to a given time while the way they are executed may change from one decade to the next. As an example, consider the nurse's role as a communicator to school staff, parents, and other health care professionals. Lina Rogers described this role in her early writings (1903). This role is considered important enough to be one of the Standards of Professional Performance in the current *Scope and Standards of Practice* (NASN, 2005) (see Chapter 4). In 1903, communication occurred in face-to-face conversations at school or in the home, in written form either hand delivered or sent by mail, or occasionally by phone. Today's nurse uses those same avenues in addition to electronic devices such as e-mail, pagers, and voice mail.

Nursing organizations, public health agencies, and educational administrators have attempted to define appropriate preparation for the school nurse since the inception of the specialty practice. One of the leaders in the district nurse movement wrote, "For district nurses a higher education and higher grade of women are required than for the hospital nurse or even hospital superintendent" (Craven, 1889/1984, p. B). To that end, leaders in public health nursing advocated for nurses to be educated within college and university programs. "The first baccalaureate degrees offered in nursing were the bachelor of science in public health nursing (BSPHN) and the bachelor of science in nursing education (BSNE)" (Ohlsom & Wood, 1999, p. 29).

Mid-century education changed from focusing only on the physical aspects of a child to recognizing the child as an entire being within the greater community. The nurse working in this environment needed to have the best possible preparation to function effectively. In 1948, NOPHN passed a resolution that stated "There is widespread belief that the nurse working with the school-age child should have a broad understanding of physical and emotional growth patterns of children and an understanding of public health and school organization and administration...The NOPHN should take steps to promote the establishment of standards of professional preparation" ("The Nurse in the School," 1949, p. 177). This editorial set forth the vision of a Massachusetts school nurse that describes the characteristics, qualifications, and role expectations of school nurses (Box 1.1).

During the convention of the American Nurses Association (ANA) in 1960, the School Nurses Branch of the Public Health Nurses Section adopted a statement that described functions and qualifications of school nurses employed as staff nurses (School Nurses Branch, 1961). The following are quotes from this statement regarding functions of school nurses employed in staff positions and recommended qualifications for school nurses employed in staff positions:

Box 1.1 ■ ■ ■

CHARACTERISTICS, QUALIFICATIONS, AND ROLE EXPECTATIONS OF THE SCHOOL NURSE–1949

- Excellent physical and mental health
- Communication skills—ability to work with school administrators, teaching staff, pupils, parents, and with community groups
- In addition to basic nurse's training, the study of child psychology is recommended
- Learn history of public school and study laws of learning, and obtain insight into teaching methods
- Understand normal growth and development
- Acquire knowledge of health education methods with groups and individuals
- Meet minimum qualifications for nurses appointed to school nursing service as described by Education Committee of the National Organization for Public Health Nursing
- To continue education by participating in in-service training at conferences and universities
- Subscribe to professional journals and periodicals
- Serve as member on the school's health education council

From The nurse in the school: Changing emphases [Editorial]. (1949). *Public Health Nursing, 41,* 177–178; used with permission.

- Schools have as their purpose the education of children and youth. They are now serving a wider age range of pupils. Programs are being developed for all pupils including those who have exceptional abilities, as well as those who are mentally and physically handicapped. Schools are confronted with many problems caused by increased enrollments, mobility of population bringing into many communities large numbers of new families without roots, and children without established friendships. School administrators, realizing the relationship of health to learning, are expanding health programs in schools so that all pupils have the opportunity to reach their maximum learning potential. School nursing services, as part of this program, must be expanded in scope and quality to meet these demands. (p. 93)
- The function of the nurse will be dependent on such factors as school policy, her own preparation and experience, pupil load, needs of particular pupils in the school, and the availability of other community services. (p. 93)
- The unique contribution of the school nurse is contingent upon her background in nursing. Her future as a school nurse depends on a sound educational background in a baccalaureate program in a collegiate school of nursing. Specialization of school nursing at the graduate level is essential for the nurse entering the field of school nursing. (p. 95)

The statement included a list of specific functions related to a school nurse staff position and a specific description of recommended qualifications. The statement then gave the same consideration to the functions and qualifications for school nurses employed in administrative and supervisory positions (School Nurses Branch, 1961). This was a significant litany of nursing functions and qualifications for its time. Many organizational publications and writings of individual nurses related to functions, qualifications, educational preparation, and standards of nursing practice are rooted in this 1960 work (ANA, 1983; Lordi, 2000; Proctor, 1993; Wold, 1981) (Box 1.2).

Bryan (1973) recommended that preservice education include a baccalaureate degree, with the academic preparation being reinforced with strong clinical experience. Possessing this body of knowledge will enable the nurse "to make decisions and

(text continues on page 20)

Box 1.2 ■ ■ ■

FUNCTIONS AND QUALIFICATIONS FOR SCHOOL NURSES EMPLOYED IN STAFF POSITIONS—1961

Functions relating to:

- *The administration of the school health program:* Gives leadership and guidance in the development and maintenance of a total school health program. Accepts a major role in the orientation, in-service education, and guidance for school personnel regarding the policies, standards, and objectives of the program. Plans with medical authority and administrative personnel within the school regarding the nurse's participation.
- *The nurse's role as a faculty member:* Serves as a faculty member in the total school program under the administrative direction of the principal.
- *The community:* Provides leadership in the coordination of the school program with the total health program of the community. Works with professional organizations, civic groups, and community agencies for the improvement or provision of health facilities for school children. Contributes to professional education in nursing, medicine, social work, education, and allied fields.
- *Evaluation and research:* Conducts studies and initiates research in the area of school health, using available resources. Evaluates the program periodically and effects needed changes.
- *Health appraisal:* Assumes a leadership role in the identification of those pupils with health needs that interfere with effective learning. Teaches others to recognize and report health deviations.
- *Counseling and guidance:* Provides counseling and guidance to pupils, parents, and school personnel to plan action for eliminating or minimizing the health problems of pupils that interfere with effective learning. Supports the promotion and maintenance of growth and development. Recognizes attitudes and cultural patterns that affect health.
- *Health education:* Contributes to the total education program of the school and community. Teaches basic principles of healthful living in relation to changing needs of individuals and groups.
- *Health protection and safety:* Studies the environment in the school, home, and community to identify elements conducive to accident, fatigue, or emotional strain. Recommends changes in the environment or in the organization of activities to eliminate or modify hazards. Gives first aid and emergency care in accordance with established policies. Teaches or arranges for instruction of school personnel in emergency care. Exercises judgment in disposition of pupils who become ill or injured at school.

Qualifications:

- Pre-service preparation in nursing
  - Graduate of an accredited school of nursing
  - Possess a current license to practice as a professional registered nurse
- Preparation for school nursing
  - Baccalaureate degree
  - Completion of a program of study, including field experience in school nursing as a part of the baccalaureate program or at the graduate level, which assures that the nurse has attained—
    - Knowledge and understanding of the total school program, specific school nursing responsibilities, factors influencing the learning process, public health, health education, and public relations.
    - Ability to interpret the school health program to others, interpret policies and procedures, contribute to the health education program, work effectively with classrooms, other school personnel, and community professionals, interpret medical recommendations, organize work effectively, provide adequate care, and evaluate own performance as a school nurse.

Excerpted from School Nurses Branch of the Public Health Nurses Section of the American Nurses Association. (1961). Functions and Qualifications for School Nurses. *American Journal of Nursing, 61,* 93–97; used with permission.

assume responsibility with complete awareness of the moral, legal, and ethical implications" (p. 18). From earlier writings to recent ones (NASN, 2002a), organized nursing has promoted the baccalaureate as minimal preparation, while describing and promoting additional studies.

Nursing practice is described in the state Nurse Practice Act in all 50 states. In some states, the state board of nursing and/or the state board of education may define specific qualifications for nurses working in schools (see Chapter 5). These qualifications may relate to academic preparation and/or to specific state or national certification. In other states there are no specific requirements for an individual functioning as the school nurse. In these states, the person in the "school nurse" position may be an unlicensed school volunteer or employee, a licensed practical nurse, or a registered professional nurse. Regardless of academic preparation, the nurse working in schools may find parameters for practice in state laws or school district policy. Throughout the history of school nursing practice, this lack of consistency in definition, qualification, and educational preparation has led to role confusion among nurses, their employers, and their clients.

PUBLICATIONS

As the specialty area of school nursing emerged in public health, books, manuals, and periodicals were published to address the provision of nursing care in schools. Printed material provided direction for the expanding programs from the cities to smaller towns and rural areas. Nurses who forged the design of school nursing practice as it has developed to meet the school health needs of the population in their local communities shared their insights and experiences as indicated by the following selections:

- Craven's (1889/1994) guide for public health nurses described preparation and characteristics for nurses working in the community. The guide lists the items to be included in a nurse's morocco (bag for writing materials, charts, pens) and trousse (case for equipment needed to provide care in the community) that were initially provided to her (Box 1.3). However, the nurse was well advised that "anything spoilt, injured, or not in good nursing order the nurse was required to replace" (p. 23). The equipment listed was essential to caring for children and adults, as the earliest public health/school nurse's assignment usually required.

Box 1.3 ■ ■ ■

CONTENTS OF A NURSE'S MOROCCO AND TROUSSE

Morocco

- 2 finger stalls
- A spare note-book for special cases when required for "notes of cases"
- 2 clean temperature charts
- Ink-bottle, ink, and pen
- 1 red, 1 blue, and 1 black lead pencils (These are for temperature charts. Sometimes a medical man wishes pulse and respiration to be drawn on the chart, as well as the temperature, with a different colour for each)
- Penknife
- Sheet of writing-paper, envelope blotting-paper, and couple of post cards (for sanitary defects, etc., it may save time for the nurse to write at once to the sanitary authorities)
- In the other pocket, for the nurse's sole use—a linen hackaback towel, nail-brush, and cake of toilet carbolic soap.

Trousse

- 1 silver probe with eye at one end
- 1 silver probe with short flattened handle
- Dressing forceps
- Small spatula for ointments
- Thermometer in case
- 1 pair sharp-pointed scissors
- Caustic in holder
- Catheters in two sizes
- Small razor and strop (to be carried in bag when required)
- Silk for sutures
- Minute sand-glass for taking pulse
- A small work bag containing: black and white cotton thread, needles, thimble, bodkin, pair of strong nail scissors, two pieces of white tape, and a yard measure

- A flat leather case, with broad leather or elastic band, to contain in 1 oz. Bottles—
  - Crystals of carbolic acid in solution
  - Carbolic oil (1 in 20)
  - Spirits of wine
  - Permanganate of potash
- In a perforated tin case: Powder, $^1/_2$ oz. oxide of zinc and $^1/_2$ oz. Prepared starch, well mixed (to be used for drying the skin after washing)
- 1 small tin of Keating's insect powder
- 1 oz. pot (with lid) simple dressing
- 1 oz. pot zinc ointment
- A large spatula for poultices
- A glass syringe in case
- A glass medicine glass in case with minim ditto
- Enema syringe with vaginal tube
- A small roll of strapping in case
- Gutta-percha tissue (a piece of)
- Two flannel and two cotton bandages
- In separate red cotton bags—
  - Small roll of tow
  - Small roll of old linen and lint
  - Small roll of cotton wool and medicated ditto

Special notes:

The best trousse for a nurse can be made by the nurse herself out of chamois or wash-leather in the shape of a large envelope with elastic bands stretched across to keep each instrument in its place. When full, the flaps can be folded over, the case rolled together, and secured with an elastic band and button.

The best cases for powders are empty tins of Keating's insect powder, as they not only have perforated lids but a movable slide under the holes, by which they can be closed when not in use.

Excerpted from Craven, D. (1889/1984). *A guide to district nurses* (pp. 18–21). New York: Garland; used with permission.

- Rogers (1908) and Kelly and Bradshaw (1918) provided lists of supplies and furnishings that were commonly available in school dispensaries. This is the list provided by the Department of Education for the use of the nurse in New York City (Rogers, 1908):

1 screen	Boric acid powder	Tr. Green Soap
1 cabinet	Collodion	Vaseline
1 table	White precipitate ointment	12 towels
Absorbent cotton	Absorbent gauze	Bandages
2 basins (white enamel)	1 glass jar (1 gallon)	1 scrap basket
Bichloride mercury tablets	1 ointment jar	2 chairs (1 high)

- Lina Rogers wrote out courses of treatment for the most frequently recurring diseases and health conditions of schoolchildren. These protocols became part of the New York City Department of Health regulations:
  - Pediculosis—Saturate head and hair with equal parts kerosene and sweet oil, next day wash with solution of potassium carbonate (one teaspoonful to one quart of water) followed by soap and water. To remove "nits" use *hot* vinegar.
  - Favus, Ringworm of Scalp—Mild cases: scrub with tincture green soap, epilate, cover with flexible collodion. Severe cases: Scrub with tincture green soap, epilate, paint with tincture iodine and cover with flexible collodion.
  - Scabies—Scrub with tincture green soap; apply sulphur ointment.
  - Impetigo—Remove crusts with tincture green soap, apply white precipitate ointment (ammon. hydrarg.).
  - Molluscum Contagiosum—Express contents; apply tincture iodine on cotton toothpick probe.
  - Conjunctivitis—Irrigate with solution of boric acid. (Struthers, 1917, p. 268)
- Helen Kelly was Superintendent of Field Nurses in the Department of Health in Chicago, Illinois, and Mabel Bradshaw was Superintendent of School Nurses with the Board of Education in Milwaukee, Wisconsin. Together they wrote that "With increasing demand for school nurses throughout the country, comes a corresponding demand for

information as to how best to organize and carry on the work" (Kelly & Bradshaw, 1918, p. vii). This was the reason they gave for coauthoring *A Handbook for School Nurses.* In Chapter III, Plan and Character of Work, they gave the following advice for routine inspections:

> Nurses should make routine inspections of all children in their schools once in two months, or oftener if possible...The eyelids, throat, skin, and hair of each pupil are examined, and the general condition as regards cleanliness, nutrition, etc., noted. In making this inspection the nurses need not touch the child, who should be instructed to open the mouth, pull down the eyelids, and show hands and wrists. In examining the hair the nurse should use two toothpicks, or if she is economically inclined, one toothpick broken in two, lifting and separating the hair so as to expose the scalp. (pp. 35–36)

There has been a proliferation of articles published over the past decades in the *American Journal of Nursing, Public Health Nursing, Journal of School Health,* and *Journal of School Nursing.* Doris S. Bryan's *School Nursing in Transition* (1973) and Susan Wold's *School Nursing: A Framework for Practice* (1981) are among the most significant independent publications describing school nursing practice in the last quarter of the 20th century. Few other books devoted specifically to school nursing are found. However, in recent years, the number published by professional organizations and private publishers in the health arena has been increasing. Woodfill and Beyrer (1991) compiled the most complete resource to date of published writings that describe the historic foundation, preparation, functions and qualifications, the teaching role dilemma, and key interpersonal relationship characteristics for the school nurse. The bibliography identifies 289 published works related to the historic perspective of the role of the nurse in the school setting.

MOVING INTO THE TWENTY-FIRST CENTURY

Today, state laws vary widely in defining preparation, qualifications, and functions for those engaged in school nursing. In some states, educational requirements must be met in order to receive mandated certification or licensure from state education or health agencies in order to practice as a school nurse. In states where there is no mandate for school health services beyond that regulated by federal legislation, local school districts may choose to hire people with a wide range of preparation for school nurse positions. Some may use parent volunteers or hire non-nurse personnel to be the "school nurse." Other districts may hire licensed practical nurses or registered nurses with varying educational and practice experience to provide health services.

Nurses, independently in their practice setting and collectively through professional organizations, have strived to interpret the scope of school nursing practice to the education community, develop an active relationship with other school personnel, and present standards to guide school administrators in the employment of nurses (Cline, 1937; NASN, 2005). Independently, nurses submit articles to school newsletters, give presentations to parent and community groups, and interact with community businesses, organizations, and agencies. Through professional organizations, nurses have promoted educational preparation, qualifications, standards of practice, and appropriate functions of school nurses through publications and presentations, and committee and task force participation at the local, state, and national level. The registered professional nurse with a baccalaureate degree has long been the minimal recommendation for the nurse engaged in this practice (Ohlsom & Wood, 1999). Leaders in nursing and public health organizations had put forth this recommendation. However, without legislation backed with funding, this recommendation has been frequently ignored or circumvented.

From this glimpse into the past, it is obvious that there continue to be themes between nurses and health agencies and physicians, community and government leaders, administrators in health and education, and even teachers, parents, and students. The difference between professional nursing organization recommendations and the actuality of state laws and local practice perpetuates the role confusion that has plagued this specialty practice of nursing since its earliest years.

Norman Hawkins (1971), a sociologist, described the school nurse as "a hybrid: expected to provide guidance in poorly defined areas, coordinate activities of which she is only vaguely a part, and cooperate in health education on terms dictated largely by others" (p. 744). From literature and from direct investigation, Hawkins suggested the following: "one tentative conclusion seems justified: that school nurses do not occupy a typical nursing role and furthermore that there is general dissatisfaction among them with many of the premises on which they are hired and certified, as well as great inconsistency and confusion among those who utilize their services" (pp. 750–751).

Throughout history, the funding for school health services has varied depending on the perceived value of the services in the community. In 1981, Wold and Dagg wrote "financial support for school nursing continues to be a problem and a political issue" (p. 6). This statement continues to be true in the 21st century. As in the early years, today's role of the school nurse focuses on a public health and wellness orientation. The school nurse's client system includes the child, the family, school personnel, and the community. The impact continues to be observable in the reduction of communicable disease, decreased absenteeism in schools, and involvement of the school nurse in daily classroom health education (Lordi, 2000; Wold & Dagg, 1981). "The highest objective of all efforts is to teach children how to be healthy and how to stay healthy" (Struthers, 1917, p. 40).

CONCLUSION

Today, school nurses recognize that their most valuable impact occurs in roles that support students' educational success (NASN, 1997). As with the first school nurse, the focus is on reducing communicable disease, increasing attendance, and providing direct and indirect care and health education. As nurses in the decades before them have done, today's school nurses "facilitate positive student responses to normal development; promote health and safety; intervene with actual and potential health problems; provide case management services; and actively collaborate with others to build student and family capacity for adaptation, self management, self advocacy, and learning" (NASN, 1999).

By understanding the practice of the pioneers in school nursing, one realizes that today's nurses have similar challenges and opportunities. School nursing today is rooted in the legacy of the articulate, dedicated, and visionary nurses who practiced in schools during the past century. Their work has significantly contributed to the recognition of school nursing as "a specialized practice of professional nursing that advances the well being, academic success, and life-long achievement of students" (NASN, 1999).

References

American Nurses Association. (1983). *Standards of school nursing practice.* Kansas City, MO: Author.

American School Health Association. (1974). *Guidelines for the school nurse in the school health program.* Kent, OH: Author.

Axelson, A. J. (1944). School nursing: What is its future? *Public Health Nursing, 36,* 441–442.

Ayling, W. E., & Johnson, E. F. (1949). The nurse-teacher in a school health program. *Public Health Nursing, 41,* 179–186.

Brainard, A. M. (1922/1985). *The evolution of public health nursing.* New York: Garland.

Breckinridge, M. (Producer). (1987). *The forgotten frontier* [Video recording]. New York: Carousel Film & Video.

Bryan, D.S. (1973). *School nursing in transition.* St. Louis, MO: Mosby.

Chayer, M. E. (1945). Guided field experiences in school nursing. *Public Health Nursing, 37,* 468–471.

Christ, E. A. (1957). *Missouri's nurses: The development of the profession, its associations, and its institutions.* Jefferson City, MO: The Missouri State Nurses' Association.

Clement, F. F. (1913). Rural nursing. *American Journal of Nursing, 13,* 520–521.

Cline, L. V. (1937). The school nurse blazes a new trail. *Public Health Nursing, 31,* 497–498.

Craven, D. (1889/1984). *A guide to district nurses.* New York: Garland.

Dilworth, L. P. (1937). School nursing—yesterday and today. *Public Health Nursing, 29,* 522–525.

Dilworth, L. P. (1944). Essential school nursing in wartime. *Public Health Nursing, 36,* 443–447.

Dock, L., & Stewart, I. M. (1938). *A short history of nursing.* New York: Putnam.

Foeller, H. (1936). The nurse in the high school. *Public Health Nursing, 28,* 617–619.

Gardner, M. S. (1924). *Public health nursing* (2nd ed.). New York: Macmillan.

Gardner, M. S. (1936). *Public health nursing* (3rd ed.). New York: Macmillan.

Goodnow, M. (1943). *Nursing history in brief* (2nd ed.). Philadelphia: W. B. Saunders.

Goodnow, M. (1948). *Nursing history* (8th ed.). Philadelphia: W. B. Saunders.

Hawkins, J. W., Hayes, E. R., & Cortliss, C. P. (1994). School nursing in America—1902–1994: A return to public health nursing. *Public Health Nursing, 11,* 416–425.

Hawkins, N. (1971). Is there a school nurse role? *American Journal of Nursing, 71,* 744–751.

Huntsman, C. (1949). A dynamic school health program. *Public Health Nursing, 41,* 538–541.

Kelly H. W., & Bradshaw, M. C. (1918). *A handbook for school nurses.* New York: Macmillan.

Lordi, S. (with Bradley, B.). (2000). *Standards of professional school nursing practice: Applications in the field.* Scarborough, ME: National Association of School Nurses.

McMaster, J. (1949). Demonstration of a modern school health program. *Public Health Nursing, 41,* 204–207.

National Association of School Nurses. (1997). *School nurses supporting student success* [brochure]. Scarborough, ME: Author.

National Association of School Nurses. (1999). *Definition of school nursing.* Retrieved July 2005 from http://www.nasn.org/about/aboutus.htm

National Association of School Nurses. (2001a). *Coordinated school health program* (position statement). Scarborough, ME: Author.

National Association of School Nurses. (2001b). *Integrated service delivery* (issue brief). Scarborough, ME: Author.

National Association of School Nurses. (2001c). *The role of the school nurse in school-based health centers* (position statement). Scarborough, ME: Author.

National Association of School Nurses. (2002a).

Education, licensure, and certification of school nurses (position statement). Scarborough, ME: Author.

National Association of School Nurses. (2002b). *School health nurse's role in education* (issue brief). Scarborough, ME: Author.

National Association of School Nurses. (2005). *School nursing: Scope and standards of practice.* Scarborough, ME: Author.

Nelson, E. A. (1944). School superintendent and school nurse. *Public Health Nursing, 36,* 240–242.

Ohlsom, V., & Wood, J. (1999). Public health and community health nursing. In T. M. Shorr (with M. S. Kennedy) (Ed.), *100 years of American nursing.* Philadelphia: J. B. Lippincott.

Palmer, M. F. (1944). Essentiality of school nursing. *Public Health Nursing, 36,* 221–222.

Pavey, A. E. (1953). *The story of the growth of nursing: As an art, a vocation, and a profession* (4th ed.). Philadelphia: J. B. Lippincott.

Pennock, M. R. (1940). *Makers of nursing history: Portraits and pen sketches of one hundred and nine prominent women.* New York: Lakeside.

Proctor, S. T. (with Lordi, S. L., & Zaiger, D. S.). (1993). *School nursing practice: roles and standards.* Scarborough, ME: National Association of School Nurses.

Randle, B. B. (1944). The changing school health program. *Public Health Nursing, 36,* 478–483.

Rhea, T. R. (1936). School health in Hawaii. *Public Health Nursing, 28,* 367–371.

Rogers, L. L. (1903). School nursing in New York City. *American Journal of Nursing, 13,* 448–450.

Rogers, L. L. (1905). The nurse in the public school. *American Journal of Nursing, 5,* 764–769.

Rogers, L. L. (1908). Some phases of school nursing. *American Journal of Nursing, 8,* 966–974.

School Nurses Branch of the Public Health Nurses Section of the American Nurses Association. (1961). Functions and qualifications for school nurses (statement). *American Journal of Nursing, 61,* 93–97.

Selekman, J. (2003). People of Jewish heritage. In L. Purnell & B. Paulanka (Eds.), *Transcultural health care: A culturally competent approach* (pp. 234–248). Philadelphia: F. A. Davis.

Steed, A. B. (1949). Getting a rural school health job done. *Public Health Nursing, 41,* 609–612.

Steward, I. M. (1943). *The education of nurses: Historical foundation and modern trends.* New York: Macmillan.

Struthers, L. R. (1917). *The school nurse.* New York: Putnam.

Swanson, M. (1939). What does a school nurse do, anyway? *American Journal of Nursing, 39,* 956–960.

The nurse in the school: Changing emphases [Editorial]. (1949). *Public Health Nursing, 41,* 177–178.

Wales, M. (1941). *The public health nurse in action.* New York: Macmillan.

Who shall administer school nursing? [Editorial]. (1938). *Public Health Nursing, 30,* 134–136.

Wold, S. J. (1981). *School nursing: A framework for practice.* North Branch, MN: Sunrise River Press.

Wold, S. J., & Dagg, N. (1981). School nursing: A passing experiment. In S. J. Wold (Ed.), *School nursing: A framework for practice* (pp. 3–19). North Branch, MN: Sunrise River Press.

Woodfill, M. M., & Beyrer, M. K. (1991). *The role of the nurse in the school setting: A historical perspective.* Kent, OH: American School Health Association.

Writers' Program of the Work Projects Administration in the State of Kansas. (1984). *Lamps on the prairie: A history of nursing in Kansas.* New York: Garland. (Original work published 1942 by Emporia, KS: Emporia Gazette Press)

Zaiger, D. S. (2000). School nursing services: The early years. *Journal of School Nursing, 16*(3), 11–19.

Chapter 2

Theories and Models of School Nursing Practice

CHARLOTTE D. BARRY ▪ SHIRLEY C. GORDON

Chapter Outline

The theory of a discipline is its most distinctive feature.

R. A. STALLONES (1980)

INTRODUCTION

Historically, Florence Nightingale asserted that nursing theories describe and explain what is and what is not nursing (Nightingale, 1859/1992, as cited in Parker, 2001). More recently, Lina Rogers taught us that school nursing was a knowledgeable endeavor and developed a framework for practice grounded in care and concern for students and communities (Rogers, 1905). Since that time, nursing knowledge and practice guides have been framed in theories and models for practice. Nursing theories and models, while structured, offer a stepping-off place for the continuing creative thinking about what nursing is and what it could be.

The study of theory in school nursing is grounded in the belief that nursing is both a discipline and a profession. "The discipline of nursing and the profession of nursing are inextricably bound and exquisitely woven aspects of the single unity of nursing. Each aspect illuminates particular duties, privileges, and realms of activity relevant to nursing as an entity" (Boykin & Schoenhofer, 2001, p. 6).

As a discipline, nursing is made up of a community of scholars who determine phenomena of interest and the domain of practice (King & Brownell, 1976). Members of a discipline commit themselves to developing knowledge that is consistent with the values and beliefs of its members. "The discipline of nursing attends to the discovery, creation, structuring, testing, and refinement of knowledge needed for the practice of nursing" (Boykin & Schoenhofer, 2001, p. 8). It is the development and refinement of a unique body of knowledge that has marked the transition of nursing from a vocation to a profession.

A discipline is a way of framing practice problems and questions. School nurses who approach their practice by asking questions such as "What is the best intervention under these conditions?" and "What is the relationship between concepts such as chronic head lice and parental involvement?" are engaged in the work of the discipline. Nurses have a unique perspective on the health care of schoolchildren. That uniqueness leads to practice questions that are fundamentally different from those of other health care disciplines such as medicine and psychology. For this reason, it is important that the discipline of nursing develop its own body of knowledge based on questions thought to be of importance to the practice of professional school nursing.

Historically, professions developed as a way to provide for the welfare of the members of social groups such as tribes, families, or communities. As the general body of what was known increased over time, groups of people began to take responsibility for the use of specialized knowledge for the good of the whole community. In 1910, Flexner identified characteristics common to learned professional groups. The most basic characteristic of a profession, according to Flexner, was the objective of addressing a unique and indispensable social need directed by a tested knowledge base.

The work of the profession of nursing is the use of knowledge in response to specific human needs (Boykin & Schoenhofer, 2001). When nursing practice is guided by a tested knowledge base, nurses are practicing professional nursing. Without a tested knowledge base to guide practice, nurses would have to rely on the knowledge of other disciplines and the uniqueness of nursing would be diminished or lost. "The viability of nursing as a profession depends on our ability to clearly articulate our unique contributions and measure the value of those contributions to those we serve" (Boykin & Schoenhofer, 2001, p. 9). Therefore, the ability to clearly document the contribution school nurses make to the health and education of students is an essential tool in safeguarding the future of school nursing.

Theory is one way to articulate what nursing is, what indispensable human need it addresses, what questions are relevant to practice, and what research is needed to develop a unique body of nursing knowledge. It is through theory that relationships are described among concepts relevant to nursing and systematically tested to determine the outcomes of those relationships in the practice of school nursing.

DEFINITIONS OF THEORETICAL TERMS

One of the first steps in understanding the value of theory to school nursing is to understand the meaning of theoretical terms. Currently there is no consensus on the definition of terms such as *concept, theoretical statement, conceptual model, theory,* and *middle-range theory.* The definitions presented in this chapter reflect the predominate usage of the terms in the nursing literature.

Concepts are the basic building blocks of theory. "A concept is a term that abstractly describes and names an object or phenomenon, thus providing it with a separate identity or meaning" (Burns & Grove, 1997, p. 139). For example, the terms *stress* and *blood pressure* are examples of abstract concepts. The use of abstract concepts and their definitions allows a shared understanding of the phenomenon under consideration to emerge and grounds communication about the relationship among concepts. Concepts are discussed through the use of theoretical statements.

Theoretical statements can be relational or nonrelational. Examples of nonrelational theoretical statements include concept definitions and statements of existence (Walker & Avant, 1995). Relational statements declare that a relationship of some kind exists between two or more concepts (Burns & Grove, 1997). They assert association (correlation) or causality (cause and effect) (Walker & Avant, 1995). Relational statements describe many characteristics of the relationship between concepts, such as direction, shape, strength, symmetry, necessity, and sufficiency (Walker & Avant, 1995). For example, a relational statement involving the concepts of stress and blood pressure might be stated as follows: as stress increases, blood pressure increases. Because both concepts move in the same direction in relationship to one another, it is considered a positive relationship. Theoretical statements are combined to form conceptual models.

A conceptual model is a set of highly abstract, related constructs (concepts) that broadly explains phenomena of interest, expresses assumptions, and reflects a philosophical stance (Burns & Grove, 1997). It provides a unique way of looking at phenomena. Conceptual models include a distinct vocabulary and lead to different questions and ways of framing clinical problems. In essence, models provide different lenses through which nursing situations can be viewed. Most disciplines have multiple conceptual models, and nursing is no exception. Models are helpful in organizing thinking about nursing situations, but, due to their level of abstraction, they cannot be directly tested in research or practice.

Theories are less abstract than conceptual models; they help organize thinking about nursing, and can be directly tested in research and practice. There are many definitions of *theory* in the literature. Some of the most commonly accepted are

> A theory is a set of interrelated constructs (concepts), definitions, and propositions that present a systematic view of phenomena by specifying relations among variables, with the purpose of explaining and predicting the phenomena. (Kerlinger, 1986, p. 9)
>
> The term theory refers to a set of logically interrelated statements of significance (concepts, propositions, definitions) that have been derived from philosophic beliefs or scientific data and from which questions or hypotheses can be deduced, tested and verified. (Silva, as cited in Moody, 1990, p. 23)
>
> A theory is a statement that purports to account for or characterize some phenomena. (Stevens, 1984, p. 1)

Theories can be categorized by their level of abstraction or generality. The most common divisions are grand theory and middle-range theory.

Grand theories attempt to describe and explain large segments of human behavior (Polit & Beck, 2004). Nursing grand theories are less abstract than conceptual frameworks so they are useful as general guides for nursing practice. However, because they are general enough to account for a large segment of human behavior, they are still difficult to test in research and practice. Nursing theorists such as Boykin and Schoenhofer and Orem and Roy have developed general theoretical systems to describe and guide the practice of nursing across settings.

Theories of the middle range are the least abstract form of knowledge structure. They generally focus on a narrow area of practice and contain fewer concepts than other levels of theory. For these reasons, they are more easily tested in research and practice. Middle-range theories can be derived from other levels of theory by specifying such factors as age of the patient, the situation, the health condition, the location, or the action of the nurse (Tomey & Alligood, 2002). Examples of nursing middle-range theories include Michel's Uncertainty in Illness theory and Locsin's Technical Competency as Caring theory.

Theories are human inventions that provide insight into understanding the world by describing, explaining, predicting, and ultimately controlling phenomena considered important to the discipline. Theories are useful in everyday school nursing practice situations, such as determining what questions are important to ask, directing observations and data collection, interpreting the meaning of data, and developing responses to student needs. It is the predictive nature of theories that enables nurses to achieve the goal of developing clinical practice that is directed by a clearly defined, unique body of knowledge (Walker & Avant, 1995).

CONCEPTUAL MODELS AND THEORIES OF SCHOOL HEALTH

Education became compulsory in the mid-19th century. For the first time in history, it was possible to have school-age children gathered together in determined places and at specific times. The roles that schools could play in reducing the spread of infectious diseases and as a vehicle for providing a wide range of health and social services were recognized.

Over time, a number of school health models and programs emerged. The basic assumptions that have underlined the development of school health models are as follows:

1. The primary goal of schools is education.
2. Education and health are linked. Educational outcomes are related to health status and health outcomes are related to education.
3. There are certain basic health needs of children and young people. These include nurturing and support; timely and relevant health information, knowledge and skills necessary to adopt healthful behavior; and access to health care.
4. The school has the potential to be a crucial part of the system to provide these basic health needs. (Allensworth, Lawson, Nicholson, & Wyche, 1997, p. 17)

In 1997, The National Institutes of Health Committee on Comprehensive School Health Programs in Grades K–12 published a report that examined a variety of school health models and programs (Allensworth et al., 1997). The report identified several predominate models: the three-component model, the eight-component model, and the Full-Service Schools model. (The Coordinated School Health Programs model is discussed in Chapter 3.)

Three-Component Model

The three-component model originated in the early 1900s. The model identified what were thought at the time to be the crucial components of school health: health instruction, health services, and a healthful environment (Allensworth et al., 1997). Health instruction focused on practices, attitudes, and knowledge that were formulated into a comprehensive health education curriculum. Health services focused on health assessment, health prevention, and remediation of existing health problems. A healthful environment included elements thought to promote a safe physical and psychological environment in which students could learn. This early model provided a tool that was useful in organizing, developing, and evaluating early school health programs. Although there was great variation in how the programs operated, school health programs generally included the three basic components of the model.

Eight-Component Model

As time passed, it became evident that the three-component program did not adequately meet the developing needs of schools and additional components were added. The three-component program was officially expanded in the 1980s to comprise health education; physical education; health services; nutrition services; health promotion for staff; counseling, psychological, and social services; healthy school environment; and parent and community involvement (Allensworth et al., 1997). This new eight-component model was thought to contain the essential requirements for and became known as the Coordinated School Health Program (see Chapter 3).

The eight-component model has been promoted by the Centers for Disease Control and Prevention (CDC) Division of Adolescent and School Health (DASH). Based on the model, DASH has published a series of documents/reports that provide guidelines for school health programs to promote healthy behavior among children and adolescents. As a result, many states have begun to adopt the model in planning school health programs. In 2000, the most recent School Health Policies and Programs Study (SHPPS) was published (CDC, 2000). The purpose of the study was to assess school health policies and programs at the state, district, school, and classroom levels. SHPPS 2000 is an example of how the eight-component model of school health has been used to structure evaluation methods. The report can be viewed at the CDC's Web site (http://www.cdc.gov/nccdphp/dash/shpps/index.htm).

Full-Service Schools Model

A recent evolution in school health programs is the model known as Full-Service Schools. The Full-Service Schools model is grounded in the original four assumptions underlying school health models. However, the assumption of the school having the potential to be a crucial part of the system to provide basic health needs was expanded to the school becoming the center for locating "a wide range of health, mental health, social, and/or family services into a one-stop, seamless institution" (Allensworth et al., 1997, p. 59). Although services offered vary from school to school, the distinguishing feature of this model is the broad scope of services offered at an individual school site through community partnerships. Services offered are in response to the unique needs of individual schools and communities and usually include health, social and legal services such as parent literacy training, individual counseling, family planning, health and dental screening, weight management programs, crisis intervention, job training, and immigration resettlement services.

Epidemiological Model

One of the earliest goals of school health programs was infectious disease prevention. For this reason, epidemiological models have been used in developing school health programs. Epidemiology is the study of the distribution of states of health and of the determinants of deviation from health in human populations (Valanis, 1999). The basic assumption of epidemiological theory is that disease does not distribute randomly in human populations (Stallones, 1980). One theoretical explanation for the distribution of disease in human populations is the epidemiological triangle, wherein there is a relationship among the concepts of host, infectious agent, and environment (Figure 2.1). Changes in one element of the triangle over time are believed to have the potential to affect the other elements and influence the risk or occurrence of disease in an individual host.

The goal of epidemiology is to understand the process by which diseases occur and progress in the human host. This process is known as the natural history of disease (Valanis, 1999). Understanding the natural history of disease leads to the develop-

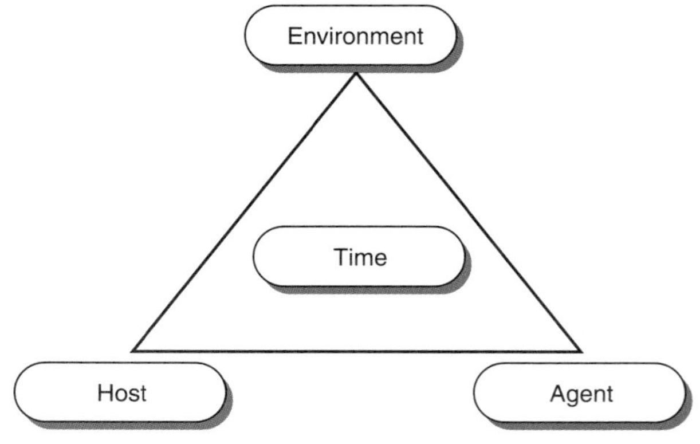

Figure 2.1 ■ The triangle of epidemiology.

ment of interventions that have the potential to prevent the adverse effects of disease before they occur (primary and secondary prevention). If disease cannot be prevented, the epidemiological goal is to limit its course and subsequent disability (tertiary prevention). TABLE 2.1 illustrates the levels of disease prevention, the focus of the interventions, and selected examples relevant to school nursing.

The epidemiological model is insufficient to serve as the sole guide in developing a program of school nursing. However, its application within a broad school health model can enhance disease prevention by encouraging school nurses and others to "think epidemiologically." Epidemiological thinking involves relating signs and symptoms of current students with those of similar cases (Valanis, 1999). Pattern knowledge of similar cases may come from previous nursing experience or the literature. Pattern recognition can alert the school nurse to the early identification of disease clusters. For example,

> An elementary school nurse thought she was seeing an increase in the number of children being treated for urinary tract infections (UTIs). When she checked the health log and medication records, she discovered that there had been an increase in the number of students taking antibiotics for UTIs as compared to the same time period the year before. Because UTIs are not thought to be communicable in school settings, she began to look at recent changes in the school environment. At the beginning of the school year, changes had been made in safety policies related to children being released from class to use the restroom. The new policy included scheduled class visits to the restrooms and discouraged individual students from being allowed to visit the restroom during nonscheduled times. When the school nurse spoke with the children who had experienced UTIs and their families, she discovered that many of the children were limiting their fluid intake and were choosing not to use the restroom at school because they were not comfortable with the new policy, did not feel they were given enough time to relieve themselves, and/or were embarrassed to go to the restroom with a large group. The school nurse took her findings to the principal and the restroom policy was amended. Students were encouraged to bring water bottles to school and to drink frequently throughout the day. In addition, the practice of allowing children to go to the restroom with a buddy was restored.

This example illustrates epidemiological thinking. The school nurse used knowledge of the usual

Table 2.1 ■
LEVELS OF DISEASE PREVENTION AND FOCUS OF INTERVENTIONS

LEVEL OF PREVENTION	GOAL	FOCUS	EXAMPLE
Primary	Promote health and prevent disease	Persons susceptible to disease with no known pathology	Diet and exercise; sports mouth protectors; hand washing instruction; immunizations; barrier contraceptives
Secondary	Detect disease in early stages in order to reverse or decrease the severity of the disease outcomes	Persons with disease who do not exhibit clinical signs	Posture and vision/hearing screenings; stress tests; height, weight, and blood pressure measurements
Tertiary	Ameliorate the course of disease; reduce disability; rehabilitate	Persons with clinical manifestations of disease	Physical therapy; cardiac and pulmonary rehabilitation programs; counseling for juvenile offenders

Adapted from Allensworth, D., Lawson, E., Nicholson, L., & Wyche, J. (1997). *Schools & health: Our nation's investment.* Washington, DC: National Academy Press; used with permission.

frequency of UTIs, combined with questions guided by an epidemiologic model. The example also points out the importance of record keeping validating the initial observation that the number of UTI cases had indeed increased.

Although the school health and epidemiology models described in this chapter are useful in developing general programs of school health, they are “other discipline” based and are therefore not sufficient in guiding the actions of school nurses. Because nursing is a unique, complex discipline, nursing models are needed that are adequate to speak to the role of nursing in school health. “Other discipline”–based models such as medicine or public health models either fail to adequately address the role of school nursing or simply list nursing as one of the components or services of the model. The next section provides insight into selected nursing models that have the potential to guide the day-to-day practice of school nursing.

Nursing Models

The selected models presented in this section are examples from the literature that provide a unique way of looking at nursing that may be useful in guiding school nursing practice. The potential use of each model to guide school nursing practice is discussed from within a nursing situation. Because nursing models present a systematic way of framing clinical interests, the nursing situations reflect what is relevant to each of the selected models. Following a presentation of a brief summary of the models and a nursing situation, a table is provided that identifies values, assumptions, foci, goals, and other important concepts that are useful to study the situation from the perspective of each of the selected nursing models. Information provided in the tables is not intended to be an exhaustive evaluation of the situation, but rather a beginning illustration of the way in which nursing models guide the types of questions that might be asked, the data that are collected, the context in which data are interpreted, and the nursing responses determined to be appropriate within specific nursing situations. Implications for the continued use of the selected models in school nursing settings are provided.

A Community Nursing Practice Model

The Community Nursing Practice model is a conceptual framework that guides practice, program development, and research (Parker & Barry, 1999) (Figure 2.2). The model, developed from essential values, is a dynamic and creative flow of concentric circles depicting the complexity and interconnection of relationships and services directed toward the well-being of individuals and communities. The essential values are respect for person and caring. Instrumental values, values that bring the core values to life, have been adopted from the World Health Organization (1978). These are access,

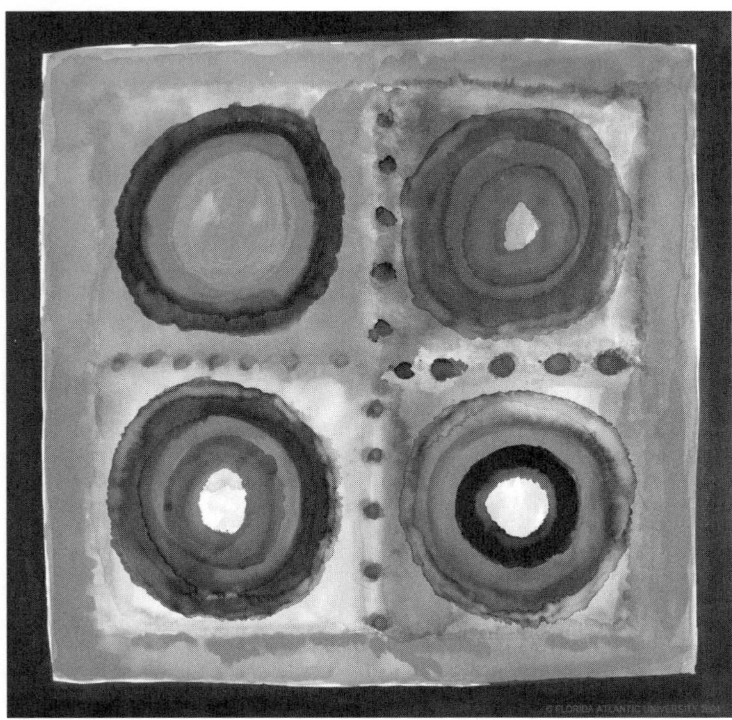

Figure 2.2 ■ Community Nursing Practice Model. (From Parker, M.E. (2006) Nursing Theories & Nursing Practice. Philadelphia, F.A. Davis.)

essentiality, empowerment, community participation, and intersectoral collaboration. Interrelated themes of person, nursing, community, and environment contribute to this model. Definitions of the key values in this model are offered for understanding:

Access is described as the ongoing and constant availability of health care that is competent, culturally acceptable, respectful, and cost-effective.

Essentiality is described from the client's view, as what is necessary for well-being. An inquiry group method has been developed and is used to guide ongoing appraisal of well-being. The guiding questions are "How do you care for yourself, family and community" and "How can I, as nurse, be helpful to you?" (Parker, Barry, & King, 2000)

Empowerment is understood as the client's awareness of making individual choices that influence health and well-being.

Community participation is described as the active engagement with members of a community fostered by openness to listen to calls for nursing and to create nursing responses that nurture well-being.

Intersectoral collaboration is the openness to seek and honor the expertise of other providers and agencies to potentiate the outcomes of services essential to well-being.

Community is described as a safe place for its members and ensures the security of being included and honored. (Peck, 1987)

Environment provides the context for understanding the wholeness of interconnected lives within a personal, communal, and global perspective. (Schuster, Chesney, Kuhns, Wallace, & Wells, 1997)

Respect and caring for persons is present in all nursing situations. Humility guides the nurse's openness to listen and learn what is essential for the other's health and well-being. The person, not the problem, disease, or disability, is the focus of nursing. A nursing response is created that nurtures and supports the other's choices for health. The school health room becomes a safe place to access care and a beginning place to reach into the community to build relationships and connections.

The model is envisioned as concentric circles around a core. The interconnectedness of the core and circles, created with watercolors in the figure, reflects the uniqueness of nursing practice and the blending of parts to form a whole.

CORE SERVICES. Core services are the services provided at each practice site. The unique lived experiences of staff and faculty with those receiving care create the substance of the core. These services provided to students, school staff, and families from the community occur in the following and frequently overlapping categories of care: (1) Design and Coordinate Care; (2) Primary Prevention and Health Education; (3) Secondary Prevention/ Health Screening/Early Intervention; (4) Tertiary Prevention/Primary Care; and (5) Nurturing Wholeness: respecting self-care practices, honoring lay and indigenous care, inviting participation and listening to clients' stories of health and well-being, and providing care that is essential for the other and culturally competent.

FIRST CIRCLE. The first circle includes persons and groups in each school and community who share concern for the well-being of persons served at the center. This includes participants in inquiry groups, parents/guardians, school faculty and noninstructional staff, after-school care groups, parent/teacher organizations, and school advisory councils. The services provided within this circle include (a) Consultation and Collaboration: building relationships and community, providing in-service and health education, and serving on school committees; and (b) Appraisal and Evaluation: conducting community assessments, appraising care provided, evaluating outcomes, and promoting programs that enhance well-being for individuals and communities.

SECOND CIRCLE. The second circle includes structured and organized groups whose members also share concern for the education and well-being of the persons served at the centers but within a wider range or jurisdiction, such as a district or county. Examples of these policy-making groups or advising groups include the school district and county public health department. The services provided in this circle include (a) Consultation and Collaboration: building relationships and community with members of these groups, contributing to policy appraisal, development and evaluation, leading and serving on teams and committees responsible for overseeing the care of students and families, and providing school nurse education; and (b) Research and Evaluation: assessing school health services, describing research findings for best practices related to school and community health, and designing research projects focused on school/community health issues and/or school/community nursing practice.

THIRD CIRCLE. The third circle includes state, regional, national, and international organization members from whom consultation or funds are sought. Services within this circle are focused on (a) Consultation and Collaboration: building relationships and community with members and collaborating about scholarship, policy, outcomes, practice, research, educational needs of school nurses and advanced practice nurses, and sustainability through ongoing and additional funding; and (b) Appraisal and Evaluation: school nursing and advanced practice faculty organizations offer a milieu for discussion and appraisal of the services provided at the centers. Examples of organizations in this circle include the state department of health's office of school health, the state Association of School Nurses, the state Association of School Health, the National Association of School Nurses, the National Organization of Advanced Practice Faculty, the Robert Wood Johnson Foundation, the Health Resources and Services Administration, the Maternal Child Health Organization, and the National Assembly of School Based Health Centers.

CONNECTION OF CORE TO CONCENTRIC CIRCLES. Connections of the core to the concentric circles of services illuminate the complexity of the practice within the Community Nursing Practice model. The core service of Consultation and Collaboration by building community relationships is a primary focus of practice beginning with nursing and social work colleagues, and extending to participating clients, families, policy makers, funders, and legislators. This service is grounded in the values of the model and is essential to the viability and sustainability of this model. It promotes the stance of humility that guides the respectful question throughout the circles: How can we be helpful to you? The answer directs the creation of individualized care and program development. Essential health care services are created within the core and extend into the first circle (Parker & Barry, 2005).

The following nursing situation illuminates the values, goal, and concepts of the Community Nursing Practice model and illustrates the circles of connections of school nursing.

Nursing Situation

Sarah, a student at a local middle school, was born with multiple birth defects, including dwarfism, a speech defect, hearing loss, and a progressive degenerative nerve disorder that has caused paraplegia. She was the sweetheart of her class and had many friends who competed to push her wheelchair through school or to bring her to the health room for assessment, medications, or a twice-daily clean catheterization. One day, the week before Christmas, Sarah told the school nurse she was thinking about posting a sign offering a reward for her lost hearing aid. She thought she had left it on her lunch tray and, although she had no money for a reward, she thought the sign might promote a search and maybe her hearing aid would be returned. When the nurse inquired further, Sarah said the hearing aid had cost $750, and then said "...not that we are poor but we would not be able to buy a new one."

Sarah's Mom was called, and she stated that insurance would not pay to replace the hearing aid and that they could not afford to buy a new one. The school nurse began to investigate community resources and did not find an agency that could help either. She mentioned this to a friend, a professor at the local university. The professor called a colleague whose husband was an audiologist. The audiologist began exploring community resources and discovered that his supplier had a special fund for such emergencies. A simple application was completed and faxed and Sarah obtained a new hearing aid.

Implications for Practice

This model provides a framework for school nursing practice grounded in the core values of respect and caring (TABLE 2.2). It guides practice by focusing on promoting the well-being of individuals and communities while reaching out to and through the circles to build and strengthen relationships and connections in the broader context. It helps explain the social and political factors that influence the health of persons and situates the school nurse in a central position to reflect on, participate with, and take action for health issues (Drevdahl, 1999). It has guided the development of four School Based Community Wellness Centers in Palm Beach County, Florida. These centers are in public schools in multicultural communities and provide services to students, families, and underserved community members (Parker & Barry, 1999).

Leininger's Theory of Culture Care Diversity and Universality

The purpose of Leininger's culture care theory is to guide nursing practice within the context of cultural beliefs and values (Leininger, 1978, 2001, Leininger & McFarland, 2002). Transcultural nursing, a specific practice model developed by Leininger (1978), provides a framework for the systematic learning about others with the intention to provide care that is culturally congruent, in that it is meaningful, appropriate, and satisfying to the persons served.

Nursing actions are directed toward culture care preservation, culture care accommodation, and culture care repatterning. (See Chapter 18 for a complete

(text continues on page 34)

Table 2.2 ■
COMMUNITY NURSING PRACTICE MODEL

Values	Respect, Caring, Access, Essentiality, Community Participation, Intersectoral Collaboration, and Empowerment
Focus	Nurturing Sarah through caring
Goal	Support of Sarah's hope for a new hearing aid
Person	Sarah is the all-important person in this situation as the nurse provides essential care for her and also delights in Sarah's independence, willingness to ask for help, trust, and cheerfulness.
Nursing	The focus of the school nurse's attention was Sarah. The nurse listened to and responded to Sarah's story of the lost hearing aid and her plans to get it back.
Community	The school nurse created a health room environment at this school where Sarah was free to be herself, to which other children felt safe to bring her, and where caring was unique for each student.
Environment	The nursing situation reveals the multiple contexts influencing Sarah's life: the school, friends, family, school nurse, health care team, and community resources. There is a natural rhythm in the story of openness, inclusion, and respect for the complexity of connections.
Connections of core and circles	Some of Sarah's essential health needs were provided through the school nursing services: nursing assessment, catheterizations, medication administration, and nebulizer treatments. Others were obtained by reaching out into the community: connecting to the audiologist, who connected to the hearing aid supplier.
First circle	The nursing situation is in the core and provides the focus for care. The school nurse coordinated Sarah's care at school in consultation with Sarah and her mother, doctor, other health care providers, and the speech pathologist. The nurse trained and supervised a health aide who provided some of the treatments and care. Ongoing appraisal and evaluation of Sarah's well-being influenced the collaborative development of a dynamic plan of care.
Second circle	The school nurse was employed by a county health care district and provided nursing care within the scope of the agency's policies, the school district's policies and guidelines for health care delivery in public schools, the local health department protocols, and the state Nurse Practice Act. Professional development and consultation were provided by the local college of nursing.
Third circle	As the circle widens, connections are developed and maintained with broader based groups and policy makers such as the state legislature, state health department, national legislature, national health initiatives, and the American Nurses Association (ANA) and the National Association of School Nurses (NASN). The influences of these groups include funding for school nursing, statutes governing care, health goals such as Healthy People 2010 (U. S. Department of Health and Human Services, 2000), Standards of Practice (NASN, 2001), and Codes of Ethics (ANA 2001; NASN, 1999).
	A question to consider here is how to influence policy change in replacing medical devices that are somehow lost or destroyed.

description of this model.) The following definitions are guides for this theory (Leininger, 2001):

Care refers to abstract and concrete phenomena related to assisting, supporting, or enabling to improve a human condition.

Culture refers to the learned shared and transmitted values, beliefs, norms, and lifeways of a particular group that guide thinking, decisions, and actions.

Culture care refers to the learned values, beliefs, and lifeways that support an individual or group to maintain their well-being, health, illness, or death.

Culture care diversity refers to the differences in values, beliefs, and lifeways regarding well-being and health, illness, or death.

Culture care universality refers to the similarities in values, beliefs, and lifeways regarding well-being and health, illness, or death.

Nursing refers to the learned humanistic and scientific profession and discipline that is focused on human care phenomena and activities in order to assist, support, or facilitate individuals or groups to maintain or regain their well-being and health or face death in a culturally meaningful manner.

Health refers to a state of well-being that is individually and culturally defined, valued, and practiced.

Culture care preservation refers to those supportive professional actions that help persons from a particular culture retain relevant care values, beliefs, and practices.

Culture care accommodation refers to those supportive professional actions that help a person from a particular culture negotiate for a beneficial or satisfying health outcome with professional care providers.

Culture care repatterning refers to those supportive actions that help persons change or modify their values, beliefs, or practices to maintain well-being and health.

The theory depicted in the Sunrise Model (Leininger, 2001) helps visualize the different dimensions of the theory and highlights factors that influence a person's beliefs about health and well-being. The Sunrise Model figure (see Chapter 18) is a metaphor for a new dawn of understanding. Although not developed for school nursing practice, this theory offers a useful model for caring for students from various multicultural backgrounds who attend school.

Nursing Situation

Magdalena had emigrated from Guatemala and was a second-grade student in Florida. Her teacher referred her to the school nurse for a distinct odor of urine that was detected by her teacher and her peers. The school nurse spoke to Magdalena and asked if she was having any problems urinating. The child was shy, spoke little English, and said she didn't know. A urine sample was obtained and gross examination revealed cloudy urine with large clumps of white matter. A home visit was arranged with the school language facilitator and the family. Both spoke Kanjobal, a Mayan dialect. The school nurse and facilitator made the visit. Magdalena's mother, Rosa, invited the home visitors in and, after hearing the nurse's concerns, explained that she too had noticed the urine odor and thought the situation would improve if Magdalena urinated less. So, she restricted Magdalena's fluids. Magdalena had been suffering for some time with painful urination, burning, frequency, and some incontinence, and so she tried not to drink. Through the language facilitator, the school nurse explained that Magdalena's symptoms were probably the result of a UTI and that the usual treatment of a UTI was antibiotics and an abundance of fluids.

Rosa and the children were on Medicaid. Their provider at the health department was three bus rides away, and, due to a language barrier, Rosa was not able to call for an appointment. Rosa shared that she was pregnant and had been going for prenatal care when she developed urinary frequency and could not successfully navigate the trip to the clinic without becoming incontinent. After hearing Rosa's story about her folk practices with Magdalena, her attempts to go to the health department, and her limited communication skills in English, the school nurse gained some understanding of this family's health beliefs, lifeways, and needs. With the mother's consent, appointments were made at the health department and a volunteer was recruited to drive them for the visits. Magdalena and Rosa were diagnosed with UTIs and were placed on antibiotic therapy. Arrangements were made with a cab company to bring Rosa for continued prenatal care, and Magdalena recovered from the UTI. The school nurse and language facilitator continued to visit to provide care and support for this family (Barry et al., 1998).

Implications for Practice

This theory provides a useful framework for school nurses grounded in the values of respect and care within the context of culture (Table 2.3). Worldwide migration has changed the faces of the students at schools and has created a challenge to understand

(text continues on page 36)

Table 2.3 ■
THEORY OF CULTURE CARE DIVERSITY AND UNIVERSALITY

Values/Assumptions	Care is essential for human growth, survival, curing, and healing. Beliefs, values, and expressions of human care may vary or may be the same among cultures. Culturally congruent care, based on the values and beliefs of an individual or group, is essential for the health and well-being of persons.
Focus	Culture care
Goal	Learning from persons about their culture care values, beliefs, and lifeways is necessary to understand their world, their needs, and the way to provide culturally competent, congruent, and responsible care practices (Leininger & McFarland, 2003). The school nurse brought a language facilitator with her to Magdalena's home. She asked to be invited in and then listened respectfully to Rosa's story about caring for herself and her daughter.
Person	Magdalena is a unique individual with values and beliefs about health, illness, and death that have been learned within the context of culture from sources such as the family, school, church, and profession. Rosa was concerned about her daughter's urinary problem and understood the link between taking in liquids and excreting them. She thought she was doing the right thing to restrict Magdalena's liquids.
Nursing	The nurse is the bridge between folk practices and professional health care services. The school nurse assessed the situation, provided care and support for Magdalena and Rosa, and connected them to primary care at the health department.
Factors Influencing Culture Values, Beliefs, and Lifeways: Technological Religious/Philosophical Kinship & Social Political & Legal Economic Educational	The Guatemalans in Florida live a subsistence life as agricultural workers. They are easily recognized by their short stature and distinctive dress. The men wear long-sleeved shirts, jeans, and baseball hats. The women dress in long skirts and wear their hair unadorned in long ponytails. Beliefs are embedded in Mayan traditions that foster family life, care of children, respect for elders, and self-respect. Education is promoted for the children, and many women attend literacy classes with their young children. Health care beliefs are broad, with use of home remedies, consultation with native curanderos, and visits to professional providers. Causes of illness are seen as a humoral imbalance or may have a spiritual connection. The political situation for Guatemalans should also be understood; the United States has not recognized the civil war in Guatemala, and many refugees are undocumented. This contributes to a reluctance to seek professional health care (Barry & Kronk, 1993; Barry et al., 1998).
Culture Care Preservation	The school nurse listened respectfully to Rosa's explanation of how she was caring for her daughter. On hearing this, the school nurse began to understand the concern this mother had for her daughter's health. The nurse supported the mother's efforts while carefully explaining, through the language facilitator, what she believed the

(continued)

Table 2.3 ■ (Continued)

	health issue was. She suggested further assessment and offered assistance with booking the appointment and arranging for transportation. Rosa said she wanted to seek her husband's advice before making any decision. The nurse supported this and asked permission to make a home visit after Rosa consulted with her husband. The school nurse supported Rosa's core values of caring for herself and her family and seeking her husband's advice on matters of importance.
Culture Care Accommodation	Keeping her language general and nonmedical, the school nurse explained the doctor's findings, instructions for antibiotic use, and need for liquids. Understanding that, in their culture, humoral imbalance expressed as too much "hot" or "cold" is associated with physical or mental illness and that ingesting hot or cold liquids assists in bringing the body back in balance (Zapata & Shippee-Rice, 1999), she explored what Magdalena liked to drink and what would be healthy in this situation. The school nurse respected the family's beliefs about the cause and cures of this health condition and negotiated the balance between professional practice and folk practice.
Culture Care Repatterning	The school nurse, with thoughtful presence, established a relationship with this family that allowed her to get to know them and their health beliefs. She became the bridge between folk and professional health practices and helped navigate the system. Magdalena recovered and returned to school feeling good about herself. Rosa continued with prenatal care and delivered a healthy baby boy. She shared that she had told her friends about how important fluids were in helping with urinary problems. One of the most important outcomes of this situation was a new cultural understanding for the school nurse and the school community. Rosa and Magdalena experienced a new understanding of professional nursing care and in particular the fullness of school nursing.

diverse and universal health care beliefs and practices. For many of these students, the school nurse is the most constant source of health care and health information. The Sunrise Model (Leininger, 1978; Leininger & McFarland, 2002) draws attention to the multiple factors that influence the health of students and to the opportunity to explore and learn. "One can begin anywhere in the Model according to one's focus" (Leininger & McFarland, 2002, p. 120), but eventually examining all the factors provides a holistic cultural assessment. Transcultural nursing fosters care that is culturally competent, congruent, and helpful.

Public Health Nursing Model

Kuss, Proulx-Girouard, Lovitt, Katz, and Kennelly (1997) developed a conceptual model for public health nursing. The purpose of the model was to describe the essential components of public health nursing. The authors based their model on several assumptions:

1. Public health nursing represents a synthesis of nursing science and public health science.
2. The primary philosophy of public health nursing focuses on the larger population, with emphasis on interaction and partnership with the community.
3. Public health nursing practice addresses the social, cultural, political, and economic contexts of the population and is not limited to the immediate surrounding of the individual.
4. Human involvement with the environment is inescapable (Buchanan, 1987).

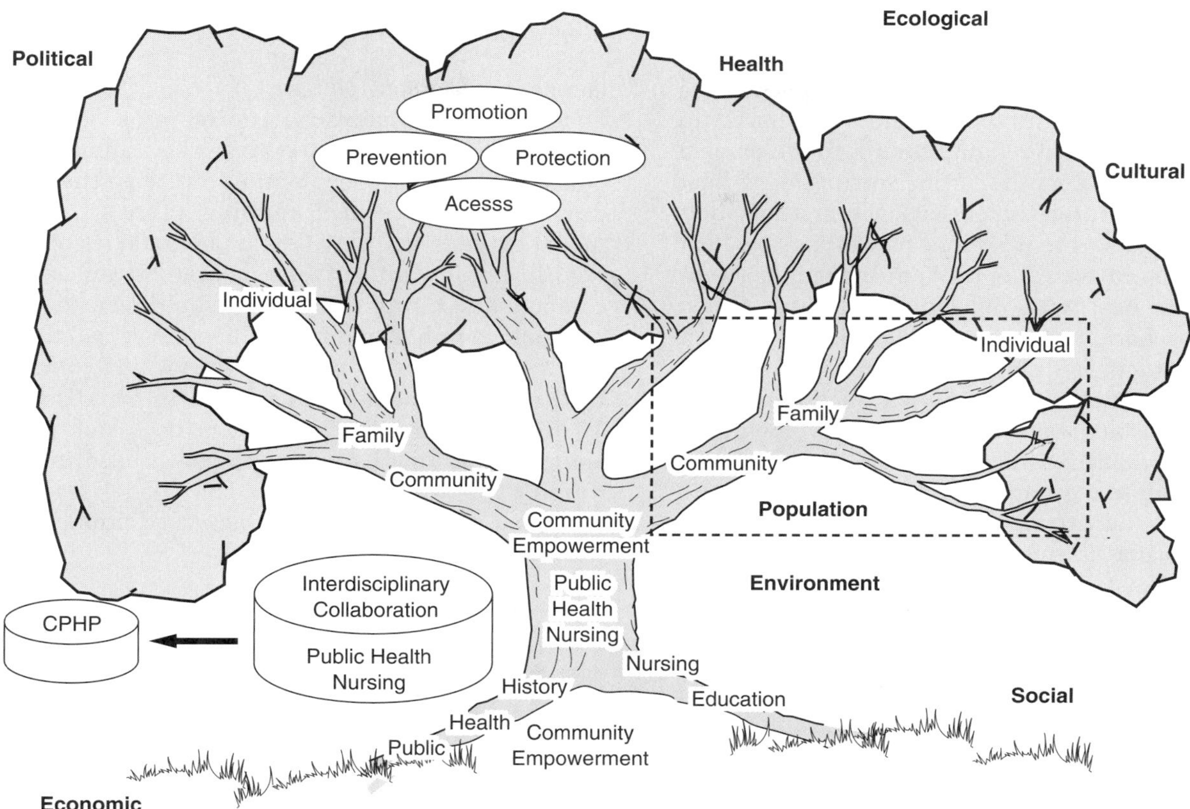

Figure 2.3 ■ Public Health Nursing model. (From Kuss, T., Proulx-Girouard, L., Lovitt, S., Katz, C., & Kennelly, P. [1997]. A public health nursing model. *Public Health Nursing, 14,* 81–91; used with permission.)

5. Members of a population, collectively and individually, make daily decisions that directly and indirectly affect the health of that population (Washington State Department of Health, 1994, as cited in Kuss et al., 1997).

The authors chose the metaphor of a flowering tree (FIGURE 2.3) to visually conceptualize the capacity of the public health nurse. The figure denotes community empowerment, defined by Wallerstein and Bernstein as "the power to act with others to effect change" (1988, p. 380), as the grass. The history of public health nursing and nursing education serve as the root system, and the trunk of the tree depicts public health nursing and core public health functions. The bifurcation point of the trunk represents community empowerment in association with public health nursing, with the branches symbolizing the focus of public health nursing services that include the population, communities, families, and individuals. The leaves of the tree represent the goals or outcomes of public health: protection, promotion, prevention, and access. The flowers of the tree are used to denote health. The area surrounding the tree symbolizes the social, cultural, political, economic, and ecological environmental forces that influence public health nursing.

The Public Health Nursing model (Kuss et al., 1997) intends to clarify, define, and broaden the term *public health nursing.* Describing the essential, complex, interrelated components of public health nursing provides a framework for nursing that may be useful to guide the practice of school nursing.

Nursing Situation

In an elementary school setting, Janice, a third grader, was sent to the health room by the teacher because her head was itching. The school nurse assessed the child and determined that she had head lice. This was the third time in 6 weeks that Janice has been diagnosed with lice. Therefore, the nurse is concerned that the infestation is becoming persistent (Gordon, 1999). The nurse was also concerned about the smell of chemicals in Janice's hair. The school nurse decided to offer the family a home visit. When a home visit was made, the mother told the nurse that she was sure that Janice was getting the lice at school and that she was doing everything she could to control the lice at home. The nurse acknowledged her efforts to treat Janice and asked her to describe how she had been treating the lice. The mother told the nurse that she had been using an insect spray on her daughter's hair before she went to school to keep her from getting more head lice. The school nurse talked with the mother about safe, effective treatment options as well as how head lice are transmitted. All of the family members were screened for lice, with no additional cases found. When the school nurse asked about Janice's neighborhood contacts, her mother acknowledged that she had heard about other children with head lice in the neighborhood but she could not identify them. The school nurse asked Janice's mother if she thought that speaking to a group of families in the neighborhood about head lice would be helpful. In response, Janice's mother offered to invite some of the other mothers over for coffee and a conversation with the school nurse about head lice.

Implications for School Nursing

For those who place school nursing as a specialty area of public health nursing, the Public Health Nursing model can be useful in directing the day-to-day practice of school nursing (Table 2.4). The model extends and clarifies the boundaries of public health nursing and serves as a guide to its essential components. Using this model would lead to a comprehensive public health approach to school nursing and suggest areas of research that would contribute to the development of knowledge in the discipline. To date, the nursing literature does not provide examples of how the model has been used in school nursing or ways in which the model has been extended or tested in the practice of public health nursing.

Table 2.4 ■
PUBLIC HEALTH NURSING MODEL

Values	Caring, Respect for Persons, Access, Community Empowerment, Interdisciplinary Collaboration
Assumption	Head lice is a community-based problem that is brought into the schools.
Focus	Interact with Janice and her family while focusing on the greater population.
Goal	Promote safe and effective treatments to treat and control the spread of head lice in the population.
Community Empowerment	The school nurse offers to meet with other community members (parents) to discuss safe and effective treatments and to identify other cases that may promote the persistent nature of the infestation in the community. By asking Janice's mother if she thought the meeting would be helpful, the nurse is starting from "where they are" (Nyswander, 1966). The meeting is facilitated by Janice's mother as a way to promote the power of others to effect change with the assistance of the public health nurse.
Core Public Health Functions	The core public health functions are to promote, protect, and restore the health of populations and to prevent disease and disability. In this situation, the use of ineffective or unsafe treatment strategies can endanger the health of students. The nurse is also trying to protect Janice (and others) from becoming educationally at risk due to excessive absences from school for head lice.

(continued)

Interdisciplinary Collaboration	In meeting with the other families in the neighborhood, the nurse brings with her knowledge of resources available in the community for the treatment of head lice. Resources in Janice's community include treatment products and combs available to students receiving free or reduced-cost lunch from the school district, a lice treatment center that provides free treatment in exchange for volunteer service, and a head lice treatment and prevention project at the local college of nursing for persistent cases. The school nurse facilitates access to these resources through a referral process.
Environmental Forces	One of the most compelling social environment forces associated with head lice is stigma. The nurse helps to promote a safe environment to discuss head lice as a community problem instead of focusing on individual students and families with head lice. The Public Health Nursing model directs the nurse to ask questions about the influence of other environmental forces (cultural, ecological, political, and economic) on the prevention and treatment of head lice in this population.

School Nursing: A Framework for Practice

Wold and Dagg (1981a) developed a conceptual framework to guide the clinical practice of school nursing. This framework is grounded in the belief that school "nursing has a vital role to play in safeguarding the health of school populations" (Wold & Dagg, 1981c, p. 18). A broad client base, duality of allegiance, and extensive roles are major components of this specialty practice that require a systematic approach to organize knowledge and provide care. The framework is composed of five overlapping strands or ideas: public health, adaptation, helping relationships, tools, and systematic process (FIGURE 2.4). The common ground is school nursing. The following definitions are guides to this conceptual framework:

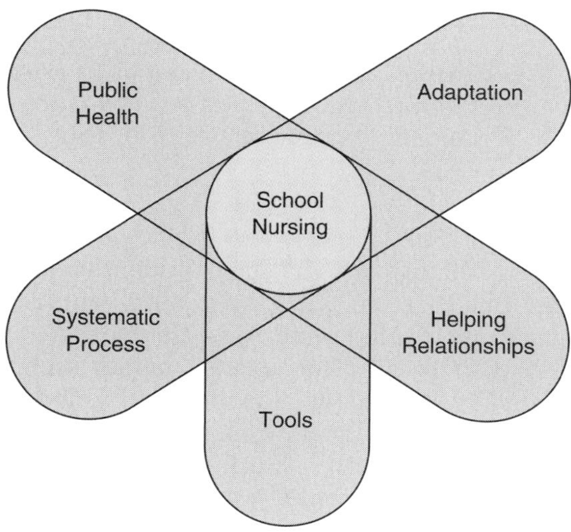

Figure 2.4 ■ Wold's School Nursing Conceptual Framework model. (From Wold, S. [1981]. *School nursing: A framework for practice.* North Branch, MN: Sunrise River Press; used with permission.)

Public Health is defined as a "continuum of activities to protect the health of the community" (Gingrich-Craff, 1981, p. 129). These activities are organized around levels of prevention: primary, secondary, and tertiary. Primary prevention is focused on health promotion and protection. Secondary prevention is focused on early detection, diagnosis, and treatment. Tertiary prevention is focused on rehabilitation and the prevention of disabling sequelae.

Adaptation is defined as "the positive, constructive end results...that occur when adjustments are made to either an internal or external environmental change" (Wold & Dagg, 1981b, p. 22). Questions to assess adaptation include:

- What limitations does the client have to cope with?
- To what degree is the client using his or her capabilities?

- How does the client evaluate his or her situation?
- What environmental resources are available and how can they be used more efficiently?

Helping Relationships are defined as helping persons achieve their goals. For the school nurse, this means a position of trust to help a student with problems.

Tools are defined as instruments useful in the practice of a profession. These tools used by the school nurses are skills, equipment, and systems such as nursing diagnosis.

Systematic Process is defined as a series of actions employed for the achievement of a certain goal. In using systematic processes, the school nurse ensures a comprehensive approach to meeting client needs. The following are identified as processes for nurses:

1. Nursing process
2. Contract-setting process
3. Health education process
4. Research process
5. Epidemiological process
6. Administrative/management process
7. Planned change process
8. Legislative process (Wold & Dagg, 1981a, p. 34)

Nursing Situation

One day, Tommy, a high school student, came to the school health room with a draining wound on his forearm. He wanted Band-Aids. He told the nurse he had had the wound for about 1 month and that it periodically opened up and drained. Upon inspection, the nurse noted the wound was the size of a half dollar, encircled with a hard, shiny, reddened area. An opening at the center was draining a moderate amount of thick, purulent exudate. When the nurse inquired if his parents had seen it, Tommy said no, that it really wasn't bothering him and that it would be all right. The nurse washed and dressed the wound and told Tommy to make sure he showed his parents because he probably needed to be seen by a health care practitioner. The nurse was concerned about spreading the infection, and she told Tommy to keep it covered and to wear a long-sleeved shirt.

Over the following days, the nurse called Tommy to the health room to see the wound. It had stopped draining but remained very inflamed. Tommy said it didn't hurt, so he had not shown it to his mother. The nurse dressed it over the next few days and, when it began to drain again, she called the parent. The following week, Tommy's condition was the same. Another call was made to the parent. After identifying herself, the nurse shared her concerns about the infection and asked how could she be helpful. The mother heard the concern in the nurse's voice and described her situation. She was divorced, had a low-paying job, had no health insurance, and cared deeply about Tommy, but was living one day at a time at best. The nurse offered to connect them to a free clinic whose providers were committed to providing compassionate care to the underserved. The mother accepted this offer for help and the nurse provided the information about the clinic. The mother was able to bring Tommy in during the evening clinic hours; he was diagnosed with a staph infection, the wound was incised and drained, and he was given antibiotics. Tommy reported back to the school nurse, who continued to provide care until the wound was healed and the antibiotic therapy was completed.

Implications for Practice

The School Nursing Conceptual Framework is the only model developed specifically for school nursing practice (Table 2.5). It is grounded in the philosophical view that school nursing is a complex practice, requiring knowledge of public health theory and humanistic theory to provide care that is competent and helpful. The model depicts school nursing in the center, symbolizing the synthesis of multiple ways of knowing and focused on providing care on multiple levels.

EVALUATING MODELS/THEORIES FOR SCHOOL NURSING

There is no "best" model/theory for establishing and evaluating a school nursing program or for guiding individual school nursing practice. It is up to school nurses to determine which of the available models/theories are most consistent with their beliefs, values, and practice. The following are questions to consider in choosing a model/theory:

1. Under what conditions is the model/theory useful to school nursing?
2. Are the goals of the model/theory important to nursing as opposed to other disciplines?
3. Does the model/theory have the potential to influence specific school nursing actions?
4. Will research based on the model/theory answer important school nursing questions? (adapted from Parker, 2001)

(text continues on page 42)

Table 2.5 ■
SCHOOL NURSING CONCEPTUAL FRAMEWORK

Values	Competence, caring, and respect
Focus	Safeguarding the health of the school population
Goal	Promotion of health for the client system
Person	Tommy is part of the client system that consists of the whole community. A unit of service may be provided to an individual, a family, a subgroup, or the community as a whole.
School Nursing	Nursing is a discipline, with a distinct body of knowledge, and school nurses have a vital role to play in the health of students.
Public Health	The nursing situation reveals the school nurse's activities focused on the secondary and tertiary levels of prevention. Her efforts focused on preventing the spread of the infection for Tommy and other students. She educated Tommy on proper hand washing and covering the wound. The nurse was concerned about the possible progression to septicemia. After determining the family had no access to health care, the nurse explored community resources and connected the family to a free clinic.
Adaptation	Tommy was adapting to his situation. The following factors were used to assess adaptation: (1) Tommy knew the school nurse was his only access to care and so he utilized the school health room. (2) He was caring for his wound with his limited resources. (3) Tommy viewed his situation as something manageable; he was getting help and thought the wound would heal. (4) The family had no access to ongoing health care, but, with the school nurse's knowledge of the community, they were able to obtain care from a local agency.
Tools	The school nurse used knowledge from basic to advanced care for this student. From assessment to evaluation of the outcomes, the nurse utilized physical assessment skills; basic equipment/supplies, such as a thermometer, gloves, soap, and dressings; and complex critical thinking skills to prioritize and develop a comprehensive plan of care.
Helping Relationships	Tommy identified the school nurse as someone who could help, and the nurse responded to his need by providing care to him and to his family, which influenced the health of the school and larger community. When the family trusted that the school nurse would help, they revealed they had no access to health care.
Systematic Process	Nursing process provided the framework. The epidemiological process focused on everything from determining the source of the infection to preventing another eruption. The systems that were useful in this situation were not static but intertwined and overlapped, forming a kind of safety net, guiding the nurse's activities directed toward Tommy and the community.

USEFULNESS OF MODELS/THEORIES FOR SCHOOL NURSING

This chapter asserts that school nursing is a distinct professional practice grounded in a unique body of knowledge. Several theories and models have been offered to guide this specialized practice focused on caring for students in schools while understanding the broader context of connections to family and community. Each model situates the school nurse as pivotal to connecting the student to resources both inside and outside the school community. Each model offers grounding in nursing values and professional practice while encouraging and supporting the development of linkages, collaborations, and partnerships beyond the school walls to demonstrate the fullness of school nursing practice (Igoe, 2000). Understanding the complexity of students' lives has been the goal and legacy of school nursing from Rogers (1905) until today. School nursing's mission is to promote health in order to enhance the potential to learn (Schumacher, 2002; Wolfe, 2002).

CONCLUSION

Theory-based school nursing practice provides a framework for school nurses to take a lead in defining the role of the school nurse and in determining what phenomena are within the legitimate boundaries of school nursing practice. Many disciplines share the goal of enhancing student learning potential. Theory provides a mechanism to articulate what school nursing is, what indispensable human need it addresses, what questions are relevant to school nursing practice, and what research is needed to develop a unique body of school nursing knowledge. Therefore, theory is the distinguishing feature of school nursing practice.

References

Allensworth, D., Lawson, E., Nicholson, L., & Wyche J. (1997). *Schools & health: Our nation's investment.* Washington, DC: National Academy Press.

American Nurses Association. (2001). *Code of ethics for nurses with interpretative statements.* Kansas City, MO: Author.

Barry, C., Bozas, L., Carswell, J., Hurtado, M., Keller, M., Lewis, E., et al. (1998, Spring). Nursing an elementary school age child provides insight to the Guatemalan culture. *Florida School Health Association Journal,* pp. 29–36.

Barry C., & Kronk, P. (1993). Nursing Guatemalan families using Leininger's Culture Care Theory. In M. Parker (Ed.), *Patterns of nursing theories in practice* (pp. 142–156). New York: National League for Nursing Press.

Boykin, A., & Schoenhofer, S. (2001). *Nursing as caring: A model for transforming practice.* Boston: NLN Press.

Buchanan, B. F. (1987). Human environment interaction: A modification of the Neuman systems model for aggregates, families, and the community. *Public Health Nursing, 4,* 53–63.

Burns, N., & Grove, S. (1997). *The practice of nursing research: Conduct, critique & utilization.* Philadelphia: W.B. Saunders.

Centers for Disease Control and Prevention. (2000). *School health policies and programs study.* Atlanta: Author. Retrieved December 22, 2003, from http://www.cdc.gov/nccdphp/dash/shpps/index.htm

Drevdahl, D. (1999). Sailing beyond: Nursing theory and the person. *Advances in Nursing Science, 21*(4), 1–13.

Flexner, A. (1910). *Medical education in the United States and Canada.* New York: Carnegie Foundation.

Gingrich-Craff, J. (1981). Structural variables: Factors affecting adaptation. In S. J. Wold (Ed.), *School nursing: A framework for practice* (pp. 128–146). North Branch, MN: Sunrise River Press.

Gordon, S. C. (1999). Factors related to the overuse of chemical pesticides in children experiencing persistent head lice. *Journal of School Nursing, 15*(5), 6–10.

Igoe, J. (2000). School nursing today: A search for new cheese. *Journal of School Nursing, 16*(5), 9–15.

Kerlinger, F. N. (1986). *Foundations of behavioral research* (3rd ed.). New York: Holt, Reinhart & Winston.

King, A., & Brownell, J. (1976). *The curriculum and the disciplines of knowledge.* Huntington, NY: Robert E. Krieger.

Kuss, T., Proulx-Girouard, L., Lovitt, S., Katz, C., & Kennelly, P. (1997). A public health nursing model. *Public Health Nursing, 14,* 81–91.

Leininger, M. (1978). *Transcultural nursing: Concepts, theories, and practices.* New York: John Wiley & Sons.

Leininger, M. (2001). Theory of culture care diversity and universality. In M. Parker (Ed.), *Nursing theories and nursing practice* (pp. 362–375). Philadelphia: F. A. Davis.

Leininger, M., & McFarland, M. (2002). *Transcultural nursing: Concepts, theories, research and practice.* New York: McGraw-Hill.

Moody, L. (1990). *Advancing nursing science through research* (Vol. 1). Newbury Park, CA: Sage Publications.

National Association of School Nurses. (1999). *Code of ethics with interpretative statements for the school nurse.* Scarborough, ME: Author.

National Association of School Nurses. (2001). *Scope and standards of professional school nursing practice.* Scarborough, ME: Author

Nightingale, F. (1859/1992). *Notes on nursing: What it is and what it is not.* Philadelphia: J. B. Lippincott.

Nyswander, D. (1966). The open society: Its implications for health educators. *Health Education Monographs, 1,* 3–13.

Parker, M. (Ed.). (2001). *Nursing theories and nursing practice.* Philadelphia: F. A. Davis.

Parker, M., & Barry, C. (1999). Community practice guided by a nursing model. *Nursing Science Quarterly, 12,* 125–131.

Parker, M., Barry, C., & King, B. (2000). Use of inquiry method for assessment and evaluation in a school-based community nursing project. *Family and Community Health, 23,* 54–61.

Parker, M. E., & Barry, C. B. (2005). Developing a community nursing practice model. In M. E. Parker (Ed.),

Nursing theories and nursing practice (pp. 389–396). Philadelphia: F. A. Davis.
Peck, S. (1987). *The different drum: Community making and peace.* New York: Simon & Schuster.
Polit, D., & Beck, C. T. (2004). *Nursing research: Principles and methods.* Philadelphia: Lippincott Williams & Wilkins.
Rogers, L. (1905). The nurse in public schools. *American Journal of Nursing, 8,* 764–773.
Schumacher, C. (2002). Lina Rogers: A pioneer in school nursing. *Journal of School Nursing, 18*(5), 247–249.
Schuster, E., Chesney, S., Kuhns, K., Wallace, C., & Wells, M. B. (1997). Discovering common ground: The future of health, healing and environment. *Advanced Nursing Practice Quarterly, 3,* 18–24.
Stallones, R. A. (1980). To advance epidemiology. *Annual Review of Public Health, 1,* 69–82.
Stevens, B. J. (1984). *Nursing theory: Analysis, application, evaluation* (2nd ed.). Boston: Little, Brown.
Tomey, A., & Alligood, M. (2002). *Nursing theorists and their work* (5th ed.). St. Louis: Mosby.
U. S. Department of Health and Human Services. (2000). *Healthy People 2010: Understanding and improving health.* Washington, DC: Author.
Valanis, B. (1999). *Epidemiology in health care* (3rd ed.). Stamford, CT: Appleton & Lange.
Wallerstein, N., & Bernstein, E. (1988). Empowerment educations: Freire's ideas adapted to health education. *Health Education Quarterly, 15,* 381–394.
Walker, L., & Avant, K. (1995). *Strategies for theory construction in nursing.* Norwalk, CT: Appleton Century Crofts.
Washington State Department of Health. (1994). *Public health improvement plan.* Olympia, WA: Author.
Wold, S. J., & Dagg, N. (1981a). A framework for practice. In S. J. Wold (Ed.), *School nursing: A framework for practice* (pp. 30–35). North Branch, MN: Sunrise River Press.
Wold, S. J., & Dagg, N. (1981b). Philosophy, roles, and goals of school nursing. In S. J. Wold (Ed.), *School nursing: A framework for practice* (pp. 20–29). North Branch, MN: Sunrise River Press.
Wold, S. J., & Dagg, N. (1981c). School nursing: A passing experiment. In S. J. Wold (Ed.), *School nursing: A framework for practice* (pp. 3–19). North Branch, MN: Sunrise River Press.
Wolfe, L. (2002). School nursing: The next hundred years. *Journal of School Nursing, 18*(5), 251–252.
World Health Organization, Alma Ata. (1978). *Primary health care.* Geneva, Switzerland: Author.
Zapata, J., & Shippee-Rice, R. (1999). The use of folk healing and healers by six Latinos living in northeast United States: A preliminary study. *Journal of Transcultural Nursing, 10,* 136–142.

Suggested Reading

School Health Programs

Allensworth, D. M., Wolford, C., & Olds, R. S. (1994). *Healthy students 2000: An agenda for continuous improvement in America's schools.* Kent, OH: American School Health Association.
American School Health Association. (1998). *School health: Findings from evaluated programs* (2nd ed.). Washington DC: U.S. Department of Health and Human Services, Public Health Service.

Epidemiology

Abramson, J. H., & Abramson, Z. H. (2001). *Making sense of data: A self-instruction manual on the interpretation of epidemiological data* (3rd ed.). New York: Oxford University Press.
Drexler, M. (2002). *Secret agents: The menace of emerging infections.* Washington, DC: Joseph Henry Press.
Harkness, G. (1995). *Epidemiology in nursing practice.* St. Louis: Mosby.
Jekel, J. F., Katz, D. L., & Elmore, J. G. (2001). *Epidemiology, biostatistics, and preventive medicine* (2nd ed.). Philadelphia: W. B. Saunders.
Katz, D. L. (2001). *Clinical epidemiology & evidence-based medicine: Fundamental principles of clinical reasoning & research.* Thousand Oaks, CA: Sage Publications.
Rothman, K. (2002). *Epidemiology: An introduction.* New York: Oxford University Press.

Health Education

Health Care Financing Administration, Medicaid Bureau. (1992). *EPSDT: A guide for educational programs.* Washington, DC: U. S. Department of Health and Human Services.
U. S. Department of Education, Office of Educational Research and Improvement. (1993). *Comprehensive school health education programs: Innovative practices and issues in setting standards.* Washington, DC: Author.

Chapter 3

Coordinated School Health Programs

ELIZABETH L. THOMAS

Chapter Outline

INTRODUCTION

Schools are charged with providing students with the knowledge and skills needed to be healthy and productive adults (Centers for Disease Control and Prevention [CDC], 2000). Since the time of the first school nurse in New York in 1902, educators have recognized that students who are healthy learn better, are more alert and physically fit, and are more likely to be present at school (Marx, 2003).

In the past, when faculty or staff in a school identified a health-related problem, such as violence, alcohol use by students, or adolescent pregnancy, it was usually up to them to find solutions. They may have taken it upon themselves to seek out others for advice, or they may have planned an assembly for students, or just dealt one-on-one with the affected student. There was no system or model in place to deal with the problem from a school-wide perspective

Because schools reach more than 95% of all youth in the United States between the ages of 5 and 17, they are often a primary focus for health promotion and disease prevention efforts (Fisher et al., 2003). Many effective programs had been developed over the years to promote healthy behaviors and address high-risk behaviors, such as HIV/AIDS awareness and fire safety. However, in 1987, Dr. Diane Allensworth and Dr. Lloyd Kolbe postulated that there could be a more effective use of time and resources if school health programs were coordinated and comprehensive, focusing on the six behaviors that resulted in early morbidity and mortality with ensuing loss of productivity and early death (Allensworth & Kolbe, 1987). The high risk behaviors identified were poor eating habits, physical inactivity, tobacco use, risk behaviors resulting in intentional or unintentional injury, abuse of alcohol and other drugs, and sexual behaviors that could result in HIV infection, other sexually transmitted diseases, or unintended pregnancy.

The eight-component Coordinated School Health Program model they proposed was published in the *Journal of School Health* in December 1987, and called the "Comprehensive" School Health Program; the model represented a framework that could be used across school settings, with minimal additional financial and human resources. The model was supported by the Centers for Disease Control and Prevention, Division of Adolescent School Health (DASH), and was referred to by DASH as the "Coordinated" School Health Program. Although the original goal was for the program to be both coordinated and comprehensive, "coordinated" was chosen to emphasize the need to avoid fragmentation and duplication of services while making each component responsible and accountable for its role (Marx, Wooley, & Northrop, 1998).

As society began to focus on health promotion and meeting the goals of the CDC's Healthy People 2000 and Healthy People 2010 initiatives, this model was seen as a possible means to achieve some of these objectives. Of the 467 objectives of Healthy People 2010, *107* are directed toward the behaviors and health of children and adolescents (Fisher et al., 2003). CDC began offering funding and technical assistance for schools, districts, and states targeting poor eating behaviors, physical inactivity, and tobacco use through coordinated school health programs (CDC, 2004a). In 2002, CDC had reported that 20 states were being supported with funding and expertise and "more than forty professional and volunteer agencies work with CDC to develop model policies [and] guidelines to assist states in implementing high quality school health programs" (CDC, 2004a).

Kolbe (2002), director of DASH and co-originator of the Coordinated School Health Program model, suggested that modern school health programs are fundamental within schools and that four goals should guide modern school health programs for students and their communities:

- Improving health knowledge, attitudes, and skills
- Improving health behaviors and outcomes
- Improving educational outcomes
- Improving social outcomes

Stating that improving educational outcomes is the fundamental purpose of schools, Kolbe (2002) asserted that the other three goals should also be fundamental, even without data to confirm the success of these goals. It is the social responsibility of schools to promote healthy behaviors and to teach personal responsibility for choices.

Implementation of the modern school health program depends on the school, the school district, and policy makers. With focus and direction, carefully planned and unduplicated health services, and a positive outlook, the modern school health program should reflect a philosophy of high standards for both health and academics. Physical, mental, emotional, and social barriers to learning will be reduced or eliminated, and attentive teaching can take place in a safe and nurturing environment (Kolbe, 2002). If coordination of school health programs does not occur, there will be a "forfeit (of) one of the most appropriate and powerful means available to improve student performance" (Kolbe, 2002, p. 10).

Coordinated school health programs are slowly being implemented, as evidenced by a publication from CDC (2002) called, "Strategies for Addressing Asthma Within a Coordinated School Health Program." CDC recommends that strategies for addressing asthma in schools be implemented using the eight-component model. Another example is Action for Healthy Kids, a highly publicized national public health chronic disease prevention initiative that is aimed at policy makers and legislators who can make sweeping changes, such as requiring that only healthy snacks be provided in vending machines; enforcing U.S. Department of Agriculture guidelines about nutritious meals; providing counseling services to students with weight issues; encouraging community-based use of school facilities for nonschool physical activity; and mandating age-appropriate comprehensive school health education to provide the knowledge and skills necessary for a healthy lifestyle as well as to affect the attitudes and behaviors related to these components of health. A healthy school environment providing these components of school health and health promotion for staff could be accomplished with the same initiative (Action for Healthy Kids, 2003). Approximately 40 national organizations promote the Coordinated School Health Program model.

COMPONENTS OF A COORDINATED SCHOOL HEALTH PROGRAM

The eight components of a Coordinated School Health Program are (1) comprehensive health education; (2) physical education; (3) school health services; (4) school nutrition services; (5) school health promotion for staff; (6) school counseling, psychological, and social services; (7) healthy school environment; and (8) parent/family and community involvement in the school community. These components are expected to be interactive with each other. They encompass "policies, procedures, and activities designed to protect and promote the health and well being of students and school staff" (National Association of School Nurses [NASN], 2001b).

The National Center for Chronic Disease Prevention and Health Promotion (NCCDPHP, 2004) offers the most current working descriptions of the components of the Coordinated School Health Program.

Health Education

Health education involves "a planned, sequential, K–12 curriculum that addresses the physical, mental, emotional, and social dimensions of health. The curriculum is designed to motivate and assist students to maintain and improve their health, prevent disease, and reduce health-related risk behaviors. It allows students to develop and demonstrate increasingly sophisticated health-related knowledge, attitudes, skills, and practices. The comprehensive health education curriculum includes a variety of topics such as personal health, family health, community health, consumer health, environmental health, sexuality education, mental and emotional health, injury prevention and safety, nutrition, prevention and control of disease, and substance use and abuse. Qualified, trained teachers provide health education" (NCCDPHP, 2004).

Physical Education

Physical education involves "a planned, sequential K–12 curriculum that provides cognitive content and learning experiences in a variety of activity areas such as basic movement skills; physical fitness; rhythms and dance; games; team, dual and individual sports; tumbling and gymnastics; and aquatics. Quality physical education should promote, through a variety of planned physical activities, each student's optimum physical, mental, emotional, and social development and should promote activities and sports that all students enjoy and can pursue throughout their lives. Qualified, trained teachers teach physical activity" (NCCDPHP, 2004).

Health Services

Health services include those "services provided for students to appraise, protect, and promote health. These services are designed to ensure access or referral to primary health care services or both, foster appropriate use of primary health care services, prevent and control communicable disease and other health problems, provide emergency care for illness or injury, promote and provide optimum sanitary conditions for a safe school facility and school environment, and provide educational and counseling opportunities for promoting and maintaining individual, family and community health. Qualified professionals such as physicians, nurses, dentists, health educators, and other allied health personnel provide these services" (NCCDPHP, 2004).

Nutrition Services

Nutrition services include "access to a variety of nutritious and appealing meals that accommodate the health and nutrition needs of all students. School nutrition programs reflect the U.S. Dietary Guidelines for Americans and other criteria to achieve nutrition integrity. The school nutrition services offer students a learning laboratory for classroom nutrition and health education, and serve as a resource for linkages with nutrition-related community services. Qualified child nutrition professionals provide these services" (NCCDPHP, 2004).

Health Promotion for Staff

Health promotion for staff includes "opportunities for school staff to improve their health status through activities such as health assessments, health education and health-related fitness activities. These opportunities encourage school staff to pursue a healthy lifestyle that contributes to their improved health status, improved morale, and a greater personal commitment to the school's overall coordinated health program. This personal commitment often transfers into greater commitment to the health of students and creates positive role modeling. Health promotion activities have improved productivity, decreased absenteeism, and reduced health insurance costs" (NCCDPHP, 2004).

Counseling and Psychological Services

Counseling and psychological services include those "services provided to improve students' mental, emotional, and social health. These services include individual and group assessments, interventions, and referrals. Organizational assessment and consultation skills of counselors and psychologists contribute not only to the health of students but also to the health of the school environment. Professionals such as certified school counselors, psychologists, and social workers provide these services" (NCCDPHP, 2004).

Healthy School Environment

The healthy school environment includes "the physical and aesthetic surroundings and the psychosocial climate and culture of the school. Factors that influence the physical environment include the school building and the area surrounding it, any biological or chemical agents that are detrimental to health, and physical conditions such as temperature, noise, and lighting. The psychological environment includes the physical, emotional, and social conditions that affect the well-being of students and staff" (NCCDPHP, 2004).

Parent/Family and Community Involvement

Parent/family and community involvement incorporates "an integrated school, parent, and community approach for enhancing the health and well-being of students. School health advisory councils, coalitions, and broadly based constituencies for school health can build support for school health program efforts. Schools actively solicit parent involvement and engage community resources and services to respond more effectively to the health-related needs of students" (NCCDPHP, 2004).

THE COORDINATED SCHOOL HEALTH PROGRAM MODEL

Figure 3.1 illustrates the interaction and interdependence of the eight components of school health identified by Allensworth and Kolbe (1987). All eight components are student centered and school specific. Even health promotion for staff is student centered because its goal is better morale and good health for the staff to reduce absenteeism, promote positive health behavior modeling, and promote commitment to the overall health program (Sinha, 2002).

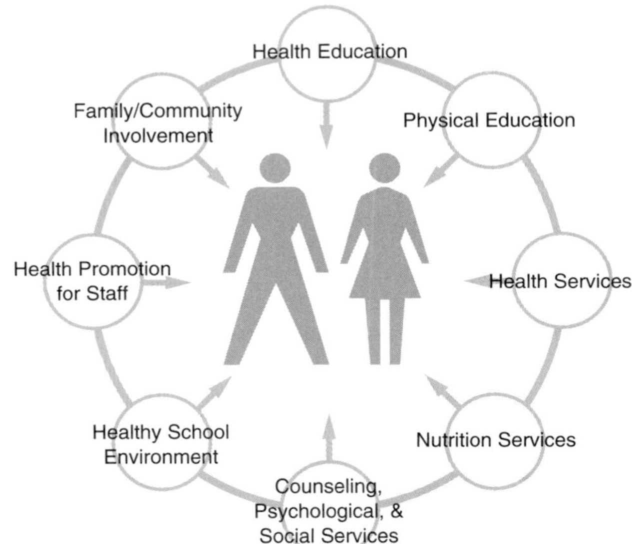

Figure 3.1 ■ The Coordinated School Health Program model. (From National Center for Chronic Disease Prevention and Health Promotion. [2004]. *Healthy Youth! Coordinated School Health Programs.* Retrieved June 29, 2004, from http://www.cdc.gov/HealthyYouth/CSHP/index.htm.)

A simple example of the way the model can be implemented follows. The school nurse and physical educator may identify a growing problem with inactivity, weight, and poor food choice habits among sixth-grade girls. With parental permission, a health club could be formed. The school counselor and the nutrition specialist might become members or advisors. Activities may include a walking program, diet diaries, inexpensive rewards for compliance with the program, community visits to a gourmet restaurant for treats, and instructions on healthy snacking. Soda and high-fat and high-sugar snacks would be removed from the cafeteria. The students might invite their parents to a volleyball game followed by healthy snacks. All components of the school health program model do not have to be included in every project, but all should be supportive of each other and of health promotion efforts in general. The framework is a tool intended to facilitate program planning at every level.

Every coordinated school health program is unique to the school and community. It should be based on all available data, perceived needs and strengths, and the culture of the school and its families, students, and staff. Many publications are offered by CDC, the Department of Health and Human Services, and the Department of Education, as well as professional organizations such as NASN, the American School Health Association, the

National Association of State Boards of Education, the American Cancer Society, and others promoting coordinated school health programs, suggesting implementation and evaluation procedures, and outlining necessary steps for success. A number of useful resources can be found at the end of this chapter that will help interested school and community partners.

HOW TO BEGIN: IDENTIFYING THE NEED OR PROBLEM

In the best of circumstances, state-level health agencies and education agencies collaborate to support and promote policy decisions conducive to and supportive of implementation of local school health programs. To that end, a school health coordinator position is encouraged to foster communication and collaboration among the state health and education agencies and school districts (Fisher et al., 2003). This position could be used to promote the role of school health programs in improving the health and academic achievement of students and to establish and maintain a statewide school health council.

The development of a school health program should begin by identifying a need of the school or community. At the state level, critical planning information can be obtained by using the Youth Risk Behavior Survey (YRBS), given every 2 years to samples of students in grades 9 through 12. The YRBS gives information about tobacco use, onset of alcohol and other drug use, lack of seatbelt use, and other risky behaviors (NCCDPHP, 2001). Another important survey useful to state policy makers is the Youth Tobacco Survey. Though not required of states, both surveys are given technical and financial support by the CDC.

Needs assessments within a school or community or just repeated observations by teachers, staff, or the school nurse may be sufficient to form the basis for a coordinated program. Reports of illness and injury may pinpoint areas of concern, as may the number of medications and treatments given or the number of health counseling and health education sessions, family and staff conferences, and outside agency referrals. Surveys and interviews can obtain information on the health and psychosocial needs of staff and students. Included in the data collection should be questions about the perceived needs of the school community, about the overall school health program, and about expectations for the role of the school in a new coordinated school health program. It is essential that coordinated school health programs focus on needs of the specific population.

The School Health Index, available free from CDC is a tool for evaluating an elementary or middle/high school in the areas of the eight components of school health. Using a questionnaire, a planning team assesses each of the eight components by asking specific questions. Scores are tabulated and areas of strength and weakness are identified. Use of the index helps to identify areas needing improvement and to prioritize needed action (CDC, 2000). "States should create a framework for coordinating state-level data-gathering and data-analysis activities and establish ongoing processes for selecting samples, collecting data, interpreting results, writing reports for state and local decision makers, and sharing data with agencies and organizations interested in improving the health of young people" (Fisher et al., 2003, pp. 9–7). State-level support for coordination and collaboration is important to the process, but lack of support does not prevent a district or school from implementing a coordinated school health program.

SCHOOL SITE HEALTH PROMOTION TEAMS: IDENTIFYING THE PLAYERS

School site health teams are highly individual. Depending on the size and location of schools, some school team members may also serve on the district school health council. In some small school districts, there could be considerable overlap because administrators may have a number of roles. School health teams need key players for a successful system of coordination and implementation of school health programs (Marx, 2003). Perhaps the most important player is an administrator who will champion the concept and the needs of the team, be a liaison with the district school health council, and articulate the value of the health program to the educational mission (Marx et al., 1998). The administrator may or may not be the team leader, but is key to the success of the team.

Leadership of the school health team depends on the strengths of the team members. A volunteer parent with strong organizational skills and discretionary time may be the team leader for a large suburban high school. He or she coordinates activities, schedules and runs meetings of the team, makes presentations to staff and students, writes letters and reports for the school district administration, and generally acts as a school health coordinator.

In some schools, it is the school nurse who leads the team. Challenged by the *Scope and Standards of School Nursing Practice* to support learning through advocacy and to provide comprehensive services in the eight components of the coordinated school health program, the school nurse is qualified to provide expertise and leadership to the school health team (NASN, 2001a). In an Issue Brief, NASN identified assuming a leadership role in health policies and programs as one of the responsibilities of the school nurse (NASN, 2002). The school nurse is acutely aware of the importance of good health for academic success as well as the importance of good health habits for the prevention of chronic conditions and their associated consequences of a limited lifespan, decreased earning power, and increased health care costs. In schools where the school nurse is on site daily and where the Healthy People 2010 recommended nurse-to-student ratio is 1:750, it seems to be a natural leadership role.

Other team members should represent their specialties for the other components of the school health team. Key leaders of the school community, such as secretaries, police liaisons, students and parents, and public health and volunteer agencies need to be included if the program is to be accepted by the school. Responsibilities of the school team "could include assessing student, family and staff needs; mapping existing and community resources that could contribute to a coordinated school health program; identifying gaps and duplications; developing action plans; and monitoring implementation" (Marx et al., 1998, p. 23).

KNOW THE COMMUNITY

In order for the team to decide on the appropriate program for the school, it will first have to know the state and district school health policies, as well as the culture and resources of the school community. School data begin with demographics. Some questions to ponder are

- Is the school urban, suburban, rural, or a combination?
- What are the health problems in the community?
- What is the quality of health agencies and community health and social centers?
- Are there strong faith-based groups in the community for help and support?
- What is the poverty level of the school community?
- What funding is available through federal and state grants?
- Is there a school health coordinator at the district level?
- Does the school board support school health initiatives?
- Is there a breakfast and lunch program that is provided and used by the students?
- What programs are currently in place?
- Are these programs effective, needed, useful, and important to the students, staff, and families?

One indicator of resources available in the community is the number of school nurse referrals that have been completed by families and returned to the school nurse; this may give clues about issues regarding access to care in the community. Another indicator that describes a community is the number of students eligible for free and reduced meals, how many actually use the program, and the number who are eligible for Medicaid.

IDENTIFYING THE TOPIC FOR THE COORDINATED PROGRAM

Using the results of the needs assessment discussed earlier, a list of problems may be identified. If more data are needed, the team should review the annual report done by the school nurse. Other sources of school data, if available, are counselor referrals, discipline reports, suspension and expulsion data, police reports and referrals, and attendance records of staff and students.

Once the list of problems or needs has been narrowed and prioritized, a survey can be designed to obtain further information about individual health practices regarding those topics. These may include dietary habits; fluid intake; physical activity; routine medical and dental evaluation and treatment; tobacco, drug, and alcohol use; sleep habits; use of sunscreen; seatbelt use; environmental safety; diagnosed chronic illness; perceived stress levels; and personal fitness goals. Questions for the staff should include professional development needs regarding school health issues, attitudes about health promotion activities, and concerns about barriers and challenges.

In determining which coordinated health program to develop and implement, it must be decided how best to use the resources, time, and commitment of the coordinated school health program team for the most positive outcomes. The decision for the program needs to involve as many stakeholders as possible for the highest level of participation (Cooper, 2003). The entire team should develop the goals and objectives.

Advocacy for needed policy changes may be important to the team. In this case, the administrator on the team may need to approach the school board regarding current practice. For example, it may be evident that physical inactivity is an issue in an inner city school where recess is a 30-minute free period in the classroom and where board games and idle chatter are the only recreation. The school health team may need to gather data on the importance of physical activity for thinking and learning (Action for Healthy Kids, 2003). At the school board meeting, the district school health council would be asked to support the policy change. A request from the board might include permission to be able to create a program of physical activity that would include classroom exercises, dancing, marching in the hallways, or more physical education classes per week. Fifteen-minute rope jumping sessions could be accomplished in small groups in the hallway. The proposal for change might include a request for financial resources for more exercise equipment or for more staff members to address safety issues so that the children could play outside. After-school recreation and intramural sports teams might be considered for additional physical activity. If the policy changes were approved, grants could be explored and written to cover the start-up fees, equipment, training, and perhaps salaries that would be needed.

In Delaware, school health teams are trained in team building, identification of health risks, and the interaction and importance of the eight-component model for coordinated school health. A School Health Leadership Institute is held for 3 days in the summer each year at a local college. School health teams composed of five specific members submit applications indicating their current level of practice and understanding of coordinated school health programs and their commitment to change. Twelve teams are selected by the state Department of Education school health coordinator. State Department of Education administrators representing the eight components of school health provide staff development by modeling the process of gathering data, planning, and implementing a coordinated school health program. School-based facilitators aid in this process along with representatives of the American Lung Association and the American Cancer Society.

Each team of five must have an administrator, a parent, a classroom teacher, and two other highly motivated staff members. The team is requested to bring as much "school data" as is available to them. Using national, state, district, and school data, the school health team is guided through the planning process to create a plan for a coordinated school health program unique to their school based on resources, needs, strengths, and commitment. Facilitators from the Department of Education, health and physical education educators, and school nurses offer expertise and support through materials, visitations, presentations, and meetings over the next 5 years. A CDC pass-through grant of $5000 is given to each team for implementation of their newly planned coordinated school health program. The mini-grant is very flexible. Funds can be used for substitutes for staff needing professional development, meals, training, meeting expenses, and disposables such as pedometers. An expectation is that this small grant is seed money to attract community financial support to further the health program goals.

One newly trained Delaware school health team purchased pedometers for all staff members, mapped a walking track, and had a contest to see how many times the entire school community could walk "around the world." Using a world map, they plotted their course and celebrated each time they arrived at a preset destination. A staff weekly weigh-in and healthy snack started each Friday morning. The state school health coordinator was invited to present the coordinated school health concept to the Parent-Teacher Association. Other inexpensive and easy-to-implement strategies used to raise health awareness included health promotion signs and posters done by students in health education classes, local news broadcast announcements, and community bulletin board notices of health competitions and slogans. Realistic school goals were posted and updated monthly. A 5- to 10-minute school-wide dance program was held 3 days each week to encourage increased physical activity. It was conducted immediately after school attendance was recorded and before students had settled down for the day. Each day a new health slogan was posted on a dry erase board in the main hallway. An e-mail on a health issue was distributed to the school staff weekly. The year's activities culminated with a health and fitness fair. The community was invited to enjoy the health fair for 2 hours after school; the central office administration was also included.

In Ohio, a school Health Improvement Team (HIT) sponsored a silver sneaker contest for a district of six schools. Students, staff, and families logged in hours exercised. HIT members kept a log of the hours, using a laminated paper sneaker for each hour's activity. The students posted the sneakers in the school hallway so that the paper sneakers "walked" around the school. Every other month, the winning school received a "silver sneaker." That silver sneaker is displayed prominently in the winning school with lots of fanfare and celebration, accompanied by positive reinforcement about the health benefits associated with physical activity. The winning school is celebrated for its commitment to good health. This simple incentive has people walking, jogging, swimming, and dancing their way to better personal fitness. After 3 years, the friendly competition is still going strong and the number of hours of physical activity and total participants have increased each year. Although data have not been gathered to document the positive effects of the HIT program, informal assessment has shown an improvement in school climate and collegiality, and an increase in physical activity (Nikkola, 2003).

The McComb School District met the challenge of a "predominantly conservative, minority, low-income district in Mississippi… fraught with low student achievement, high dropout rates and student disciplines" (Cooper, 2003, p. 1) with a coordinated school health program that began with community input and buy-in. The focus is having students ready to learn through a coordinated school health program. Some of the components of the program include

- Emphasizing early identification and intervention
- Placing a health clinic at each school site with a full-time Registered Nurse and Mental Health Counselor/Interventionist
- Establishing a centralized health office for the district with a Health Service Supervisor to administer
- Establishing a full-time "Health and Wellness Student Assistance Team" at each school site to address student needs utilizing a pro-active prevention approach
- Implementing model programs with proven results
- Providing a safe learning environment conducive to learning with landscaped and renovated facilities, security officers on-site, and a customer friendly staff with a motivating attitude
- Encouraging parent training in literacy, parenting, family violence prevention and in helping their children with schoolwork
- Implementing comprehensive school health education programs to enhance a student's opportunity and ability to develop skills for independent thinking and decision-making
- Utilizing behavioral interventionists to provide prevention training and implement interventions to address behavior issues at each school site
- Providing a child psychiatrist and licensed social worker charged with providing direct services to youngsters experiencing emotional difficulties
- Collaborating with state and local child-servicing agencies in order to coordinate services across the community spectrum (McComb School District, 2002, pp. 7–8)

Relying on community leadership for a needs analysis and comprehensive plan was a critical element of the success of the program (Cooper, 2003). Funding for the program was secured from federal sources such as the No Child Left Behind act (Title VI), as well as local, state, and private partnerships. Cooper acknowledged the impact of a proactive leader who knows how to listen to all the vested parties. Implementation of the program was accomplished over time by focusing on a few components each year. After 5 years, reading readiness dramatically improved, as did state test scores, attendance, graduation rates, and discipline referral rates (Cooper, 2003). Cooper urged that schools and districts bear in mind that schools must "create an environment in which every teacher can teach and every student can learn" (p. 6).

THE ROLE OF THE SCHOOL NURSE

NASN (2001b) issued a position statement on the role of the school nurse in a coordinated school health program. Although the school nurse can provide leadership for the team, he or she may also play a role in some or all of the eight components. These roles include the following activities (NASN, 2001b):

School health services: assessing student health status, providing emergency care, ensuring access to health care, and identifying and managing barriers to student learning

Health education: providing resources and expertise in developing health curricula and providing health information

Health promotion for faculty and staff: providing health information and health promotion activities, monitoring chronic conditions, and maintaining records

Counseling, psychological, and social services: collaborating with counseling staff to identify student psychosocial problems and to provide input and intervention

School nutrition services: providing education about nutritious foods, monitoring menus and food preparation, and encouraging the inclusion of healthy foods on menus, in vending machines, and for classroom snacks

Physical education programs: collaborating with physical educators to meet physical education goals, providing information to students about physical activity, and helping to design appropriate programs for students with special health concerns

Healthy school environment: monitoring, reporting, and intervening to correct hazards, collaborating to develop a crisis intervention plan, and providing adaptations for students with special needs

Family and community involvement: taking a leadership role in collaborating with community agencies to identify and provide programs to meet the physical and mental health needs of children and families

SCHOOL DISTRICT ADMINISTRATION LEADERSHIP: IDENTIFYING THE ADVISORY COMMITTEE

A district-level school health council is an ideal support for the local school health team. A district school health council has the function of analyzing the health strengths and needs of the school community in order to establish a framework for coordinated school health programs within the individual schools. The council should be representative of local businesses, faith-based groups, local elected officials, the school board, central school district administration, parent groups, and staff and students from individual schools (Marx et al., 1998). The council should be diverse and reflective of the community in race, ethnicity, socioeconomic status, and religion, and should have members with both expertise and influence over policy makers. A district school health coordinator's job description should include demonstration of research-based health programs; provision of national, state, and local data for comparison (also called 'benchmarking') and planning; management of the district school health council; consultation services for local school teams; and advocacy for school health programs (Ottoson, Streib, Thomas, Rivera, & Stevenson, 2004).

EVALUATION OF THE COORDINATED SCHOOL HEALTH PROGRAM

Evaluation of the coordinated school health program should be continuous. Implementation should be incremental, and small successes celebrated. Questionnaires, such as those found in the School Health Index, could be helpful in measuring progress. Surveys may be useful tools to assess the impact of individual health promotion efforts. Some schools use surveys as part of their school improvement plan, so questions targeting the coordinated school health program might be inserted into those surveys.

Simple evaluation forms, such as "I wish you had done___________ differently" or, "Please consider including___________ next time" are not threatening, and can measure the effectiveness of the program. A review of attendance records for staff and students is important to see if there is an impact. There may be short-term impacts of the well-designed program, such as better diets, higher levels of daily activity, less stress, reduced or eliminated smoking, and better school attendance, as reported by participants. Longer term effects may show less obesity and hypertension, less need for medications to treat chronic illness, and less reporting of excessive alcohol use (Fisher et al., 2003).

Evaluation is a part of the improvement process. If outcomes of the school health program are successful, then new goals can be set. If outcomes are not positive, then re-evaluation and more planning must occur for programs to be successful. Both process evaluations and outcome evaluations can be used to measure success and provide information for planning and revision of future programs; they also can evaluate the use of human and financial resources (Fisher et al., 2003). An example of the total process is depicted in FIGURE 3.2.

CONCLUSION

Coordinated school health programs are cost-effective, unduplicated efforts to improve health and academic achievement, leaving no child behind. Health problems disrupt both education and the future productivity of both students and staff. Some health issues are improving, but some, such as obesity and physical inactivity, are getting worse (Cross, 2002). If schools are to be held "accountable for their entire mission of education and promotion of successful child development…then coordinated school health programming is a fundamental piece of this larger mission" (Cross, 2002, PowerPoint slide). "Only when schools consider coordinated school health programs to be as essential as history, social studies or language arts will they be able to maximize academic achievement and positive health outcomes among the children and youths they serve" (Tyson, 1999, p. 12).

It is hoped that school health programs will be both coordinated and comprehensive. It is a process

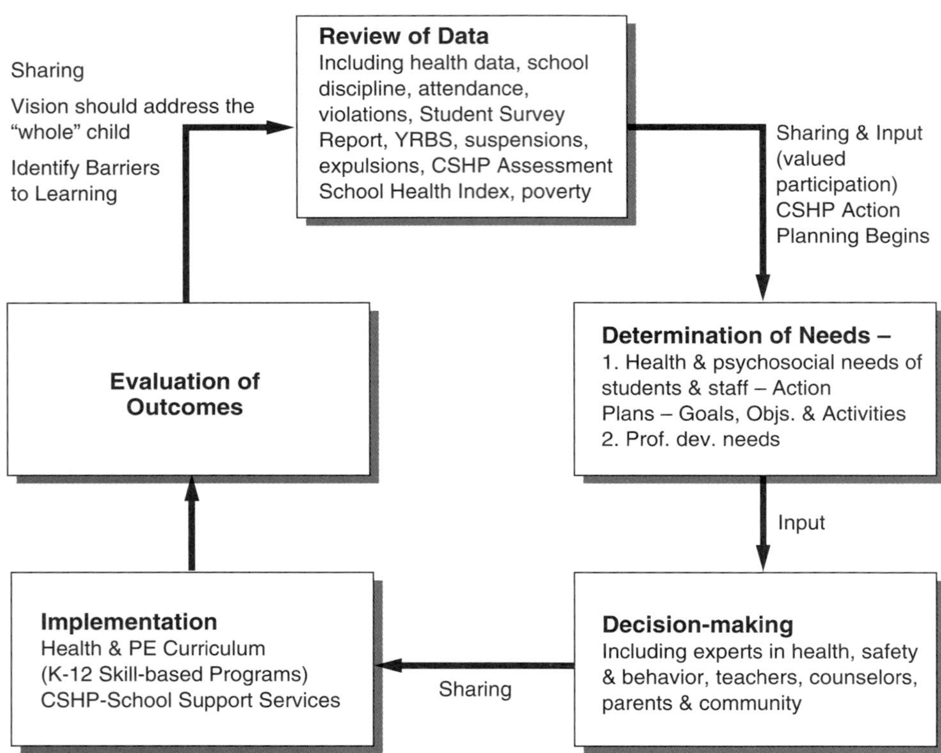

Figure 3.2 ■ School improvement process. (CSHP, Coordinated School Health Program; PE, physical education; YRBS, Youth Risk Behavior Survey.) (From Arns Ray, J. [2003, March 31]. *Delaware school board presentation: Coordinated school health programs* [unpublished PowerPoint presentation]. Retrieved May 15, 2003, from http://jaray@doe.k12.de.us; used with permission.)

that promotes effective interdisciplinary communication; recognizes the strengths of multiple professionals, each with their special body of knowledge; involves the entire school community; and keeps the health of the students and staff at its core.

RESOURCES

The following list of resources may be helpful to individuals, school health teams, or district health councils planning for implementation of a coordinated school health program.

- Action for Healthy Kids (2003) is a national initiative responding to the epidemic of obesity. Believing that healthy schools produce healthy students, Action for Healthy Kids promotes good nutrition and daily physical education by changes in policy and practices. Information is available at the initiative's Web site (http://www.actionforhealthykids.org/html/main.htm).
- *Health is Academic* (Marx et al., 1998) ties health to academics and illustrates how a coordinated school health program can have a lifelong effect on positive health behaviors.
- A school wellness Web site is available with news, statistics, and information about available programs (http://www.cdc.gov/healthyyouth/index.htm).
- The School Health Index is a self-assessment and planning guide developed by the CDC to "identify strengths and weaknesses of your school's health promotion policies and programs for promoting health and safety, develop an action plan for improving student health, and involve teachers, parents and students and the community in improving school policies, programs, and services" (CDC, 2004b, p. 1). It has versions for both elementary and middle/high school and uses the Coordinated School Health Program model to address physical activity, healthy eating, a tobacco-free lifestyle, and a wide range of safety-related behaviors. The School Health Index is available free in elementary and secondary editions by fax at 1–888–282–7681 or can be downloaded free from the CDC's Web site (http://www/cdc.gov/nccdphp/dash/SHI/index.htm).
- *Stories from the Field* (Marx, 2003) was developed as a resource for schools beginning

coordinated school health programs. It demonstrates the many differences effective school health programs can have, plus the barriers, challenges, and successes. Asserting that the work is always ongoing and can be improved, the document offers lessons learned, hope, reassurance, and practical advice. It is available free from CDC.

References

Action for Healthy Kids. (2003). *Taking action for healthy kids: A report on the Healthy Schools Summit and the Action for Healthy Kids Initiative.* Healthy Schools Summit. Retrieved July 2005 from http://www.actionforhealthykids.org/devel/pdf/the_report.pdf

Allensworth, D. D., & Kolbe, L. J. (1987). The Comprehensive School Health Program: Exploring an expanded concept. *Journal of School Health, 57,* 409–412.

Arns Ray, J. (2003, March 31). *Delaware school board presentation: Coordinated school health programs* [unpublished PowerPoint presentation]. Retrieved May 15, 2003, from http://jaray@doe.k12.de.us

Centers for Disease Control and Prevention. (2000). *School Health Index for physical activity, healthy eating and a tobacco-free lifestyle: A self assessment and planning guide.* Atlanta: Author.

Centers for Disease Control and Prevention. (2002). *Strategies for addressing asthma within a coordinated school health program* [booklet] (pp. 1–8). Atlanta: Author.

Centers for Disease Control and Prevention. (2004a). *Programs in brief.* Retrieved June 29, 2004, from http://www.cdc.gov/programs/health1.htm

Centers for Disease Control and Prevention. (2004b). *School Health Index: A self-assessment and planning guide.* Atlanta: Author.

Cooper, P. (2003, January). Our journey to good health. *The School Administrator [web edition],* 1–6. Retrieved February 23, 2003, from http://www.aasa.org/publications/sa/2003_01.Cooper.htm.

Cross, A. W. (2002, October 3). *Health and academics: The price of high stakes testing* (presentation to American School Health Association at Charlotte, North Carolina). Retrieved April 18, 2003, from http://across@unc.edu

Fisher, C., Hunt, P., Kahn, L., Kolbe, L., Patterson, B., & Wechsler, H. (2003). Building a healthier future through school health programs. In *Promising practices in chronic disease prevention and control* (pp. 9–1–9–21). Atlanta: Centers for Disease Control and Prevention.

Kolbe, L. J. (2002, Autumn). Education reform and the goals of modern school health programs. *The State Education Standard,* pp. 4–11.

Marx, E. (2003). *Stories from the field: Lessons learned about building coordinated school health programs.* Atlanta: Centers for Disease Control and Prevention.

Marx, E., Wooley, S. F., & Northrop, D. (1998). *Health is academic: A guide to coordinated school health programs.* New York: Teacher's College Press.

McComb School District. (2002). *McComb Healthy Schools Project.* McComb, MS: Author.

National Association of School Nurses. (2001a). *Position statement: Coordinated school health program.* Retrieved August 22, 2004, from http://www.nasn.org/positions.htm

National Association of School Nurses. (2001b). *Scope and standards of professional school nursing practice.* Washington, DC: NASP Press.

National Association of School Nurses. (2002). *School nursing services role in health care: Role of the school nurse [issue brief].* Retrieved July 2005 from http://www.nasn.org/issues.htm

National Center for Chronic Disease Prevention and Health Promotion. (2001). *Youth Risk Behavior Surveillance System: Information and results / Youth 2001 online.* Retrieved May 5, 2003, from http://www.cdc.gov/nccdphp/dash/yrbs/2001/youth01online.htm

National Center for Chronic Disease Prevention and Health Promotion. (2004). *Healthy Youth! Coordinated School Health Programs.* Retrieved June 29, 2004, from http://www.cdc.gov/HealthyYouth/CSHP/index.htm.

Nikkola, N. (2003, March 31). *School health team (HIT Team)—unpublished notes.* Retrieved March 31, 2003, from http://nnikkola@earthlink.net

Ottoson, J., Streib, G., Thomas, J., Rivera, M., & Stevenson, B. (2004). Evaluation of the National Health Coordinator Leadership Institute. *Journal of School Health, 74,* 170–176.

Sinha, D. (2002). *A framework for strengthening health promotion programs for school staff: Strengthening coordinated school health programs.* Columbia, MD: Mid-Atlantic Division, American Cancer Society.

Tyson, H. (1999, January). A load off the teacher's backs: Coordinated school health programs. *Kappan,* pp. 1–14.

Chapter 4

Standards of Practice: What They Are and How to Use Them

SUSAN PROCTOR

Chapter Outline

A professional organization has a responsibility to its membership and to the public it serves to develop standards of practice.

AMERICAN NURSES ASSOCIATION (2004a, p. 1).

INTRODUCTION

The National Association of School Nurses (NASN) and the American Nurses Association (ANA) have recently developed an updated version of practice standards for school nursing (NASN & ANA, 2005). Based upon generic standards of practice crafted for all registered nurses by ANA (2004a), this effort is the latest in a long line of evolutionary conceptualizations regarding school nursing as a specialty within nursing.

Standards of practice are the professional expectations that guide practice. The extent to which nurses access these standards and, more particularly, structure their practice around them, is unknown. One reason for this is that standards are global, general statements in need of some explication and illumination to render them practical and utilitarian in the work setting. Second only to a definition of nursing and a statement of philosophy, standards are the *beginning,* not the end, of a comprehensive description of nursing practice. To fully operationalize practice standards, they need to be reflected in position descriptions and vacancy announcements, performance evaluation tools, and practice competencies, as well as competencies for the education of nursing professionals. This chapter discusses the sometimes elusive subject of standards with a particular spotlight on standards of practice for the school nurse. Specifically, this chapter seeks to identify, discuss, and amplify the meaning and use of practice standards, explore the history of nursing standards in general and school nursing standards in particular, examine the several standards statements and their meanings, reinforce and legitimatize their considerable importance in school nursing, offer practical and realistic suggestions on their use, and suggest areas for research.

STANDARDS OF PRACTICE: WHAT THEY ARE AND WHAT THEY ARE NOT

Prior to considering the formally adopted standards of practice and their role in the life of the specialty of school nursing, it is useful to briefly examine and understand other standards that also impact on school nursing.

Kinds of Standards

There are different kinds of standards of interest to the school nurse. Some apply strictly to nursing, some to the world of prekindergarten through grade 12 education. Because school nurses inhabit both universes, they are affected and influenced by both. Standards that exist for clients and their welfare, nursing and its practice, and the integrity of nursing as a discipline are, of course, applicable to all nurses in active practice regardless of their venue. However, depending upon the state and the school district, school nurses may also be affected by standards in place for schools, teachers, or school staff within the field of public education.

Standards Relevant to the Practice of Nursing

There are formal and informal standards; in large part, the difference is determined by their degree of legality (Schwab, Gelfman, & Cohn, 2001). Within nursing, standards may be *practice standards, legal standards, a standard of care,* or *educational standards.* TABLE 4.1 outlines and contrasts the kinds of standards designed for or expected of the school nurse as a practicing health care professional. Collectively, they have considerable influence in affecting, guiding, and influencing the practice of the school nurse.

Practice Standards

Practice standards are those that set the tone for what is expected of the practitioner: they *broadly subscribe the scope of practice* of a profession or discipline, or a specialty within that discipline. In subscribing a scope of practice, they set the stage for the clarification, delineation, interpretation, and implementation of a nursing practice role on the one hand, and its subsequent accountability and evaluation on the other. Practice standards may be clinical, pertaining to a clinical specialty or unique clinical role (e.g., those for school nursing, diabetes nursing, or hospice nursing), or functional, addressing areas of nursing practice that span the scope of the discipline and affect all clinical specialties or roles (e.g., administrative nursing or nursing informatics) (ANA, 2004b). Further, practice standards are increasingly being used to substantiate a community "standard of care" (see later) (Schwab, Hootman, & Gelfman, 2001).

Legal Standards

Legal standards are those that are grounded in law or statutory regulations. They are most often state law but also may be federal law. State law guides the licensure of registered nurses in all 50 states, and regulations promulgate the implementation of licensure and other practice-related law (see Chapters 12, 13, and 14).

Standard of Care

Often termed a *community standard,* a standard of care (note that "standard" is used as a singular noun) refers to what is expected of a nurse within a given community, large or small, at a given time, under certain conditions. If a nurse is sued for nursing actions or the absence of nursing actions in the performance of school nursing practice, the "standard of care" will be that which is inferred from the current level of practice in a community; professional publications, including textbooks, journals, and position statements; district policies, protocols, and procedures; often, and importantly, the school district's position description of the nurse's job; and the specifics or context of the nurse's work situation. Schwab, Gelfman, and Cohn (2001) noted that pupil-to-nurse ratios have an impact here; a nurse with responsibility for large numbers of students (in the thousands) would not be held to the same standard of care as would a nurse employed full time in one school with an enrollment of less than 500. *Context* is therefore critical in determining a community standard of care for a particular situation.

Educational Standards for Nursing Practice/Qualification

Standards or something akin to standards, addressing the necessary educational preparation of a nurse to successfully practice nursing, exist in every state. Each of the state boards of nursing prescribes some

(text continues on page 60)

Table 4.1 ■

NURSING-RELATED STANDARDS AND THEIR USE

TYPE	DEFINITION	AUTHOR	USE	REMARKS
Practice	Authoritative statements by which the profession or nursing specialty describes its practice and related accountability.	Usually a professional organization.	Guide role development, position descriptions, & performance evaluation, among other functions.	Broad scope of practice statements that necessitate elaboration with specifics for optimal use. May have a clinical focus (e.g., school nursing) or a functional focus (e.g., administration).
Legal	Statements of knowledge, skill, and performance required for the practice of nursing contained or reflected in statutes of law or regulations.	Law-making bodies (state legislatures, U.S. Congress) as well as governmental agencies assigned to develop/administer regulations and carry out law.	Protect the public through assurance of competence and the appropriate practice of nursing; assess the competence of nursing practice and its congruity with legal benchmarks.	Most laws and regulations governing nursing practice in the United States are at the state level.
(Standard of [Community]) Care	The expected level of practice within a community. A Community Standard of Care serves as the norm for nursing care in a particular setting or context.	Various authors or no author. Represents the current practice in a community. May be based on publications, policies, position descriptions, and the nurse's educational preparation.	May be used separately or together with legal statutes and regulatory codes to determine negligence or the lack thereof in lawsuits.	Usually used as a singular noun i.e., *the Standard of Care*; assesses what would be usual and expected practice in a particular setting by a specific person under these circumstances. Context is often key.
Educational	Required or recommended educational preparation for the practice of nursing or a nursing specialty.	Required standards: usually a state legislation or a state governmental agency; recommended standards: professional organizations.	Guide the acquisition of knowledge/skill necessary for the practice of nursing or a nursing specialty. Improve quality of care.	Found in only some states. Although all states prescribe the educational content for nursing in general, not all do so for school nursing as a specialty.

fundamental content that must be attained and achieved by all persons before licensure. States are in remarkable agreement on this content because licensure is predicated on passing the national licensing examination known as NCLEX (National Council on the Licensure Examination for Registered Nurses) (National Council of State Boards of Nursing, 2003).

In the case of the specialties within nursing, educational standards *describe the body of knowledge* that a nurse entering a particular specialty should have. There is no agreement on what constitutes a "body of relevant knowledge" for the many specialties within nursing, in part because the job of educational standards development is left to the individuals teaching nursing in the various specialties, and it is, or will be, their efforts that will spur the development of national standards of educational preparation within a given specialty.

There currently exist no national standards of *educational* preparation for school nursing practice, that is, a set of broad, global statements that would set down what must be learned or mastered by a nurse in order to successfully practice nursing within schools. There is an NASN-endorsed group of competencies described for the school nurse, which includes a Bachelor of Science degree in nursing (BSN). These competencies, a result of a research effort by the Southern Regional Education Board (SREB, 2000), hold considerable promise for conversion to or as a stimulus for the development of a national set of educational standards for the BSN nurse. A position paper of the National Consortium of School Nurse Educators (1998) briefly describes some principles and content areas for the educational preparation of the school nurse at the master's level.

Several states, such as Ohio, Massachusetts, Minnesota, Indiana, California, and others, individually prescribe educational standards, content, or competencies for the practice of school nursing (see Chapter 5). Although educational standards for the preparation of school nurses may vary from state to state, most educational requirements bear close resemblance to standards of practice or nationally accepted definitions of practice.

Standards That Apply to the K–12 Educational Setting

Because school nurses practice in two worlds, those of health care and education, standards affecting or imposed on public (or private) education may also impact the practice of nursing in the schools. Therefore, standards expected of professionals in schools (teachers, administrators, and others) may also apply to the nurse. An example would be state audits of public school programs such as those serving special education populations.

What Standards of Practice Are Not: The Story of Limbs, Branches, and Leaves

It is useful to briefly discuss what professional practice standards *are not* or should not be, before proceeding to define them and examine their use. First, as broad scope statements, standards of practice are usually not helpful used *alone* as a position or job description for a school nurse; that is to say, importing the 16 primary standard statements and the four "sub" standards, and using them with no further explanation of the nursing role in a given district or setting, does not serve nursing practice in that school or district well. This is because the roles and activities in which the nurse engages, particularly as the nurse uses the nursing process, are state and/or district specific, and the uniqueness of the position cannot be fully understood, comprehended, or appreciated through the use of standards statements *by themselves.*

Second, the language of a standards statement does not lend itself well to use within a performance evaluation instrument without the accompanying measurement criteria and the addition of sub-objectives or criteria that bring the meaning of the standard into the specific context of the school, district, or setting for which it is intended (see Chapter 11). The scope of school nursing practice is so broad that performance evaluation must consider the context. For example, a nurse employed full time in special education, responsible for the care of children with severe disabilities, will and should have his or her practice evaluated differently from the nurse in regular education. Also, the standards statements do not serve the nurse or the schools well as a *comprehensive and refined* listing of competencies essential to practice without further development and explication. Their language, intentionally broad, would not inform an uninitiated reader as to the specific expectations of practice without considerably more elucidation. To put it simply, the standards are the trunk, major limbs, and to some extent the branches, but not the small twigs or leaves, of a tree.

A Definition

Now one can ask, what really *are* professional standards? The official, most recent, and best definition of a nursing standard of practice is that issued in 2004 by ANA:

> Standards are authoritative statements by which the nursing profession describes responsibilities for which its practitioners are accountable. Consequently, standards reflect the values and priorities of the profession. Standards provide direction for professional nursing practice and a framework for the evaluation of this practice. Written in measurable terms, standards also define the nursing profession's accountability to the public and the outcomes for which nurses are responsible. (2004a, p. 1)

Applying this definition to school nursing standards, one can peruse the preceding definition, identify concepts, and extrapolate them to the practice of school nursing. Key concepts appear to be:

- Authoritative statements
- Description of responsibilities
- Reflection of the values and priorities of the [specialty]
- Provision of direction for practice
- Framework for practice evaluation
- Language written in measurable terms
- Accountability to the public
- Accountability for client outcomes

TABLE 4.2 provides an analysis of how the key concepts of the definition are anchored within the practice of school nursing, and hence, within school nursing practice standards.

Table 4.2 ■

ELUCIDATION OF KEY CONCEPTS OF THE ANA'S "STANDARDS OF PRACTICE" DEFINITION WITHIN SCHOOL NURSING STANDARDS

KEY CONCEPT	HOW MANIFESTED WITHIN SCHOOL NURSING	REMARKS
Authoritative statements	The language of the standards' statements reflects original ANA language and thereby carries the weight and impact of this professional organization. The words used to construct each standard are consistent with those used throughout nursing, intentionally chosen and crafted to connote specific meaning, agreed upon by leaders in the specialty of school nursing, endorsed by the NASN and the ANA, and included so as to promote clarity and reduce ambiguity about the practice of school nursing.	The authors of the school nursing standards carefully deliberated as to the impact of each standard statement and its measurement criteria before authorship. Possible impacts and influences on practice and on school districts were carefully considered.
Description of responsibilities	Responsibilities are broadly outlined, consistent with the purpose and role of a standard. Previously published and endorsed documents, including standards of practice and treatises addressing the comprehensive role of the nurse in the school, were combined with the views of the authors to reflect the contemporary school nursing role and its future projections.	Publications of a variety of professional nursing organizations were employed in the development of school nursing standards. The authors represented these groups well as well as a variety of roles within school nursing.

(continued)

Table 4.2 ■ (Continued)

KEY CONCEPT	HOW MANIFESTED WITHIN SCHOOL NURSING	REMARKS
Reflection of values and priorities	The standards (1) adhere to the principles of nursing in general and are built on the nursing process; (2) speak to what is essential in school nursing practice for the safe and competent care to children and families; (3) recognize the dynamic of the health care delivery system and its impact on the specialty; (4) recognize the current political and economic climates within public education; and (5) expect the same caring, competent care from school nurses as is expected of nurses in other practice settings.	The authors made every effort to acknowledge, consider, and incorporate political, economic, and social factors influencing the practice of school nursing while not compromising the integrity of the practice.
Provision of direction for practice	There is a reciprocal relationship between standards of practice and practice itself. First, national standards have solidified conceptualizations of practice; similarly, experience in practice has led to the revision of standards. Second, standards have influenced the direction of practice by shaping and directing the content of nursing curricula; in turn, nursing curricula have contributed to formulation and clarification of the language of standards.	Competency identification for school nursing should flow from standards of practice.
Framework for practice evaluation	Standards of practice can effectively serve as a springboard for development of performance evaluation instruments. Together with more particularistic treatises such as practice guidelines and position descriptions, standards can be a conceptual framework for a performance evaluation instrument.	NASN is interested in utilizing standards to develop a nationally available performance evaluation instrument. Such instruments have been previously developed and published by NASN (Ackerman, 1995; Lordi, 2000).
Written in measurable terms	Each standard statement is accompanied by several measurement criteria that serve as benchmarks or indicators of competent practice. The criteria allow assessment of the degree to which a school nurse has met or is meeting the spirit of a standard statement.	The measurement criteria can be used in conjunction with a rating scale such as a Likert scale that allows for both quantitative and qualitative assessment of the meeting of the standard.

(continued)

KEY CONCEPT	HOW MANIFESTED WITHIN SCHOOL NURSING	REMARKS
Accountability to the public	The standards reflect what is considered optimal nursing practice through their grounding in the nursing process, a critical thinking framework expected of all nurses in all settings at all times. The public is further protected and accountability ensured through the infusion of additional standards that complement the nursing process and ensure competent practice.	The standard have two sections: the *Standards of Practice* (formerly Standards of Care), and the *Standards of Professional Performance.* Together, they provide assurance to the public that a nurse, practicing by these standards, will deliver safe, appropriate, and competent care.
Accountability for client outcomes	The standards are written in such a way that responsibility to the client is paramount. The standards and their measurement criteria are further designed to facilitate a focus on the outcomes of nursing interventions in order to quantify and justify nursing time in schools.	The nursing process, as a *Standards of Practice* section, was reformulated in the early 1990s to include a sixth step: "Outcomes Identification" (ANA, 1991). The inclusion makes fluid the requisite that the nurse look for and measure client outcomes and that the result of nursing interventions be apparent and documented.

THE HISTORY OF PRACTICE STANDARDS WITHIN SCHOOL NURSING

Practice Standards for Nursing

General standards of nursing practice preceded the development of standards for the various specialties. Throughout the first half of the 20th century, the focus of professional nursing in the United States was on the care of the single individual in a hospital setting. In the 1960s, ANA, examining and writing about the nature and scope of nursing practice, determined that a set of national standards for nursing was needed. These standards developed by ANA were generic and spoke generally to the role of the nurse, laying down an expected framework for any nurse in any setting. General or generic standards have been published four times by ANA: in 1973, 1991, 1998, and most recently 2004.

After authoring the 1973 standards, ANA recognized that "specialty" standards were needed for nurses practicing in differing care areas within hospitals as well as for those practicing outside the acute setting, and that a generic or general set, while laying down overall principles, presented some "fit" problems across the wide spectrum and scope that was modern nursing. They urged the development of specialty standards by the professional organizations representing each of the nursing specialties at the time.

In school nursing, determining which organization represented the specialty was an important question. When nurses began to describe their practice for schools, they spoke with many voices. Documents and publications were forthcoming from at least four organizational perspectives during this time: the School Nurses Branch of ANA; the Department of School Nurses of the National Education Association (NEA); the Committee on School Nursing Policies and Practices of the American School Health Association (ASHA); and the National Council for School Nurses of the American Association of Health, Physical Education, and Recreation. Regrettably, communication among and between them appeared to be rare. One has to wonder whether the disparity of effort among several groups, all claiming to represent the interests of school nursing, helped or hindered the progress of the specialty.

It was not until 1983 that a *universally endorsed* set of standards for school nursing was written, synthesizing the views of the several groups (ANA, 1983). This landmark publication closely paralleled the *Standards of Nursing Practice* (ANA, 1973) in both language and format.

Practice Standards for School Nursing: The History

Early attempts at role definition consisted of lists of tasks, largely organized around the physical assessment of the child, with particular attention to the developmental parameters of height, weight, vision, and hearing. Definitions of school nursing and/or components of school health were proposed by non-nurses with input from school nurses. Among the non-nurse groups weighing in on nursing practice in schools was a coalition group of the National Education Association and the American Medical Association. The American Association of School Administrators also offered their perspective as to the role (ASHA Committee on School Nursing Policies and Practices, 1959; Basco, 1963; Wilson, 1964).

Even before ANA generated a set of standards for nursing, school nurses continued, as they had for much of the 20th century, to define and articulate their practice, especially to school administrators. Efforts were eventually forthcoming from nurses that prescribed philosophies, practice guidelines, and role definitions and presented, with remarkable clarity, the role of the nurse in the school. A history of the key documents of school nursing practice standards, with the names of nurses who authored them, is provided in Table 4.3. Key components of the history of practice standards are listed chronologically in this section; the publisher of each document follows the title in parentheses.

Table 4.3 ■

SIGNIFICANT DOCUMENTS AND THEIR CONTRIBUTORS: SCHOOL NURSING STANDARDS DEVELOPMENT

YEAR	DOCUMENT TITLE	AUTHOR(S)	PUBLISHER
1955	*Functions, Standards, and Qualifications for Public Health Nursing*	Public Health Nurses Section of the American Nurses Association (ANA)	ANA
1956, 1957, 1959	*Recommended Policies and Practices for School Nursing*	Committee on School Nursing Policies and Practices of the American School Health Association (ASHA) • Eunice Lamona RN, Chair, 1956 • Lyda Smiley RN, Chair, 1957 • Irma Fricke RN, PHN, Chair, 1959 *Plus* 62-nurse member committee from 25 states	JOSH (ASHA)
1963	*Evaluation of School Nursing Activities: A Pilot Project Using a Scoring System and Accepted Standards of School Nursing*	Delores Basco RN, PHN, Maryland	*Nursing Research*
1964	*Functions and Qualifications in the Practice of Public Health Nursing* (2nd ed.)	Public Health Nurses Section of the ANA	ANA

(continued)

YEAR	DOCUMENT TITLE	AUTHOR(S)	PUBLISHER
1966	*Functions and Qualifications of School Nurses*	School Nurses Branch, Public Health Nurses Section of ANA	ANA
1966	*School Nursing*	School Nurses Branch, Public Health Nurses Section of ANA	ANA
1970	*Standards for School Nurse Services*	National Commission on Standards, Department of School Nurses of the National Education Association (NEA; later the National Association of School Nurses [NASN]) • Gemma Jean RN, BS, Chair, New Hampshire • Helen Brion RN, MS, New York • Allie Cable RN, BS, Oklahoma • Ann Garber RN, MEd, Connecticut • Zorada Hodge RN, BS, Minnesota • Rowena McAllister RN, BS, Texas • Beatrice Shaffer RN, BS, Pennsylvania • Ruby Wheatly RN, BS, Iowa • Sally Williams RN, MS, California	NEA
1973, 1975	*Standards of Nursing Practice* and *A Plan for Implementation of the Standards of Nursing Practice*	Committee of ANA	ANA
1974	*Guidelines for the School Nurse in the School Health Program*	School Nurse Subcommittee of ASHA • Virginia Thompson RN, MPH, Chair, Texas • Mary Lou Brand RN, MA, Colorado • Helen Brion RN, MS, New York • Marguerite Cobb RN, MS, Washington • Virginia DePuy RN, BS, Pennsylvania • Marion Fleck RN, MPH, PhD, New Mexico • Ann Hill RN, MPH, JD, California • Marion Landgraf RN, BS, Maryland • Dee MacDonald RN, MA, Tennessee • Joan Olden RN, MA, Missouri • Edith Vincent RN, MA, Delaware	ASHA
1981	*Guidelines for a Model School Nursing Services Program*	Study Committee on Professional Standards of NASN • Helen Weber RN, MA, Chair, Nebraska • Judy Beck RN, MA, PNP, California	NASN

(continued)

Table 4.3 ■ *(Continued)*

YEAR	DOCUMENT TITLE	AUTHOR(S)	PUBLISHER
		• Helen Brion RN, MS, New York • Delora Brown RN, MA, California • Regina Eddy RN, BS, California • Pauline Fenelon RN, MA, Rhode Island • Anne Garber RN, MEd, Connecticut • Edia Harris RN, BS, Louisiana • June Heckel RN, BS, Missouri • Gemma Jean King RN, BS, New Hampshire • Maureen Robinson RN, Michigan • Beatrice Shaffer RN, MS, Pennsylvania • Lorrine Sheehan RN, BS, Iowa • Jean Smith RN, BS, Washington • Eleanor Thelander RN, BS, Minnesota • Sally Williams RN, MA, California	
1983	*Standards of School Nursing Practice*	• Georgia Macdonough RN, MA, SNP, Chair (NASN) • Victoria Hertel RN, MS, SNP (ASHA) • Ruth Hutchinson RNC, MS (ANA Division on Community Health Nursing Practice) • Susan Lordi RN, MS, PNP (National Association of Pediatric Nurse Associates and Practitioners) • Carol Stade RN, MN (ANA Division on Maternal Child Health Nursing Practice) • Eleanor Thelander RN, BS (NASN) • Jean Wood RN, PhD (Public Health Nursing Section of the American Public Health Association)	ANA
1990	*Guidelines for a Model School Nursing Services Program*	Susan Proctor RN, MPH, California	NASN
1991	*Implementation Guide for the Standards of School Nursing Practice*	Implementation Guide Committee, ASHA • Alicia Snyder RN, MA, New Mexico • Bernice Baxter RN, MEd, CAN, Pennsylvania • Nela Beetem RN, SNP, Missouri	ASHA

(continued)

YEAR	DOCUMENT TITLE	AUTHOR(S)	PUBLISHER
		• Ann Eastman RN, MS, Texas • Mary Ellen Gillette RN,C, MEd, Florida • Victoria Hertel RN, MSN, Colorado • Dorothy Oda RN, DNSc, California	
1991	*Standards of Clinical Nursing Practice*	ANA Practice and Guidelines Committee Representatives from Nursing Organization Liaison Forum (NOLF): • Donna Zaiger RN, BS, represented NASN	ANA
1993	*School Nursing Practice: Roles and Standards*	Susan Proctor RN, MPH, California with Susan Lordi RN, MS, PNP, California Donna Zaiger RN, BS, Missouri	NASN
1997	*Standards of Clinical Nursing Practice* (2nd ed.)	ANA Task Force with NOLF input	ANA
1998	*Standards of Professional School Nursing Practice*	Standards of Practice Task Force: • Charla Dunham RN, MEd, Chair (Chair, NASN Standards & Practice Committee) • Nancy Birchmeier RN, BS (NASN Standards & Practice Committee) • Linda Edwards RN, DrPH (American Public Health Association, Public Health Nursing Section) • Tona Leiker RN, MN (ANA) • Judith Maire RN, MN (National Association of State School Nurse Consultants) • Susan Proctor RN, DNS (Author, NASN Standards Writings) • Genie Wessel RN, MS (ASHA) • Linda Wolfe RN, MEd (Past-Chair, NASN Standards & Practice Committee) • Doris Luckenbill RN, MS, CRNP (NASN President) (Ex-Officio Member)	NASN
2000	*Standards of Professional School Nursing Practice: Applications in the Field*	Susan Lordi RN, MS, PNP with Beverly Bradley RN, PhD	NASN

(continued)

Table 4.3 ■ (Continued)

YEAR	DOCUMENT TITLE	AUTHOR(S)	PUBLISHER
2001	*Scope and Standards of Professional School Nursing Practice*	Standards/Practice/Issues Committee, NASN (short scope statement added to 1998 standards)	NASN
2005	*School Nursing: Scope and Standards of Practice* (2nd ed.)	Standards of Practice Task Force • Elizabeth "Libby" Thomas, Chair, RN, MEd (NASN) • Roberta Bavin, RN, MN, CPNP (National Association of Pediatric Nurse Practitioners and Associates) • Carol Bickford, RN, BC, PhD (ANA) • Charlotte Burt RN, BC, MSN, MA (ASHA) • Julia Cowell, RNC, PhD (American Public Health Association, Public Health Nursing Section) • Linda Davis-Alldritt RN, MA (National Association of State School Nurse Consultants) • Maria Rivera RNC, MSN, MA (National Center for School Health Nursing) • Janis Hootman RN, PhD (NASN President) (Ex-Officio Member)	NASN/ANA

1955: Functions, Standards, and Qualifications for Public Health Nursing (ANA)

Though increasingly numerous as school district employees, many school nurses in the mid-20th century were public health nurses employed by local health departments. The proportion of their time spent in schools was substantial. Acting in response to a need by public health nurses for standards of practice that included services to children in school, the Public Health Nurses Section (PHNS) of ANA published their public health nursing standards (ANA-PHNS, 1955).

1956, 1957, & 1959: Recommended Policies and Practices for School Nursing (ASHA)

Beginning in 1952, the Committee on School Nursing Policies and Practices of the ASHA responded to a member challenge for the creation of "guidelines setting up standards for school nursing" (ASHA Committee on School Nursing Policies and Practices, 1959, p. 388). The committee worked for 4 years under the leadership of Eunice Lamona and Lyda Smiley and was composed of 62 nurses from 25 states. Using the annual conferences of ASHA as meeting opportunities, the leadership of the committee presented their results to ASHA's Governing Council in 1955. The first version was published in the *Journal of School Health* in early 1956 (ASHA Committee on School Nursing Policies and Practices, 1956) and was in such demand that a second printing of four thousand additional copies was exhausted in a short time (ASHA Committee on School Nursing Policies and Practices, 1957). A second edition was published in 1959 following brief revisions by the ASHA Governing Council.

1963: Evaluation of School Nursing Activities: A Pilot Project Using a Scoring System and Accepted Standards of School Nursing (Nursing Research)

A remarkable research paper, published in 1963 by the journal *Nursing Research,* incorporated both the ASHA Committee on School Nursing Policies and Practices work (1959) and ANA's public health nursing standards (ANA, 1955) into the development of a research questionnaire. The author, Delores Basco, was a supervising public health nurse for the Bureau of Public Health Nursing, Baltimore City Health Department, at the time and supervised 160 public health nurses, 71 of whom delivered services in schools ranging from 2.5 to 18 hours per week. Although not a standards document as such, it is the first published attempt during this era to use in-print accounts of school nursing functions as a framework for understanding and evaluating school nursing practice (Basco, 1963).

1964: Functions and Qualifications in the Practice of Public Health Nursing (2nd ed.) (ANA)

A second edition of the public health nursing standards was published in 1964. School nurses representing the School Nurses Branch of the Public Health Nurses Section sat on the executive committee. A footnote in the second edition reads "For more specific functions and activities for the public health nurse assigned to a school, ... refer to statements of functions and qualifications prepared by the School Nurses Branch, Public Health Nurses Section ... of the American Nurses Association" (ANA-PHNS, 1964, p. 6).

1966: Functions and Qualifications of School Nurses (ANA) and School Nursing (ANA)

Independent work by the School Nurses Branch of the ANA-PHNS produced two additional publications in 1966. The first paralleled its parent document, the public health nursing standards issued in 1964 by ANA (ANA-PHNS, 1966a). A second document, authored by the same group, appears to be a statement of philosophy/description of services (ANA-PHNS, 1966b).

1970: Standards for School Nurse Services (NEA)

By late 1968, another national group, also representing the interests of school nursing, was meeting (G. Durgin, personal communication, November 3, 2003). This group, the Department of School Nurses of NEA, later became NASN. In 1970, their National Commission on Standards published a paper enumerating 10 functional areas that reflected content from earlier work but in a different format (NEA Department of School Nurses, 1970). The commission, chaired by Gemma Jean of New Hampshire, scribed the identified functional areas as statements with behavioral objectives beneath each. A brief document of 11 pages and one of the earliest of the Department of School Nurses' publications, it stood on par with the standards/role statements previously developed by the ASHA Committee on School Nursing Policies and Practices (1959) and ANA-PHNS (1964) and compared favorably with both

1973: Standards of Nursing Practice (ANA) and 1975: A Plan for Implementation of the Standards of Nursing Practice (ANA)

The *Standards of Nursing Practice* (ANA, 1973) were the first formal and authentic practice standards for use in nursing "at large." Largely designed for use in the acute care setting, their issuance began the era of accountability to the patient and quality of care (Pohlman, 2001). An implementation guide followed 2 years later (ANA, 1975).

1974: Guidelines for the School Nurse in the School Health Program (ASHA)

ASHA weighed in again in 1974 with *Guidelines for the School Nurse in the School Health Program.* Developed by a subcommittee of the school nursing section of that organization with national representation and some inter-organizational constituency, these guidelines were significant, because, for the first time, school nursing was conceptualized using role concepts such as Health Manager and Deliverer of Health Services. By speaking conceptually, it described large areas of role responsibility without resorting to an inventory of tasks and duties.

The book also addressed educational qualifications for school nurses, evaluation of school nurses, supervision in school nursing, and guidelines for employment and supervision of health assistants. Of interest is the fact that school nurse is referred to generically as "school nurse practitioner" throughout the document. Its reference list is also illuminating; it indicates that, in addition to ANA, ASHA, and the NEA Department of School Nurses, the American Association of Health, Physical Education, and Recreation's National Council on School Nursing was also writing and publishing documents on the role of the school nurse.

1981: Guidelines for a Model School Nursing Services Program (NASN)

NASN was in its infancy as an independent organization, barely 2 years after its breakaway from NEA, when it produced a second edition of the 1970 *Standards for School Nurse Services* titled *Guidelines for a Model School Nursing Services Program* (NASN, 1981; G. Durgin & P. Roberts, personal communication, November 3, 2003). Enumerated within its covers were 16 content areas, each supplemented with an education-related goal for the student.

Further, each of the content areas was expanded upon through the inclusion of knowledge/competency and performance criteria written in measurable terms.

The work was the product of the Study Committee on Professional Standards, chaired by Helen Weber of Nebraska and supported by a grant from NASN awarded through a competitive process. Comprised entirely of NASN members, the composition of the committee allowed for geographic diversity (see Table 4.3). The book was somewhat task- rather than process-oriented and reflective of a medical (systems) model; nonetheless, it continued an era of serious contributions to the role literature within school nursing.

1983: Standards of School Nursing Practice (ANA)

Without a doubt, the cornerstone publication for school nursing standards was the release in 1983 of the *Standards of School Nursing Practice.* Unlike either the earlier efforts by ASHA (1974) or NASN (1981), this text used the 1973 ANA *Standards of Nursing Practice* as a template, thus bringing school nursing into harmony with the larger profession. The book was process-oriented and provided the practicing nurse with eight standard statements around which to organize and evaluate one's practice. *Each standard statement was accompanied by a rationale, structure criteria, process criteria, and outcome criteria.* A glossary appended the standards. *Structure criteria* were defined as

> Criteria that focus on the environment [school nurse practice environment] and its resources. They include consideration of the purpose of the institution, agency, or program, and its legal authority to carry out its mission; organizational characteristics; physical resources and management; qualifications of health professionals and other workers; physical facilities and equipment; and status with regard to accreditation, certification, or approval by appropriate voluntary or governmental bodies. (ANA, 1983, p. 17)

In other words, the structure criteria provided the nurse with yardsticks to examine the extent to which the work setting, its members, and its accoutrements supported and allowed for quality nursing practice. An example of a structure criterion for Standard II, "Program Management," was "The school setting provides an environment conducive to the privacy, confidentiality, and efficiency of school nursing practice" (ANA, 1983, p. 4).

Process criteria were also helpful to the practicing nurse. The working group defined process criteria as "criteria that focus on the major sequence of events and activities in the delivery of care" (ANA, 1983, p. 17). The process criteria provided some of the "leaves on the tree" that the broader language of the standards could not (and should not) elucidate, listing many appraisal statements that could readily be used in performance evaluation. An example of a process criterion serving Standard III, "Nursing Process," Part D, "Intervention," was "The nurse intervenes appropriately for individuals and populations at risk for preventable, potential health problems" (ANA, 1983, p. 9).

Refreshingly, *outcome criteria* were also included, reflecting the 1973 ANA *Standards of Nursing Practice.* Outcome criteria were defined as "Criteria that focus on the end result of nursing care; a measurable change in the state of the client's health or the end product of the professional process" (ANA, 1983, p. 17). If, however, the inclusion of outcome language was meant to direct the nurse's (and the school district's) attention to the ultimate goal of nursing, which was maintenance or improvement of health and the optimal education of the child, the criteria in the 1983 document did not do so. Regrettably, outcome criteria were largely a measure of nursing activities rather than client outcomes. An example of an outcome criterion for Standard V, "Health Education" was "Health education activities are documented" (ANA, 1983, p. 13). Nonetheless, the endowment of this document to the specialty was so significant that it is among the most influential contributions to the school nursing literature of the 20th century.

Unlike the 1974 ASHA work and the 1981 NASN document, which were largely developed by a single professional organization, the genesis of the 1983 standards was one in which representation was sought from several nursing and health organizations interested in school nursing and school health. The small but effective working group was chaired by Georgia Macdonough of Arizona, who represented the National Association of State School Nurse Consultants. Other organizations at the table were ANA (two divisions), the American Public Health Association, ASHA, the National Association of Pediatric Nurse Associates and Practitioners, and, of course, NASN. Member names are noted in Table 4.3.

1990: Guidelines for a Model School Nursing Services Program (NASN)

Responding to a call from the membership in 1989, Susan Lordi, then NASN President, solicited an author to rewrite and update the 1981 *Guidelines for a Model School Nursing Services Program* document. Unlike earlier NASN versions (NEA, 1970; NASN, 1981), a link was made with existing standards of practice and all eight of the 1983 school nursing standards were infused into the book, either using the precise language or with moderate adaptations. This revised edition of the *Guidelines* combined the eight ANA school nursing standards with two standards formulated in California for the educational preparation of school nurses (Proctor, 1990).

Each of the 10 standards was explicated with a central theme definition, rationale for the standard, measurement criteria, and a narrative titled "Building Toward This Standard." The standards, in turn, were nested within six role concepts, borrowed from the nursing arm of the Western Interstate Commission on Higher Education (1985) and coincidentally similar to role concepts proffered by ASHA (1974) and Wold and Dagg (1981) several years earlier. The six roles for the school nurse were Provider of Client Care, Communicator, Planner and Coordinator of Client Care, Client Teacher, Investigator, and "Role Within the Discipline of Nursing."

Reflective of the national standards of school nursing practice, the revised version of the *Guidelines* was actually an *implementation* guide for the standards. It continued the effort to describe the school nursing role in terms of concepts rather than duties and was a broad statement of the considerable breath and scope of contemporary school nursing practice. In keeping with the position of the NASN Publications Committee, the title was not changed from that of the first version.

1991: Implementation Guide for the Standards of School Nursing Practice (ASHA)

Unbeknownst to NASN, the School Nurse Study Committee of ASHA was, at the same time as the revisions were being made to the *Guidelines* document described previously, also engaged in the development of an implementation guide for the 1983 *Standards of School Nursing Practice.* The project, conceived in 1984, was delayed in its development and publication. Unfortunately for the school nursing community, the book was not issued until a year after NASN's revision of the 1990 *Guidelines* text appeared in the literature.

Structured around the school nursing standards of practice, a narrative of two to three single-spaced pages was interspersed after each standard statement. The narrative did not address measurement criteria but rather discussed the use of the standard in practical terms, leaving it to the reader to apply to his or her own setting. The book also came replete with a section titled "Contemporary Issues" that featured papers on issues of the day (e.g., HIV), several of which were authored by committee members. There were also appendices with sample forms.

The committee, chaired by Alicia Snyder of New Mexico, was a relatively large group in contrast to the size of some of the other working groups in this trajectory (see Table 4.3). The product of their work was a scholarly, useful, and meaningful contribution to the school nursing literature. Most importantly, it spoke directly to the national standards of practice and endeavored to translate the standards into a user-friendly context for the practicing school nurse.

1991: Standards of Clinical Nursing Practice (ANA)

The ANA's Practice and Guidelines Committee undertook the development of new generic standards of practice applicable to all nurses in all practice setting in 1990. These were to supplant the 1973 *Standards of Nursing Practice* and were intentionally retitled *Standards of Clinical Practice* to differentiate them from nursing standards developed for nonclinical practice settings or roles. Realizing that there was a long-standing recognition of the need for specialty standards, the ANA, in its wisdom, invited representatives of the Nursing Organization Liaison Forum (NOLF), to work with them. The NOLF's membership consisted of nurses from over 40 specialties within nursing. Donna Zaiger of Missouri was the NASN representative on NOLF. ANA's charge to this group was to "define the nature and purpose of standards of practice for nursing and the relationship of quality assurance activities and standards of practice to specialization in nursing practice, credentialing, and implications for nursing information systems" (ANA, 1991, p. v).

The result was a new set of *generic* standards that differed from the 1973 work in two significant ways. First, the standards were divided into "Standards of Care," sequestering the nursing process into one section, and "Standards of Professional Performance," gathered into a second section describing a "competent level of behavior in the professional role" (ANA, 1991, p. 3). Standards of Professional Performance were further explained thusly: "All nurses are expected to engage in professional role activities appropriate to their education and position. Ultimately, nurses are accountable to themselves, their patients [clients], and their peers for their professional activities" (ANA, 1991, p. 3). The second important difference from the first set of generic standards was that a sixth step, Outcome Identification, was added to the nursing process ("Outcome" was used in the singular at this point in time). The document was written in such a way that it could and would serve as a template for nursing specialty organizations in the development of revised specialty standards.

1993: School Nursing Practice: Roles and Standards (NASN)

Susan Lordi, as past president of NASN, invited the author of the revised NASN *Guidelines* book, Susan Proctor, to work with her and then NASN President, Donna Zaiger, on retrofitting the NASN's *Guidelines for a Model School Nurse Services Program* (Proctor, 1990) to align with the 1991 *Standards of Clinical Nursing Practice* (ANA, 1991). As noted, Donna Zaiger had been involved in the development of the ANA *Standards of Clinical Nursing Practice,* representing NASN by way of NOLF. During these deliberations, she sensed a strong push from ANA for NASN and other specialty groups within nursing to make specialty standards more reflective of the 1991 ANA standards' language and format.

The group of three took the *Guidelines* book and, with no change to the body of the document, inserted all six of the ANA Standards of Care (nursing process) and applicable Standards of Professional Performance beneath each of the 1990 standards statements, but preceding the narrative text for each of the 10 standards. Further, Susan Lordi authored an introductory chapter to provide explanation of the ANA *Standards of Clinical Nursing Practice* and the reason for the "retrofit," and Donna Zaiger developed a glossary for the book. The content of the remainder of the book did not change from the format of the 1990 *Guidelines,* with the 10 standards statements retaining their language and not reverting to the language, structure, and format of the ANA template. The new work, published in 1993 as *School Nursing Practice: Roles and Standards,* became known as the NASN standards (Proctor, 1993). This was perhaps an unfortunate title, as the book was really a streamlined version of the 1990 *Guidelines* designed to fit the 1991 ANA generic standards and not a *universally endorsed* set of standards for school nursing.

1998: Standards of Clinical Nursing Practice (2nd ed.) (ANA)

Refining their 1991 work, ANA, in 1998, made minor changes to the language of one of the standards and added several measurement criteria throughout the document. The revised work continued the use of Standards of Care and Standards of Professional Performance. Most specialty organizations in nursing were converting or had converted their specialty standards to the ANA template by the time the second edition appeared. (*Note:* This book was the second edition using this title but actually the third published set of generic standards.)

1998: Standards of Professional School Nursing Practice (NASN)

With the publication of the second edition of the *Standards of Clinical Nursing Practice* (ANA, 1998), there was considerable encouragement from ANA and others to develop standards for school nursing that were *completely* consistent and consonant with the ANA work. ASHA school nurse member Victoria Hertel circulated a draft of proposed revisions to the 1991 ANA standards speaking to school nursing (Hertel, 1996).

A small task force was assembled in 1997 by the then NASN president, Doris Luckenbill, to begin work on the standards format revision. Again, as in the case of the 1983 standards effort, representation was interorganizational. Representation was garnered from NASH, ASHA, the American Public Health Association's Public Health Nursing Section, ANA, and the National Association of State School Nurse Consultants (see Table 4.3). Charla Dunham of Washington, Chair of the Standards/Practice/Issues Committee of NASN, chaired the committee. True to the form of the clinical standards of practice, both Standards of Care and Standards of Professional Performance were included. In contrast to the 1983 standards, which had structure, measurement, and outcome criteria, however, this set contained only measurement criteria; structure and outcome measures were subsumed within the measurement criteria. Much of the language of the 1993 NASN implementation book (Proctor, 1993) was retained. Also, in contrast to the 1983 standards, "professional" was added to the title.

The 1998 ANA *Standards of Clinical Nursing Practice* was used as a template. Within the Standards of Care section, the six steps of the nursing process as Standards I through VI were reconstructed to accommodate the practice of school nursing. Similarly, the eight standards that constituted the Standards of Professional Performance section were reworded to characterize school nursing, and three new standards were added. In the end, ANA approved and endorsed 17 standards, and they were published by NASN in 1998 as the *Standards of Professional School Nursing Practice.*

2000: Standards of Professional School Nursing Practice: Applications in the Field (NASN)

As noted at the beginning of this chapter, standards are designed to be used as overriding principles and require some explication prior to unfettered use. So it was not a surprise that, less than 2 years following publication of the NASN *Standards,* an implementation manual appeared. Susan Lordi authored the implementation book, assisted by Beverly Bradley, then President-Elect of ASHA. The "Applications" book, as it is known, reiterated the standards and their measurement criteria but also elucidated two additional sections within each standard: "Institutional Support" and a discussion of the meaning of the standard. The Institutional Support section listed criteria for evaluating the extent to which the *school district* supported the nurse in the attainment of a given standard in his or her practice. The discussion section provided the nurse with a greater understanding of the meaning of the standard and suggested ways that the standard might be achieved. An extensive glossary was appended that included a sample evaluation tool based upon the standards, for use in the performance evaluation of a nurse by a non-nurse (Lordi, 2000).

2001: Scope and Standards of Professional School Nursing Practice (NASN & ANA)

The NASN Standards/Issues/Practice Committee, noting the ANA's incorporation of scope language into various related works, believed that the 1998 NASN standards document needed a "scope" statement as a preface. A "scope statement describes the who, what, where, when, why, and how of the specialty" (NASN & ANA, 2001, p. vii). A 7-page scope statement was inserted as a preface to the 1998 standards. The language of the standards statements and the measurement criteria *were unaltered* from the 1998 edition.

2004: Nursing: Scope and Standards of Practice (ANA)

In December 2003, ANA published a substantively revised version of their generic standards of practice, this edition with a scope statement and, conveniently, appending all prior versions/editions of the generic standards (ANA, 2004a). The book also appended a scope statement originally scribed in the mid-1980s (ANA, 1987). For the first time, the practicing registered nurse had a document that combined all earlier versions of both standards and scope statements with the most recent standards of nursing practice and scope of nursing practice statement, painting a picture of the evolution in the conceptualization of the practice of nursing. A second printing was issued in June 2004.

The 2004 version of the scope and standards of nursing practice departed from earlier editions by addressing some functional roles for nurses within the scope statement as well as within the Implementation standard. Specifically, the document addressed aspects of the advanced-practice nursing role: coordination, health teaching/education and health promotion, consultation, and prescriptive authority and treatment. It also changed "Standards of Care" to "Standards of Practice" (Praeger, 2005). Further, an index catalogued content from all versions of the generic standards as well as the 1987 scope statement (ANA, 1973, 1987, 1991, 1998, 2004a). A comprehensive and highly useful document, it serves, as did its predecessors, as a ready template for specialty standards development within the many nursing areas of expertise.

2005: School Nursing: Scope and Standards of Practice (2nd ed.) (NASN & ANA)

In 2004 and 2005, a task force was convened by NASN and ANA to develop a new edition of the scope and standards for school nursing practice. The group, chaired by Libby Thomas of Delaware, had a constituency that represented the diversity of prior school nursing standards' task forces: NASN, ASHA, ANA, the Public Health Nursing Section of the American Public Health Association, the National Association of Pediatric Nurse Practitioners and Associates, the National Association of State School Nurse Consultants, and the National Center for School Health Nursing (see Table 4.3). The product reflected the template laid down by ANA (2004a). It is expected that NASN will subsequently author an implementation manual not unlike earlier documents (Lordi, 2000; Proctor, 1993).

THE STANDARDS: WHAT ARE THEY AND WHAT DO THEY MEAN?

The standards of school nursing practice (NASN & ANA, 2005) are made up of "Standards of Practice" (formerly "Standards of Care") and "Standards of Professional Performance." Each standard has a *standard title, statement* (the actual language of the standard), and *measurement criteria.* The criteria, benchmarks or indicators of competent practice, allow the standard to be evaluated. Although the language of standards statements may remain fairly constant across time, measurement criteria often flux and change in keeping with changes in role and practice. The standards are addressed individually in this section within the context of Standards of Practice and Standards of Professional Performance. The standards, without their measurement criteria, may be found in TABLE 4.4.

Standards of Practice

The Standards of Practice, as the components of the nursing process, *describe a competent level of nursing care for all practicing registered nurses, regardless of practice setting.* Although the content and nature of the assessment may vary from that in other areas of nursing practice, there remains the same legal responsibility to execute the nursing process in accordance with the standard of care expected of a school nurse in a particular community and in congruence with the state Nurse Practice Act. The nursing process is depicted in FIGURE 4.1.

When the nursing process was reconceptualized in 1991 and a sixth step was added, ANA-identified themes were infused throughout all the steps of the

Table 4.4 ■
STANDARDS OF SCHOOL NURSING PRACTICE*

STANDARD NUMBER	STANDARD TITLE	STANDARD LANGUAGE
Standards of Practice		
1	Assessment	The school nurse collects comprehensive data pertinent to the client's health or the situation.
2	Diagnosis	The school nurse analyzes the assessment data to determine the diagnoses or issues.
3	Outcomes Identification	The school nurse identifies expected outcomes for a plan individualized to the client or situation.
4	Planning	The school nurse develops a plan that prescribes strategies and alternatives to attain expected outcomes.
5	Implementation	The school nurse implements the identified plan.
5A	Coordination of Care	The school nurse coordinates care delivery.
5B	Health Teaching and Health Promotion	The school nurse provides health education and employs strategies to promote health and a safe environment.
5C	Consultation	The school nurse provides consultation to influence the identified plan, enhance the abilities of others, and effect change.
5D	Prescriptive Authority and Treatment	The advanced practice registered nurse uses prescriptive authority, procedures, referrals, treatments, and therapies in accordance with state and federal laws and regulations.
6	Evaluation	The school nurse evaluates the progress toward attainment of outcomes.

(continued)

STANDARD NUMBER	STANDARD TITLE	STANDARD LANGUAGE
Standards of Professional Performance		
7	Quality of Practice	The school nurse systematically enhances the quality and effectiveness of school nursing practice.
8	Education	The school nurse attains knowledge and competency that reflects current school nursing practice.
9	Professional Practice Evaluation	The school nurse evaluates one's own nursing practice in relation to professional practice standards and guidelines, relevant statutes, rules, and regulations.
10	Collegiality	The school nurse interacts with and contributes to the professional development of peers and school personnel as colleagues.
11	Collaboration	The school nurse collaborates with the client, family, school staff, and others in the conduct of school nursing practice.
12	Ethics	The school nurse integrates ethical provisions in all area of practice.
13	Research	The school nurse integrates research findings into practice.
14	Resource Utilization	The school nurse considers factors related to safety, effectiveness, cost, and impact on practice in the planning and delivery of school nursing services.
15	Leadership	The school nurse provides leadership in the professional practice setting and the profession.
16	Program Management	The school nurse manages school health services.

*From the National Association of School Nurses and American Nurses Association. (2005). *School Nursing: Scope and Standards of Practice.* Silver Spring, MD: Nursesbooks.org/American Nurses Association.

nursing process reflecting responsibilities for and to all clients. The themes are

- Providing age-appropriate as well as culturally and ethnically-sensitive care
- Maintaining a safe environment
- Educating patients [clients] about healthy practices and treatment modalities
- Assuring continuity of care
- Coordinating the care across settings and among caregivers
- Managing information
- Communicating effectively
- Utilizing technology (ANA, 2004a, p. 4)

The themes are reflected in measurement criteria associated with each standard. There are six standards of practice.

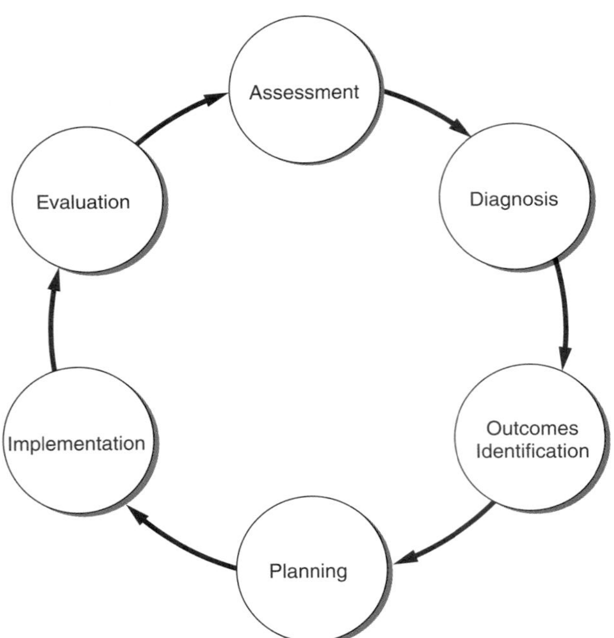

Figure 4.1 ■ Steps of the nursing process, illustrating the continuous and circular nature of the process. Beginning at the top with Assessment, the process is ongoing.

Standard 1: Assessment

The school nurse collects comprehensive data pertinent to the client's health or the situation.

Assessment has been a step in the nursing process since its inception (Yura & Walsh, 1973). Assessment can be a one-time procedure or a progressive process that is continuous, evolves, and has many facets. Indeed, in school nursing, it is not unusual for assessment to be ongoing for months or even years. Assessment data may be voluminous after long periods of time and, in themselves, may require management to be readily retrieved and apprehended.

The essence of the Assessment standard and its measurement criteria is that

- Diagnosis involves systematic assessment, comparing and contrasting clinical findings with normal and abnormal parameters.
- All relevant constituencies and sources are included in data collection.
- Data are collected in a manner that designates priority.
- Data are collected using evidence-based techniques.
- Analytical models and problem-solving tools are used in data collection.
- Data are documented in a retrievable form.
- Patterns and variances are gleaned from the synthesis of data.
- The Advanced Practice Registered Nurse (APRN) initiates and/or interprets diagnostic tests as part of assessment.

Standard 2: Diagnosis

The school nurse analyzes the assessment data to determine the diagnoses or issues.

When the nursing process was first conceived in the 1970s, before the days of complex evaluations and advanced practice nursing, assessment was simpler and the nurse could usually come to a ready conclusion of what was happening with the client (Yura & Walsh, 1973). However, as the world of nursing, its levels, and scope expanded, the need for nursing diagnoses became apparent. Due, in part, to the work of Marjory Gordon, Lynda Carpenito, and others, diagnoses were offered that were separate from assessment and further differentiated nursing from medicine. The North American Nursing Diagnosis Association (NANDA) was founded in the 1970s with a self-designed mission to develop a taxonomy of universal diagnoses to be used by nurses (Hootman, 1996). NANDA annually publishes the most current listing of diagnoses with definitions and classifications approved by the organization (NANDA, 2005).

There is scarcely a school nurse who is not familiar with nursing diagnoses. Indeed, school nurses have been urged to use standardized diagnoses for some time, especially by NASN (Hootman, 1996). Initially, nursing diagnoses accepted and approved by NANDA were problematic for school nurses because, although they dealt adequately with the individual client with a health problem, they came up short with regard to wellness and health promotion diagnoses, and for any client group numbering more than one. Thanks to Marge Lunney and colleagues, NANDA approved the first wellness diagnoses gleaned from and for the practice of school nursing (Lunney, 1996; Lunney, Cavendish, Luise, & Richardson, 1997; NANDA, 2005).

The essence of the Diagnosis standard and its measurement criteria is that

- Diagnoses or issues flow from all collected assessment data.
- Diagnoses may, from time to time, necessitate validation from the client, the school staff, or other providers.
- Diagnoses need documentation in such a

manner that they facilitate the identification of outcomes and a nursing plan.

- Diagnoses are expressed in standardized language (i.e., taxonomy) so that they are readily retrievable.
- The APRN compares and contrasts assessment data in arriving at both a medical and a nursing diagnosis.
- The APRN uses complex data and assists others in the diagnostic process.
- The APRN assists staff to develop and maintain diagnostic competence.

Standard 3: Outcomes Identification

The school nurse identifies expected outcomes for a plan individualized to the client or situation.

A new step of the nursing process added in 1991 by ANA, originally a singular "Outcome" but now "Outcomes Identification," is a stage to which nurses are still becoming accustomed. Formalized outcomes identification came about as a natural extension of diagnosis because of the need to consider goals *prior* to planning, and the contemporary emphasis on promoting and measuring outcomes of care as quality assurance indicators (see Chapter 11). Evidence-based practice also emphasizes outcomes (Costante, 2001).

A focus on outcomes facilitates a perspective that promotes evaluation of the effectiveness of nursing plans and interventions. National research priorities within school nursing have ranked the linking of nursing services to favorable educational outcomes for children as the most needed and critical area of research (Brainerd, 2000; Edwards, 2002). Stock, Larter, Kieckehefer, Thronson, and Maire (2002) recently enumerated several studies in which positive outcomes for children were correlated with nursing services in schools. The impetus for identifying and accounting for outcomes is prominent at the present time; many school nursing leaders have underscored the importance of an outcomes focus in contemporary practice (Cavendish, Lunney, Luise, & Richardson, 2001; Costante, 2001; Denehy, 2000; Igoe, 2000; Wolfe, 2002).

Like diagnoses, outcomes have been standardized and are available for use in any nursing setting as a result of efforts of the Center for Nursing Classification at The University of Iowa. An outcomes book, like the annual diagnoses book from NANDA, titled *Nursing Outcomes Classification (NOC)* (Moorhead, Johnson, & Maas, 2004) is updated and published periodically and is available in software format as well (Dochterman & Jones, 2003). Each outcome *may actually be measured* using one of 11 standard measurement tools (per the 2004 edition). These measurement tools, together with indicators developed by the authors, assist the nurse or others in evaluating the outcome. Further, outcomes are conveniently linked to corresponding diagnoses for ready consumption in a book by M. Johnson, Bulechek, Dochterman, Maas, and Moorhead (2001).

The essence of the Outcomes Identification standard and its measurement criteria is that

- Outcomes flow from the diagnosis(es).
- Outcomes are formulated in concert with the client and his or her family as well as school staff and community members, as necessary.
- Outcomes are culturally appropriate.
- Outcomes consider risks, benefits, costs, scientific evidence, and clinical expertise.
- Outcomes consider client and family values, ethics, and the client and family environment.
- Outcomes set realistic timelines for attainment.
- Outcomes ensure continuity of care.
- Outcomes are modified as necessary.
- Outcomes require documentation as measurable goals so that their attainment, or lack thereof, may be noted.
- Outcomes are expressed in standardized language (i.e., taxonomy) so that they are readily retrievable.
- The APRN formulates outcomes using scientific evidence and the outcomes are achievable through the use of evidence-based practice.

Standard 4: Planning

The school nurse develops a plan that prescribes strategies and alternatives to attain expected outcomes.

The development of a plan for an individual student or for a family is an important nursing function. A written plan might be an Individualized Health Care Plan (IHP), an Individualized Education Program, an Individualized Family Service Plan, a 504 Plan, or an emergency plan of care (see Chapter 9). Many examples of plans are available throughout the school nursing literature, especially in NASN publications or via publishers focused on school nursing.

The essence of the Planning standard and its measurement criteria is that

- In order to achieve the outcomes specified, there must be a plan.
- The plan is specific to the client or family under consideration; is developmentally, culturally, and environmentally appropriate; and seeks to promote health and prevent disease.
- The plan is developed collaboratively with the client, family, school personnel, and others.
- An IHP is developed for clients with special health care needs as part of the total education and care program.
- The plan provides for continuity of care.
- The plan specifies timelines for implementation.
- The plan prioritizes outcomes collaboratively with significant constituents.
- The plan provides direction to other members of the school team.
- The plan reflects current statutes, rules, regulations, and standards.
- The plan incorporates current research and practice trends.
- The plan considers the economic impact of its implementation.
- The plan is expressed in standardized or recognized language so that its elements are readily retrievable.
- The APRN incorporates research, diagnostic strategies, and expert clinical knowledge into the plan.
- The APRN designs a plan to meet the needs of complex clients.
- The Nurse in a Role Specialty (NIRS) designs multidisciplinary plans.
- The NIRS supports the planning process with organizational/system development efforts.
- The NIRS integrates clinical, human, and financial issues into the plan.

Standard 5: Implementation

The school nurse implements the identified plan.

Synchronous with the use of universal diagnoses and outcomes, standardized interventions have likewise been developed. The Center for Nursing Classification at The University of Iowa has identified numerous interventions. *Nursing Interventions Classification (NIC)* (Dochterman & Bulecheck, 2004) articulates with both the NANDA and NOC taxonomies, and revisions are published periodically. Each intervention is accompanied by *activities* that allow the nurse or others to implement the intervention. Conveniently, interventions are linked to NANDA diagnoses and NOC outcomes within an available "linkages" text (M. Johnson et al., 2001) and in software as well (Dochterman & Jones, 2003). An excellent guide to using and linking NANDA, NOC, and NIC is *Using Nursing Languages in School Nursing Practice* (Denehy, 2004).

An extensive compendium of nursing interventions for use in the school setting has been prepared by Hootman (2004). The interventions, all NIC-formatted, address a wide variety of physical and emotional health problems of children and represent an extraordinary compilation of appropriate and possible nursing actions.

The essence of the Implementation standard and its measurement criteria is that

- Implementation is linked to and flows from the plan, and is therefore consistent with it.
- Implementation of the plan is done in a timely and safe manner.
- Implementation changes, modifications, or omissions in the plan are documented.
- Implementation uses diagnosis/problem-specific interventions.
- Implementation of the plan utilizes community systems and resources.
- Implementation is collaborative with nursing colleagues and other significant parties.
- Interventions are based upon the current standards of school nursing practice (NASN & ANA, 2005).
- Interventions are expressed in standardized language (i.e., taxonomy) so that they are readily retrievable.
- The APRN implements the plan by facilitating utilization of community resources and systems.
- The APRN supports the collaborative efforts of the nurse and others in plan implementation.
- The APRN monitors care practices and contributes new knowledge to school nursing care practices if outcomes are not met.
- The NIRS uses management and systems concepts in implementing the plan.
- The NIRS supports plan implementation through strengthening relevant organizational systems.

Note: Standard 5 has four subsections, most or all of which may apply depending upon circumstances.

Standard 5A: Coordination of Care

The school nurse coordinates care delivery.

Coordination of care has long been a staple of public health nursing, and hence, school nursing practice (Cary, 2000). Coordination, in the parlance of community health nursing, is defined as "The conscious activity of assembling and directing the work efforts of [a group of health] providers so that they can function harmoniously in the attainment of the objective of client care" (Stanhope & Lancaster, 2000, p. G-7). Much of the practice of school nursing is engaged in working with others in the school or community setting to facilitate implementation of a plan. This is particularly true when a plan is implemented for the child with special needs.

The essence of the Coordination of Care substandard and its measurement criteria is that

- Care coordination is part of implementation.
- Implementation involves the creation and coordination of an IHP for the client with special health needs.
- Coordination of care is documented as part of implementation.
- The APRN imparts leadership for care coordination.
- The APRN coordinates care through a synthesis of all available and relevant data.
- The APRN coordinates care and care delivery across the continuum of systems and resources.

Standard 5B: Health Teaching and Health Promotion

The school nurse provides health education and employs strategies to promote health and a safe environment.

Health education includes more than classroom health instruction. Aspects of health education are common to the nursing role in other settings. Among these are individual client education, family and group education, faculty and staff in-service, and community education. This standard, however, further advocates for the nurse to serve as an evaluator of health curricula for accurate and appropriate content, and to suggest and provide health resources to teachers as needed.

Nurses are not usually prepared to do classroom education for students without additional educational preparation. Although a nurse may successfully engage in guest appearances, delivering selected health content such as family life education or communicable disease content, this is quite different from serving as the faculty member of record, a role wherein the nurse would engage in the assessment of individual learners, structure and organize curricula for optimal delivery, evaluate student learning through such techniques as test construction, and successfully manage a large group of child or adolescent learners.

Some states have an option for nurses to become teachers or, specifically, teachers of health. In these instances, state statutes usually stipulate that nurses learn about educational pedagogy and methods, teaching strategies, learner evaluation, and classroom management.

Health promotion is central to all of nursing practice but is particularly integral to community health nursing practice. It is again one of the cornerstones of public health nursing and has been a focus of school nursing since its inception with Lillian Wald and Lina Rogers (Kulbok, Laffrey, & Goeppinger, 2000; Zaiger, 2000).

The essence of the Health Teaching and Health Promotion substandard and its measurement criteria is that

- Health education is an integral part of the practice of the school nurse.
- Health promotion should permeate all aspects of the school nursing role.
- Care implementation involves classroom teaching or expert consultation.
- Health instruction addresses contemporary developmental, lifestyle, social, or self-care issues and topics.
- Health promotion and health teaching techniques in which the nurse engages are developmentally and culturally appropriate.
- Care implementation for the school community involves safety and self-care education.
- Health principles are promoted through the coordinated school health program.
- The effectiveness of health education and health promotion activities is pursued by the nurse through feedback from relevant parties.
- Needs assessments are conducted to ascertain the health instruction and health promotion needs of a school community.
- Health education extends to individual and group health counseling.
- Design, implementation, and evaluation of health education, health curricular, and health promotion materials and activities are an extension of this standard, as appro-

priate to the educational preparation of the nurse.

- Teachers and other staff are provided with consultation on health education issues.
- The APRN uses contemporary information and research of the pedagogy of education in designing, developing, and evaluating health educational activities.
- The APRN designs health information in a developmentally, culturally, and educationally effective manner.
- The APRN evaluates various health informational sources for accuracy, readability, and quality.

Standard 5C: Consultation

The school nurse provides consultation to influence the identified plan, enhance the abilities of others, and effect change.

In community nursing, consultation is sometimes difficult to differentiate from coordination and collaboration. Nonetheless, it is included as a substandard under Implementation because it is seen as critical to the implementation process for any client or family; a plan cannot be implemented without expert sharing of knowledge by the nurse with those in need of the information, such as the client, family, or other providers or caregivers.

The essence of the Consultation substandard and its measurement criteria is that

- All relevant data and current scientific evidence are included as part of consultation, as appropriate.
- Stakeholders are involved in any decision making that occurs through, or as a result of, nurse consultation.
- Effective consultation moves the plan and implementation forward and contributes to change.
- The APRN synthesizes all clinical data and evidence and incorporates theoretical frameworks in the provision of consultation.
- The APRN involves the client and family in decision making as appropriate.
- The APRN provides consultation that facilitates change.

Standard 5D: Prescriptive Authority and Treatment

The advanced practice registered nurse uses prescriptive authority, procedures, referrals, treatments, and therapies in accordance with state and federal laws and regulations.

The definition of the APRN may vary somewhat depending upon the organizational or government entity defining it. Alternately used is the designation Advanced Practice Nurse (APN). In general, the APRN is a Clinical Nurse Specialist (CNS), a Nurse Practitioner (NP), a Certified Nurse-Midwife (CNM), or a Certified (Registered) Nurse Anesthetist (CNA or CRNA).

ANA defines APRNs as

> RNs who have acquired specialized clinical knowledge and skill to provide health care. These nurses are expected to hold a master's or doctorate degree. They build on the practice of registered nurses by demonstrating a greater depth and breadth of knowledge, a greater synthesis of data, increased complexity of skills and interventions, and role autonomy. (ANA, 2004a, p. 14)

NASN noted that "The term Advanced Practice Registered Nurse (APRN) is being increasingly used by legislative and governing bodies to describe the collection of registered nurses that practice in a role beyond the normal role of basic registered nursing" (NASN, 2003, p. 1).

It is common in today's schools to find APRN's practicing as school nurses in the traditional role, in the role of primary care delivery, or both. This substandard devotes itself to the role of the school nurse as an APRN *in primary care* ministration.

The essence of the Prescriptive Authority and Treatment substandard and its measurement criteria is that

- The APRN uses clinical knowledge and skill and laboratory or diagnostic tests, as necessary, to prescribe therapies and treatments appropriate to the client and his or her needs, and evaluates their therapeutic and nontherapeutic effects.
- The APRN's pharmacological prescriptions are based on current knowledge and practice.
- The APRN informs the client and family about the prescribed therapies, including intended and adverse effects, costs, and alternatives.

Standard 6: Evaluation

The school nurse evaluates progress toward attainment of outcomes.

Evaluation is continuous. It is also systematic and criterion based. It is further said that evaluation is a circular phenomenon that begins at the beginning of a process. The notion here is that an awareness of whether care has been successful should be considered *from the outset* and that evaluation should neither be neglected nor "tacked on" as a step to the nursing process. The questions to be answered are "Is what I (we) did making a positive difference?" "Were the goals or the objectives of the endeavor successful?" and "Could anything have been done differently?"

The essence of the Evaluation standard and its measurement criteria is that

- Outcomes are systematically evaluated in relation to the elements of the plan and its timeline.
- Evaluation involves all who are affected by the plan, implementation, and outcomes, including the client, the family, school staff members, community providers, and others as appropriate.
- Evaluation appraises client responses to, and attainment of, outcomes in order to assess the effectiveness of strategies used.
- The results of the evaluation are documented.
- Evaluation employs ongoing assessment to revise diagnoses, outcomes, plans, and interventions as necessary.
- Evaluation disseminates evaluative results to relevant parties per client wishes, relevant policy, regulation, or statute of law.
- The APRN engages in evaluation of the diagnosis and its accuracy and the interventions and their effectiveness, both in relation to expected outcomes.
- The APRN and the NIRS use evaluative data to assess the impact of the plan on all constituencies, including communities and institutions.
- The NIRS uses evaluation data to implement policy or procedural change, as necessary.

Standards of Professional Performance

It is not enough to competently use the nursing process as a solo practitioner with students, families, and staff. Professional nursing practice also demands that the nurse meet the Standards of Professional Performance. Professional performance standards extend to self and to other professionals and staff, as well as to school nursing as a specialty within the nursing profession. The Standards of Professional Performance may be categorized into four areas:

1. *The maintenance and competency of practice,* that is, how well the nurse attends to the quality of his or her practice (Standards 7, "Quality of Practice"; 8, "Education"; 9, "Professional Practice Evaluation"; and 13, "Research")
2. *Contributions to the profession,* that is, whether the nurse "gives back" (Standards 10, "Collegiality"; and 15, "Leadership" [the practice-centered aspect of the standard])
3. *Integrity in practice,* that is, how "principled" the nurse is (Standard 12, "Ethics")
4. *Advocacy and stewardship,* that is, how effective the nurse is in working with others, in using resources maximally and optimally for the benefit of students and families, and in leading and managing (Standards 11, "Collaboration"; 14, "Resource Utilization"; 15, "Leadership" [the profession-focused aspect of the standard]; and 16, "Program Management")

TABLE 4.5 illustrates these category-standard relationships and identifies the meaning of each of the standards of professional performance.

There are 10 professional performance standards, 9 prescribed by ANA, and 1 developed specifically for school nursing. The reader is encouraged to access *Standards of Professional School Nursing Practice: Applications in the Field* (Lordi, 2000) as a guide to implementation of the 1998 version standards, both by the nurse and by the school district. Susan Lordi's implementation text will be helpful until a successor is available to articulate with the newest standards (NASN & ANA, 2005).

Standard 7: Quality of Practice

The school nurse systematically enhances the quality and effectiveness of school nursing practice.

This standard is the *quality assurance* component often missing in school nursing, particularly when schools are contrasted with health care settings such as those accredited by the Joint Commission on Accreditation of Healthcare Organizations. The Quality of Practice standard requires the nurse to stand apart from practice and the practice environment long enough to "see the forest for the trees," and to put measures in place to monitor and assure effectiveness of both individual nursing practice and the whole of the school health program.

The essence of the Quality of Practice standard and its measurement criteria is that

- Quality assurance of both nursing care and the school health program is an expected part of the school nursing role.
- Health policy, procedures, and practice guidelines that are contemporary and realistic contribute to the likelihood of improved quality.

(text continues on page 83)

Table 4.5 ■

CATEGORIES WITHIN THE STANDARDS OF PROFESSIONAL PERFORMANCE

STANDARD NUMBER	STANDARD TITLE	MEANING OF THE STANDARD
Maintenance and Competency of Practice		
7	Quality of Practice	The practice environment must be continually evaluated as a means of quality assurance and a basis for improvement of school nursing services.
8	Education	The nurse must periodically and regularly access educational sources in order to maintain currency in relevant school nursing knowledge and skills.
9	Professional Practice Evaluation	The nurse is responsible for evaluating his or her own practice in accord with professional standards, state and local law, and district policy.
13	Research	Research is promoted in practice and relevant research is reviewed and utilized.
Contribution to the Profession		
10	Collegiality	There is a professional duty to contribute positively toward the development of nurses and others in the school setting.
15	Leadership	The nurse is expected to exercise leadership within the specialty of school nursing.
Integrity in Practice		
12	Ethics	Professional and honorable behavior is always the norm for the school nurse.
Advocacy and Stewardship		
11	Collaboration	Inclusive and functional networks and relationships must be cultivated to provide effective care.
14	Resource Utilization	Safety, efficacy, and cost must be considered when ascertaining the best use of available human and material resources.
15	Leadership	The nurse, as the only health care professional in the school, is expected to be a leader in health and child advocacy issues.
16	Program Management	Contemporary practice in school nursing requires management skill, both formal and informal.

- Quality of practice measures, following appropriate application of the nursing process, are documented in an accountable, ethical, and responsible manner.
- Quality improvement activities are used to initiate meaningful changes in the practice of a single nurse, a group of nurses, and the school health program as a whole.
- Quality of practice implementation employs creative and innovative techniques to improve care delivery.
- Quality of practice incorporates new knowledge and approaches if desired outcomes are not attained.
- A wide array of quality improvement activities are enumerated as examples for nursing involvement. They are contained within the measurement criteria for Standard 7 (NASN & ANA, 2005).
- The APRN and the NIRS maintain expertise and certification in the area of the specialty.
- The APRN and the NIRS design quality improvement proposals and activities.
- The APRN and the NIRS implement quality improvement activities.
- The APRN and the NIRS evaluate the need for practice or program change.
- The APRN and the NIRS identify areas for the use and conduct of research, and evaluate both the quality of nursing care and the practice environment.

Standard 8: Education

The school nurse attains knowledge and competency that reflects current school nursing practice.

Professional development is a notion long familiar to school nurses. Many states have continuing education requirements for registered nurse license renewal. Several states also stipulate higher education requirements that must be completed for state school nurse certification. Regardless of a state's requirements or lack thereof, this standard exhorts nurses to assume the responsibility for keeping themselves current, particularly if the school district does not facilitate professional development for all its employees.

There is scarcely an area in all of nursing in which a nurse can be become obsolete as quickly as can occur in school nursing. The reasons for this are obvious. First, often there are no other nurses with whom to consult/commiserate about clinical or practice issues. The nurse is therefore prone to professional isolation. Second, the nurse works in a non–health care delivery setting wherein the language and the mission of the organization do not consider the health of children as the primary focus of activity. Medical and nursing terminologies, important dimensions of keeping current, are typically not used. The result is the nurse who is naively out of date and engaged in practices that may be obsolete or counterproductive. In addition, many school nurses are not involved with local, state, or national school nursing organizations.

The essence of the Education standard and its measurement criteria is that

- Nurses serving children and families in schools are held to the same standard of currency as are nurses in other practice settings.
- Education is regular, ongoing, and related to appropriate and relevant knowledge bases and professional issues.
- Education is a lifelong commitment, emanating from self-identified learning needs arrived at through self-reflection.
- Education is pursued that maintains and expands skills and competence and reflects current practice.
- Educational knowledge and skill acquired are specific to the specialty and to its roles, settings, or situations.
- Records, as evidence of higher and continuing education, are retained.
- Other learning activities are pursued for the maintenance and expansion of clinical and professional knowledge.
- The APRN and the NIRS utilize research findings and other evidence to increase expert knowledge, expand role performance, and enhance the awareness of professional issues.

Standard 9: Professional Practice Evaluation

The school nurse evaluates one's own nursing practice in relation to professional practice standards and guidelines, relevant statutes, rules, and regulations.

Closely related to education is the issue of self-evaluation of the quality of one's nursing practice. Traditional performance evaluation, wherein a supervising nurse appraises the performance of a practicing nurse, is often a problem for nurses within the school setting; nurses who work alone, or those who are supervised by a non-nurse, face particular challenges in having their performance as a registered nurse appropriately and adequately appraised (see Chapter 11). Further, many nurses begin their tenure in school districts with little or no orientation. Non-nurse administrators assume that because a nurse is a Registered Nurse, he or she must know all that is required to do the job. As most school nurses know, nothing could be further from the truth.

In the absence of external evaluation, this standard holds the nurse to self-evaluate in accordance with the "standard of care" in the particular community (see Standard of Care discussion earlier in this chapter). A nurse with a large pupil-to-nurse ratio, for example, would not be held to the same standard of care as would a nurse with a lower ratio and, therefore, fewer students (Schwab, Gelfman, et al., 2001). Self-appraisal should be conducted utilizing criteria that reflect accepted and agreed-upon role definitions *congruent with the nurse's practice situation,* such as position descriptions; evaluation instruments; district policy; national, state, or local role statements; or state or federal law. The subject of performance evaluation is further explored later in this chapter.

The essence of the Professional Practice Evaluation standard and its measurement criteria is that

- As available, self-evaluation uses written criteria based on contemporary, accepted, and applicable indicators for school nursing.
- The care and services the nurse provides are developmentally, culturally, and ethically sensitive and competent.
- The nurse identifies strengths and areas for improvement in periodic self-evaluation.
- Self-evaluation involves seeking feedback from others, such as clients, families, and peers.
- The nurse invites and participates in peer evaluation, as appropriate.
- Goals are established during the self-evaluative process that are subsequently acted on for self-improvement.
- The nurse examines his or her rationale for practice decisions and actions as part of self-evaluation.
- The APRN and the NIRS seek formal evaluation from all relevant constituencies.

Standard 10: Collegiality

The school nurse interacts with and contributes to the professional development of peers and school personnel as colleagues.

This standard exhorts nurses to behave in a collegial way, interact with and support school colleagues in a manner that will enhance their practice, and promote the profession. Lordi (2000) made the point that sharing with others empowers not only the recipients of the sharing but the nurse and health program in the district as well. She further noted that collegiality extends to inquiries about family members of school staff and to participation in faculty/staff social functions so that the nurse is perceived as part of the "team."

Three key attributes of this standard are worth noting: (1) the duty to share relevant clinical knowledge with nursing staff as well as with teachers and other school staff, as needed; (2) the duty to guide and mentor nursing and other health care students; and (3) the duty to contribute to the profession through participation in professional nursing and other organizations.

The essence of the Collegiality standard and its measurement criteria is that

- Being fully professional involves sharing knowledge and skill, formally or informally, to help others function and grow in their respective roles.
- The provision of feedback and beneficial counsel to peers is an aspect of collegiality.
- Professional interaction with peers and colleagues enhances the nurse's practice, as well as the health of the school community.
- Peers and colleagues are treated with caring and compassion by the nurse.
- The practice environment created by the nurse is conducive to the education of nursing and health care professionals, as well as the school community.
- Collegiality includes efforts to make the school and/or the school district an emotionally healthy place for persons to work and children to learn.
- Participation, membership, or leadership in local, state, and/or national school nurse organizations is essential to advancing the specialty.
- The APRN models expert practice to team members and others.
- The APRN and the NIRS mentor nursing students, nurse colleagues, and others, as appropriate.
- The APRN and the NIRS participate with multi- and interdisciplinary teams to advance role development and nursing services.

Standard 11: Collaboration

The school nurse collaborates with the client, family, school staff, and others in the conduct of school nursing practice.

This standard reminds the nurse that no professional is an island. In all but the simplest circumstances, it is necessary to communicate plans, outcomes, and the like to relevant persons. Written plans are part of this collaborative effort. IHPs, Individualized Education Programs, Individualized Family Service Plans, 504 Plans, and emergency plans specify the nurse's role, and often the role of others, and allow other parties to assist and be collaborative in care. Collaboration comes naturally to most nurses, as this has been a component of successful nursing practice for decades. In fact, in some situations in schools, care cannot be delivered without considerable collaboration.

The essence of the Collaboration standard and its measurement criteria is that

- Communication with the client, family, and providers is critical to good care.
- Written plans are collaboratively developed that focus on outcomes as well as care-related decisions, and document relevant communication with all concerned.
- Cooperation and partnering with others is necessary to bring about positive outcomes and needed change for the client.
- Referrals are documented, including strategies for continuity of care.
- The APRN and the NIRS collaborate with others through inter- and multidisciplinary efforts that may involve research, management, technology, consultation, and education.
- The APRN facilitates interdisciplinary cooperation with other health care providers.

Standard 12: Ethics

The school nurse integrates ethical provisions in all areas of practice.

This standard asks the nurse to behave ethically. This means placing the child and the family before oneself or one's employer. It also means behaving morally and honestly in all matters pertaining to the child and his or her family. Many nurse practice acts *require* the registered nurse to be an advocate for his or her client. Therefore, in these states, there is a *legal responsibility* to be a client advocate.

The essence of the Ethics standard and its measurement criteria is that

- The *Code of Ethics for Nursing with Interpretive Statements* (ANA, 2001) and the *Code of Ethics with Interpretive Statements for School Nurses* (NASN, 1999) are used to guide practice decisions, when necessary.
- Care is delivered in a manner that protects client autonomy, dignity, and rights.
- The maintenance of confidentiality, within the context of legal and regulatory parameters, is essential to ethical practice.
- Client advocacy and the promotion of client self-advocacy are central to competent and ethical practice.
- Professional role boundaries are respected, and appropriate professional and therapeutic nurse-client relationships are maintained.
- Ethical practice includes maintenance of the self, physically, emotionally, and socially.
- Ethical practice involves assisting others in ethical decision making and involvement in ethically related activities, such as serving on an ethics committee, as appropriate.
- Incompetent, dangerous, or unethical practice by others is reported.
- Ethics resources are used to assist in ethical decision making as necessary.
- The APRN apprises clients and families of the risks, benefits, and expected outcomes of health care.
- The APRN and the NIRS participate in interdisciplinary/multidisciplinary teams that address ethical issues.
- The NIRS apprises administrators of the risks, benefits, and expected outcomes of health care.

Standard 13: Research

The school nurse integrates research findings into practice.

Research, here, means everything from published findings to statistical data used or collected by the nurse as part of everyday practice (see Chapter 8). As more and more nurses are engaging in research, the body of knowledge about what is best practice in school nursing is growing. Evidence-based practice necessitates that nursing actions be based on sound theory and research.

The essence of the Research standard and its measurement criteria is that

- Research findings and the best available evidence are used in guiding practice.

- Support for and participation in research should be commensurate with a nurse's education. Examples of participatory activities are listed within the measurement criteria for Standard 13 (NASN & ANA, 2005).
- The APRN and the NIRS generate nursing knowledge through research-related activities that improve health care practices.
- The APRN and the NIRS disseminate relevant research findings to nursing staff and others through a variety of means.

Standard 14: Resource Utilization

The school nurse considers factors related to safety, effectiveness, cost, and impact on practice in the planning and delivery of school nursing services.

This broad standard encompasses a wide array of issues, including cost containment, efficacy of services, and client safety. This standard also may be seen as an extension of the previous discussion of the Ethics standard regarding the legal duty of client advocacy. The language of this standard makes it clear that the nurse is to choose the best for clients, and help clients or their parents make the best decisions based on services needed. "Best" refers to resources (people, goods, services) that are *safe and efficient,* offer the client or the district the *most reasonable cost,* and are possible within the context and parameters of the role, as manifested in a particular setting. As noted, the resources may be material resources such as equipment, medication, or other supplies, or human resources, in which case the nurse may assign or delegate persons to provide aspects of care while a student is at school, or assist and direct the family in finding accessible, safe, and cost-effective care in the community. Resources also may be a menu of services available elsewhere in the community that are deemed the best for this client at this time.

The essence of the Resource Utilization standard and its measurement criteria is that

- Factors such as safety, effectiveness, and cost-benefit issues are evaluated when choosing interventions or practice options in order to attain expected outcomes.
- Assistance is provided to the client and family in selecting and securing the best services to address client needs.
- Assignment or delegation of nursing tasks to unlicensed assistive personnel (UAPs) or others is not automatic. If allowed by state law, the nurse considers the circumstance and condition of the client, the potential for harm to the client in the delegation/assignment of the task to an unlicensed person, the complexity of the task, the designee's ability to safely and effectively perform the task, and the probability of the anticipated outcome. The prudent nurse should always analyze whether delegation or assignment of certain procedures is prudent *regardless* of what state law or regulation may say.
- Informed consumers are more likely to commit to a plan and follow prescribed activities than are those who are uninformed. The nurse engages in educating clients and families about risks, benefits, costs, school health services, and prescribed interventions.
- The APRN utilizes community and organizational resources to design inter- and multidisciplinary plans of care.
- The APRN formulates innovative client care solutions that address quality maintenance and effective resource utilization.
- The NIRS obtains appropriate resources for nursing interventions using innovative strategies and solutions.
- The NIRS acquires organizational resources to create a work environment conducive to achieving the plan and outcomes.
- The NIRS designs evaluative methodologies to measure the effectiveness and safety of interventions and outcomes.
- The NIRS supports activities that facilitate the informing of others about the risks, benefits, and the costs of care, or of the plan and solution.

Standard 15: Leadership

The school nurse provides leadership in the professional practice setting and the profession.

The standard of Leadership is new with the 2004 edition of generic nursing standards. ANA saw the wisdom of designating leadership—professional, moral, and personal—as intrinsic to the practice of every nurse. It is of interest that, of the 19 standards in *Nursing: Scope and Standards of Practice* (ANA, 2004a), none except Standard 7, "Quality of Practice," is as detailed in its descriptions of measurement criteria. The Leadership standard is broad in its intent and ambitious in its scope. Its school nursing counterpart is equal in its stateliness and meaning.

Leadership refers to both formal and informal leadership. This standard expresses the value that the school nurse need not be a formal leader in order to engage in and exercise leadership. Rather, leadership is expected of the nurse all of the time he or she is acting in a professional capacity.

The essence of the Leadership standard and its measurement criteria is that

- Teamwork, both team building and team cooperation, is inherent in the role of the school nurse.
- Leadership involves the nurse in the creation and maintenance of healthy working environments in all communities of care.
- A clear vision, with accompanying clarity of goals and implementation strategies, is part of the role of nurse as leader.
- There is a commitment to lifelong learning for self and others.
- A sense of responsibility to others is expressed by assisting them to succeed through teaching or mentoring.
- The nurse is flexible and creative in times of change.
- A passion for quality work, energy, and excitement are part of the leadership qualities of the nurse.
- Acceptance of mistakes by self and others builds an environment in which risk-taking is safe.
- Employees who are valued by the nurse are inspired to loyalty and greater productivity.
- Leadership engages the nurse in overseeing and supervising the practice of UAPs or others according to state law or district policy.
- Representation of nursing and health services entails participation on councils, committees, task forces, and administrative teams.
- Promotion of the profession and the specialty of school nursing is accomplished through engagement in professional nursing, school nursing, and/or school health organizations.
- Knowledge of the mission, purpose, and curricula, as well as programs of the school district, is essential for the nurse as an informed and supportive employee.
- Knowledge of the roles and responsibilities of other school professionals and personnel is expected of the nurse as team member.
- The roles and responsibilities of adjunct school health personnel are coordinated by the nurse.
- The APRN improves client care through working to influence decision makers.
- The APRN enhances the effectiveness of the health care team by providing direction.
- The APRN recognizes changes in care needs and addresses emerging problems by developing or revising policies or protocols reflective of evidence-based practice.
- The APRN and the NIRS advance the profession through publication and presentations for both professional and lay audiences.
- The APRN and the NIRS effect change in practice and outcomes through the creation and development of innovations.
- The NIRS improves client care, health services, and school policy through professional involvement that influences decision makers.
- The NIRS enhances the effectiveness of the interdisciplinary team by providing clear direction.

Standard 16: Program Management

The school nurse manages school health services.

The Program Management standard is unique to school nursing. It is not among the standards put forth by the ANA in its most recent generic document (ANA, 2004a). As one of the broadest and most encompassing of all the standards, Program Management in school nursing embraces a concept of management that extends from case management of the individual child to running a large health services program. Depending upon the preparation of the nurse, his or her position in a school district, pupil-to-nurse ratios, and the size of the district, management responsibilities can vary widely. It was apparent to the authors of the latest school nursing standards document that, without some program management skills, most school nurses would be rendered ineffectual (NASN & ANA, 2005).

Program management, at its best, includes needs assessment, program planning, budgeting, fund raising, policy analysis and development, and the supervision and training of health UAPs. As noted, the extent of the nurse's responsibility in these areas depends upon individual credentials and preparation, position, and the practice environment.

The essence of the Program Management standard and its measurement criteria is that

- The school nurse is expected to manage aspects of or the whole of the school health program, depending upon practice environment, position, and education.

- School health needs assessments are conducted to ascertain existing problems and determine the need for new programs.
- A program planning process is used in implementing health programs.
- Program management involves knowledge of existing and emerging child health trends as well as the sources of funds for school health services, with their related laws, as appropriate.
- Policies and procedures are developed in collaboration with school administration, the board of education, and, as necessary, the board of health.
- Ongoing evaluation of existing programs is conducted and results are communicated to administrators and boards of education.
- The orientation, training, supervision, and evaluation of UAPs and other health-related personnel are ongoing.
- Changes in programs are initiated based on results of program evaluations and quality-of-care activities.
- Environmental health and safety factors are monitored, prevention issues addressed, and prevention strategies implemented.
- Technology is used to support nursing and health program activities.

PUTTING STANDARDS TO USE

As noted earlier, using the standards as they are stated, without amplification or measurement criteria, may present problems: (1) the standards language is of sufficient breadth as to render ready application difficult, particularly for the non-nurse; and (2) the standards may not lend themselves to uniform application, even with a single school district. That is to say, in some districts, a nurse may be able to meet the intent of some of the standards, but not all of them, due to excessive pupil-to-nurse ratios, inadequate educational preparation, unique assignment or role, or the particulars of the work environment itself. Similarly, the standards, as written, necessitate the use of a graduated measurement tool, such as a Likert scale, with numerical values or word descriptors, to assess the degree or extent to which a nurse meets a particular standard. This is why the standards should be used as a framework and "customized" to individual work settings or environments.

There are seven primary ways in which standards of practice may be used in the school setting: (1) in the development of *position descriptions*; (2) as a framework for the development of *performance evaluation* instruments; (3) for use in *discussion with school district administrators* unfamiliar with the role of the nurse; (4) as a framework for a *quality assurance* program to evaluate the entirety of the school health program; (5) as a guide in *competency identification* for school nursing practice; (6) as a framework for *database development and data collection*; and (7) as a quasi-*legal standard* for use in cases of litigation against school nurses. Often, the first three of these are interrelated.

Other uses include their application in the development of guidelines or agency-specific policies, protocols, or procedures, all of which allow for more specificity and tailoring to a practice setting. Standards may further serve as guideposts for quality improvement and as a basis for clinical ladders in health care delivery settings (Dean-Barr, 2001).

Position Descriptions

Standards can guide the development of position or job descriptions. They are also useful in revising existing position descriptions. Typically, a position description is a statement that stipulates the duties or functions of an individual within an organizational structure. Job descriptions prescribe the authority, accountability, and responsibility of the individual (Ellis & Hartley, 2004) and may serve as a basis for performance evaluation, depending upon how they are constructed.

Constructing a Position Description

Whereas some position descriptions may be broad, general statements outlining conceptual areas of practice without listing specific duties or functions, others may be composed of specific role competencies interspersed with broader language (Ellis & Hartley, 2004). To use the standards as a basis for a position or job description, a commitment has to be reached that the standards do, indeed, reflect the mission and philosophy of health services of the school district. "The link between the work environment and the nurse's ability to deliver care and services is recognized and employers must provide an environment supportive of nursing practice" (NASN, 1998, p. 2). Position descriptions usually begin with broad statements such as "Working within the auspices of this school district, the nurse shall provide health care services to pupils as determined by state statute and in accordance with school district policies and the state nurse practice act." It may continue with equally broad statements of role function taken from state or national professional organizations or other sources, and go on to itemize specific responsibilities or competencies within the context of the larger statements. It may mention the national standards of practice as an entity, specifying that nursing practice in the district is to be in accordance with the standards. Conversely, it may list each standard individually and nest related duties or functions beneath the standard. As an example, under Standard 1, "Assessment," a position description might add "Assesses children for illness, injury, and emotional distress. Performs a brief assessment of children during screening activities." There is a plethora of published material on the role of the school nurse that can and should be used in the development of position descriptions.

Performance Evaluation

One of the most helpful roles that standards can play is that of guiding the development of performance evaluation instruments. Although position descriptions paint the nursing role with a broad brush, they may not contain information specific enough to serve as an evaluation tool. Performance evaluation is also termed *performance appraisal, performance review,* or *performance assessment.*

Congruence with the district's position description is critical. A nurse hired under a position description that varies markedly from the instrument used to evaluate his or her performance is disadvantaged in that there is a "disconnect" between what is initially expected and put forth and what is expected and appraised during routine evaluation. Whatever the framework for evaluation, performance appraisal must minimally look at the nurse's critical thinking, interpersonal skills, and clinical and technical skills.

Past and Present Efforts

Several nationally published evaluation tools have been developed in the past 20-plus years, all modeled on one or another version of the standards of practice. The most recent was published in 2000.

- 1985: *An Evaluation Guide for School Nursing Practice Designed for Self and Peer Review* (NASN, 1985) promoted self and peer evaluation of clinical and technical knowledge and skills about which a nurse would be familiar and would expect of another nurse, but which would not be known or apparent to a school administrator.
- 1987: *Evaluating School Nursing Practice: A Guide for Administrators* (ASHA, 1987) was addressed directly to administrators, both nursing and non-nursing, to facilitate ready evaluation of staff school nurses based upon the 1983 ANA school nursing standards. The document contains several versions of evaluation instruments with short and long forms of each.
- 1995: *Job Performance Evaluation Guidelines for School Nurses* (Ackerman, 1995) drew upon the work of Stronge (1994) and Stronge and Helm (1991) in providing not only an instrument for evaluation but some principles of good performance evaluation in an educational setting. As with its predecessors, a Likert scale was used in designing the appraisal instrument. This instrument is sufficiently broad that use by nurses and non-nurses alike is possible. It addressed the 1993 school nursing standards (Proctor, 1993).
- 2000: *A Sample School Nurse Evaluation Tool for the Non-Nurse Administrator Based on the 1998 Standards of School Nursing Practice* is the latest in the succession of instruments. Incorporated as an appendix into *Standards of Professional School Nursing Practice: Applications in the Field* (Lordi, 2000), it employed a 4-point Likert scale rather than a 5- or 6-point scale, as had the earlier tools. It was developed for the 1998 NASN school nursing standards.

Application

FIGURE 4.2 illustrates how a nurse's performance in school vision screening might be appraised using the *Standards of Professional School Nursing Practice* (NASN, 1998). Adapted from an earlier evaluative model (Proctor, 1986), the Standards of Care, as the nursing process, and some of the Standards of Professional Performance serve as a framework from which other objectives may be developed in order to evaluate even the smallest functions and components of the school vision screening program and its process.

As may be seen in Figure 4.2, objectives within the model are on three levels: Level I includes the standards themselves, which serve as macro-objectives to be used at the program level and as a framework for the development of "finer," more position-specific objectives. Level II objectives are the measurement criteria, the language of which should be taken directly from the NASN and ANA standards (2005). Specific to each standard, measure-

(text continues on page 91)

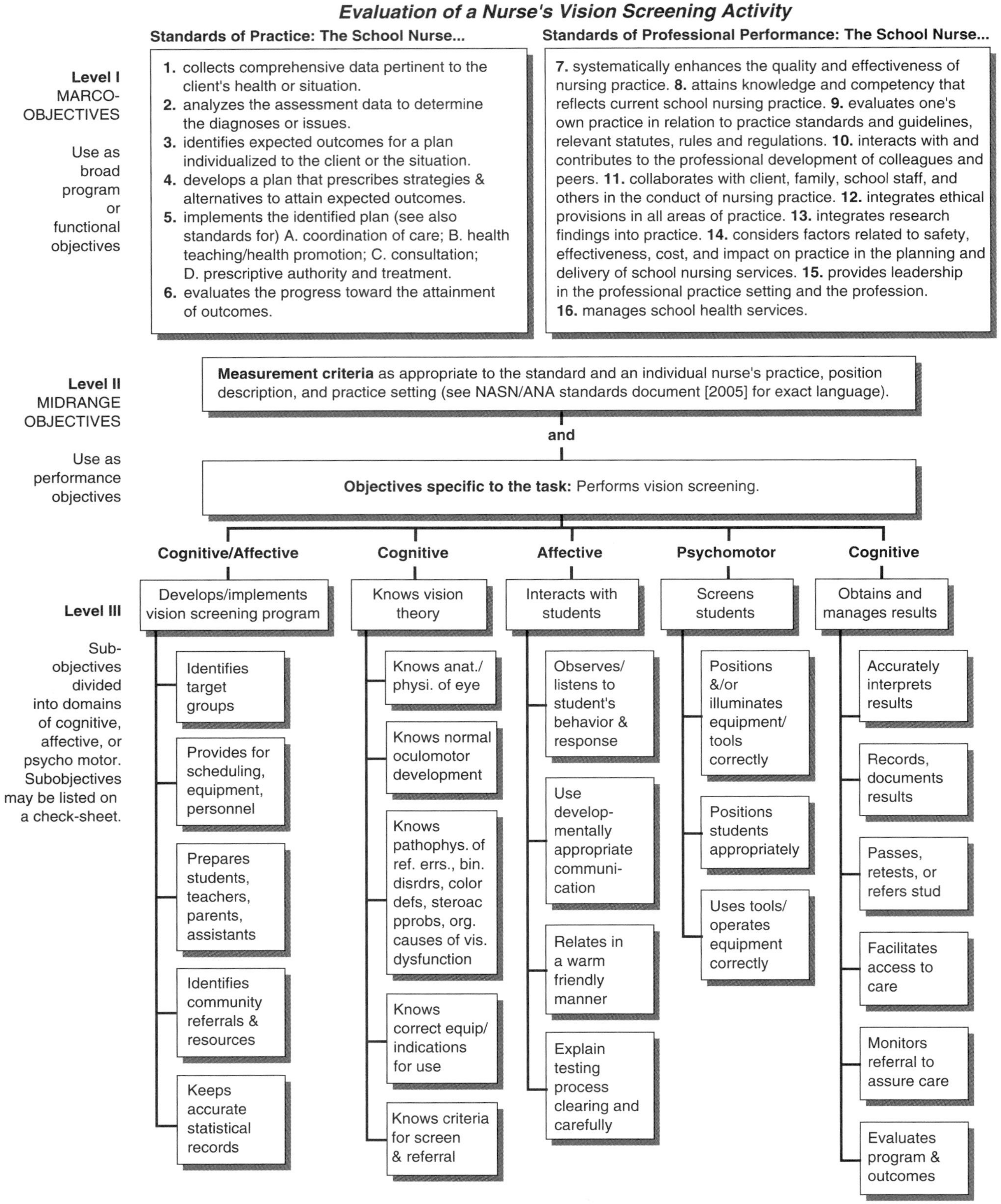

Evaluation of a Nurse's Vision Screening Activity

Level I MARCO-OBJECTIVES

Use as broad program or functional objectives

Standards of Practice: The School Nurse...

1. collects comprehensive data pertinent to the client's health or situation.
2. analyzes the assessment data to determine the diagnoses or issues.
3. identifies expected outcomes for a plan individualized to the client or the situation.
4. develops a plan that prescribes strategies & alternatives to attain expected outcomes.
5. implements the identified plan (see also standards for) A. coordination of care; B. health teaching/health promotion; C. consultation; D. prescriptive authority and treatment.
6. evaluates the progress toward the attainment of outcomes.

Standards of Professional Performance: The School Nurse...

7. systematically enhances the quality and effectiveness of nursing practice. **8.** attains knowledge and competency that reflects current school nursing practice. **9.** evaluates one's own practice in relation to practice standards and guidelines, relevant statutes, rules and regulations. **10.** interacts with and contributes to the professional development of colleagues and peers. **11.** collaborates with client, family, school staff, and others in the conduct of nursing practice. **12.** integrates ethical provisions in all areas of practice. **13.** integrates research findings into practice. **14.** considers factors related to safety, effectiveness, cost, and impact on practice in the planning and delivery of school nursing services. **15.** provides leadership in the professional practice setting and the profession. **16.** manages school health services.

Level II MIDRANGE OBJECTIVES

Use as performance objectives

Measurement criteria as appropriate to the standard and an individual nurse's practice, position description, and practice setting (see NASN/ANA standards document [2005] for exact language).

and

Objectives specific to the task: Performs vision screening.

Level III

Sub-objectives divided into domains of cognitive, affective, or psycho motor. Subobjectives may be listed on a check-sheet.

Cognitive/Affective — Develops/implements vision screening program
- Identifies target groups
- Provides for scheduling, equipment, personnel
- Prepares students, teachers, parents, assistants
- Identifies community referrals & resources
- Keeps accurate statistical records

Cognitive — Knows vision theory
- Knows anat./physi. of eye
- Knows normal oculomotor development
- Knows pathophys. of ref. errs., bin. disrdrs, color defs, steroac pprobs, org. causes of vis. dysfunction
- Knows correct equip/indications for use
- Knows criteria for screen & referral

Affective — Interacts with students
- Observes/listens to student's behavior & response
- Use develop-mentally appropriate communi-cation
- Relates in a warm friendly manner
- Explain testing process clearing and carefully

Psychomotor — Screens students
- Positions &/or illuminates equipment/tools correctly
- Positions students appropriately
- Uses tools/operates equipment correctly

Cognitive — Obtains and manages results
- Accurately interprets results
- Records, documents results
- Passes, retests, or refers stud
- Facilitates access to care
- Monitors referral to assure care
- Evaluates program & outcomes

Figure 4.2 ■ An example of the use of standards of school nursing practice in evaluation of nurse school vision screening performance.

ment criteria are designed to be used as performance objectives. Level III provides examples of "finer" sub-objectives that may be used in performance evaluation as well. The sub-objectives fall into one of three domains or combination of domains: *cognitive,* which are measures of knowledge and critical thinking, including the use of the nursing process; *affective,* which are measures of valuing, interpersonal skill, and demeanor; and *psychomotor,* which are measures of technical skill.

Anticipated Efforts

An NASN task force is being formed to revisit the issue of a nationally available performance evaluation instrument based on the latest version of the standards. Using developed competencies as a basis for the design of a performance appraisal instrument (Bobo, Adams, & Cooper, 2002), they hope to integrate and align competencies with various standards as well as make the instrument more fluid and adaptable to a variety of settings.

Discussions with Non-Nurse School Administrators

Understandably, non-nurse administrators rarely if ever appreciate the latitude of the nursing role in the schools. The standards may be used in interactions with such individuals to facilitate their general education about the capabilities of nursing and to assist them in supporting and guiding the implementation of nursing services within school districts. Like most members of the public who are not health care professionals, non-nurse school administrators take their view of nursing from the media, mostly television. The school nurse who has the misfortune to succeed a nurse who was particularly unimpressive in his or her practice may find the standards a valuable ally in breaking down lingering negative impressions of the nurse role and nursing within a given school or school district.

Quality Assurance

Recalling the ANA's original purpose in standards development, one of the roles of standards, both for nursing as a whole and for the specialties within nursing, was to accomplish quality assurance (ANA, 1991). The 20 standards (16 general standards plus 4 "sub"-standards) may also then be used to appraise nursing function across the whole of the school health program. Despite the categorization imposed on the school health program by depictions such as that of the Coordinated School Health Program model (Allensworth, 1995, as cited in McKenzie & Richmond, 1998), the reality in most school districts is that nurses are almost always central to the school health program and are not constrained by artificial boundaries such as "Health Services," or exclusively relegated to one or another component of the coordinated model.

Nurses provide direct nursing services, coordinate the delivery of other health services, provide health instruction, manage the school health program, engage in resolving issues regarding the school environment and nutrition, offer health counseling, confer and collaborate with physical education personnel, collaborate with families and community agencies, are involved with employee health, and generally are the "glue" that holds school health entities together. Indeed, as Ackerman noted, evaluating nursing practice, in itself, may constitute evaluation of the school health program: "The evaluation of the school nurse concomitantly evaluates the school health program. If the objectives of the school health program are defined and clarified, the extent to which program objectives have been met reflects the performance of the school nurse" (1995, p. 1). Further, the involvement of school nursing in management, health education, counseling, and other areas strengthens the value of the school nurse and enhances job security.

The standards certainly advocate for evaluation of the whole of the school health program by the nurse. Outcomes Identification (Standard 3) speaks specifically to the intent of the standards that the nurse take responsibility for quality assurance of the *whole* of the school health program. Quality of Practice (Standard 7) states that nursing practice, regardless of the focus, be evaluated and that a responsibility in the domain of quality of care is the assurance of the quality in the totality of the school health program, depending upon one's role and scope of practice. Program Management (Standard 16) directs the nurse, within measurement criteria, to evaluate the whole of the school health program.

Competency Identification and Development

Another exceedingly important use of standards is to guide the development of competencies. It is recognized that this relationship is a reciprocal one; that is, competencies explain and clarify standards and promote their adaptation, and standards illuminate possible competencies and serve as a guidepost to competency discovery, recognition, and development.

Competency Definition

Competency is defined as "the application of knowledge and the interpersonal, decision-making, and psychomotor skills expected for the [school] nurse's practice role within the context of public health, welfare, and safety" (National Council of State Boards of Nursing, as cited in Bobo et al., 2002, p. 279). Although there are numerous other definitions of competency in the nursing and related literature, such as those given in Poster and Marcontel (1999), Bobo and colleagues preferred that of the National Council of State Boards of Nursing, presumably because of its holistic language.

The Work of the Southern Regional Education Board

Competency development based upon national standards has surged forward on three significant fronts in recent years. First is the exhaustive work of the SREB's Council on Collegiate Education for Nursing, a consortium of nursing schools from colleges and universities in the southeastern United States. Their effort, the identification of competencies for the baccalaureate-prepared school nurse, provided a solid compilation of the roles, knowledge, skills, and behaviors that should be characteristic of the school nurse entering practice with a minimum of a BSN (SREB, 2000). Using an extensive focus group methodology, analysis of SREB data resulted in the identification of 69 (59 primary + 10 sublevel) competencies. Of these, 59 were linked with or nested under one of the steps of the nursing process and reflected five of the six then-standards known as "Standards of Care" (now Standards of Practice); only Outcomes Identification was not represented. Ten additional competencies, *not* linked to one of the Standards of Care, were grouped independently under a category titled "Professional Development." These spoke directly or indirectly to some of the 11 "Standards of Professional Performance" in place at the time, though not to all. Although not all of the 1998 standards of practice were represented, the SREB effort nonetheless gave great impetus to further work on competency identification in refinement and further alignment with the NASN standards, in development of an evaluation tool based on the SREB competencies, and in spearheading efforts at advanced practice competency detection, discovery, and development.

National Competency Forum

NASN convened a Competency Forum in 2001 under the leadership of Nichole Bobo, the organization's Education Coordinator. Members of this group subsequently identified competencies associated with *all* of the standards contained in the documents in place at the time (NASN, 1998; NASN & ANA,2001) and formatted their developing product per the then-recognized Standards of Care and Standards of Professional Performance (Bobo et al., 2002).

Advanced Practice Competency Development

Efforts are under way by members of the National Consortium of School Nurse Educators to identify and refine advanced practice competencies expected of the nurse holding a minimum of a master's degree. Following in the footsteps of SREB and building upon the SREB competencies, five focus groups were held in geographically diverse areas, nationally. Data gathered by these focus groups are currently being analyzed (Proctor, Baucom, & Griffin, n.d.).

Database Development and Data Collection

Nursing practice in schools can be effectively monitored and documented through the development of a database that uses the standards as a conceptual and categorical framework. Such a database can subsequently guide the collection and analysis of data related to nursing and health care activities within school districts, important for demonstrating outcomes, sharing nursing activities with school administration and boards of education, and generating substantiation for new nursing positions and activities in schools. Most school districts respect and look to national standards for validation of professional activities. Using national standards of nursing practice as a framework, or documenting and reporting nursing activities, would certainly enhance the professional status of nursing as a discipline within schools.

Legal Standard

The last way in which standards may be used is as a legal gauge. Although standards are not laws, statutes, or regulations, they nonetheless carry substantial weight, particularly in the *absence* of any legal source. If a nurse's practice is called into question, several resources, in addition to local or state laws or regulations, may be used to determine the degree of innocence or culpability of a school nurse. Among these are professional organization statements/position papers; journals and texts; nursing education curricula; clinical practice guidelines; district position descriptions and/or performance evaluation instruments; school board/district policies, protocols, and procedures; and *standards of practice,* both generic and specialty standards (Schwab, Gelfman, et al., 2001).

In these instances, national standards of practice could be introduced into a court dispute and witnesses or a defendant asked to attest to the soundness of the standards as describing a scope of practice for the school nurse. In this case, the standards would be used in concert with a school district's position description, any district policy governing nursing action, and state practice guidelines.

In theory, the standards would be influential in a courtroom because they were developed and deliberated over by nurse leaders nationally, representing a wide swath of nursing organizations. Additionally, the standards have been concluded to be *a realistic and essential* set of statements about the practice of school nursing in the United States. Finally, they were approved and endorsed by the boards of directors or representative committees of two national organizations, NASN and ANA.

RESEARCH ON THE USE OF STANDARDS OF PRACTICE

A few studies have investigated the degree to which school nurses practice according to standards of practice. Delores Basco's work was the first published account of congruity between nursing practice and nursing standards. Basco (1963) found a high degree of agreement between "participants' perception of their work achievements and the ANA and ASHA standards of care [in place] at the time of this research" (L. F. Johnson, 2003, p. 10). L. F. Johnson (2003) also compared three research studies to NASN's standards of practice. Using the 1998 NASN standards, her findings noted that (1) White's 1985 "clusters" of care activities of school nurses were not assessed as congruent with standards of practice; (2) Lowe and Miller's 1998 study of chronic health problems of students in schools showed that the activities of school nurses in one state could easily correspond to 9 of the 11 Standards of Professional Performance; and (3) Guilday's 2000 study (built on White's work) used an instrument that queried school nurses about their practice, and concluded that standards of practice aligned with questionnaire items in all but one instance (all as cited in L. F. Johnson, 2003).

L. F. Johnson's own work (2003) surveyed school nurses in one state in order to assess the proximity of their practice with the "Professional Performance" standards contained in the 1998 edition of the NASN standards of practice. The state was one in which pupil-to-nurse ratios were judged less than optimal, using NASN's recommendation for staffing (NASN, 1995). Nurses in the sample (n = 221) reported that they practiced according to 5 of the 11 professional performance standards 50% or more of the time. The five standards were Collegiality, Ethics, Collaboration, Resource Utilization, and Communication. The standard least likely to be attended to was Performance Appraisal, followed by Research. These results suggest that high pupil-to-nurse ratios may impact on the degree to which a nurse can practice in concert with national standards of practice.

CONCLUSION

Standards are living, dynamic language statements about the scope of practice of persons practicing as registered nurses in the United States. Standards may be generic or specific to a nursing specialty; they have a 50-year history of evolution and refinement, a process that continues and is not stagnant.

Standards have practical and not just esoteric value. They are valuable allies for the school nurse in developing position descriptions, crafting performance appraisal instruments, evaluating the quality of the school health program, communicating with non-nurse school administrators, and describing the role of the nurse in legal proceedings. Finally, they can set the stage for badly needed competency identification and development.

References

Ackerman, P. L. (1995). *Job performance evaluation guidelines for school nurses.* Scarborough, ME: National Association of School Nurses.

American Nurses Association. (1973). *Standards of nursing practice.* Kansas City, MO: Author.

American Nurses Association. (1975). *A plan for implementation of the standards of nursing practice: A report of the Congress for Nursing Practice of the American Nurses Association.* Kansas City, MO: Author.

American Nurses Association. (1983). *Standards of school nursing practice.* Kansas City, MO: Author.

American Nurses Association. (1987). *The scope of nursing practice.* Washington, DC: American Nurses Publishing.

American Nurses Association. (1991). *Standards of clinical nursing practice.* Washington, DC: American Nurses Publishing.

American Nurses Association. (1998). *Standards of clinical nursing practice* (2nd ed.). Washington, DC: American Nurses Publishing.

American Nurses Association. (2001). *Code of ethics for nursing with interpretive statements.* Washington, DC: American Nurses Publishing.

American Nurses Association. (2004a). *Nursing: Scope and standards of practice.* Washington DC: American Nurses Publishing.

American Nurses Association. (2004b). *Scope and standards for nurse administrators* (2nd ed.). Washington, DC: American Nurses Publishing.

American Nurses Association, Public Health Nurses Section. (1955). *Functions, standards, and qualifications for public health nursing.* New York: American Nurses Association.

American Nurses Association, Public Health Nurses Section. (1964). *Functions and qualifications in the practice of public health nursing* (2nd ed.). New York: American Nurses Association.

American Nurses Association, Public Health Nurses Section, School Nurses Branch. (1966a). *Functions and qualifications for school nurses.* New York: American Nurses Association.

American Nurses Association, Public Health Nurses Section, School Nurses Branch. (1966b). *School nursing.* New York: American Nurses Association.

American School Health Association. (1974). *Guidelines for the school nurse in the school health program.* Kent, OH: Author.

American School Health Association. (1987). *Evaluating school nursing practice: A guide for administrators.* Kent, OH: Author.

American School Health Association. (1991). *Implementation guide for the standards of school nursing practice.* Kent, OH: Author.

American School Health Association, Committee on School Nursing Policies and Practices. (1956). Recommended policies and practices for school nursing. *Journal of School Health, 26*(1), 13–26.

American School Health Association, Committee on School Nursing Policies and Practices. (1957). Recommended policies and practices for school nursing. *Journal of School Health, 27*(1), 3–11.

American School Health Association, Committee on School Nursing Policies and Practices. (1959). Recommended policies and practices for school nursing (3rd pub., 2nd ed.). *Journal of School Health, 29*(1), 388–395.

Basco, D. (1963). Evaluation of school nursing activities: A pilot project using a scoring system and accepted standards of school nursing. *Nursing Research, 12,* 212–221.

Bobo, N., Adams, V. W., & Cooper, L. (2002). Excellence in school nursing practice: Developing a national perspective on school nurse competencies. *Journal of School Nursing, 18*(5), 277–285.

Brainerd, E. (Ed.). (2000). *Health of America's children at school: Developing a nursing research agenda.* (Proceedings of an Invitational Summit Meeting on School Nursing Research, Elkridge, Maryland, March, 1999.) Washington, DC: National Nursing Coalition for School Health.

Cary, A. (2000). Case management. In M. Stanhope & J. Lancaster (Eds.), *Community and public health nursing* (5th ed., pp. 380–399). St. Louis: Mosby.

Cavendish, R., Lunney, M., Luise, B. K., & Richardson, K. (2001). The Nursing Outcomes Classification: Its relevance to school nursing. *Journal of School Nursing, 17*(4), 189–197.

Costante, C. C. (2001). School [health] nursing: Framework for the future (Part II). *Journal of School Nursing, 17*(2), 64–72.

Dean-Barr, S. L. (2001). Standards and guidelines: Have they made a difference? In J. M. Dochterman & H. K. Grace (Eds.), *Current issues in nursing* (6th ed., pp. 234–240). St. Louis: Mosby.

Denehy, J. (2000). Measuring outcomes of school nursing practice: Showing that school nurses do make a difference. *Journal of School Nursing, 16*(1), 2–4.

Denehy, J. (2004). *Using nursing languages in school nursing practice.* Scarborough, ME: National Association of School Nurses.

Dochterman, J. M., & Bulecheck, G. M. (2004). *Nursing Interventions Classification (NIC)* (4th ed.). St. Louis: Mosby.

Dochterman, J. M., & Jones, D. A. (2003). *Unifying nursing languages: The harmonization of NANDA, NIC, and NOC.* Washington, DC: American Nurses Publishing.

Edwards, L. H. (2002). Research priorities in school nursing: A Delphi process. *Journal of School Nursing, 18*(3), 157–162.

Ellis, J. R., & Hartley, C. L. (2004). Preparing for workplace participation: Job descriptions. In *Nursing in today's world* (8th ed., pp. 454–489). Philadelphia: Lippincott Williams & Wilkins.

Hertel, V. (1996). *Draft for the revision of standards of school nursing practice to meet format of ANA's standards of clinical nursing practice.* Unpublished manuscript. Denver, CO.

Hootman, J. (1996). Nursing diagnosis: A language of nursing; a language of powerful communication. *Journal of School Nursing, 12*(4), 19–23.

Hootman, J. (2004). *Quality nursing interventions in the school setting: Procedures, models, and guidelines* (2nd ed.). Scarborough, ME: National Association of School Nurses.

Igoe, J. B. (2000). School nursing today: A search for new cheese. *Journal of School Nursing, 16*(5), 9–15.

Johnson, L. F. (2003). *Congruity between current school nursing practice and national standards of practice.* Unpublished master's thesis, Division of Nursing, California State University, Sacramento.

Johnson, M., Bulechek, G., Dochterman, J. M., Maas, M., & Moorhead, S. (Eds.). (2001). *Nursing diagnoses, outcomes, and interventions: NANDA, NOC, and NIC linkages.* St. Louis: Mosby.

Kulbok, P. A., Laffrey, S. C., & Goeppinger, J. (2000). Community health promotion: An integration model for practice. In M. Stanhope & J. Lancaster (Eds.), *Community and public health nursing* (5th ed., pp. 284–303). St. Louis: Mosby.

Lordi, S. L. (with Bradley, B.). (2000). *Standards of professional school nursing practice: Applications in the field.* Scarborough, ME: National Association of School Nurses.

Lunney, M. (1996). The significance of nursing classification systems to school nursing. *Journal of School Nursing, 12*(2), 6–8.

Lunney, M., Cavendish, R., Luise, B. K., & Richardson, K. (1997). Relevance of NANDA and health promotion diagnoses to school nursing. *Journal of School Nursing, 13*(5), 16–22.

McKenzie, F. D., & Richmond, J. B. (1998). Linking health and learning: An overview of coordinated school health programs. In E. Marx & S. F. Wooley (with D. Northrup) (Eds.), *Health is academic: A guide to coordinated school health programs* (pp. 1–14). New York: Teachers College Press/Education Development Center, Inc.

Moorhead, S., Johnson, M., & Maas, M. (2004). *Nursing*

Outcomes Classification (NOC) (3rd ed.). St Louis: Mosby.

National Association of School Nurses. (1981). *Guidelines for a model school nursing services program.* Scarborough, ME: NASN.

National Association of School Nurses. (1985). *An evaluation guide for school nursing practice designed for self and peer review.* Scarborough, ME: NASN.

National Association of School Nurses. (1995). *Caseload assignments* [position statement]. Retrieved November 9, 2003, from http://www.nasn.org/

National Association of School Nurses. (1998). *Standards of professional school nursing practice.* Scarborough, ME: Author.

National Association of School Nurses. (1999). *Code of ethics with interpretive statements for school nurses.* Scarborough, ME: Author.

National Association of School Nurses. (2003). *Position statement: The role of the advanced practice registered nurse in the school setting.* Retrieved July 2005 from http://www.nasn.org/positions/2003psadvanced.htm

National Association of School Nurses and the American Nurses Association. (2001). *Scope and standards of professional school nursing practice.* Washington, DC: American Nurses Publishing.

National Association of School Nurses and the American Nurses Association. (2005). *School nursing: Scope and standards of practice.* Silver Spring, MD: Nursesbooks.org/American Nurses Association.

National Consortium of School Nurse Educators. (1998). *Position statement: Educational preparation of school nurses.* Unpublished manuscript. (Available from Barbara Zimmerman, Department of Nursing, Millersville State College, Millersville, PA.)

National Council of State Boards of Nursing. (2003). *NCLEX examination.* Retrieved September 25, 2003, from http://www.ncsbn.org

National Education Association, Department of School Nurses. (1970). *Standards for school nurse services.* Washington, DC: National Education Association.

North American Nursing Diagnosis Association (NANDA). (2005). *Nursing diagnoses: Definitions and classification 2005–2006.* Philadelphia: NANDA International.

Pohlman, K. J. (2001). Legal framework and accountability for school nursing practice. In *Legal issues in school health services: A resource guide for school administrators, school attorneys, and school nurses* (pp. 95–121). North Branch, MN: Sunrise River Press.

Poster, E. C., & Marcontel, M. (1999). School nursing role and competence. *Journal of School Nursing, 15*(2), 34–42.

Praeger, S. (2005). Changing standards: Implications for school nurse educators. *NASN Newsletter, 20*(1), 16–20.

Proctor, S. E. (1986). Evaluation of nursing practice in schools. *Journal of School Health, 56*(7), 272–275.

Proctor, S. E., Baucom, T. E., & Griffin, J. M. (n.d.). *School nursing APN competency study.* Unpublished raw data. Division of Nursing, California State University, Sacramento.

Proctor, S. T. (1990). *Guidelines for the model school nurse services program.* Scarborough, ME: National Association of School Nurses.

Proctor, S. T. (with Lordi, S. L., & Zaiger, D. S.). (1993). *School nursing practice: Roles and standards.* Scarborough, ME: National Association of School Nurses.

Schwab, N. C., Gelfman, M. H. B., & Cohn, S. D. (2001). Fundamentals of U.S. law. In N. C. Schwab & M. H. B. Gelfman (Eds.), *Legal issues in school health services: A resource guide for school administrators, school attorneys, and school nurses* (pp. 55–79). North Branch, MN: Sunrise River Press.

Schwab, N. C., Hootman, J., & Gelfman, M. H. B. (with Gregory, E. K., & Pohlman, K. J.). (2001). School nursing practice: Professional performance issues. In N. C. Schwab & M. H. B. Gelfman (Eds.), *Legal issues in school health services: A resource guide for school administrators, school attorneys, and school nurses* (pp. 123–165). North Branch, MN: Sunrise River Press.

Southern Regional Education Board. (2000). *Curriculum and faculty development in community-based care: School nurses and nurse educators collaborate.* Atlanta: Author.

Stanhope, M., & Lancaster, J. (2000). *Community and public health nursing* (5th ed.). St. Louis: Mosby.

Stock, J. L., Larter, N., Kieckehefer, G. M., Thronson, G., & Maire, J. (2002). Measuring outcomes of school nursing services. *Journal of School Nursing, 18*(6), 353–359.

Stronge, J. H. (1994). Individual/institutional balance in evaluation. In A. McConney (Ed.), *Toward a unified model: The foundations of educational personnel evaluation* (pp. 17–32). Kalamazoo, MI: Center for Research on Educational Accountability and Teacher Evaluation (CREATE).

Stronge, J. H., & Helm, V. M. (1991). *Evaluating professional support personnel in education.* Newbury Park, CA: Sage Publications.

Western Interstate Commission on Higher Education. (1985). *The preparation and utilization of new nursing graduates.* Boulder, CO: Author.

Wilson, C. C. (1964). *School health services: NEA-AMA Joint Commission on Health Problems in Education.* Washington, DC: National Education Association/American Medical Association.

Wold, S. J., & Dagg, N. V. (1981). A framework for practice. In S. J. Wold (Ed.), *School nursing: A framework for practice* (pp. 30–35). North Branch, MN: Sunrise River Press.

Wolfe, L. C. (2002). School nursing: The next hundred years. *Journal of School Nursing, 18*(5), 250–251.

Yura, H., & Walsh, M. B. (1973). *The nursing process: Assessing, planning, implementing, and evaluating* (2nd ed.). New York: Appleton-Century-Crofts.

Zaiger, D. S. (2000). School nursing services: The early years. *Journal of School Nursing, 16*(3), 11–19.

Chapter 5

Requirements for School Nursing Practice and Certifications

CAROL COSTANTE

Chapter Outline

INTRODUCTION

School nursing, like other nursing specialties, has its roots in general nursing practice, most specifically, public health nursing. All of nursing shares the same basic legal framework so that licensure and practice regulations apply equally, as do the general principles of certification and nursing education. Upon this foundation rest the core values that define the school nursing specialty practice, such as its scope and standards, competencies, essential educational preparation, professional certification, and school nurse qualifications. This chapter addresses general nursing practice regulations, as well as qualifications, academic preparation, and certification related specifically to school nursing.

For the purposes of this discussion, unless otherwise noted, "nurse" refers to a licensed, registered nurse, and "nursing" denotes the scope of professional practice for a registered nurse. A "school nurse" is considered, at minimum, a registered nurse, although it is recognized that this is not universally accepted. In some states, a licensed practical nurse may qualify for the title "school nurse." "General nursing" refers to the practice of diagnosing and treating human responses to actual and potential health problems (Schwab & Gelfman, 2001b, p. 618). According to the National Association of School Nurses (NASN) (1999a): "School nursing is a specialized practice of professional nursing that advances the well being, academic success, and lifelong achievement of students. To that end, school nurses facilitate positive student responses to normal development; promote health and safety; intervene with actual and potential health problems; provide case management services; and actively collaborate with others to build student and family capacity for adaptation, self management, self advocacy, and learning."

NURSING LICENSURE

Prior to 1903, only training schools taught the art of nursing; there were no performance standards for these schools, and anyone could care for the sick. No regulations governed "nursing." In 1903, North Carolina became the first state to adopt a mandatory nursing licensure law, quickly followed by New Jersey, New York, and Virginia in that same year (Kerr, 2003). Thus began the professionalization of contemporary nursing.

The power to regulate licensure is reserved for states. Each state possesses what is known as "parens patriae" power under which it can create laws to protect the public's health, safety, and welfare (Pohlman, 2001). The regulatory method of licensure is used when the indicated activities are complex and require specialized knowledge, skill, and independent decision-making. "Licensure is the process by which an agency of state government grants permission to an individual to engage in a given profession upon finding that the applicant has attained the essential degree of competency necessary to perform a unique scope of practice" (National Council of State Boards of Nursing [NCSBN], 2004d).

The NCSBN (2004e) explains further that professional nursing licensure requirements define what is necessary for one to be able to practice nursing safely and what validates that the applicant meets those requirements. In addition to ensuring that a specified scope of practice is performed legally only by licensed individuals, licensure provides title protection for those roles, for example, "registered nurse." The disciplinary action authority allowed under licensure further protects the public's health, safety, and welfare when legal provisions are violated.

Nursing licensure in the United States is conferred on successful completion of a written examination after a candidate graduates from an accredited basic nursing education program with either a Nursing Diploma, an Associate of Arts degree (AA), or a Bachelor of Science degree in nursing (BSN). All states require new graduates to take the National Council Licensing Examination for RNs (NCLEX-RN), but each state's Board of Nursing (BON) regulates its own licensure process. Once licensed, a registered nurse may practice only in the state in which she or he is licensed, unless the state is part of the compact agreement; however, one may gain licensure in another noncompact state through the process of reciprocity. Assuming that the requirements for licensure are similar, reciprocity generally consists of applying for licensure in another state and paying the licensure fee.

Interstate Compact

In 1997, the National Council of State Boards of Nursing unanimously endorsed a "mutual recognition" model of nursing regulation, which allows a nurse who holds a license in his or her state of residency to practice in any state that has signed onto the interstate compact (NCSBN, 2004e). Box 5.1 lists the various reasons that NCSBN cites to support the mutual recognition model (NCSBN, 2004b).

The NCSBN (1999) promotes uniform core licensure requirements because it believes that increased consistency in licensure requirements is an appropriate direction for regulation in a highly mobile and increasingly global society. Since a national nursing licensure examination has been

Box 5.1 ■■■

RATIONALE FOR THE MUTUAL RECOGNITION MODEL OF NURSING REGULATION

- The growing need for nursing practice to occur across state lines.
- The variety of settings in which nurses work and the technologies they use that may cross state lines.
- The expectation and desire by consumers to have access to qualified nurses (based on national competencies) regardless of state lines.
- The need for more expedient and efficient authorization to practice.
- More uniformity in laws and approaches to new technology and practice modalities across states.
- It may be more cost effective.

(NCSBN, 2004b)

available to all jurisdictions for years, NCSBN proposes that other nursing licensure requirements be more consistent from state to state. Not only would uniform licensure requirements be less confusing for nurses and the public, they would also assist the implementation of the mutual recognition compact by diminishing concerns over disparate qualifications for licensure in compact states. The elements of the proposed core licensure requirement would include nursing education requirements; assessment of competence through examination, practice, and continuing education; and the bases for professional conduct and disciplinary actions (NCSBN, 1999). Such uniform licensure requirements would necessitate legislation in most states.

Historically, nursing has had difficulty in coming together over major issues, and mutual recognition is no exception. One of the main areas of disagreement is the minimum preparation requirement for nursing. For example, North Dakota requires a Bachelor of Science degree in Nursing (BSN) for entry into professional nursing practice (Pohlman, 2001). If North Dakota signed onto the interstate compact, would RNs in all other participating states be permitted to practice there irrespective of their educational preparation? Then there are the conditions for relicensure that differ across states, such as continuing education requirements.

Despite the challenges, in 1999 Maryland became the first state to sign the interstate compact, and by September 2005, the number of interstate compact states totalled 18 (Table 5.1) (NCSBN, 2005). Three additional states have endorsed, but not implemented, the interstate compact.

School nurses must first be properly licensed as nurses in the states in which they practice; this is also true for advanced practice nurses who may work in school settings. Most states require RN licensure for qualification as a school nurse, but one-third of the states also allow licensed practical nurses (LPNs) to practice in a school setting (NASN, 2004). The mutual recognition model of nursing licensure would allow school nurses who reside in border communities to practice in neighboring states without seeking reciprocity as long as both states are "compact" states, and if the nurse meets the state's requirements to be a school nurse. The compact would also serve to support the telenursing

Table 5.1 ■
INTERSTATE COMPACT STATES

STATES IMPLEMENTING THE COMPACT		STATES PENDING COMPACT IMPLEMENTATION
Arizona	Nebraska	New Jersey
Arkansas	New Mexico	New Hampshire
Delaware	North Carolina	South Carolina
Idaho	North Dakota	
	South Dakota	
Iowa	Tennessee	
Maine	Texas	
Maryland	Utah	
Mississippi	Wisconsin	
Virginia		

Source: NCSBN (2005).

that is practiced in some rural areas, including nursing in schools. The NCSBN (1997) describes telenursing as "the practice of nursing over distance using telecommunications technology." From a licensure standpoint, the issue is not the type of technology used—for example, telephone, email, video conferencing or interactive television—it is the practice of nursing across state lines. The interstate compact alleviates that conflict.

NURSE PRACTICE ACTS AND BOARDS OF NURSING

State legislatures enact a Nurse Practice Act for each state and the State Board of Nursing (BON) is charged with regulating nursing through this statute. Boards of Nursing are state governmental agencies with the responsibility "to protect the public through the regulation of individual licensed nurses" (NCSBN, 2004a). Nurse Practice Acts apply to all nursing roles in every setting, including school nursing. Box 5.2 defines functions of the Nurse Practice Act according to the NCSBN (2004c).

The BON is usually responsible for defining the requirements for entry into practice. The Board also sets license renewal requirements, including continuing education in those states where the nurse practice act mandates continuing education credits for relicensure. In addition, many BONs regulate nursing education programs, often requiring accreditation from an authorized body such as the National League for Nursing Accrediting Commission (NLNAC) or the Commission on Collegiate Nursing Education (CCNE). In some states, nursing education programs are also subject to the general standards of the regulatory body for the specific educational institution (Pohlman, 2001).

Furthermore, BONs are authorized to develop administrative rules and regulations to clarify the Nurse Practice Act. Once enacted, these rules and regulations have the force and effect of law (NCSBN, 2004c). Declaratory Rulings are "issued by an administrative agency that interprets the law, regulations, or policies of the agency; such rulings are often issued in response to a question" (Schwab & Gelfman, 2001b, p. 610). "While not binding *per se*, such rulings may be considered 'standards of practice' within the state and may be cited as such in a civil suit" (Schwab, Gelfman, & Cohn, 2001, p. 60). These written opinions of the BON may be particularly useful in states that have very general nurse practice acts and for specialties such as school nursing in which the issues change rapidly in response to societal and healthcare delivery changes. For example, the Connecticut Board of Examiners of Nursing issued a declaratory ruling on Delegation by Licensed Nurses to Unlicensed Assistive Personnel in 1995 (Schwab et al., 2001). BONs generally keep licensees apprised of these declaratory rulings through their regular communication system to nurses in their states. See Box 5.3 for examples of school nursing questions that have resulted in declaratory rulings.

Box 5.2 ■ ■ ■

THE FUNCTIONS OF STATE NURSE PRACTICE ACTS

- Defines the authority of the Board of Nursing, its composition and powers.
- Defines nursing and the scope of nursing practice.
- Identifies types of licenses and titles.
- States the requirements for licensure.
- Protects titles.
- Identifies the grounds for disciplinary action.

(NCSBN, 2004c)

Box 5.3 ■ ■ ■

SAMPLE SCHOOL NURSING QUESTIONS THAT RESULTED IN DECLARATORY RULINGS

By the Maryland Board of Nursing

- May a registered nurse accept responsibility for supervising, instructing, monitoring or evaluating an unlicensed person performing nursing acts that are assigned by other non-nursing individuals/entities in the school setting? (1990a)
- May licensed nurses act on verbal orders transmitted through a third party? (1997)
- May school health nurses delegate tracheostomy suctioning and tracheostomy tube change/replacement to certified nursing assistants? (2003)

By the Iowa Board of Nursing

- Does state law allow registered nurses to administer over-the-counter medications to children enrolled in the public school system upon parental request? (1985)
- May non-nursing staff discontinue a nasogastric tube in a school setting after the school nurse has inserted the tube and started the feeding and medication? (1988)
- May a teacher, instructed and supervised by an RN, insert a catheter into and/or remove one from a patent gastrostomy for the purpose of administering liquids? (1989)

In addition, BONs may respond in a simpler written fashion to issues of practice for which there is already case law or Declaratory Rulings available. One example is a letter from the Maryland BON to a school nurse who inquired whether and how subcutaneous glucagon administration could be delegated to an unlicensed person in the school setting (B. Newman, personal communication, October 22, 1993).

CONFLICTS IN STANDARDS AND PRACTICES

In general, the State Nurse Practice Act should not conflict with other state statutes governing school nursing practice. To adapt to the nature of the school environment, however, some school nursing procedures or processes on the local or state level may counter normal nursing practice. For example, it is common practice for school nurses to refrain from documenting extremely sensitive health-related information in student health records, such as a diagnosis of human immunodeficiency virus/acquired immunodeficiency disease (HIV/AIDS). Because health records in schools are part of the educational records and the confidentiality of educational records cannot be guaranteed in the same way that health records in health institutions are protected, in school nursing it may be considered best practice to exclude this type of health information. The data can be safely maintained in personal notes that are kept locked in the school health office, and on a health problem list to which only the nurse and a substitute would have access.

If the school nursing community in the state has an ongoing relationship with the Board of Nursing, the Board should be kept apprised of the nuances of this specialty practice so that revisions to the Nurse Practice Act, which occur annually in most states, will consider the unique nature of school nursing. The process of Declaratory Rulings may also be used to address specialty-specific issues, as demonstrated in the previous section.

There is a greater likelihood that education standards or practices will be incompatible with school nursing principles (Costante 2001a,b; Institute of Medicine, 1997; Pohlman, 2001; Schwab et al., 2001). This may arise because the missions of the health and education disciplines are dissimilar, and because the laws and regulations governing their programs are sometimes contradictory, as they are developed by different governmental agencies.

These ".... inconsistencies between federal and state laws addressing health and education" (National Task Force on Confidential Student Health Information, 2000, p. 7) have been a long-standing challenge. The problems caused by such discrepancies may have a greater impact in those school districts where the education agency contracts school nursing services from a health entity such as a private hospital or public health agency. Nurses not employed by education agencies may be less understanding of, and may perceive a reduced allegiance to, the mission of education (Costante, 2001a) in addition to their usual practice of operating under a different set of standards regarding records maintenance and information sharing (NASN, 2002b). However, the federal statute that governs all student health records (FERPA) pertains to school employees as well as contracted employees who provide school health services (NASN, 2002b). The federal Family Educational Rights and Privacy Act (FERPA) of 1974 governs any education records in public and private schools that receive federal financial assistance (NASN, 2002b).

In recent years, however, positive gains have been made in aligning health and education regulations, goals, and outcomes. An emphasis on coordinated school health programs and frequent collaborations between health and education agencies around student health issues have been positive forces in shaping this synchrony (Marx & Wooley, 1998; National Task Force on Confidential Student Health Information, 2000).

Confidentiality

Nevertheless, conflicts remain in some important areas such as in treatment, counseling, and assessment and referral services for students with drug or alcohol abuse problems or family planning issues.

Disagreement exists between the specific federal law that stipulates confidentiality regarding drug and alcohol treatment centers and FERPA regarding parental access to student records (Gelfman & Schwab, 2001; NASN 2002b). Conflicts also exist in some states where minor consent-to-treatment laws, albeit variable, protect the rights and the privacy of students accessing the healthcare services identified in the law. The confounding problem is that any record of a referral or related discussion with the student for services covered under the minor consent regulation by a school health professional is also subject to FERPA, permitting parents to access all of their minor children's school records (NASN, 2002b; Schwab & Gelfman, 2001a).

Confidentiality and the maintenance of health records is a recurrent area of discord for school health professionals because health records are not distinguished from other types of education records, and because in some ways FERPA is less stringent than the laws that protect health records in a healthcare setting (NASN, 2002b; National Task Force on Confidential Student Health Information, 2000). There are "...conflicts between the policies, practices and administrative directives of local schools, legal obligations and ethical standards of practice of school health professionals" (National Task Force on Confidential Student Health Information, 2000, p. 7). FERPA does allow access to education records by anyone with a "legitimate educational interest"; however, confusion reigns because it is left up to school districts to define the limitations and there is no penalty if FERPA is not followed (Bergren, 2001; NASN, 2002b).

School staff may believe that they have a right, and indeed a responsibility, to have knowledge of student health issues because they perceive that it supports their ability to provide the most appropriate and inclusive services to students. Conversely, health-related information in schools should be shared only on a need-to-know basis and parents have the ultimate right to decide what is shared and with whom (National Task Force on Confidential Student Health Information, 2000). For example, there is no absolute educational reason for a teacher to know that a student is HIV positive. School nurses have a vital role in helping families determine which information on their child's health status impacts on the school setting and to inform them of their rights.

School nurses, as all nurses, are bound by professional and ethical standards to protect clients' privacy and confidentiality regarding personal health information (American Nurses Association [ANA]; 2001; NASN, 1999b, 2001). As a result, at times school nurses may feel compromised by competing sets of principles. The federal Health Information Portability and Accountability Act (HIPAA) of 1996 does not govern school health records (NASN, 2002b): "...school health records were excluded from the definition of protected health information with the explanation that Congress protects the privacy of these records through FERPA" (Bergren, 2001, p. 337). Indirectly, HIPAA affects schools because it can impede them from obtaining identifiable student information from healthcare providers, even though the law specifically excludes communication between healthcare professionals (including school nurses) for the purpose of coordinating care. HIPAA does apply to "...school-based health centers (SBHCS) administered by covered entities,.... and most school-based healthcare providers employed by an agency other than a school district or university" (NASN, 2002b). HIPAA impacts SBHCs inasmuch as they are primary healthcare clinics within schools and their student healthcare records are not considered education records. The issues surrounding FERPA versus HIPAA continue to be examined in the health and education arenas with the goal of protecting student health information while not imposing artificial barriers. More information on FERPA and HIPAA is in Chapter 13.

PREPARATION AND QUALIFICATIONS FOR SCHOOL NURSING

The various entry levels into nursing, with their respective arrays of competencies, create enormous confusion on the part of the public. In addition, it is not reasonable to expect, or demand, the same performance standards and accountability from nurses with varying levels of preparation. Even more problematic is the fact that the public does not understand the purely adjunctive role of technically prepared, licensed healthcare assistants such as practical (LPN) or vocational (LVN) nurses. Inequality in services to children results when healthcare providers with different levels of preparation and licensing are charged by school districts to provide equivalent nursing services in schools (Costante, 2001a).

The professional school nursing organization (NASN, 2002a) has established that minimum preparation for school nursing is a baccalaureate degree. School nursing is a complex specialty with a broad scope of practice necessitating specific skills and extensive knowledge in an unusually wide range of areas (NASN, 2001, 2002a; Proctor, 1998; Wold, 2001). The independent nature of the practice and the advanced skills and complex judgments that are required in amorphous and demanding situations command this minimum level of educational preparation (Costante, 2001a,c; NASN, 2001, 2002a). The primary rationale for requiring a BSN is the inclusion of the principles of public health nursing in the curriculum, which promotes an aggregate and population focus. These are generally not included in Diploma and Associate Degree educational programs. Despite the pervasive belief that baccalaureate preparation is necessary, currently only 18 states, plus the Department of Defense schools, require a bachelor's degree for qualification as a school nurse (NASN, 2004). On the other hand, some school districts, certain employers, and school nursing roles maintain the baccalaureate standard even in the absence of a state requirement (NASN, 2004). "While there are national standards of practice, there are not national standards of education for nurses who practice in schools" (Proctor, 2001, p. 476).

Some school nurse leaders purport that master's degrees should be required of those entering school nursing (Wold, 2001). Although graduate education is both justified and desirable based on the nature of school nursing practice, it is at present impractical to enforce it as an entry requirement. Neither education or health budgets, nor the numbers of qualified nurses educated at the master's level, could support this quality of healthcare personnel for all schoolchildren in the United States. For nurses in management, supervisory, or consultant positions, however, a master's degree should be an essential requisite (Costante, 2001a,c). "Equity of school nurse qualifications across school districts and states—at a minimum of the bachelor's degree entry into practice—should, perhaps, be the first priority, along with making such qualified school nurses available to every school-age child in the country" (Costante, 2001a, p. 498).

However, in school districts with few school healthcare resources, employing a nurse with a master's degree who delegates appropriately with a focus on health promotion and disease prevention could be an effective, cost-efficient way to impact the health and wellness of school communities. Even though advanced assessment skills and analytical reasoning are vital in school nursing, a master's-prepared nurse practitioner is not necessary, or cost-effective, for a general school health services program (Costante, 2001a,c; Proctor, 1998). Given the budgetary implications and human resource realities, advanced practice nurses may best be utilized in school-based health centers, where their abilities to diagnose and treat are essential.

Attainment of an advanced degree is the accepted norm for professional school personnel after a state-designated period of time so the same requirement ultimately should be expected of school nurses (Costante, 2001a,c). This value on higher education sets an expectation that professional colleagues working toward complementary goals have similar educational requirements. "For the nurse to be less well prepared than other school colleagues reduces his or her effectiveness and diminishes professional credibility" (Proctor, 2001, p. 474). The acquisition of post-baccalaureate education demonstrates a respect for learning that translates into a high functioning workforce, as well as providing ample leadership and mentoring (Costante, 2001a,c).

Continuing education in school health–related fields, even if it does not result in a master's degree, should be ongoing to ensure that skills are up to date. In addition, because school nurses provide services in conjunction with their education peers in an environment whose mission is learning, they are obligated to keep current with education issues and trends. For example, the Federal No Child Left Behind Act of 2001 demands sweeping education reforms, which have implications for school nurses, that is, requiring accountability for results and focusing services on students who are disadvantaged or have limited English language proficiency.

The uniqueness of school nursing requires that "school nurses need to be 'bilingual'; that is, they must be well versed in both the disciplines of health and education and have special expertise regarding the role of health on student learning" (Costante, 2001c, p. 66). This dual expertise is necessary for healthcare services to contribute to the student's learning process, and to be regarded as equal to other services provided by schools. To achieve this status, knowledge beyond the baccalaureate level is vital in areas such as principles of education, family systems, community health, special education, advanced nursing assessment, and health education (Costante, 2001a,c; NASN, 2002a; Poster & Marcontel, 1999; Proctor, 1998; Wold, 2001).

Graduate education is intended to translate to higher-level competencies, particularly if the curriculum is competency-based. According to the National Council of State Boards of Nursing, standards of competence must be applicable to all nurses in a practice role and address the continuum of practice levels from entry to continued competence (Poster & Marcontel, 1999). "Competency is the application of knowledge and the interpersonal, decision-making, and psycho-motor skills expected for the [school] nurses' practice role within the context of public health, welfare, and safety" (NCSBN, 1996). Inherent in this definition is that the school nurse not only must possess knowledge and skills, but also needs to be able to apply these to advance the health and educational success of the school-age child (Bobo, Adams, & Cooper, 2002). This is the ultimate goal and the rationale for requiring school nurses to possess a minimum of a BSN that includes public health theory and practice.

NASN, in conjunction with the Southern Regional Education Board Council on Collegiate Education for Nursing, collaborated to identify entry-level competencies and align them with the Scope and Standards of Professional School Nursing Practice (Bobo et al., 2002) (see Chapter 11). The development and recognition of school nursing competencies provide guidance for the academic programs that design curricula to prepare school nurses and for the practice settings that hire and evaluate school nurses, as well as for competency-based certification examinations.

SCHOOL NURSING CERTIFICATION

Professional certification is prescribed by professional nursing organizations to indicate "a level of competence above the minimum criteria for licensure and verify that an individual has met certain standards of preparation and performance" in a specialized area of practice (Schwab, Hootman, Gelfman et al., 2001, p. 139). Competency consists of critical thinking and logical, safe, and evidence-based decision making (National Board for Certification of School Nurses [NBCSN], 2003a). According to the American Board of Nursing Specialties (ABNS) (2003), the ultimate goal of certification is to assist consumers in making informed choices regarding their healthcare practitioners. The NBCSN (2003b) asserts that professional "certification assures a national standard of preparation, knowledge and practice."

Certification is formal recognition that an individual has mastered a specified body of knowledge or proficiency, and met certain standards (Schwab & Gelfman, 2001b, p. 609). Two types of certification exist for school nurses: (1) professional certification and (2) state certification. Unlike almost any other professional nursing certification, the national certification for school nurses is an acknowledgement of excellence in practice.

Professional certification for school nurses requires a baccalaureate degree, licensure as an RN, and current employment in school health services or school-related services; the NBCSN recommends that the applicant have at least 3 years of experience in school nursing practice. The 4-hour exam is a competency-based written examination (Costante, 2002). This nationally derived certification purports to measure the knowledge and judgment required for expertise in clinical school nursing practice. NBCSN is the only professional body that currently certifies school nurses. The American Nurses' Credentialing Center (ANCC), affiliated with the ANA, certified school nurses until 2000, but now only recertifies its existing credentialed school nurses through ongoing continuing education requirements.

The content of the NBCSN examination includes health appraisal (25%), health problems and nursing management (30%), health promotion/disease prevention (20%), special health issues (10%), and professional issues (15%) (Professional Testing Corporation, 2004). Recertification occurs every 5 years, with documentation of 75 hours of continuing education in subjects related to school nursing practice being the primary focus. National certification may be revoked if one falsifies the application, if the RN license is revoked, or if the individual misrepresents the certification status (Professional Testing Corporation, 2004).

Other than certification examinations, no nationally established and universally accepted knowledge, content, and skills that school nurses must be able to demonstrate for safe or optimal practice have been identified (Schwab et al., 2001). As a result, individual states determine the skills and knowledge that school nurses must possess in their respective jurisdictions. Consequently, across and within states, such variability in standards creates significant disparity in role expectation, services delivered to schools, and preparation and competency of the providers of school health services. Unfortunately, some states have no system of professional accountability or mentoring for nurses working in schools.

State education agencies may stipulate requirements that licensed nurses must meet to function in the role of school nurse in a particular state (Duncan & Igoe, 1998; Schwab et al., 2001). Several states have developed standards through teacher certification requirements, in addition to the other state laws or state agency or school district guidelines that regulate the qualifications to be a school nurse. In some states, state school nursing organizations have promulgated recommended competencies for practice within the state (Schwab et al., 2001).

State certification for school nurses, sometimes called teacher certification or licensure, generally mandates minimum educational requirements for employment, as well as specifies continuing education and/or graduate education requisites for ongoing certification (Costante, 2002). These state-specific employment standards for school nurses are usually regulated by the state education agency, although they may not be monitored by these agencies. Requirements sometimes parallel those for other student support services personnel in schools, such as guidance counselors, social workers, and psychologists. Because state certification involves employment standards only, it in no way conflicts with professional certification, which measures specific nursing knowledge and skills (Gregory & Marcontel, 2000). NASN (2002a) supports both state and professional certification in the specialty practice of school nursing. Currently, 50% of U.S. states, as well as the U.S. Department of Defense schools, have some form of certification process (NASN, 2004). However, extreme variability reigns in regard to which nursing certification applies, its requirements, and whether it is mandated versus optional. According to surveys of states with certification, school nurse certification apparently holds tangible advantages both to individual school nurses and to school health services programs. These benefits are summarized in Box 5.4 and Table 5.2.

In some cases, school nurse certification mirrors the teachers' certification process, but in other cases, the criteria are less stringent (Costante, 2002). Based on data from a survey of the states with certification (Costante, 2002) and information provided by states annually to NASN (2004), there appears to be great disparity among states regarding the various parameters of certification, such as:

- *To whom the requirement applies:* All nurses in the state; certain categories of nurses only; or leaving it up to school districts to decide whether to hire only certified school nurses.
- *Educational preparation required:* Baccalaureate in nursing only; baccalaureate with public health theory and practice; baccalaureate degree in nursing or related field; diploma or associate degree in nursing; being a licensed practical nurse; or, master's degree (ultimately).
- *Certification requirements:* coursework requirements and types or levels of certification.
- *Continuing education (CE) requisites:* Some states stipulate ongoing education for maintenance of the state license, but credentialing bodies may require specific continuing

Box 5.4 ■ ■ ■

STATE SCHOOL NURSE CERTIFICATION

Advantages to School Health Services Programs:

- Establishes a standard of practice and an expectation of that standard.
- Ensures adequately prepared school nurses to actualize a coordinated school health practice.
- Supports role-appropriate and similar preparation for all school nurses.
- Demonstrates commitment to quality school health services for all children.
- Affirms the connection between health and education for students.
- Raises awareness of child health needs and the ability to address them in the school community, thereby increasing the likelihood that children's health needs will be met.

(Costante, 2002)

Table 5.2 ■

PERCEIVED PERSONAL BENEFITS OF MANDATED STATE CERTIFICATION

IMMEDIATE	LONG TERM
Increases salary or justification for professional salary	Usually results in better retirement benefits
Generates confidence in practice	May require school districts to hire certified nurses
Enhances educational credibility	Potentially promotes an interest in professional certification
Promotes respect from education faculty and families	Supports higher personnel standards
Recognizes professional status	Provides job security
	Establishes universal credentialing for all education personnel
	Improves professional growth opportunities
	Legitimizes the specialty
	Assists with lobbying efforts
	Eases job transfers between jurisdictions

Source: Costante (2002).

education for recertification; the types and content of the CE vary considerably.

- *Remuneration:* Compensation in parity with certified teachers or wages determined by the school district irrespective of certification.

Other examples of differences include North Carolina, which is the only state to use the NBCSN professional certification as its state certification, whereas Arizona's certification for school nurses is administered and granted by their State Board of Nursing.

By creating state standards, certification helps to minimize the disparity of services in schools and ensure that all students have access to services from equally prepared and competent providers (Costante, 2001a). Many school nurse leaders agree that states would benefit from establishing standards for the school nurse, just as they do for teachers and other professional school staff (Costante, 2001b,c; Proctor, 2001; Wold, 2001). Nevertheless, states cite numerous barriers and challenges to instituting state certification for school nurses (Costante, 2002). These include:

- *Varied school nurse employers*. Although educational systems are the most common employer of school nurses (NASN, 2004), in many states public health nurses or private contractors, for example, hospitals, home health agencies, or private consultants, provide school nursing services. It may be complicated to achieve consensus for certification requirements that are aligned with teacher requirements where there are a variety of employers of school nurses.
- *Lack of awareness of the impact of health on learning*. There are still some who believe that "School nurses provide services that may be regarded as having a lower value and priority than those provided by teachers and other school employees" (Wold, 2001, p. 34). If the educational system does not regard health as a vital component of learning, there is little incentive on its part to establish certification. This constitutes one of the greatest challenges for school nurses who want to make a positive difference in this specialty. Further, it demonstrates the continued need for school nurses to conduct research that demonstrates the efficacy of their practice and to distribute this vital information to the public.
- *Role expectations*. According to Wold (2001) and others, it seems that a large number of states are unable to define their expectations of school nurses. With confusion about the role of contemporary school nurses, the various educational programs that lead to a nursing license, and the different types of healthcare providers in schools, the uniqueness of school nursing that merits a certification requirement is often unclear to educators and the public. In addition, states may believe that certification is unwarranted where mandates for licensure already exist. The school nursing community bears the responsibility to adequately define the role, including the competencies required, and to market its value.
- *Lack of state mandates*. An inverse relationship appears to exist between states that have regulations mandating school nurses and certification requirements that are nonexistent, weak, or optional. According to NASN (2004), only one-third of the states, the District of Columbia, and schools within the U.S. Department of Defense mandate on-site school nurses, even though "nearly every state has law that mandates some health services in schools" (Proctor, 2001, p. 476). However, mandates are meaningless without ratios. In those states with mandates for school nurses, the ratios of nurse to students are either not specified in law, or range from 1:500 to 1:11,500. Currently only 16 states meet the recommendation of Healthy People 2010 of one nurse for every 750 students (Personal communication, NASN, October 2005; U.S. Department of Health and Human Services [USDHHS], 2000).
- *Impact on employment*. Many nurses may be disinclined to promote school nurse certification if the requirements are beyond their current qualifications and if they feel that their livelihoods may be jeopardized by the implementation of such regulations. If public health agencies or private contractors can legally be hired to provide school nursing services without the necessity of certification, school districts may choose this lesser route to avoid the potentially higher salary obligation that usually accompanies mandated certification.
- *Lack of constituency support*. Promulgating certification regulations is generally dependent on grass roots initiation. It may be difficult to garner support where currently employed nurses feel threatened, in states with small school nurse numbers or rural geography, in jurisdictions where school

nurse positions are volatile and budget dependent, or where the additional requirements are not associated with higher remuneration.

- *Recruitment issues.* Increased employment requirements demanded by certification coupled with noncompetitive salaries for nurses, nontraditional work environments, or lack of access to higher education institutions in which to obtain requisite courses may be detriments to an adequate supply of qualified school nurse candidates.
- *Maintaining certification.* State regulations such as school nurse certification, being politically derived, are always subject to scrutiny and reinterpretation. Because of its budgetary implications, demonstrating positive student outcomes related to having well-qualified school nurses is essential to sustaining certification.

CONCLUSION

School nurses are governed by the same nursing standards as are other nurses; however, they also are guided by the school nurse specialty guidelines and standards. Because of the independent nature of the practice, the clinical judgments required in the school community setting, such as variable resources and demanding situations, and the focus on health promotion, prevention of disease, and case management services in a community setting, a baccalaureate degree is generally considered the minimal requirement for entry into school nursing. As with other nursing specialties, certification denotes competency. School nursing is recognized as a complex nursing specialty with a wide scope of practice demanding specific skills and a broad knowledge in both the health and education disciplines.

References

American Board of Nursing Specialties (ABNS). Accreditation standards. Retrieved September 7, 2003 from http://www. nursingcertification.org/standards.htm.

American Nurses Association (ANA). (2001). *Code of Ethics for Nurses with Interpretive Statements.* Washington, DC: Author.

Bergren, M. D. (2001). HIPAA hoopla: Privacy and security of identifiable health information. *Journal of School Nursing, 17*(6), 336–341.

Bobo, N., Adams, V. M., & Cooper, L. (2002). Excellence in school nursing practice: Developing a national perspective on school nurse competencies. *The Journal of School Nursing, 18* (5), 277–285.

Costante, C. C. (2001a). Future challenges for school health services and the law: A manager's perspective. In N. Schwab & M. Gelfman (Eds.), *Legal issues in school health services: A resource for school administrators, school attorneys and school nurses* (pp. 489–507). North Branch, MN: Sunrise River Press.

Costante, C. C. (2001b). School health nursing: Framework for the future, Part I. *Journal of School Nursing, 17,*(1), 3–11.

Costante, C. C. (2001c). School health nursing: Framework for the future, Part II. *Journal of School Nursing, 17*(2), 64–72.

Costante, C. C. (2002). State certification for school nurses. *Journal of School Nursing, 18*(2), 102–116.

Duncan, P., & Igoe, J. B. (1998) School health services. In Marx, E. & Wooley, S.F. (Eds.) with Northrup, D. (1998). *Health is academic.* New York City: Teachers College Press.

Gelfman, M. (with Schwab, N.). (2001). School health records and documentation. In N. Schwab & M. Gelfman (Eds.), *Legal issues in school health services: A resource for school administrators, school attorneys and school nurses* (pp. 297–316). North Branch, MN: Sunrise River Press.

Gregory, E. K., & Marcontel, M. (2000). National school nurse certification, Part II: Questions and answers. *Journal of School Nursing, 17*(3), 157–161.

Institute of Medicine, Committee on Comprehensive School Health Programs in Grades K–12. (1997). In D. Allenworth, E. Lawson, L Nicholson, & J. Wyche (Eds.), *School health: Our nation's investment.* Washington, DC: National Academy Press.

Iowa Board of Nursing. (July 25, 1985). *Declaratory ruling No. 3. Administration of OTC medications by school nurses.* Retrieved February 20, 2004 from http://www.state.ia.us/nursing/pdf_files/ruling3.pdf.

Iowa Board of Nursing. (January 27, 1988). *Declaratory ruling No. 19. Removal of NG tube.* Retrieved February 20, 2004 from http://www.state.ia.us/nursing/declaratory_index.html.

Iowa Board of Nursing. (December 7, 1989). *Declaratory ruling No. 47. Teacher inserting gastrostomy tube in a continent gastrostomy.* Retrieved February 20, 2004 from http://www.state.ia.us/nursing/declaratory_index.html.

Kerr, T. (2003). Old Dominion's centennial. *Advance for Nurses,* 5(11 D.C.), 14.

Maryland Board of Nursing. (December 18, 1990[b]). *Declaratory ruling No. 90-21. Registered nurses accepting responsibility for supervising, instructing, monitoring and evaluating unlicensed persons performing nursing functions assigned by other non-nursing individuals/entities in the school setting.* Retrieved February 20, 2004 from http://www.mbon.org/practice/pdf/90-21/pdf.

Maryland Board of Nursing. (February 25, 1997). *Declaratory ruling No. 97-5. Licensed nurses acting on verbal orders (oral or telephone), or on a modified written order.* Retrieved February 20, 2004 from http://www.mbon.org/practice/pdf/97-5/pdf.

Maryland Board of Nursing. (July 29, 2003). *Declaratory ruling No. 2003-2. School health nurse, registered nurse supervision and monitoring of certified nursing assistants in the performance of tracheostomy suctioning and tracheostomy tube change/replacement.* Retrieved February 20, 2004 from http://www.mbon.org/practice/pdf/2003-2/pdf.

Marx, E., & Wooley, S. F. (Eds.) with Northrup, D. (1998). *Health is academic.* New York City: Teachers College Press.

National Association of School Nurses (NASN). (1999a). *Definition of school nursing.* Retrieved February 20, 2004 from http://www.nasn.org.

National Association of School Nurses (NASN). (1999b). *Code of ethics with interpretive statements for the school nurse.* Brochure. Scarborough, ME: Author.

National Association of School Nurses (NASN) & the American Nurses Association (ANA). (2001). *Scope and standards of professional school nursing practice.* Scarborough, ME: Author.

National Association of School Nurses (NASN). (2002a). *Education, Licensure, and Certification of School Nurses.* Position statement. Scarborough, ME: Author.

National Association of School Nurses (NASN). (2002b). *School health nurse's role in education: Privacy standards for student health records.* Issue brief. Scarborough, ME: Author.

National Association of School Nurses (NASN). (2004). *2003 annual state affiliate report summary.* Report. Scarborough, ME: Author.

National Board for Certification of School Nurses (NBCSN). (2003a). *School nurse certification. Position statement.* Retrieved September 7, 2003 from http://www.nbcsn.com/pscertification.htm.

National Board for Certification of School Nurses (NBCSN). (2003b). *Home page.* Retrieved September 7, 2003 from http://www.nbcsn.com/.

National Council of State Boards of Nursing (NCSBN). (1996). *Definition of competence.* Retrieved February 24, 2004 from http://www.ncsbn.org/resources/ncsbn_competence_two.asp#Definition%20of%20Competence.

National Council of State Boards of Nursing (NCSBN). (1997). *Telenursing: A challenge to regulation.* Retrieved March 1, 2005 from http://www.ncsbn.org/resources/complimentary_ncsbn_telenursing.asp.

National Council of State Boards of Nursing (NCSBN). (1999). *Uniform core licensure requirement.* National Council Paper. Retrieved March 3, 2004 from http://ncsbn.org/regulation/nursingpractice_nursing_practice_licensing.asp

National Council of State Boards of Nursing (NCSBN). (2004a). *Nursing regulation.* Retrieved March 9, 2004 from http://www.ncsbn.org/regulation/nursingpractice.asp.

National Council of State Boards of Nursing (NCSBN). (2004b). *Nurse licensure compact.* Retrieved March 3, 2004 from http://www.ncsbn.org/pdfs/NLCA_Fact_Nov02.pdf.

National Council of State Boards of Nursing (NCSBN). (2004c). *Nursing regulation.* Retrieved February 20, 2004 from http://www.ncsbn.org/regulation/index.asp.

National Council of State Boards of Nursing (NCSBN). (2004d). *Nursing regulation.* Retrieved March 8, 2004 from http://ncsbn.org/regulation/nlc.asp.

National Council of State Boards of Nursing (NCSBN). (2004e). *Nursing regulation.* Retrieved March 8, 2004 from http://www.ncsbn.org/nlc/rnlpvncompact.asp.

National Council of State Boards of Nursing (NCSBN). (2005). *Nurse licensure compact implementation.* Retrieved October 15, 2005 from http://ncsbn.org/nlc/rnlpvncompact_ mutual_recognition_state.asp.

National Task Force on Confidential Student Health Information. (2000). *Guidelines for protecting confidential student health information.* Kent, OH: American School Health Association.

Pohlman, K. J. (2001). Legal framework and financial accountability for school nursing practice. In N. Schwab & M. Gelfman (Eds.), *Legal issues in school health services: A resource for school administrators, school attorneys and school nurses* (pp. 95–121). North Branch, MN: Sunrise River Press.

Professional Testing Corporation. (2004). *Certification Examination for School Nurses: Handbook for Candidates.* New York: Author.

Poster, E. C., & Marcontel, M. (1999). School nursing role and competence. *Journal of School Nursing, 15*(2), 34–42.

Proctor, S. E. (1998). Identifying a "critical mass" of specialty content for school nursing. *Journal of School Nursing, 14*(3), 2–4.

Proctor, S. E. (2001). The educational preparation of school nurses: Implications for hiring and liability protection. In N. Schwab & M. Gelfman (Eds.), *Legal issues in school health services: A resource for school administrators, school attorneys and school nurses* (pp. 473–482). North Branch, MN: Sunrise River Press.

Schwab, N. C., & Gelfman, M. (2001a). Confidentiality: Principles and practice issues. In N. Schwab & M. Gelfman (Eds.), *Legal issues in school health services: A resource for school administrators, school attorneys and school nurses* (pp. 261–295). North Branch, MN: Sunrise River Press.

Schwab, N. C., & Gelfman, M. (Eds.) (2001b). Glossary. *In Legal issues in school health services: A resource for school administrators, school attorneys and school nurses* (pp. 607–623). North Branch, MN: Sunrise River Press.

Schwab, N. C., Gelfman, M., & Cohn, S. D. (2001). Fundamentals of U.S. law. In N. Schwab & M. Gelfman (Eds.), *Legal issues in school health services: A resource for school administrators, school attorneys and school nurses* (pp. 55–79). North Branch, MN: Sunrise River Press.

Schwab, N. C., Hootman, J. & Gelfman, M. (with Gregory, E. K. & Pohlman, K. J.) (2001). School nursing practice: Professional performance issues. In N. Schwab & M. Gelfman (Eds.), *Legal issues in school health services: A resource for school administrators, school attorneys and school nurses* (pp. 123–165). North Branch, MN: Sunrise River Press.

U.S. Department of Health and Human Services (USDHHS). (2000). *Healthy people 2010: National health promotion and disease prevention objectives.* Washington, DC: U.S. Department of Health and Human Services, Public Health Service.

Wold, S. (2001). School health services: Origins and trends. In N. Schwab & M. Gelfman (Eds.), *Legal issues in school health services: A resource for school administrators, school attorneys and school nurses* (pp. 7–54). North Branch, MN: Sunrise River Press.

PART II

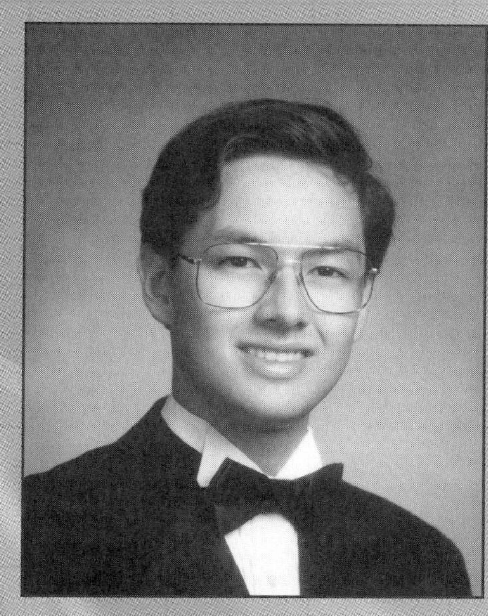

Roles and Functions of the School Nurse

Chapter 6

Roles of the School Nurse

LINDA C. WOLFE

Chapter Outline

INTRODUCTION

School nursing has a rich history of supporting both education and health initiatives to promote the health and well-being of children. More than 100 years ago, founder Lillian Wald envisioned a role for the nurse within the community to serve all, regardless of economic or social status or national origin. Her vision to "contribute our sense of community to what seems an alien group [immigrants]" (Duffus, 1938, p. 35) logically led her to embrace and merge public health goals (to ensure freedom from communicable disease), educational goals (to eliminate absenteeism), and social goals (to build literate and productive citizens).

> The concept of a nurse ready to give her services in the home to all who needed them, making no distinction between those who could pay and those who could not, allied with no religious group, seeking to educate as well as to heal, was waiting to be born. Lillian Wald and Mary Brewster brought it into being. It was time. (Duffus, 1938, p. 37)

Unlike the medical model of school health that initially focused on exclusion of students with infection, the school nursing model has fostered since its inception the inclusion of all children in the school setting: "... the addition of the nurse to the staff made it possible to reverse the object of medical inspection from excluding the children from school to keeping the children in the classroom and under treatment" (Wald, 1915/1991, p. 52).

In the 21st century, the school nurse continues to support children in meeting the universal goals of education and health for academic success and optimal wellness, respectively. In successful school nurs-

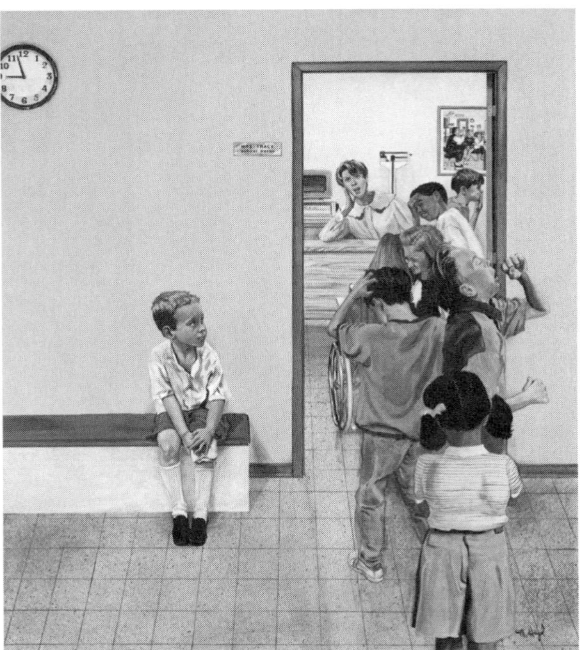

A day in the life of the school nurse—1993. (School Health Corporation)

ing practices, these goals weave seamlessly together to create a safety net and springboard for children to grow into healthy and successful citizens. The school nurse's ultimate goal is articulated in the mission of the National Association of School Nurses (NASN): "to advance the well being and life-long achievement of students" (National Association of School Nurses [NASN], 1999). School nurses accomplish this by assisting students to improve or manage their current health status. Although this goal or outcome of school nursing practice has remained consistent and fairly easily articulated over the last century, there have been challenges in articulating the "role" of the school nurse in terms of nursing service expectations. Both internally (among school nurses) and externally (among the school health, nursing, and medical communities), changes in school nursing service delivery have resulted in changes to role definitions.

Changes in client profiles, school demographics, and nursing skills have all influenced role definitions and task expectations of the school nurse. If, however, differences in geography, resources, institutional settings, employers, educational preparation and tradition are erased from the equation, the question "What is the role of the School Nurse" can be easily answered. ***The role of the school nurse is to ensure the child enters the classroom in optimal health and is ready to learn.*** The more challenging questions remain, that is, "What is a school nurse?", "What are the responsibilities of a school nurse?" and "How does a school nurse assure optimal wellness and readiness to learn?"

DEFINITION OF SCHOOL NURSING

The definition of school nursing metamorphosed over the past century to accommodate changes in the needs of the student and to incorporate the enhanced knowledge and skills of the nurse. These changes, along with wide differences among practice settings, challenged authors and experts to clearly address the issue of role clarity. TABLE 6.1 demonstrates changes as observed through definition during the past century.

As late as 1995, authors were still perplexed concerning the role of the school nurse. An exhaustive review of the professional literature on school nurse evaluation by one cohort of educators concluded that "the role of the school nurse has not been clearly defined and delineated, not necessarily because of the nurses themselves, but because of the changing and sometimes contradictory expectations of society and educators" (Stronge, Helm, & Tucker, 1995, p. 121). In a 1993 NASN document, the "essence" of school nursing as a "specialty branch of professional nursing" was explored through the identification of global standards of practice (Proctor, Lordi & Zaiger, 1993, p. 11). In 1999 the NASN Board approved a comprehensive definition of school nursing and in 2001 NASN and the American Nurses Association jointly released the *Scope and Standards of Professional School Nurse Practice*, which includes the 1999 definition.

> School nursing is a specialized practice of professional nursing that advances the well being, academic success, and life-long achievement of students. To that end, school nurses facilitate positive student responses to normal development; promote health and safety; intervene with actual and potential health problems; provide case management services; and actively collaborate with others to build student and family capacity for adaptation, self management, self advocacy, and learning. (NASN, 1999)

Within school nursing practices throughout the United States and internationally, great diversity

(text continues on page 114)

Table 6.1 ■
DEFINITIONS OF SCHOOL NURSING

DATE	ORGANIZATION	DEFINITION
1902	Lillian Wald, reflections from *The House on Henry Street* (pp. 48–49)	" … with her [school nurse] assistance [to the school physician], few children would lose their valuable school time and that it would be possible to bring under treatment those who needed it."
1918	Helen W. Kelly and Mabel C. Bradshaw, *A Handbook for School Nurses* (p. 32)	"The function of the school nurse is threefold. She assists in the *prevention* of contagion and in the *correction* of physical defects, and is responsible for the *education* of children, and sometimes of their parents in the principles of personal and public hygiene."
1937	Mary Ella Chayer, *School Nursing* (p. 26)	"The primary purpose of the school nurse is education in healthful living."
1955	National Education Association (NEA) and the American Medical Association (AMA) *The Nurse in the School* (p. 10)	"The qualified nurse working in the school can help the school to meet its health obligation… The nurse usually serves as liaison between the home, the school and the community resources for health services."
1967	National Education Association, National Council of School Nurse Organizations, Policy Statement (as cited in "Professional School Nursing Termed 'Dynamic Discipline'", p. 3)	"The primary function of the school nurse is to strengthen the educational process through improvement of the health status of children and youth."
1982	National Association of School Nurses Policy Statement, Philosophy of School Health Services and School Nursing (NASN, 1989)	"The specialized school nurse, employed by a board of education, enhances the educational process and potential of the student."
1993	National Association of School Nurses, Roles & Standards of School Nursing Practice for School Administrators and Community Leaders (NASN, 1993)	"School nursing is a specialty branch of professional nursing that seeks to prevent or identify student health or health-related problems and intervenes to modify or remediate those problems. A comprehensive school health program includes delivery of health services and health education which directly contributes to the student's education as well as the health of the family and community."
1999	National Association of School Nurses Board of Directors (June 1999, http://www.nasn.org)	"School nursing is a specialized practice of professional nursing that advances the well being, academic success, and life-long achievement of students. To that end, school nurses facilitate positive student responses to normal development; promote health and safety; intervene with actual and potential health problems; provide case management services; and actively collaborate with others to build student and family capacity for adaptation, self management, self advocacy, and learning."

exists relative to such issues as student-to-nurse ratios, delegation and supervision of care, prescribed educational nurse preparation, and local needs. References to role confusion in the past perhaps would be more accurately described as "task confusion," which is directly related to the absence of a standardized model for the delivery of school health services. Three main factors are frequently cited as contributors: "(a) their [school nurses'] status as boundary dwellers in the school setting; (b) lack of clear, appropriate, and agreed-to role expectations; and (c) role conflict within the school and school health team" (Wold, 2001, p. 34). However, the *essence* of the practice, that is, the role of the school nurse, has remained relatively stable over the years. It is the responsibilities and tasks that continue to change and evolve in order to meet the clients' ever-changing needs.

WHAT IS A SCHOOL NURSE?

Perceptions and Reality

School nurses will readily confirm that students, families, and the general public often ask, "Are you a real nurse?" Even questions such as, "What do you do?" are not unusual. The public's presumptions are often based on personal experience as a student or as the parent of a student.

When children are asked to describe the school nurse, they often use words that portray the nurse as a guardian, a provider of first aid, a safe haven, or a surrogate parent. Parents will use words that indicate that the school nurse is a primary care provider or a health advocate. Healthcare providers see the school nurse as a gatekeeper to the school system or a link in the continuity of care. Teachers see the school nurse's primary roles as planner/coordinator, care provider, and communicator (Leier, Cureton, & Canham, 2003, p. 5). School nurses respond with a laundry list of duties, from managing the "Lost and Found" to providing skilled nursing care of a medically fragile child.

In response to the question "What do school nurses do?" the author composed a poem for School Nurse Day 2002 (Box 6.1).

Box 6.1 ■ ■ ■

THAT'S WHAT SCHOOL NURSES DO

How many times have they asked me? I wonder.
My answers leave much to desire.
How do YOU answer the question inquired,
"*What* do School Nurses do?"

I remember the time when I stayed way past seven.
His throat and his forehead ablaze – poor Devin!
His mother had promised to come at eleven
And That's What School Nurses Do.

Glen was just five and in cancer remission.
He didn't like doctor *or* school nurse attention.
Discreetly I watched for exposures or symptoms
And That's What School Nurses Do.

She was going on ten. She was oh so embarrassed.
She'd wet in her pants and was soaked. Alas!
So I washed, changed and powdered. Then she skipped back to class
And That's What School Nurses Do.

The band teacher came in with shortness of breath.
"The doctors found cancer throughout," he said.
So, we cried and we laughed and we lived – 'til his death
And That's What School Nurses Do.

A rare skin disorder was Juan's diagnosis.
What in the world was epidermolysis?
It took the whole school team to keep him from crisis
And That's What School Nurses Do.

They came off the buses in tears. They had heard.
Their classmate was dead from a gun, was the word.
To my door they brought grief and remorse and anger
And That's What School Nurses Do.

Their glasses need fixing. Their zippers get broken.
Their hearts yearn for healing. Their needs go unspoken.
My office is open to let them all come in.
Well, That's What School Nurses Do.

(Wolfe, 2002, p. 3)

Demographics

Little research specific to the demographics of school nursing has been carried out. In 2000, the U.S. Department of Health and Human Services (USDHHS), Bureau of Health Professions, Division of Nursing conducted a national survey of registered nurses. This survey estimated that 83,269 nurses were working in Student Health Services. Of this number, 66.5% worked full time (TABLE 6.2). This includes registered nurses hired for public and private schools, colleges, and other school health services.

Historically, descriptions of school nursing have limited the number of practitioners to those providing direct services to children in grades K–12 or those employed by Boards of Education. Today's definition of school nursing lends itself to a larger cohort of "students" and employers, including those in preschool through college settings. The practice of school nursing is not limited to the grassroots school nurse who provides hands-on or direct oversight of the care of students. School nurses also include school nurse administrators, school nurse consultants, researchers, instructors of school nurses, and other nurses who contribute to students' educational success with limited or indirect student contact.

Changes in membership demographics of the National Association of School Nurses reflect a more diverse and educated workforce, as does the national Registered Nurse Population survey from 2000. TABLE 6.3 shows current data from this latter survey. Registered nurses responding to the survey who self-identified as working in "Student Health Services" listed a variety of positions not typically considered roles of the school nurse. One example is the certified nurse anesthetist, but the typical school nurse continues to be one who considers him- or herself a staff nurse with primary responsibilities to students within assigned schools. Almost 58,000 registered nurses working as a staff nurse in 2000 used the title "school nurse." Table 6.3 shows the diversity of titles within the field.

Educational Preparation

The diversity of job titles parallels the diversity of educational preparation of school nurses. A 2002 Position Statement of the National Association of School Nurses established minimum educational criteria for the school nurse:

> It is the position of the National Association of School Nurses that every school-aged child deserves a school nurse who is a graduate of a baccalaureate degree program from an accredited college or university and licensed by that state as a registered nurse. These requirements are the minimal preparation for the skills needed at the entry level of school nursing practice. Additionally, NASN supports state certification, where required, and promotes national certification of school nurses through NBCSN [National Board for Certification of School Nurses]. (NASN, 2002)

Table 6.2 ■
REGISTERED NURSES PROVIDING SCHOOL HEALTH SERVICES, 2000

	NUMBER IN SAMPLE	TOTAL IN UNITED STATES (ESTIMATED)	PERCENTAGE OF TOTAL (ESTIMATED)
Student Health Services	1,106	83,269	3.8
Board of Education (public schools)	745	56,239	2.6
Private or parochial schools	66	5,132	0.2
College or university	219	16,379	0.7
Other school health service	72	5,519	0.2

Source: The Registered Nurse Population, U.S. Division of Health and Human Services, 2001, p. 51, portion of Table 13. Employment setting of primary positions of registered nurses employed in nursing: March 2000.

Table 6.3 ■

TITLES OF REGISTERED NURSES IN STUDENT HEALTH SERVICES, 2000

EMPLOYMENT SETTING	TOTAL
Student health services	83,269
Administrator or assistant	2,707
Certified nurse anesthetist	213
Clinical nurse specialist	1,033
Consultant	589
Head nurse or assistant	1,240
Instruction	3,505
Nurse clinician	333
Nurse practitioner, midwife	4,035
Private duty	93
Researcher	673
Staff nurse	64,871
Supervisor or assistant	410
Other	2,884

Source: The Registered Nurse Population, U.S. Division of Health and Human Services, 2001, p. 60, portion of Table 22. Employment setting and type of position of employed registered nurses: March 2000.

Although NASN defines a school nurse as a registered nurse with a baccalaureate degree, many locales require nurses to exceed this minimal preparation and others loosely use the term "school nurse" for employees required to minimally hold certification in First Aid. TABLE 6.4 provides an overview of the diversity of educational backgrounds from the Registered Nurse Population survey. A 2002 NASN membership survey found similar results with "just over half having at least a baccalaureate and 29% with a diploma" (Maple Alley Market Research, 2002, p. 3). The number of those using the title "school nurse" without meeting nationally recognized minimal standards is unknown.

It should be noted that NASN, along with many states and diverse employers, identifies the baccalaureate degree for entry level into practice. This should not be interpreted as the extent of the school nurse's education. The need for ongoing continuing education specific to this specialty practice is paramount. Because the school nurse works in an independent setting, often without medical or nursing supervision, his or her nursing skills must necessarily be exceptional and current.

The demographics of school nurses are important in examining the tasks and abilities of the school nurse. Higher levels of educational preparation have been correlated with increased quality of nursing care and higher levels of ethical decision-making (Proctor, 2001, p. 474). With approximately 60% of school nurses holding a minimum of a baccalaureate degree (USDHHS, 2001, p. 57) and 51% of states having specific educational requirements for entry into school nursing (Brenner et al., 2001, p. 298), the public can assume there exists a relatively large work force with advanced skills and knowledge. This bodes well for the future of school nursing, as increased competencies will surely be needed to meet the growing need for specialized medical and nursing care.

Table 6.4 ■

EDUCATIONAL PREPARATION OF THE SCHOOL NURSE, 2000

DIPLOMA	ASSOCIATE DEGREE	BACCALAUREATE	MASTERS	DOCTORATE
18.8%	22.9%	41.3%	16.8%	0.1%

Source: The Registered Nurse Population, U.S. Department of Health and Human Services, 2001, p. 57, developed from Table 19. Employment setting and highest nursing-related educational preparation of registered nurses employed in nursing: March 2000.

WHAT ARE THE RESPONSIBILITIES OF THE SCHOOL NURSE?

School nurse responsibilities and school health services models are as diverse as the clients and the communities served. The need to individualize care is intrinsic to the practice. Nurses are adept at nursing diagnosis and intervention for individual clients. School nurses become adept at nursing diagnosis and intervention for cohorts of clients within the school community. Specific responsibilities and duties are dictated by client needs, but are refined by the external influences of the school community and the boundaries of the practice and the capacity of the nurse.

Client Needs

The needs of clients cover the entire spectrum of acute illness, injury, chronic conditions, and mental health needs for school-age children and adolescents. TABLE 6.5 describes six major categories of student health status that require nursing assessment and intervention. The school nurse is responsible for all of the students within the school community, unlike other specialists who provide services to a defined, specific caseload (NASN & ANA 2001b, p. 1). As the needs of the children and adolescents continue to grow and become more complex, it behooves the school nurse to be an effective team member and collaborator to ensure the health and well-being of the student population. In 1999, a local journalist described the issue thus:

> And it's true that a modern school nurse's repertoire still includes a hefty dose of old-school classics: sprains, lice, stomachaches and skinned knees. But some of the roles school nurses tackle today…were practically unknown in school 25 years ago. (Isaacs, 1999, p. 1)

Students today are affected by diminished access to comprehensive healthcare services; physical and emotional abuse/neglect; bullying; increased rates of cancer; increased exposure to communicable diseases; poor dental care; domestic violence; dysfunctional, homeless, illiterate, or unemployed families; environmental factors affecting health status, such as poor indoor air quality; health illiteracy; mental health conditions resulting in depression and suicide; nontraditional families, including single parents, gay couples, grandparents, and guardians raising children; nutritional alterations illustrated by obesity and the resulting type 2 diabetes and eating disorders; preventable injuries; early sexual activity evidenced by sexually transmitted diseases and teen pregnancy; substance abuse of illicit drugs, tobacco, and alcohol and misuse of medications; technology resulting in advanced medical equipment in the classroom; telehealth; and armed conflict, with its implications for fear, uncertainty, bioterrorism, and broken families. In 1989, the Carnegie Corporation of New York released a landmark study on education. A key finding, relative to health, is described in the following statement: "School systems are not responsible for meeting every need of the student, but, when the need directly affects learning, clearly the school must meet the challenge. So it is with health" (Carnegie Corporation, 1989).

Often the school nurse is the only health professional within the school system with the educational preparation to take leadership on health issues. When health is the primary issue, the school nurse is uniquely positioned within the school to serve as advocate, liaison, and provider of care.

With the passage of the Individuals with Disabilities Education Act (Public Law 94-142) in 1975, every child gained the right to a free education in the least restricted environment. As a result, children previously excluded from school now receive educational services through age 21 to 27, depending on state statute. The numbers of children with chronic conditions, including physical disabilities, appear to continue to rise. In 1998 the National Center at the American Nurses Foundation (as cited in Periard, Knecht, & Birchmeier, 1999) estimated that 10% to 20% of American school-age children have chronic social, emotional, or health problems. Another authority estimates that 9% to 14% of children in the community have functional limitations (Benedict & Farel, 2003). The school nurse addresses the child's healthcare needs that interfere with full access to the classroom. In addition, the school nurse is responsible for management of the child's medical and safety needs (Hootman, 1994). Management encompasses the provision or oversight of nursing care during school hours and the coordination of care through supervision and the development of necessary Individualized Healthcare Plans and Emergency Care Plans.

The 1999 Supreme Court decision in *Cedar Rapids Community School District v. Garret F.* further supports the responsibility of the school to provide nursing services when necessary for the child to have full access and benefit from school programs (NASN, 2001). Services can range from peak flow monitoring to intensive wound care management, depending on the needs of the child. Nebulizers, glucose monitoring, catheterizations, and tube feedings are commonly used in schools today.

Table 6.5 ■
RELATIONSHIP OF STUDENT HEALTH STATUS TO SCHOOL NURSING SERVICES

STUDENT HEALTH DESCRIPTION	NURSING ASSESSMENT/INTERVENTION
Well Student	• Perform nursing assessment of immunization and tuberculosis status. • Screen for deviant health findings (e.g., vision, health, dental). • Refer to community healthcare providers for diagnosis and resolution of identified findings. • Reinforce positive self-health management measures. • Provide health education for enhancing self-health management.
Students with Urgent Health Needs Problems are usually related to illness/injury (e.g. trauma, communicable disease) or concerns over altered health status.	• Perform nursing intervention for stabilization/resolution of urgent health concerns. • After assessment, return students to classroom and/or refer to community providers for further medical follow-up.
Students with Chronic Health Problems Students who are usually mainstreamed into the regular school population (e.g., asthma, diabetes). These students may present with routine issues or with occasional acute episodes.	• Manage chronic and ongoing health problems in cooperation with parents and community healthcare providers. • Educate school personnel and students in appropriate health management measures, develop health management plans, delegate appropriate nursing procedures and train/monitor school personnel regarding activities related to student health.
Students with Psychosocial Problems For example, alcohol/drug use/abuse, evidence of physical/sexual abuse, or other mental/emotional/physical issues. Students may present with frequent or chronic complaints or urgent/emergent issues.	• Offer crisis intervention and referral to community healthcare providers for students presenting with mental health/alcohol/drug crisis. • Provide ongoing health counseling for nonacute problems or follow-up activities.
Students with Medically Fragile Conditions For example, cardiomyopathy requiring transplant, unstabilized diabetic reaction. These students may receive special education in a contained classroom or may be "mainstreamed" into regular classrooms. They may require multidisciplinary/health/education team management. They may present with "routine" problems or acute episodes related to their chronic health issues.	• Conduct ongoing, intensified, involved nursing management. • Delegate nursing procedures to non-nursing personnel and monitor these personnel. • Collaborate with community healthcare providers and case management and/or coordinate care between parent/educators and health disciplines.

(continued)

STUDENT HEALTH DESCRIPTION	NURSING ASSESSMENT/INTERVENTION
Technology-Dependent Students with Multiple Health Problems These students are the most fragile and cannot maintain daily school attendance without some direct intervention from licensed personnel. The National Task Force on Technology-Dependent Children defines these students as: • Having a chronic disability • Requiring the routine use of a medical device to compensate for the loss of life-sustaining body function • Requiring daily, ongoing care and/or monitoring by trained personnel.	• Direct clinical nursing services required to provide treatment/support necessary for the student to attend school.

Source: Adapted from Hootman (1996), pp. 1–4 and 1–5.

"Students" are more broadly defined today and extend beyond the traditional student in a public school, grades K–12. Today, school nurses work in settings such as preschool, college campuses, boarding schools, drug rehabilitation facilities, schools for the deaf, incarceration sites, international programs for children of those in the armed forces and alternative schools. School nurses are adept at working with all children, regardless of their school setting or their socioeconomic backgrounds, ages, gender, sexual orientation, nationality, faith, and so forth.

The School Community

Along with the client needs and the boundaries of the practice, the school community impacts on how school health services are operationalized. The school community includes not only the personnel and facilities of the school but also the surrounding community of people in terms of commerce, culture, and services. To treat a child holistically, the school nurse must consider the school community's unique strengths and challenges. These variables mold the individual practice of each school nurse.

School nurses are hired by a variety of employers, including Boards of Education (public, private, and parochial schools), public health agencies, hospitals, and independent nursing service agencies. They care for infants in preschool programs, youngsters in elementary settings, adolescents in secondary education, young adults in university settings, and developmentally delayed adults in extended schooling programs. In some states, the school nurse also provides health-related services to school staff (see Chapter 45). Management goals and budget constraints differ across this diverse spectrum of environments. The school or governing authority, such as the legislature, dictates the number of hours the school nurse will be on-site, the nurse-to-student ratio, and the level of support services for nursing services.

The school nurse must meet the expectations of multiple hierarchies of supervision over his or her practice. It is a challenge to simultaneously please boards of health, education, and nursing, in addition to the local building principal who may likely complete the school nurse's annual performance evaluation. In states with a State School Nurse Consultant (working at either the state Department of Education or Department of Health), the conflicting expectations can be addressed and resolved at the state level. In addition, the Consultant can advocate for uniformity in areas such as minimum hiring credentials, caseload assignments, and job descriptions.

In 2000, 76.8% of schools had a full or part-time school nurse who provided health services (Brenner et al., 2001). On a local level, the school will determine the level of authority the school nurse has over aspects of the environment that influence children's health status. For example, the school nurse who identifies a safety hazard on the playground may have the authority to direct a custodian to make adaptations to the playground equipment to improve its safety or the school nurse may need to seek school board approval. Schools may have a staff physician or school nurse supervisor for consultation or oversight of the school health program. In these schools, services are enhanced by the establishment of uniform guidelines for practice and for professional supervision and evaluation of the school nurse's performance. Some schools may offer school-based or school-linked services to augment those of the school nurse, but generally the school nurse is the only healthcare professional within the school setting. This physical isolation from other nursing and healthcare colleagues and resources, necessitates that the school nurse be comfortable and skilled with the independent management of his or her health office and client caseload.

Needs assessments of communities reveal individuals who are not able to access healthcare services, nor can they identify the reasons for seeking care. Although some locales are proactive in providing preventative services, others are more inclined toward responding to presenting complaints. Physician and hospital services may be within walking distance yet unaffordable or services may be free at a clinic, which is hundreds of miles from the student and family in need. In those communities where nurses are available within the school setting, the school nurse often fills the void in providing care or linking families with the necessary resources to obtain care. Clearly, the greatest challenge to the school nurse "is determining how best to use one's resources" (Hootman, 1994, p. 8).

Boundaries of the Practice

While the need of the client and the community will directly influence the school nurse's intervention, external influences and expectations from the school community along with boundaries of practice will also create variances amongst job expectations and duties. Boundaries are created by laws and regulations related to nursing and education, community needs and resources, and the school environment.

The federal Individuals with Disabilities Act (IDEA) (see Chapter 14) insures that all children receive educational services and requires that all children receiving special education have an Individualized Educational Program (IEP). The school nurse is an important team member in understanding how medical needs will impact on educational goals. Similarly, Section 504 of the Rehabilitation Act of 1973 requires all public entities to make accommodations to buildings or programs to allow physical access to the programs. The school nurse can be a strong advocate and educator for the team in identifying appropriate accommodations.

In states where delegation to unlicensed assistive personnel (UAP) is prohibited, school systems must hire nurses to provide direct care. UAPs do not hold licensure, but work within some schools performing nursing or assigned nurse's aides tasks, ideally under supervision and after training. In the same way, the scope of practice within a state Nurse Practice Act directs what duties can be performed by nurses (inclusive of APNs, RNs, and LPNs) and what level of educational preparation is required to practice school nursing. Differences among states result in differences in individual practice as the school nurse has limited or expanded responsibilities for caring for children. For example, if a child enters school without the prerequisite immunizations, the intervention will vary amongst practice settings. In one state, the school nurse will personally provide the inoculations. In another state, the school nurse will be responsible for ensuring compliance through referral and follow-up. In yet another state, the school nurse will have no accountability because the tracking is delegated by the educational administrator to a secretary. Education mandates may further expand the school nurse responsibilities by assigning responsibilities for emergency care and preventative health.

Even within a single district in a single town, two school nurses will engage in different daily tasks based on the student demographics, the individual attributes of the school nurse, and the on-site administration. As educational reform and medical technology continue to advance, the public can expect that the responsibilities of the school nurse will continue to expand. School nurses must constantly adapt to the ever-changing clients, school community, and laws. Changes within any of these will directly impact the priorities and tasks of the school nurse. In any example, from direct care of a child who is technology dependent to the one who is contemplating suicide, the type and quality of services provided by the school nurse is directly impacted by a number of variables.

School Nurse Capacity

Another key influence in addressing client needs is the *capacity* of the school nurse. Capacity is the ability of the school nurse to meet the volume of client needs within the scope of school nursing practice. The numbers of students continue to grow, as do their healthcare needs. Clearly, the child's well-being is impacted by the nurse-to-student ratio and daily accessibility (Fryer & Igoe, 1995, p. 13). A 1:750 ratio is the national recommendation of both the National Association of School Nurses (NASN, 1995) and the U.S. Department of Health and Human Services (health objective 7.4, USDHHS, 2000). Currently only 17.6% of schools have an established minimum ratio, and of these, only 22.9% meet the 1:750 recommended ratio (Brenner et al., 2001, p. 296). The case mix and the time allotted to each school also influence the role of the school nurse (Jones & Clark, 1993). Interestingly, an inverse relationship was observed between the number of schools a school nurse serves and the number of students seen by the school nurse (Jones & Clark,

1993, p. 15). In some schools, the addition of health aides and clerks may support school nursing services.

HOW DOES A SCHOOL NURSE ENSURE OPTIMAL WELLNESS AND READINESS TO LEARN?

There are no step-by-step instructions or magic formulas for student success. Each client, setting, and challenge is unique. Success in ensuring that a student has optimal wellness and enters the classroom ready to learn is dependent on the school nurse's ability to adapt to the needs of the client as an individual and to creatively assume and blend a myriad of roles on behalf of the client.

Adapting to the Needs of the Student

School nurses must constantly adapt to changes in client needs. One school year, let alone one school day, is never like the previous one. Success is measured through meeting of established expected outcomes. Thus, school nurses achieve successful client management when the student is able to participate successfully in the educational process. Change (e.g., new students, new diagnoses, new medical technology, new community stressors) is inevitable and will continue to alter short-term goals that are aimed at student wellness and educational success. Nurses are adept at using the nursing process and applying it in the school setting. Through data collection and analysis, school nurses effectively identify new needs, provide new interventions, and articulate new outcomes.

The specific needs of clients and communities change as the political, social, economic, and cultural environments change around them. While Maslow's Hierarchy of Needs (FIGURE 6.1) is applicable to all clients, the specific needs change; thus, the interventions of the school nurse change. For example, in the early 20th century the basic need for "food" was manifested by emaciated children who were hungry, even starving, because of the lack of food. The school nurse intervened to help families gain access to food sources through community charity. Today, children continue to have a basic need for "food." Many present with symptoms of overweight, obesity, and lowered immune systems resulting from the diminished intake of healthy foods. Today's school nurse intervenes to help families to access and understand the importance of making dietary choices to create balanced and nutritional meals.

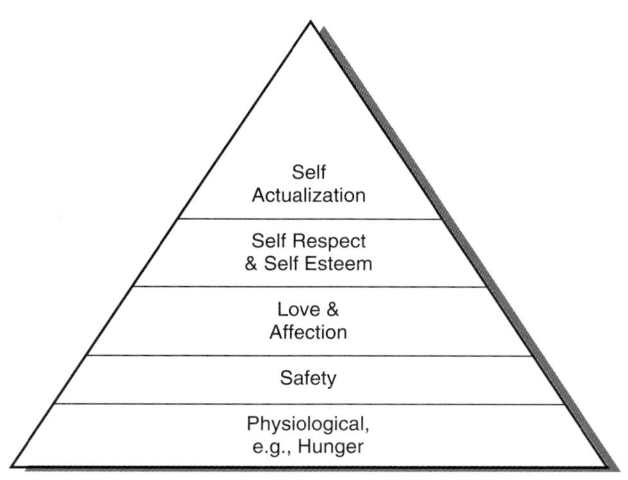

Figure 6.1 ■ Maslow's hierarchy of basic human needs.

Many "Roles" Within School Nursing

School nurses assume many roles to meet the needs of their clients. Many of these are explored further throughout this text. It is perhaps the breadth of nurse activities subsumed within school nursing and the unique non-medical practice setting that creates this specialty practice and differentiates it from other nursing specialties. Throughout school nursing history, the roles of skilled **clinician, advocate, social worker, health educator,** and **liaison** have been the foundation for the development of programs and services for children and for creating and maintaining school nurse positions.

Clinician

The school nurse is a skilled clinician prepared to provide or supervise the delivery of daily nursing care and case management during school hours. Early detection, daily nursing care, and monitoring support the client's overall health status. Quality of care is dependent on exceptional assessment skills, the ability to make effective nursing diagnoses, competence in choosing sufficient but practical interventions, and the wisdom to identify outcomes. By using the nursing process, the school nurse provides a continuum of care through screening, assessment, intervention, referral, and follow-up. Common activities include development of individualized healthcare plans, administration of medications or treatments, and monitoring for compliance or meeting expected outcomes.

> Hootman cites three compelling examples of the impact of school nursing services related to the nurse's clinical skills (Hootman, 1994, p. 7):

1. It is not uncommon for school nurses to see students who have waited through the weekend with acute health issues because their parents had no one else to turn to for their health care.
2. One school … nurse reported that students brought her an unconscious student who had just been involved in an auto accident occurring off campus.
3. In Oregon's Multnomah County schools there has been an 85% decrease in surgeries for scoliosis since the implementation of spinal screening by the school nurses in all public middle and high schools. The impact of the screening can be seen when one considers the time of recuperation, the discomfort of the surgery, and the average local rate of $100,000 per treatment.

As a clinician, school nurses perform interventions and provide nursing services that parallel those of their colleagues. In the school setting, these are provided without direct cost to students and staff, that is, they are not individually charged for the care they receive; however, in hospitals and community medical services, such tasks are billable services. In the 1990s, school systems began to explore ways to be compensated for expenses related to federal- and state-mandated services (see Chapter 44). One program that has received attention is the ability to bill for school nursing services provided to students covered by Medicaid.

Advocate

As an advocate, the school nurse's goal is not constrained by existing limitations of the nurse or community resources. Rather, the primary goal is to meet the needs of the client, through whatever means are required, and to provide a school environment that is physically and emotionally safe. This may utilize existing programs or require the creation of new ones. On a local level this often entails working against the status quo to get equipment or services for a child in order for him or her to be safer or healthy in the school setting. This can also mean advocating for system changes to meet the health needs of the student population as a whole, for example, improved air quality, scheduled daily physical activity, and nutritional school meals.

Good advocacy and negotiating skills are required if the nurse is going to meet with success on behalf of the student by convincing the school system to commit additional funds or a social agency to increase services. Lillian Wald, founder of school nursing, used her political connections to advocate for child labor laws, ungraded classes, decent housing, parks and playgrounds and improved public health (Duffus, 1938, p. 303).

Today's school nurse knows that advocacy sometimes takes place outside of the school in order to address more global issues impacting a student's health and well-being. Effective advocacy occurs when school nurses demonstrate professional accountability and participate in professional organizations, such as NASN, in order to articulate common goals and speak with one voice. In recent years, school nurses have effectively worked with national organizations and used grassroots efforts to change local and national legislation on issues such as affordable health care, access to services, enhanced services under IDEA, and improving the student-to-school nurse ratio.

Fundamental to having influence as an advocate is being a **leader**. School nurses combine their knowledge and passion about school health with keen communication skills to work proactively in affecting the future of school nursing and school health. As a leader, the school nurse is proactive in such activities as developing crisis response plans and leading school crisis teams in ensuring the school community is prepared for emergencies or disasters. The skills required to prepare effectively for a crisis response and emergencies are presented in Chapter 10.

Social Worker

The role of social worker is closely woven into school nursing practice. A child cannot be treated in isolation. Family and community support is essential to the child's health. Health status is affected by conditions other than disease and disability. As observed by Maslow (see Figure 6.1), basic needs include food, shelter, and clothing. These needs must be addressed prior to, or simultaneously with, other health interventions. Teaching communicable disease prevention through handwashing and hygiene instruction is impossible if the child does not have access to running water and a clean home environment.

As a social worker, the school nurse can be described as a **navigator**, who helps families to identify local resources and negotiate complex medical systems to connect the family with healthcare services, financial resources, shelter, food, and health promotion. In this role, the school nurse may assume the responsibilities of a **case manager** or **team leader/member**. As a case manager, the school nurse coordinates care between school, home, and community. All too often, the school nurse is the only health professional who is aware of all the services and agencies involved with the client's care. As a team leader/member, the school nurse brings together and facilitates the collaboration of a multidisciplinary team to develop ways to improve the health of a child, the staff, or the community.

Health Educator

As a health educator, the school nurse uses numerous opportunities within the school setting for individual and group education. Chapter 7 explores the multiple components of the school nurse's role as an educator. Today's school nurses are like the first school nurses who provided follow-up home visits after the physician examined the child and prescribed a medication or treatment to ensure compliance was not compromised by lack of understanding or resources. Today's education and follow-up regarding treatment begins when the school nurse works directly with the family to assure they have the resources to obtain the prescription and are capable of understanding and following prescribed treatments. Consultation can take place anywhere—at school, at home, on the telephone, or on email. However, the role of health educator is dependent on the amount of time the school nurses spends in a particular school on a daily or weekly basis.

Health education extends beyond care of the child with an acute illness who requires short-term prescriptive intervention. Children with chronic conditions, such as asthma, often have a knowledge deficit regarding their condition, its control, and its prognosis. School nurses address this need by directly providing individual or group education in the school setting, inviting a qualified expert to come to the school to work directly with the students or referring the family to local educational resources.

Complementary to this is health education to faculty and support personnel. Successful management of a child with diabetes or other chronic conditions will necessitate education of school personnel including food service personnel, instructional staff, and specialists who work with the child throughout the day. Anticipatory guidance relative to age, activities, chronic conditions, and so forth is a part of overall health education.

The general school population and educational staff need information and guidance on health promotion/protection and disease prevention. School nurses promote health by speaking to classes or at faculty meetings (e.g., classroom instruction on reproductive health or faculty instruction on standard precautions for bloodborne pathogens); arranging for school speakers and community resources (e.g., a dietitian to speak on healthy food choices or the American Cancer Society to speak on self breast exams); and sponsoring student and adult programs (e.g., Prom Promise, where students pledge not to drink on prom night, or the Great American Smokeout, where smokers pledge to abstain from smoking for one day). In some states the school nurse's title is School Nurse Teacher. In these regions of the country, the school nurse is required to have both nursing and educational preparation to teach the required Health Education course within the school curriculum.

Liaison

Serving as the health liaison to the community, the school nurse is a skilled **translator** of educational and medical goals and a **coordinator** between the school and medical communities. The school nurse is a part of a student's overall healthcare team, which includes the healthcare provider, emergency services, medical specialists, and home services. When the school nurse is not included as a part of the continuum of care, health care can become fragmented. As a member of two divergent communities (educational and medical/nursing), it is necessary for the school nurse to have the ability to communicate fluently with practitioners from both fields and to use every opportunity to promote and clarify the role of the school nurse as an influential and effective partner. Ideally, the school nurse takes the lead in preventive care (through health education and early detection) and provides follow-up (through implementation of medical prescriptives and monitoring for compliance, adverse effects, and success.)

Other Roles

The primary roles listed in the preceding paragraphs are complemented by other roles depending on the many factors described in previous sections of this chapter. Common roles include:

- **Catalyst** (being a change agent)
- **Collaborator** (working effectively with others in a synergistic fashion as in teams [Chapters 9 and 10] or through the Coordinated School Health Program [Chapter 3])
- **Counselor** (providing mental health intervention, ongoing support, and a safe haven for troubled or insecure clients) (Chapters 34, 38, 39, and 40)
- **Emergency nurse** (being a first responder to injury/tragedy; providing first aid and triage) (Chapters 10 and 22)
- **Epidemiologist** (participating in public health surveillance, identifying health/safety risks) (Chapters 20 and 21)

- **Gatekeeper** (providing primary screening, assessment and referral) (Chapter 20)
- **Health expert** (acting as a resident health resource and consultant to students, faculty, and community)
- **Manager** (overseeing the health office and the assigned school(s)' health services program) (Chapter 46)
- **Mentor** (serving as a role model and preceptor)
- **Policy/guidelines maker** (participating in discussion, recommendation, and writing of policy/regulatory change)
- **Researcher, evaluator** (evaluating in a formal or informal manner the effectiveness of school nurse interventions; participating/directing research activities) (Chapter 8)
- **Safety inspector** (assessing the school environment and student behaviors to identify safety risk factors; making recommendations for appropriate change)
- **School entry overseer** (representing school authorities in monitoring and intervening to ensure student compliance with requirements for immunizations, health status reports, school attendance)
- **Surrogate parent** (providing emotional support)
- **Team member** (serving on IEP, crisis, and other school teams related to the health, safety and well-being of students and staff) (Chapters 9 and 10)

NASN ISSUE BRIEF ON THE ROLE OF THE SCHOOL NURSE

In 2002, the National Association of School Nurses released an Issue Brief entitled "School Health Nurse's Role in Education, Role of the School Nurse" (NASN, 2002b). The Issue Brief is intentionally broad and applicable to all practice settings and all levels of practice. It separates the role into seven components, based on the 1999 definition of school nursing.

1. The school nurse provides health care to students and staff.
2. The school nurse provides leadership for the provision of health services.
3. The school nurse provides screening and referral for health conditions.
4. The school nurse promotes a healthy school environment.
5. The school nurse promotes health.
6. The school nurse serves in a leadership role for health policies and programs.
7. The school nurse serves as a liaison between school personnel, family, community, and healthcare providers.

The seven overarching roles provide a complete, yet complex, picture of the school nurse's role. They apply to school nurses at all levels of practice, in all geographical settings and with all clients. The conclusion of the Issue Brief encapsulates the role of the school nurse as one who supports the "physical, mental, emotional, and social health of students and their success in the learning process" (NASN, 2002b).

Application to the Nontraditional School Nurse

The "traditional" school nurse is the school nurse who provides or oversees direct care to clients within the school. As school nursing numbers have grown and health services have become an essential and valued component of a comprehensive school program, positions for school nurse administrators on the district, local (district, city, or county) and state level have been created. The role of these administrators also falls within the seven general roles outlined in the NASN Issue Brief. While administrators do not provide direct care, they are involved in setting policy, evaluating school nurses and Health Services programs, and providing for continuing education. The effectiveness of the administrator directly impacts on the quality of Health Services delivered within the school setting. (See Chapter 46.)

Higher education faculty and researchers are also members of the specialty practice of school nursing at large. They promote and enhance the specialty practice through their work with undergraduate and graduate students choosing a school setting for clinical experience and the sharing of new research and best practice for school nurses. They may also be responsible for developing and teaching programs leading to state certification of the school nurse or participate in advanced degrees leading to the Masters of Science in Nursing with a specialty in School Nursing.

The roles identified in this chapter are applicable to all levels of practice. Direct care staff, supervisors, consultants, researchers, and educators assume and promote the various roles as they care for students, supervise care of students, or identify best practice for the care of students.

CREATIVE ROLE DESCRIPTIONS

New school nurses are often intrigued and overwhelmed by the plethora of roles required of them. The following are conceptual pictures and descriptions of the "Role of the School Nurse" created by newly hired school nurses.[1]

- Hats—A common depiction of the school nurse is one with many hats. "What hat shall I wear today?" asked one (FIGURE 6.2). Another drew a picture of a school nurse with hats piled on her head like Dr. Seuss' infamous "Cat in the Hat" (Seuss, 1957).
- Octopus—Another common theme shows the school nurse as an octopus. Each arm is busy with a different task and still there aren't enough appendages to cover all the responsibilities.
- Puzzle or Chain—Many new school nurses see themselves as a piece in a larger puzzle or chain link of school health. Others compartmentalize their role into pieces of a puzzle or links of a chain. One wrote, "The puzzle is *not* complete without 'all' the pieces."
- Quilt—This concept depicts the various roles of the school nurse as pieces of a quilt. One school nurse described her various roles like the squares of her grandmother's soft, old quilts that held all the best pieces (memories) of her life. The school nurse quilt weaves together all the necessary roles and skills to protect and nurture students.
- Bridges—All types of bridges are used to describe the school nurse. Typically the bridges link the school with the community, but in many cases the school nurses used covered bridges to depict the protective nature of the role.
- Twister—While most descriptions of the school nurse role are extremely positive, using a game icon is not unusual. The Twister game depiction uses all the colored circles to indicate roles. The school nurse must successfully move over and under the other "players" to connect the circles and win the game. Another "game" showed the school nurse rolling the dice to move across a board. Moving from "eye safety" to "asthma teaching" to "vision screening" are just some of the beginning tasks. Midway through the board, a stop sign appears reading, "Do Not STOP. There is more." Then passing items such as "teen pregnancy" and "handwashing," the school nurse arrives at the finish line labeled "Happy, Healthy Kids." This is likened to the school nurse who depicted herself as The Little Engine That Could (Piper, 1930).
- Cheerleaders—Advocating is another common theme. The cheerleader, a lighthouse, or a handshake all seek success for students.
- Maslow's Hierarchy—New school nurses often categorize their roles based upon Maslow's theory (see Figure 6.1).

  Level One, Physiological Needs: The school nurse is an advocate, clinician, emergency nurse, and team member.

  Level Two, Safety: The school nurse is a case manager, collaborator, coordinator, epidemiologist, health educator, navigator, safety inspector, and school entry overseer

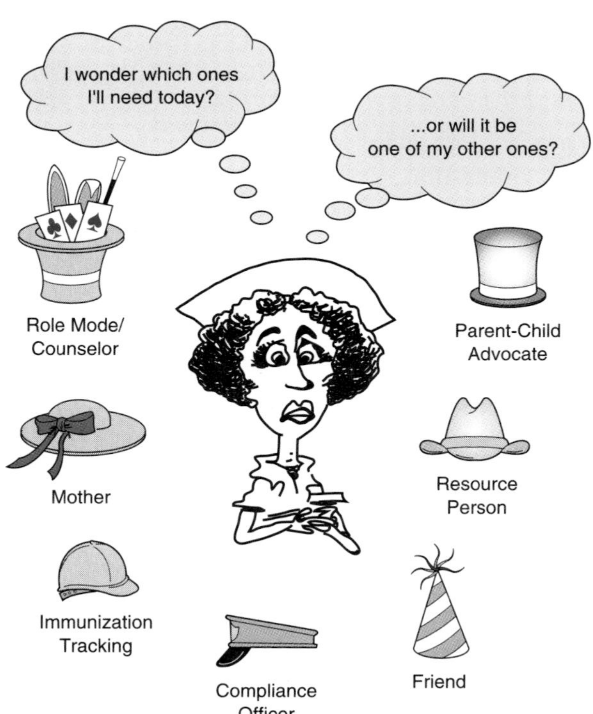

Figure 6.2 ■ I wonder which ones I will need.
Created by Rita McCommons, RN

[1]Students were school nurses working toward certification in Delaware between the years of 1998 and 2003. The Delaware Department of Education's Orientation class is required for state certification.

Level Three, Love and Affection: The school nurse is a liaison, social worker, and surrogate parent.

Level Four: Self-Respect and Self-Esteem: The school nurse is a counselor and health expert.

Level Five: Self-Actualization: The school nurse is a catalyst and mentor

CONCLUSION

Healthy children are successful learners. The school nurse has a multifaceted role within the school setting, one that supports the physical, mental, emotional, and social health of students and their success in the learning process (NASN, 2002b).

The 1989 Carnegie Report's identification of schools' responsibility to address the healthcare needs of students is compelling today. Much of this work falls within the expanding role of the school nurse. Perhaps the Carnegie (Carnegie Corporation, 1989) findings can be rephrased for school nurses in this way: The school nurse cannot be responsible for every need of every child, faculty member, and community; yet, when the need directly influences the learning ability of the student in the school setting and the school nurse has the authority and resources to intervene, meeting that need becomes the role of the school nurse.

References

Benedict, R. E., & Farel, A. M. (2003). Identifying children in need of ancillary and enabling services: A population approach. *Social Science & Medicine, 57*(11), 2035–2047. Abstract retrieved January 2, 2004 from Occupational Therapy News & Events at http://www.soemadison.wisc.edu/kinesiology/ot/newsevents/.

Brenner, N. D., Burstein, G. R., DuShaw, M. L., Vernon, M. E., Wheeler, L., & Robinson, J. (2001). Health services: Results from the School Health Policies and Programs Study. *Journal of School Health, 71*(7), 294–304.

Carnegie Corporation. (1989). *Turning points: Preparing American youth for the 21st century. The report of the Task Force on Education of Young Adolescents.*

Chayer, M. E. (1937). *School nursing: A contribution to health education.* New York: G. P. Putnam's Sons.

Duffus, R. L. (1938). *Lillian Wald: Neighbor and crusader.* New York: The Macmillan Company.

Fryer, G. E., & Igoe, J. B. (1995). A relationship between availability of school nurses and child well-being. *Journal of School Nursing, 11*(3), 12–14, 16, 18.

Hootman, J. (1994). Nursing, our most valuable natural resource: School-age children. *Nursing Forum, 29*(3), 5–17.

Hootman, J. (1996). *Quality nursing interventions in the school setting.* Scarborough, ME: National Association of School Nurses.

Issacs, B. (1999). *Good medicine: Today's school nurse faces medical needs unheard of 25 years ago.* Lexington Herald-Leader. Retrieved September 9, 1999 from http://www.kentuckyconnect.com/heraldleader/news/090799/livingdocs/schoolnurse07.htm.

Jones, M. E., & Clark, D. (1993). A study of school nurse utilization. *Journal of School Nursing, 9*(2), 10–17.

Kelly, H. W., & Bradshaw, M. C. (1918). *A handbook for school nurses.* New York: The Macmillan Company.

Leier, J. L., Cureton, V. L., & Canham, D. L. (2003). Special day class teachers' perceptions of the role of the school nurse [electronic version]. *Journal of School Nursing, 19*(5), 292–300.

Maple Alley Market Research. (2002). *Market research report: Overview & Longlook, Inc. NASN Member Survey Project.*

National Association of School Nurses (NASN). (1989). *Philosophy of school health services and school nursing* [brochure]. National Association of School Nurses.

National Association of School Nurses (NASN). (1993). *Roles & standards of school nursing practice for school administrators and community leaders* [brochure]. Scarborough, ME: National Association of School Nurses.

National Association of School Nurses (NASN). (1995). *Position statement: Caseload assignments.* Retrieved January 2, 2004, from http://www.nasn.org/positions/caseload.htm.

National Association of School Nurses (NASN). (1999). *Definition of school nursing.* Retrieved January 6, 2004, from http:www.nasn.org.

National Association of School Nurses (NASN). (2001). *Issue brief: Impact of Cedar Rapids community school district vs. Garret F. on school nursing services.* Retrieved January 2, 2004, from http://www.nasn.org/briefs/briefs.htm.

National Association of School Nurses (NASN). (2002a). *Core purpose / mission statement.* Retrieved January 6, 2004, from http:www.nasn.org/about/aboutus.htm

National Association of School Nurses (NASN). (2002b). *Issue brief: School health nurse's role in education, role of the school nurse.* Retrieved January 6, 2003, from http://www.nasn.org/briefs/role.htm.

National Association of School Nurses (NASN) & American Nurses Association (ANA). (2001a). *Position statement: Education, licensure, and certification of school nurses.* Retrieved October 31, 2003, from http://www.nasn.org/positions/education.htm.

National Association of School Nurses (NASN) & American Nurses Association (ANA). (2001b). *Scope and standards of professional school nurse practice.* Washington, DC: American Nurses Publishing.

National Education Association (NEA) & American Medical Association (AMA). (1960). *The nurse in the school* (2nd ed.) Report of the Joint Committee on Health Problems in Education. Washington, DC: National Education Association.

Periard, M. E., Knecht, L. D., & Birchmeier, N. (1999). A state association surveys school nurses to identify current issues and role characteristics. *Journal of School Nursing, 15*(4), 12–18.

Piper, W. (1930). *The little engine that could.* New York: Platt & Munk Publishers.

Proctor, S. E. (2001). The Educational Preparation of School Nurses: Implications for Hiring and Liability Protection. In N. C. Schwab & M. H. B. Gelfman (Eds.),

Legal issues in school health services. North Branch, MN: Sunrise River Press.

Proctor, S. T., Lordi, S. L., & Zaiger, D. S. (1993). *School nursing practice: Roles and standards.* Scarborough, ME: National Association of School Nurses.

Professional School Nursing Termed "Dynamic Discipline". (March, 1969), Editor, *The School Nurse, 1*(1), 3.

Seuss, Dr. (1957). *The cat in the hat.* Boston: Houghton Mifflin.

Stronge, J. H., Helm, V. M., & Tucker, P. D. (1995). *Evaluation handbook for professional support personnel.* Kalamazoo, MI: CREATE, The Evaluation Center.

U. S. Department of Health and Human Services (USDHHS).(2000). *Healthy People 2010, understanding and improving health, 1.* Retrieved on January 6, 2004 from http://www.healthypeople.gov/document/HTML/Volume1/07Ed.htm#_Toc490550856.

U.S. Department of Health and Human Services, Health Resources and Services Administration (USDHHS). Bureau of Health Professions, Division of Nursing. (2001). *Registered Nurse Population, March 2000.* Washington, DC: U.S. Department of Health and Human Services, Health Resources and Services Administration. Bureau of Health Professions, Division of Nursing.

Wald, L. (1991). *The house on Henry Street.* New Brunswick, NJ: Transaction Publishers. (Original work published 1915)

Wold, S. J. (2001). School Health Services: History and Trends. In N. C. Schwab & M. H. B. Gelfman (Eds.), *Legal issues in school health services.* North Branch, MN: Sunrise River Press.

Wolfe, L. C. (2002). President's letter. *NASN Newsletter, 17*(1), 3.

Chapter 7

The School Nurse's Role as a Health Educator

SUSAN G. PRAEGER

Chapter Outline

INTRODUCTION

Good teaching makes a difference. School nurses can be either more or less effective in the classroom regarding health promotion based on the way they teach. In 1996 the National Commission on Teaching and America's Future asserted that the single most important factor in student learning is the quality of the teacher. The work of the commission led to a decade of focusing on what teachers know (content) and can do (pedagogy). According to Whitehurst (2002), research indicates that good teachers do make a difference in terms of student achievement. If school nurses are going to help students learn about the importance of good health behaviors and if they are going to help students learn to choose and perform positive health promotion activities, then how (pedagogy) they teach students will be as important as what they teach (content). If the message is not delivered effectively, if school nurses are not effective teachers, then the chances of learning taking place are considerably lower.

In the monograph *How Teaching Matters* (2000), Wenlinsky notes that teacher knowledge of the subject matter through professional preparation programs and good verbal skills correlates with higher student achievement. When teachers emphasize higher-order thinking skills and hands-on learning activities, their students outperform peers whose teachers did not use these approaches. Also, students who were regularly tested on the material tended to outperform peers who were assessed using portfolio or project activities.

What do these findings mean for school nurses? First, professional preparation in the specialty of school nursing is essential in order to be an effective teacher of topics relevant to school health. Understanding and becoming proficient in the methods of effective teaching, which include critical thinking skills, how to engage students in relevant hands-on activities, as well as skills in appropriate testing measures are essential to being ready to implement the role of school nurse as an educator. In other words, knowing the content is only half of the equation.

The purpose of this chapter is to familiarize the school nurse with the professional performance role of educator as it relates to the school setting. The objectives of this chapter are that the school nurse will be able to:

- Define the national imperatives for education in schools.
- Describe the context in which education takes place in schools.
- Describe the role of the school nurse as reflected in professional nursing standards.
- Analyze how the components of teaching can be applied to the school nurse's role as educator.

IMPERATIVES FOR EDUCATION

World, national, professional, and state goals, standards, and rules are in place to guide programs and individuals in determining not only competencies for educational performance but also priorities for education. The United Nations Millennium Development Goals, Healthy People 2010 and the National Education Goals all contribute to understanding the framework in which school nurses can make a difference in promoting health for students in schools. These overarching goals define where we, as members of the global community and as a nation, want to place our emphasis in terms of helping students become healthy citizens. The goals have been agreed on by world leaders in the case of the Millennium Development Goals, and by all levels of leaders and citizens in the case of national health goals. Professional standards from the National Association of School Nurses (NASN) and the American Nurses Association (ANA) as well as state regulations define the context and expectations for professional performance related to the school nurse's role in education.

GLOBAL AND NATIONAL IMPERATIVES FOR HEALTH EDUCATION

The Millennium Development Goals (Millennium Project, 2000) outline the priorities for action to promote a healthy sustainable world population with a special focus on the world's children. Addressing the major leading causes of morbidity and mortality, the goals provide the framework for school nurses to meet the needs of children from a global perspective. Although all of the goals have relevance to school nursing practice, the ones that relate to the role of school nurse as educator include achieving universal primary education, promoting gender equality, reducing child mortality, improving maternal health, and combating human immunodeficiency virus/acquired immunodeficiency syndrome (HIV/AIDS), malaria, and other diseases. Each of these areas has implications for school nurses in terms of content to be addressed when educating both students and communities.

The Global School Health Initiative is a project of the Health Promotion Department in the Social Change and Mental Health Cluster of the World Health Organization (WHO, 2003). The Global School Health Initiative is designed to promote health promotion and education activities to improve the health of students, school personnel, families, and other members of the community through schools.

With an emphasis on health-promoting schools, the goals of the initiative include fostering health and learning; engaging all of the stakeholders in efforts to make school a healthy place; striving to provide a healthy environment, school health education, and school health services; implementing policies and practices that respect an individual's well-being and dignity, provide multiple opportunities for success, and acknowledge good efforts and intentions as well as personal achievements; striving to improve the health of school personnel, families, and community members as well as pupils; and working with community leaders to help them understand how the community contributes to, or undermines health and education. The Global School Health Initiative has implications for school nurses in its emphasis on appropriate pedagogies, comprehensive multidisciplinary education efforts, and humanistic approaches that support positive outcomes.

Both the Millennium Development Goals and the Global School Health Initiative are consistent with WHO principles supporting health (complete physical, mental, and social well-being) as the fundamental right of every human being with value to all citizens. Health is fundamental to peace and security and requires informed opinion and active cooperation. A basic premise is that inequality is a danger to all.

The emphasis on equality is resonated in the Healthy People 2010 (HP2010) (USDHHS, 2000) goals of the United States, which focus on eliminating disparities in health care and increasing the quality and quantity of life for all citizens to promote health and prevent illness, disability, and premature death. Divided into 28 focus areas with specific objectives, the HP2010 objectives give specific guidance on primary health problems that need to be addressed. The focus areas and the leading health indicators should be used by school nurse educators who are interested in addressing the major problems faced by youth in our nation (TABLE 7.1). The goal of the "educational and community based programs" focus area is to "increase the quality, availability and effectiveness of educational programs designed to prevent disease and improve health and quality of life" (USDHHS, 2000). The school setting is specifically identified as needing to increase high school completion rates as a means of avoiding the consequences on uninformed health choices that contribute to risky behaviors of young people.

The emphasis on high school completion in HP2010 and universal education in the Millennium Development Goals is consistent with the National Education Goals set forth by the National Education Goals Panel (2002). The goals include readiness to learn, high school completion, achievement, competency, adequate instruction, safe and drug-free schools, parental participation, and health literacy.

The U.S. Department of Education (2002) has continued to support the national goals as indicated in its strategic planning process to: create a culture of achievement; improve student achievement; improve the quality of teachers; and establish disciplined and drug-free education environments.

These global and national agendas suggest that health promotion strategies through effective health education programs are essential to meet global and national goals for healthy living. School nurses, representing one healthcare provider group in the com-

(text continues on page 135)

Table 7.1 ■

HEALTHY PEOPLE 2010 GOALS: INCREASE QUALITY AND YEARS OF HEALTHY LIFE AND ELIMINATE HEALTH DISPARITIES

28 FOCUS AREAS WITH GOALS AND SELECTED SCHOOL-RELATED OBJECTIVES

1. Access to Quality Health Services
Goal: Improve access to comprehensive, high-quality healthcare services.
- 1–1 Persons with health insurance
- 1–2 Health insurance coverage for clinical preventive services
- 1–3 Counseling about health behaviors
- 1–11 Rapid prehospital emergency care
- 1–14 Special needs of children

2. Arthritis, Osteoporosis, and Chronic Back Conditions
Goal: Prevent illness and disability related to arthritis and other rheumatic conditions, osteoporosis, and chronic back conditions.

3. Cancer
Goal: Reduce the number of new cancer cases as well as the illness, disability, and death caused by cancer.

4. Chronic Kidney Disease
Goal: Reduce new cases of chronic kidney disease and its complications, disability, death, and economic costs.

5. Diabetes
Goal: Through prevention programs, reduce the disease and economic burden of diabetes, and improve the quality of life for all persons who have or are at risk for diabetes.
- 5–1 Diabetes education
- 5–17 Self-blood-glucose-monitoring

(continued)

Table 7.1 ■ *(Continued)*

6. Disability and Secondary Conditions
Goal: Promote the health of people with disabilities, prevent secondary conditions, and eliminate disparities between people with and without disabilities in the U.S. population.

6–2	Feelings and depression among children with disabilities
6–9	Inclusion of children and youth with disabilities in regular education programs

7. Educational and Community-Based Programs
Goal: Increase the quality, availability, and effectiveness of educational and community-based programs designed to prevent disease and improve health and quality of life.

7–1	High school completion
7–2	School health education
7–3	Health-risk behavior information for college and university students
7–4	School nurse-to-student ratio
7–11	Culturally appropriate and linguistically competent community health promotion programs

8. Environmental Health
Goal: Promote health for all through a healthy environment.

8–16	Indoor allergens
8–20	School policies to protect against environmental hazards
8–21	Disaster preparedness plans and protocols

9. Family Planning
Goal: Improve pregnancy planning and spacing and prevent unintended pregnancy.

9–1	Intended pregnancy
9–3	Contraceptive use
9–4	Contraceptive failure
9–5	Emergency contraception
9–6	Male involvement in pregnancy prevention
9–7	Adolescent pregnancy
9–8	Abstinence before age 15 years
9–9	Abstinence among adolescents age 15 to 17 years
9–10	Pregnancy prevention and sexually transmitted disease (STD) protection
9–11	Pregnancy prevention education

10. Food Safety
Goal: Reduce foodborne illnesses.

10–1	Foodborne infections
10–4	Food allergy deaths
10–5	Consumer food safety practices

11. Health Communication
Goal: Use communication strategically to improve health.

11–1	Households with Internet access
11–2	Health literacy

12. Heart Disease and Stroke
Goal: Improve cardiovascular health and quality of life through the prevention, detection, and treatment of risk factors; early identification and treatment of heart attacks and strokes; and prevention of recurrent cardiovascular events.

(continued)

13. HIV
Goal: Prevent HIV infection and its related illness and death.
- 13–6 Condom use

---

14. Immunization and Infectious Diseases
Goal: Prevent disease, disability, and death from infectious diseases, including vaccine-preventable diseases.
- 14–22 Universally recommended vaccination of children age 19 to 35 months
- 14–23 Vaccination coverage for children in day care, kindergarten, and first grade
- 14–24 Fully immunized young children and adolescents
- 14–25 Providers who measure childhood vaccination coverage levels
- 14–26 Children participating in population-based immunization registries
- 14–27 Vaccination coverage among adolescents
- 14–28 Hepatitis B vaccination among high-risk groups

---

15. Injury and Violence Prevention
Goal: Reduce injuries, disabilities, and deaths due to unintentional injuries and violence.
- 15–16 Pedestrian deaths
- 15–18 Nonfatal pedestrian injuries
- 15–19 Safety belts
- 15–20 Child restraints
- 15–21 Motorcycle helmet use
- 15–22 Graduated driver licensing
- 15–23 Bicycle helmet use
- 15–29 Drownings
- 15–30 Dog bite injuries
- 15–31 Injury protection in school sports
- 15–33 Maltreatment and maltreatment fatalities of children
- 15–35 Rape or attempted rape
- 28–17 Sexual assault other than rape
- 28–18 Physical assaults
- 15–38 Physical fighting among adolescents
- 15–39 Weapon carrying by adolescents on school property

---

16. Maternal, Infant, and Child Health
Goal: Improve the health and well-being of women, infants, children, and families.
- 16–2 Child deaths
- 16–3 Adolescent and young adult deaths
- 16–19 Breastfeeding
- 16–22 Medical homes for children with special healthcare needs
- 16–23 Service systems for children with special healthcare needs

---

17. Medical Product Safety
Goal: Ensure the safe and effective use of medical products.

---

18. Mental Health and Mental Illness
Goal: Improve mental health and ensure access to appropriate, quality mental health services.
- 18–1 Suicide
- 18–2 Adolescent suicide attempts
- 18–7 Treatment for children with mental health problems

(continued)

Table 7.1 ■ *(Continued)*

19. Nutrition and Overweight
Goal: Promote health and reduce chronic disease associated with diet and weight.
- 19–3 Overweight or obesity in children and adolescents
- 19–4 Growth retardation in children
- 19–15 Meals and snacks at school

20. Occupational Safety and Health
Goal: Promote the health and safety of people at work through prevention and early intervention.
- 20–9 Worksite stress reduction programs
- 20–10 Needlestick injuries

21. Oral Health
Goal: Prevent and control oral and craniofacial diseases, conditions, and injuries and improve access to related services.
- 21–12 Dental services for low-income children
- 21–13 School-based health centers with oral health component

22. Physical Fitness and Activity
Goal: Improve health, fitness, and quality of life through daily physical activity.
- 22–6 Moderate physical activity in adolescents
- 22–7 Vigorous physical activity in adolescents
- 22–8 Physical education requirement in schools
- 22–9 Daily physical education in schools
- 22–10 Physical activity in physical education class
- 22–12 School physical activity facilities

23. Public Health Infrastructure
Goal: Ensure that Federal, Tribal, State, and local health agencies have the infrastructure to provide essential public health services effectively.

24. Respiratory Diseases
Goal: Promote respiratory health through better prevention, detection, treatment, and education efforts.
- 24–1 Deaths from asthma
- 24–2 Hospitalizations for asthma
- 24–3 Hospital emergency department visits for asthma
- 24–4 Activity limitations
- 24–5 School or work days lost
- 24–6 Patient education
- 24–7 Appropriate asthma care

25. Sexually Transmitted Diseases
Goal: Promote responsible sexual behaviors, strengthen community capacity, and increase access to quality services to prevent sexually transmitted diseases (STDs) and their complications.
- 25–11 Responsible adolescent sexual behavior
- 25–12 Responsible sexual behavior messages on television

26. Substance Abuse
Goal: Reduce substance abuse to protect the health, safety, and quality of life for all, especially children.

(continued)

26–6 Adolescents riding with a driver who has been drinking
26–9 Substance-free youth
26–10 Adolescent and adult use of illicit substances
26–14 Steroid use among adolescents
26–15 Inhalant use among adolescents
26–16 Peer disapproval of substance abuse
26–17 Perception of risk associated with substance abuse

27. Tobacco Use
Goal: Reduce illness, disability, and death related to tobacco use and exposure to secondhand smoke.
27–2 Adolescent tobacco use
27–3 Initiation of tobacco use
27–4 Age at first tobacco use
27–7 Smoking cessation by adolescents
27–9 Exposure to tobacco smoke at home among children
27–10 Exposure to environmental tobacco smoke
27–11 Smoke-free and tobacco-free schools
27–14 Enforcement of illegal tobacco sales to minors laws
27–15 Retail license suspension for sales to minors
27–16 Tobacco advertising and promotion targeting adolescents and young adults
27–17 Adolescent disapproval of smoking
27–18 Tobacco control programs
27–19 Preemptive tobacco control laws

28. Vision and Hearing
Goal: Improve the visual and hearing health of the Nation through prevention, early detection, treatment, and rehabilitation.
28–2 Vision screening for children
28–4 Impairment in children and adolescents
28–9 Protective eyewear
28–12 Otitis media
28–14 Hearing examination
28–15 Evaluation and treatment referrals
28–16 Hearing protection
28–19 Noise-induced hearing loss in children

Source: U.S. Department of Health and Human Services. (2000). *Healthy People 2010: Understanding and improving health* (2nd ed.). Washington, DC: U.S. Government Printing Office, November 2000.

munity, are challenged to "inform, educate, and empower people about health issues," one of the essential public health services described by the Centers for Disease Control (1994).

PROFESSIONAL AND STATE IMPERATIVES FOR EDUCATION

Leading organizations in the United States have much to say regarding what should be done to make a difference in our nation's schools. Global and federal initiatives have established the importance of health promotion through world and national goals that specifically address the health of persons in the school setting; the next step is to understand what is being proposed as the guidelines for meeting these goals. This section presents some of the guides from leading decision-makers in education in the United States.

In the education arena, school nurses need to interface with professionals whose expertise in and commitment to education provide a foundation for understanding the educational climate in the schools and who understand the role the school nurse can play in promoting health through educational interventions. Although much of what is done in nursing is considered the exclusive province of the nursing profession, school nurses are engaged in the educational world as part of the school health team, and it is essential to speak the language of education and meet their standards for educational performance while in the school setting. If school nurses are committed to improving the health of students in their schools, and committed to improving the health of the nation, then understanding and appreciating the standards that guide educators are essential in preparing for the role as educator in the schools.

Each U.S. state is mandated to provide public education for children and youth that is supported through state funding. Because education expenses consume large portions of state budgets and much of it is tax-based, there is considerable concern about providing accountability for educational expenditures. To be good stewards of citizens' money, states use a variety of mechanisms to be accountable for their educational endeavors. This accountability occurs through professional organizations and by state and national agencies and programs.

The main professional organizations related to teaching in schools in America are the American Federation of Teachers (AFT) and the National Education Association (NEA). The AFT (2004) mission includes improving the quality of the services provided by educators. The National Education Association (NEA, 2002) mirrors this commitment to improving teacher quality through strengthening classroom teaching in each component of the teacher development continuum, from quality teacher education programs to quality novice and experienced teachers.

According to the National Board for Professional Teaching Standards (NBPTS), "the fundamental requirements for proficient teaching are relatively clear: a broad grounding in the liberal arts and sciences; knowledge of the subjects to be taught, of the skills to be developed, and of the curricular arrangements and materials that organize and embody that content; knowledge of general and subject-specific methods for teaching and for evaluating student learning; knowledge of students and human development; skills in effectively teaching students from racially, ethnically, and socioeconomically diverse backgrounds; and the skills, capacities and dispositions to employ such knowledge wisely in the interest of students" (NBPTS, 2002, p. 2).

NBPTS (2002) has specified five core propositions for good teaching that are echoed by other professional groups. Good teachers are: (1) committed to students and their learning; (2) knowledgeable about the subjects they teach and how to teach; (3) responsible for managing and monitoring student learning; (4) systematically reflecting and improving their practice; and (5) members of learning communities.

How does one become a good teacher? Teacher education preparation occurs predominantly at the college level. Accountability for teacher preparation and performance rests both with the preparation programs for teachers as well as in the performance of teachers in the classroom. Accountability approaches vary by teacher preparation program and by state. The National Council for Accreditation of Teacher Education (NCATE, 2004) is the teaching profession's largest recognized accrediting body and its work, similar to the accreditation process for schools of nursing, has resulted in increased standards for teacher preparation. NCATE accreditation assures that good pedagogy (the methods of teaching), content mastery, the ability to work with diverse learners, and clinical experience are all part of the process to prepare classroom teachers to work in a democratic society.

In addition to professional organization commitment to excellence, states are responsible for ensuring educational accountability. Each state requires that teacher preparation programs are approved by the state department of education. This approval process may be based on inspection and observation by the state itself, or on documentation of accreditation by an accrediting body, most often NCATE. In other words, the NCATE process may be used by states to guide their own observation, states may use other criteria, or they may accept the accreditation process formulated by NCATE as evidence of a quality teacher preparation program.

The federal government, under Title II, requires the annual reporting of the scores of education graduates on state licensing or certification examinations. As a result of the combined efforts of NEA, AFT, the Association of Curriculum Supervision and Development (ASCD) and educational leaders, the Educational Testing Service (ETS, 2004) has developed a series of testing processes, similar to the NCLEX-RN for licensing registered nurses, to determine content and pedagogy mastery of teachers. PRAXIS II is a standardized test administered by ETS to determine content mastery of the aspiring teacher. More than 70% of states use PRAXIS II to determine content proficiency of its entry-level teachers. A few states require performance-based assessment to determine competency of an entry-level teacher in the classroom. Cost in terms of evaluators' time is a major issue in states deciding to mandate teaching proficiency once they are hired and in practice. However, the trend toward accountability in practice may eventually outweigh the concerns of cost in terms of evaluation as educational reform is discussed and demanded at the local, state, and national levels.

What do these tests mean in terms of teacher preparation? Professional educators consider national goals and directives, state requirements, professional standards (NCATE), and the two high-stakes tests of PRAXIS II and PRAXIS III when preparing teachers for the classroom. PRAXIS I is a basic skills test that some programs use as an entry-level requirement to a teacher education program to determine mastery of reading, writing, and math; this is similar to the requirement that certain courses be taken in order to enter nursing school. The PRAXIS Series: Professional Assessments for Beginning Teachers® includes summative tests to determine the end product or quality of the teaching preparation program. Many states use PRAXIS I: Computer-Based Academic Skills Assessment and PRAXIS II: Subject Assessments to grant an initial teaching license. PRAXIS III: Classroom Performance Assessments is utilized in assessing actual teaching skills and classroom performance.

To help education students prepare for professional practice as teachers, the profession has worked to align the standards, preparation, and feedback into a cohesive model to ensure success of teachers in the classroom, accreditation of programs, and accountability to the public in terms of the quality of education that children and youth are receiving. As with nursing, the formative component of professional preparation (the opportunity to learn, receive feedback, and improve over time) is essential to mastering the complicated process of teaching. This alignment has resulted in the support of an evidence-based conceptual framework adopted by many teacher education programs designed to provide a model for getting ready to be in the classroom that parallels PRAXIS III. PATHWISE is the formative process model developed by the Educational Testing Service to help teacher preparation programs organize experiences for effective teaching. PATHWISE includes the components of what are considered to be good teaching. School nurses can use this framework to understand what teachers are trying to accomplish in the classroom as well as for developing the skills necessary to be an effective health educator with students, staff, families, communities, or administrators in groups or one-on-one.

A CONCEPTUAL MODEL FOR EFFECTIVE TEACHING

In *Enhancing professional practice: A framework for teaching,* Danielson (1996) details a framework for helping teachers meet the expected standards that will prepare them for PRAXIS and for helping colleges of education be prepared for NCATE evaluation. In other words, Danielson's work was designed to clarify the criteria of good teaching and provide an evidence-based framework to meet the need for quality teachers prepared to assume responsibility for the nation's youth. Her work was based on formal analyses of the tasks of teaching, reviews of research, analyses of state regulations for teacher licensing, and extensive pilot testing of the criteria in her framework. Other influences on the framework include the National Board for Professional Teaching Standards (NBPTS), the work of multiple educators, analyses of the conceptions of teacher duties, and research on the pedagogical implications of constructivist learning (Danielson, 1996). Constructivist learning refers to the theoretical proposition that learning takes place when a learner is able to construct the meaning of the experience to the real world around him or her—in other words, moving from simple to complex, concrete to abstract, and directional to comprehensive. This allows learners the opportunity to learn within the context of the world around them. Developmental variations, individual learning styles, and environmental factors all need to be considered when helping a learner see the world from a new perspective.

Since the late 1970s, educators have felt increased pressure to help students attain more complex outcomes. By the 1990s, every state had adopted "report cards" on how children and youth in schools were performing on a range of desirable school achievement goals. The federal 2001 No Child Left Behind acts have only accelerated this accountability trend. Educators moved to emphasize critical thinking, problem solving, lifelong learning, collaboration, and deeper understanding in the learning process. This change entailed a shift from behaviorist perspectives to a view on learning derived from cognitive learning theory. More attention was given to the interplay among content, the teacher, the learner, and the context. The objective was to achieve deep understanding (Danielson & McGreal, 2002). The conception of learning and hence good teaching has thus gradually shifted from a behaviorist to a more constructionist view.

A constructionist approach to learning emphasizes that learning takes place when the learner is able to make sense of the concepts for themselves. This differs for each student based on his or her own worldview, experiences, and cognitive structures. In other words, each person brings his or her own unique learning style, repertoire of skills and experiences, as well as individual goals to the learning experience. When combined with the emotional maturity and motivation of the student, learning takes place. This means that each learner will learn what is relevant to him or her and it may not necessarily be what other learners are learning.

For example, school nurses are often called on to teach about the pubertal changes related to growth and development. Students respond to the same learning situation in a variety of ways. Some interpret the information as too much or too scientific; others say it was helpful in understanding who they are and what is happening to them; some are perplexed by the whole topic and others interpret the class to each other and their parents as a talk about sex. The constructionist approach challenges the teacher to recognize that the learners need to make sense of the experience themselves. They have to examine the meaning and its applicability and make a decision as to how this can be used to change their behavior. For example, the school nurse lists the top four reasons to avoid unprotected sexual activity. The students cite those reasons back to you. However, this does not mean that they will avoid unprotected sexual activity when making health choices. The school nurse needs to consider a learning environment where students can explore the meaning of unprotected sexual activity, how it could impact their lives, what choices they have, and what skills they need in order to make a decision about this information. Danielson's (1996) framework clarifies the conditions that should be considered when planning and implementing learning experiences and how to evaluate the outcomes.

School nurses can use Danielson's framework when implementing the role of educator in the school because nursing is about sharing knowledge and helping individuals, families, and communities apply that knowledge in the pursuit of health. The clarity and simplicity of the framework make it transferable to any teaching situation and it is supported by the premises of major learning theories.

THE SCHOOL NURSE AS EDUCATOR: PROFESSIONAL IMPERATIVES

Both the American Nurses Association (ANA) and the National Association of School Nurses (NASN) address current standards of professional performance. ANA standards are the minimum expectations for professional performance and accountability. NASN standards also address the minimum expectations for the school nurse. The following NASN standards of professional performance clearly describe the expectations for performance of the school nurse in the area of health education (NASN & ANA, 2001).

Standard XI. Health Education

The school nurse assists students, families, school staff, and community to achieve optimal levels of wellness through appropriately designed and delivered health education. Measurement criteria include the expectation that the school nurse:

- Participates in the assessment of needs for health education for students and the school community.
- Provides developmentally appropriate formal health instruction within the classroom based on sound learning theory.
- Provides individual and group health teaching and counseling for and with clients.
- Participates in the design and development of health curricula.
- Participates in the evaluation of health curricula, health instructional materials, and other health education activities.
- Acts as a resource person to school staff regarding health education and health education materials.
- Furthers the application of health promotion principles within all areas of school life, for example, food service, custodial, and so forth.
- Promotes self-care and safety through the education of staff regarding their own health and that of their students.

In the ANA standards (2003), the role of the nurse as an educator is addressed in Standard V of the Standards of Practice, the implementation phase of professional practice. Inherent in the ANA standards is the expectation that all of the measurement criteria for the standard will be met by the nurse in practice. In terms of the overall standard related to implementation, it is expected that nurses use evidence-based interventions, community resources, collaboration strategies, and systems management approaches while documenting all interventions. In addition to the broad standard related to implementation, ANA specifies secondary standards related to implementation, including Standard 5B: Health Teaching and Health Promotion. Measurement Criteria related to this standard specify that the nurse:

- "Provides health teaching that addresses such topics as healthy lifestyles, risk-reducing behaviors, developmental needs, activities of daily living, and preventive self-care.

- Uses health promotion and health teaching methods appropriate to the situation and developmental level, learning needs, readiness, ability to learn, language preference, and culture.
- Seeks opportunities for feedback and evaluation of the effectiveness of the strategies used" (p. 28).

This emphasis on teaching in the professional nursing standards indicates that good teaching is considered a critical component of nursing practice. The expectation is that all nurses use health teaching to promote health in professional practice. The question, however, is what does this consist of and how does one go about being a good teacher who can make a difference? The next section of this chapter outlines a nationally recognized approach to preparing effective teachers. This approach is used to prepare teachers in classrooms across America and can be useful in helping the school nurse be an active, accepted, and effective member of the health education team in schools.

A FRAMEWORK FOR TEACHING

Danielson's (1996) Framework for Teaching simplifies the complexities of teaching by considering four major aspects or domains that are essential to the role of educator. Each domain includes several components or activities that a teacher needs to consider in order to be effective. These domains and components (Table 7.2) provide a framework for planning, implementing, and evaluating the effectiveness of the school nurse in the role of health educator. In other words, the framework addresses the what, who, when, and how of implementing the role of educator in school nursing practice. The domains include planning and preparation, the classroom environment, instruction, and professional responsibilities.

Table 7.2 ■
ESSENTIAL DOMAINS TO THE ROLE OF EDUCATOR

Domain	Components
Domain 1: Planning and Preparation	Demonstrate knowledge of content and pedagogy Demonstrate knowledge of students Select instructional goals Demonstrate knowledge of resources Design coherent instruction Assess student learning
Domain 2: The Classroom Environment	Create an environment of respect and rapport Establish a culture for learning Manage classroom procedures Manage student behavior Organize physical space
Domain 3: Instruction	Communicate clearly and accurately Use questioning and discussion techniques Engage students in learning Provide feedback to students Demonstrate flexibility and responsiveness
Domain 4: Professional responsibilities	Reflect on teaching Maintain accurate records Communicate with families Contribute to the school and district Grow and develop professionally Show professionalism

Source: Danielson (1996).

Domain 1: Planning and Preparation

Demonstrate Knowledge of Content and Pedagogy

Before beginning teaching, the school nurse needs to decide what to teach. This is determined through a number of venues. The health education curriculum that has been decided by a local district or mandated by the state directs many of the educational experiences that need to be included in the schools. While some states have not reached consensus on what the approved health curriculum ought to be, the American Alliance for Health, Physical Education, Recreation and Dance (AAHPERD) (http://www.aahperd.org), the largest organization of professionals supporting and assisting those involved in physical education, leisure, fitness, dance, health promotion, and education, has developed standards for health education. The overall goal of the National Health Education Standards for youth is to achieve health literacy. This means being able to obtain, interpret, and understand basic health information and services in order to enhance health. In 1995, national standards for developmentally appropriate, planned, and sequential health instruction in the nation's preschool, elementary, and secondary schools were developed and published by a coalition of organizations and agencies (American Cancer Society, 1995). Therefore, in addition to HP2010 objectives, clear guidelines are available for developing school health education programs when state or local guidelines are absent or incomplete.

The school health program, with input from teachers, administrators, staff, parents, students, community members, and school nurses should reflect the priorities for health promotion and disease prevention in the community and direct health education interventions. Topics that are relevant to the school population, the community, or the nation based on student needs, trends in the population, or community concerns are often added to reflect priorities on a timely basis. The need to prepare for and accommodate students with possible anaphylaxis reactions in the school, a rise in unintended pregnancies, the prevalence of bullying or violence, or recent morbidity or mortality from diseases or injuries might trigger the need for health education programs in the school that are beyond the established health education curriculum.

When planning topics that are potentially controversial, the school nurse and members of the school health team need to be aware of any district policies as well as consider how to develop support from constituent groups before embarking on potentially controversial areas such as those related to drugs, alcohol, sexual behavior, family values, assault prevention, and other similar topics. While many states mandate health education topics for students, they also include the provision that parents have the right to be notified about certain topics, as well as the right to review materials, to be present during the class or to exclude their student from the learning experience if they so desire. It is important for the school nurse to be familiar with local and state policies regarding health education content.

Content expertise depends not only on one's profession but also on being current in and able to appreciate the nuances of the concepts inherent in the topic and the evidence-based data that support the topic. While school nurses are clearly one of the team members in the school who are expert in health content, there may be other teachers, school staff, and community members who can contribute to a topic either as a team or individually. If assigned to teach about a particular topic, it is essential that the school nurse prepare well in advance to identify current information, data, and recommendations about the particular health behavior. Being expert in the topic is important, but equally important is knowing how to teach it—the pedagogy of education. This means possessing an understanding of teaching methodologies based on learners' developmental levels, cognitive strengths, and needs. School nurse preparation programs need to build on the basic foundation that includes theory and practice in teaching and learning that is core in most prelicensure nursing programs. Because school nursing takes place in schools, as opposed to at the bedside or in staff meetings, school nurse preparation programs need to include an understanding and opportunity to practice classroom management skills that are developmentally appropriate when teaching in the school setting. The planning phase affords the school nurse the opportunity to consider the best way to approach the material.

Demonstrate Knowledge of Students

School nurses need to be prepared to work with all age and developmental groups. Knowing who the audience is, together with the experiences, expectations, and aspirations of the individuals, is essential in the planning process in order to build on the students' previous levels of knowledge and skill and to address any misconceptions or behaviors that might interfere with health-promoting activities. When planning educational experiences in the classroom, knowing the student's developmental level, the courses that they have been studying, and how they function as a class can help the school nurse prepare for experiences that will be relevant and appropriate. Consultation with the classroom teacher in advance can provide information about the class and student dynamics. It is important to be aware of any students with special learning or behavioral concerns in the class who will need accommodations or alternative approaches that need to be considered in the planning.

Working with parents and community members can be challenging because the school nurse has to anticipate the demographics, needs, abilities, and motivation of the audience. In presenting a series on adolescent development to parents of seventh-grade students, the nurse understands that parent and guardian expectations will vary depending on how many have older children, how many are experiencing adolescents in the home for the first time, and the kinds of problems or concerns they are encountering in their parenting approaches. Whether the learner is a student or a staff, family, or community member, standards of cultural competency need to be the hallmark of the planning process. In other words, the school nurse needs to consider language barriers, literacy issues, values that influence the receptivity to the message, and stereotypes or biases on the part of the school nurse that might interfere with the delivery of an effective learning experience. Cultural expectations regarding teen dating vary widely among groups and individuals living in the same community. Presenting information about "typical" adolescent behavior may not represent the norms and expectations of the learners. It is important for the nurse to be prepared to accommodate, acknowledge, and affirm the value of cultural differences in the group and the right of every person to make his or her own decisions based on a combination of informed decision-making, values, and goals.

Select Instructional Goals

The goals to be selected in planning for instruction, whether for an individual or a group, need to reflect the outcomes that will be relevant for the individuals, the school, or the community. Using Healthy People 2010 or the Millennium Development goals ensures that the goals are supported by the broader community and reflect the needs of large numbers of individuals. Problems in a district may also direct the selection of goals. For instance, when problems of teasing and bullying occur in the school community, this may indicate the need (goal) for a safe school community. Rising rates of unintended teen pregnancies and subsequent school dropouts may lead to a goal to increase high school completion rates of pregnant and parenting teens. A recent teen death due to illegal substance use and the rise in illegal drug transactions in the area may warrant a goal of safe and drug free schools. Each of the goals described thus far is important and not likely to be achieved in one or two classroom sessions. The school nurse needs to consider the overall goal or outcome of the instructional process and then specifically plan the steps to achieve these goals.

Goals are the broad conditions that can be achieved. Specific outcomes or objectives are the measurable components of the learning process. It might take a long time to demonstrate that teaching interventions resulted in higher pregnant and parenting teen graduation rates, but the number of pregnant and parenting teens who know how to accurately identify signs of impending illness in an infant that require healthcare interventions, thereby avoiding unnecessary absences from school, could be measured.

When planning instruction, the school nurse should specify the learning objectives to be achieved as a result of the learning experience. The objectives should include who the learner is (student, parent, staff, community members, etc.), what he or she will be able to do as a result of the learning experience, and when he or she should be able to do this. The objectives should be realistic, measurable, achievable, and meaningful.

Realistic refers to the relationship between teaching and learning. A lesson that explores the risks related to drug and alcohol use does not prepare students with the skills to avoid such use. However, a lesson designed to give students an opportunity to role play and discuss and debrief how to deal with pressures related to peer drug or alcohol consumption might realistically have an objective that the learner will be able to demonstrate three ways to avoid the use of drugs or alcohol when faced with peer pressure.

Measurable, as one of the components of an objective, refers to the aspect of being able to document that learning has occurred at some level. In this safe and drug-free school example, measurement could occur through post-lesson scenarios when students are asked to describe what they would do when faced with a peer pressure situation. Students can be given a role play or case study after the learning experience to determine their level of appropriate response.

Achievable refers to the possibility of being able to accomplish the learning objective in the stated time frame with the expected level of competency. Having adequate time to set the stage for the learning experiences, to involve the students and get them motivated, as well as to give them opportunities to practice the skills needed to meet the objectives is required in order to accomplish this objective. In other words, a short class period where students passively listen to content, or only one or two students participate in a role play, is not going to be adequate in order to help students achieve the objective. More than likely, the learning experience will require several sessions in order to achieve the objective. This is not to say that a school nurse needs to plan lessons for multiple class times, but rather that he or she needs to be realistic about what can be achieved in the period of time available and match that to the learning objective.

Finally, the most important criterion of the learning objective is that it be *meaningful* in relation to the goal and the learner. For instance, a lesson designed to help a student identify the health risks of illegal drugs that measures the outcome by having the students name drugs and their potential risk of harm will not determine if the students know how to choose the correct health promoting behavior. In this case, the school nurse would not be able to demonstrate or document that the learning activity was meaningful. Keep in mind, however, that being able to demonstrate the appropriate skill when faced with a challenging health decision does not necessarily mean that the learner will choose to use that skill, only that he or she has it in his or her repertoire of responsible behaviors.

What does this mean for school nurses? Each time a lesson is prepared, the school nurse needs to consider what the outcomes will be and if they are realistic, achievable, measurable, and meaningful. How hand washing is taught to kindergartners will be different from how it is taught to seventh graders because it will be tied into different objectives and consequently different teaching strategies and outcome measures. The goals for each session may be the same (to reduce the spread of disease), but the approaches will include all of the variables that need to be considered when planning a lesson.

Demonstrate Knowledge of Resources

Once the school nurse has identified the health problem, understands the learners, and has determined the expected goal and objectives, the "how to" of planning begins. This entails identifying resources necessary for implementing the plan, including people, materials, and processes. People resources refer to identifying the best person or persons for the job. Experts in the community, peer teachers, teams of teachers, parents, students, and community members or school nurses may be the right persons to implement the lesson. Involving more people has both advantages and disadvantages. Going back to the example of promoting safe and drug-free schools, the school nurse might contact a local law enforcement agent with the narcotics task force. This person might be an expert in drug identification, prevalence of use, and related risk behaviors. This expertise may be much more than the school nurse possesses and brings an added and realistic dimension to the lesson. Peer teachers, those who are also students but have special training in sharing knowledge, have the advantage of the "identification factor": students can more readily identify with their peers than with the school nurse. However, disadvantages need to be assessed. Does the person understand and value the goals that you are trying to achieve? Does he or she have other goals that might conflict or compete with the stated goals? Is he or she able to achieve the intended outcomes? Does he or she value and understand the school community and cultural diversity represented in the learners?

Teaming with classroom teachers, other members of the school health team or community experts has the advantage of bringing in experts while still allowing the school nurse to maintain an active role in meeting the goals of the learning experience. Team work requires planning, which means additional time to collaborate, coordinate, and sometimes practice and refine an integrated learning experience.

Material resources have the potential, as with people resources, to drive a learning experience. Materials provided free by educational, commercial, or professional ventures may stimulate the school nurse to consider implementing the program because of its availability. Although free, available, well-packaged materials are tempting to use, the educational goal based on a need or problem should drive the learning experience and choice of materials. Consideration of a resource should be made on the basis of how well it meets the learning objectives and how it engages the learner to be actively involved and thinking critically (which is different than its entertainment factor). Box 7.1 lists some of the criteria that the school nurse should consider when selecting resources.

Materials that reflect the cultural diversity of the community, including illustrations of the community's racial, ethnic, gender, and socioeconomic diversity, need to be used or the school nurse must build in opportunities to discuss how cultural differences could impact the problem-solving and decision-making process. A media resource that portrays young people as having access to automobiles and unsupervised time may be inconsistent with community values and cause concern from parents who hear about it from their children. Presentations

Box 7.1 ■ ■ ■

CRITERIA FOR SELECTING TEACHING RESOURCES

When selecting teaching resources, determine how well they meet the learning objectives and actively engage learners. For example, resources should be:

- Compatible with instructional objectives
- Supportive of school health plan
- Consistent with community values
- Culturally sensitive
- Developmentally appropriate
- Financially affordable
- Visually appealing
- Used to promote critical thinking
- Accurate
- Time efficient

on topics related to reproduction, faith, family values, drugs, tobacco and alcohol, sexuality and risk taking behavior all need to be carefully screened first. Organizing a school health team that includes parents, students, community members, and school staff members can provide an opportunity to jointly evaluate resources and help the school nurse consider strategies for community buy-in prior to use.

Process resources include the kinds of experiences in which learners might engage to meet the learning objectives. For instance, kindergartners might need to practice hand washing, accessing drying systems (paper or air) and disposing of any waste in order to learn the techniques of good hand washing. Where, when, and how this will occur requires planning on the part of the school nurse in collaboration with the classroom teacher (and possibly the custodial staff) to manage a class of kindergartners. Third-grade students might be very willing to sit in their seat and observe a brief demonstration, but seventh-grade students may prefer a more hands-on approach. Some topics are better suited to small group discussion and others require students being able to move around the room. Being aware of the facility is essential to planning. This means that moving of furniture, accessing technology and support for its use, and organizing the learners into different configurations needs to be decided in advance; the space and resources need to be able to accommodate the kinds of approaches that are included in the plan.

Design Coherent Instruction

At this point in the planning process, the school nurse organizes how the learning experience will come together. Keep in mind that learners vary in their abilities to learn, in how they process information and in their motivations. The instruction needs to be organized to allow for this variation. Inform the learner of how the experience is going to be organized. A simple approach for designing instruction, regardless of the length of the lesson or the audience, is to consider set, body, and closure when planning and implementing the lesson.

Set refers to setting the stage for the learning to occur. It might start with something as simple as "Today we are going to learn three ways to prevent tooth decay." An impact statement, on the other hand, might be more effective in motivating the learners for the lesson. The school nurse could display a picture of a child whose face is swollen from a dental abscess and who is in considerable pain, or a picture of decayed teeth. Questions such as "How might this person be feeling?" or "How would you like it if your teeth looked like this?" help learners focus on what the lesson might mean to them. Impact statements, common or recent problems, analogies to other situations, and relevance to the learner's world can all be used in setting the tone for understanding the objectives of the lesson. After the students claim that they wouldn't want to experience these problems, then the school nurse can tell them that they will be learning ways (the objective) to avoid this from happening to them (the goal).

Body refers to the body of the lesson. This is the knowledge, beliefs, and skills that the learner needs to have in order to demonstrate the new behavior. Often called the cognitive, affective, and psychomotor domains, these aspects of learning tie together the lesson so that learners can understand, practice, and incorporate the knowledge into their world view. Students might understand (cognitive domain) the fact that drinking alcohol is related to impaired decision-making with consequences such as motor vehicle injuries and unprotected sexual activity. They might also have had opportunities to practice (psychomotor domain) being in situations in which refusal skills can be used. However, if they do not believe (affective domain) that it could happen to them, then they might not put that knowledge and those skills into action when choosing to drink alcoholic beverages.

Designing coherent instruction refers to the plan that the school nurse has for helping the learners achieve the goal. It is systematic and orderly; helps learners understand the problem, content, or issues; and gives them opportunities to think critically about the content in terms of achieving the objectives. The body of the lesson can be organized according to skills, concepts, or problems. It can be organized by moving from the simple to the complex, from the concrete to the abstract, or from the beginning to the end if there is a timeline related to the learning, or it may be an analogy to something else they know and can relate to.

For instance, when considering instructional design, the analogy of making a sandwich might be useful: The school nurse as educator needs to lay the foundation for what is going to happen, similar to setting down the bun or piece of bread on which the rest of the sandwich rests. "Boys and girls, have you ever thought about what it would be like to not be able to see? Wouldn't this make it hard for you to learn some things in the classroom? As the school nurse, one of my jobs is to begin to find students who might need help seeing better. Today we are going to talk about and practice how you can be ready to have your eyes tested during vision screening tomorrow. By the end of class today, you will know what to expect when you have your eyes tested and what you need to do." This is the set: letting learners know what will happen, what to expect, and what they will achieve. Continuing with the sandwich analogy, a bun by itself would be inadequate as a meal. It needs the filler: the burger, the vegetables, and the condiments. The body is the filler: the content that helps the learner master the knowledge, skills, and attitudes. In the case of vision screening for kindergarten or first-grade students, it is a matter of simple explanation, clear instructions, demonstration, and practice while building their confidence so that they will be ready for this experience.

Closure (putting on the top bun) lets the learner know what they have achieved and what they are now able to do. It is the time to summarize, to make the points of the lesson, to tie it together for the learners based on what they have learned. No new content is introduced at this time as the lesson is pulled together into a coherent whole. "Girls and boys, you have done a great job today. You have practiced recognizing your shapes (or letters) and saying them clearly out loud. You have seen how I will move my hand over your eyes without touching them and you did this while keeping your eyes very still…".

How the school nurse decides to organize the learning experience depends on many factors: time, needs, learner abilities, learning styles, the objectives of the experience, the complexity of the content and skills, and the school nurse's own comfort level with the content, the audience, and the plan. The more time devoted to planning, the more likely it is that the school nurse will be prepared, comfortable, and confident in the educator role.

Assessing Student Learning

Planning requires that the school nurse consider what behaviors would best demonstrate that learning has occurred as a result of the learning experience. If the objective was that kindergarten students were able to demonstrate correct hand washing technique, then it would be appropriate to observe them doing the washing before meals or after toileting rather than having them tell you what they would do. Psychomotor skills are easily observable except in risk-taking situations when adults are not usually present to observe the behavior. In these cases it might be more appropriate to assess the learning through presentation of case studies and asking students how they would behave in a given situation. Role play also affords the opportunity to demonstrate learning. It's important to continue to consider the meaningfulness of the assessment. A paper-and-pencil test or survey responses may elicit the correct answers but does not assure the teacher that the student will use the behavior in a given situation. Establishing the assessment process during the planning phase allows the school nurse to consider what needs to be done in creating an environment where the behavior can be learned, practiced, mastered, and then assessed to determine the value of the learning activity.

Domain 2: The Classroom Environment

Create an Environment of Respect and Rapport

General consensus among learning, developmental, and social theorists suggests that people learn better when they are in an environment free from fear, threat, and ridicule. Humanistic theorists such as Carl Rogers and Abraham Maslow have long advocated that unconditional positive regard, the sense of accomplishment, and opportunities to succeed motivate learners to do better and risk more. If learning is a change in behavior, then that implies an inherent risk: the giving up of old behaviors for new ones. Learners, whether children or adults, need to feel safe to take that risk to consider, try, and practice new behaviors. Only in an environment of respect can this take place. Implications for the school nurse include knowing the rules of the classroom if visiting a teacher's classroom or establishing clear rules of behavior if setting up a course as part of the school nurse role.

When working with adults, it helps to establish the expectations at the beginning of the experience, whether the learners are parents, staff, or community members. For instance, if an after-school or evening series on understanding and living with adolescents is offered, the planning process should take into consideration that there might be professionals and nonprofessionals, those who are confident or intimidated when entering a school environment, and experts or misinformed about the topic. Added to this mix, there might be individuals who like to talk, listen, dominate, or challenge what you are saying. As mentioned earlier, the mix of adult learners may be difficult to assess during advance planning and the school nurse needs to be prepared for a variety of learners with a range of personal needs. Creating an environment of respect and rapport with adults follows the same principles as when working with children and youth: be clear about the guidelines for the learning experience and establish a time frame.

Establish a Culture for Learning

While the classroom teacher is primarily responsible for this and the next three components (managing classroom procedures, managing student behavior, and organizing physical space), the school nurse can be instrumental in contributing to learner success by working closely with the classroom teacher to support the learning environment or to make modifications as needed. School nurses who are either assigned to the classroom as health teachers or who have opportunities for extended classroom contact need to consider the learning culture as part of their responsibilities.

An important variable to consider is whether or not the school nurse is expected to be available for healthcare crises while engaged in teaching a lesson. If this is the case, additional planning needs to take place to make sure that the classroom teacher is able to resume responsibility for the class, that the students understand that their learning needs are important but that you have responsibilities that might interfere with the class, and that the school staff are supportive of your teaching activities and will interrupt only in emergency situations. This planning contributes to the climate of learning because it lets the students know that your time with them is important and that their learning is valuable to them and their health. According to Danielson (1996), some of the basic principles to consider when establishing a learning climate include feeling valued and safe, mutual respect, caring, rapport, and cultural sensitivity.

Manage Classroom Procedures

Working with the classroom teacher in advance will help ensure a smooth transition to your presence in the classroom. If students are expected to sit in assigned seats, take turns in responding to questions, or required to raise their hands and wait for acknowledgement before answering, then you need to be aware of these procedures and continue with them or explain how and why the procedures might be different for the lesson. In any classroom setting, the school nurse needs to be familiar with the plan and prepared for emergency evacuation in case of fire, tornado, or other drills that might take place in the classroom location.

Manage Student Behavior

The topics that a school nurse typically presents in the classroom are related to health and therefore of a personal nature. Students tend to relate the content to themselves, their friends, and their family members when seeking generalization of the content and validating what they are learning. This should be encouraged in terms of promoting critical thinking and being able to conceptualize the consequences of action. However, it can also lead to potential problems. For instance, when talking about growth and developmental changes, students may feel embarrassed. Topics related to mental health may promote introspection and reflection on feelings of decreased self-esteem, depression, or suicide. Discussions about behaviors and the health risk consequences can lead to concerns about relatives' health and fears that the student might have for their family members. Anything discussed by a school nurse could have relevance to the personal lives of the students. One of the goals is to make the content relevant. However, it can also result in students disrupting the class because of their concerns, their embarrassment, and their feelings. Topics related to sexual behavior, drugs, alcohol, bullying, violence, and self-esteem can provoke inappropriate comments, use of street language or slang, personal derisions about other students or individuals, and personally revealing information that should be held confidential. The school nurse needs to think about how to handle these situations in advance and be prepared to deal with them.

One solution might be to let students know during the "set" that you want and value their input and realize that the content in the lesson will have personal implications. You might speak about the importance of confidentiality and how difficult that is to maintain. You might suggest that all questions related to the content, unless it is for clarification purposes, be written down on pieces of paper that you will read and answer either toward the end of the class or at another time. This way students who are uncomfortable asking questions have an opportunity to ask in a nonthreatening manner, students who might be prone to repeated monopolizing of the classroom can be helped to channel their energy by adhering to the written question approach, and as the school nurse, you can monitor questions so that they are framed in an appropriate manner. For example, fifth- and sixth-grade boys often ask about genital development and use common slang terminology. As the school nurse, you can read those questions and respond by saying, "There were several excellent questions about the growth of genitals. While some of you used terminology that you might have heard, we are going to use the correct scientific or anatomic terminology when referring to body parts. I am going to put several questions together to answer this next question." In this way, you acknowledge their questions but do not have to read them verbatim, thereby managing effectively student participation, and potentially disruptive behavior.

Meeting with the teacher ahead of time allows you to determine if there are classroom problems that need to be monitored and strategies that are in place and should be followed. This is a good time to establish the classroom teacher's role during the class. Unless this is a class period where the teacher is scheduled not to be present, there are certain advantages to having the teacher available in the room. It will help if you are called out unexpectedly. In addition, you will have an experienced teacher in the room who will be hearing the lesson and you will be able to collaborate on strategies to include follow-up about the lesson in subsequent classes.

Typical problem behaviors that the school nurse might encounter are frequent interruptions, monopolizing of content, inappropriate comments, distracting behavior, disruptive behavior, and student inattention. Each of these behaviors can be dealt with in a variety of ways. For consistency and in order to promote learning, the teacher's response to these problem behaviors should be considered in light of the classroom climate for learning. Recognize students as valuable members of the learning community, encourage them to be motivated to learn, and follow basic principles of engaging students and treating them with respect; how problem behaviors are dealt with should reflect the goals that enhance learning. For example, if the classroom climate is established that everyone has the right to learn and you notice that several students are passing notes, or talking to each other during the class, this could be interpreted as either a distracting or disruptive activity that interferes with other students' ability to learn.

Several strategies might work to limit this behavior and use of the strategies will depend on one's comfort level, the extent of the disruptive behavior, what has happened previously, and the goals for the learning climate. Visual contact or close physical proximity to the involved students may be adequate to let them know that you are aware of their behavior and do not approve of it. Engaging those students who are not paying attention can help them refocus on the point of the lesson. This can be problematic if they are asked to summarize the discussion so far or to repeat a pertinent point. The question that needs to be asked is whether humiliation or embarrassment will motivate a student to participate better in the future or only serve as an impediment to being engaged because of the extent of the embarrassment.

Another approach is to redirect the classroom activities to involve the students in more active participation through structured group work followed by a brief report. If any students are talking to each other or passing notes, they can be put in separate working groups. This can be done by assigning groups or having the students count off into groups by numbers. If the activity occurs near the end of the class and there will be another session, tell the students of your concern about their behavior and the need to be respectful of other students in subsequent classes. Pointing out student problem behavior in class lets other students know that you are committed to maintaining a positive climate in the classroom that is respectful of all of the students in the class.

Organize Physical Space

Depending on the objectives of the class and the methods to help students achieve those objectives, the school nurse needs to consider how the classroom is set up and how the physical space can best be organized. In an attempt to have students learn to make decisions about negotiating risky situations such as withstanding peer pressure related to alcohol consumption, then students need to have the opportunity to participate in face-to-face interaction with their peers. A lecture style format with all of the desks and chairs facing the front would be appropriate for a demonstration of this activity and for two or three students to enact a role play for the entire class, but it would not allow each of the students the opportunity to practice for themselves. In this case, the school nurse needs to determine how this can best be achieved. Moving the desks and chairs so that dyads or triads of students can work together will help meet the objective better than a lecture style format. If a goal is to have student–student interaction, then the classroom needs to be set up so that all of the students can see each other, either in a circle or a horseshoe formation. If students need practice skills such as teen parents practicing feeding techniques, then the room needs to be set up so that students can realistically practice the skills. When teaching staff how to be prepared for an anaphylactic reaction, they need practice with epinephrine-injectable trainers. Not only do they need to be able to see the demonstration clearly, but there must be adequate numbers of trainers; the room must be set up so that they can practice the technique and the school nurse is able to observe their technique in order to provide appropriate feedback.

Other physical environment considerations include adequate ventilation in the classroom and lighting that is adequate for illuminating materials but avoids direct sunlight that can be distracting to students. Lighting consideration is also important in the use of overhead, slide or LCD projectors, video monitors, or computers in the classroom to make sure that everyone is able to see the projection. Position the students and equipment so that direct sunlight is not an issue. Avoid having the room so dark that students' behavior, as well as their reactions to the material, cannot be monitored.

Domain 3: Instruction

The domain of instruction is the actual delivery of the lesson. It includes the set, body, and closure of the lesson. All of the planning leads to the effective delivery of the material so that the students are able to meet the objectives. The components of the instruction domain include communicating clearly and accurately, using questioning and discussion techniques, engaging students in learning, providing feedback to students, and demonstrating flexibility and responsiveness. Each of these is important to consider with all learners, whether students, staff, or community members.

Communicate Clearly and Accurately

Communication in the classroom takes the form of verbal, nonverbal, visual, and auditory communication. Verbal communication requires skills in elocution, or speaking and enunciating clearly so that students are able to understand you. If you have a regional accent, a physical speech impediment, or a tendency to talk fast, then it is important to establish practices that allow students to understand your spoken word. This can be done by supplementing your oral presentation with visual cues on slides, handouts, or using the board in the classroom. If you are a fast talker and are unable to consciously slow your pacing, it often helps to write on the board or overhead as you speak so that you need to slow down to keep pace with your writing. Watch students' visual responses to your presentation. Are they frequently asking you to repeat things, asking you to slow down, or asking how to spell words? These are clues that they are having difficulty understanding you.

Nonverbal communication in the classroom can add to the lesson by expressing your positive regard for the students and their ability to learn. Attentive listening to their questions and concerns, and asking or using their names lets students know that you value them as learners and their input. If you do not know all of the students' names in a class and want to be able to respond to them by name, you can start the class by providing them with trifold name cards on which they write their name along with a few key words to describe how they feel about the lesson for the class, what they hope to get out of the class, or a visual that describes something about them or the topic. Instruct the students to place these facing forward so you and others can see them and you can make reference to their beginning thoughts, experiences, or personal goals during the class and as part of the closing summary.

How you respond to an incorrect contribution from a student can also impact the instruction. Facial expressions of disbelief, distaste, or boredom convey negative messages to the learners. Neutral, smiling, or encouraging facial expressions allow the students to feel more confident as they work through trying to respond or think critically. Keeping your eye on the clock, writing notes, watching other students, and impatience when a student is trying to formulate a response can be interpreted by all students as an attitude that students and learning are not important to you.

Visual communication needs to be considered when planning and delivering a lesson. Written material needs to be clear, legible, grammatically correct, spelled correctly, and appropriate to the age, developmental level, reading skills, and culture of the learner. A good rule to follow on materials that are displayed on slides, overheads, or on computer screens is to keep it short and simple. Use key words to highlight the major concepts. Use no more than seven lines of text with less than six words per line. Preferably, just include the key concepts and use a font that is easy to read (Courier, Times, or Arial) and large enough to be read from a distance. Contrasting colors for the font and background help highlight the text. Decisions as to what kind, how much, and the size of graphics and background templates should take into consideration the purpose of the lesson. Graphics or templates that illustrate the theme of the lesson can be useful. Too many details can be distracting and using no graphics at all can be boring.

The sounds that you use are also important. If your voice does not project well, or if there is background noise, then you need to consider strategies such as a microphone or conscious voice projection. Changing the tempo and volume of your voice can maintain student interest if used properly. Silence can be a powerful and effective communication tool. Silence can also help learners who have lost the pace of the lesson refocus.

Use Questioning and Discussion Techniques

Giving students time to think and process information allows them to formulate questions, consider applications and sort through any discrepancies or concerns they might have. Asking questions and promoting discussion allows learners to listen to each others' responses, opinions, and perspectives that they might not have considered themselves, thus expanding their understanding that not everyone views the same information from the same perspective. "When teachers use skilled questioning, they engage their students in an exploration of content. Carefully framed questions enable students to reflect on their understanding and consider new possibilities" (Danielson, 1996, p. 92).

Instructional goals reflect what it is hoped the learner will achieve. If the goal is that students come to school well rested and ready for a day of active learning, and the audience is elementary school parents at a parent meeting, the objective will be that parents provide structure and opportunities for adequate rest and nutrition at home for their children. When considering the learning environment, let parents know that their ideas are important, that there is no one solution, and that what they share will be respected and valued. Asking them to identify why a good night's sleep is important, or rapid-fire questions about facts related to rest, nutrition, and productivity might alienate or disengage those parents who do not know the answers, or it might allow some parents to take over the session as they do know all of the answers.

Good questioning engages learners in exploration. Ask them what it is that they want to know. What happens when their children do not seem to get enough sleep at night? Do some of them have the same experiences or do their children respond differently? When are they likely to see these behaviors? How does it affect their lives when one of their children acts this way? What are some of the things that seem to cause their children to be tired? A good teacher engages all of the learners in the discussion and focuses questions to eventually discover and explore possible solutions. What seems to work best? How can you do this? What seems to get in the way of making it work? Does anyone want to comment on this idea? Are there any other ways of doing this? Having a handout of tips or strategies can be given as a supplement to the meeting but first let the learners think through alternatives, consider other perspectives, and become engaged in finding solutions. Additional suggestions are listed in TABLE 7.3.

Everyone likes to feel that his or her contribution is valued. Each time learners give an answer they want some validation that it was valued. This can be done with positive feedback about the contribution and how it ties into the learning activity. However, the school nurse may be faced with learners who provide erroneous information, give a wrong answer to a question, or go off on an irrelevant tangent. Acknowledging the learner's response while providing correct information, respecting the learners, and staying focused on the learning objectives can be challenging. You do not want to reinforce incorrect information nor do you want the person who contributed that information to feel that his or her input is not valued. Help the learner problem solve why he or she provided that information. You can thank the person and then ask other learners if there are other options to consider. After the discus-

Table 7.3 ■

QUESTIONING AND DISCUSSION TECHNIQUES

Avoid Yes/No questions.
Give time to think before expecting a response.
Encourage all students to participate.
Acknowledge contributions.
Seek clarification: "Can you give an example?"
Encourage learners to comment on others' answers.
Request further elaboration.
Encourage participation.
Discourage domination.
Show respect for learners.
Use learner's questions to focus a discussion.

Source: Danielson (1996).

sion has continued, go back and summarize the common misconceptions, noting how they are held by a number of people, and mention the learners have done a good job in problem solving to consider all aspects of a problem. A comment such as, "Wrong! Does anyone else have the correct answer?" does not create a learning environment conducive to feeling safe and respected.

Another concern is the learner who wants to answer all of the questions even when none have been posed. When one learner tends to dominate the discussion, the school nurse can acknowledge his or her contribution and then ask others in the room to comment on their experiences or to provide another perspective. When establishing a culture for learning, the school nurse can clarify the expectation that everyone will have a chance to speak and participate and remind students of this when necessary with comments such as, "You have a lot of ideas to contribute today and I would like to hear more about it, but let's hear from others in the class and perhaps we can meet later to discuss your ideas some more." Questioning techniques and leading a discussion are at the heart of helping learners understand the application of the material to their own lives and health. Highlighting possible questions as part of the planning process can remind the school nurse to incorporate those questions at appropriate places in the lesson. In summary, discussion can be engaging and promote critical thinking when it is based on questions formulated to encourage active participation, considers a variety of perspectives, and applies the discussion to real-life situations.

Engage Students in Learning

According to Danielson (1996), this component is the most important in learning. It is the reason for teaching and when it does not occur, the consequences in terms of student inattention and disengagement or even disruptions become obvious. "What is required for student engagement is *intellectual involvement* with the content, or active construction of understanding. School, in other words, is not a spectator sport" (p. 95). Engagement does not mean keeping busy in the classroom or staying on task but that learners are actively participating in and invested in the learning experience. In other words, they want to be learning so that they will learn something that is meaningful to them. A variety of strategies can be used to achieve this engagement but audio–visual materials, physical activity, hands-on experiences, or student participation do not necessarily guarantee learning if the learner is not fully engaged in the experience.

School nurses can contribute to learner engagement, both through care provided in the health office and content taught in the classroom. For instance, if a student is hungry, feeling afraid of being bullied, pregnant, worried about a sick family member, or having difficulty breathing, he or she is not going to be able to be fully engaged. School nurses can identify these students and help them meet their needs so that they can be ready to learn. If this is, as Danielson purports, the core of teaching and learning, then school nurses need to be vigilant in identifying students who are at risk from not being able to fully participate in the learning environment.

Provide Feedback to Students

Formative and summative feedback are essential in the learning process. Learners need intermittent feedback so that they have a chance to determine how they are doing and what they need to do to meet the learning objectives. This kind of feedback is formative; it helps learners determine if they are on target and what needs to be done next. Summative feedback, on the other hand, occurs at the end; this kind of feedback measures how one has done in meeting the objectives. It is often reflected in a grade or a certificate of completion. When the school nurse is a guest presenter in a health class, feedback is usually formative, providing informal feedback to students about their understanding of the concepts and processes discussed.

The classroom teacher would most often be responsible for assessing the outcome measures as described in the course plan. There are times, however, when the school nurse provides summative feedback. For instance, after teaching a class on first aid, babysitting care, or CPR, the learners might have to perform on certain measures, either written, verbal, or behavioral to demonstrate their knowledge and skill in order to receive a certificate of attendance. If the school nurse is assigned to teach a health course that requires a grade at the end of the term, then summative feedback in the form of a grade will be necessary. If the school nurse is conducting evaluation research regarding the outcomes of certain educational interventions, end of program measures such as scores on standardized tests or a demonstration of proficiency might be included in the funding and documentation process for grant reporting purposes.

Feedback is helpful in guiding learners to understand their progress toward mastery as well as to indicate what areas need continued work. Some of the principles related to feedback include significance, appropriateness, comprehensiveness, constructiveness, and timeliness. All learners should get feedback, not just those who excel and not just those who are having difficulty. Learners who have worked hard to achieve need positive reinforcement for their work and guidance on ways to improve; learners who are struggling also need direction. Feedback should be proportional to the significance of the work. Learners who invest more time or more effort on heavily weighted assignments deserve more feedback than activities in which less investment occurs. Keeping in mind the learning goals and stated objectives, feedback should be geared to helping learners determine their progress toward meeting the objectives. For instance, when working with students on objectives to increase their physical activity, helping them gauge how much their endurance has improved is more appropriate than testing their understanding of pulse rates.

Feedback should involve as much of the learning experience as possible. A written test that only measures vocabulary related to bones but ignores decisions about carrying books in a back pack or the importance of calcium does not let the learner appreciate the scope of what was learned. Finally, feedback needs to be timely and constructive. Timeliness is important so that the learner is able to relate the feedback to his or her current perceptions and behaviors in order for change to take place and it needs to be constructive in order to motivate the learner to continue to learn (Danielson, 1996; Danielson & McGreal, 2002).

Demonstrate Flexibility and Responsiveness

School nurses quickly learn the importance of flexibility and responsiveness in all aspects of the role of school nurse. This is especially true in the role of educator. Imagine that you have planned for weeks to present a talk to the middle school parent–teacher organization on pubertal changes as the first in a series on understanding adolescents. That same week it was learned that three classmates had been suspended because of illegal substance use. Parents come to the meeting concerned about the incidence of illegal substance use in the community, the role of the school in curbing this problem, and the need to vent their fears, concerns, and frustrations in working with teens. While your plan had included a systematic approach to understanding adolescents by first talking about the physical changes of puberty followed by the cognitive and social changes, leading into risk behaviors and communicating with the adolescent, you quickly realize the importance of responding to the needs of the audience, in this case parents who are worried and teachers who feel they cannot be responsible for all of the behaviors of adolescents. The plan may have to be put aside for another time or tied into the concerns of parents and teachers. In other words, the school nurse needs to be responsive to the needs of the learners and flexible in adapting to those needs.

During a class, the school nurse may be needed elsewhere in the building or district for emergency needs. Planning in advance to accommodate such situations requires the school nurse to be flexible. Sharing with students your disappointment at not being able to finish the topic and the plan for either completing the lesson or providing supplemental materials if the lesson cannot be made up communicates to the learners that their learning is important, that you care about them being able to learn it, and that you will follow through with your commitment to help them learn.

Some situations may not be easily anticipated. The student who has lost a family member to a tragic death may want to talk about it in the middle of a class on another topic. Knowing how to be both sensitive to the individual student while supporting the needs of the entire class requires responsiveness and flexibility as well as a clear understanding of school policies on working with students who are experiencing crisis. No one, not even the school nurse, can be expected to do personal counseling, teach a class, and maintain confidentiality all at the same time. In this situation of crisis, the school nurse can stop the lesson for a moment and instruct the students to do some reflective work such as drawing or writing on a pertinent question related to the topic for a few minutes. Once the class is focused on the activity, the school nurse can facilitate helping the student in crisis to the appropriate source of support according to school policy.

Domain 4: Professional Responsibilities

Inherent in the NASN and the ANA standards are explicit guidelines for the professional responsibilities of the school nurse in all areas of practice. Specific reference to the professional responsibilities of the school nurse as educator include assessment of needs for health education; individual and group health teaching; design, develop and evaluate health curricula and health instructional materials; be a resource person; promote school-wide health; educate staff; apply evidence-based interventions; access community resources; collaborate; and document all interventions, relevant health promotion teaching, appropriate methods, feedback, and evaluation. The standards should be used to guide school nurses in being accountable for practice.

Reflect on Teaching

Developing a lesson plan includes a reminder to evaluate the effectiveness of the lesson. Did it meet the intended goals? Were the learners able to achieve the objectives? Were the strategies effective? Were the materials appropriate? Did the timing work? Were there questions that can be incorporated into a similar class in the future? In other words, the school nurse as educator needs to consider what worked, what did not work and what strategies will make it more effective in the future. Although there may be a tendency to put a lesson aside until the next time, reflection offers the school nurse the opportunity to consider successes and areas for improvement while the experience and feedback are still fresh.

Maintain Accurate Records

Many schools require that teachers maintain and submit lesson plans so that schools are able to be accountable for the content taught and experiences provided. Depending on school policy, the school nurse might not be held to the same standard of accountability of daily lesson plans. Even if documentation of school nurse activities as educator is not required, adequate documentation is necessary to account for time spent and impact made on health promotion activities. A lesson plan can take many forms depending on the school nurse's organizational preferences. Some school nurses prefer a narrative format, others an outline format, and some a timeline. Regardless of the format, the components should include a listing of the title of the lesson, the intended audience, the goal of the lesson, and the learner objectives in behavioral and measurable terms. Also included should be an outline of the lesson, materials needed, time frame, and measurement tools to determine that the learner has met the objectives. A simple format (FIGURE 7.1) is a one-page plan similar to those required by professional nursing organizations for approving continuing education efforts. Comments can be written at the bottom of the table or on the back of the sheet or maintained in a lesson database.

Documentation should include copies of the materials used, including notes, handouts, electronic files, slides, and in the case of borrowed materials, their source, as well as costs involved and which staff or parents reviewed the materials. The accountability involved with maintaining these records can be useful to school nurses in documenting their contribution to the education of learners, time spent out of the health office, and impact on the community. It can also be used as part of a portfolio of materials for evaluation of the school nurse.

Communicate with Families

Letting families know what goes on in the classroom serves several important purposes. First, it informs them about what is taught so that they are knowledgeable about their children's education. This knowledge allows them to support and build on that learning within the context of family values and expectations. It also helps families to be partners in the educational process of the school community leading to more buy-in and support. The school nurse can accomplish this by letting families know in advance what topics are going to be addressed. School newsletters and teachers' notes can prepare families for different topics that might be discussed. Additional readings available at the school, in the public library, and on Web sites can be included. Written tips that empower parents to feel that they are active participants in their child's education help establish a climate where reinforcement can take place. For instance, in the case of hand washing, send home a brief note explaining that hand washing was taught in order to reduce the spread of germs. "Today, students learned how to wash their hands before meals, before touching babies, after toileting, after coughing, sneezing or blowing their noses, and after touching pets. They were taught to sing the ABC alphabet song so that they would learn to wash for a long-enough period of time. They were encouraged to have a paper towel ready before washing so that they do not have to touch the towel dispenser or faucet when in a public bathroom. Please ask your child to demonstrate this skill for you and encourage them to use it at home and when they are away from home. Good hand washing can reduce the spread of germs and decrease the number of sick days that children experience. Thank you for your support."

State and district regulations may dictate how to inform parents of upcoming topics that might be considered controversial for which they have the right to exclude their child from the learning experience. Specific topics may include assault prevention; pubertal topics; drug, alcohol, and tobacco prevention programs; information on sexually transmitted diseases; and any other topic that members of the community and/or the school have indicated might be of concern to parents.

Some parents do not receive, nor are they able to read the messages that are sent home. School nurses must make every effort to inform parents and give them the opportunity to be prepared to answer questions that their children might raise regarding health topics discussed in school. For instance, in a lesson on decision-making regarding alcohol use, a student might go home and ask his or

Title of Lesson				
Goal				
Intended Audience			Dates	
Objectives	Topical Outline	Methods	Materials and Time	Evaluation
Comments:				

Title of Lesson: Bicycle Helmet Safety				
Goal: HP 2010: Reduce injuries, disabilities, and deaths due to unintentional injuries and violence. 15. Injury and Violence Prevention: 15–23 Bicycle helmet use				
Intended Audience Grades 2–5			Dates: Start of school year. Could be one 35 minute session or three brief lessons	
Objectives	Topical Outline	Methods	Materials and Time	Evaluation
Understand why helmets are important in reducing injury	Impact demonstration Facts What it means to them	Question and answer session Demonstration with student participation	5 minutes Eggs, Jell-O brain molds, ramp for collision demonstration	Able to list reasons why helmet use reduces injury
Practice wearing helmets	Proper fit Proper use Common problems	Demonstration Practice	10 minutes Donations from local merchants, police, PTO or children's hospital	Demonstrate proper technique
Wear helmets when riding bikes to school	Resistance Making it OK	Discuss Design activity "Helmet show"	5 minutes Groups prepare for helmet fashion show	Increased number using helmets when riding to school
Comments: Make brain mold with extra gelatin to keep form. Provide bandanas, stickers and hair ties for design activity. Consider having two groups present the pros and cons of helmet wearing and then discuss what each group thought of the other's ideas. Put notice of lesson in school newsletter and local community newspaper to reinforce the topic. Consider donation sources for any student without a helmet.				

Figure 7.1 ■ Sample lesson plan format.

her parents why they drink alcohol and parents who are not informed about this topic may feel that the school is interfering with their personal lifestyle choices. Knowing in advance gives families the opportunity to place the learning within the context of the family and allows the family members to become better informed about health choices at the same time that their children are learning about making healthy choices.

School policies about informing parents and obtaining informed consent need to be clearly communicated with parents or guardians on an annual basis. If negative consent is used (in other words, if parent do not want their child to participate in a learning activity, they must notify the school) there needs to be clear guidelines so parents know about this option. Extraordinary efforts are made to make sure that all parents receive adequate and timely notice so that they can obtain additional information and make an informed decision in advance of the learning experience. For instance, sending notes home with students about an upcoming puberty talk the next week may not be effective if the note does not make it out of the student's book bag until after the class. If the family wanted to talk to their child about puberty before the class, then this could be distressing to the parents and upsetting to the student, and could jeopardize the relationship of trust between the family and the school. Clear policies about parental notification should be established, in place, and communicated clearly before any controversial activities are undertaken. If they are not in place, the school nurse can advocate for their inclusion.

Contribute to the School and the District

Danielson (1996) speaks about the importance of the school community and the responsibility of professionals to make a contribution beyond their day-to-day jobs. For school nurses, this means being involved in the life of the school: getting along with other members of the school community, fostering a positive environment and identifying ways to meet the goals of the school that are beyond the health office walls. For example, on a basic level, the school nurse participates in school events, such as an evening orientation for new students and their families. The more proficient school nurse may identify information to help new parents and students make the transition to the school by volunteering to prepare materials and a brief motivational presentation at an open house meeting. Assuming a leadership role in promoting school or district wide health through student or employee fitness programs is an example of distinguished performance in contributing to the school and the district. Implementing a walk to school day that engages community members in making their sidewalk areas and neighborhoods safe and has students learning and practicing safe walking habits can make a substantial contribution to a healthy community and students arriving safely at school.

Grow and Develop Professionally

The NASN standards of professional practice (NASN & ANA, 2001) indicate a clear expectation that school nurses will continue to pursue professional development throughout their careers whether or not this is required by employers or state licensing boards. Professional growth in the role of school nurse as educator requires attendance at professional meetings, reading evidence-based peer reviewed journals, and getting feedback on your performance. Each of these activities helps you grow by keeping you current with the latest trends and findings that can impact school health. Keeping track by maintaining documentation of professional development activities provides evidence to licensing organizations as well as your employer of efforts toward continued growth as a school nurse.

Show Professionalism

Although an important member of the education team, school nurses are often autonomous in daily practice while simultaneously working as colleague, consultant, health educator, and researcher. In the classroom, on teams, and in the health office, the school nurse is able to show professionalism while simultaneously informing colleagues, parents, students, and the community about the professional roles of school nurses. Using the criteria described by Danielson (1996), the school nurse can implement health education interventions that are consistent with the professional standards of teachers across the United States. Being able to communicate about the educational process and the role of the school nurse in that process will help clarify the professional responsibilities of the school nurse as well as potentially increase the recognition value of having school nurses as active, participating members of the health education team in schools.

TEACHING OPPORTUNITIES FOR SCHOOL NURSES

As already suggested in this chapter, there are numerous opportunities for school nurses to function in the role of educator and learners can be any individual or group of students, staff, teachers, administrators, board members, colleagues, parents/guardians, families, and community members. Teaching can take place on a one-on-one basis; in small groups; in medium to large size classes; in school assemblies in formal and informal settings; in staff and professional meetings; or through print, online, or other electronic media.

The most obvious and often implemented role of the school nurse occurs in relationship to the standards of care for school nurses when using the nursing process to educate clients and their families about their health conditions, options for health promoting behavior and strategies to improve health. Small group teaching occurs when there is a special group interested in learning about a health-related topic. For example, teachers in second grade might want to learn how to work with students with allergies in their classroom. The lesson plan would be developed around their needs to identify triggers and signs and symptoms, and to provide emergency care. Students who are pregnant may be in a small group and learning about infant feeding options.

Classes in health are obvious places where the school nurse can implement the role of educator. Other opportunities exist in government classes as a venue for talking about legal rights and responsibilities of minors in relation to health care; in math classes for learning about calculating the body mass index (BMI); in language classes for learning how to ask for healthcare help when speaking to persons in another language; in English classes to learn about strategies for communicating about health concerns and studying about themes related to health in literature; in history classes to discuss the evolution of healthcare concerns and what can be done to make changes for the future; in art or music classes to share strategies for relaxation and health promotion; and of course, in science classes that relate to almost all topics of health.

Establishing your role as educator may take time and can be accomplished in small increments. Requesting just a few minutes at all-school assemblies to share a brief, relevant, and well-delivered health message can make an impact on the entire school in a short time while increasing your visibility and recognition as a health educator. Brief messages (similar to public service announcements) can be delivered along with the daily announcements that are either read in the classroom or projected over a whole school sound system. Some schools have televised announcements and school news broadcasts. These approaches can be used to share health messages to the entire student population. Myths on Monday, Tips for Tuesday, Wellness Wednesday, Thoughts on Thursday, or Facts on Friday can be the focus of health messages centered around the school's health goals, Healthy People goals, national health observances, or current health issues of concern in the school or community.

Regular, brief messages about health can become institutionalized in the school under the leadership of the school nurse so that students and staff begin to anticipate health messages. Health topics can be reinforced through a variety of venues to strengthen the support of the message and to help educate others about the importance of the topic. This can be done in the classroom with follow-up activities provided to classroom teachers, notes home to parents, and notices in the school newsletter, the community newspaper, or local cable access television.

In addition to being a guest speaker in a class, school nurses might develop of series of classes to meet with students who are overweight, have reactive airway disease, or another topic of interest. These series might be held outside the regularly scheduled class sessions, as brown bag lunches, during common study hall periods, or before or after school. They may involve students, parents or a combination of both depending on the topic.

In some schools, the expectation is that the school nurse is in the classroom to address health promotion strategies to improve health behaviors. In these situations the school nurse needs to develop a plan that is congruent with the mission of the school and consistent with the expectations for classroom preparation and performance of all teachers in the school. School nurses may be asked to share their expertise in professional meetings with other school nurses. Principles for teaching and learning apply regardless of the audience. Sharing with other school nurses is an important mechanism for promoting dialogue to improve school nursing practice, as the professional exchange that takes place allows the school nurses present to consider different approaches and to validate or question their practice.

School board meetings and community meetings are an important venue for advocating for health policy change, supporting health promotion programs, and increasing understanding of the scope and responsibilities of school nursing practice. Preparing for these meetings using the four domains and associated components described by Danielson (1966) allows school nurses to be well prepared and confident in delivering messages.

ISSUES IN THE ROLE OF SCHOOL NURSE AS EDUCATOR

School nurses need to be actively involved in the educator role. However, there are several issues that need to be considered when implementing the role of health educator. These include time, access to students, controversial topics, confidentiality, expertise, and evaluation. A major consideration is time. When will there be enough time to prepare, much less implement a lesson plan? How can you be assured that it will be uninterrupted? Addressing these issues in advance of agreeing to teach or accepting a teaching assignment is crucial. If teachers in your school have assigned planning periods and are represented by the same organization as school nurses, then school nurses need to ascertain if their contract also allows for a planning period. If not, then clarify the expectation for being able to have time to prepare and how other activity expectations will be adjusted. For example, if the school expects the health office doors to be open to students from the beginning to the ending bell each day, when can uninterrupted time to do the planning necessary for an effective lesson be scheduled?

A different issue is access to students. With the emphasis on accountability and demonstrating proficiency, some schools and teachers limit the school nurse's access to classes. Strategies to deal with this issue include several approaches. At the beginning of the year, distribute a list of topics to all teachers that you would be willing to discuss in the classroom, letting teachers know of your availability and time constraints. Knowing the school curriculum can help plan appropriate topics in advance so that they complement ongoing curriculum endeavors. At weekly staff meetings, mention national health observances that are being planned or taking place and suggest strategies that teachers can use to incorporate those topics in their classes. Volunteer to be available to come into class to talk about the topic or to provide teachers with relevant resources so they can incorporate it into their existing lessons. Demonstrating a willingness to be involved, identifying the needs of classroom teachers, limiting the time spent in a classroom by being well prepared and delivering an effective message may result in teachers requesting your services more in the future.

Keep in mind, however, that some of the topics that may be relegated to the school nurse are those controversial topics that classroom teachers do not want to be responsible for addressing. In addition to sometimes being beyond the teacher's area of expertise, some of the topics might clash with family and community values, or they might provoke disruptive responses by students. All potentially controversial topics should be planned well in advance. Include as many key partners in the planning as possible.

Teachers can help determine when best to tie the topic into the existing curriculum and can collaborate to develop strategies for transitioning to the topic. Teachers should plan to be present during any controversial lessons so that there is additional support in the classroom. For instance, when teaching about growth and development to fifth- and sixth-grade students, having a respected male figure or female figure in the classroom can help maintain order and also has the benefit of allowing the school nurse to link the topic to the on-going curriculum and support services in the school. While there might not be enough time to address all of the questions that the topic generates, the school nurse can leave a question box in the class and let students know that questions will be addressed at another time with the support of the classroom teachers.

Parents need to be involved so that they can support the lessons taught and be informed themselves so they are prepared to address questions that students are likely to bring home after a controversial topic. This planning includes the opportunity to preview materials and understand how the class will be approached. Many schools and states allow parents the option to remove their students from classes that are potentially controversial. In order to do this, parents need to know well in advance what is going to be taught, how it will be addressed, when it will be happening, as well as what alternative learning experience may be provided to their child. Incorporating messages throughout all health lessons that encourage students to talk to their parents or guardians about these topics and to determine how their family values might influence their behavior now that they have been provided with this information and skill is essential for linking schools and communities together. It also has the added advantage of providing health information to a wider network of persons who can reinforce and role model positive health behaviors. In addition to notes sent home in advance of controversial topics, newsletter announcements and follow-up information can help to reduce the mystique of the topic and what has been discussed in class. Parent-teacher meetings in advance of topics can help parents learn about the topic, strategies for talking about it at home, and approaches to promote resiliency and reduce risk factors in youth.

Another aspect about controversial topics is the worry about how some students may respond to topics discussed in class. Relating personally to any health topic is important in order to consider the value of the health behavior in relationship to the self. However, students who are emotionally fragile, who have been abused, who have experienced loss, or who have family members or close friends who have experienced health concerns may be vulnerable to emotional stress when these topics are raised in class. School nurses and teachers need to anticipate this possibility in advance, review the school crisis plan, and establish a mechanism for identifying students at risk and providing the appropriate support for them when sensitive issues are raised.

Sensitive issues are often private issues and respect for individual privacy needs to be preserved. As Danielson (1996) pointed out, the role of the school nurse as educator includes knowing the learners, being aware of resources to assist students, and creating an environment of respect and rapport that includes caring. Inherent in teaching about health and discussing health-related topics is the importance of confidentiality. Students have a right to know that their private health information can remain private. This is sometimes challenging when students share their own and family members' health information in a classroom setting. The school nurse can help students understand the importance of respecting confidentiality and help set up guidelines in the classroom about how confidentiality principles will be implemented. A school-wide discussion with staff and administrators can help develop strategies to teach and protect the rights to privacy regarding health information.

Evaluation is another potentially controversial topic related to the role of the school nurse as educator. Evaluation that determines the value of the learner's experience should be part of the planning process. Evaluation of the school nurse as an educator needs to be addressed in advance of the teaching-learning process. For instance, you need to know if your teaching will be observed and evaluated by administrative staff in the school and for what purposes this information will be used: formative to help you improve your performance as an educator or summative to determine the efficacy of this aspect of your role as school nurse with potential job assignment or merit considerations. In either case, the school nurse may feel threatened by this process if it has not been part of the expectation during the planning process. Anticipating the need for evaluation can help one be an active and willing participant in this institutional process of personnel evaluation and educational accountability.

Another problem related to evaluating the role performance of the school nurse as an educator is who does the evaluation. The American Nurses Association (2004) implies that the profession is able to monitor itself and has the processes in place to conduct such monitoring to assure the safety of the public. Nurse administrators are expected to supervise and evaluate other professional nurses in their role performance. However, many school districts do not have nurse administrators. In addition, there may be collective bargaining constraints about who is able to conduct the evaluation of members of the collective bargaining unit. In other words, it might be possible that only administrators are allowed to supervise and evaluate. More on this topic of school nurse evaluation is given in Chapter 11.

It is also important to consider licensing regulations. Some states specifically state in their nurse practice acts that the practice of nursing can be evaluated only by another professional nurse. In other words, only another nurse can determine the value of nursing practice provided by a professional nurse. This discrepancy (the lack of school nurse supervisors who are nurses and the need to be evaluated by another professional nurse) can be controversial. School nurses can address this issue proactively by informing their representatives in the educational system of any relevant legislation that defines the nature of evaluation for a professional nurse and seeking acceptable solutions. For instance, evaluation of the school nurse in the role of educator can be done by an educator who is evaluating the school nurse in terms of the components of professional practice as described by Danielson. That evaluator would need to be skilled and knowledgeable in the role of educator and the content area covered. However, it would be inappropriate for that same person to evaluate the clinical nursing practice of the school nurse in terms of assessing, diagnosing, planning, determining outcomes, implementing and evaluating school nursing practice if he or she is not a professional nurse. School districts might want to consider a cooperative relationship with a neighboring district to have school nurse supervisors from other districts contribute to the evaluation process of the school nurse in the role of educator, or to have another school nurse serve as a consultant on the evaluation team in order to provide the professional perspective required by some state regulations.

A final perceived issue related to the school nurse in the role of educator is expertise. Both the school nurse and the school system, which includes teachers, parents and administrators, may believe that "a nurse is a nurse and not a teacher." They may not recognize the contribution that a school nurse can and should make to the education and health of the school and community. They may not be aware of the educational background that the school nurse brings to the school setting, including an understanding of educational principles, supervised practice in the role of educator, and an appreciation for the components of professional teaching practice. It is up to the school nurse to advocate to be able to function in the role of educator both as mandated by professional standards of practice and health goals. School nurses who lack the expertise in the role of the school nurse as educator can seek supervised experiences or course work in the foundations of education and teaching strategies to help develop the skills and confidence to implement this role with expertise.

References

American Cancer Society, Inc. (1995). *National health education standards.* Atlanta, GA: American Cancer Society, Inc. (95-50M-No. 2027).

American Federation of Teachers (AFT). (2004). *Mission statement.* Washington, DC: American Federation of Teachers, AFL-CIO. Retrieved August 2, 2004 from http://www.aft.org/about

American Nurses Association (ANA). (2003). *Nursing: Scope and standards of practice.* Washington, DC: Author.

American Nurses Association (ANA). (2004). *Scope and standards for nurse administrators* (2nd ed.). Washington, DC: Author.

Centers for Disease Control and Prevention (CDC). (1994). *The essential public health services.*

Atlanta, GA: Centers for Disease Control and Prevention. Retrieved August 2, 2004 from http://www.phppo.cdc.gov/nphpsp/10EssentialPHServices.asp

Danielson, C. (1996). *Enhancing professional practice: A framework for teaching.* Alexandria, VA: Association for Supervision and Curriculum Development.

Danielson, C., & McGreal, T. (2002). *Teacher evaluation to enhance professional practice.* Princeton, NJ: Educational Testing Service.

Educational Testing Services. (2004). *The Praxis series: Professional assessments for beginning teachers®.* Princeton, NJ: Author. Retrieved on August 2, 2004 from http://www.ets.org/praxis/index.html

Millennium Project. (2000). *Millennium development compact in human development goals—A compact among nations to end human poverty.* United Nations. Retrieved August 2, 2004 from http://www.unmillenniumproject.org/documents/MDC.pdf

National Association of School Nurses (NASN) & American Nurses Association (ANA). (2001). *Scope and standards of professional school nursing practice.* Washington, DC: Author.

National Board for Professional Teaching Standards (NBPTS). (2002). *What teachers should know and be able to do: The five core propositions of the national board.* Arlington, VA: Author. Retrieved August 2, 2004 from (http://www.nbpts.org/about/coreprops.cfm#knowdo)

National Commission on Teaching and America's Future (NCTAF). (1996). *What matters most: Teaching for America's future.* Washington, DC: Author. Retrieved on August 2, 2004 from http://www.nctaf.org/article/?c=4&sc=42

National Council for Accreditation of Teacher Education (NCATE). (2004). *Standards.* Washington, DC: Author. Retrieved on August 2, 2004 from http://www.ncate.org/ncate/m_ncate.htm

National Education Association (NEA). (2002). *About NEA: What is the National Education Association?* Washington, DC: Author. Retrieved August 2, 2004 from http://www.nea.org/aboutnea.html

National Education Goals Panel. (2002). *Building a nation of learners: Goals.* Washington, DC: Author. Retrieved August 2, 2004 from http://www.negp.gov/

U.S. Department of Education (USDOE). (2002). *Strategic plan 2002–2007.* Washington, DC: U.S. Department of Education. Retrieved August 2, 2004 from http://www.ed.gov/about/reports/strat/plan2002-07/plan.pdf

U.S. Department of Health and Human Services (USDHHS). (2000). *Healthy People 2010: Understanding and improving health* (2nd ed.). Washington, DC: U.S. Government Printing Office.

Wenlinsky, H. (2000). *How teaching matters: Bringing the classroom back into discussions of teacher quality.* Princeton, NJ: Policy Information Center, Educational Testing Service and Milken Family Foundation. Retrieved August 2, 2004 from http://www.ets.org/research/pic/teamat.pdf

Whitehurst, G. (2002). *Research on teacher preparation and professional development.* White House Conference on Preparing Tomorrow's Teachers. Washington, DC: U.S. Department of Education. Retrieved on August 2, 2004 from http://www.ed.gov/admins/tchrqual/learn/preparingteachersconference/whitehurst.html

World Health Organization (WHO). (2003). *Global school health initiative.* Geneva: WHO. Retrieved August 2, 2004 from http://www.who.int/school_youth_health/gshi/en/

Chapter 8

The School Nurse's Role Related to Research

JUDITH VESSEY

Chapter Outline

INTRODUCTION

School Nursing Research is the systematic investigation and application of knowledge to improve the health of students while fostering school nursing practice. Research uses the process of scientific inquiry to answer questions and solve problems. Generating new knowledge, however, is only the beginning. Disseminating and using school nursing research findings helps demonstrate that school nursing practice is accountable, clinically efficacious, and cost-effective. In today's educational arena, community leaders, legislators, and parents are concerned about student academic performance, school safety, and fiscal responsibility. These concerns have led to calls for improved educational accountability. For school nurses to be seen as a requisite, integral part of the education system, they must show that school nursing makes a difference in students' academic performance. Moreover, evidence-based practice helps ensure that students receive the best possible care, and that school nurses contain costs and demonstrate the clinical efficacy of school nursing practice (Denehy, 2003; Hootman, 2002).

The National Association of School Nurses (NASN) recognizes this challenge and seeks to advance the delivery of professional school health services to promote optimal student learning through initiating, supporting, participating in, and utilizing outcome-based research that validates school nursing practice. Two marks of a profession are its research scholarship and the way its members use the evidence of scholarship to shape its practice. Together these help define a profession's area of expertise and its contributions to society. Research scholarship involves three tasks: generation, dissemination, and utilization of knowledge.

Conducting research and implementing research findings into practice are not easy tasks;

research activities are resource-intensive processes. Adequate personnel, expertise, money, time, and access to students are necessary to successfully complete a single study. School nursing research, however, can be advanced through an individual's specific interests and through creative partnerships with others. This chapter provides a brief overview of the trajectory of research activities and includes models for conducting research projects in school settings.

OVERVIEW OF RESEARCH ACTIVITIES

The research trajectory involves three basic steps: the discovery of knowledge through the conduct of research studies, dissemination of that knowledge to professionals and interested public, and the utilization of new knowledge by practitioners in the clinical arena. Each of these activities is performed in concert with the others. Conducting research generates new knowledge, while the dissemination and utilization of that knowledge provide the foundation for evidence-based practice. Although the scope of this chapter does not permit a thorough explication of these diverse research activities, a brief description of each is provided. A list of selected texts that provide detailed information about the various steps of the research process can be found in Box 8.1.

Box 8.1 ■ ■ ■

RESEARCH AND REFERENCES

The books listed below are all used as undergraduate and/or graduate texts for research courses. Several authors (e.g., Burns & Grove, 2002; Polit & Beck, 2003) offer study guides as well. Texts and their accompanying study guides provide an excellent introduction to research and are suitable for self-study or to use as a reference. Consulting university faculty and/or reading book reviews in nursing research journals and less formal reviews published on Amazon.com and other Internet sites will help individuals determine the appropriate text to meet their needs.

Critiquing Research

Burns, N., & Grove, S. K. (2002). *Understanding nursing research* (3rd ed.). Philadelphia: W. B. Saunders.

Burns, N., & Grove, S. K. (2002). *A study guide for understanding nursing research* (3rd ed.). Philadelphia: W. B. Saunders.

Fain, J. A. (2004). *Reading, understanding, and applying nursing research* (2nd ed). Philadelphia: F. A. Davis.

Girden, E. R. (2001). *Evaluating research articles from start to finish* (2nd ed.). Thousand Oaks, CA: Sage Publications.

Conducting Research

Burns, N. (2001). *The practice of nursing research: Conduct, critique & utilization* (4th ed.). Philadelphia: W. B. Saunders.

Polit, D. F., & Beck, C. T. (2003). *Nursing research. Principles and methods* (7th ed.). Philadelphia: Lippincott, Williams, & Wilkins.

Polit, D. F., & Beck, C. T. (2004). *Nursing research. Principles and methods: A study guide* (7th ed.). Philadelphia: Lippincott, Williams, & Wilkins.

Data Analysis

Munro, B. (2005). *Statistical methods for healthcare research* (5th ed.). Philadelphia: Lippincott, Williams, & Wilkins.

Presenting Research

Garson, A., Gutgesell, H. P., Pinsky, W. W., & McNamara, D. G. (1986). The 10-minute talk: Organization, slides, writing, and delivery. *American Heart Journal, 111,* 193–203.

Discovering New Knowledge

There is an unlimited potential and need for school-based nursing studies. The majority of healthcare practices are not evidence based; it is estimated that no more than 20% of all medical practice is supported by evidence (Kongstvedt, 2001) and considerably less research has been done to identify "best practices" in nursing. This requires that school nurses demonstrate what they do, how they do it, and how it helps keep students healthy and available for learning.

Types of Research

Even if school nurses do not have any plans to conduct a study, they will be using research evidence in their practices. Being able to identify a study's research methodology is the first step to critiquing it. Research is classified in a number of different ways, such as by the type of method used, or whether an intervention was tested. The most common types of research methodologies are briefly described below.

Qualitative and Quantitative Research: Studies may be labeled "qualitative" or "quantitative" depending on the types of data collected and the analytic techniques employed. In *qualitative research,* the goal is to discover important underlying dimensions of a phenomenon or patterns among its relationships with other phenomena. Knowledge is generated by using methods of inquiry, such as in-depth unstructured interviews or serial observations. Such techniques emphasize the meaning of the experience for the individual. Narrative (nonnumeric) data are then subjectively interpreted using a set of rules for the specific qualitative methodology used. Qualitative methods often used by nurse researchers include case studies, ethnographies, phenomenology, or historical research. Almost all qualitative research is *nonexperimental* (see below). An example of qualitative research can be found in Box 8.2.

Quantitative Research: Quantitative research seeks to generate knowledge using highly structured investigative approaches that rely on the statistical analysis of empirical (numerical) data. In quantitative research, this includes data that are already numbers, such as heights, weights, or body mass indexes (BMIs). It also includes data that are collected in such a way that they can be labeled numerically, such as survey item choices that are labeled never (0), sometimes (1), or always (2). These numerical data can then be manipulated statistically to describe relationships of interest. Certain decisions about the phenomena of interest are made prior to constructing a questionnaire or designing an experiment. While virtually all experimental research is quantitative, some types of nonexperimental research, such as surveys or evaluation studies, also use quantitative techniques. Examples of specific types of quantitative research may be found in Boxes 8.3, 8.4, and 8.5.

Traditionally, studies have used a single methodology. However, many current studies use *mixed methods*—a combination of qualitative and quantitative approaches. Mixed methodologies allow investigators to better answer the research question. For example, a comparison of health visits of cheerleaders and football players provides information about

Box 8.2 ■■■

ABSTRACT OF A QUALITATIVE STUDY

Kelly, M., McCarthy, A., & Mordhorst. M. (2003). School nurses' experience with medication administration. *The Journal of School Nursing, 19*(5), 281–287.

Purpose: To report school nurses' experiences with medication administration

Design: A qualitative analysis of written surveys and focus groups

Sample: Random sample of written comments from 649 NASN members who completed a survey on medication administration

Method: A qualitative analysis was conducted on the eight survey items that had the most written comments. In order to clarify information obtained from the survey, two focus groups with local school nurses were conducted. A constant comparative method of analysis was used. Six categories of concern emerged: delegation of medication administration, comfort with delegation, self-administration of medication, medication administration errors, storage of medication and administration policies.

Results: The findings suggest that school nurses across the country have similar concerns regarding the administration of medications in the school setting.

Conclusion: Considering that 4% to 6% of children receive medication at school during a typical day, many concerns are emerging and prompting schools to change their policies regarding medication administration. Results from this nationwide survey describe a conjunction of circumstances that lead to professional unease and the potential for medication errors. These findings suggest a significant unmet need for access to health-care services in schools with only 2-day/week nurses. School nurses may be able to use this study to advocate for increasing the number of school nurses in their school district.

Box 8.3 ■■■

ABSTRACT OF A DESCRIPTIVE QUANTITATIVE STUDY

Lohse, J. (2003). A bicycle safety education program for parents of young children. *The Journal of School Nursing, 19*(2), 100–110.

Purpose: To examine the parental perceptions of the benefits and barriers to bicycle helmet use and their level of knowledge about bicycle safety issues.

Design: A quasi-experimental design. Pender's Health Promotion Model was used as the theoretical framework.

Sample: Parents of first and second grade students in three elementary schools. Two-hundred and fifty-one Bicycle Helmet Questionnaires were returned and used in the study

Method: The instrument used was the Bicycle Helmet Questionnaire (BHQ). The first 15 questions included demographic data and general bicycle helmet information, questions 16–21 focused on parental perceptions of the barriers and benefits of helmet use, questions 23–27 examined parental safety knowledge, and the last question determined parental support for helmet legislation. In addition, a bicycle safety program was taught in two of the elementary schools prior to the distribution of the BHQ. The BHQ from those two schools was then compared to the third school that did not receive any education prior to completing the survey.

Results: The study determined that parents of children in schools that received the education intervention prior to completing the questionnaire had significantly higher knowledge level scores and were in favor of helmet legislation for children.

Conclusion: This statistic in conjunction with the results from this study indicate the importance of a bicycle safety education intervention as well as the need for legislation.

Box 8.4 ■■■

ABSTRACT OF A CORRELATIONAL QUANTITATIVE STUDY

Lenz, B. (2003). Correlates of young adult tobacco use: Application of a transition framework. *The Journal of School Nursing, 19*(4), 232–237.

Purpose: To identify factors to serve as targets for anticipatory guidance prior to high school graduation to reduce tobacco initiation among young adults after graduation.

Design: Secondary analysis of cross-sectional sample

Sample: Two hundred and three randomly selected freshmen and sophomore students at a major Midwestern university

Method: A survey was completed by the students that included questions about tobacco use, drug use, mental health issues, stress, smoking, environment, and other lifestyle choices.

Results: The study found that students who used marijuana and alcohol were more likely to use tobacco. Implications for the importance of starting health promotion programs at the high school level were also drawn from this study.

Conclusion: Anticipatory guidance has traditionally been used throughout the nursing profession to help people during times of transition. During this period of instability and vulnerability between high school and young adulthood, anticipatory guidance can have a significant impact.

the type and number of injuries whereas interviews with injured athletes will provide information about why the injuries are occurring.

Nonexperimental versus Experimental Research: Nonexperimental research primarily differs from experimental research based on how much the data are manipulated. In *nonexperimental research,* the researcher collects and interprets data about the natural state of affairs. The researcher does not introduce or seek to measure the effects of an intervention (Polit & Beck, 2003) and has little control over a study's variables.[1] Nonexperimental quantitative research, such as surveys or questionnaires,

[1]A *variable* is a characteristic or attribute of a person or object that varies (Polit & Beck, 2003).

Box 8.5 ■ ■ ■

ABSTRACT OF A QUANTITATIVE EXPERIMENTAL INTERVENTION STUDY

Telljohann, S., Price, J., Dake, J., & Durgin, J. (2004). Access to school health services: Difference between full-time and part-time school nurses. *The Journal of School Nursing, 20*(3), 176–181.

Purpose: To compare the number of student visits to the school nurse for health reasons and the number of nurse-led classroom health education activities to whether the school nurse was part time (2 days/week) or full time (5 days/week).

Design: Quasi-experimental

Sample: A stratified random sample of schools from an inner city school district in a large Midwestern city; seven schools with 5-day/week nurses and seven schools with 2-day/week were used.

Method: The 14 school nurses participating in this study were asked to track the number of student visits for an entire academic year by using a form developed by the director of health services for the district. This assessed both the number and type (30 types of visits/health services were identified) of student visits. Independent sample t tests were then conducted on the demographic and background variables for the school in the 5 day/week nurse group vs. those in the 2 day/week group.

Results: Of the 30 health conditions/activities investigated, 28 were statistically significantly higher with full-time school nurses than part-time school nurses. It was hypothesized that 5-day/week nurses would be involved in health service activities 2.5 times as often as the 2-day/week nurse. However, this study found that 21 of the 30 health service activities in schools with 5-day/week nurses were accessed by students more often than the expected 2.5 times.

is by far the most common type conducted by school nurses. There are several reasons for this. First, sufficient data exist to analyze. Second, a number of variables in which researchers are interested cannot be manipulated (i.e., age, gender, socioeconomic status). Third, it may be impractical or unethical to conduct an intervention study. Two common types of nonexperimental research are descriptive and correlational.

Descriptive research seeks to systematically describe aspects of individuals, groups, or situations and the frequency with which they occur. No attempt is made to explain or predict how the circumstances may change in the future (Fain, 2004). Two examples would be tracking incomplete immunization records or describing patterns of absenteeism. Surveys, interviews, questionnaires, and observations are common methods used in descriptive research. A sample abstract of a descriptive study can be found in Box 8.3.

Correlational research examines interrelationships between and among identified variables (Fain, 2004). A correlation coefficient, the statistical index that describes the strength of the relationship, and whether that relationship is positive or negative, is calculated. No active interventions occur at the time of study. Although information from correlational research is helpful in explaining phenomena, it can never be used to assume a cause-and-effect relationship. An example of correlational research includes determining whether school absenteeism is correlated with teasing in school-age youths. Even if a positive relationship is demonstrated, there is not enough to say that one caused the other. A sample abstract of a correlational study can be found in Box 8.4.

Nonexperimental research is also classified by different time dimensions. *Prospective research* examines data collected in the present (e.g., class surveys) while *retrospective research,* uses previously collected data (e.g., health records). Although retrospective data are readily available, these data are rarely as good as prospective data because the researcher has not had any control over how the data were collected or how the variables were identified and defined.

Intervention or Experimental Research: *Intervention or experimental research* is used when an investigator seeks to test the effect of a new procedure or intervention, such as whether an asthma education program administered by a school nurse results in better student adherence to their medication regimens. Unlike nonexperimental research, the researcher is an active participant in intervention studies rather than a passive observer (Polit & Beck, 2003). Hunches and ideas are refined into measurable hypotheses and then tested using the scientific method.

Characteristics of experimental research are threefold. First, the investigator does something to, or for, a group of participants. This process is referred to as manipulation. Second, the experimenter uses a control group. This group of subjects does not receive the intervention. This allows the investigator to evaluate the effectiveness of the intervention by measuring the differences in outcomes between the groups receiving and not receiving the intervention. Third, the experimenter assigns participants to intervention or control groups randomly or without systematic bias. There are many different designs that can be used for conducting intervention research; they vary in their rigor according to the attention each gives to the three fundamental characteristics—manipulation, control, and randomization. A sample abstract from an intervention study can be found in Box 8.5.

Needs Assessments and Evaluation Research: Two research methods commonly used by school nurses are *needs assessments,* or studies that collect data about the needs of a group, and *evaluation research* that determines how well a program or policy works. School nurses often perform a needs assessment when contemplating a new program or evaluation research to assess the success of an ongoing program. They also frequently participate in larger school district needs assessment or evaluation projects. Performing quality needs assessments or evaluation research is difficult but is an important skill for school nurses as such studies help validate school nursing.

The Research Process

Regardless of the type of research being conducted, all studies use a similar scientific process. The research process is a way of thinking about the phenomena of interest. It consists of a series of decisions and related activities that help investigators refine their initial hunch into a measurable question or hypothesis allowing for formal testing and analysis. The research process, depicted in FIGURE 8.1, is a dynamic one; researchers often move back and forth between the two steps as they construct and implement their project. Many researchers, for example, alter their initial question based on information discovered during the literature review, or search for additional literature support when designing the study's methodology.

Step 1: Identifying the Question/Defining the Problem. The investigator(s) first must select the area in which they are interested in studying. There is no shortage of questions. School nurses encounter clinical questions every day that beg to be investigated, such as: What are common asthma triggers in the classroom? or Does the school lunch program contribute to student obesity? Multiple sources provide guidance for potential areas of research in the school setting. Some NASN priority areas include the impact of nursing interventions on students'

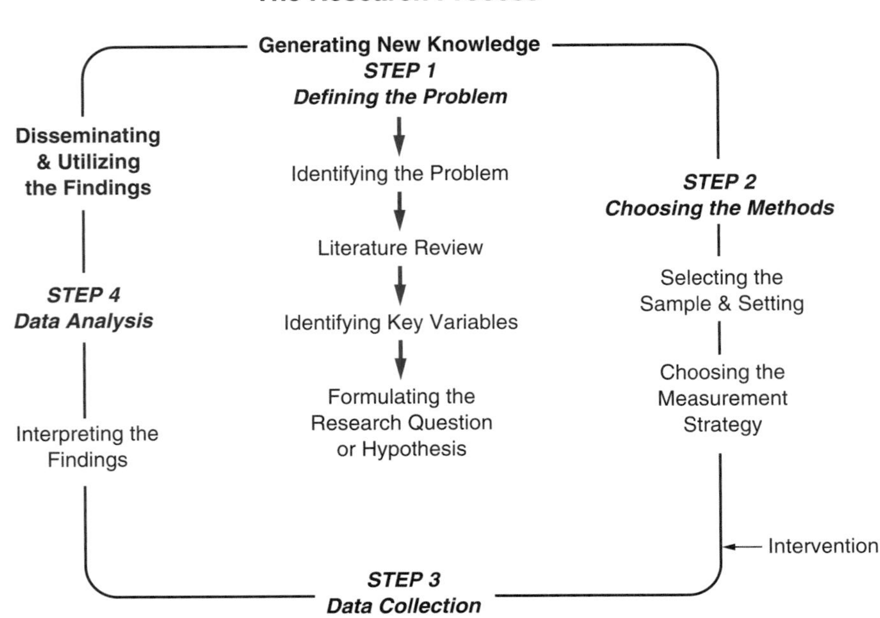

Figure 8.1 ■ The research process. (©Vessey, 2004, with permission.)

Box 8.6 ▪▪▪

A RESEARCH AGENDA FOR SCHOOL NURSING

Rank	Research Issue
1	Impact of school nurse services on student health
2	Relationship between school nurse practice and educational outcomes
3	Benefits and cost effectiveness of school health services
4	Value of school health services to the educational system
5	Predictors of outcomes for students, including special needs students
6	Nursing interventions for mental health promotion
7	Characteristics of successful school nurse interventions
8	Prevention and interventions for children with chronic diseases
9	Core elements of school nursing practice
10	Nursing interventions in violence and substance abuse prevention

From: Edwards, L. H. (2002). Research priorities in school nursing: A Delphi process. *Journal of School Nursing, 18,* 157–162.

management of their chronic conditions and on mental health issues of students and staff. The National Nursing Coalition for School Health, through the use of the Delphi Process with school nursing leaders, identified and agreed upon an agenda of school nursing research priorities; these can be found in Box 8.6 (Edwards, 2002). Using the eight components of the coordinated school health model (Chapter 3) is another avenue for identifying questions of specific interest to school nursing. Sample questions related to school absenteeism and academic performance are provided in Box 8.7. Finally, another source of questions or problems can be found in the *Healthy People 2010* (http://www.healthypeople.gov) specific objectives relevant to school health.

After determining the area of interest, the investigators carefully review the published literature to orient themselves to what is known about the topic of interest. The literature review also informs the researcher whether the problem has been studied before, and if so, when, where,

Box 8.7 ▪▪▪

AREAS OF STUDY AND SAMPLE RESEARCH QUESTIONS SPECIFIC TO REDUCING ABSENTEEISM AND/OR BETTER ACADEMIC PERFORMANCE USING THE COORDINATED SCHOOL HEALTH MODEL

Healthcare Services

- Does intensive, in-school management of students' asthma result in fewer exacerbations, less absenteeism, and better academic performance?

Health Education

- Do overweight students who successfully participate in weight reduction programs demonstrate improved academic performance?

Safety

- Do video cameras in school buses reduce harassment and related absenteeism?

Counseling

- In children with chronic illnesses, does proactive, in-school counseling improve therapeutic adherence and decrease disease flare-ups?

Nutrition

- When students participate in the federal free/reduced breakfast program, do they report less psychosomatic illnesses than prior to their participation?

Physical Education

- Do youths who engage in daily physical education have less absenteeism due to illness?

Staff Wellness

- Does offering health monitoring services (e.g., blood pressure screening) reduce staff absenteeism?

Parent and Community Involvement

- What difference do free eyeglass programs sponsored by the Kiwanis Club and Wal-Mart make in the academic performance of needy children's learning?

and by whom. Information about previously used research approaches, variables selected, instruments employed, and design strengths and weaknesses can be gleaned. Lastly, reviewing the literature helps the investigators refine the research question.

The literature review can include articles indexed on on-line data bases (e.g., PubMed, CINAHL), government reports, and sources identified from bibliographies or reference lists of other published articles. Both data-based research and conceptually driven articles are noted. Literature may be drawn from nursing research and specialty nursing literature, theoretical works (e.g., Piaget), methodological sources (e.g., research textbooks), and databased articles from related disciplines. The literature can be retrieved from the Web, university libraries, or inter-library loan.

After collecting the literature, each reference is screened for its relevance to the area of interest. By reading the title and abstract and scanning for key words, the researcher selects those citations that are useful for refining the research question and study methodology. Theoretical literature provides a conceptual foundation for the study; methodological sources help determine an appropriate methodology for the study; and data based, content-specific articles inform the researchers as to what has previously been done. The information from key articles is critiqued as to its quality and its contribution to the phenomena of interest.

From the literature review, the researcher(s) are able to identify the key variables. These are used in formulating the research question or hypothesis. The research question is "a concise, interrogative statement that is written in the present tense and includes one or more concepts (variables)" (Fain, 2004, p. 95). A hypothesis is a statement that predicts the expected relationship among the variables. Hypotheses take different forms and are categorized as simple or complex, non-directional or directional, and research or statistical. A standard format that is described in any research text is used for constructing hypotheses and including the variables to be examined, their expected relationships with each other, and the measures used.

Step 2: Designing the Methodology. A study's methodology is partially determined by whether the research seeks to identify or describe a phenomenon or to predict what will happen in response to selected interventions. For example, if the researcher wanted to determine (i.e., identify) whether obesity is a problem in the district's elementary school population, the school nurse would conduct a descriptive study, collecting and analyzing BMIs for the entire student body and noting the percentage that were above recommended cut-offs. To better describe the characteristics of students who were overweight, the school nurse could correlate the students' BMI scores with information about race/ethnicity, socioeconomic status, and/or participation in various extracurricular activities. The choice of which variables should be correlated is based on the literature review or clinical observation. If, however, the school nurse wanted to predict whether the weight of obese youths could be reduced, she could track students' BMIs prior to and after eliminating "junk food" in the cafeteria and vending machines. Numerous possibilities of methodologies can be employed, depending on the research question. Each methodology has different rules regarding sample size, instrumentation, and analyses.

Phase 3: Data Collection. Data collection refers to the gathering of information needed to address the research question (Polit & Beck, 2003). It is structured according to the research question, the methods, and numerous situational variables. It generally follows a specific, carefully defined plan. A variety of approaches can be used to collect the data depending on the study's objectives and selected methodology. Behavioral data may be collected through observation or self-report, psychological data may be collected using valid and reliable scales or questionnaires, and biophysical data may be collected using instrumentation ranging from electronic sphygmomanometers to complex biochemical analyses. Whenever possible, instruments that have established reliability and validity appropriate for the study participants should be selected over ones that are investigator-derived.

A second important component of data collection is accessing subjects in an appropriate and ethical fashion. First and foremost, this requires that the study has been reviewed and approved by the appropriate ethics committee or Institutional Review Board (IRB). In part, the IRB will ensure that the research addresses all HIPAA and FERPA regulations (see Chapter 13). IRB approval is required for all federally funded research and by many other entities that sponsor research; regardless of whether IRB approval is mandated, it is always an excellent idea as it protects the rights of students. If there is no access to an IRB, at the very least, signed approval for the study by school administrators is required.

After IRB approval is given, informed consent is collected from all participants prior to data collection. There are several key elements of informed consent. Participants, and for most school-based studies this includes students and their parents, must be told about the study both orally and in writing and in a fashion that they will understand (i.e., written at a low enough reading level) and participation must be voluntary (i.e., students can never be forced to participate) (Polit & Beck, 2003). Information about the study includes what will be done, by whom, the amount of time involved, any real or potential risks or benefits, whether there is any compensation, and that the participant may withdraw at any time without penalty. Questions about the study are then addressed. Parents are asked to sign a consent form and students can agree verbally, sign assent on the same form as their parents, or sign a separate, simplified assent form, depending on an IRB's determination as to the most appropriate method. The individual collecting the consent then witnesses the form. Obtaining informed consent should never be taken lightly. Because students are considered a vulnerable population and their rights must be protected, and because ethical considerations may affect the study design, it is important to consider them from the study's inception.

Equally important but seemingly more mundane in the data collection process is ensuring that the data are collected in the purest way possible. Potential problems range from not planning for alternative testing days in case of snow, to having broadcast announcements interfere with focus group taping (Horowitz et al., 2003). The school nurse is instrumental in helping to identify potential problems so that they may be addressed prior to data collection.

Phase 4: Analyzing the Results. The first step in data analysis is to enter the data into the appropriate software package. Computer software packages exist for both qualitative and quantitative data. Making sure that the database is as error free as possible, the data are analyzed according to the plan determined in the study's methodology. For quantitative studies, descriptive statistics are calculated to organize, summarize, and describe the data. Inferential statistics are then used to allow the investigator to infer as to the likelihood that the relationship found in the study sample is the same as in the larger population. In qualitative analysis, there are few universally accepted analytic procedures. However, the goal is to synthesize the large amounts of narrative data so that general conclusions can be drawn around the research question.

Phase 5: Disseminating and Utilizing Research Findings. The last step of the research process is to share the study's results with interested constituencies. This includes the professional nursing community, school administrators, and students and their parents. The dissemination and utilization of knowledge comprise the second and third parts of the research tripartite.

Disseminating New Knowledge

Research findings are disseminated to professional colleagues through two major portals—publications and presentations. The "gold standard" is to publish a databased article in a refereed publication such as the *Journal of School Nursing.* This way, the largest intended audience is reached with the study's results and findings are available to anyone reviewing the literature at any point in time. Because all manuscripts are initially critiqued by experts in the area prior to being accepted, publishing in a refereed journal denotes the quality of the study. Each journal has its own submission process and author guidelines. Researchers are advised to go online to the journals' websites to obtain this information and follow it carefully when drafting their manuscripts. For example, the author guidelines for the *Journal of School Nursing* can be found at: http://www.nasn.org/josn/authorguides.htm.

Research findings also may be conveyed in podium or poster presentations at national professional conferences. Generally, investigators submit an abstract that is peer-reviewed by a panel of experts. Investigators whose research studies or research utilization projects are deemed appropriate, both in their rigor and salience to the conference audience, will be asked to present.

Podium Presentations

Research presentations are generally short, only 10 to 15 minutes in length, so it is important to be as concise and organized as possible. The best presentations begin with a well-written abstract that serves as the outline for the presentation. The presentation follows a standard format: introduction, study purpose and significance, methodology, results, summary and conclusions, and recommendations for further study and/or implementation of results (Garson, Gutgesell, Pinsky, & McNamara, 1986)

PowerPoint presentations are used in most research presentations and these slides may be prepared into a handout for the audience. When preparing PowerPoint slides, they should be specific to the content being presented. Generally, the allotted time is one slide per minute. Data displayed by graphs and charts are helpful in presenting results to participants. Some suggestions for preparing PowerPoint slides can be found in Box 8.8.

For an effective delivery and to stay within the allotted time constraints, the presenter should rehearse the presentation. Immediately prior to the presentation, inspect the facility. Check out the placement of the podium and its relationship to the screen, type of microphone and audio–visual equipment, and how to adjust the lighting. Lastly, introduce yourself to the session convener and the audio–visual support personnel. Thorough preparation will help ensure that the research results are conveyed as effectively as possible.

Box 8.8 ■ ■ ■

POWERPOINT SLIDE PRESENTATION SUGGESTIONS

Text

- Give each slide a title.
- Follow the Golden Rule: no more than seven lines, seven words wide per slide.
- Use key words only.
- Make sure each slide contains an independent thought.

Design

- Use no more than two different fonts.
- Use upper- and lowercase letters.
- Use color, highlights, underlining, borders, and slide transition features judiciously.
- Use symbols and graphs wherever appropriate.
- Highlight major points—use bullets rather than numbers.
- Avoid overuse of abbreviations.

Presentation Layout

- Introduction (1–2 slides): "What made me think of this?"
- Study purpose and significance (1–2 slides): "Why did I do it?"
- Methodology (2–4 slides): "How I did it"
- Results (2–4 slides): "What I found out"
- Summary and conclusions (1–3 slides): "What I learned" and "What it means"
- Recommendations (1 slide)

Poster Presentations

Posters provide a concise presentation of the most pertinent information about a study. This medium also allows presenters to directly interact with interested parties. When preparing your poster, it is important to first ascertain the type and size of the display area. Although most venues will provide boards, some require freestanding posters to be used on table tops. The dimensions of the presentation area also vary. "Landscape" layouts are usually used in the United States whereas "portrait" layouts are used in most other countries.

Consultation with a graphic designer or educational media specialist is useful in conceptualizing how key information can be presented in a unified style. The total message needs to communicate the study's major points clearly and logically. Major message pieces include the research objectives/questions, significance, methodology, results, conclusions, implications, and key references. Pictorial and graphic illustrations are useful in clarifying the message. The reader should be able to grasp the key content in approximately five minutes and the text needs to be readable from approximately six feet (Van Hoozer, Mitchell, & Shaw, 1993). Design your poster so that it is readily portable and always come prepared with the necessary implements for displaying the poster. Because the exhibiting surfaces vary, the presenter should bring a small tack hammer, push pins, thumbtacks, double-sided tape, and Velcro with adhesive backing.

Posters are generally mounted for a full day of display with a scheduled session when the presenter is in attendance. The presenter then stands directly next to the poster to readily engage in direct dialog with interested parties, addressing issues and questions of importance to each. One advantage of a poster presentation is that it can be reused to communicate information about the study to additional groups.

Regardless of the form, however, research findings need to be disseminated to other school nurses, the school district's administration, the local school board, school staff, parents, and/or the student body. Relevant information can be presented at local and state school board and home and school association meetings or student assemblies, emphasizing the specific constituency's role in the research project. An overview of the study can also be published in school newsletters or the local newspaper. Not only will this keep key constituencies informed, it will help with "buy-in" for utilizing research findings.

Utilizing Knowledge

Research utilization is the third major step in the research trajectory. Although the purpose of conducting research studies is to generate knowledge that will improve nursing practice, it is often a decade or more before research findings are operationalized in the clinical arena (King, as cited in Bock, 1990). Research utilization helps bridge this research-practice gap. *Research utilization* refers to the successful transference of practice-based research knowledge into evidence-based clinical practice. It requires that a series of thematic studies be critiqued for their veracity and pragmatic utility for clinical innovation. The body of knowledge is then synthesized into a single conceptual area and evidence-based protocols are then derived. Personnel are educated, the protocol is operationalized, and its success is evaluated. If necessary, replication studies in the school setting can be conducted. Specific steps in completing a research utilization project are listed in Box 8.9.

Research utilization is both an individual and organizational responsibility (Melnyk, 2002). Utilization of knowledge begins when school nurses read and critique research studies in a common area of interest. It helps them stay abreast of questions that are being asked about nursing and school health, innovations that are being tested, and the potential for applying reported findings to their practice setting. To accomplish this effectively, nurses need to know research terminology, understand the research process, be able to critique the appropriateness of studies for their setting, and have the authority to change practice. District or statewide projects may be the most feasible way to engage in these activities.

State school nurse consultants and professional organizational initiatives can help advance research utilization by actively endorsing and providing training and consultation on the research utilization process. Professional organizations and federal and state school health personnel can then use the research utilization process in developing evidence-based clinical guidelines. These guidelines, in turn, standardize practice decisions to improve the quality of school health services. As new research findings emerge, protocols can then be modified accordingly. Frequently, the research utilization process will lead to a new research question that needs investigation. Research utilization initiatives are most likely to be effective when the importance of a project is transparent to all participants. Developmental activities that can promote research utilization may be found in Table 8.1.

Box 8.9 ■■■

COMPLETING A RESEARCH UTILIZATION PROJECT

Step 1. Identify an area of concern.

Step 2. Assign responsibility for each phase of the project.

Step 3. Search the literature for relevant research reports.

Step 4. Collect and organize the data.

Step 5. Evaluate the evidence; examine the veracity of the studies and their clinical relevance for school nursing.

Step 6. If evidence is sufficient, design practice applications: policies, protocols, or guidelines for clinical care. (If evidence is insufficient, consider implementing a research study.)

Step 7. Identify expected outcomes after implementation and design evaluation tool.

Step 8. Provide in-service education to all involved parties.

Step 9. Monitor clinician adherence.

Step 10. Evaluate the project's effectiveness; use Continuous Quality improvement mechanism, if appropriate.

Step 11. Document the project's success.

Step 12. Disseminate the results of the project to local constituencies and interested professionals.

Step 13. Monitor implementation and determine the next steps.

MODELS FOR CONDUCTING RESEARCH PROJECTS

Depending on a study's complexity, a variety of models can facilitate research activities. Smaller, discrete studies may be executed by a single individual who has appropriate training while complex studies,

Table 8.1 ■

DEVELOPMENTAL ACTIVITIES FOR UTILIZING RESEARCH FINDINGS

AREA FOR DEVELOPMENT	INDIVIDUAL OR SMALL GROUP ACTIVITIES	ORGANIZATIONAL OR PROFESSIONAL ACTIVITIES
Awareness of Current Literature	Read articles independently. Participate in journal clubs. Learn literature search techniques.	Include in job description, career ladders. Make literature available. Publish selected critiques in newsletters. Sponsor online "grand rounds."
Educational Opportunities	Enroll in continuing education or formal research courses.	Offer continuing education courses, tuition remission. Provide release time.
Resources	Peer support Improve practice efficiency.	Arrange for consultation services. Improve standards of care.

such as those that are multisite, longitudinal, or use numerous sophisticated methodologies, are best done by a team with organizational support.

Simple, Discrete Projects

Simple, discrete projects are those that ask a single research question at one point in time and are limited to one school or school district. Examples would include surveying teachers' attitudes regarding asthmatic students carrying their own inhalers or evaluating what students know about the dangers of illicit substance use. Such projects are ideal for studies of limited scope such as surveys that examine questions relevant to the immediate constituency. For a single-site study to be successful, the school nurse must have the necessary skill sets (e.g., inquisitiveness, perseverance, research training) and resources (e.g., statistical software) to conduct research or access individuals who can support the endeavor. Many resources and supplies, such as secretarial support and copying and postage, may be in-kind contributions from the school. Larger school districts with a separate testing and evaluation division employ methodologists and statisticians who may be able to support a project. Because a small, quality research project requires almost as much planning as a larger one, partnering with other individuals or groups is often beneficial.

Collaborative Research Projects

Collaborative research endeavors of intradisciplinary or interdisciplinary groups have significant advantages over single venue studies but they are more difficult to implement. Ideally, such studies will be implemented by national or state professional organizations, state school nurse consultants, or school district leadership. No nurse can do this alone. But by capitalizing on the combination of experiential and knowledge expertise and resources of numerous participating sites, properly designed research using more diverse samples can result. Resulting data may be scrutinized and interpreted more thoroughly by individuals with differing backgrounds working together (Hootman, 2002). Ultimately, there is greater generalizability of the findings and the evidence is more valid for determining whether the clinical efficacy of nursing interventions is enhanced.

The Role of Professional Organizations

NASN recognizes the challenge to advance the delivery of professional school health services through initiating, supporting, participating in, and utilizing outcome-based research that validates school nursing practice as detailed in the *Scope and Standards of Professional School Nursing Practice* (NASN & ANA, 2001). To that end, NASN supports a small grants program, requires materials such as *Position Statements* and *Issue Briefs* to be data-based whenever possible, and identifies priorities for school-based research. NASN also partners with other organizations such as the American School Health Association and the American Public Health Association (Hootman, 2002). This coalition serves as the advisory board for the National Center for School Health Nursing which helps set the agenda for research needed in school health. NASN research priorities may be found at: http://www.nasn.org/resources/research.htm.

Many professional organizations such as the American Association of Critical Care Nurses and the Association of Women's Health, Obstetric, and Neonatal Nurses embrace collaborative, multisite research and research utilization projects as methods for more rapidly advancing nursing theory and evidence-based nursing practice (Bratt, 2000). Such multi-site studies ensure that questions important to an organization's constituency are asked and investigated. To date, NASN has not sponsored multi-site research studies that draw on the expertise of the membership, but may do so in the future.

Partnering with Academic Institutions, Professional Organizations, and Community Agencies

Partnerships between school nurses and academic researchers for conducting research are ideal ways of advancing the science related to school-based health care. Many collegiate schools of nursing routinely use schools for student clinical experiences with school nurses serving as preceptors. Ideally, this relationship can be extended to include research and other scholarly endeavors through joint projects of interest to both school nurses and nursing faculty. While school nurses may see the actual conduct of research as a daunting task, academic nurse researchers can be equally put off by the difficulty accessing students in schools.

Designing Successful Research Partnerships

Conducting quality studies requires organizational support, careful planning, attention to detail, forthrightly addressing partners' competing agendas, flexibility of the research team members, and a shared vision that research makes a difference in school health outcomes. Many good studies have faltered when these key factors have been ignored or underestimated. Studies that are mutually conceived and conducted with respect to each party's desires and needs are destined for better success.

First, a shared and sustained vision among participating agencies (e.g., professional organizations, colleges, school districts), the principal investigators, and other site participants as to the study's potential for contributing to the knowledge base of school nursing practice must be shared by all stakeholders. Discussions among potential research partners (i.e., school nurses and faculty) are needed to discern what potential research or evaluation projects are of interest to all parties. Beginning with a simple, straightforward yet meaningful study is more likely to lead to success. Yet even simple projects are likely to take several months. Multi-site projects should be avoided unless there is sufficient infrastructure; these are long-term endeavors that as are likely to be logistically complex and may take several years from conception to completion (Broome, 1999). Discussing a study's potential time line is important; school personnel need to understand the length of the study and when the various components are expected to be completed and who is responsible for each part. Partners must understand each others' positions about research, their skill sets, and the differences in their work milieus. Clear lines of communication are required. Designing the study's methodology should be a joint endeavor of the research team.

Each player's level of participation, whether as a co-investigator who is intimately involved in the study's conduct or as a primary support person, must be realistically determined prior to initiating the study. Because school nurses have intimate knowledge as to how their school operates, their input is invaluable during the study design phase. Information concerning administrators' attitudes toward research activities, the demographic composition of the student body, and other logistical factors (e.g., school schedule and calendar) are critically important in determining the appropriate sample characteristics and data collection methods. School nurses also can help determine the correct timing for formally approaching administrators and "selling" them on the study. As the insider, the school nurse can present the reasons as to why participating in this study is particularly salient to the mission of the school. For example, highlighting the benefits of implementing research on improving the identification of students who are bullies or being bullied reinforces that the school district is serious about their school safety campaign. Sometimes school policies help determine a school nurse's role. For example, a district may require having an "inside" investigator; the school nurse may serve as a co-investigator even though the day-to-day involvement with the study may be quite small.

Adequate resources must be available, as many methodologically fine studies have faltered when these have been underestimated. The necessary personnel, supplies, support services, and funding for all steps of the research project need to be in place. Support for appropriate research review and human subjects protections must be in place; ideally, the lead organization will have its own Institutional Review Board (IRB). If not, partnering with a university will ensure access to an IRB. Seeking approval of school administrators should be the minimum approval sought in the absence of an IRB.

Small grants from community groups or professional organizations such as the state school nurses association, local Sigma Theta Tau International chapter or the Junior League can help defray research expenses. Planning ahead for funding is important. Not only is there a several month timeline between the due date for applications and awarding grant monies, the processes are always competitive. Each granting agency has its own requirements. They range from requiring membership in a particular group to funding only novice researchers or research within a specific focus area. Start with small, local grants and build a successful track record before seeking large, national grants. When negotiating with external researchers, the school nurse needs to look for ways that both parties can benefit from the process. For example, the Lion's Club is interested in vision research while the local chapter of the American Heart Association would more likely fund obesity research. Budgetary issues require special consideration in multisite studies as each group of stakeholders needs to have their financial needs addressed.

Protocols for data ownership and reporting results need to be in place. Ownership conveys responsibility for disseminating the findings, being responsible for its long-term storage and security, and answering any questions about the research from participants or their families, the IRB, funding agencies, or school administrators. A formal dissemination plan should include clear authorship and presentation guidelines. Areas to be addressed are data rights and access, manuscript generation and clearance, abstract and presentation policies, and publicity information. In addition to professional publications and presentations, other research dissemination activities should be considered. For example, teachers can use selected data sets as a "real life" experience for teaching math or science. The possibilities are endless—restricted only by the imagination and willingness of the parties to work together (Vessey, 2002a).

Using Consultants

As healthcare professionals, school nurses frequently consult with specialists when children present with complex medical problems that are outside the school nurses' scope of practice. Similarly, school nurses who engage in research may benefit from the expertise of one or more consultants when designing and implementing a research study. The information garnered from consultants helps enrich the researcher's understanding of the phenomenon to be investigated by offering advice as to how to improve the study design or conduct statistical analyses. No one is an expert in all phases of the research process; virtually all investigators benefit from the advice of a consultant on selected aspects of a research project.

Ideally, consultants are consulted at the beginning of the project to ensure that the literature review is complete and the methodology is appropriate for the question to be asked, or troubleshoot for potential problems. For example, although drafting a questionnaire may seem deceptively simple, a bad design can significantly influence the validity of the results. Do the questions cover all of the major content areas of interest to the investigator? Are the questions asked in such a way that their intent is clear to the participant? If the survey uses multiple-choice responses, is the full range of responses included? Are items numbered in such a way that they facilitate data entry and analysis? Are open-ended questions appropriate for a study's sample size, or will the amount of data generated be too onerous to interpret? The more complex the study, the more potential pitfalls there are.

Unfortunately, some investigators may only seek consultation after a problem occurs. Sometimes a problem can be corrected or ameliorated, such as increasing the number of participants or using different statistical analyses in interpreting the data. However, sometimes a fatal flaw has occurred and little can be done to fix the problem. For example, forgetting to gather information about students' heights when evaluating students' risk for hypertension invalidates the data analysis. Studies that used measures where the instruments were developmentally or culturally inappropriate or the design so onerous that an inadequate number of subjects cannot be recruited are two such examples. Consultants who are most likely to be helpful to school nurses conducting research are:

- *The Librarian:* can instruct researchers in accessing on-line databases, identifying relevant literature, and obtaining articles.
- *A Content Expert:* knowledgeable about the work already done in the area; can help researchers identify relevant constructs to be examined and the studies that still need to be conducted.
- *A Methodologist:* helpful in designing the study, determining the necessary sample size, evaluating data collection tools, and designing an analytic plan.

- *A Statistician:* helpful in designing, conducting, and interpreting appropriate statistical analyses.
- *An Editor:* can edit drafts of manuscripts to help enhance the likelihood of their publication by a refereed professional journal.

School nurses may be able to access some or all of these individuals within the school district, neighboring universities, or the community. They may also be accessed via the Internet using national organizations for the condition being studied (i.e., the state chapter of the American Lung Association, NASN or the School Nurse Consultants group). The scope of the work and the consultants' interest in the project will determine the extent, if any, of consultant fees. If the consultants are invested in the project (e.g., an area of interest, having a child in the district, etc.), many will provide advice for free or for a nominal fee. Some consultant fees can range up to several hundred dollars per hour for complex projects. In such cases, it is imperative that the consultant's ability to provide the services be evaluated in the beginning. Good consultants, though, are worth the expense, and will likely save you time and money while enhancing the project's success in the long run.

PERSONAL RESPONSIBILITIES

One of NASN's core values is to support the "(c)ontinuous critical exploration and utilization of knowledge and involvement with the sustenance of a healthy learning environment" (http://www.nasn.org/about/aboutus.htm). This requires that all school nurses consider it their personal responsibility to proactively advance evidence-based practice in whatever way is appropriate for their backgrounds. Admittedly, everyone reading this chapter has a different level of research expertise and a different level of interest in research, but there are specific strategies in which all school nurses can engage. These include the following:

- *Learn to question.* Much of what school nurses do is based on tradition, intuition, or authority rather than on knowledge garnered through the scientific method. For some, it is easier to be "told what to do" rather than interpreting and employing new knowledge. In part, this is a reflection of school nurses' education since many have never had formal academic research training. For example, more than two thirds of nurses think that the statistics in research articles are not understandable (Funk, Champagne, Wiese, & Tornquist, 1991). Books such as *Statistics for dummies* (Rumsey, 2003), continuing education programs, or graduate school courses can help school nurses develop expertise in interpreting research evidence. Regardless of one's level of expertise, however, all school nurses need to question how they practice, question what school nursing knowledge is based on, and to think about what research evidence might improve it (see Boxes 8.6 and 8.7 for examples).
- *Critically read or learn about topics related to school health.* By reading the professional research and evidence-based clinical articles from nursing and related disciplines, school nurses can keep abreast of new knowledge such as pharmacological breakthroughs in asthma management, the replacement of standard height and weight measurements with BMI calculations for determining childhood obesity, or how the reauthorization of IDEA (Individuals with Disabilities in Education Act) will influence school nursing services to students with special healthcare needs. School nurses should also read lay articles or watch media coverage to know what healthcare information their constituencies are receiving. By doing so, school nurses can help debunk front page coverage of such topics as "the dangers of immunizations" and "herbal lice cures," substituting evidence-based findings whenever possible. Subscribing to a professional journal in addition to the *Journal of School Nursing* in an area of interest—such as asthma, violence prevention, or nutrition—helps increase a school nurse's area of expertise within a selected domain. Appropriate literature may also be reviewed through Web-based scanning subscriptions such as that offered for a nominal fee to members of Sigma Theta Tau International. Participating in a journal club with others interested in school health is a beneficial approach to critiquing the research literature in a given area. Attending nursing and interdisciplinary conferences also helps one keep current about school health information.
- *Ensure that school health policies and protocols are evidence-based and up-to-date.* All school health policies need to be reviewed and updated on a regular, planned schedule. The review schedule should be determined depending on how rapidly knowledge is

emerging in a given area. For example, immunization protocols should be reviewed at least once a year, while asthma protocols might be reviewed every two years and general first aid policies reviewed every three to five years. Reading recent position statements, policies, protocols, and guidelines that are released from NASN, state and federal agencies, and other professional groups will help keep school nurses abreast of new information and provide templates for policy and procedure development. Becoming Internet savvy also helps school nurses be aware of emerging evidence-based practices. The Web site http://www.guidelines.gov compiles the latest evidence from a variety of international professional health and medical organizations and federal agencies and has some guidelines, such as those on asthma, that would be useful for school nurses. Another not-for-profit organization that has updated evidence-based healthcare databases is the Cochrane Library (2005). Their systematic reviews may be useful for school nurses. Examples from their library are provided in Box 8.10.

Box 8.10 ■ ■ ■

SELECTED TITLES RELEVANT TO SCHOOL HEALTH IN *COCHRANE DATABASE OF SYSTEMATIC REVIEWS*

- Educational interventions for children with asthma (Wolf, Gueavara, & Grum et al.)
- Family therapy for asthma in children (Panton & Barley)
- Growth monitoring in children (Panpanich & Garner)
- Interventions for educating children who attended the emergency room for asthma (Haby, Waters, & Robertson)
- Interventions for treating head lice (Dodd)
- Interventions aimed at improving immunization rates (Szilagyi, Vann, & Bordley et al.)
- Interventions for treating obesity in children (Summerbell, Ashton, Campbell, Edmunds, Kelly, & Waters)
- Community-based interventions for the prevention of burns and scalds in children (Turner, Spinks, & McClure)
- School-based programs for preventing smoking (Thomas)
- Community interventions for preventing smoking in young people (Sowden, Arblaster, & Stead)
- Complex behavioral and educational interventions for nocturnal enuresis in children (Glazener, Evans, & Peto)
- Primary prevention for alcohol misuse in young people (Foxcroft, Ireland, & Lister-Sharp)
- Alarm interventions for nocturnal enuresis in children (Glazener, Evans, & Peto)
- Antibiotics for acute otitis media in children (Glasziou, Del Mar, & Sanders)
- Antibiotics for persistent nasal discharge (rhinosinusitis) in children (Morris & Leach)
- Exercise to improve self esteem in children and young people (Ekeland, Heian, & Hagen)
- Interventions for preventing eating disorders in children and adolescents (Pratt & Woolfenden)

Source: The Cochrane Library. (2005). Alphabetical list of the Cochane Reviews. Issue 2. Retrieved August 2005 from http://www.cochrane.org/cichrane/rerbstr/mainindex.htm

- *Share "the evidence" on topics of interest.* School personnel and parents benefit from being educated on research evidence that improves their ability to better serve students. Posting relevant articles on faculty and staff bulletin boards, editing a column in the school newsletter, and contributing to home and school meetings or staff in-services are all ways that interesting research findings may be conveyed to others. By having all constituencies educated, the willingness to participate in studies or adopt evidence into practice will be enhanced.
- *Join or support a research project team.* School nurses need to proactively facilitate school health research activities within their schools. They can help establish a supportive climate for research in their schools. School

nurses can take the initiative in approaching schools of nursing as to what role they might play in facilitating research studies. Helping researchers access school populations is important but bringing local knowledge concerning school operations and clinical expertise to the research team is invaluable. School nurses can help shape the research conducted in their schools to ensure that key questions address ways to improve school nursing practice. By formalizing their relationships with respective schools of nursing, other academic units, or community agencies, school nurses become aware of their research or evaluation interests. Studies that are mutually conceived are destined for better success. School nurses also can choose products that will be useful for potential research endeavors, even if the inception of a study is not imminent. For example, when selecting software vendors, products should be evaluated as to whether they have the capabilities for collecting data of interest, downloading data into basic statistical packages or spreadsheet software for analysis, and have sufficient security to meet the IRB subject protections standards (Vessey, 2002b). If active participation in research projects is not possible, school nurses can support research activities by donating to local or national nursing research foundations.

CONCLUSION

School nurses have the responsibility to ensure that their practice is as evidence-based as possible. This requires that they engage in all phases of the research process—knowledge generation, dissemination and utilization. While not all school nurses will actively participate in all phases of research processes all the time, all school nurses can adopt a positive attitude about the role research plays in ensuring that students receive the best possible care available and demonstrating the clinical efficacy of school nursing.

References

Bock, L. R. (1990). From research to utilization: Bridging the gap. *Nursing Management, 21,* 50–51.

Bratt, M. M. (2000). Collaborative institutional research. *Journal of Child and Family Nursing, 3,* 251–258.

Broome, M. (1999). Collaborative research: The art of negotiation. *Journal of Child and Family Nursing, 2*(1), 1–2.

Denehey, J. (2003). Developing a program of research in school nursing. *Journal of School Nursing, 19,* 125–126.

Edwards, L. H. (2002). Research priorities in school nursing: A Delphi process. *Journal of School Nursing,* 18, 157–162.

Fain, J. A. (2004). Reading, understanding, and applying nursing research (2nd ed). Philadelphia: F. A. Davis.

Funk, S. G., Champagne, M.T. Wiese, R. A., & Tornquist, E. M. (1991). Barriers to using research findings in practice: The clinician's perspective. *Applied Nursing Research, 4,* 90–95.

Garson, A., Gutgesell, H., Pinsky, W., & McNamara, D. (1986). The 10-minute talk: Organization, slides, writing, and delivery. *American Heart Journal, 111,* 193–201.

Hootman, J. (2002). The importance of research to school nurses and school nursing practice. *Journal of School Nursing,* 18, 18–24.

Horowitz, J. A., Vessey, J. A., Carlson, K. L., Bradley, J. F., Montoya, C., & McCullough, W. (2003). Conducting school-based focus groups: Lessons learned from the CATS Project. *Journal of Pediatric Nursing,* 18, 321–331.

Kongstvedt, P. R. (2001). *Essentials of managed health care* (4th ed.). Gaitersburg, MD: Aspen Publications.

Melnyk, B. M. (2002). Strategies for overcoming barriers in implementing evidence-based practice. *Pediatric Nursing, 28,* 159–161.

National Association of School Nurses (NASN) & the American Nurses Association (ANA). (2001). *Scope and standards of professional school nursing practice.* Washington, DC: American Nurses Publishing.

Polit, D. F., & Beck, C. T. (2003). *Nursing research. Principles and methods* (7th ed.). Philadelphia: Lippincott, Williams & Wilkins.

Rumsey, D. (2003). *Statistics for dummies.* Hoboken, N.J.: John Wiley & Sons.

The Cochrane Library. (2005). *Alphabetical list of titles of Cochrane Reviews.* Issue 2. Retrieved August 2005 from http://www.cochrane.org/cochrane.org/cochrane/revabstr/mainindex.htm

van Hoozer, H., Mitchell, S., & Shaw, C. L. (1993). The scientific "research" poster presentation. *Reflections, 19*(3), 34–35.

Vessey, J. A. (2002a). Partnering with schools of nursing to promote research. NASN *Newsletter, 16*(3), 15.

Vessey, J. A. (2002b). An evaluation of commercial school health software for use in multisite research studies. *Journal of School Nursing, 18,* 95–100.

Vessey, J. A., & McGowan, K. (2005). Evidence-based practice. In C. Silkworth, M., M. Arnold, J. Harrigan, & D. Zaiger. *Individualized healthcare plans for the school nurse.* MN: Sunrise River Press.

Chapter 9

Student Health and Education Plans

BARBARA ZIMMERMAN

Chapter Outline

INTRODUCTION

The increased rates of chronic conditions in children have resulted in a great demand for school health services. As a result of increasing technological advances, many students with multiple complex healthcare needs are able to attend school. This has created a greater need for technological skill and adaptive services with accommodations. In addition, schools are required to provide a free, public education in the least restrictive environment to special groups of students, as specified by Federal Law P.L. 105–17, the Individuals with Disabilities Education Act (IDEA). Section 504 of the Rehabilitation Act of 1973, P.L 93–112 requires access to the school or learning program of qualified students with disabilities and mandates that accommodations be made to assist them in their educational endeavors (see Chapter 14). The school nurse is in a pivotal role to provide the needed care for these students, empower them to take responsibility for their own care, teach staff and faculty about the special needs of these students, and advocate for services so students can achieve an optimal level of functioning and maximize their learning. This communication is best facilitated by the development of written plans of care.

There are many types of plans; some are required by professional standards of practice, such as Individualized Health Plans (IHP) and Emergency Action Plans (EAP) and are initiated by the school nurse, while others are mandated by federal laws. IDEA mandates the development of the Individualized Education Program (IEP) and Section 504 of the Rehabilitation Act recommends the development of a 504 Accommodation Plan. These plans can be initiated by the coordinator for special education or any other multidisciplinary educational team member, including the school nurse. These plans are discussed in detail later. Depending on the criteria of each of the above plans, the accommodations needed by students are the key elements to assist them to have full access to an education by promoting their well-being and optimizing their learning.

COMMON LANGUAGE

Using a standardized language in writing the various plans provides a means for school nurses to communicate to school administrators, faculty, staff, and parents. It also enables the school nurse to use a common database from which to view trends, conduct research, and obtain reimbursement for services (Arnold & Silkworth, 1999). The standardized language of the North American Nursing Diagnosis Association (NANDA), the Nursing Interventions Classification (NIC), and the Nursing Outcomes Classification (NOC) are research based and developed inductively based on existing practice (NANDA, 2001). This language of the nursing profession (NANDA, NIC, NOC) is one approach to assist nurses in decision-making skills using a systematic methodology for determining nursing diagnoses and the appropriate interventions to meet client needs, as well as the outcomes to demonstrate the effectiveness of the interventions. There are also other systems that have their own "common language," such as the Omaha System.

The standardization of language facilitates accessing reimbursements based on interventions; these include Medicaid, Maternal and Child Health Grants, Early Periodic Screening, Diagnosis and Treatment (EPSDT), or Children's Health Insurance (Lowe & Miller, 1998). A common language also provides a database for research and documentation regarding nursing practice (McCloskey & Bulechek, 2000). These reasons more than validate the need for school nurses to speak a common language, such as NANDA, NIC, and NOC, in the documentation of student health care and services.

The National Association for School Nurses (NASN) has embraced the use of NANDA, NIC, and NOC (NASN, 2003). NIC includes any treatment based on clinical judgment and knowledge that a nurse performs to enhance client outcomes (McCloskey & Bulechek, 2000). In NIC, 514 interventions are categorized into 6 domains; all are coded for computer information systems toward reimbursement (McCloskey & Bulechek, 2000). The most frequently used nursing interventions by school nurses, using NIC, are shown in Box 9.1. An example of school nurse interventions divided by domain is in Box 9.2.

Nursing Outcomes Classification (NOC) defines the client's status resulting from nursing interventions (Moorhead, Johnson, & Maas, 2004). These outcomes are stated in neutral terms so that hopefully the client's status will move in the desired direction. NOC consists of 330 outcomes divided into domains, such as physiological health, psychosocial health, and health knowledge (Moorhead et al., 2004). The outcomes are not goals; instead they are variable concepts so the client status can be monitored for change, thereby providing an effective means to evaluate nursing interventions. A goal is either met or not met. The NOC outcomes assess the actual state at any given point in time using a five-point scale. More than one NOC outcome may be relevant for a NANDA diagnosis. An example of NANDA, NIC, and NOC is shown in Box 9.3.

A recent addition to a NOC outcome label is "Student Health Status," which has 32 indicators relating to the health status of students (Denehy, 2003). This outcome classification can be most relevant to school nurses in showing the effectiveness of their care. By measuring outcome effectiveness of the intervention, school nurses have a vehicle to demonstrate accountability to school administration and parents (see Chapter 11).

According to Denehy (2003), outcome measurement and documentation are imperative if school nurses are to show that they make a contribution to the health and well-being of students. California school nurses demonstrated this accountability when the outcome of an intervention was that 99% of students treated (some 7,000) returned to class (Awbrey & Juarez, 2003). The protocol developed by these school nurses addressed the well-being of students and academic achievement.

School nurses must demonstrate that what they do leads to the academic success of students. School nurses work in tandem with faculty to promote student learning by keeping them in the classroom in a state of health and ready to learn. With the use of a standardized language, the school nurse can begin to show the value of school nursing services in the educational setting (Denehy, 2003). The proof is in the "evidence" of the student's optimal level of functioning and academic achievement.

Multidisciplinary Educational (MDE) Teams, otherwise known as the Instructional Support Team, Pupil Services Team, and Building Resource Team, can easily understand and use the standardized language of school nursing because it describes the interventions needed and the student's response. The interventions describe the team members' roles for the services needed and can be very easily incorporated into many of the plans. Should a school district be computerized, this standardized language would provide a means for tracking and analyzing outcome data.

Box 9.1 ■ ■ ■

MOST FREQUENTLY USED NURSING INTERVENTIONS BY SCHOOLS NURSES

McClosky & Bulechek (2000).

- Abuse protection support: child
- Active listening
- Allergy management
- Analgesic administration
- Anger control assistance
- Anticipatory guidance
- Anxiety reduction
- Bleeding reduction
- Bleeding reduction: wound
- Calming technique
- Caregiver support
- Contact lens care
- Coping enhancement
- Counseling
- Crisis intervention
- Decision-making support
- Delegation
- Documentation
- Emergency care
- Emotional support
- Eye care
- Family integrity promotion
- Family involvement
- Family support
- Fever treatment
- First aid
- Grief work facilitation
- Health care information exchange
- Health education
- Health screening
- Health system guidance
- Heat/cold application
- Humor
- Infection control
- Learning facilitation
- Learning readiness enhancement
- Medication administration: oral
- Medication management
- Multidisciplinary care conference
- Nutritional counseling
- Pain management
- Parent education: adolescent
- Parent education: childbearing family
- Patient rights protection
- Referral
- Self-esteem enhancement
- Skin surveillance
- Socialization enhancement
- Spiritual support
- Substance use prevention
- Suicide prevention
- Support group
- Teaching: individual
- Telephone consultation
- Touch
- Triage
- Values clarification
- Vital signs monitoring
- Wound care

Box 9.2 ■ ■ ■

NIC NURSING INTERVENTIONS USED BY SCHOOL NURSES (EXAMPLE)

DOMAIN 1	DOMAIN 2	DOMAIN 3	DOMAIN 4	DOMAIN 5	DOMAIN 6
Physiological: Basic	**Physiological: Complex**	**Behavioral**	**Safety**	**Family**	**Health System**
Urinary catherization: intermittent	Medication administration	Active listening	First aid	Teaching: infant care	Referral
Heat/cold application	Seizure precautions	Emotional support	Crisis intervention	Developmental enhancement	Multidisciplinary care conference
Pain management	Seizure management	Behavior management: overactivity/ inattention	Suicide prevention	Family integrity promotion	Documentation
	Airway management	Health education	Health screening	Family support	Telephone consultation
		Anticipatory guidance	Immunization/ vaccination administration	Normalization promotion	Delegation
		Substance use prevention	Latex precautions	Parent education: childbearing family	Staff supervision
		Teaching: sexuality	Risk identification		Supply management
		Self-esteem enhancement			Preceptor student

DISCUSSION QUESTIONS:

1. List NIC interventions used in your school nursing practicum according to domain.
2. Compare the different domains used.
3. What NANDA nursing diagnoses would trigger these interventions?
4. What NOC outcomes could be used to evaluate the effectiveness of these interventions?
5. What skills and education would the school nurse need to perform these interventions?
6. How would you document these interventions?

Example of a completed form used to help undergraduate students completing a practicum in a school setting at the University of Iowa to identify frequently used interventions, November 1998. This form could be adopted for use in any setting. (Submitted by Janice Denehy, PhD, RN. Used with permission.)

THE NURSING PROCESS IN THE SCHOOL SETTING

Components of the Nursing Process

The development of all plans incorporates the components of the nursing process. The nursing process involves several components. The first component is *assessment*. It provides key information for which critical thinking and decision-making lead to a nursing diagnosis. Assessment is a process of data collection of both subjective and objective information. The assessment starts with an interview of the student/family, including the following topics: parent and student knowledge of illness and treatment; current health status; and the student's perception

Box 9.3 ■ ■ ■

AN EXAMPLE OF NANDA, NIC, AND NOC

Ineffective Breathing Pattern (1.5 1.3) related to asthma as evidenced by coughing and shortness of breath. One NIC is Airway Management (3140); some examples include: (1) use fun techniques to encourage deep breathing for children, (2) assist with peak flow monitoring, (3) auscultate breath sounds, and (4) teach patient how to use prescribed inhalers. An example of a NOC is Asthma Control (0704) which includes 17 indicators, three of which are: (1) initiates action to avoid personal triggers (070401); (2) sleeps through the night with no nocturnal cough (070406); and (3) reports symptom free state with minimal medication regimen (070409) (Moorhead et al., 2004).

of his or her condition and its impact on activities of daily living (ADL) and on socialization and barriers to self-care. Other aspects of the assessment include review of current and past medical records; collaboration with healthcare providers (primary and community) with parental permission; physical assessment findings; interview with relevant school staff; review of attendance records; observation of the student in the classroom and on the playground; and observation of student adherence and competency of the therapeutic regimen.

During the process of assessment, the school nurse must be sensitive to the cultural aspects of the student's healthcare practices. Assessing the student's (family's) health beliefs and practices in a culturally sensitive manner is critical to the plan development and the success of student outcomes (see Chapter 18). Culturally congruent care provides for the use of rituals, folk medicine, ancient practices such as acupuncture, or herbs (that are not harmful or contraindicated) in addition to accommodating modern healthcare practices into the plan. In this way, trust and respect between the student and family and the school nurse can be built and strengthened. With an increasingly diverse community, the school nurse must develop knowledge about the cultures within his or her practice in order to conduct a culturally sensitive health assessment and provide culturally congruent care.

The second component of the nursing process is *nursing diagnosis*. Through the process of critically analyzing the data, the school nurse formulates a nursing diagnosis (Praeger, Zickler, & Mosca, 2002). A nursing diagnosis is a means by which to classify the human response patterns to illness. NANDA has developed a diagnostic classification system that results in the clinical judgment about clients' responses to actual or potential health problems based on the assessment data (NANDA, 2001). According to Hootman (1996b), "Nursing diagnoses describe the complexity of students' responses and the unique focus of the nurse's service. The diagnostic labels succinctly describe the professional issues the nurse identifies and manages so that non-nurses can understand our focus of service" (p. 6).

The nursing diagnosis has three parts: label, etiology, and signs/symptoms. The *label* is the nursing diagnosis statement or the stem. The *etiology* includes the contributing factors that lead to the problem. The interventions developed must modify, remove, or control the etiology. The etiology can be pathophysiology (such as that which causes asthma or diabetes), situational (parental divorce/death, homeless, etc.), environmental (communicable disease or unsafe access), age related (developmental stages), or personal stressors (lack of nutrition or sleep or use of drugs) (Hootman, 1996a). The third part includes *signs and symptoms* that are indicators to validate the diagnostic label.

The five types of nursing diagnosis levels within NANDA include: (1) *actual*, in which the state has been clinically validated by characteristics; (2) *risk or potential for*, in which the student is vulnerable to develop the problem; (3) *possible*; (4) *wellness*, the client desires to move to a higher level of wellness or potential for enhanced; and (5) *syndrome*, a cluster of actual and "at risk for" diagnoses.

In the third component of the nursing process, *goals or outcomes are identified*. The goals are mutually formulated with the student, family, or faculty and describe the overall desired outcomes. They need to be realistic in relation to the student's abilities and obtainable within the school setting/resources. Keeping the educational setting in mind, goals should reflect the optimal level of functioning so that fewer school days are missed and an overall availability for learning can occur. The outcome criteria for evaluation are developed from the goals (and nursing diagnoses). The goals should be stated in clear, concise, and measurable terminology that can be understood by relevant school staff and have some element of time attached to them.

The fourth component of the nursing process is the plan using *nursing interventions*. Nursing interventions validate each nursing diagnosis and are developed from etiological factors. In the "actual" nursing diagnosis, interventions should decrease or eliminate the contributing factors or promote a higher level of wellness or monitor the status. In the "potential for" nursing diagnosis, the interventions must be developed to reduce or eliminate the risk factors. Part of the interventions include in-service to staff and faculty about the illness and potential crises that may occur or the special services needed to accommodate the student in the classroom/program.

The fifth component, *evaluation*, is key in the nursing process. This component consists of determining if the goals have been met, if the interventions need to be modified, and if the nursing diagnosis still exists or a new one has developed. Should changes be needed, the school nurse can revise the interventions as needed by adding and dating the additional changes in the plan. Should an outcome be met, a date with resolution of that problem should be placed in a tickler file for reevaluation at a later date. Evaluation is a very important component for both the student and the school nurse. The student moves to a more optimal level of functioning or learning (if met) and the school nurse demonstrates professional accountability.

THE INDIVIDUAL HEALTH PLAN AND THE EMERGENCY ACTION PLAN

The school nurse often functions as a case manager for students with special health needs. The school nurse assesses the student and determines the needs and barriers relating to student safety or well being; collaborates with a parent (and perhaps primary care provider); coordinates care (and adaptive needs) during the school hours; educates the faculty about the student needs (as well as signs of impending crisis); and supports the student with coping and learning how to integrate the regimen (condition) into daily life activities. The documentation of this process is an Individualized Healthcare Plan (IHP) for managing the health needs of students (American Academy of Pediatrics [AAP], 2001). IHPs have both an administrative and clinical purpose in promoting comprehensive, coordinated, continuity of care, and evaluation (NASN, 2003). They also promote communication of those needs with school staff, administration, students, and parents (NASN, 2003). Using a standardized language related to interventions and outcome will assist school nurses to determine the effectiveness of their care in meeting the health needs of school-age youth.

Some chronic conditions have the potential to develop into a medical crisis and require an Emergency Action Plan (EAP). This plan stems directly from the IHP and provides all staff with the necessary steps for action should a crisis result (NASN, 2003). IHPs and EAPs provide data for evidence-based practice and are required as part of the Professional Standards of Care for School Nurses (NASN & ANA, 2001).

The school nurse uses her professional judgment to determine if students require an IHP and initiates the IHP to meet the student's health needs. The purpose of the IHP/EAP is to ensure that the student is able to maximize the learning opportunities by achieving an optimal level of functioning. This differs from the Individual Education Program (IEP) mandated by the federal IDEA law, which is educationally based to meet special education needs or services for the student with disabilities. Should a student require health-related services or have a condition that impacts on his or her ability to learn, the school nurse plays a very important role in the IEP development. The school nurse also has an essential role in the 504 Accommodation Plan by using assessment skills in evaluating if the student has a mental or physical impairment that limits a major life activity. Other key roles include provision of services or care, primary prevention interventions, and case management (Arnold & Silkworth, 1999). Yet, for the student who may have the IEP or 504 plan, the IHP (and EAP, if needed) remains the first step in the process.

The IHP is developed by the school nurse to provide for the needs or services of students with health problems. These plans are developed cooperatively with the student, family, and primary care provider. The IHP provides a means for the school nurse to identify healthcare needs, document the provision of care and progress toward achieving outcomes to optimize student learning. The IHP also provides communication so continuity of care is maintained.

The format of the IHP aligns with the nursing process and the NASN Standards of Care for School Nurses (NASN, 2003). School nurses, especially those responsible for large numbers of students, must prioritize health needs that occur on a daily basis. The priority for IHP development is especially important for students who are medically fragile, require complex health services on a daily basis, have an illness that could result in a health crisis, or have an IEP or 504 Accommodation Plan (Arnold & Silkworth, 1999). Part of the interventions of the IHP necessitates the development of an EAP. The plan requires school nurses to distribute the EAP to individuals who may be in contact with the student and teach them how a crisis may appear and what action to take.

Process of Development

Many types of formats exist for IHP development and can be tailored to fit the documentation formats of the school health office. *Individualized Healthcare Plans for the School Nurse* edited by Silkworth, Arnold, Harrigan, and Zaiger (2005) provides comprehensive resources for the school nurse. In addition, NASN's publication list has resources for special healthcare needs and IHP development (http://www.nasn.org). Utilizing resources for NANDA by Wilkinson (2000), NIC by McCloskey and Bulechek (2000), and NOC by Moorhead et al. (2004) will promote communication.

Standardized IHPs (computerized and printed versions) are a good starting point but must then be tailored to meet the specific needs of the student. If computerization is utilized, always have documentation in a retrievable form that is password protected to ensure student privacy. Computerization makes it easier for ongoing evaluation to measure the student outcomes.

The format must be easy to use and facilitate documentation. One format that may be helpful is seen in Box 9.4. Because many school nurses have a large student-to-school nurse ratio, the process for IHP development must be simplified and practical. One suggestion would be to develop a packet for each of the most common chronic conditions (especially those that could result in a health crisis, i.e., allergy, asthma, diabetes, seizures, etc.). Each packet would contain a health assessment sheet with specific questions relevant to that illness; a letter to the parent explaining the need for the development of an IHP, and permission to contact primary providers for health information related to the learning process if needed; teaching sheets about the illness or treatment regimens (for student and family); an IHP form; and an emergency action plan form. Preparing IHP packets can be a time saving feature for the school nurse.

The development of an assessment sheet, specifically for asthma, seizures, allergy, or diabetes, can incorporate illness-related questions that provide the parent the opportunity to incorporate their child's specific signs (such as, peak flow, blood glucose levels, cough or wheeze, lightheadedness or tingling) of crisis. The assessment form provides a forum to share the school's procedure for handling the crisis and the district's medication policy. Obtaining a parent signature validates the approval of the procedures or indicates the need for individual changes based on their child's need. The NASN publication entitled *Care of Students with Special Needs* provides sample letters to parents whose child has special healthcare needs or requires care during school hours, a letter to healthcare providers, and letters seeking asthma information or updates for the emergency action plan (Praeger et al., 2002).

When emergency contact cards are returned at the beginning of the school year and the student has been identified as having a chronic condition, the process can begin by mailing the assessment sheets to the parents or interviewing the student and parent. For those students who had an IHP and EAP from the previous year, a copy can be made and sent to the parent for any updating in treatment or medications. This also provides a means for parents to sign and indicate approval of the plan.

Priority for IHP and EAP development must be given to those students with medically fragile or chronic conditions that may result in a health crisis. For this population of students, the IHP and EAP must be developed quickly for the safety of the student and the education of faculty and staff who may need to recognize and deal with the health crisis. Boxes 9.5 and 9.6 are examples of an IHP with two types of format for Asthma and Peanut Allergy.

The EAP is developed for school faculty/staff who may come in contact with the student, so that they will know how to recognize a health crisis and intervene appropriately. The EAP must be written in very clear, succinct terminology that could be understood by all school staff (including cafeteria and playground aides and those who provide transportation). The format can be simply a statement such as: "If (name) looks like this:...... Do this immediately:........."

The EAP should contain emergency contact information and emergency actions that are to be taken in a health crisis. The school nurse must determine which students require an EAP. Some criteria to use in the decision-making include stability of the condition, potential for an urgent or life-threatening situation to develop, students who require regular medical procedures at school, and parent request (Harrigan, 2002). The EAP should be approved by the parent and distributed to the appropriate individuals, such as the teacher, playground, or cafeteria aide, bus driver, and so forth. A list of all individuals who have a copy of the EAP must be noted on the form.

One suggestion is to attach the student's school picture to the form and, on the back of the form, include a basic fact sheet about the illness/crisis that could result. In this manner the school nurse would be providing that staff person with a basic understanding of the illness and what to expect for the individualized student. An in-service program

(text continues on page 188)

Box 9.4

IHP FORMAT

ASSESSMENT DATA

- Interviews:
  - Student
  - Parent
  - Staff/faculty
- Review of records (past and present)
  - Medical
  - Nursing and IHP and EAP
  - Educational and IEP and 504 Accommodation Plan
  - Attendance patterns
- Consultation:
  - Providers (parental consent)
- Assessment:
  - Physical
  - Screening
  - Management skills of therapeutic regimen
  - Knowledge:
    - Chronic illness/disability
    - Health crisis symptoms
  - Barriers to adaptation
    - Treatment regimen
  - Coping
  - Normalization

NURSING DIAGNOSIS

- NANDA nursing diagnosis
- Patient diagnostic statement must be accurately derived from assessment data.
- Nursing diagnosis = Problem + Etiology
- Must have:
  - "Related to" evident in assessment data.
  - "Signs and symptoms" evidence in assessment data to verify "defining characteristics"
- Nursing diagnosis statement is realistic for current status and setting.
- Types:
  - Actual
  - risk for
  - wellness

STUDENT GOALS

- Student-focused describing the desired outcome
- Clear, concise, and measurable
- Developed from nursing diagnosis
- Origin for outcome criteria NOC
- Timeline

NURSING INTERVENTIONS

- Nursing Interventions (NIC) are derived from or pertain to diagnostic statement and outcomes
- NIC written in student specific format including:
  - Who (staff, faculty, gym teacher, etc)
    - What
    - How
    - Should address:
    - The holistic needs including nursing strategies designed to assist the student to meet the outcome criteria
- Include: ongoing assessments, student teaching, collaborative activities, faculty-staff in-service, development of Emergency Action Plan (EAP)
- In "actual" NANDA diagnosis:
  - Interventions should decrease or eliminate the contributing factors or promote a higher level of wellness or monitor status.
- In "risk for" NANDA diagnosis:
  - Interventions must reduce or eliminate the risk factors.

EXPECTED OUTCOMES

- Nursing Outcomes Classification (NOC)
- Appropriate related indicators are selected and current level of achievement is supported by assessment data.
- NOC scales identified student desired outcome derived from and specific to diagnostic statement.
- Stated in neutral terms with rating scale
- Realistic and achievable

(Adapted from Arnold & Silkworth [1999]).

Box 9.5 ■ ■ ■

IHP OF ASTHMA

Name: Address: Date of birth:
Parent(s): Address: Telephone: (h) (w)

DIAGNOSIS: Sara is a 10-year-old child who was recently diagnosed with asthma following hospitalization for a crisis.

ASSESSMENT:

SUBJECTIVE DATA

- States she is scared and doesn't want to feel like an elephant is sitting on her chest again; also states she is afraid when she begins to get short of breath; doesn't understand how to use the inhaler, pathology, or triggers.
- Lives with mom and siblings, ages 17, 14, and 12. The mother works and gets home at 5:30; Mother is trying to understand the illness and use of inhalers.
- Teacher states concern for child, "She seems preoccupied, isn't concentrating, and has missed a lot of work due to absences, seems to cry easily."
- The gym teacher states she has been unable to keep up with the rest of the class activities, and coughs frequently.
- Sara states that she feels like her friends don't like her anymore because she can't play and is always coughing.

OBJECTIVE DATA:

- Demonstrates difficulty using the inhaler; needs assistance with inhaler administration, demonstrated a lack of understanding of disease, medications, triggers, or actions to take with a crisis. Lung sound wheezes RLL and LLL, cough dry and nonproductive, SOB upon exertion. Peak flow meter reading = 125 on 2/20; WEIGHT LOSS of 6 pounds (2.72 kg) on 9/19 = 56 lb (25.40 kg), 2/20 = 50 lb (22.68 kg).

NURSING DIAGNOSIS:

1. KNOWLEDGE DEFICIT RELATED TO NEW DIAGNOSIS OF ASTHMA EVIDENCED BY A LACK OF UNDERSTANDING OF ASTHMA, TRIGGERS, MEDICATION USE, ACTIONS FOR CRISIS. (8.1.1)

   GOAL: Sara will develop knowledge and understanding of disease, etiology, triggers, medications, administration, crisis symptoms, and actions.

   INTERVENTIONS: NIC—Teaching: Disease Process (5602). Provide education on: what is asthma, triggers, crisis warning signs, crisis action, medications, administration techniques, peak flow meter use, contact person in a crisis.

   - Assist student with administration of medications, demonstrate techniques, and use visual aids. Use role play and observe technique and reinforce behavior.

   OUTCOME: NOC—Knowledge: Disease Process (1803) Description of: disease (180302), risk factors or triggers (180304), treatments (180308), crisis (180310): none–1; limited–2; moderate–3; substantial–4; extensive–5

2. INEFFECTIVE COPING, RELATED TO ANXIETY FROM NEW DIAGNOSIS OF ASTHMA (NANDA 5.1.1)

   GOAL: Improved coping, decrease anxiety, return to premorbid social activities.

   NIC INTERVENTIONS: Coping Enhancement (5230)

   - Encourage student to verbalize feelings.
   - Promote decision-making skills.
   - Assist the student to identify coping techniques used, role play using various strategies.
   - Encourage her to participate in social activities.
   - Communicate with the mother to utilize community services including support group.
   - Share asthma information with her classmates when she is ready.

   NOC OUTCOME: Coping (1302) Verbalizes sense of control (130203); seeks information concerning illness and treatment (130206); Uses effective coping techniques (130212): Never–1; Rarely–2; Sometimes–3; Often–4; Consistently–5 Participates in two social activities in 6 months.

(Continued on the following page)

Box 9.5

IHP OF ASTHMA *(Continued)*

3. ALTERED ROLE PERFORMANCE RELATED TO UNCONTROLLED ASTHMA EVIDENCED BY INABILITY TO KEEP UP NORMAL ROUTINE (3.2.1).

GOAL: Understand and participate (initiate) asthma management plan to improve optimal level of functioning and minimal school time lost.

GOAL: She will use adaptive PE, and class schedule adjustment as needed to decrease absentee days and in order to improve her academic performance.

INTERVENTIONS: Normalization Promotion (7200)

- Keep log of symptoms, triggers, crisis symptoms, and treatment.
- Keep log of peak flow readings for 2 weeks, with permission to collaborate with the physician.
- Promote her self-care skills in such a way that integrate them into daily schedule.
- Make new or renew friendships/social activities as stamina improves.
- Develop management plan, gaining authorization of medications and treatment from healthcare provider.
- DEVELOP ACTION PLAN—list locations of plan.
- IN-SERVICE PERSONNEL—list individuals who received in-service and date received.
- Assist teacher to recognize child's tolerance levels and crisis symptoms.
- Assist the teacher with an adapted class schedule, if needed.
- Assist physical education (PE) teacher with adapted PE activities; educate PE teacher on limitations, signs of crisis, and inhaler use.

OUTCOME: Asthma Control (0704)

Monitors peak flow when symptoms occur (070411): never–1; rarely–2; sometimes–3; often–4; consistently–5

Initiates action to manage personal triggers (070402): never–1; rarely–2; sometimes–3; often–4; consistently–5

Self-manages exacerbations (070415): never–1; rarely–2; sometimes–3; often–4; consistently–5

Participates in age-appropriate activities (070405), that is, participates in gym and classroom activities to her optimal level: never–1; rarely–2; sometimes–3; often–4; consistently–5

Box 9.6

INDIVIDUALIZED HEALTHCARE PLAN—PEANUT ALLERGY

Name:
Date of birth:
Parent(s):
Emergency contact:
Primary care provider:
Hospital:
Medical diagnosis:
Allergies:

Address:
Grade:
Telephone: (h) (w)
Telephone:
Telephone:
Insurance:
PRN Medications/treatment:

ASSESSMENT DATA:

HISTORY: Allergic to peanuts; diagnosed (month/year); reactions began as mild to moderate—treated with Benadryl; family vigilance increasing; asthma diagnosis 3 years ago.

CURRENT STATUS AND MANAGEMENT: Primary care provider; knowledgeable about reaction, treatment and trigger foods; lack of knowledge about trigger effects in air and other foods; last reaction resulted in ER visit related to breathing difficulty; EpiPen prescribed.
SELF CARE: Knows the feeling of oncoming reaction; seeks school nurse for medication.
PSYCHOSOCIAL STATUS: Mother and student have growing concern of increasing severity of reactions; fear event will occur again; knows friends who eat peanut butter sandwiches at lunch; mother wants child isolated in classroom to eat, child doesn't agree but is fearful in the cafeteria; student doesn't want to be singled out.
ACADEMIC ISSUES: Regular attendance; regular education; 504 needed for school compliance; teacher notes lack of concentration and decrease in socialization with friends and playground activity.

NANDA NURSING DIAGNOSIS	STUDENT GOAL	NIC INTERVENTIONS	NOC OUTCOMES	EVALUATION/ RESOLUTION OR REVIEW DATE
Ineffective Breathing pattern r/t Peanut allergy evidenced by SOB, cough and tightness in throat (1.5.1.3)	Student will identify reaction and seek help and treatment immediately.	Airway Management (3140) Monitor breathing/ airway; Administer EpiPen; Repeat EpiPen 15 min. prn Give Benadryl after crisis resolves. Notify parent EAP in place.	Respiratory Status: Ventilation (0403) Ease of Breathing (040305) 1– Extremely compromised 2– Substantially compromised 3– Moderately compromised 4– Mildly compromised 5– Not compromised	
Knowledge Deficit r/t peanut allergy evidenced by new treatment with EpiPen and signs of more severe reaction (8.1.1)	In 2 months the student will learn to self-administer EpiPen; carry medication at all times; be able to describe the first signs of a reaction.	Teaching: Prescribed medication (5616) Learn to recognize distinct, subtle change in first minutes of reaction. Instruct on self-medication. Instruct on action of med and time for effectiveness; back up EpiPen location. Educate school staff and kitchen staff on peanut-free table; cross contamination of foods.	Knowledge: Treatment regimen (1813) Description of self-care responsibilities for emergency situations (181303) 1–none; 2–limited; 3–moderate; 4–substantial; 5–extensive Performance of treatment procedure by student (181312) 1–none; 2–limited; 3–moderate; 4–substantial; 5–extensive	

(Continued on the following page)

Box 9.6 ■ ■ ■

INDIVIDUALIZED HEALTHCARE PLAN—PEANUT ALLERGY *(Continued)*

Fear R/T peanut allergy evidenced by worsening severity of reactions (9.3.2)	Student demonstrates less fear and resumes social contacts in 3 months.	Coping enhancement (5230). Have student involved in EAP development. Encourage student to share perspective of "fear". Encourage decision-making. Encourage social activities.	Plans coping strategies for fearful situation (140405). Maintains role performance (140410). Maintains social relationships (140411). Maintains concentration (140412). Using scale: 1–never demonstrated; 2–rarely demonstrated; 3–sometimes demonstrated; 4–often demonstrated; 5–consistently demonstrated

Parent________________ Date _______ School nurse _______Date _______
EAP: ____ yes; no____ Located at ____
Copy to: ___ Teacher ____ Lunch aide ____ Playground aide ____ Bus driver ____ Principal _____ Kitchen staff _______
504 Plan: _______yes _______ no

can be given prior to the start of school where the school nurse provides a basic overview of the most common illnesses that could result in a crisis and describe the use of the fact sheet/EAP. On completion, the EAP can be distributed to the appropriate faculty and staff. This technique can allay staff fears of the unknown, provide safety for the student, and allow for the distribution of the information to be in a confidential, yet informative manner. See Boxes 9.7, 9.8, and 9.9 for examples of EAPs.

Whereas the IHP and EAP are initiated by the school nurse as part of professional practice, two other types of plans are mandated by federal law. The IEP is a plan based on educational objectives while the 504 Accommodation Plan provides equal access to the educational program. Although both are part of federal laws, only the IEP comes with a small share of federal funding; the 504 is strictly financed by the school district.

INDIVIDUALS WITH DISABILITIES ACT (IDEA)

The Individuals with Disabilities Education Act (IDEA), P.L. 105–17 amended in 2003 provides special education, related services and assistive technology devices to those students who are "eligible." (See Chapters 14 and 27 for more detail.) IDEA provides for an appropriate evaluation, an individualized education program in the least restrictive environment that is free, and involvement of the parents in decision-making. IDEA also provides the parents with procedural safeguards. The federal regulations provide definitions for eligibility criteria and related services, yet each state interprets the federal law in a way that fits into the educational infrastructure of that state. Every state has

(text continues on page 191)

Box 9.7

EMERGENCY ACTION PLAN—ASTHMA

Name: Sara　Date of birth:　Grade:
School:　District:
Parent/guardian:
Emergency contact:　Telephone (h)　(w)
Healthcare provider:　Telephone:

KNOWN ALLERGIES: Dust mites, pollen, animal dander, ragweed
HEALTH PROBLEM: Asthma and eczema
SPECIAL TRANSPORTATION: No
PICTURE OF SARA:

In a health emergency, Sara looks like:

Has difficulty in getting breath.

Looks scared, fearful.

States that it feels like "an elephant sitting on my chest."

States: "I can't breathe."

Sits, leaning forward, doesn't talk.

Coughs, can't stop or no relief.

Skin color change around lips—gray, blue.

Please do the following:

Call school nurse, or administration if school nurse is not available.

Allow Sara to use inhaler; provide assistance if needed.

If her inhaler is in the school health office send someone to notify the school nurse or retrieve the inhaler. Do not leave Sara alone.

Encourage Sara to slowly breathe out through partially closed lips.

Stay with Sara and try to keep her calm.

If symptoms:

Decrease after 15 minutes, return to class (check peak flow in health office)

Remain the same in 10 to 15 minutes, repeat inhaler use, contact parent.

Increase in severity, Call 911 and report location and problem.

Parent_________________ Date ________ School nurse ________Date________
Copy to: ___Principal ___ Secretary ___ Parent ____Playground aide _____Cafeteria aide
____Teacher _____Other:
___Health file _____Site 504 coordinator _____Substitute teacher

Box 9.8

EMERGENCY ACTION PLAN—PEANUT ALLERGY

Student:　Date of birth:　Grade:
School:　District:
Parent/guardian:
Emergency contact:　Telephone: (h)　(w)
Healthcare provider:　Telephone:

(Continued on the following page)

Box 9.8 ■ ■ ■

EMERGENCY ACTION PLAN—PEANUT ALLERGY *(Continued)*

KNOWN ALLERGIES:
HEALTH PROBLEM: Peanut allergy—severe

PICTURE OF STUDENT:

Asthmatic _____Yes ____No (Asthma may increase the severity of an allergic reaction.)

In a health emergency, the student looks like:

Complains of nasal stuffiness—quick onset.

Palms of hands become reddened and very itchy.

Lips become itchy.

Short of breath.

States: "I can't breathe."

"It is hard to swallow."

"It feels like a lump in my throat."

Coughs, can't stop.

Looks scared, fearful.

Feels nauseous.

Please do the following:

Remove student from area (because of peanut fumes).

Call the school nurse, or administration if the school nurse is not available.

Allow student to use EpiPen, give assistance if needed.

Know locations of EpiPen in school (school health office, administration office, cafeteria).

Do not leave the student alone.

Encourage the student to breathe slowly.

Keep the student calm.

If symptoms:

Decrease after 15 minutes, return to health office, contact parent.

Remain the same in 15 minutes, repeat EpiPen use, contact parent.

Increase in severity, call 911 and report location and problem.

(Note: Request advanced life support, as many ambulances do not carry epinephrine.)

After crisis subsides, troubleshoot reason for occurrence.

Parent________________ Date ________ School nurse _______________Date ______
Copy to: ___Principal ___ Secretary ___ Parent ____Playground aide _____Cafeteria aide _______Kitchen staff ____Teacher _____Other:
___Health file _____Site 504 coordinator _____Substitute teacher

Box 9.9 ■ ■ ■

EMERGENCY ACTION PLAN—PANIC ATTACK

Student: Date of birth: Grade:
School: District:
Parent/guardian: Telephone: (h) (w)
Emergency contact: Telephone:
Healthcare provider: Telephone:

KNOWN ALLERGIES:
HEALTH PROBLEM: Panic attack

PICTURE OF STUDENT:

SYMPTOMS: Although there is no threat of harm, the student is reliving the event and his body is experiencing it as if it were real. The attack is a discrete period of intense fear. It begins abruptly and usually peaks within 10 to 15 minutes, gradually disappearing in minutes to an hour.

In a health emergency, the student looks like:

He is in a panic state.

Sweating

Trembling

Pounding heart

Nauseous

Short of breath

Sense of impending doom

Please do the following:

Separate the student from the other children, to rear room or nurse's office if possible or call the school nurse.

Do not leave the student alone.

Encourage the student to breathe slowly.

Keep the student calm.

Reassure that the trauma is not present and try to make the student comfortable.

Work with student on the prescribed relaxation techniques from therapist (guided imagery) [attach directions if needed]. Assist the student to try to identify the trigger for that episode, and communicate with the school nurse about the episode.

Parent_________________ Date ________ School nurse _______________Date ______
Copy to: ___Principal ___ Secretary ___ Parent ____Playground aide _____Cafeteria aide _______Kitchen staff ____Teacher _____Other:
___Health file _____Site 504 coordinator _____Substitute teacher

regulations to ensure compliance with the provisions of IDEA.

Students may be eligible for services if the disability impacts on their ability to learn. A multidisciplinary educational team determines eligibility and identifies the services needed. The school nurse is a key member to this team, since many students who meet the eligibility will have chronic and special health needs. The health assessment and interventions are crucial in the identification of services and placement (NASN, 2002). Based on the evaluation of the team, students are provided services that enable them to safely take part in the educational program. These are written into an individualized educational program (IEP).

Multidisciplinary Educational Team

Each school district has a team to evaluate students and develop IEPs. The 1997 amended IDEA requires a special education teacher, a regular teacher, trained and qualified persons representing the related services, an administrator, someone familiar with general curriculum, and a parent to be on the multidisciplinary educational team. Qualified personnel are defined as "personnel who have met the State's educational agency recognized certification or licensing requirements that apply to the area of related services in which they provide" (CFR 300.24 Related Services). "Related services" are those services—transportation and such developmental, corrective, and other supportive services—as are required to assist an exceptional child to benefit from special education. Some examples include art therapy, music therapy, occupational, recreational or physical therapy, counseling, school psychological services, social services, speech and language services, transportation, and healthcare services. Although the school nurse is not specifically named, she should be a permanent member of the team, since all students will use her services at some point. The school health services are those nursing services that are necessary for the student to benefit from special education (Zaiger, 2001).

It is beneficial for the school nurse to initiate a discussion with the school administration regarding the value of her presence as a core member of the school team that meets to discuss students, as the school nurse has a unique perspective and a separate body of knowledge related to health issues. The school nurse is one of the few school professionals who not only sees every student in his or her scope of practice in the school setting, but is also responsible for their care.

Evaluation Procedure

The team receives a referral from a teacher, parent, or school nurse and begins the process of evaluation for eligibility, after parental permission for the evaluation is received. In some schools, the school professional team will offer the teacher strategies to use in the classroom before a full evaluation is recommended. However, often the initial evaluation is a complete individualized evaluation. The purpose is to determine whether the student is a "child with a disability" (as defined under IDEA 602(3)) and what needs require interventions. The evaluation is carried out by the multidisciplinary educational team using a variety of assessment tools and strategies to gather relevant functional, health and developmental information, including information provided by the parent who may assist in determining whether the student is a "child with a disability."

Information is also collected to determine how the student is to be involved in and progress through the general curriculum. No single procedure can be used as the sole criterion for determination, and technically sound instruments and screening tools are used to determine the contribution of cognitive, behavioral, physical, or developmental factors that impact on the student's ability to learn. The student is assessed in all areas of the suspected disability using strategies that provide relevant information that directly assist in determining the educational needs of the student (IDEA, sec. 614, 50).

Components and Process of IEP Development

The school nurse must be an active member of this team because he or she is one of the only individuals who can determine if the impairment or health problem will impact on the ability or availability to learn. There is a health assessment component in the evaluation process that can be completed only by the school nurse. The assessment includes a complete health history review, a physical assessment including an in-depth neurological exam, an interpretative review of medical records, hearing and vision assessment, school health records review, interview with a parent, classroom observation, and a review of the student's attendance pattern.

The multidisciplinary educational team of qualified professionals and the parent of the child make the determination of eligibility. The evaluation summary report includes the category in the definition under which the student is eligible; the student's present level of performance and educational needs; whether the student needs special education and related services; and what modifications are needed in order to meet the measurable annual goals in the IEP. The components of the IEP include:

- A statement of the student's present level of educational performance
- A statement of annual goals
- A statement of short-term instructional objectives
- A statement of specific education and related services to be provided
- A description of the extent to which the child will participate in regular education programs and a description of the program to be provided
- The projected dates for initiation of services and the anticipated duration of services

Objectives, evaluation procedures, and a schedule for determining, on at least an annual basis, achievement of the short-term instructional objectives must be noted. The annual goal is a broad, general statement that describes the outcome for that student at the conclusion of that academic year. Then the short-term objectives must follow as clear, concise statements that describe each step used to achieve the goal. The objectives must be behavioral and measurable, stating what the student will need to do. Certain criteria should be addressed in these objectives, such as the following; identify who is to perform the objective; list the specific observable behavior; describe the result of the performance; list relevant conditions for performing the behavior and list the acceptable criteria for evaluation at the minimal level of performance (IDEA, sec. 614).

In addition to the annual goal and objectives, a description of the specific related services must be completed as well as dates for initiation and duration of these services. An annual review for the purpose of updating goals and objectives is mandated by law. A reevaluation of the student is required every 3 years or sooner if requested by the parent or required by a State's interpretation (IDEA, sec. 614). For example, Pennsylvania requires annual reevaluation of all students with mental retardation.

Health Component of the IEP

The school nurse documents the present level of performance and any interpretation of results related to the health condition. The *present level of performance* (health) is a summary of pertinent data from the IHP and the impact on the student's ability to learn or participate in the educational program. A *statement for special education needs* should reflect the nursing services that are needed by the student to benefit from special education and meet the IEP goals. The *special education* needs would be equivalent to the nursing interventions in the IHP. In addition, if modifications or adaptations are needed to eliminate any health-related barriers, these should be noted in the special education needs (Arnold & Silkworth, 1999). The *annual goal* can be the goal in the IHP. The *short-term (instructional) objectives* would be the outcome measures of the IHP (Box 9.10).

Box 9.10 ■ ■ ■

INDIVIDUALIZED EDUCATIONAL PROGRAM

Student name: Address: Date of birth:
Parent(s) name: Address: Telephone: (h) (w)

Eligible for special education and related services: Learning disability and seizures

STATEMENT OF PRESENT LEVEL OF EDUCATIONAL PERFORMANCE (AS IT RELATES TO HEALTH):
Student receives medication administration two times during the school day. Often the student forgets or is preoccupied with other tasks. The student does not understand the effects that seizures have on daily life or the implications of skipping medication doses. Seizure activity has not been controlled well. Following a seizure the student is tired and needs to sleep for 30 minutes. Interrupting class for the student to take a missed dose of medication and experiencing seizures decreases the student's ability to learn from the special education program.

STATEMENT OF ANNUAL GOALS:

- Increase responsibility for management of seizures, that is, medication administration.
- Increase knowledge and understanding about seizures and the need to take medications regularly to decrease the number of seizures.

STATEMENT OF SHORT-TERM INSTRUCTIONAL OBJECTIVES:
The student will use the cues or reminders to go to health office for medication administration; by December, the student will have missed only five medication doses or less and by the end of the academic year, the student will not miss any medication doses.

The student will be able to explain what a seizure is and why it happens and if he or she has certain triggering events. By the end of the academic year, he or she can draw a sketch of where in the brain it happens and how the medication prevents it from happening.

At the conclusion of the academic year, the student will be able to describe what it feels like just before a seizure and prepare for it by telling someone.

STATEMENT OF SPECIFIC EDUCATION AND RELATED SERVICES TO BE PROVIDED:
SN: Develop a behavior plan with cues and reminders for student to take medication and rewards for adherence.
SN: From the Individualized Health Plan (IHP) develop an Emergency Action Plan (EAP) for seizures and in-service appropriate faculty and staff members.
SN: Administer medication.
SN: Communicate with parent or healthcare provider as to medication adherence update and record of seizure activity.
Teacher communicates with SN and parents as to changes in behavior or attention.
Teacher communicates with SN and parents as to schedule of all day class outings and request for parent to attend for medication administration.
SN/teacher/administration: Develop crisis plan for student.
Initiation of services date: September 1st
Duration of services: June 10th

Role of the School Nurse: Students with Special Needs

The role of the school nurse on this IEP team is crucial. Only the school nurse can provide a holistic perspective on the impact of the student's health on his or her ability to learn. In addition, the school nurse may provide nursing services as part of the IEP's "related health services." The school nurse determines if health services are needed during the school day to maintain the health status of the student and/or allow the student to participate in the special education program. These interventions/services should be documented on the IHP, which further validates the need for the IEP health component. Examples of "related health services" for students with ADHD include medication administration, memory cues, and behavior modification with social skills to allow the student to benefit from the special education program; for students with seizures, interventions might include medication administration and EAP training of staff to ensure a safe environment that allows the student to benefit from the education program.

The school nurse has a diverse role as part of the multidisciplinary educational team. As one of the "related service providers," she renders health services, identifies eligible students, assesses the student's functional and physical health status, develops an IHP and EAP, assists in the development of the IEP, aids parents in connecting with community resources, helps parents and teachers to remove health-related barriers to learning; provides in-service education to teachers and staff about the student's needs; delegates or supervises personnel providing special health services; evaluates the effectiveness of the health components of the IEP; and maintains a collaborative relationship with health providers and services within the community (NASN, 2002). These roles include case management, education, collaboration, coordination, and advocacy for the student's needs.

The school nurse is responsible for periodically updating the student's health status and noting any changes needed in health services. Interventions are listed as direct or indirect. All direct nursing services would indicate direct nursing care or teaching while the indirect nursing services would include case management activities, development of the plans (IHP, EAP, and the health component of the IEP), and in-services for staff and faculty. This update is also important for the purpose of reimbursement. States have various methods for documenting related services for reimbursement. School nurses should check with their school administration. By integrating the IHP into the health component of the IEP, school nurses may be able to receive reimbursement (Arnold & Silkworth, 1999). This process validates a component of school nurse accountability for practice that is evidenced by nursing services having direct impact on student achievement.

Individualized Family Service Plan (IFSP)

For the child with a disability prior to age 5, IDEA mandates the development of an IFSP to ensure provision of early intervention services to the family (IDEA, Part 300 Federal Legislation, 1999). Each state is required to have policies and procedures in place that meet the "child find" requirements. Child find is a public outreach awareness system to locate and identify children thought to be eligible for special education within the school district's jurisdiction. A public notice through various means (newspapers or other media) provides residents of the school district with information about children younger than 5 years of age with disabilities who may need special education or related services. The state must have policies and procedures to ensure that those children identified are evaluated. As part of an initial evaluation and any reevaluation, a group that includes the individuals described as qualified professionals should review existing data (IDEA, Federal Regulation 300.52–300.53).

Each state provides early intervention services through special education units within the school district or contracts with local educational agencies depending on each state's regulations. The school nurse may be involved in screening vision and hearing, developmental assessment using standardized screening tools, as well as physical/functional assessments. Components of the IFSP are similar to the IEP. When the child is age 5, the case manager contacts the home school district for a final IFSP evaluation report to transition the child to kindergarten.

Transition Services and Plans

Transition plans are mandated by IDEA. For the student with a disability who is age 14 and no later than age 16, a transition plan must be developed and placed in the IEP. Interventions and services need to reflect the transition to work, vocational training, or post-secondary education. Often the student is included, along with the parent, to plan experiences and study to prepare the student for post-school activities. The role of the school nurse is equally important in transition plans regarding the impact that the disability may have in the new setting as well as the health-related knowledge or skills the student may need to be successful in his or her next endeavor, that is, self-catheterization, knowledge of the influence of activity on insulin needs, and so forth. For students beginning to transition to work–study and internship experiences, the school nurse must determine how and when to implement the treatment regimens and what changes would be needed. The student's independence and adherence in the treatment regimen would also need to be evaluated (IDEA, Part 300.347–300.348, Federal Regulations, 1999).

504 ACCOMMODATION PLAN

Another federal mandate to provide services to students with disabilities is Section 504 of the Rehabilitation Act 1973 which requires all public educational agencies to "protect" handicapped students' rights for equal opportunity to access and participation in the school program and extracurricular activities. The school must provide aides, services, or accommodations needed for the student to have an equal opportunity to participate in and benefit from school programs. The intent of Section 504 is to "accommodate" for differences within the regular education environment (34 CFR Part 104).

Although this is a federal law, no federal funding or state allocations are mandated for Section 504, so all costs for reasonable accommodations must be funded by the school district. Each state has interpreted the federal law and developed regulations for compliance within the infrastructure of the state educational department. In some states, the person responsible for compliance with the law is referred to as the 504 Coordinator. The principal and/or guidance counselor are often the designees in Pennsylvania schools (Chapter 15, PA School Code, 1991). There is no multidisciplinary educational team as there is for those eligible for services under IDEA.

Section 504 Definitions

While the term "disabled" is reserved for students who are eligible for services under IDEA, the term handicapped is usually associated with Section 504. The individual with a *handicap* is one who has a physical or mental impairment that substantially limits one or more major life activities. The physical or mental *impairment* includes (A) "any physiological disorder, cosmetic disfigurement or anatomical loss affecting one or more of the following systems: neurological; musculoskeletal; special sense organs; respiratory, including speech; cardiovascular; reproductive; digestive; genitourinary; hematologic and lymphatic; skin; and endrocrine or (B) any mental or psychological disorder such as mental retardation, organic brain syndrome, emotional or mental illness and specific learning disabilities" (34 Code of Federal Regulations Part 104.3). Examples of disorders may include juvenile rheumatoid arthritis, HIV, asthma, allergy, diabetes, seizures, ADHD, panic disorder, temporary medical conditions (fractures, surgery), amputation, spinal cord injury, and behavior disorders (Conduct Disorder or Oppositional Defiant Disorder). Also, children who have adaptive physical education (but do not need an IEP, such as for scoliosis or cardiac repair), those who receive Occupational Therapy and Physical Therapy (but do not need an IEP, such as for rheumatoid arthritis), and those with a temporary or long-term injury that affects mobility are additional examples of students who may qualify. Examples of access and accommodations consist of those related to transportation to and from school, barriers into or throughout the building, adaptive aids, or services during school hours, and extracurricular activities.

Section 504 Procedures

Teachers, guidance counselors, the school nurse, the individual student, or the family can refer a student for an evaluation. A written request is needed from the parents to the school or vice versa. Although parental consent is not required for the evaluation, it is highly recommended. The designated Section 504 school official would coordinate the relevant staff or personnel. The type of handicap present and the type of services that may be needed determine the evaluation process and who is part of the evaluation group, the composition of which may vary dependent on the health need of the child). The evaluation may consist of a parent meeting, classroom observation, teacher input, and review of medical records. The evaluation must be complete and accurate in order to assess the nature of the handicap and how it impacts on the student's ability to access the school and the educational program. For example, a student may have fused spinal bones that prevent a student from leaning over a desk to write so the evaluation may consist of a parent and student interview and physical/functional assessment.

The recommendations for the types of services, aids, or accommodations must be made by a group of individuals who are knowledgeable of Section 504 and the student's needs. The 504 group reviews the nature of the handicap, the impact on the student's education, and the services that would be needed. Examples of 504 Student Accommodation Plans are shown in Boxes 9.11, 9.12, and 9.13.

Box 9.11 ▪▪▪

SECTION 504 STUDENT ACCOMMODATION PLAN—PEANUT ALLERGY

Student name: Date of birth: Grade:
Parent name: School: Date of meeting:

1. *Describe the nature of the concern*:
   Allergic to peanuts; diagnosed over summer break; reactions began as mild to moderate—treated with Benadryl; asthma diagnosis 3 years ago with current status stable; has knowledge about reaction, treatment and trigger foods; lack of knowledge about trigger effects in air and other foods; last reaction resulted in ER visit resulting in breathing difficulty; EpiPen prescribed; confusion with asthma versus severe reaction at onset of symptoms.
2. *Describe the basis for the determination of the handicap*:
   Mother and student express growing concern of increasing severity of reactions; fear of event occurring again; knows friends who eat peanut butter sandwiches at lunches; mother wants child isolated in classroom to eat, child doesn't but is fearful in the cafeteria; student doesn't want to be singled out by carrying lunch and sitting separately. Having difficulty concentrating due to food in classroom. Student frequently visits school nurse to rule out the presence of a reaction and for reassurance.
3. *Describe how the handicap affects a major life activity:*
   - Ineffective breathing pattern related to peanut allergy evidenced by shortness of breath, cough and tightness in throat when in contact with the smell, touch or taste of peanuts. (including utensils or surfaces that might have come into contact with nuts of any kind)
   - Knowledge deficit related to peanut allergy evidenced by new treatment, EpiPen and signs of more severe reaction or anaphylaxis emergency
   - Fear related to peanut allergy evidenced by worsening severity of reactions and lack of concentration in class.
4. *Describe the reasonable accommodations that are necessary:*
   - Develop emergency action plan (EAP) for school staff (cafeteria, kitchen, playground, teachers, bus drivers, parent volunteers).
   - School nurse will educate staff for signs of crisis and how to administer EpiPen, if delegated in the EAP.
   - School nurse and cafeteria/kitchen staff will develop allergy free eating area and methods to prevent contamination and cross-contamination. Signage states "catchy title or privileges" consisting of "free of nuts"…. Review food handling non-latex glove use and reasons.
   - School parent–teacher organization financially supports school in-service for students (or just that grade but more than one class).
   - Teacher develops integration of allergy-free concepts when appropriate in class—reading books, writing, science, and so forth.
   - Administration sends letters to parents regarding allergy-free school procedures including list of items not to be sent to school (latex balloons, food with nuts or milk or wheat, etc.).
   - Teacher communication with school nurse/parent regarding trips, outings for medication administration arrangement.
   - School nurse assists with administration of EpiPen; teaching procedure for self-administration, types/reasons for use, how to determine crisis, differentiate allergic crisis from asthma crisis, and action in crisis plan; troubleshoots with various settings or situations.
   - Student demonstrates self-care or health maintenance and ability to make appropriate decisions in managing allergy symptoms.
   - School nurse communicates with parent/physician as to changes or problems in allergy management plan; emergency responders for provisions of care in emergency.

Review date: 2 months:__________ then November and January of academic year or, as warranted
Participants: (name/title) Date:
Copy to:_____ Health file _____ Site 504 coordinator _____ Parent _____ Case manager_____ Other

Box 9.12

SECTION 504 STUDENT ACCOMMODATION PLAN—PANIC ATTACK

Student name: Date of Birth: Grade:
Parent name: School: Date of meeting:

1. *Describe the nature of the concern*:
   Student experienced a very traumatic event 6 months ago. Since that time he has had difficulty sleeping, frequent headaches, and withdrawal from social activities. His concentration is interrupted by flashbacks. When this occurs, he goes into a panic state, exhibiting sweating, trembling, pounding heart, nausea, shortness of breath, and sense of impending doom. Although there is no threat of harm the student is reliving the event and his body is experiencing the memory as if it were real.
2. *Describe the basis for the determination of the handicap:*
   The attack is a discrete period of intense fear. It begins abruptly and usually peaks within 10 to 15 minutes, gradually disappearing in minutes to an hour. The panic attack is a result of the diagnosis of posttraumatic stress disorder. The trigger that causes these events to occur can be subtle. It can be a sound, smell, or flashback of the traumatic episode. The student cannot control what is happening and after the event is very embarrassed and tired. The student takes medication and has psychotherapy sessions to help with the episodes. The student loses concentration and class time and feels stigmatized by his panic episodes. The student has withdrawn from the other children, especially at recess and lunch.
3. *Describe how the handicap affects a major life activity:*
   - Ineffective breathing pattern related to panic evidenced by shortness of breath, sweating, and nausea
   - Fear related to traumatic event evidenced by panic state and lack of concentration in class.

   These occurrences have disrupted the learning process, socialization, and the ability of the student to experience a day without the fear of an attack.
4. *Describe the reasonable accommodations that are necessary:*

   Teacher: Separate the student from other children, to rear of the room or the nurse's office if possible.

   Teacher and school nurse: Encourage him to tell you his own thoughts.

   Teacher: Reassure that the trauma is not present and try to make the student comfortable.

   Teacher and school nurse: Work with the student on the prescribed relaxation techniques from his therapist (guided imagery).

   School nurse: Assist the student to try to identify the trigger for that episode.

   School nurse: Maintain communication to parent and therapist regarding medications, techniques to dissipate the reaction.

   School nurse: Administer medication and practice role playing what to do when it starts, help student to learn how to gain control.

   Teacher: Assist the student to ease gradually into new situations, preparing the student with what to expect ahead of time.

   School nurse: Encourage the student to share with a friend (about the panic attack) and begin to develop social contact.

   School nurse (teacher): It is emotionally difficult for others to see this occur, so explain that this is an illness and that the student is working hard to get better.

Review date: 2 months: ______________ then, as warranted
Participants: (name/title) Date:
Copy to: _____ Health file _____ Site 504 coordinator _____ Parent _____ Case manager _____ Other

***Dependent on each state practice act, certain parts may be delegated.

Box 9.13 ■ ■ ■

SECTION 504 STUDENT ACCOMMODATION PLAN—ASTHMA

Name: Sara Date of birth: Grade:
School: Date of meeting:

1. *Describe the nature of the concern*:
Sara has just been diagnosed with asthma within the past 2 months and has difficulty understanding what asthma is, how to complete the treatment regimen, how to recognize a crisis, and fearful when she becomes short of breath because of hospitalization.

2. *Describe the basis for the determination of the handicap*:
Sara is unable to keep up with the gym class requirements without becoming short of breath, coughing, and experiencing fatigue. She has missed 8 days in 2 months due to an asthma crisis and hospitalization. Academic performance has dropped due to anxiety, absence, and inability to concentrate (failed two tests and homework not complete). Lung function less than 75% normal. Sara has to use the inhaler medications frequently throughout the day and has difficulty with the administration of the inhalers.

3. *Describe how the handicap affects a major life activity:*
   - Unable to complete gym activities.
   - Requires medication administration; uses inhalers frequently.
   - Unable to take part in all class activities (trips, activities due to fatigue or triggers to asthma).
   - Has school absences due to asthma crises.

4. *Describe the reasonable accommodations that are necessary:*
   - Gym teacher and nurse develop adaptive (but inclusive) gym.
   - In-service gym teacher regarding limitations, signs of crisis, inhaler administration
   - Develop programs building up to normal endurance, incorporating ability and stamina as asthma management improves.
   - The school nurse assists with inhaler administration, teaching procedure, types/reasons for use, peak flow meter reading to determine crisis so that Sara can demonstrate self-care or health maintenance and be able to make appropriate decisions in managing asthma symptoms.
   - Teacher communication with the school nurse/parent regarding trips, outings for medication administration arrangement. Teacher to incorporate "fish" or "ant farm" instead of furry animals.
   - Teacher develops a "missed class work plan" for absences, arranges for one-to-one help or new concepts that were missed, and provides adequate time for make up work to be handed in.
   - School nurse to educate teacher for signs of crisis and provide emergency action plan (EAP).
   - School nurse to review with Sara: triggers, adherence schedule of inhalers, crisis plan, how to recognize the symptoms of a crisis.
   - School nurse to communicate with parent/physician as to changes or problems in asthma management plan; recommend support group for Sara.

Review date: 2 months:_________then September and January of academic year or as warranted
Participants: (name/title) Date:
Copy to:_____ Health file _____ Site 504 coordinator _____ Parent _____ Case manager _____ Other

For example, a student with arthritis might require the use of a word processor to provide a quicker, less painful means of writing. For the student with AIDS, Section 504 may address administration and monitoring of medication or a class schedule modification to address the student's stamina. Services for the student with ADHD may include modification of the regular classroom with special assistance from an aide or special directions needed by the faculty, having an extra set of textbooks at home, developing a behavior plan, monitoring of medication, and counseling. In all of these cases, the Section 504 services would allow the student an equal opportunity to learn.

504 Accommodation Plan Components

The 504 Accommodation Plan consists of the following components: (1) description of the nature of the concern; (2) description of the basis for the determination of the disability; (3) description of how the disability affects a major life activity; (4) description of supplementary aids, services, and accommodation needed; (5) review/reassessment date; and (6) participants' names/titles; name of case manager. Also included in the 504 Accommodation Plan are lists of the types of services, aids, and accommodations as well as the dates for the initial agreement and when services are to be initiated and terminated (34 CFR, Part 104).

Types of interventions that enable access to or participation in the educational program or activities include instructional interventions (classroom-small group); tools (writing, computer, augmentative, or sensory access); procedures (schedules or routines); and services (medical, interpretation, personal care, or transportation). Examples of medical services might be dispensing medication or catheterization; personal care could involve assistance with daily personal needs or assistance with ambulation or transferring from a wheelchair. There may be a need to modify the classroom to accommodate specific allergic reactions, a plan for evacuation for a wheelchair-bound student, or accommodations for special diets or an emergency action plan for a student with a peanut allergy. For many of the accommodations, in-service for faculty or staff is part of the process and should be identified in the plan.

School Nurse's Role in a 504 Student Accommodation Plan

The school nurse's role is critical to the development of Student Accommodation Plans. Students who may qualify for Section 504 may be having their needs met through the IHP. On the other hand, it may take the authority of the Section 504 to obtain all the necessary accommodations from other staff or faculty. The IHP can be incorporated into a Student Accommodation Plan (Arnold & Silkworth, 1999).

The school nurse can easily incorporate the IHP and EAP into the 504 Accommodation Plan (Table 9.1). The *assessment data* for the IHP can be used for the Section 504 "description of the nature of the concern" and the "description of the basis of the determination of the disability"; the *Nursing Diagnosis* can be the Section 504 "description of how the disability affects a major life activity"; and the *Nursing Interventions* can serve as Section 504 "description of instructional aids, services, and accommodations" (29 U.S.C. sec. 794). If a student qualifies for Section 504, there must be an IHP and an EAP (if relevant) on file in the health office. If the student has an EAP, it must be incorporated into the 504 Accommodation Plan or attached to it. Once it is completed and signatures are obtained, the faculty and/or staff in-service can be completed.

Differences Between IDEA and Section 504

All individuals who are disabled under IDEA are also considered to be handicapped and therefore protected under Section 504. However, all individuals who have been determined to be handicapped under Section 504 may not be disabled under IDEA. Students who qualify for a 504 plan usually are in

Table 9.1 ■
COMPONENTS OF IHP AND 504 ACCOMMODATION PLANS

ASSESSMENT DATA	NURSING DIAGNOSIS	NURSING INTERVENTIONS	EXPECTED OUTCOMES
Description of the "nature of the concern" Description of the "basis of the determination of the disability"	Description of "how the disability impacts a major life activity"	Description of "instructional aids, services and accommodations" and EAP if needed	

Source: Arnold & Silkworth (1999, p. 44).

regular education and receiving the regular curriculum. Students who are not eligible for IDEA services but are "handicapped" may need reasonable accommodations in order to access the educational program. Often, a student may qualify under both, yet the school district will provide an IEP due to advantages with funding and service resources.

Whereas IDEA limits eligibility only to students who have certain specified types of disabilities that may need special education, Section 504 protects all handicapped students who have any physical or mental impairment that limits one or more major life activities (learning), even if they do not need special education. An example of a student who would qualify under Section 504 and not IDEA is one with juvenile arthritis who does not need special education. This student may need adaptive aids to assist in note taking or writing because of painful joints, but does not need any assistance in "learning."

Both IDEA and Section 504 are federal laws but are carried out for different reasons. IDEA comes to the state with a baseline funding with the sole purpose to supply the "eligible" student with an IEP that enables the student to be involved in and progress in the general curriculum while meeting their educational needs that result from the student's disability. Should the "child with a disability" be eligible under the criteria, an initial evaluation is conducted by the multidisciplinary education team to determine eligibility and develop a statement of the special education and related services needed for the modification of the education program.

IDEA requires states to set up a process to comply with the law regarding process and procedures. As a result, each state has developed a structure for their IDEA educational process to fit that state's infrastructure. Therefore the IDEA process will vary among states. IDEA has general criteria for states to interpret and develop policy and procedure for compliance with the law, that is, initial evaluation, reevaluation, and components of the IEP. It also provides safeguards, that is, due process, grievance and appeals to the board of special education (Council of Administrators of Special Education [CASE], 1998).

On the other hand, Section 504 is a result of a civil rights law with the sole purpose to prevent discrimination on the basis of a handicap. This law provides for reasonable accommodations to be made for individuals who are "protected handicapped" persons. The student who qualifies as a "protected handicapped student" has a disability that interferes with the ability to benefit from or gain access to his or her educational program and needs accommodations in order to learn Just as students without the disability. The student should not need special education.

Some aspects of both laws are similar with regard to free, appropriate public education. By meeting the regulations for IDEA, schools also meet Section 504. Yet in other aspects, the laws differ. IDEA defines "eligible" students who have certain types of disabilities and as a result of that disability need special education or specially designed instruction. Section 504 "protects" all handicapped students who have a physical or mental impairment that substantially limits one or more major life activities, including learning but do not need special education (TABLE 9.2).

There are many protections for safeguarding the procedure for the IEP but very few with the 504. IDEA provides for due process and hearings/grievances through an Office of Special Education while the violations for Section 504 are reported directly to the Office of Civil Rights and can be taken directly to the regional civil rights court without first going through an administrative hearing (CASE, 1998).

Table 9.2 ■

COMPARISON OF THE IEP VS. SECTION 504 ACCOMMODATION PLAN

IDEA	CRITERIA	SECTION 504
IDEA, Part 300—Right to a Free Appropriate Public Education for students with special needs. Active identification, "child find" required of each Local Education Agency (LEA) for ages 3 years and older.	Federal Regulations	Section 504 (Rehabilitation Act of 1973)—Prohibits discrimination on the basis of a handicap (Civil rights legislation). Deals with providing reasonable accommodations for students who are handicapped.

(continued)

IDEA	CRITERIA	SECTION 504
To ensure that all children with disabilities have available a free appropriate public education that emphasizes special education and related services designed to meet their unique need and prepare them for employment and independent living.	Purpose	To ensure that "protected handicapped" students have equal opportunity to participate in school programs and extracurricular activities to their maximum extent appropriate to the ability of the student.
A. "A child with a disability" is considered a child with mental retardation, hearing impairment, vision impairments, speech or language impairments, deaf-blindness, emotional disturbances, orthopedic impairment, autism, traumatic brain injury, other health impairments, specific learning disability, and who, by reason thereof, needs special education and related services. B. Child aged 3 through 9—"child with a disability" may include a child experiencing developmental delays.	To qualify	"Protected handicapped students" have a disability that substantially limits participation in or access to the school, education program or extracurricular activities. Protected is a handicapped student who has a physical or mental impairment that substantially limits a major life activity
Student requires specially designed instruction and related services to benefit from the education.	Special or regular education	Appropriate education is comparable to the education provided to non-handicapped students, requiring that reasonable accommodation be made.
Federal funding set base amount per eligible student.	Funding	No funding
Requires modification to provide access to FAPE.	Accessibility	Regulations require building and program be accessible via reasonable accommodations
Informed consent required before evaluation. Multidisciplinary team must have special education teacher, regular teacher, administrator, individual related services for membership, and parent.	Process	Informed consent not required but recommended. Designated 504 individual and any other staff that may have input about the barriers. Composition varies with each case.
Full comprehensive evaluation required assessing all areas related to the suspected disability. Must be variety of sources. Reevaluation every 3 years or less.	Evaluations	Information from a variety of sources that demonstrates the impact the condition has on access to the building or program.

(continued)

Table 9.2 ■ *(Continued)*

IDEA	CRITERIA	SECTION 504
Interpretation of evaluation data by MDT must result in an IEP. IEP must contain specific components involving learning objectives and goals.	Placement or services document	Service agreement contains the list of reasonable accommodations and dates of services. Must include an Accommodation Plan describing what the assessment found and how that impacts on the accessibility to the program.
Grievance procedure, due process, administrative hearing, at Office of Special Education	Procedural safeguards	Due process or Office of Civil Rights and discrimination court case.

Source: Council of Administrators of Special Education (1998, pp. 4–7).

To assist in better understanding of the two federal regulations, the school nurse can obtain information from the Office of Special Education and Office of Civil Rights. More importantly is the need to obtain the interpretation of the regulations from the state's department of education. On the local level, contact the individuals who are appointed within the school district to comply with these federal regulations.

CONCLUSION

The number of students with special needs in the schools is increasing. Students with special needs, due to either a chronic condition or disability, are at higher risk for academic failure and dropping out of school, at a rate almost two times that for students without disabilities (*Federal Register*, 1997). These students are more likely to become unemployed or incarcerated (*Federal Register*, 1997). Often students from minority backgrounds are not placed appropriately in the educational system. Even with the two federal laws in place since 1973 (Section 504) and 1975 (IDEA), many students have not benefited from the services that are available (*Federal Register*, 1997). The 1997 Revisions of IDEA and those being developed in 2005 are directed at improving these results and making schools accountable to their state for improving the education of students with special needs. The expectation of students with disabilities are to be integrated into the general education program, ensuring their access when appropriate and providing the necessary accommodations to promote a higher level of success with a more meaningful educational program. To prepare these students for employment and independent living changes, an outcome approach is needed to ensure accountability for better results for children with disabilities.

School nurses strive to promote the development of students with special health needs towards independence in their own care. This includes becoming knowledgeable about all aspects of their disability and treatment, empowered to advocate for oneself, and motivated to become proactive with their disability. The school nurse must demonstrate leadership within the educational team so students with special needs can achieve these goals.

The NASN Standards of Care require the use of the nursing process when providing care for school age youth (NASN, 2003). The IHP is just one example of this. The school nurse has a responsibility to be proactive and advocate for the students with special needs; she or he can do that best by being a member of the multidisciplinary education team and a member of the Section 504 team. The school nurse is the only individual "qualified" (IDEA Part 300.23) to provide an interpretation of a student's health status and the impact on the ability to learn.

Theoretically, with health-related needs, the IHP should do what Section 504 does. With an IHP in place, the 504 Accommodation Plan is not needed if the IHP can provide all the necessary accommodations. It is this area of practice that designates the school nurse as an invaluable part of the educational team. One of the main goals for the school nurse is to promote and maintain the health of students at an optimal functioning level in order to maximize student learning. Proactively developing the IHP and serving as a regular member of the multidisciplinary educational team demonstrates the school nurse's accountability for practice.

The IHP enhances communication among the members of the team so they might better understand the student's health status and its impact on their learning. It ensures safety for students in health crises and decreases anxiety among faculty and staff in case of health emergencies. In many cases, the IHP provides the accommodations that every school should do regardless of the federal mandate in Section 504. This is just one of numerous roles for the school nurse but is possibly the most critical in ensuring the safety of students and their ability to succeed in today's society.

References

American Academy of Pediatrics (AAP). (2001). *Policy statement: The role of the school nurse in providing school health services.* Elk Grove Village: IL:AAP.

Arnold, M., & Silkworth, C. (1999). *The school nurse's source book of individualized healthcare plans* (Vol. II). North Branch, MN: Sunrise River Press.

Awbrey, L. M., & Juarez, S. M. (2003). Developing a nursing protocol for over-the-counter medications in a high school. *Journal of School Nursing, 19*(1), 12–15.

Council of Administrators of Special Education, Inc. (1998). Student access: A resource guide for educators. *Section 504 of the Rehabilitation Act of 1973.*

Denehy, J. (2003). Documentation dilemma: What to record and why. *Journal of School Nursing, 19*(4), 187–190.

Harrigan, J. (2002). *Overview of school health services.* Castle Rock, CO: NASN.

Hootman, J. (1996a). *Nursing diagnosis: Application in the school setting.* Scarborough, ME: NASN.

Hootman, J. (1996b). Nursing diagnosis: A language of nursing. *Journal of School Nursing.* 12(4), 5–9.

Individuals with Disabilities Education Act (IDEA) Code Federal Regulations (CFR), Part 300. (1999).

Lowe, J., & Miller, W. (1998). Students with chronic health problems. *Journal of School Nursing,* 14(5), 4–16.

McClosky, J., & Bulechek, G. (2000). *Nursing intervention classification.* St. Louis: C. V. Mosby.

Moorhead, S., Johnson, M., & Maas, M. (2004). *Nursing outcomes classification.* St. Louis: C. V. Mosby.

National Association of School Nurses (NASN). (2003). *Position statement: Individualized health care plans.* Available at: http:www.nasn.org/positions/careplans.htm

National Association of School Nurses (NASN). (2002). *Issue brief: School nurses and the Individuals with Disabilities Education Act (IDEA).* Available at: http:www.nasn.org/briefs/idea.htm

National Association of School Nurses (NASN) & the American Nurses Association (ANA). (2001). *Scope and standards of school nursing.* Scarborough, ME: Author.

North American Nursing Diagnosis Association (NANDA). (2001). *NANDA Nursing diagnoses: Definitions and classification 2001–2002.* Philadelphia: NANDA.

Praeger, S., Zickler, C., & Mosca, N. (2002). *Care of students with special needs in schools.* Castle Rock, CO: NASN.

Section 504 of Rehabilitation Act 1973 (29 U.S.C.A. –794).

Silkworth, C., Arnold, M., Harrigan, J., & Zaier, D. (2005). *Individualized healthcare plans for the school nurse.* North Branch, MN: Sunrise River Press.

U.S. Department of Education (USDOE). (1997). *Federal Register, 62*(204), 55028–55092.

Wilkinson, J. (2000). *Nursing diagnosis handbook with NIC interventions and NOC outcomes.* Upper Saddle River, NJ: Prentice-Hall.

Zaiger, D. (2001). *School nursing practice: An orientation manual* (2nd ed.). Scarborough, ME: NASN.
34 Code of Federal Regulations Part 104.3
Chapter 15. Protected Handicapped Students. (1991). Public School Code of PA.

Chapter 10

Emergency Management, Crisis Response, and the School Nurse's Role

BETTY FITZPATRICK

Chapter Outline

INTRODUCTION

Ten years ago, the thought of devoting a chapter of a text about school health to Emergency Management and Crisis Planning might have been perceived as far-fetched, but this is no longer true. From the era of school shootings to snipers on the loose to threats of bioterrorism, school children are confronted with unimaginable traumas and fears of catastrophe. How should schools prepare themselves to provide necessary supports? What is the role of the school nurse? Are there ways to spot troubled youth and intervene to avoid violence in the school setting?

In 1996, the nation became familiar with school shootings when a student in Moses Lake, Washington killed one teacher and two students. Soon after, communities in Pearl, Mississippi, West Paducah, Kentucky, Jonesboro, Arkansas, and Springfield, Oregon suffered similar tragedies. Then on April 20, 1999 two students entered Columbine High School shooting and killing 12 students and one teacher and injuring 23 others before killing themselves. The entire nation and world reacted. Columbine entered the lexicon of the English language. Never more would the first image conjured up in someone's mind when they heard the word Columbine be a beautiful, resilient, alpine flower.

Forever more it would bring images of terrorized students fleeing a school and parents frantically searching and waiting to hear from their sons and daughters. The country was fixed to TV screens as a 4-hour drama unfolded before their very eyes. A nation was left to wonder, what went wrong? Columbine High School had joined the club that no school wanted to be part of—school districts and communities that have experienced crisis. This chapter discusses the school nurses' role in emergency management (including natural and man-made disasters), crisis response, short-term and long-term needs after traumatic events, early identification of troubled youth, and the school nurse as first responder.

School violence has not been confined to the United States or to this past decade. In Dunblane, Scotland, a crazed man entered a primary school and killed 16 children and their teacher; in Osaka, Japan, a crazed man entered an elementary school and killed 8 students and injured 18 others in a knife attack; and in 2004, Chechen rebels crammed 1,200 children, parents, and teachers into a gymnasium on the first day of school and held them for 52 hours before killing 349, 172 of whom were children, and wounding 542.

In Bath, Michigan in May of 1927, Andrew Kehoe, a farmer and treasurer of the local school board, detonated dynamite in the school building, killing 38 children and 5 adults, and injuring 58 others. Mr. Kehoe was angry about new taxes levied to support the school. While many have never heard of this tragedy, this small community remembers the event and its aftermath 75 years later. While many communities believe "it couldn't happen here," these events illustrate it could happen anywhere. It is incumbent on schools to plan for any type of disaster.

The events of September 11, 2001 and the sniper assaults in the Washington, DC area only emphasize this. The impact of tragedy on the role of the school nurse is significant. The school nurse is looked to for the first response, for physical or psychological first aid, crisis response, emergency management, bioterrorism and communicable disease expertise, and for long-range support. The educational background and clinical expertise of the school nurse prepares her or him to play a critical role in all these arenas.

This chapter provides guidelines and suggestions for the nurse to carry out this role. It is divided into sections on emergency management, crisis response, risk assessment of the troubled student, and the school nurse as a first responder with first-hand accounts from the author's experience at Columbine High School, the World Trade Center terrorist attack, and cluster suicides at one high school. Implications for school nursing practice are discussed.

For the purposes of this chapter, a disaster is any incident that results in multiple human casualties or essential public health services or any incident that requires an increased level of response beyond the routine operating procedures, including increased personnel, equipment, or supply requirements (Maloney, Fitzgerald, Elam, & Doyle, 2000). Disasters include but are not limited to hurricanes, floods, tornadoes, nuclear accidents, fires, civil riots, shootings, hostage situations, and biochemical emergencies. They are difficult to anticipate and react to when they happen. Awareness and planning are crucial to minimize the effects of disaster on a community.

EMERGENCY MANAGEMENT

Emergency Management is not a new concept. It originated in the early 1970s when the Forest Service experienced many large forest fires in the California area. Multiple agencies organized together to respond efficiently and effectively to an emergency without duplication of services or resources. This is known as the "Incident Command System" (ICS). Over the years, it has become the standard by which communities respond to large-scale disasters, both natural and man-made.

Typically, when a disaster strikes, multiple agencies respond. Communities that plan, prepare, and use the ICS process find that they are better able to respond successfully to their crisis. A critical incident in the school is an event that overwhelms a person's ability to cope and negatively affects the school and classroom behavior (Johnson, 2004). School districts across the nation are developing Emergency Management Plans and teams utilizing ICS as a way to respond to any crisis that may occur (Jefferson County Schools, 2000). The school nurse plays an important role on the team.

Safe Schools

As school officials develop emergency plans, one of the primary goals is to assure students, staff, parents, and communities that their school is safe. Students will learn and grow only in an environment where they feel safe. Superintendents and all school officials should have a primary responsibility to ensure that all of their schools are safe. Components of school safety should include the following:

A focus on academic excellence

Partnerships

Prevention

Intervention

Crisis intervention

School climate survey/assessment

All of these components will include a multidisciplinary team approach and a commitment by school boards and legal counsel to develop a systematic framework that is broad and encompassing for any emergency. Each component has many pieces and will take extensive work to develop fully. One component of the intervention has been previously discussed under the guise of Emergency Management and the ICS. The school nurse can participate effectively in all of these pieces and assume a leadership role.

The school nurse is the key person in the school community who is knowledgeable of the physical and emotional needs of the students served by the school. She or he is also familiar with the staff, parent, and community that encompass the school. It is critical, therefore, that the school nurse be a resource in the planning, implementation, and execution of the disaster plan. The school nurse is particularly important in the areas of crisis response and being a first responder to the public health crisis, first aid/CPR (response and training), staff development for responding to a crisis, including bioterrorism, developing community outreach/partnerships, and implementing short- and long-term mental health and physical health support on site. The role of the school nurse in crisis intervention and partnerships is one for which the school nurse is particularly skilled and prepared.

Before discussing emergency plans and the role of the school nurse, it is necessary to examine the ICS, as it relates to specific school emergency plans. As school districts have adapted to the ICS as the format for their own school's plan, many communities have signed agreements that all agencies involved will use the ICS system. When multiple agencies are required to coordinate a response to a disaster, they may choose to use the Unified Command Center where all agencies responding are represented.

The Incident Command System

Incident Command is a complex job that requires effective planning and organization. Its purpose is to mitigate, plan, respond, and recover. The system is designed on the following concepts:

- Establishes common organizational structure, terminology, and operating procedures.
- Reduces confusion.
- Provides for tasks to be performed quickly/effectively.
- Establishes one person in charge of the total emergency operation.
- Provides an effective span of control related to who is in charge.
- Provides effective communication/coordination of response agencies/school district.
- Provides effective transition of responsibility/authority during emergency situation.

Incident Command Team

The Incident Command Team is composed of school staff members who are preidentified and includes an Incident Commander (IC); Liaison Officer; Public Information Officer (PIO); Financial Officer; and Operations, Documentation, and Logistics personnel. The functions of the team are to:

- Assume emergency responsibilities and report immediately to the Command Center,
- Control immediate emergency response by providing leadership,
- Have primary and backup personnel for each leadership responsibility,
- Relinquish control when law enforcement/fire personnel arrive,
- Become part of the Unified Command Structure, and
- Coordinate both emergency response and communication with law enforcement/fire personnel.

There are several different models evolving for teams. Agencies might change the name of team members. For example, some agencies use the Liaison Officer and Safety Officer interchangeably. Documentation Personnel might also be called Planning/Intelligence Personnel.

The Incident Commander (IC) is solely responsible for emergency/disaster operations and should remain at the Command post to direct all emergency operations. At the school site, this is usually the principal. The school incident commander should be ready to turn over the command to law enforcement or other agency heads if, for example, the emergency's nature changes to that of a crime scene or hazardous material spill. During the Columbine shootings there was confusion that did not settle out until all agencies responding cooperated and formed a Unified Command Center. It was critical that the school principal be included in this center as he was the one most knowledgeable about the school layout, number of staff and students inside, and district staff available for support and planning.

The IC is responsible for the following tasks:

- Assess the emergency situation; determine the threat to human life or the site.
- Decide on implementing appropriate responsibilities and procedures.
- Authorize information release through the PIO and District Communications.
- Authorize the release of students to parents/guardians during or after the emergency.
- Determine when to release staff after the emergency situation.
- Ensure that the emergency response is documented for legal/financial reasons.
- Monitor how well or poorly the plan worked.

The *Liaison Officer* responds directly to the IC and responsibilities include:

- Report to the command center immediately.
- Seal off emergency area.
- Keep unauthorized persons from entering area.
- Coordinate with law enforcement/fire and emergency responders.
- Attend briefings with IC.
- Assume responsibilities of IC, if necessary.
- Provide building blueprints/site maps, and so forth.
- Assign staff/support personnel to the duties of:
  media supervision
  traffic control
  parent supervision
  first aid support
  student supervision (evacuation and reunification)

The *Public Information Officer* (PIO) reports directly to the IC and responsibilities include:

- Set up official news media site (away from command site).
- Act as official spokesperson.
- Coordinate joint press releases.
- Monitor news broadcasts regarding the emergency.
- Correct misinformation immediately.
- Communicate with parents, community, and so forth.

Documentation Personnel responsibilities include:

- Maintain written documentation of emergency and other phone calls and events
- Compile student attendance records.
- Identify absent/missing students.
- Account for all staff.
- Forward copies of written documentation after the emergency is over.
- If there is a death(s): remove student name from mailers, computers, autodialers, mailing lists, and so forth.

The *Logistics Person* is responsible to:

- Report to the command center immediately.
- Give the appropriate emergency signal (lockdown, evacuation, etc.).
- Immediately contact appropriate emergency personnel and district officials.
- Notify the Crisis Response Team.
- Contact school transportation.
- Contact community partners (Mental Health, Red Cross, etc.).
- Monitor use of the phone.
- Distribute supplies and equipment.
- Coordinate witness information.
- Coordinate supplies, staffing, and facilities' needs.

Operations Personnel are responsible to:

- Report to the Command Center for instructions.
- Wait for police/fire at the main entrance.
- Turn off gas/electricity as directed by the IC.
- Report location of injured.
- Report building damage.
- Direct and support fire, police, and rescue workers.
- Extinguish small fires immediately.
- Coordinate building activities (i.e., lockdown,

evacuation, sealing windows, structural damage, etc.).
- Check every classroom, restroom, and building area.
- Work with Logistics Personnel related to staff, supplies, facilities, and communications.

The *Finance Office* or Administrator is responsible for financial activities such as keeping track of expenditures, payment records, overtime, purchasing, and contracting for services.

This structure is a modular structure that can be fluid to adjust to the expanding or shrinking needs of the emergency, as well as the size and type of facility. Each box in FIGURE 10.1 notes a function…not a person. A variety of personnel can fill these roles: administrator, counselor, school nurse, psychologist, social worker, teachers, secretary, aides, custodian, or other support staff.

Team members should have the desire to be on the team. They should possess such personal characteristics as a calm demeanor; good leadership, crisis, and communication skills; and a sense of compassion. An effective team usually ranges from a minimum of four members to a maximum of eight members. Key duties will include medical/nursing intervention, debriefing, counseling, security, administrative duties, and communication at many levels.

School nurses are uniquely qualified to participate in all aspects of emergency management and crisis response. She or he has the experience to participate in all aspects of planning, responding, mitigation, recovering, and evaluating.

The recovery phase includes "engaging in short-term efforts to restore people to physical and mental health and vital systems to minimum operating conditions; and long-term efforts to restore entire disaster areas to previous conditions" (Schools and Terrorism, 2004, p. 48). Mitigation includes "activities that eliminate or reduce the chance of occurrence or the effects of a disaster" and include changes in policies and security practices (i.e., checking bookbags, keeping school door locked) (Schools and Terrorism, 2004, p. 50).

The school nurse is vital in direct response as in planning first aid response, triage techniques, evacuation plans for students with special needs, direct treatment of students and or staff, and emotional support to traumatized students and staff. *Disaster Preparedness Guidelines for School Nurses* (Doyle & Loyacono, 2002), prepared for the National Association of School Nurses, has specific guidelines that all school nurses should follow.

INCIDENT COMMANDER (IC)
Name ____________
Phone # ____________

PUBLIC INFORMATION OFFICER
Name ____________
Phone # ____________

DISTRICT COMMUNICATIONS
Name ____________
Phone # ____________

SCHOOL ADMINISTRATOR
Name ____________
Phone # ____________

District Security Personnel
Name ____________
Phone # ____________

District Crisis Response
Contacts & Numbers

LIAISON OFFICER
Name ____________
Phone # ____________

OPERATIONS Personnel
Name ____________
Phone # ____________

DOCUMENTATION Personnel
Name ____________
Phone # ____________

LOGISTICS Person
Name ____________
Phone # ____________

Staff without students to supervise

Staff with students Supervisory Duties

Staff with First Aid Responsibility

Custodial Staff

Figure 10.1 ■ Sample emergency management system.

What Should a School Emergency Plan Include?

The first step is to develop a school emergency plan. Key players on the crisis team should be involved in the development and implementation. Each school should determine the make-up of their teams based on who is available as resources. Key players include but are not limited to the principal or assistant principal, school nurse, psychologist or social worker, guidance counselor, teaching staff, secretarial staff, classified staff, food services personnel, and custodial staff. Additional members might include community members, parents, students, or members of school decision-making committees.

The plan needs to include the following:

- An outline of a predetermined response plan
- Provision for trained individuals with knowledge and skill to act as emergency responders
- Provisions to minimize the risk of serious injury, death, or property damage
- Provision for immediate first aid to those in need
- Provision for counseling and support for staff, students, parents, and community members during and after the crisis
- Exercises and drills to determine if the plan works
- Provision for accurate, up-to-date information to be given to parents, the community and the media
- Guidelines for responding to the media during a crisis
- Guidelines for how to utilize community resources and create partnerships to assist in the response
- Debriefing procedures for crisis teams
- Guidelines for how to evaluate the response and revise the plan as necessary
- A goal to return the school to its normal level of function as soon as possible
- Development of a "post emergency plan" for the aftermath of any disaster

The goal is to facilitate effective communication, decision-making, and coordination of services between the school and emergency responders and the school community. Once a plan is developed, there should be an assessment, as each emergency situation is unique and many decisions will need to be made at the individual site as the situation unfolds. Emergency plans should include a comprehensive list of situations and be reviewed annually. Training should also take place annually with mock drills practiced several times a year.

Schools are challenged by disaster and crisis. A proactive approach that includes detailed planning is important. Will there be enough resources in place? Are community partnerships in place? The time to forge alliances is not during or after an emergency. Community partnerships and collaborations need to be forged early in order to have a successful outcome. Make sure all the players are included. The list of community participants should be reviewed annually. Since 9/11 and the threat of all types of terrorism, it is critical that new partnerships be developed with public health, emergency preparedness, and other agencies. In emergency and crisis situations, individuals will respond as they are trained! Training should be thorough, complete, and ongoing.

Communities that do not respond effectively to mass tragedy experience multiple sequelae. These include:

- Increase in death by suicide and accidents
- Increase in family dysfunction, domestic violence, and divorce
- Higher rates of substance abuse and depression
- Increase in dropout rate and decreases in staff retention

Unfortunately, those at highest risk usually do not seek treatment (Pfefferbaum, 1999).

Developing a "Go Box"

It is imperative that each school creates a "**Go Box**" that contains essential information and equipment. This should be portable and accessible and something that an assigned person can grab and take with them as soon as the emergency is declared. The school nurse can be a critical person in compiling the "Go Box." Its recommended contents are shown in TABLE 10.1.

Most schools are now planning for 24 to 72 hours of lockdown. This means that the school needs to have enough supplies for medical treatments and medications to last until the students are reunited with their parents.

SCHOOL NURSES AND CRISIS RESPONSE

The school nurse is a natural leader and integral partner as plans are developed for first aid, evacuation, care for special needs students, triage responsibilities, staff education, and surveillance for

Table 10.1 ■
"GO BOX" CONTENTS

Student list
Staff list
Significant health problem list: Students Staff
Medication list: Students Staff
Blueprints of school, school yard, and outside buildings
Emergency evacuation plans for special education/special needs students
Two- to three-day supply of medication for these students
Walkie-talkie/cellular phone/bullhorn
Copy of emergency plan/flip chart
Flashlight/extra batteries
Pictures of students/staff (yearbook)
Local and district phone books and other important numbers.
Master keys for buildings
Markers, pens, legal pads, name tags

possible infectious diseases (Doyle & Loyacono, 2002). School nurses are key to medical planning, surveillance, and reporting; they are effective communicators and educators regarding health risks and providers for immediate crisis support and links to mental health for long-term support. They are an important link to the medical/public health community and to parents.

School nurses have long been important members of their school crisis teams. Usually, these teams are familiar with single incident responses, that is, the death of a student or staff member or, on occasion, a multiple fatality accident. Crisis team members must prepare themselves to respond to a situation where there are hundreds of victims. School nurses must have preparation in both the short- and long-term crisis response. Typically, short-term response includes the period from the start of the emergency until several days thereafter. Long-term response can continue years after the disaster or crisis.

Short-term needs include:

- First aid
- "Psychological first aid"
- Defusing and debriefing
- Establishing a sense of safety
- Establishing a sense of normalcy

Long-term needs include:

- Grief support
- Ongoing psycho-education
- Community outreach
- Identification of posttraumatic stress disorder (PTSD), anxiety, and depression
- Outside referrals
- The principles of interventions are as follows:
- There is no right or wrong way to respond. Each individual will have his or her own unique way to react and almost all responses are normal.
- There is no accurate, predetermined timetable for recovery.
- The incident cannot be erased. How we integrate this memory is crucial to our mental well-being.
- Be aware of developmental differences in reaction to crisis and loss.
- Be sensitive to cultural/ethnic differences in grief response.
- The response to a human-caused catastrophe is different from that to a natural disaster.
- Some who have been affected may have ongoing problems.

It is imperative that the school nurse and all members of the crisis teams understand reaction to loss. Loss is a normal reaction to an abnormal situation. The victim of trauma or loss will react based on a variety of influences: life history, personality, social support systems, previous losses, closeness to the threatening event, coping strategies, age, and current developmental stage (Table 10.2).

Table 10.2 ■

DEVELOPMENTAL STAGES OF POSSIBLE REACTIONS TO ILLNESS OR DEATH

AGE	CONCEPTS OF DEATH	FEELINGS	BEHAVIORS	HOW TO HELP
Birth–2 years	• Separation/ absence • Reacts to change in routine and emotional climate	• Miss and ache for sound, smell, sight or feel of someone • Fears being abandoned • General anxiety	• Thrashing, Rocking, throwing • Crying • Sucking, biting • Sleeplessness • Indigestion	• Physical contact and reassurance • Attend to immediate physical needs • Maintain routines • Include the child in process of mourning when possible and appropriate • Be patient
2–5 Years	• Death is temporary and reversible • Finality of death is not evident • To be dead is to be sleeping or on a trip • May wonder what deceased is doing • Magical thinking and fantasies, often worse than realities • Understanding is limited	• Sad • Anxious • Insecure • Withdrawn • Confusion • Angry • Scared • Cranky (feelings acted out in play) • Agitated	• Crying • Fighting • Interested in dead things • Acts as if death never happened • Regressive behaviors • Repetitive questions • Expressing strong feelings in his/her sleep and dreams • Expressing feeling through play	• Answer repetitive questions • Give simple and truthful answers to questions • Include child in family rituals and in mourning process • Provide safe ways to express feelings • Maintain structure and routines • Encourage children to play and to have fun • Tolerate the child's needs to regress for awhile (being held, sleeping with others, thumb sucking etc.) • Physical contact • Let the child cry • Talk

(continued)

AGE	CONCEPTS OF DEATH	FEELINGS	BEHAVIORS	HOW TO HELP
6–9 Years	• Thinks about the finality of death • Thinks about the biological processes of death • Death is associated with bodily harm, mutilation and disintegration • Personify death—a spirit, monster, death man, ghost gets you when you die • Who will care for me if my caregiver dies • My actions or words caused the illness or death • Death is a punishment	• Sad • Anxious • Withdrawn • Confusion • Angry • Scared • Cranky (feelings acted out in play)	• Aggressive acting out • Withdrawal • Nightmares/sleeping disturbances • Act as if the death never happened • Lack of concentration • Declining or greatly improved grades • Regressive behaviors • Specific questioning—looking for detail	• Answer questions truthfully • Look for confused thinking • Encourage expression of feelings • Offer physical outlets • Encourage drawing, reading, playing, art, music, dance, acting, sports • Physical contact • Have intentional times to grieve together • Let child choose how to be involved in the death and mourning process • Find peer support for the child • Work with school to tailor workload • Talk
9–12 Years	• Understanding of the finality and universality of death • Death may happen again • What will happen if my caregiver dies • My actions and words caused the illness or death	• Vulnerable • Anxious • Scared • Lonely • Confused • Angry • Sad • Abandoned • Guilty • Fearful • Worried • Isolated • Shock • Denial • Emotional turmoil heightened by physical changes	• Aggressive acting out • Withdrawal • Talks about physical aspects of illness or death • Acts like illness or death never happened • Does not show feelings • Nightmares/sleep disturbances • Lack of concentration • Declining or greatly improved grades • Regressive behaviors	• Answer questions • Expect and accept mood swings • Give choices about how to be involved in death and mourning rituals • Find peer support groups • Encourage expression of feelings • Encourage reading, writing, art, music, sports • Talk

(continued)

Table 10.2 ■ *(Continued)*

AGE	CONCEPTS OF DEATH	FEELINGS	BEHAVIORS	HOW TO HELP
			• Changing behavior • Acting out role confusion	
12 years and older (teenagers)	• Understanding the finality of death • If I show my feeling I will be weak • I need to be in control of my feelings • Can sense own impending death • Self-centered and thus have an exaggerated sense of their own role in regards to the death	• Vulnerable • Anxious • Scared • Lonely • Confused • Angry • Sad • Abandoned • Guilty • Fearful • Worried • Isolated • Shock • Denial • Depression • Highly self-conscious about being different due to grief	• Impulsive behavior • Fighting, screaming, and arguing • High risk behavior • Grieving for what might have been • Acts like the illness or death never happened • Lack of concentration • Changes in grades • Sleep disturbances • Changes in eating patterns • Changes in peer group • Acting out role confusion • Conflict within teen about moving to independence and remaining dependent	• Expect the thoughts and feelings of the teen to be contradictory and inconsistent • Allow their coping behavior in covering up their grief if it is basically harmless to themselves and others • Encourage expression of feelings • Look for high risk behaviors • Encourage relationships with other supportive adults • Listen • Display honest grief, share in discussions • Answer questions truthfully • Give choices about involvement in death and mourning rituals • Encourage peer support groups • Talk

Source: Jefferson County Schools (1997).

The school nurse must be aware of all the potential losses that students and staff may bring into the crisis situation with them. This will greatly influence how they react to the present crisis.

Death and serious losses will trigger the act of grieving. Grieving is a process that will assist the individual to move forward and integrate this life event in a meaningful and healthy way that will allow him or her to once again function at a productive level. Kubler-Ross (1969) suggested five stages of reaction to death: denial and isolation, anger, bargaining, depression, and acceptance. All literature and studies since are a variation of her seminal work on death and dying. There is no set timetable to spend or resolve each stage. Nor is there a specific sequence, and many people will move back and forth through different stages. Fatigue, insomnia, generalized somatic complaints, eating problems, distractibility, and restlessness are a few common physical symptoms. Unresolved grief can manifest itself many years later. Individuals with unresolved grief pay a high price in mental distress and illness. Grief that is not paid attention to can lead to other serious problems, such as substance abuse, risky behaviors, anxiety, panic disorders, clinical depression and psychosomatic illnesses (Herman, 1997). It is imperative that school nurses keep these points in mind as they monitor students after they have been impacted by a major disaster. The school nurse should be aware of appropriate developmental stages and how individuals in each stage react to death, the variety of ways a student may react to loss, cultural differences, exterior and interior supports of individual students, and the anticipated grief reactions. He or she is then prepared to be a contributing member of the crisis team and emergency response plan.

Prior to the event, crisis teams should have determined what type of debriefing system should be used for student and staff as psychological first aid. There are a variety of methods, such as NOVA (National Organization of Victims' Assistance) [Box 10.1], CISM (Critical Incident Stress Management), and the Sanford Model developed by Nancy Sanford from the Los Angeles Unified School District. It is essential that victims be encouraged to participate in debriefing groups but this must always be voluntary. No matter what method is used, it will be helpful to understand a person's immediate reaction to a crisis [Box 10.2].

Box 10.1 ■ ■ ■

STAGES OF CRISIS INTERVENTION

Safety and Security	= physical safety, emotional security
Ventilation and Validation	= tell the story, validate the crisis
Prediction and Preparation	= anticipate the future, prepare to cope

(NOVA, 1999)

Box 10.2 ■ ■ ■

IMMEDIATE CRISIS REACTION

Physical Reactions	Emotional Reactions
Immobilization (frozen flight)	Shock, disbelief, denial (emotional numbness)
Mobilization (flight, fight, adapt)	Cataclysm of emotions (Anger, fear, confusion, shame, frustration, humiliation, grief)
Exhaustion	Reconstruction of life equilibrium

No matter which method of debriefing is utilized, all the above stages should be followed. The debriefing should be guided by a skilled facilitator; group norms are agreed to; everyone should have a chance to speak; individuals may pass; and confidentiality is assured, unless, of course the facilitator feels a group member is in danger of hurting himself or others. Mary Schoenfeldt's training manual, *School Crisis Response Teams: Lessening the Aftermath*, describes the five phases of a debriefing session (Schoenfeldt, 1993). They are:

Introductory Phase: Explain process, establish guidelines, introduce participants, and establish safety.

Facts Phase: Dispel rumors, establish known facts, provide students with an opportunity to share their experience with the event.

Reactions Phase: Allow students to talk about their feelings and normalize their feelings. Emphasis is placed on the feelings. There is no right or wrong way to feel. Also included is discussion of feelings and reactions after the event was "over." Again, it is important to stress that all reactions are normal responses to an abnormal situation/event. This phase will also address how this event may have affected the student's friends, family, and the community.

Teaching Phase: The facilitator summarizes facts; clears up misconceptions; explains what to expect next; and explains typical trauma reactions, including behavioral, physical, emotional, and cognitive symptoms. Risk-taking behavior should be discussed and discouraged. Healthy coping skills should be discussed as well as other helpful outside supports and resources.

Closure Phase: This final phase helps affirm the value of the group process and group cohesiveness. Reviewing intense feelings and the way group members can assist each other is essential to closure. Reminding the members that what was shared in the group should remain confidential is an important step. Thank the students for their participation and willingness to share their feelings. Discuss next steps and proactive plans and determine if there is a need for further meetings. Finally, go around the group and do a check by asking each student to share what they learned. Facilitators should let students know that they are available for individual conferencing, if desired. After students leave, it is imperative that the school nurse and any cofacilitator debrief each other. What went well, and what could be improved? Are there any students about whom the school nurse is concerned and needs to follow further? The school nurse can be the key to organizing the groups and keeping track of those students who still need debriefing or have declined.

While the immediate care of traumatized students is being undertaken, many other matters need to be addressed by other crisis team members simultaneously. They include:

- Have district administrators organize necessary internal and external support.
- Establish a communications system for internal systems as well as public media announcements and briefings.
- Request additional services if needed.
- Coordinate with other schools if they are affected.
- Communicate the crisis team plan to other staff members.
- Determine what information will be shared with different groups.
- Create fact sheets, memos to parents, press releases, letters to the community, and so forth.
- Designate a safe room for students.
- Designate a place for crisis coordination (include food/drink for crisis team).
- Designate a meeting place for parents, if necessary (can be off campus).
- Coordinate community resources.
- Plan for parent/community meetings.
- Debrief all crisis team members at the end of the day.
- Plan for additional responses.

Remember that crisis counseling or debriefing is NOT therapy. Most victims will be able to resolve their reaction to the crisis/disaster with their normal coping skills and the support of their family, friends, and church or community groups. However, a long-term response should also be planned.

Parents are a key link to returning the school to its normal routine. Communication is essential, with short, frequent communications that support what is happening at school. Box 10.3 contains recommendations for a communication with parents.

Another helpful resource for parents is one developed by Nancy Rich (Box 10.4), entitled "Critical Incident Stress Reactions," which was used with great success after the Columbine school shootings.

Box 10.5 provides parents with guidance regarding when their child's reaction to the crisis is atypical and requires the intervention of professional therapists.

Box 10.3 ■ ■ ■

QUICK TIPS FOR PARENTS AFTER A CRISIS

- Provide comfort and reassurances that their child is safe.
- Be honest and open about the disaster/tragedy.
- Assist parents to encourage their children to express their feelings through talking, drawing or playing.
- Limit TV viewing (especially if there is media coverage of the disaster).
- It is okay to let them see that you are feeling sad in response to the disaster/tragedy.
- Return to normalcy; try to maintain daily routines as much as possible.
- Seek help for yourself if necessary.

Box 10.4 ■ ■ ■

CRITICAL INCIDENT STRESS REACTIONS

Over the next few weeks you may experience normal reactions to the kind of experience you've been through.

Physical	Cognitive	Emotional	Behavioral
Fatigue/ exhaustion	Lack of concentration	Fear	Change in activity
Insomnia	Flashbacks	Guilt	Change in communication
Sleep disturbances	Difficulty in making decisions	Emotional numbing	Withdrawal
Over-/under activity	Memory disturbances	Oversensitivity	Suspiciousness
Nightmares	Amnesia	Anxiety	Hyperalertness
Change in appetite	Confusion	Depression	Startle reaction
Digestive problems	Poor problem solving	Feeling helpless	Change in sexual behavior
Physical problems	Disturbed thinking	Anger	Emotional outbursts
Headaches	Poor abstract thinking	Irritability	Scapegoating
Nausea	Change in alertness	Frustration	Pacing

These reactions are normal and, although painful, are part of the healing process. There is not a lot anyone can do to make you not experience these uncomfortable feelings but there are some things you can do to feel more whole.

THINGS TO TRY:

- Within the first 24 to 48 hours, periods of strenuous physical exercise alternating with relaxation will alleviate some of your physical reactions.
- Structure your time—keep busy.
- You're normal and having normal reactions—don't label yourself crazy.
- Talk to people—talk is the most healing medicine of all.
- Beware of numbing the pain with drugs or alcohol. You don't need to complicate this with a substance abuse problem.
- Reach out—people do care.
- Keep your lives as normal as possible.
- Spend time with others.

(Continued on the following page)

Box 10.4 ■ ■ ■

CRITICAL INCIDENT STRESS REACTIONS *(Continued)*

- Help those around you as much as possible by sharing feelings and checking out how they are doing.
- Give yourself permission to feel rotten.
- Keep a journal—write your way through those sleepless hours.
- Do things that feel good to you.
- Realize those around you are also under stress.
- Accept offered help.
- Eat nutritious, well-balanced meals high in carbohydrates and low in sugar.
- Avoid excessive use of caffeine.
- Don't make any big life changes.

(Nancy Rich, MA, LPC, CTS, 1999. Reprinted with permission of author)

Box 10.5 ■ ■ ■

WHEN TO CALL FOR HELP

Any significant change in your child's normal behavior

Suicide threats, direct or indirect

Unexplained crying, sadness, feelings of worthlessness

Preoccupation with death

Dramatic change in personality or appearance

Irrational, bizarre behavior

Changed eating or sleeping patterns

Severe decline in school performance

Isolation

Taking unnecessary risks

Use of alcohol or drugs

Withdrawal from friends and family

Withdrawal from activities of previous interest

Giving away belongings

Cutting or burning oneself

(Jefferson Center for Mental Health, 2000)

Long-Term Response

Immediate severe reactions need to be referred as soon as possible; however, symptoms that last over a 1-month period need to be monitored or referred for evaluation. Issues arise regarding resiliency versus vulnerability. It is necessary to assess what positive protective factors victims have in place and the degree of exposure of the event to the victim. Successful treatment of trauma victims has been achieved with a variety of therapies, including medication and cognitive therapy, to mention a few. School nurses are in a unique position to evaluate and observe students as they present with increasing numbers of physical and emotional symptoms, such as anxiety, depression, and posttraumatic stress disorder and syndrome (Fletcher, 1996) in order to provide support and to refer as necessary (see Chapter 34). School health professionals can also be key in assisting the educational staff in providing appropriate supports as trauma victims return to the classroom. A comprehensive school plan that involves all school staff needs to be in place that successfully reintegrates students back to school and their school day. Staff should be aware that students will return as changed individuals. Their definition of normal has been altered but a "new normal" can be achieved, and they can be successful.

Again, communication with parents is essential. FIGURE 10.2 helps illustrate the circles of concern of victims following a tragedy. This will help

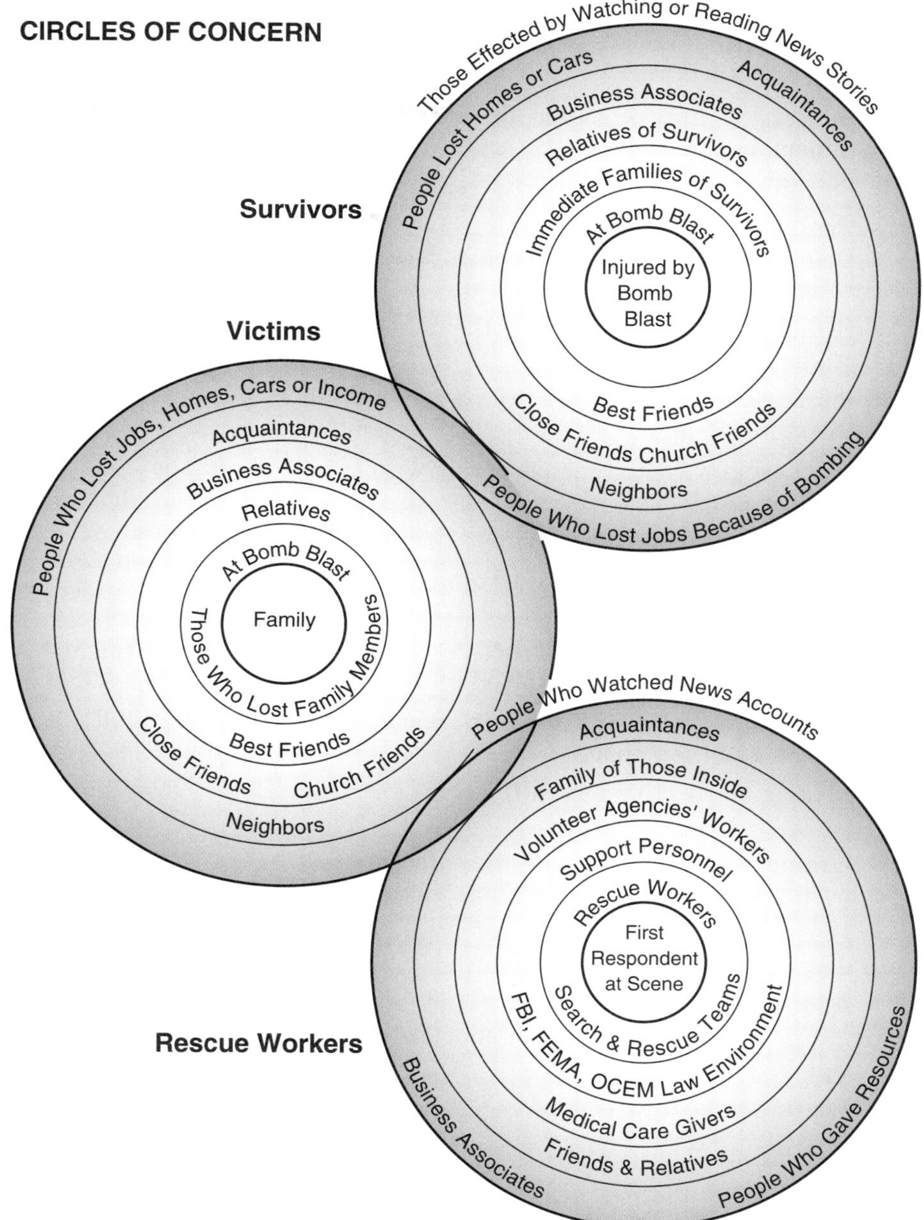

Figure 10.2 ■ Circle of concern. (*Source*: Jefferson Center for Mental Health, 1999.)

support personnel identify those students who could be at risk. It uses a bombing as the event but any disaster could be substituted.

PROVIDING ASSISTANCE TO TEACHERS

Many teachers will look to members of the crisis team for guidance on appropriate classroom activities. The school nurse has the education and experience to be a resource to the classroom teacher for suggested guided activities. Suggestions for classroom activities after a loss include the following:

- Writing a eulogy
- Designing a tribute for a yearbook
- Posting a sympathy card for all to sign and send to family
- Writing stories about the victim and or the incident
- Drawing pictures that describe your feelings around the incident
- Composing a song in memory of the victim/victims
- Creating a sculpture

- Debating controversial issues
- Investigating laws governing similar incidents
- Building a fitness course or brick path to remember the event
- Planting a garden or tree to remember the event
- Donating books to the school library in the name of the student
- Establishing a scholarship in the name of the student
- Participating in a community run or event in the student's name
- Discussing ways to cope positively with traumatic events
- Discussing the stages of grief
- Conducting a mock trial (if laws were broken)
- Starting a new school activity, such as Students Against Destructive Decisions (SADD) if alcohol was involved in the event
- Encouraging students to keep a journal of events and their reactions
- Placing a collection box in the class for notes to the family
- Urging students to write the things they wish they could have said to the victim
- Discussing alternatives to coping with depression if suicide was involved
- Analyzing why people take drugs and suggest ways to help abusers if substance abuse was involved
- Writing a reaction paper
- Writing a "Where was I when it happened" report
- Discussing historical precedents about issues related to the crisis
- Reading to the class appropriate and related stories
- Encouraging mutual support
- Discussing and preparing the students for the funeral
- Directing energy to creative pursuits, physical exercise, or verbal expression when anger arises
- Creating a class story or drama relevant to the issue
- Designating a few responsible students to stay in touch with the victim's family and invite the family to class events
- Remembering the students on holidays and anniversaries of the event

SCHOOL VIOLENCE RESULTING IN CRISIS

School violence has captured the attention of society. While it captures headlines and is certainly a crisis for the schools in which it occurs, in actuality, the incidence is small. In 1999, the year of the Columbine shootings, the odds of a child being killed on campus were 1 in 2 million. In the year 2000, the odds of a child being killed on campus were 1 in 3 million (The Justice Policy Institute, 2002; Ziedenberg, Brooks, & Schiraldi, 2000). The following graphs (FIGURE 10.3) demonstrate information about school shootings and causes of death in young persons.

From 1991 to 1997, the number of ninth- to twelfth-graders who brought a weapon to school fell from 26% to 18%; those involved in a fight and needing treatment by a nurse or doctor decreased from 4.4% to 3.5%. However, the report from the 1999 FBI symposium on school violence (including college campuses) revealed:

> 3 million incidents of violence a year on U.S. campuses,
>
> 282,000 students attacked each month,
>
> 100,000 incidents of students carrying guns to school on a daily basis, and
>
> A doubling of the incidence of youth homicide in the past 20 years.
>
> (Federal Bureau of Investigation, 1999)

The Justice Policy Institute's report on school violence (Ziedenberg et al., 2000) demonstrated the difference between public perceptions versus reality (FIGURE 10.4). The information clearly demonstrates the challenges educators and especially school nurses face in assuring students, staff, parents, and local communities that school is a safe place.

Early Warning Signs of Potential Violence in School Children

There has been much discussion about how to identify those students who might be likely to perpetrate violent acts against others or themselves. Groups such as the Secret Service, FBI, U.S. Department of Justice, and U.S. Department of Education have studied this issue extensively. In August of 1998, the U.S. Department of Education and the U.S. Department of Justice released a publication entitled *Early Warning, Timely Response*. This was sent

REASONS FOR DEATH

School Year	Accidental	Bully-Related	Drug-Related	Gang-Related	Hate Crime	Interpersonal Dispute	Robbery	Sexual Motivated	Suicide	Unknown
1993-1994	4	1		8		11	1	1	7	22
1994-1995				4		6			4	7
1995-1996	1	3		1		10	2		6	13
1996-1997	1	2		2		11		1	1	8
1997-1998		4		6		15		1	9	9
1998-1999	1	1		1	15	3			5	5
1999-2000	3			1		6			9	13
2000-2001	2			1		1	3		6	11
2001-2002						1	1		2	1
2002-2003				1		7			9	4
2003-2004				3		8			3	9
Totals	12	11		28	15	88	7	3	61	102

LOCATIONS OF DEATHS

School Year	Athletic Field	Restroom	School Bus	Cafeteria	Classroom/ Office	Hallway	Library	Near School	On Campus	Play-ground	Parking Lot
1993-1994	4	1	5	1	4	5		7	19	1	8
1994-1995	1	1			2	5		8	3		1
1995-1996	2	1	6		6	8		5	4		4
1996-1997	4	1	2		1	6		6	5		1
1997-1998	2	3	1	1	1	2		11	17		6
1998-1999	1	4	2		2	2	7	4	8		1
1999-2000		5		1	3	1		12	6	2	2
2000-2001		5			1			7	3		8
2001-2002					2	1		1			1
2002-2003	1	4	2	3	1	2		3	2		3
2003-2004	3	1	3					7	6	1	2
Totals	18	26	21	6	23	32	7	71	73	4	37

Figure 10.3 ■ Reasons for deaths.

to every school in the United States. Two subsequent reports were published—*The School Shooter, A Threat Assessment Perspective*, by the FBI (O'Toole, 2000), and *The Final Report and Findings of the Safe School Initiative*, by the U.S. Secret Service (Vossekuil et al., 2002).

Seven school districts where school shootings had taken place were invited to a week-long dialogue with law enforcement, justice officials, behavioral specialists, educators, and mental health experts. This extensive body of work has emphasized that a profile of a school shooter does not exist.

Public Perception vs. Reality: Data and Polling in Context

40%	The decrease in school associated violent deaths between school year 1997-1998 and 1998-1999
49%	The increase in poll respondents who fear a school shooting in their community from 1998 to 1999
1 in 2 Million	The chance that a school-aged child would die in a school in 1998-1999
71%	The portion of poll respondents who thought a school shooting was "likely" to happen in their community
56%	The decline in juvenile homicide arrests between 1993 and 1998
62%	The portion of poll respondents who believe that juvenile crime is on the increase
4%	The portion of juvenile homicides that occur in rural areas
First	The rank of rural parents in fear for their children's safety in schools vs. urban and suburban parents

Figure 10.4 ■ Public perception vs. reality: Data and polling in context.

While all these documents do agree on commonalities shared by school shooters, there is not one profile that would allow institutions to identify the student who might be capable of these acts. There are some warning signs and safeguards that schools can put in place to allow them to intercede early, identify troubled students, and have procedures in place that would decrease a violent act occurring in their school. However, profiling can stereotype innocent students. It can also exclude students who do not "fit" the profile but may pose a risk for targeted violence. Profiling can create bias against students who are different because of appearance, ability or disability, race, sexual preference, and religious beliefs, to name a few. It may also open the door to litigation (Vossekvil et al. 2002).

A Secret Service Report studied 37 school shootings involving 41 attackers. They interviewed 10 attackers. The U.S. Secret Service and the U.S. Department of Education (2002) reported on the findings of their safe school initiative. Their 10 key findings were:

1. Incidents of targeted violence at school rarely were sudden, impulsive acts.
2. Prior to most incidents, other people knew about the attacker's idea and/or plan of attack.
3. Most attackers did not threaten their targets directly prior to advancing the attack.
4. There is no accurate or useful "profile" of students who engaged in targeted school violence.
5. Most attackers engaged in some behavior prior to the incident that caused others concern or indicated a need for help.
6. Most attackers had difficulty coping with significant losses or personal failures. Moreover, many had considered or attempted suicide.
7. Many attackers felt bullied, persecuted, or injured by others prior to the attack.
8. Most attackers had access to and had used weapons prior to the attack.
9. In many cases, other students were involved in some capacity.
10. Despite prompt law enforcement responses, most shooting incidents were stopped by means other than law enforcement intervention (U.S. Secret Service, 2002, pp. 11–12).

Violence is the product of an interaction between the perpetrator, situation, target, and the setting. There is a distinction between making a threat and posing a threat (Reddy, 2000).

There are early warning signs or "red flags." Schools need to be proactive and have safety nets in place in order to identify troubled students and provide support and interventions prior to tragic events. Educators should strive to form partnerships with parents, community, and support resources so that a system is in place when there are indicators that a student may need help. In this way, school systems can act responsibly and in a caring manner to intervene before problems escalate. All care must be taken to avoid misinterpretation and misuse of these early warning signs. The following principles are offered to guide professionals:

- Do no harm—these signs should not be used to misidentify, stereotype, isolate, or punish. All schools are required by law to have professional staff and a plan to evaluate students for potential disabilities. Confidentiality laws remain in place and parental consents should be obtained.
- Understand violence and aggression within a context—what else is going on in school, home, peers, and outside social environments (including work and church) that may

influence the student? What are his or her strengths and weaknesses?

- Avoid stereotypes—preconceived stereotypes can interfere with the ability to fairly and professionally assess a situation and can do irreparable harm.
- View warning signs within a developmental context—staff should be aware of typical developmental behavior so as to avoid misinterpretations.
- Understand that children typically exhibit multiple warning signs—research has demonstrated that students who commit violence against themselves or others usually exhibit multiple warning signs.

(U.S. Department of Education, 1998)

The early warning signs include:

- Social withdrawal
- Excessive feelings of rejection
- Excessive feelings of isolation and being alone
- Being a victim of violence
- Feelings of being picked on and persecuted
- Low school interest and poor academic performance
- Expression of violence in writings and drawings
- Uncontrolled anger
- Patterns of impulsivity and chronic hitting, intimidating, and bullying behaviors
- History of discipline problems
- Past history of violent and aggressive behavior
- Intolerance for differences and prejudicial attitudes
- Drug use and alcohol use
- Affiliation with gangs
- Inappropriate access to, possession of, and use of firearms
- Serious threats of violence

(U.S. Department of Education, 1998)

This list is not inclusive and students who exhibit some of these signs will not necessarily go on to commit violent acts against themselves or others. Good judgment, common sense, professional assessment teams, knowledge of laws, and school board policies and appropriate intervention plans will go a long way to assist a school in ensuring safety nets that protect students and staff alike.

Imminent signs are those that indicate a student is close to acting in an injurious way to themselves or others and MUST be acted on immediately. They include:

- Serious physical fighting with peers or family members
- Severe destruction of property
- Severe rage for seemingly minor reasons
- Detailed threats of lethal violence
- Possession and/or use of firearms and other weapons and threatening to use it
- Other self-injurious behaviors or threats of suicide
- Detailed plans (time, method, place) to harm or kill self or others

Developing the Plan

In an effort to be proactive, many school districts have established a plan to respond to concerns that a student may be potentially dangerous to him- or herself or others. These plans should be formulated within the framework that already exists in schools to allow for interventions for students. They should be consistent with guidelines, regulations, policies, and laws that currently exist to provide for equal access to education for all students, prohibit discrimination, ensure appropriate confidentiality, allow for sharing of information as deemed necessary, and ensure safety of all. The following is a partial list of such regulations that must be considered as risk assessment plans are developed:

Americans with Disabilities Act (ADA)

Individuals with Disabilities Education Act (IDEA)

Family Educational Rights and Privacy Act (FERPA)

Mandatory Child Abuse Reporting Laws

Gun Free Schools Act of 1994

Privacy Laws

OSHA requirements (state and federal)

Laws regulating disclosure of information related to juveniles

State campus safety legislation

Laws related to civil commitments of juveniles

Fourth Amendment

Fifth Amendment

Local and educational policies and procedures

Case law

Risk Assessment

Risk assessment is the process of assessing and managing a threat directed at an individual, a group, or one's self. A threat is defined as a situation in which the individual or group of individuals poses or has made a threat that may impact a person's physical safety or emotional status. Risk assessment involves the gathering and analyzing of various pieces of information about the individual(s) making the threat, determining if the potential for violence is real, and assessing the seriousness and imminence of the threat. The intent of this process is to design and implement intervention and management strategies that reduce or eliminate the potential for risk. Risk assessment supports schools in successfully managing the potential for violence. This process can also be used for identifying those students who are at risk for harming themselves (suicidal students).

A risk assessment team is a group of appropriate individuals representing the school, school district, mental health, law enforcement, and district legal counsel. Risk assessment teams are comprised of appropriate school and outside support personnel who can identify risk factors and have the knowledge and expertise to make further plans and interventions for the student. The school nurse is a natural member of this team. As mentioned previously, teams can be school level or district level.

The risk assessment team will be responsible for the following activities:

- React to potentially violent situations and gather and evaluate appropriate information.
- Locate resources to help manage a potential threat.
- Develop, implement, and monitor intervention strategies for the threat maker.
- Develop, implement, and monitor both short-term and long-term reintegration plans for the threat maker.
- Advise district administrators on the variables for risk potential.
- Maintain written documentation about the process.
- Forward violence risk concerns and information to the appropriate district level and/or law enforcement so that measures can be implemented to ensure safety.
- Follow appropriate laws, policies, and procedures.
- Conduct a preliminary investigation, including an interview of the student, review of student records, and interviews of other appropriate parties, including staff, students, parents, etc.).
- Determine the level or risk and seriousness of the threat.
- Determine response actions.

Response actions may include school consequences, law enforcement actions, mental health involvement, social services involvement, safety management plan, parental involvement, and a reentry plan. If risk assessment determines that the threat situation is serious and imminent, 911 and law enforcement should be called immediately.

There are five levels of risk assessment, with 1 being the highest and 5 the lowest. The following is a brief description of the levels.

Level 1: High risk of potential violence (qualifies for immediate arrest/hospitalization)

- Imminently dangerous to self and/or others
- Detailed threats of lethal violence
- Possession/use of firearms or other weapons
- Serious physical fighting
- Displayed significant early warning signs
- Significant existing risk factors and/or precipitating events
- Few, if any, stabilizing factors present

Level 2: High risk of potential violence that does not qualify for immediate arrest or hospitalization but requires referrals and active case management

- Displayed significant early warning signs
- Significant existing risk factors and/or precipitating events
- Few stabilizing factors may be present.
- Individual is going to hurt someone or self if some designated or inferred event occurs or does not occur in the future.
- Threat may or may not be explicit.
- Threat may be made and/or posed for future harm.

Level 3: Insufficient evidence for violence potential—sufficient evidence for repetitive and/or intentional infliction of emotional distress on others

- Displayed some early warning signs.
- Some existing risk factors and/or precipitating events
- Some stabilizing factors may be present.
- Threat of violence intended to cause others emotional distress
- Threat of violence rather than act of violence
- Threat of violence involving intimidation
- At-risk person may deny intention to cause distress but repeated actions are sufficient enough to cause distress in others.

Level 4: Insufficient evidence for violence potential/sufficient evidence for unintentional infliction of emotional distress on others

- Some early warning signs may be present.
- Little record of serious risk factors or dangerous behaviors
- Stabilizing factors reasonably well established
- Threat of violence does occur and could cause emotional distress.
- Single threat does occur but at risk person does not have intent.
- Individual can acknowledge the impact of his or her behavior.
- Individual can acknowledge the behavior is unacceptable and will not occur again.

Level 5: Insufficient evidence for violence potential/insufficient evidence for infliction of emotional distress on others

- Unfounded allegation and no risk of harm
- Story made up and untrue

(Adapted from Jefferson County Schools, Golden, Colorado, Risk Assessment Guidelines 2002)

The risk and stabilizing factors discussed in the above are described in Box 10.6. Stabilizing factors are essential to a student's mental health and stability. Risk factors and stabilizing factors should be examined at the same time. Figure 10.5 is a flow chart that demonstrates how decisions are made relative to risk assessment for one district; every school district should review the information and customize it for its particular needs.

Involving the Players

Safety should always be the number one consideration and schools will have to involve law enforcement, parents, child and family services, and mental

(text continues on page 227)

Box 10.6 ■ ■ ■

RISK VERSUS STABILITY FACTORS

Factors that increase or reduce the possibility of violent behavior

Place an "x" in the appropriate box for indicators that are identified as Risk and Stability factors

RISK FACTORS

Peers

- Behaviors on the part of peers that may give the at-risk student an excuse or rationalization to commit violence, acts as catalyst and/or justification for violence (perceived bullying, harassment, teasing, etc.)
- Perceived disparities in peer treatment—special groups get special treatment, favoritism toward certain peer groups or individuals
- Peer encouragement of violent acts
- Peer accomplices for violent acts

STABILITY FACTORS

Coping Skills

- Balance important issues simultaneously and without difficulty.
- Manage multiple life issues
- Responsible and values commitments to others

Interpersonal Skills

- Multiple friendships
- Ability to mix well with a variety of others
- Sense of self and self-worth
- Connections with friends and family

(Continued on the following page)

Box 10.6 ■ ■ ■

RISK VERSUS STABILITY FACTORS *(Continued)*

RISK FACTORS

Family

- Parents divorced/separated, having an affair
- Violence in the home
- Emotional, physical, sexual abuse
- Excessive harsh/severe discipline
- Substance abuse/dependency
- Neglectful and/or ineffective parenting
- Weak or absent same sex parent

Psychological Issues (if documented in medical/mental health records)

- Mental disorder(s)
- Depression/bipolar disorder
- Narcissistic, antisocial, paranoid, schizoid personality

Substance Abuse/Dependency

- Chemical/drug dependency and use

Self-Esteem

- Feelings of inadequacy, no self-worth
- Sense of being powerless, shame, isolation, inadequacy

Non-Acceptance of Responsibility

- Blames others
- Externalizes responsibility

Attachment Issues

- Intense and/or absent attachments
- Unwillingness to let go of attachments/relationships

Academic Issues

- Identified learning disabilities
- ADHD resulting in impulsive behaviors
- History of poor academic performance

STABILITY FACTORS

Mental Health Resources

- Avail themselves in a meaningful, productive, therapeutic relationship
- Therapy used to facilitate change
- Participates in drug/alcohol intervention programs
- Participates in self-help programs

Spirituality

- Positive spiritual belief system
- Use of positive prayer
- Actively believes and participates in his/her positive spiritual belief system

Peer Support

- Has law abiding pro-social friendships
- Has numerous friendships not limited to one social group

Rules and Boundaries

- Student accepts consequences appropriately
- Student understands difference between right and wrong
- Student follows school rules and expectations

Family

- Positive parental involvement
- Parents care about student's performance at school, respect for authority, exposure to drugs and alcohol, types of friends, type of media student is interested in
- Parents set and implement limits
- Effective and appropriate parenting skills and modeling exhibited
- Control and restrict access to weapons

RISK FACTORS	STABILITY FACTORS
Fantasy Life	
• Fantasies with violent themes, power and control components	
Spiritual Issues	
• Anti-God and anti-religious feelings	
• Satanism	
Birth Order	
• Successful older siblings may contribute to feelings of inadequacy, and so forth	
Background Issues	
• Geographical mobility	
• Early initiation of behavior problems	
• Criminal background	
• Poverty	
• History of bullying behaviors	
• Previous suicide attempts/threats	
Precipitating Events (catalyst for violent acting out)	
• Victim of bullying, ridicule	
• Significant personal rejection	
• Loss of romantic or personal relationships	
• Disciplinary action/investigation	
• Extreme jealousy	

health services in any of the above situations. Partnerships with all these groups will help to create safer schools and communities. While schools have many good, comprehensive prevention programs that begin in elementary school and continue through high school, they also must have successful intervention practices and plans. These interventions include:

- Coordinated services and partnerships that include all the players: school staff, parents, and community members
- Continuous communication with parents that is two-way. Staff should be willing to listen and to inform of the progress or lack thereof of their children.
- Maintenance of confidentiality and parents' right to privacy (FERPA) except when the responsible party determines there is an imminent danger
- Empowering students, staff, and families to intervene
- Supporting students in being responsible for their own actions
- Simplifying staff requests for urgent assistance

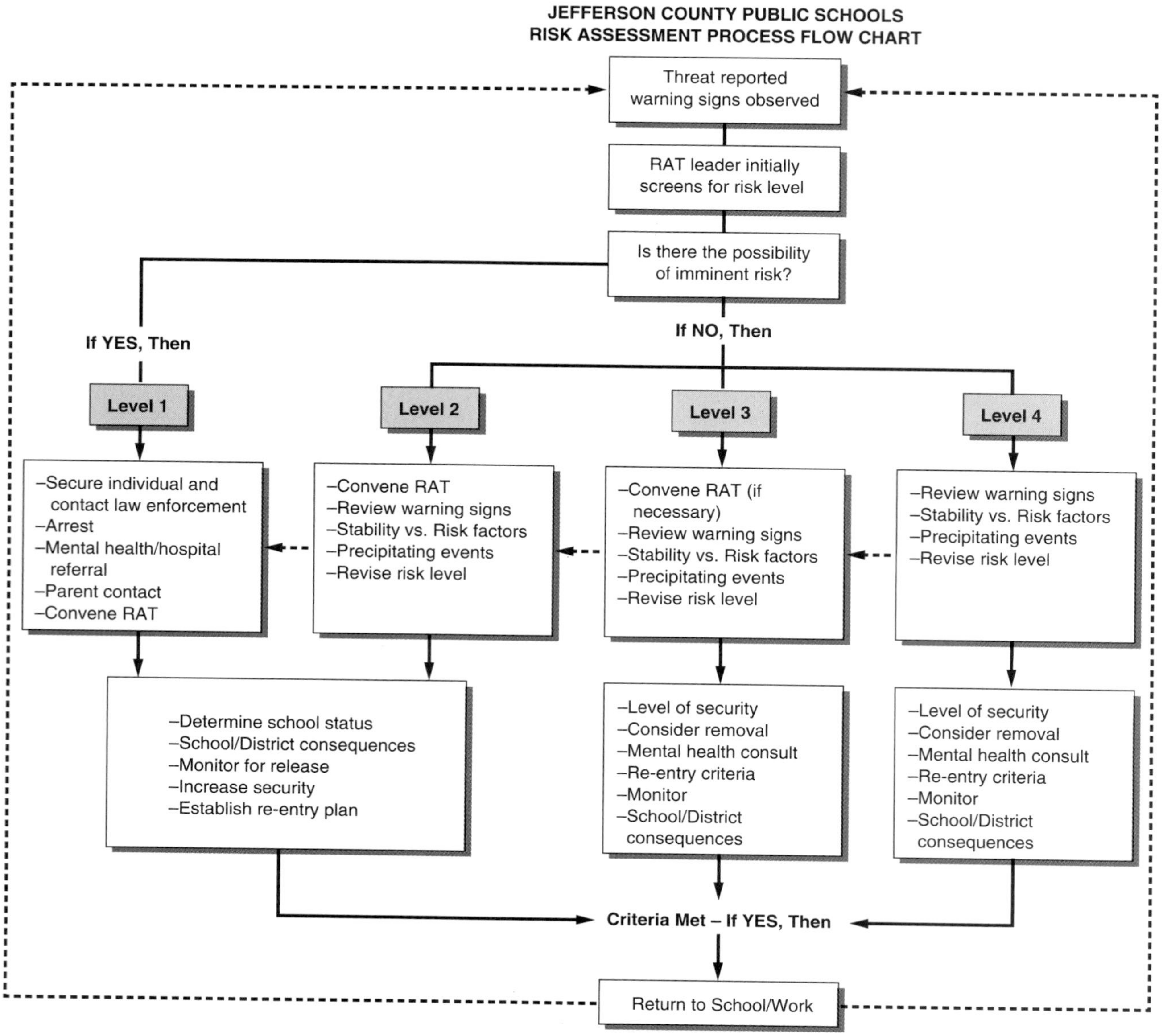

JEFFERSON COUNTY PUBLIC SCHOOLS
RISK ASSESSMENT PROCESS FLOW CHART
Threat reported warning signs observed
RAT leader initially screens for risk level
Is there the possibility of imminent risk?
If YES, Then
If NO, Then
Level 1
Level 2
Level 3
Level 4
–Secure individual and contact law enforcement
–Arrest
–Mental health/hospital referral
–Parent contact
–Convene RAT
–Convene RAT
–Review warning signs
–Stability vs. Risk factors
–Precipitating events
–Revise risk level
–Convene RAT (if necessary)
–Review warning signs
–Stability vs. Risk factors
–Precipitating events
–Revise risk level
–Review warning signs
–Stability vs. Risk factors
–Precipitating events
–Revise risk level
–Determine school status
–School/District consequences
–Monitor for release
–Increase security
–Establish re-entry plan
–Level of security
–Consider removal
–Mental health consult
–Re-entry criteria
–Monitor
–School/District consequences
–Level of security
–Consider removal
–Mental health consult
–Re-entry criteria
–Monitor
–School/District consequences
Criteria Met – If YES, Then
Return to School/Work

Figure 10.5 ■ Jefferson County public schools risk assessment processing flow chart.

- Making interventions available as early as possible
- Using sustained, multiple, coordinated interventions
- Analyzing the contexts in which violent behaviors occur
- Building upon and coordinating internal school resources

The following is a brief description of one school district's plan and procedures around risk assessment (Jefferson County Schools, 2002). Plans will depend on size, resources, community partnerships, and so forth.

Jefferson County Schools is the largest school district in Colorado, with more than 88,000 students and 156 schools. Each school has a school building team. Those teams can utilize the resources of the district level team, which includes community resources and law enforcement. It is important to remember that risk assessment is a parallel process that does not prevent the usual suspension/expulsion procedures from taking place. Disciplinary action may be occurring at the same time the risk assessment team is evaluating a student.

The risk assessment procedure used in Jefferson County Schools was developed after extensive training by Dr. Kris Mohandie, a Los Angeles

Police Department psychologist who has authored several books on violence including *School Violence Threat Management*. Readers are encouraged to refer to this resource for more detailed information on school violence and threat management (Mohandie, 2000).

BIOTERRORISM

While the discussion thus far has focused on violent events, most of the planning today revolves around the threat of bioterrorism. Bioterrorism refers to agents that can inflict a disproportionately large number of injuries and fatalities. The acronym CBRNE is used to refer to agents that fall into this category: chemical, biological, radiological, nuclear, and explosives.

Biological agents, also referred to as biological warfare, include toxins (botulism and ricin), viral hemorrhagic fevers (i.e., Ebola), plagues (i.e., bubonic), anthrax, smallpox, infected vectors (i.e., mosquitoes), and contaminated food and water. Chemical agents include nerve agents (either in vaporized or liquid form), blister agents, and industrial chemicals. TABLE 10.3 lists information regarding the most anticipated biological agents.

All of these produce a variety of symptoms. As students present to the school nurse, it is his or her

Table 10.3 ■
BIOLOGICAL AGENTS

DISEASE	SYMPTOMS	INCUBATION	PERSON-TO-PERSON TRANSMISSION
Anthrax			
Inhalation	Flu-like symptoms. Appears to improve, then rapid respiratory failure and shock	1 day to 6 weeks	None
Cutaneous	Intense pruritis, followed by painless papular/vesicular lesions. Develops into eschar surrounded by edema. Initially resembles insect bite	1–12 days	Direct contact with lesion
Gastrointestinal	Abdominal pain, nausea, vomiting, diarrhea, GI bleeding	1–7 days	None
Botulism	Afebrile, excess mucus in throat, dysphagia, dizzy, difficulty moving, descending weakness, flaccid paralysis	12–80 hours	None
Smallpox	Prodromal symptoms. Papular/vesicular rash distal to proximal; rash is all at same stage.	7–17 days	Airborne; droplet nuclei lesions are contagious.

Source: Delaware Department of Health and Social Services, 2004.

responsibility to "monitor unusual symptoms or signs, recognize patterns of symptom presentation, act to protect against spread of communicable diseases, and provide immediate treatment and decontamination for members of the school community" (NASN, 2002). The student should be questioned as to whether other members of the family are ill with similar symptoms. Are the student's friends also affected? If there is any suspicion of a possibility of an outbreak or if the symptoms are suspicious, public health officials should be notified immediately, and they will provide guidance as to the next steps to take.

One of the possible steps is to "lock down" the school to prevent anyone from entering or leaving. The goal is to keep outside threats from entering the building and internal conditions from affecting the community. The same planning system discussed earlier will be enacted. This is one of the reasons why schools are now preparing for being "parental custodians" for 48 to 72 hours. At the start of every school year, a letter should be sent to parents that explains the lockdown protocol. Designated staff should know and practice their roles in securing the building, getting the "go-box" and supplies, and getting students to safety.

Planning needs include preparations for meeting the students' and staff's needs for safety, clean air, toileting, nutrition, and sleeping. This includes medical supplies and a supply of student medications. In addition, there needs to be a system in place to count heads, a system for discharge to parents, and arrangements for transportation to another facility if need be. The students' emotional needs must be addressed and supplies should be available for some activities. Teachers and staff need to be aware of their responsibilities to the students and have made arrangements for their own families' safety. The same after-care measures can be used as discussed earlier in this chapter.

LESSONS LEARNED FROM THE COLUMBINE SHOOTINGS AND OTHER MAJOR DISASTERS THAT AFFECT SCHOOLS

There is now, tragically, a wealth of information that describes the long-term effects of crisis on school children. While crisis planning and support were created in response to natural disasters, it is apparent that human-caused disasters create different challenges that can cause more serious and enduring psychological sequela than ever realized.

A report following the bombing of the Federal Building in Oklahoma in 1995 (Pfefferbaum & Call, 1999) demonstrated that more than one third of youth in a large sampling of Oklahoma City middle and high school students reported knowing someone killed in the blast. The study was part of a clinical assessment completed 7 weeks after the bombing designed to provide information to school personnel organizing support services following the bombing. The report demonstrated that female sex, relationships to victims, and television exposure predicted posttraumatic stress symptomatology at 7 weeks (Pfefferbaum, Call, & Sconzo, 1999).

At Columbine High School, attempts were made to survey students after the shooting as they started a new school year in the fall of 1999. Complications arose with the process and the outside agency involved with the survey was unable to use the data gathered. It can be anecdotally reported that a similar number of students (33%) reported significant symptoms of emotional distress (Report to Jefferson County School Board, January, 2000 from School District Crisis Team).

Several other significant events retraumatized the same population of students in a 12-month period following the shootings. They included the suicide of the mother of one of the shooting victims, an Internet threat from another state that closed Columbine High School for several days, a nonrelated abduction and murder of a young boy who lived in the surrounding area, another unrelated murder of two teenagers (both Columbine students) who were working in a sandwich shop near the high school, and a suicide of a popular basketball player at the high school. The tragedy that surrounded the students created a situation that made recovery difficult.

The challenges that confronted the school district following the shooting were enormous. All 2,000 students and 170 staff members were designated victims of crime by the county District Attorney. This allowed all included to apply for Victims' Services, including counseling. Many families utilized private counseling services and also the services of their church counseling and support services. But most students, staff, and parents looked to the school and district staff for guidance.

Thousands of individuals were served by the community services for up to 2 years after the event; more than 2,500 received mental health services during this time. These costs do not include the additional cost of school district support services. In addition to mental health services, medical support was also required for those students who were physically injured. Four students returned paralyzed and in wheelchairs while 25 others had injuries of varying degrees that needed medical management. In addition, many students who were psychologically traumatized required individual academic support.

During the school year following the shootings, 52 students required the services of homebound teachers before they could return to school full-time (Fitzpatrick, 2000). Additional support was available to school staff, as necessary. Special attention was required at the school, as the school had to undergo extensive physical repair. Special attention was given to details in the project; even the sound of the fire alarm was altered so it did not mimic the sound that students who were trapped in the building that day heard for hours on end. Safety drills and fire drills had to be planned with great caution, so as to not retraumatize students and staff. Great attention was paid to significant holiday and anniversary events. It was necessary to continue support in the school years following the shooting. The graduating class of 2002 was the last class to have been present on that day in April. But school children of all ages remember that day and school districts must be aware and responsible as they acknowledge the effect of any major disaster on their student population.

School nurses had a major role in delivering care and support to students throughout the school district following the tragedy both directly at Columbine High School and in the other 150 schools in the district. The model to deliver health services to the students of Jefferson County is different than that for many school districts. The nurses coordinate services for five or six schools with the assistance of clinic aides. A full-time nurse was assigned to Columbine High School to coordinate health services. A full-time clinic aide was also present. The school nurse was a vital source in giving emotional support and referring students to mental health personnel. She was a resource and a major force in conducting educational opportunities for students, staff, and parents around what to expect, both physically and emotionally, after the events of the tragedy as they began to recover.

Another major tragedy that has demonstrated research on the effects of such events on school children is that of the terrorist acts on September 11, 2001. In May of 2002, an initial report was given to the New York City Board of Education. Key findings of significance to school districts were:

- An estimated 75,000 children in NYC (10.5%) have symptoms consistent with posttraumatic stress disorder (PTSD).
- An estimated 190,0000 (26.5%) New York City public school children in grades 4 to 12 have at least one of the assessed mental health problems (excluding alcohol abuse) and require some form of intervention
- Each of the mental health problems (probable psychiatric disorders) assessed exceeded the expected rates, based on pre-9/11 non-NYC community estimates
- The mental health impact is observed citywide; the prevalence of disorders is elevated all over the city, with effects not limited to Ground Zero schools.
- At least two-thirds of children with probable PTSD following the 9/11 attacks have not sought any mental health services from school counselors or from mental health professionals outside the school.
- Virtually all children in Ground Zero schools were personally physically exposed to one or more effects of the attack, including 73% who were in or near the cloud of smoke and dust.
- Two-thirds of children in the remainder of the city also experienced personal physical exposure to the effects of the attack.
- Eleven percent of NYC public school children had a family member or close friend exposed to the attack and 1% had a family member who was killed in the attack.
- Almost two-thirds of NYC public school children spent much of their time learning about the attack from the television.
- Nearly two thirds of NYC public school children had been exposed to one or more traumatic events prior to 9/11 (these included seeing someone killed or seriously injured, seeing the violent/accidental death of a close friend or family member).

It is clear that the challenges to school nurses to support students in schools that have experienced disasters and tragedies are enormous. Another example of crisis involved hundreds of thousands of students in the Washington D.C., Virginia, and Maryland areas who were traumatized and in lockdown for many days as a sniper went on a rampage in the fall of 2002.

CONCLUSION

It is incumbent on school nurses and their leadership to take a major role in the educational system to continue to be advocates for the physical and mental well-being of all students and to actively lobby both locally and nationally for appropriate support and resources. School nurses are in a pivotal position. They are trusted and respected. Their comprehensive and broad education provides an excellent background for being a first responder. "It is the position of the National Association of School Nurses that school nurses should be designated and recognized as, and given the authority to act as, first responders to mass casualty emergencies, including those resulting from bioterrorist events" (NASN, 2002).

School nurses are key to medical planning for schools. They are important for disease surveillance and reporting. School nurses are the link to the public health community. They are looked to as major communicators to student, staff, and parent groups regarding health risks, and they are a link to the mental health community. School nurses will be looked on increasingly by school districts and the medical community to provide support for any type of disaster/tragedy that occurs to the school-age population. It is an awesome responsibility but one that they are very capable of fulfilling.

SOME HELPFUL WEB SITES

American Academy of Child and Adolescent Psychiatry
http://www.aacap.org/publications.fadstam/disaster.html

American Academy of Pediatrics
http://www.aap.org/terrorism/index.html

American Counseling Association
http://www.counseling.org

American Psychological Association
http://www.apa.org/therapy/traumatic.stress

Centers for Disease Control
http://www.bt.cdc.gov

Center for Effective Collaboration and Practice
http://www.air-dc.org/cecp/

Center for Mental Health Services Knowledge Exchange network
http://www.mentalhealth.org/index.htm

Emergency Services and Disaster Relief Branch Center for Mental Health
http://www.mentalhealth.org/cmhs/emergencyservices

Federal Emergency Management Agency (FEMA)
http://www.fema.org/kids

Federal Government Substance Abuse and Mental Health
http://www.samhsa.org

Helping Children Cope with Disaster, National Parent Information Network
http://www.npin.org/library/2001/n00563.html

Helping Children and Adolescents Cope with Violence and Disasters
http://www.nimh.nih.gov/publicat/violence.cfm

High School for Heroes
http://www.hs4heroes.org

Jefferson County Schools
http://www.jeffco.k12.co.us

Johns Hopkins University
http://www.hopkins-biodefense.org

National Association of School Nurses
http://www.nasn.org

National Association of School Psychologists
http://www.nasp.org

National Center for Posttraumatic Stress Disorder
http://www.ncptsd.org/what is new.html

National Institute of Mental Health
http://www.nimh.nih.gov/publicatio/ridence.cfm

Posttraumatic Stress Disorder (PTSD), Trauma, Disasters and Violence
http://www.nimh.nih.gov/anxiety.ptsdmenu.cfm

Sesame Workshop
http://www.sesameworkshop.org/parents

Talking with Children When Disaster Strikes
http://www.tpt/org/TPTspecialedition/walsh.html

Ten Tips to Help Your Kids Deal with Violence, Parenting Press
http://www.parentingpress.com/resp 10 tips.html

Terrorism and Children, Purdue University Extension
http://www.ces.purdueedu/terrorism/children/index.html

University of Oklahoma, Department of Pediatrics
http://pediatrics.ouhsc.edu/

U.S Department of Education of Education
http://www.ed.gov

U.S. Department of Justice
http://www.usdoj.gov/

U.S. Government Information and Resources in Response to September 11th Events
http://www.firstgov/gov/featured/usgresponse.html

References

Delaware Department of Health and Social Services. (2004). *Biological agents. Division of Public Health. Dover Delaware.*

Doyle, J., & Loyacona, T. (2002). *Disaster preparedness guidelines for school nurses.* Scarborough, ME: National Association of School Nurses.

Federal Bureau of Investigation. (1999, July). *Symposium on the school shooter.* Quanitco, VA.

Fitzpatrick, B. (2000). *Report to school board, Jefferson County schools.* Golden, CO: Author.

Fletcher, K. (1996). Childhood posttraumatic stress disorder, in E. Marsh & R. Barkley, *Child psychopathology (pp. 330–371).* New York: The Guilford Press.

Herman, J. (1997). *Trauma and recovery.* New York: Basic Books.

Jefferson Center for Mental Health. (1999). *Training manual for first Responders.* Handouts for staff training after Columbine shooting Arvada, CO

Jefferson Center for Mental Health. (2000). *Parent guide to warning signs.* Arvada, CO.

Jefferson County Schools. (1997). *Crisis response team training manual.* Golden, CO. Author.

Jefferson County Schools. (2000). *Emergency management training manual.* Golden, CO. Author.

Jefferson County Schools. (2002). *Risk assessment training manual.* Golden, CO. Author.

Johnson, K. (2004). *Classroom crisis: The teacher's guide.* Alameda, CA: Hunter House.

Kubler-Ross, E. (1969). *On death and dying.* New York: Macmillan.

Maloney, P., Fitzgerald, S., Elam, K., & Doyle, J. (2000). *Managing school* emergencies III. Scarborough, ME: NASN.

Mohandie, K., (2000). *School violence threat management.* San Diego:

National Association of School Nurses. (2002). *Position statement: School nurse role in bioterrorism emergency preparedness.* Retrieved October 22, 2004 from http://www.nasn.org/positions/bioterrorism.htm

National Organization of Victims' Assistance. (1999). *Training manual.* Washington, DC.

New York City Board of Education Report. (2002, May). *Effects of the World Trade center attack on NYC public school students.* Prepared by Applied Research and Consulting, LLC. & Columbia University Mailman School of Public Health.

O'Toole, M. E. (2000, August). *The school shooter: A threat assessment perspective.* Association of Threat Assessment Professionals Annual Convention. Anaheim, CA. Retrieved August 2002 from http://www.fbi.org

Pfefferbaum, B. (1999). Presentation to Jefferson County school officials to assist in planning mental health services to students following school shootings at Columbine HS. Littleton, CO, April 1999.

Pfefferbaum, B., & Call, J. (1999). Lessons from the first two years of project heartland: Oklahoma's mental health response to the 1995 bombing, *Psychiatric Services, 50*(7), 953–955.

Pfefferbaum, B., Call, J., & Sconzo, G. (1999). Organizing the mental health response to human-caused community disasters with reference to the Oklahoma city bombing. *Psychiatric Services, 50*(7), 966–968.

Reddy, M. (2000). *Evaluating risk for targeted violence in schools: Comparing risk assessment, threat assessment, and other approaches.* National Threat Assessment Center, United States Secret Service.

Rich, N. (1999). *Critical incident stress reactions.* Jefferson Center for Mental Health, Arvada CO.

Schoenfeldt, M. (1993). *School crisis response: Lessening the aftermath.* Renton, WA: Schoenfeldt & Associates.

Schools and Terrorism: A supplement to the report of the National Advisory Committee on children and terrorism. (2004). *Journal of School Health, 74*(2), 39–51.

The Justice Policy Institute. (2002). *Study on school violence.* Washington, DC: Author.

U.S. Department of Education (USDOE). (1998). *Early warning, timely response; A guide to safe schools.* Washington, DC: U.S. Department of Justice.

U.S. Department of Health and Human Services. (2005). Bioterrorism Hospital Preparedness: CBRNE: HRSA. Retrieved May 2005 from www.hrsa.gov/bioterrorism/CBRNE/index.htm

Vossekuil, B., Fein, R., Reddy, M., Borum, R., & Modzeleski, W. (2002). *The final report and findings of the safe school initiative: Implications for the prevention of school attacks in the United States.* Washington, DC: U.S. Department of Education and U.S. Secret Service, National Threat Assessment Center.

Ziedenberg, J., Brooks, K., & Schiraldi, V. (2000). *School house hype: Two years later.* Justice Policy Institute. Retrieved May 5 from http://www.justicepolicy.org

Chapter 11

Evaluation of School Nurse Practice

PATRICIA GUILDAY ▪ JANICE SELEKMAN

Chapter Outline

INTRODUCTION

School nurses usually work independently, frequently as the only healthcare provider in their school. They have multiple responsibilities and are expected to meet the competencies of school nursing practice. Yet how are they evaluated and how do school nurses demonstrate the efficacy of their practice? Because they are usually not directly supervised by a nurse or evaluated by one, it is important to know who evaluates them and by what criteria. This chapter explores the evaluation of practice, especially as it relates to identifying and using outcome measures.

Florence Nightingale introduced science into the delivery of nursing care (Denehy, 2002). She was the first to note a relationship between nursing interventions and patient outcomes. These connections set the stage for the body of modern nursing research. The art and science of nursing continue to evolve. The "art" of nursing often defines itself by what nurses do and by the number of tasks and interventions performed. It is the "science" of nursing, however, that not only determines "best practice" and validates practice but also measures the results or outcomes of nursing interventions.

Nursing has created an environment in which the clinician who can perform the most tasks efficiently is the one most respected (Hill, 1999). Yet, a method is not yet in place that allows nurses in any setting to demonstrate and document that they perform skills and other tasks accurately and appropriately according to the gold standard of practice. This task-oriented role definition does not allow nurses, in particular school nurses, to evaluate the impact they have on the students entrusted to their care or on the state of health within the school and the school community. It also does not validate the importance or relevance of those tasks.

Maintaining the health and safety of students is a priority for school nurses (Stock, Larter, Kieckehefer, Thronson, & Maire, 2002). The presence of school nurses is meant to ensure that student health will be maintained, and consequently, that students will be more successful in school. School nurses use the phrase "school nurses do make a difference" (Denehy, 2000, p. 2) to validate their existence, yet, until recently, nurses were not being asked to demonstrate their effectiveness or to validate the difference they made. The recent emphasis on measuring outcomes challenges school nurses to show that they positively influence the health of children. It is also hoped that they will have an indirect positive effect on educational outcomes (Denehy, 2000).

If education is linked to health, then what is it about health services that ensures optimal student performance? Research should support the relationship between quality nursing services and positive outcomes in students' health. School nurses are often the only contact school-age children and adolescents have with the healthcare system. A model that delineates exemplary school nursing practice should seek to identify the connection between student interventions made by expert nurses and positive student outcomes (Pulcini, Couillard, Harrigan, & Mole, 2002).

FACTORS INFLUENCING SCHOOL NURSE EVALUATION

The clinical services that school nurses deliver are influenced by many variables:

- Educational preparation of the nurse (A bachelor's degree in nursing should have exposed the nurse to the principles and resources of community health as well as an introduction to nursing research.)
- Size of the school and the ratio of school nurse to students (The National Association of School Nurses recommends the nurse/student ratio be 1:750.)
- Ages of the students
- Baseline health status of students
- Community standards and expectations, such as the community's perception of the school nurse as simply an acute care provider in the school setting or as a valued member of the healthcare community
- Health care resources in the community, such as the availability of primary care and referral sources
- Administrative support from the school, the district, the Board of Education, and the Board of Public Health
- Amount of time the nurse spends in each school
- Ancillary duties assigned to the nurse, such as being responsible for late arrivals to school, absence lists, and truants
- Supervisory expectations, especially in states where one school nurse is responsible for multiple schools with the caregiving tasks delegated to non-nurses.

A task-oriented approach has opened the door for ancillary personnel being employed in schools under the direction of a school nurse. The supervising nurse may be assigned multiple schools or she may be the only nurse employed by a district. In this model, the professional nurse delegates direct care to a non-nurse who is employed in the school on a daily basis. This scenario severely limits the amount of time that the nurse has to interact with students and assess, or therapeutically manage student health problems. Consequently, the presence of unlicensed assistive personnel makes it difficult to determine which positive results are attributable directly to the actions of the school nurse.

WHO EVALUATES SCHOOL NURSES?

Since nurses are often the only healthcare professionals in a non-medical education setting, evaluations may be conducted by non-nursing personnel using non-nursing evaluative measures. An informal survey of practicing school nurses in 2003 revealed that most are evaluated by their principal or non-nurse education supervisor. Occasionally, a nurse in a supervisory capacity for the district or state Department of Education may be responsible for evaluating and monitoring school nurse practice.

School administrators may not have a clear understanding of the role of the school nurse. For any evaluation tool to have meaning for those performing the evaluation and to those being evaluated, it is the responsibility of school nurses to discuss their roles and responsibilities with those who supervise or coordinate school health services (Grabeel & Zaiger, 1998) and to differentiate their roles from those of other school personnel.

CURRENT METHODS OF EVALUATION

In addition to role confusion, evaluation tools are rarely specific to measure the efficacy of school nurse practice, as most of the criteria were designed to evaluate teachers. School nurses not only provide care for students within the school, but they also may engage in classroom health teaching, grant writing for school programs, policy development, participation on multidisciplinary teams, monitoring of the quality of the school environment, and outreach with the community No one else in the school performs all of these duties, yet these activities may not be evaluated.

There is a dearth of literature supporting that practicing school nurses are evaluated in a manner that is relevant to their practice, one that reflects the nursing skills of critical thinking, interpersonal relationships, and technical skills. There are currently multiple ways by which nurses are evaluated. Nurses, including those who work in schools, utilize peer review, self-evaluation, and continuing education to determine personal competence. Rarely is it reported that employers or supervisors of school nurses utilize any of these measures in their evaluative process. Therefore, many nurses are evaluated by standards or measures that may include such teacher-relevant categories as lesson planning, classroom management, test scores, instructional strategies, student-teacher interaction, effective communication with parents, providing prompt feedback to students regarding their performance, keeping records of student performance, and evaluation of student progress.

Others are evaluated on the criteria used for special personnel, such as guidance counselors, disciplinarians, psychologists, speech and language pathologists, and other support staff. These evaluation measures may include:

- Interacting with students and staff
- Establishing appropriate goals and objectives
- Using time efficiently
- Using appropriate methods and activities effectively
- Evaluating student performance
- Maintaining accurate records
- Complying with policies

Nurses have even reported being evaluated on the same form used for the custodians and clerical staff, on such criteria as the following:

- Job knowledge (job descriptions that are often developed by non-nurses)
- Quality of working relationships
- Attendance
- Use of sick or personal time
- Quality of work, as measured by neatness, thoroughness, absence of errors and safety violations; forms filled out accurately; or following the appropriate chain of command
- Number of tasks completed (number of students seen and referrals made to outside agencies)
- Ability to adjust to new assignments, including attitude

Some school nurses are evaluated solely on the number of tasks they perform. This includes the number of students seen, treatments completed, vision and hearing screenings completed, and medications administered. While this method certainly documents what the school nurse does, it does not speak to the quality and efficacy of these tasks nor the impact they have on students. In this modality, the school nurse is asked to keep lists or tabulations of what she does (TABLE 11.1).

A review of school nursing literature yields an abundance of articles related to identifying and itemizing nursing services. Numerous quantitative studies define school nursing practice by compiling a list of the most frequent interventions used in the school health office (Guilday, 2000; Telljohann, Price, Dake, & Durgin, 2004). The quality of these interventions or their impact on the students is not taken into consideration. Nursing makes a poor argument for having a professional school nurse available on a daily basis in every building if the only justification for this nursing presence is how many "tasks" that nurse is able to accomplish. Many of these tasks can be taught to ancillary personnel, much like parents are taught to perform medical therapies for their children. The major difference, however, is that parents are only taught to perform the skill to meet their child's needs. They are not educated in the variability of skills nor provided with the knowledge to determine when a skill should not be done. In addition, performance of some skills by non-nurses (such as administration of medication) is contrary to the Nurse Practice Acts in some states.

Traditionally, educational systems have asked school nurses to evaluate and measure their practice by providing lists of services. This process of listing services, that is, number and types of procedures performed, number of student visits, and counts of screenings and referrals, results in impressive lists that are perceived as important to legislators, school administrators, and parents. Nowhere in these reports are the outcomes of nursing services addressed, nor is there any indication of whether the task was performed accurately. A task-based focus of school health delivery does not provide the information necessary to support growth of the specialty.

Table 11.1 ■
EXAMPLE OF A SUMMARY OF SCHOOL HEALTH SERVICES

District: Centerville
School: Public School #1
Start Date: 09/01/04 End Date: 06/13/05

Care of Sick and Injured	Total	Referred	Follow-up
Illness—Acute	2,694	9	0
Illness—Chronic	196	2	0
Injury—In school	1,056	3	0
Injury—Outside of school	331	1	0
Injury—Ongoing wound care	16	0	0
Miscellaneous	1,600	2	0

Health Procedures	Total	Procedures	Total
Medications given	7,912	Stoma care	0
Catheterizations	0	Blood glucose	0
Tube feedings	97	Blood pressure	20
Trach care	0	Wound care	0
Suctioning	0	Peak flow	69
Nebulizer	129	Other treatments	57
Cast care	0		

Conferences	Total
Parents	2,301
Students	2,003
Staff	8
Community agency	18
Home visits	0
Medical consultations	0
Other consultations	51

COMPETENCIES

A more appropriate focus in the evaluative process is to evaluate the school nurse not only by what she does and how many times she does it, but also on the quality of her performance. School nurses are judged by using competencies, standards, performance indicators, or some other type of criteria determined by the school or hiring organization (Box 11.1). Competencies are considered to be professional expectations. Competence "implies the use of knowledge and skill in the context of the client's needs and welfare (and)...effective use of personal, cognitive, psychomotor, and affective abilities" (Poster & Marcontel, 1999, p. 34).

The National Association of School Nurses (NASN) has adopted competencies proposed by the Southern Regional Education Board that relate to the NASN standards of practice (2001) and describe what school nurses do, with the ultimate goal of improving school nurse practice (Aiken, 2000; Bobo, Adams, & Cooper, 2002; Tustin, Canham, Berridge, Braden, & Starke, 2002) (Table 11.2). Competence emphasizes that the school nurse must possess knowledge and skill; it implies that the application of this knowledge and skill will benefit the health and educational success of the school-age child and adolescent (Bobo et al., 2002). Competencies are a major component of certification programs. The National Council of State Boards of Nursing (NCSBN, 1996) defines the elements of competence as a specific knowledge base, awareness of practice standards, psychomotor skills, decision-making skills, communication skills, experience, and attitude. Competency monitors are designed to document and monitor the ability of

Box 11.1 ■■■

KEY TERMS

- **Competency**—The application of knowledge and the interpersonal, decision-making and psychomotor skills expected for the (school) nurses' practice role within the context of public health, welfare and safety (National Council of State Boards of Nursing, 1996).
- **Performance Indicators**—Identified behaviors that are reflective of job responsibilities
- **Outcomes**—The impact of the results of interventions on the client. In a health application, outcomes reflect a change in the status of a client as a result of nursing interventions.
- **Standards**—Authoritative statements that reflect the values and priorities of the nursing profession and provide direction for professional nursing practice. These standards recognize nursing's accountability to the community and delineate the client outcomes for which nurses are responsible (ANA, 1991).

professionals to perform safely and effectively in a given setting.

The problem with this means of evaluation is that the nurse is evaluated only by how competent or skilled and knowledgeable she is in the performance of her job description and not by the impact of those interventions or even whether the interventions/activities are relevant, necessary, or appropriate to the situation. It is easy to identify what the nurse does and how well she does it. It does not reflect how the level of expertise affects the student population, the family, or the school.

MEASURING OUTCOMES

In the continuum of measuring efficacy of practice, the next step, then, is to validate not only what was done and how well it was done, but also to examine the impact of the nurse's skills and knowledge with measurable, observable outcomes. Outcome measurements provide objective evaluative evidence related to the healthcare process. Outcome measurement refers to collecting and analyzing data using predetermined outcome indicators (Duffy & Korniewicz, 1999).

(text continues on page 245)

Table 11.2 ■

LINKING SREB CCEN COMPETENCIES WITH *SCOPE AND STANDARDS OF PROFESSIONAL SCHOOL NURSING PRACTICE*

STANDARDS OF PROFESSIONAL SCHOOL NURSING*	EXAMPLES OF EXPECTED COMPETENCIES OF SCHOOL NURSES**
Standard I. Assessment	
The school nurse collects client data.	Collect aggregate data-characteristics of the population, health statistics, health-related learning needs, and the population's readiness to learn.
	Collect data on individuals and families and develop comprehensive histories.
	Perform physical assessment and specific screening tests using protocols defined by agency policies and federal and state mandates.
	Assess the community, school, and home for risk factors.
	Assess students' health based on the problem they report.

(continued)

Table 11.2 ■ *(Continued)*

STANDARDS OF PROFESSIONAL SCHOOL NURSING*	EXAMPLES OF EXPECTED COMPETENCIES OF SCHOOL NURSES**
Standard II. Diagnosis	
The school nurse analyzes the assessment data in determining nursing diagnoses.	Validate the assessment data from individuals, families, and groups.
	Establish priorities based on assessments.
	Use standardized universal language.
Standard III. Outcome Identification	
The school nurse identifies expected outcomes individualized to the client.	Define and create situation-specific ways to measure results.
	Identify resources and establish time frames and criteria to measure results.
	Use standardized universal language.
Standard IV. Planning	
The school nurse develops a plan of care/action that specifies interventions to attain expected outcomes.	Develop a plan to promote health and reduce risk factors.
	Plan aggregate interventions, teaching strategies in collaboration with the school system and community resources.
	Collaborate with the school system and community to plan health-related activities for groups.
	Use standardized universal language.
Standard V. Implementation	
The school nurse implements the interventions identified in the plan of care/action.	Perform health teaching and counseling activities.
	Intervene with aggregates (families, classes, teachers, community groups) as stated in plan of action.
	Delegate responsibility.
	Document interventions accurately in retrievable format.
	Maintain confidentiality.
	Provide care that is culturally and ethnically sensitive.
	Help clients obtain resources and services.

(continued)

STANDARDS OF PROFESSIONAL SCHOOL NURSING* **Standard V. Implementation *(cont'd)***	EXAMPLES OF EXPECTED COMPETENCIES OF SCHOOL NURSES**
	Respect rights of students and families in making decisions.
	Understand professional standards.
	Adhere to state regulations.
	Base practice on up-to-date knowledge, theory, and research.
	Use technology to get up-to-date information and expand teaching skills.
	Participate in ongoing research activities.
	Assess the economic, legal, and political factors that influence the delivery of health care.
	Delegate and supervise delivery of care by other approved providers.
	Collaborate with community agencies to reduce duplication of services and to expand resources.
	Coordinate care to meet the health needs of students, families, and vulnerable populations.
	Develop strategies to promote healthy communities.
	Use creative problem-solving techniques.
	Develop community partnerships.
	Use various local, state, and national resources.
	Orient other health care providers.
	Use various methods and adapt them to students' needs.
	Be sensitive to the impact of nonverbal communication.
	Clarify students' needs and preferences.
	Help students and families interpret health information.
	Keep communication focused on facts.

(continued)

STANDARDS OF PROFESSIONAL SCHOOL NURSING*	EXAMPLES OF EXPECTED COMPETENCIES OF SCHOOL NURSES**
Standard V. Implementation *(cont'd)*	
	Provide developmentally appropriate programs to promote health and prevent disease.
	Inform students and parents of available resources and help them access services.
	Understand and explain to others the boards and organizations that influence the delivery of health services.
Standard VI. Evaluation	
The school nurse evaluates the client's progress toward attainment of outcomes.	Monitor the progress of clients toward desired results.
	Check health status at specified intervals.
	Revise plan of care (if warranted).
	Participate in quality assurance for activities such as development of policies and procedures.
	Evaluate delivery models for health care.
	Appraise performance through constructive comments from peers, self-assessment, and adherence to relevant regulations.
STANDARDS OF PROFESSIONAL PEFORMANCE	
Standard I. Quality of Care	
The school nurse systematically evaluates the quality and effectiveness of school nursing practice.	Participate in quality assurance activities such as development of policies and procedures.
Standard II. Performance Appraisal	
The school nurse evaluates one's own nursing practice in relation to professional practice standards and relevant statutes, regulations, and policies.	Develop personal goals for professional development.
	Appraise performance through constructive comments from peers, self-assessment, and adherence to relevant regulations.
Standard III. Education	
The school nurse acquires and maintains current knowledge and competency in school nursing practice.	Complete an orientation program.
	Attend relevant continuing education programs.
	Work toward certification as a school nurse.

(continued)

STANDARDS OF PROFESSIONAL SCHOOL NURSING*	EXAMPLES OF EXPECTED COMPETENCIES OF SCHOOL NURSES**
Standard IV. Collegiality	
The school nurse interacts with and contributes to the professional development of peers and school personnel as colleagues.	Interact with peers and multidisciplinary team members.
	Participate in professional organizations.
	Participate in community organizations that deal with educational issues.
Standard V. Ethics	
The school nurse's decisions and actions on behalf of clients are determined in an ethical manner.	Maintain confidentiality.
	Provide care that is culturally and ethically sensitive to clients.
	Act as client advocate in obtaining resources and services.
	Respect student and family autonomy and rights.
	Demonstrate understanding of professional standards.
	Adhere to state regulations.
	Inform clients and parents of their rights.
Standard VI. Collaboration	
The school nurse collaborates with the student, family, school staff, community, and other providers in providing student care.	Demonstrate good written and verbal communication with parents, teachers, staff, school-age children, and other providers.
	Articulate clearly the value and role of the nurse in the school setting.
	Understand the organizational structures that influence the delivery of health services.
Standard VII. Research	
The school nurse promotes use of research findings in school nursing practice.	Base practice on current knowledge, theory, and research.
	Use information technologies to maintain currency of knowledge base and expand teaching modalities.
	Participate in ongoing research activities.
	Interact with nurse educators who engage in research.
	Collaborate with multidisciplinary teams in developing research proposals.

(continued)

Table 11.2 ■ *(Continued)*

STANDARDS OF PROFESSIONAL SCHOOL NURSING*	EXAMPLES OF EXPECTED COMPETENCIES OF SCHOOL NURSES**
Standard VIII. Resource Utilization	
The school nurse considers factors related to safety, effectiveness, and cost when planning and delivering care.	Assess economic, legal, and political factors that influence health care delivery in schools and communities.
	Delegate and supervise delivery of care.
	Collaborate with other community agencies to reduce duplication and to expand use of resources.
Standard IX. Communication	
The school nurse uses effective written, verbal, and nonverbal communication skills.	Communicate clearly.
	Use varied modalities.
	Be sensitive to influence of nonverbal cues.
	Clarify client needs and preferences.
	Help clients interpret health information.
	Keep communication focused on facts.
Standard X. Program Management	
The school nurse manages school health services.	Coordinate care to meet health needs of client, families, and vulnerable populations.
	Develop strategies to promote healthy communities.
	Use creative problem-solving techniques.
	Develop community partnerships.
	Use wide range of resources.
	Orient other health care providers.
	Evaluate health care delivery models.
Standard XI. Health Education	
The school nurse assists students, families, the school staff, and community to achieve optimal levels of wellness through appropriately designed and delivered health education.	Provide developmentally appropriate programs to promote health and prevent illness.

* National Association of School Nurses & American Nurses Association. (2001). *Scope and standards of professional school nursing practice.* Washington, DC: Author.
** Southern Regional Education Board. (2001). *Curriculum and faculty development in community-based care: School nurses and nurse educators collaborate.* Atlanta, GA: Author.

The movement to the model of evaluation of nursing services known as outcomes measurement began in the 1970s. The focus at that time shifted to the economics of healthcare and quality assurance, performance improvement, and outcome measurement programs. The measurement of outcomes is essential in demonstrating the effectiveness of nursing care delivery (Hill, 1999).

Outcome measure can be defined as a measure of change—the difference from one point in time (usually before an intervention) to another point in time (usually following an intervention). It is important for nurses to identify what they do (nursing interventions) in response to various client conditions (nursing diagnoses) and to note the specific effects of those interventions (nursing outcomes). Duffy and Korniewicz, writing on quality indicators, stated that "nursing…has a social and professional responsibility to provide evidence or data that help to guide and improve care" (1999, p.2).

It is no longer satisfactory for a teacher to say "But I taught that in the classroom"; the more important question to ask is, "What did the student learn because of how and what the teacher taught?" Similarly, it is one thing to say that the school nurse monitored X and referred Y, but toward what end? It is much more important and effective to be able to demonstrate the impact the intervention had on the health of the student or on some other variable.

In an attempt to standardize the language used and to develop a documentation system, The Center for Nursing Classification at the University of Iowa, College of Nursing spearheaded the development of the Nursing Interventions Classification (NIC) and the Nursing Outcomes Classification (NOC). These were developed to correspond to the North American Nursing Diagnosis Association (NANDA) diagnostic system (see Chapter 9 and Box 11.2). NANDA, NIC, and NOC (referred to as N3) are the only American Nurses Association (ANA) recognized languages that represent all nursing specialties (Keenan, Killeen, & Clingerman, 2002).

Standardized language is needed in order to develop a body of research that documents the outcomes of nursing interventions. By using these indicators, data can be collected and entered into an understandable and workable electronic data entry system that will facilitate statistical analysis of the input. These data will form the basis for what is referred to as a Minimum Data Set.

In 1999, NASN adopted a position statement supporting the need for a formal structure for electronic data sets to support nursing care and the use of a standardized language.

> NASN promotes the teaching and implementation of standardized nursing vocabulary as recognized by the ANA…. These languages provide common terms for the nursing care elements of the NMDS [Nursing Minimum Data Set]. The languages that have met these standards include the North American Nursing Diagnosis Association (NANDA), Nursing Interventions Classification System (NIC), and the Nursing Outcomes Classification System (NOC). (NASN, 1999)

Box 11.2 ■ ■ ■

NANDA, NIC, AND NOC

NANDA The North American Nursing Diagnosis Association promotes the use of nursing diagnoses as clinical judgments "about individual, family, or community responses to actual or potential health problems/life processes" (NANDA, 2001).

NIC: Nursing Intervention Classifications is a comprehensive standardized language to describe treatments that nurses perform, including physiological and psychosocial. A defined set of these 514 interventions has been identified as relevant to school nursing.

NOC: Nursing Outcomes Classification is a comprehensive standardized language to describe 330 patient outcomes following nursing interventions. The NOC taxonomy focuses on patient behavior status and perceptions with an attempt to classify these behaviors into classes that match NANDA and NIC systems (Moorhead, Johnson, & Maas, 2004).

In 2001, NASN's position statement was updated to reflect the importance of standardized documentation to support the impact of school nursing services: "With the advent of computers, the use of agreed upon terms to record data is necessary. To document, store, aggregate and retrieve nursing care data accurately and consistently, fields and data elements must be equivalent within and between student health record databases" (NASN, 2001). This process will help define nursing practice.

The Use of NANDA and NIC in the School Setting

School nursing research related to the use of N3 has been conducted by Cavendish, Lunney, Luise, and Richardson (1999, 2001). They began their work with a 1997 study that looked at the relevance of

NANDA to school nursing (Lunney, Cavendish, Luise, & Richardson, 1997). Subsequent studies by this group have focused on NIC and NOC in the school setting. In making their case for the use of N3, these researchers acknowledge the demand for outcome data that support the quality and cost effectiveness of school nursing services.

One drawback of N3 is the fact that none of the field studies to develop the taxonomies were conducted in the school setting. The trend in school nursing research is to correlate student academic success and student well-being with quality nursing services. So it is necessary for research in this area to translate the taxonomy that was originally hospital/service-based for use in the outpatient and community settings.

School nurses do not routinely document using NANDA taxonomy. Many school nurses have found it difficult to identify nursing diagnoses of students in the school setting, especially since the system was originally designed for use in the adult acute care setting (Lunney et al., 1997). These researchers compiled a list of NANDA diagnoses that were relevant to school nursing practice. The most commonly identified diagnoses identified by school nurses are in Table 11.3.

Table 11.3 ■

NANDA DIAGNOSES USED MOST FREQUENTLY IN THE SCHOOL SETTING

Self-esteem disturbance
Altered nutrition: more than body requirements
Ineffective individual coping
Pain
Impaired social interaction
Impaired physical mobility
Diarrhea
Altered nutrition: less than body requirements
Anxiety
High risk of infection
Altered growth and development
Chronic low self-esteem
Situational low self-esteem
Impaired verbal communication
Bathing self-care deficit
Body image disturbance
Fear
Altered family processes
Fatigue
Dressing/grooming self-care deficit

Source: Lunney et al. (1997).

The Nursing Interventions Classification (NIC) is a taxonomy of 514 nursing interventions organized into 7 domains and 30 classes. Each intervention consists of a label, code for computerization, a definition, and a list of activities (University of Iowa, 2004). Documentation using NIC could be one way to demonstrate comprehensive care in the educational setting and to facilitate communication among healthcare providers.

The use of standard NIC terminology may alleviate time-consuming paper documentation once nurses are familiar with the terminology, and support the use of computer data collections. Cavendish, Lunney, Luise, and Richardson (1999) identified 163 interventions used by school nurses. Table 11.4 lists the 12 most frequently used interventions (used on the average from once a week to every day).

Documentation, as the most frequently identified intervention, mandates the utilization of a standardized language system. The other frequently used interventions involved student/family interactions. Some interventions not included on the list but identified by the participants include community outreach, grant writing, health record maintenance, routine screening, healthcare plan development, and health curriculum development (Cavendish et al., 1999).

A second study demonstrated that school nurses use 114 interventions in the school setting at least monthly. Daily interventions include active listening, documentation, first aid, health education, infection control, and medication administration and management (Pavelka, McCarthy, & Denehy, 1999). However, the highest frequency of interven-

Table 11.4 ■

COMMON INTERVENTIONS USED IN THE SCHOOL SETTING

1. Documentation
2. First aid
3. Medication management
4. Medication administration: oral
5. Medication administration
6. Infection control
7. Health screening
8. Health education
9. Telephone consultation
10. Heat/cold application
11. Presence
12. Emotional support

Source: Cavendish et al. (1999).

tions was from the behavioral domain with the intent to facilitate life-style changes in students.

Identification of Outcomes of School Nursing Practice

As Denehy stated in an editorial in the *Journal of School Nursing*, "School nurses need to be proactive in systematically measuring the outcomes of their care. Providing concrete data on the contributions school nurses make to the health and educational outcomes of children will solidify nursing's position in the school setting" (2000, p. 4). The effective school nurse, aware of trends in healthcare, responds to changes in the school and community. Responsible clinical practice demands that school nurses describe what they diagnose and treat in the school communities and detail the outcomes of their practice (Hootman, 2002). The identification of nursing interventions and their impact on measurable outcomes can change the common misperception of educators and policy makers that nurses are in schools only to provide first aid, ensure compliance with immunization requirements, and perform tasks that could be delegated to assistive personnel.

The results of a Delphi study conducted to develop a school nursing research agenda (Edwards, 2002) ranked the "impact of school nurse services on student health" as the number one issue to be addressed. Number two was the "relationship between school nurse practice and educational outcomes" (p. 16). These two agenda items speak loudly for the need for outcomes regarding school nurse practice. Others areas identified for research included:

- Benefits and cost-effectiveness of school health services
- Value of school health services to the educational system
- Predictors of outcomes for students, including special needs students
- Nursing interventions for mental health promotion
- Characteristics of successful school nurse interventions
- Prevention and interventions for children with chronic diseases
- Core elements of school nursing practice
- Nursing interventions in violence and substance abuse prevention

Nurses need to establish a connection between interventions and outcomes. This fits well with the nursing process: assessment, identification of the problem, planning, intervention, and evaluation. Nurses, and especially school nurses, need to refine and expand on the evaluation of the intervention. Use of the scientific method for data collection and analysis allows for the measurement and evaluation of outcomes (outcome measurement). Measurement has been defined as the assignment of numbers to phenomena according to specific rules (Polit, Beck, & Hungler, 2001). School nursing is just beginning to define the phenomena unique to their practice. What is lacking are data about the effectiveness of school nursing services (Hootman, 2002).

Leaders in school health are not accustomed to focusing on outcomes of school nurse interventions beyond reporting anecdotal and case history information. Previous data reported included frequency, type, and duration of nursing interventions; number of students served; number and type of chronic conditions of students; and frequency or disposition type for students seen by a school nurse. Initial attempts in identifying outcome measures often focused on special populations and specific goals that could be met by health education. Examples include higher scores on posttests of knowledge related to specific content on sexuality, health concepts, asthma, and the harm of secondary smoke; lowered smoking rates; identification of eating disorders by teachers; improved peak flow and inhaler technique; improved immunization rates; increased physical activity rates; lower injury rates; decreased anxiety and depression; increased self esteem; and increased environmental safety compliance (Stock et al., 2002). There was no identified logic as to why these outcomes were chosen other than to meet an identified need.

The "School Nurse Corps" created by the Health Services Program of the Washington State Office of Superintendent of Public Instruction has become one of the leaders in developing school nurse outcome measures (Maire, Larter, & Stock, 2001). Their task force has done extensive literature review and is building an infrastructure for measuring outcomes. As part of their research, they asked the question, "What are the most important outcomes of school nursing services?" Their results are in TABLE 11.5; however, they determined that the development of an infrastructure that documented the impact of school nursing also needed support from educational administration and school nurse supervisors as well as having appropriate software for data entry and assistance in data analysis (Stock et al., 2002).

NOC evaluates the status of clients following nursing interventions. "The standardized outcomes were developed to measure the effects of nursing interventions and are used in all settings and with all client populations" (NASN, 2001, p. 2). The seven NOC domains include functional health, physiologic

Table 11.5 ■

OUTCOMES OF SCHOOL NURSE INTERVENTIONS—WASHINGTON STATE

- Children are physically and emotionally healthy.
- Decreased visits to the emergency room.
- Decreased accidents in school.
- Obesity reduction.
- Decrease in tobacco use.
- Decrease in adolescent pregnancy.
- Decrease in HIV infections.
- Families enrolled in health insurance.
- Families have resources they need for their child.
- Decrease in visits to school nurse among students who have received early identification of a health need.
- Students and families show progress in managing student healthcare needs.
- Healthcare of children with chronic conditions is managed.
- Mandated screenings are completed.
- Individual Education Plans reflect school nurse input.
- Academic success.
- School environment is nurturing, caring, healthy.
- Improved attendance.
- Readiness to learn (in class, attentive, emotionally and physically healthy).

Source: Maire, Larter, & Stock (2001).

health, psychosocial health, health knowledge and behavior, perceived health, family health, and community health. It is hoped that the outcomes that result (NOC) will validate the interventions or strategies used by nurses (NIC) in a variety of settings.

NOC and the analysis of client outcomes can be used to examine the quality of healthcare, influence health policy, identify resource needs, develop educational initiatives, and support clinical decision-making. Outcomes and their relevance to school nursing reflect a practice focus of health promotion, health protections, and disease and illness management. In one survey, Cavendish et al. developed a list of the 190 NOC outcomes available at that time; school nurses were asked to indicate the percentage of children or families for whom they affected each outcome, with a scale of 0% to 100%. "For 8 outcomes, the mean percentage ratings were over 50%. For 33 outcomes, the mean percentage ratings were over 40%. For 90 outcomes, the mean percentage ratings were over 30%" (2001, p. 193).

The researchers compiled a list of 40 outcomes that were identified as relevant to school nursing practice, even though the sample was small and the percentages were low (TABLE 11.6). The N3 school-nursing core reflects the range of services school nurses provide in the areas of health promotion, health protection, and disease management. The researchers acknowledge that future studies need to be conducted to identify outcomes related to academic performance, school attendance, and extracurricular activity participation. There are now 330 identified possible outcomes.

Cavendish et al.'s study used a deductive approach by using a predetermined set of outcomes (NOC) and asked nurses to select those that were applicable to their practice. Selekman and Guilday (2003) used focus groups with a national group of practicing school nurses to inductively identify those indicators that best reflected the desired outcomes by which their practice could be evaluated. Ten themes of desired outcomes were identified and prioritized (TABLE 11.7).

- Students have increased time in the classroom.
- Students receive first aid, emergency services, and services for their acute care needs.
- Students receive needed competent health-related interventions (procedures, medications).
- Students with chronic health conditions have their healthcare needs met.
- Wellness promotion and disease prevention enhanced the overall health of the school.
- Students receive appropriate referrals related to the assessments made.
- Students learn in a safe environment.
- Community outreach to meet student needs is enhanced.
- School nursing services are cost effective.
- Parents, teachers, administration, and staff express satisfaction with health-related services (Selekman & Guilday, 2003).

Study participants identified 62 quality indicators by which the desired outcomes could be measured. The large number of quality indicators allows for options for school nurses practicing in various settings to demonstrate that desired outcomes had been met. The indicators could be operationally defined in whichever ways best fit a given school environment.

Table 11.6 ■
OUTCOMES FOR USE IN THE SCHOOL SETTING (N = 227)

Immunization behavior**	Knowledge: disease process*
Health-promoting behavior**	Hope*
Knowledge: infection control**	Compliance behavior*
Growth**	Health beliefs: perceived resources*
Health-seeking behavior**	Oral health*
Knowledge: medication**	Adherence behavior*
Knowledge: personal safety**	Knowledge: diet*
Knowledge: health behaviors**	Physical maturation: male*
Self-esteem*	Well-being*
Knowledge: health resources*	Decision-making*
Comfort level*	Child development: middle childhood*
Vital signs status*	Participation: health care decisions*
Health beliefs: perceived control*	Tissue integrity: skin and mucous membranes*
Body image*	Identity
Health beliefs*	Risk detection
Treatment behavior: illness or injury*	Risk control: Tobacco use
Health beliefs: perceived ability to perform*	Social support
Physical maturation: female*	Information processing
Health orientation*	Communication ability
Risk control*	Health beliefs: perceived threat

** 50% to 73%
*40% to 49%
The remainder were below 40%.
Source: Cavendish et al. (2001, p. 194).

Table 11.7 ■
DESIRED OUTCOMES AND POTENTIAL QUALITY INDICATORS

DESIRED OUTCOME: THEME 1

Students have increased time in the classroom or learning environment (decreased time lost from class; increased seat time) related to health needs.

Potential Quality Indicators

1. Minutes out of class (and where students go to meet their health needs [health office, administrative office, home, other]).
2. Number and percent who go home, return to class, stay in school but not in class.
3. Attendance rates (decreased absenteeism for health-related issues).
4. Number and percent of students who are able to complete the school day after receiving medical or psychosocial interventions.
5. Nurse-determined exclusions from school due to communicable disease and missing immunizations.

DESIRED OUTCOME: THEME 2

Students receive first aid, emergency services, and services for their acute health care needs.

Potential Quality Indicators

1. Minutes until first aid is provided.
2. Minutes until intervention for acute needs.

(continued)

Table 11.7 ■ *(Continued)*

Potential Quality Indicators *(cont'd)*

3. Appropriateness of services provided (and who provided them).
4. Interventions that are based on assessment findings (decision making).
5. Evaluation of treatments provided.
6. Decreased time to diffuse crises (because of crisis management, debriefing).
7. Decrease in staff injuries and attention to acute health needs of staff (decreased absences for health-related reasons).
8. Appropriate decisions to call 911 or parent (number of times emergency medical service is called and by whom).

DESIRED OUTCOME: THEME 3

Students receive needed competent health-related interventions (procedures, medications).

Potential Quality Indicators

1. Increased medication compliance (accuracy of dose or medication, safety of medication storage and administration, students are knowledgeable about their medications, increased compliance of caregiver having ordered medication available to the school).
2. Accuracy of medication or treatment orders (written authorization, charting of administration, interpreting physician orders).
3. Evaluation of the efficacy of medication and treatments (and communicating findings to parents and primary health care providers).
4. Safe performance of health-related procedures (catheterization, dressings changes, chest physiotherapy, nasogastric feeding, ostomy care, tracheotomy care; monitored for adverse reactions and treatment efficacy; knowledge of assessments needed prior to skill; knowledge of when skill should not be performed based on assessments; number of procedures performed and by whom).

DESIRED OUTCOME: THEME 4

Students with chronic conditions have their health care needs met.

Potential Quality Indicators

1. Development and implementation of 504 accommodations, ensuring student needs are met (health-related accommodations are included; nurse has input into the 504, if applicable; modifications are made as needed).
2. Individualized Health Plan is developed, implemented, and evaluated.
3. Individualized Education Program is developed with input from the nurse when health care needs must be included.
4. Student knowledge about treatment plan.
5. Compliance with treatment regimen (self-care).
6. Time in the classroom (for children with chronic conditions).
7. Case management (coordinate services, as reflected in decreased lost time from classes; coordinated access to services; liaison between family, health care provider, and health care system).
8. Knowledge of staff related to the needs of children with chronic conditions.
9. Decreased morbidity (complications; increased early identification of potential or real problems; fewer hospitalizations).

DESIRED OUTCOME: THEME 5

Overall health of the school is enhanced by wellness promotion and disease prevention measures.

Potential Quality Indicators

1. Identification of children who require further intervention based on health screening results (vision, hearing, scoliosis, height and weight, blood pressure, health history, pregnancy)

(continued)

2. Increased immunization rates (audit status of students and staff).
3. Increased infection control (number of children sent home not immunized, demonstrating signs of communicable disease, or at risk from sequelae of infection; actions taken to decrease spread [flu shots]; increased hand washing).
4. Increased knowledge by students related to health promotion measures (infection control, nutrition, exercise, sleep; health teaching; anticipatory guidance; have healthy babies).
5. Increased knowledge among staff related to health promotion measures.
6. Increased staff awareness of environmental conditions that spread or exacerbate illness (e.g., asthma triggers).
7. Increased mental health status (increased communication skills [socialization, refusal skills, mediation skills, anger management]; increased self-esteem; participation in grieving and anticipatory grieving; staying in school [decreased truancy]; lower suicide and homicide rates; decrease in eating disorders; decrease in disruptive students in the classroom; fewer discipline problems; decreased violence to self and others).
8. Decreased high-risk behaviors (make more positive choices); (decrease in smoking, alcohol use, drug use, pregnancy rate, sexually transmitted diseases).
9. Increased number of students with a medical home.
10. Recording of child's health history and pattern of need for health care.

DESIRED OUTCOME: THEME 6

Students receive appropriate referrals related to the assessments made.

Potential Quality Indicators

1. Decreased time from screening to referral.
2. Facilitation of appropriate referrals (problems are referred appropriately; number of referrals made and services accessed; appropriate use of community health resources).
3. Increased follow-up on referrals and recommendations.
4. Increased access to care including health care providers, resources, and services.

DESIRED OUTCOME: THEME 7

The environment in which students learn is safe.

Potential Quality Indicators

1. Decrease in accidents (safe physical plant [playground safety, school safety, bus safety, food safety], active on safety committee, data collection and injury tracking to identify where and when they occur and what kinds occur, decreased litigation related to accidents).
2. Decreased adverse effects from environmental risk factors (made recommendations related to air-quality safety, toxic chemical storage and use, allergen-free environment [foods, carpets, latex, animals, use of aerosol sprays, and air quality in school]).
3. Increased staff safety awareness (knowledge provided in injury prevention programs).
4. Increased medication safety (decreased errors; proper storage and labeling; monitoring system and notation of side effects; accountability for Class II medications).
5. Development and implementation of crisis and evacuation plans (participated on Emergency Preparedness Team or Crisis Intervention Team, developed safety plan for children with special needs).
6. Have emergency medications that are covered by standing orders.

DESIRED OUTCOME: THEME 8

Overall health of the school is enhanced by community outreach.

Potential Quality Indicators

1. Increased linkages between the school and community (interdisciplinary committees: child study team, school health advisory teams; collaboration with the schools of nursing [student nurses and gradute students assist with physicals, screenings, medications, classroom education, etc.]).

(continued)

Table 11.7 ■ *(Continued)*

Potential Quality Indicators *(cont'd)*

2. Increased use of community resources by families (help children and families navigate the health system, help families with appropriate use of the system; increase access to services, home visits).
3. Nurse is seen as a consultant and health expert (for calls related to student health issues).
4. Increased development of school health policies based on data collection and research findings.
5. Increased advocacy for families (decreased barriers related to cultural diversity; facilitated increased compliance with the law).

DESIRED OUTCOME: THEME 9

School nursing services are cost-effective.

Potential Quality Indicators

1. Decreased absences of staff (decreased needs for substitutes).
2. Increased student attendance.
3. Decreased cost to the community (related to appropriate use of community resources, e.g., emergency room, medical home).
4. Increased Medicaid reimbursement for qualified students.
5. Increased grant monies received.

DESIRED OUTCOME: THEME 10

Parents, teachers, administration, and staff express satisfaction with health-related services.

Potential Quality Indicators

1. Use of nurse as resource for health questions and acute health care needs.
2. Availability of staff training related to health issues.
3. Reports of decreased stress because of decreased classroom disruption.
4. Parent reports of taking fewer sick days from work or increased productivity because of increased health of child.
5. Parent reports of feeling more empowered (having increased health-related knowledge).
6. Parent reports of confidence in the nurse as their child's advocate.

The potential outcomes identified represented the vast scope of school nursing practice as well as the breadth of student services provided. All components of the health continuum were identified: health promotion, disease prevention, care of students with acute and chronic health needs, and the needs of families and staff as well as the multiple interdisciplinary roles in which nurses engage. While some of the outcomes are similar to those in NOC, others are more concise and specific to the school environment.

The usefulness of outcome measures is multidimensional. Practitioners need to know that their care makes a difference; taxpayers want to know what they are getting for their money; and organizations and healthcare agencies want to benchmark their performance (Hill, 1999). The responsibility to measure these outcomes rests with practicing nurses. As clinicians, nurses have the responsibility to do more than define their practice; they must show that it makes a difference. Outcome measurements are a way to demonstrate accountability and effectiveness to those served by school nurses and those who employ them. The search for outcomes will promote responsibility on the nurse for better selection of interventions and of documenting both the interventions and the outcomes. This requires follow-up with the client and changes the focus from the process and activities to the outcomes or impact of the activities on the student.

Tools

A tool that is comprehensive and outcome-focused has not yet been developed to evaluate school nurses and school nursing services. To adopt a standard means of evaluation, it is necessary to determine what it is that school nurses believe would best reflect the efficacy of their practice. Do they want to evaluate how many services they can deliver within the school year or how competent and skilled they are in the delivery of these same services, or do they want to identify trends in school health and document school nurses' response to these trends? The answer is "YES" to all of these questions, but these are not enough. Tustin et al. (2002) developed a tool that uses the NASN standards as an appraisal framework, indicating the degree to which the school nurse meets the standards. Ultimately, however, to validate practice, competent nurses responding to trends in school health need a means to demonstrate how their interventions affect the student population and the school.

Using Outcomes in Research

Outcomes are often associated with research. Research is an important component of school nursing practice (see Chapter 8) and yet it is often frightening to the practicing nurse. The National Association of School Nurses includes the application of and involvement in nursing research in its Standards of Professional School Nursing Performance, identifying it as an integral component of school nursing practice. It states that school nurses contribute "to nursing and school nursing through innovations in practice and participation in research or research related activities" (NASN & ANA, 2001, Standard IX). Without data that support school nursing services, school nursing may not continue to exist.

In addition, decisions about the quality and cost-effectiveness of care are relative to the diagnoses, the interventions provided, the outcomes of the services, and how these data compare to data from similar populations (Cavendish et al., 1999). Inferences about outcomes must be based on valid, reliable data and the assurance that interventions were properly and appropriately delivered (Stock et al., 2002). Thus research can result in the provision of cost-effective services, as well.

CONCLUSION

The movement toward demonstrating competence, accountability, and outcomes is reflective of a national healthcare trend. The trend is toward data collection that clearly documents quality outcomes. Changes in healthcare organizations, financing, and regulatory reform have had a substantial effect on the practice of healthcare professionals and the systems that establish competence in practice. Managed care organizations, employers and the government recognize that competence affects both cost and quality of care. Competent practice resulting in positive client outcomes relies on tools that enable school nurses to quantify and define quality nursing care.

Development of a means of quantifying observable outcomes is an area for further research. Ultimately, a comprehensive evaluation of school nurse practice would include an accounting of the number and type of nursing tasks/skills performed, competencies that guide the responsibilities of the nurse, and outcome measures that reflect the effect the nurse has on the school community. Inclusion of quality outcomes, however, needs to become an essential part of that evaluative process.

School nurses may have difficulty shifting their focus from tasks to outcomes. The need to measure outcomes can be framed by the question, "Towards what ends do you perform those tasks?" As stated by Korniewicz and Duffy in their Outcomes Module for ANA, "although quality healthcare is associated with the absence of negative outcomes…, quality itself cannot always be assured. However, methods to assess or improve patient care can be measured" (2003, p. 5).

There is ongoing discussion as to the outcome measures that would demonstrate the efficacy of school nurse practice. Use of outcome measurements is only one component of a multifaceted evaluation process, although an important one. Thus, a complete evaluation of school nursing services should include the processes (doing the right thing and doing it correctly), the structure (having the right tools) and the outcomes (having the right things happen) so that they benefit students, families, the school, and the community.

Evaluation of one's practice will bring school nursing into compliance with the NASN standards (NASN & ANA, 2001) and assist in validating the efficacy of school nurses in the schools. School nurses "do it all"; evaluation of their role should be comprehensive and reflect the wide spectrum of their role, with the ultimate outcome being the improved health of children and adolescents in order for optimal learning to occur.

References

Aiken, E. (2000). *Curriculum and faculty development in community-based care: School nurses and nurse educators collaborate.* Atlanta, GA: Southern Regional Education Board, Council on Collegiate Education for Nursing.

American Nurses Association (ANA). (1991). *Standards of clinical nursing practice.* Kansas City, MO: American Nurses Publishing.

Bobo, N., Adams, V., & Cooper, L. (2002). Excellence in school nursing practice: Developing a national perspective on school nurse competencies. *Journal of School Nursing, 18*(5), 277–285.

Cavendish, R., Lunney, M., Luise, B., & Richardson, K. (1999). National survey to identify the nursing interventions used in school settings. *Journal of School Nursing, 15*(2), 14–21.

Cavendish, R., Lunney, M., Luise, B., & Richardson, K. (2001). The nursing outcomes classification: Its relevance to school nursing. *Journal of School Nursing, 17*(4), 189–197.

Denehy, J. (2000). Measuring the outcomes of school nursing practice: Showing that school nurses do make a difference. *Journal of School Nursing, 16*(1), 2–4.

Denehy, J. (2002). A tribute to nurses and Florence Nightingale. *Journal of School Nursing, 18*(3), 125–127.

Duffy, J., & Korniewicz, D. (1999). *Quality indicators: Outcomes measurement using the ANA safety and quality indicators.* Retrieved April 2003 from http://nursingworld.org/mods/working/QY/ceomfull.htm

Edwards, L. (2002). Research priorities in school nursing: A Delphi process. *Journal of School Nursing, 18*(3), 157–162.

Grabeel, J., & Zaiger, D. (1998). Utilizing standards of nursing practice for effective school nursing management. *Journal of School Nursing*, 14(2), 47–48.

Guilday, P. (2000). School nursing practice today: Implications for the future. *Journal of School Nursing*, 16(5), 25–31.

Hill, M. (Fall, 1999). Outcomes measurement requires nursing to shift to outcome-based practice. *Nursing Administration Quarterly*, 24, 1–16.

Hootman, J. (2002). The importance of research to school nurses and school nursing practice. *Journal of School Nursing, 18*(1), 18–24.

Keenan, G., Killeen, M., & Clingerman, E. (2002). NANDA, NOC, and NIC: Progress toward a nursing information infrastructure. *Nursing Education Perspectives, 23*(4), 162–163.

Korniewicz, D., & Duffy, J. (2003). *Essential concepts for staff nurses: The outcomes imperative.* Retrieved June 2004 from http://www.ana.org

Lunney, M., Cavendish, R., Luise, B., & Richardson, K. (1997). Relevance of NANDA and health promotion diagnoses to school nurses. *Journal of School Nursing, 13*(5), 16–22.

Maire, J., Larter, N., & Stock, J. (2001). *School nurse outcome measures.* Washington: Center for Children with Special Needs, State Office of Superintendent of Public Instruction.

Moorhead, S., Johnson, M., & Maas, M. (2004). *Nursing outcomes classification (NOC)*. St. Louis, MO: C. V. Mosby.

National Association of School Nurses (NASN). (1999). *Position statement: Nursing minimum data set for school nursing practice.* Retrieved May 2003 from http://www.nasn.org

National Association of School Nurses (NASN). (2001). *Position statement: Nursing classification systems: North American Nursing Diagnosis Association (NANDA), Nursing Interventions Classification (NIC), and Nursing Outcomes Classifications (NOC).* Retrieved June 2004 from http://www.nasn.org

National Association of School Nurses (NASN) and the American Nurses Association (ANA). (2001). *Scope and standards of professional school nursing practice.* Washington, DC: American Nurses Publishing.

National Council of State Boards of Nursing (NCSBN). (1996). *Assuring competence: A regulatory responsibility* [Position paper]. Chicago: Author.

North American Nursing Diagnosis Association (NANDA). (2001). *Nursing diagnosis definition and classifications 2001–2002*. Philadelphia: Author.

Pavelka, L., McCarthy, A. M., & Denehy, J. (1999). Nursing interventions used in school nursing practice. *Journal of School Nursing, 15*(1), 29–37.

Polit, D., Beck, C., & Hungler, B. (2001). *Essentials of nursing research.* Philadelphia: Lippincott.

Poster, E., & Marcontel, M. (1999). School nursing role and competence. *Journal of School Nursing, 15*(2), 34–42.

Pulcini,J., Couillard, M., Harrigan, J., & Mole, D. (2002). Personal and professional characteristics of exemplary school nurses. *Journal of School Nursing, 18*(1), 33–40.

Selekman, J., & Guilday, P. (2003). Identification of desired outcomes for school nursing practice. *Journal of School Nursing, 19*(6), 344–450.

Stock, J., Larter, N., Kieckehefer, G., Thronson, G., & Maire, J. (2002). Measuring outcomes of school nursing services. *Journal of School Nursing, 18*(6), 353–359.

Telljohann, S., Price, J., Dake, J., & Durgin, J. (2004). Access to school health services: Differences between full-time and part-time school nurses. *Journal of School Nursing, 20*(3), 176–181.

Tustin, J., Canham, G., Berridge, J., Braden, D., & Starke, T. (2002). Professional development and appraisal system for school nurses. *Journal of School Nursing, 18*(4), 229–236.

University of Iowa. (2004). Center for Nursing Classification and Clinical Effectiveness. Retrieved June 2004 from http://www.nursng. uiowa.edu/cnc

PART III

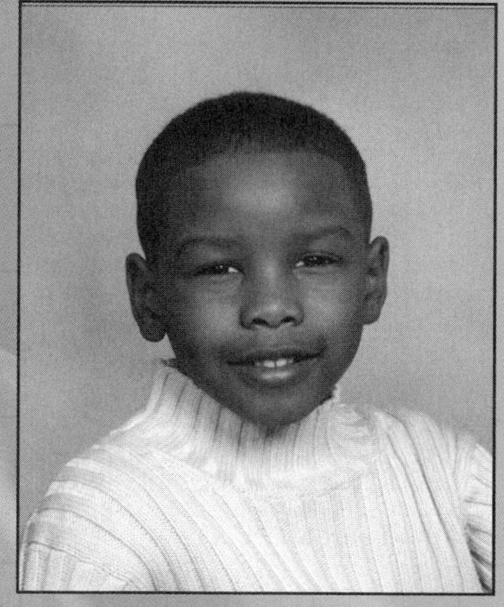

Legal Concerns

Chapter 12

Legal Issues Related to School Nursing Practice: The Foundation

LYNN ROSSI-SCOTT ▪ JANET SOBEY BUBERT

Chapter Outline

INTRODUCTION

This chapter provides insight into the general foundations for the numerous legal issues confronted by school nurses in their daily work. Because laws in each state vary, and because court decisions applicable in one jurisdiction may not apply in another, the school nurse is well advised to study the statutes, regulations, and court decisions applicable to the practitioner's geographical location. However, the general legal principles that guide these individual laws and decisions are, for the most part, the same, and can serve as a guide to an understanding of the specific legal duties and responsibilities of the school nurse. Therefore, this chapter addresses the general foundations of the U.S. legal system; the resultant standard of care expected of a school nurse; and the potential civil, criminal, and administrative consequences of violating that standard of care. Some insight into financial and liability protection for the school nurse is provided next. Finally, this chapter addresses legal proceedings in which the school nurse is not a party, but, rather, is a witness giving testimony about third-party matters as a result of the nurse's work in the school environment.

LEGAL FOUNDATIONS

The U.S. legal system is built on an organized framework of legal principles established in the federal constitution, which are then further established and implemented in each of the 50 states through state constitutions. Under both the federal and state frameworks, the legal foundation is the constitution itself that establishes the government and its powers and responsibilities and that establishes the legal protections and rights afforded individuals living within the government's jurisdiction. Statutes, based on the powers and responsibilities in the constitution, are then written, enforced, and, ultimately, interpreted by divisions of the government through regulations. Finally, courts interpret the statutes and the constitution in individual disputes to determine whether the laws themselves are legal, constitutional, and enforceable, and to determine whether an individual's or organization's actions violated an established law or responsibility. Therefore, the major sources of law are the federal and state constitutions, statutes, and regulations, and federal and state court decisions.

Constitutional Law

United States Constitution

The United States Constitution essentially establishes the federal government and its rights and responsibilities, and then establishes the methods by which individuals are protected from that same government. For example, while Article I of the Constitution establishes the United States Congress and its ability to make laws, the First Amendment to the Constitution prohibits Congress from making laws that require citizens to practice a certain religion, prevent citizens from exercising their religions of choice, or abridge citizens' rights to free speech.

There are provisions in the United States Constitution that may also be of particular relevance to the school nurse. The Fourth Amendment prohibits unreasonable searches and seizures. The Fifth Amendment provides for an individual's right against self-incrimination in the criminal context, and protects an individual from being deprived by the government of life, liberty, or property without due process of law. The Tenth Amendment reserves to the states any power not specifically delegated in the Constitution to the federal government. Amendment Fourteen prohibits any state government from making or enforcing any law that abridges the privileges and immunities provided by the U.S. Constitution, and requires that no state government can deprive an individual of life, liberty, or property without due process of law. Finally, the Fourteenth Amendment also prohibits any state from denying any person equal protection of the laws.

Three Branches of Government

The United States Constitution establishes the three branches of the federal government: Legislative, Executive, and Judicial. The Legislative branch consists of Congress, which is divided into the Senate and the House of Representatives. Congress's responsibility is to make laws necessary for carrying out its specified powers. Congress cannot make laws that would exceed its constitutional authority. For example, because the First Amendment prohibits the establishment of religion, Congress could not establish an official national religion. These federal laws are codified in books known as the United States Code (USC).

Interestingly, none of Congress's enumerated powers relate to education or health care. Therefore, for the most part, both education and health care are state functions, rather than federal functions. However, Congress often uses other avenues to regulate areas not specifically enumerated among its powers. For example, the "commerce clause" of Article 1, Section 8 of the Constitution allows Congress to regulate commerce among the states. Congress also often ties the receipt of federal funds to a recipient's agreement to comply with federal laws. Using one of these methods, then, Congress has implemented a number of significant federal laws affecting health and education, which are discussed below.

The Executive branch consists of the Office of the President and all executive departments and federal agencies. Under Article II of the Constitution, the President is responsible for the faithful execution of all federal laws. Of specific importance to the school nurse are the U.S. Department of Education and the U.S. Department of Health and Human Services. The U.S. Department of Education, among other things, oversees civil rights issues related to students, such as discrimination claims of unequal treatment by school employees; oversees the federal confidentiality protections related to students' records; oversees grant programs which may include the provision of nursing services; and drafts regulations related to the school nurses' services to students who are disabled. The U.S. Department of health administers grants related to school health services. Both of these federal agencies draft and enforce regulations designed to implement federal laws and provide guidance and opinions regarding compliance with federal laws. For example, all of the federal laws referenced below have regulations that interpret and implement those laws. Most often, the federal regulations are much more detailed than the federal laws they interpret.

The third branch of federal government established under Article III of the U.S. Constitution is the Judicial branch, which consists of a system of federal courts designed to provide interpretations of laws and analyses of actions to determine their compliance with federal laws and responsibilities. The U.S. Supreme Court reviews the appealed decisions of the Circuit Courts of Appeal, each of which cover several states. These Circuit Courts of Appeal, in turn, review the appealed decisions of the federal district courts within the geographical territories they cover.

State Constitutions

State constitutions operate very similarly to the federal constitution—they establish state governments, define the governments' powers and responsibilities, and detail the rights of individuals as they relate to their state governments. Because health care and education are reserved to the states by virtue of the Tenth Amendment to the U.S. Constitution, state constitutions often have many provisions about health care and education. Of course, the provisions vary widely among the states. However, in general, state constitutions allow their legislatures to write laws regulating the practice of health care, regulating public health matters, and establishing and regulating public education, and sometimes, to a degree, private education. State constitutions usually establish state education agencies and health departments, which then interpret and enforce those state laws through the agencies' regulations.

Statutory Law

Federal and State Laws

Statutes are bills that are passed by either the U.S. Congress or the state legislatures and then signed by the president or the state governors, as appropriate, to become law. Laws are designed to establish specific rules of behavior, rights, and responsibilities for governmental agencies, organizations, businesses, and individuals. Federal laws generally apply to all U.S. citizens and, sometimes, to visitors to the United States. State laws, on the other hand, apply to state residents and, often, to non-state residents who are visiting, doing business, or traveling in the state.

Examples of federal laws of particular importance to the school nurse include the following: the No Child Left Behind Act of 2001 (NCLB), 20 USC § 301 et seq., establishes federal accountability standards for public school districts; the Individuals with Disabilities Education Act (IDEA), 20 USC § 1400 et seq. (Chapter 14) guarantees that students who are disabled and in public schools will receive a free appropriate public education at public expense; the Asbestos Hazard Emergency Response Act (AHERA), 15 USC § 2641 et seq., requires public and private schools to inspect school buildings for asbestos and to implement appropriate responses when asbestos-containing material is found; the Rehabilitation Act, known as "Section 504," 29 USC § 794 et seq. (Chapter 14) prohibits discrimination on the basis of disability in the provision of public services, including education; the Family Educational Rights and Privacy Act (FERPA), 20 USC § 1232g, (Chapter 13) protects the confidentiality of student records and allows parents access to their children's student records in public schools and private schools that receive federal funds; the Stewart B. McKinney Homeless Assistance Act, 42 USC § 11431 et seq., ensures that homeless children have access to public education; the Americans with Disabilities Act (ADA), 42 USC § 12101 et seq., (Chapter 14) prohibits discrimination on the basis of disability in the provision of public services by public entities, including public school districts; the Family and Medical Leave Act (FMLA), 29 USC § 2611 et seq., allows 12 weeks of unpaid leave for an employee with an eligible medical condition or for an employee to care for a sick family member; Medicaid, 42 USC § 1396a, provides for compensation for medical expenses incurred by eligible individuals; and the Health Insurance Portability and Accountability Act (HIPAA), 42 USC § 300gg & 42 USC § 1301 et seq., (Chapter 13) protects the confidentiality of medical records and prevents lapses in insurance. All of these laws impact public school districts, while some also have an impact on private schools.

State laws, on the other hand, because of the states' exclusive role in establishing public education and regulating health care, tend to be much more specific regarding education and health issues. Each state has a series of statutes establishing its public education system, often addressing issues such as curriculum, student admission and attendance, employee rights and responsibilities, student rights and responsibilities, student discipline, school finance, accountability standards, graduation standards, construction of school facilities, purchasing, administration of medications at school, sex education, and school health programs. Typically, state statutes establish a state education agency to oversee the public education system in the state. Each state also has a series of statutes addressing state health issues, usually including nursing practice, medical records management and confidentiality, consent to medical treatment, child consent to medical treatment, child abuse reporting, child immunizations, communicable disease prevention and control, and do not resuscitate orders. State statutes typically establish a state board or agency that oversees the practice of nursing and a state agency or department that oversees public health issues and programs throughout the state.

Civil and Criminal Laws

There are two general kinds of federal and state laws: criminal laws and civil laws. Criminal, or penal, laws make it a crime to commit certain actions. Federal criminal laws address mostly federal topics, such as alteration of U.S. currency or mail fraud (18 USC § 331; 18 USC § 501). State criminal laws of concern to the school nurse normally address issues such as mandatory child abuse reporting, assault, kidnapping, theft, fraud, controlled substances, records tampering, and practicing nursing without a license.

Civil laws, on the other hand, normally address the rights of individuals or groups to seek monetary or other compensation or to stop (or seek an injunction against) some action. Federal civil laws of concern to the school nurse are the federal laws such as Family Medical Leave Act (FMLA), Individuals with Disabilities Education Act (IDEA), Americans with Disabilities Act (ADA), Family Educational Rights and Privacy Act (FERPA), and Medicaid. State civil laws of concern to the school nurse are generally the laws that regulate the practice of nursing, establish and regulate public education, and regulate public health.

Conflicts of Laws

Because there are so many different laws, federal and state, civil and criminal, education and health, sometimes the provisions of one law may conflict with those of another law. Often it is up to a court to determine whether there actually is a conflict between the laws and, if so, which law prevails in a particular conflict. These conflicts sometimes make it difficult for the school nurse to follow all laws applicable to the nursing profession. A school nurse living in one state and working in another, or who works with children who reside in more than one state, may also be faced with conflicting statutory requirements. Sometimes, the laws of one state may conflict. When such conflicts arise, it is important for the school nurse to receive careful legal advice from counsel knowledgeable about both education and health law, and to seek interpretive guidance from the proper legal authorities.

Conflicts between state laws are often informally interpreted by state attorneys general, who are the state officials who advise and represent state agencies, and, in that capacity, issue opinions designed to assist in implementation of state laws. On a much more formal basis, courts are often called on to interpret apparent conflicts between laws. While each specific situation is open to an individualized interpretation, some general principles normally apply. When they must resolve such issues, the courts and attorneys general will first try to interpret both statutes so that they do not conflict. When that is impossible, in general, federal statutes control over state statutes, a doctrine known as "preemption." Further, neither federal nor state legislatures can exceed the scope of their constitutional authority when passing laws. When two state statutes conflict, the most recent or the most specific statute often prevails over an older or more general statute.

When a state law conflicts with a federal law, the first consideration is whether the preemption doctrine applies. If it does, then the federal law supersedes the state law. The U.S. Supreme Court, in 1992, in *Cipollone v. Liggett Group, Inc.*, ruled that a federal law may expressly preempt a state law. The court further held that preemption is implied if the scope of the federal statute indicates that Congress intended its law to be the exclusive determiner of the subject of the law, or if the state law actually conflicts with the federal law. In *Freightliner Corporation v. Myrick*, in 1995, the U.S. Supreme Court further held that state law presents an actual conflict with federal law when: (1) it is impossible for a private party to comply with the requirements of both a state and federal law; or (2) the state law obstructs the purpose and objectives that Congress intended with the federal law. When preemption applies, federal law controls, and a plaintiff is precluded from bringing an action under the state law.

Conflicting Laws: Implications for School Nurses

The Texas Attorney General was recently called on to interpret three apparently conflicting statutes of special importance to school nurses. Federal law requires that children who are homeless must be admitted to public schools without regard to the availability of immunization records (McKinney Homeless Assistance Act). However, Texas law requires that, within 30 days of school enrollment, a child's parent must provide the child's immunization record or proof that the child is exempt from the statutory requirement (Tex. Educ. Code § 25.002). Texas law further requires that all students must be fully immunized, unless exempt. Provisional admission is allowed if a child begins the necessary immunizations and continues receiving them as rapidly as medically feasible (Tex. Educ. Code § 38.001).

The Texas Education Agency and the Texas Department of Health interpreted these statutes differently. The two state agencies did agree, however, that, because federal law preempts state law, homeless students must be admitted regardless of immunization status. They disagreed on another important point, however. The Texas Education Agency's position was that every child must be admitted for 30 days in order to begin immunizations, secure medical records or prove exemption. The Texas Department of Health's position was that children who have not started immunizations may be prohibited from enrolling in school, unless they can immediately prove an exemption. Therefore, both agencies asked the Texas Attorney General to resolve the conflict.

In 2004, the Attorney General examined the two statutes and the agencies' positions and determined that the two laws could be read together so that they do not conflict because they have different purposes: 25.002 addresses only the documents necessary for school admission in order to promote consistency in the school enrollment of children; 38.001 establishes immunization requirements necessary to promote students' health. Therefore, the Attorney General opined, only the Texas Department of Health has the authority to regulate provisional school admission, not the Texas Education Agency, and the Texas Department of Health can establish a rule prohibiting a nonimmunized, nonexempt student from enrolling in school, even for the provisional 30 days. The Attorney General further pointed out, however, that the Texas Department of Health could not restrict the right of a parent, whose child is fully or partially immunized, from having 30 days to produce the required immunization documentation (Tex. Att'y Gen. Op. No. GA-0178 (2004)) (Box 12.1).

Box 12.1 ■■■

A school nurse attempting to resolve the apparent conflict between two apparently conflicting laws is well advised to follow the same analytical process as the courts and attorneys general:

1. Can both statutes be interpreted so that they both have meaning and do not conflict?
2. Is one a federal law, which would preempt a state law?
3. Is one law a constitution, which would preempt a statute?
4. Is one law much more specific on the conflicting point?
5. Is one law much more recently implemented?
6. Is one law applicable to residents of a state or to any person who happens to be located, even transitorily, in a state?

While this analysis is not a substitute for competent legal advice, it can provide guidance on an informed analysis of such conflicts.

Regulatory Law

Regulations, on the federal and state levels, are designed to interpret and assist in the implementation of federal and state statutes. Regulations, however, are not supposed to exceed the parameters of the laws they interpret. Federal and state agencies draft regulations, rules, and guidances to assist in the implementation and interpretation of statutes. After the initial drafting, regulations and rules are generally subject to an opportunity for the public to review and comment on them prior to their adoption by the agency that drafted them. The federal laws described above all have regulations. Examples of state regulations may include child immunization requirements, communicable disease notification procedures, communicable disease prevention procedures, health screenings, school-based health center requirements, medication administration requirements, requirements for consents to medical treatment, confidentiality protections, and nurse practice standards.

Typically, these state and federal agencies also are responsible for reviewing contested cases, which may arise from a variety of issues, including discipline of a professional, termination of employment, revocation of licensure, and other matters about which a party is complaining or contesting some adverse impact. For example, a state nursing board may be responsible for determining the eligibility requirements for nursing licenses, for bestowing those licenses on eligible individuals, and for revoking nursing licenses based on improper conduct. As another example of a contested case, an education agency may review a school district's termination of a school nurse's employment contract.

Figure 12.1 shows the general statutory and regulatory impacts on health and public education. Generally, the chart shows that the U.S. Congress enacts federal laws, which are signed by the President. Those laws are then interpreted and enforced by federal agencies through regulations,

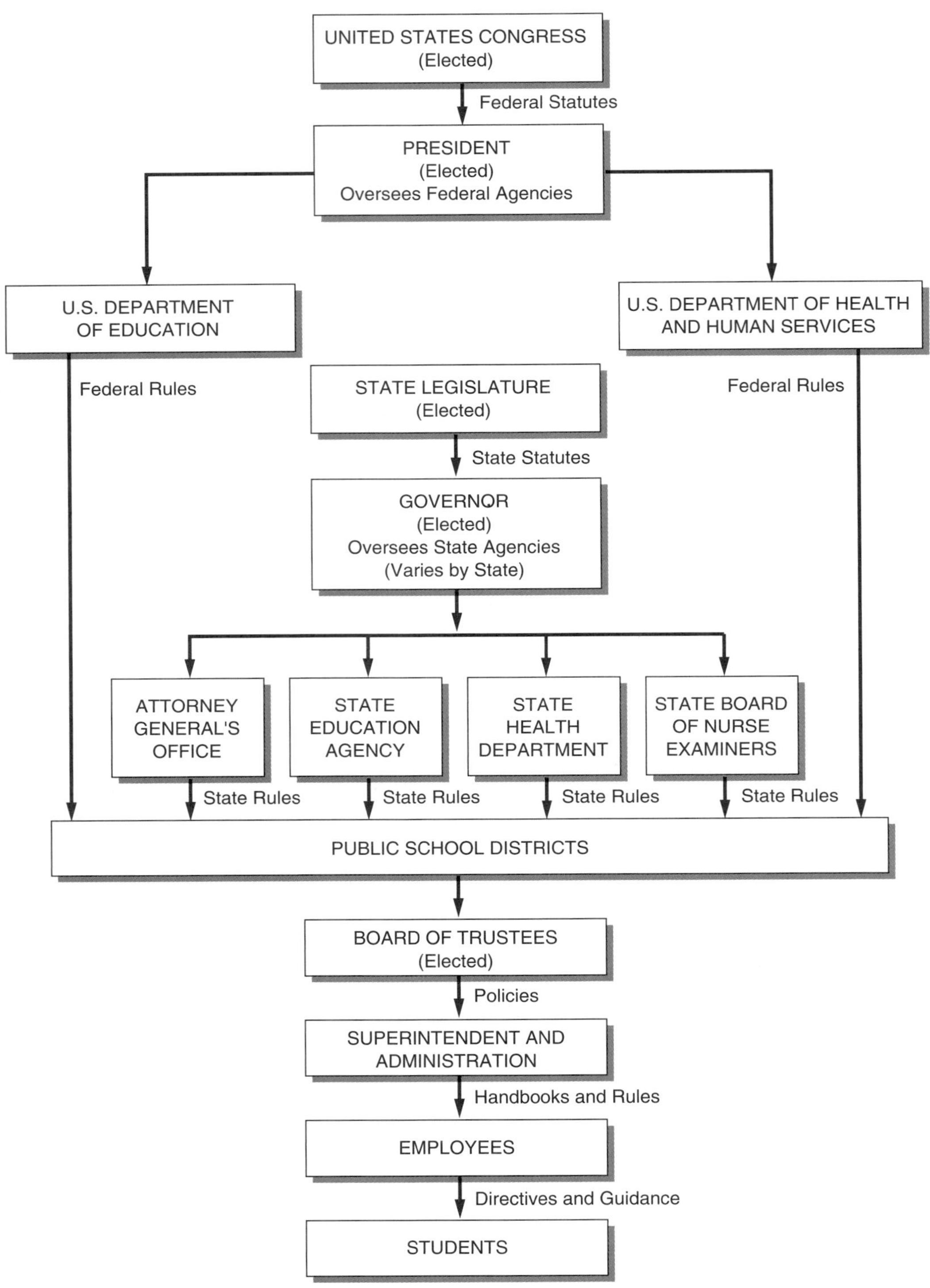

Figure 12.1 ■ Statutory and regulatory impacts on health and public education.

which directly impact public schools, and sometimes those private schools that accept federal funds or engage in interstate commerce. Each state also has a state legislature that enacts state laws regarding health and public education, which are then signed by the state's governor. State agencies, including education agencies, health departments, and state nursing boards, then draft regulations that interpret and implement the statutes passed by the state legislature. State Nursing Boards draft regulations that apply to nurses in general, regardless of their work setting, and regulations that apply specifically to school nurses. School nurses, however, have employers who are not healthcare professionals, as shown by Figure 12.1.

Public school districts are typically overseen by elected school boards made up of citizens who oversee the management of the districts, usually by establishing board policies to guide the activities of their staff. Private schools normally have appointed boards that also make policies. Those board policies must comply with all applicable federal and state laws and regulations. Superintendents of schools and their supporting administrators then implement those policies. The administrators, in turn, supervise all employees who perform the day-to-day operations involving the education and care of students. All activities of these employees, including the school nurses, must, likewise, comply with federal and state laws and regulations.

Common Law

Elements of a Lawsuit

Common law, or case law, results from decisions made by judges and juries in the court system. A lawsuit results when a complainant or "plaintiff" files a "complaint" or "petition" with a court, complaining of the actions of a "defendant," and notifies the defendant of the complaint. The plaintiff must allege what is known as a "cause of action," which is a statement of facts that represent a violation of some law or legal responsibility and which gives the plaintiff the right to seek a judicial remedy. After the plaintiff files a complaint or petition, the defendant must then file an "answer" or response to the complaint. The defendant's answer usually establishes the defendant's responses to the allegations, any immunity claimed, and any legal defenses to the action.

After both parties have explained their preliminary positions to the court, the parties engage in what is known as "discovery," a sometimes lengthy and extensive process in which both parties have the opportunity to obtain documents and other evidence from each other and from third parties and to require individuals to answer questions under oath. This may involve a few documents and witnesses or may involve thousands of documents and a large number of witnesses. Usually after discovery is complete, the parties will then file dispositive motions with the court, which dispose of preliminary matters by allowing the judge to rule on certain issues before trial. The judge may rule on preliminary matters, such as whether or not the court has "jurisdiction," or authority to hear the case, or whether the plaintiff can prove sufficient facts to establish the plaintiff's cause of action. If the entire case is not disposed of through dispositive motions, then the case is set for trial.

At trial, each party is allowed to prove its case through the testimony of witnesses, the presentation of evidence, and the display of exhibits. All of a party's witnesses are subject to cross-examination by the other party. Parties may object to questions asked by the other party and to the admission of evidence and exhibits attempted to be introduced by the other party. Attorneys representing the parties, or the parties appearing on their own, known as *pro se*, may be allowed to make opening and closing arguments or to submit written arguments, or briefs, on the merits of the case.

Trials may be held before judges or juries. If a trial is before a jury, the jury decides all questions of fact, but the judge decides all questions of law. In a trial before a judge, the judge decides all questions of fact and law. A question of fact is a conclusion reached regarding a factual dispute, and usually relates to making a decision about specific actions that occurred in a given situation, such as, for example, whether a school nurse reported a positive result of a pediculosis screening to the student's parents. A question of law, on the other hand, resolves the application or interpretation of a law to the specific facts, as decided. A question of law often relates to the elements of a constitutional or statutory violation, whether the specific facts decided constitute a legal violation, or whether a statute comports with the constitution such that it is constitutional. For example, a question of law would be whether a school nurse has a legal responsibility to notify parents of the results of a pediculosis screening. Often, questions of fact and law are intertwined.

After a judge, with or without a jury, makes a final decision in a case, that decision is reduced to writing and may be published in a set of books so that others can research those decisions. Court decisions can also be appealed to and reviewed by higher courts, usually a court of appeals and a supreme court.

Court Systems

A court's jurisdiction is a very important concept, as a court can only consider issues it has the authority to consider and its decisions are controlling only in the geographical area that the court covers. There are two court systems: the state court system and the federal court system. State courts cover all issues related to state laws (state questions) and may cover issues related to federal laws (federal questions). Federal courts have jurisdiction to cover all cases related to federal laws (federal questions) and cases involving parties from more than one state (diversity jurisdiction). A person filing a lawsuit must show why the court in which the lawsuit is filed has jurisdiction. Certain federal laws may preempt state laws in a particular area of law; which may require a plaintiff to bring a claim related to that area of law only in federal court, because the federal court has what is known as "exclusive jurisdiction." For example, in *Jass v. Prudential Health Care Plan*, the federal Court of Appeals for the Seventh Circuit, in 1996, ruled that when a person has a complaint related to medical services covered by an insurance plan, any complaints the patient has that a nurse or other professional acted negligently may be covered by the Employee Retirement Income Security Act of 1974 (ERISA). The court in *Jass* ruled that if ERISA covers the claim, then the complaining patient is required to bring the case in federal court and may not bring the claim in state court.

Both the federal and the state court systems establish local courts that conduct trials and hear cases, and a series of appellate courts that have increasingly broader geographical jurisdiction and review the appealed decisions of the lower courts. Typically, a local district court case can be appealed to an appeals court that may oversee the decisions of hundreds of courts within a larger geographical area. That appeals court case can then be appealed to the supreme court of the state in which the lawsuit arose, if it is a state case, or the U.S. Supreme Court, if it is a federal case.

For example, a decision in a Tarrant County, Texas state district court case, which is only binding in Tarrant County, can be appealed to the state court of appeals in Fort Worth, Texas, which covers a portion of north Texas. That appellate court decision can then be appealed to the Texas Supreme Court, which covers the entire state of Texas. The Texas Supreme Court's decision, then, is controlling law in Texas. However, once a case has gone all the way through a state's appeal process, the state Supreme Court decision may be appealed to the United States Supreme Court, if it involves a federal question. In the federal court system, the federal trial would be held in one of the federal district courts in the Northern District of Texas and would be subject to be appealed to the Fifth Circuit Court of Appeals, which covers all appeals of all federal district court cases in the states of Texas, Louisiana and Mississippi. The Fifth Circuit's decision then is controlling law only in Texas, Louisiana, and Mississippi, the geographical area the Fifth Circuit covers. That Fifth Circuit decision can then be appealed to the U.S. Supreme Court, which selectively hears appeals from all of the Circuit Courts of Appeals throughout the United States. A Supreme Court decision applies to the entire country, and is the only court decision that does so.

It is, therefore, important to know what court jurisdictions control a school nurse's practice. Different courts in different jurisdictions may reach different decisions on issues that are very similar. Only if the school nurse knows which jurisdictions cover the nurse's geographical area will the nurse be able to understand which court decisions are controlling law. For example, in 1999, state courts in Connecticut and New York were each asked to consider the state's respective education law that mandated scoliosis screening for public school students. In each state, a parent attempted to bring a private cause of action against a school district for failing to provide scoliosis screening. In both cases, the school districts moved to dismiss the lawsuit because the laws in question did not expressly provide for a private right of action by an individual. When a statute is silent as to whether an individual can sue another party in a tort (or personal injury)-type action for violating the statute, the courts must determine whether a private cause of action is implied.

In *Uhr v. East Greenbush Central School District*, the New York state court concluded that no private cause of action was allowed, because it was inconsistent with the statute's legislative scheme, which included an immunity provision for liability that arose as a result of conducting the screenings. Focusing on the state's interest in protecting state entities from financial liability, the New York court rejected the plaintiff's argument that the legislature, by implication, intended to hold school districts liable for a failure to screen because it provided express immunity only for the results of screenings.

The Connecticut court, however, reached a completely different result in *Doe v. Voluntown Board of Education*. The Connecticut statute does not include any immunity provisions. The Connecticut court concluded that, although there was no statutory language authorizing a private cause of action, it was up to the legislature to include language to expressly prohibit a private cause of action. Focusing on the state's interest in achieving the statute's purpose, the court determined that allowing an individual to sue a school district for its failure to provide mandatory screenings is consistent with the legislature's purpose to promote early detection of scoliosis.

These cases underscore how separate courts may interpret the same statutory duty very differently. Therefore, it is important for the school nurse to understand fully the controlling law in the nurse's geographical area.

While the state in which the school nurse works will normally serve to identify for the nurse which court cases are applicable to the nurse, it is more difficult to determine with the federal circuit courts of appeal, because each court covers a multistate area. To assist in understanding which federal circuit court decisions are controlling law in a particular geographical area, the attached map at FIGURE 12.2 shows the federal circuit courts and their geographical jurisdictions.

Court cases have what is known as "precedential value"; in other words, they serve as precedent to guide citizens and courts that are seeking answers to conflicts in other cases. However, different facts in different cases can result in different decisions. Further, given the large number of courts, decisions among courts may conflict. It is, therefore, often important for an appellate court to review appealed cases to resolve the conflicts between cases in order to provide further and more refined guidance.

FIGURE 12.3 describes how a local action or decision can be reviewed by the court system. A cause of action arising from an alleged violation of state or federal law or some legal duty may initially be heard by the governing body of the school or district, a process known as "exhaustion of administrative remedies." The Board of Trustees' decision, then, can be appealed to either the state's education agency or some other state or federal agency with jurisdiction to hear a contested case, in certain limited circumstances, again known as "exhaustion of administrative remedies." However, if no administrative remedies need to be exhausted, a lawsuit can be filed in state or federal court, depending on which court properly has jurisdiction. The district court conducts the trial and decides the case. The trial court's decision can then be appealed to an appellate court or to the state or U.S. Supreme Court. State Supreme Court cases are usually final, unless they involve substantial federal issues, which require appeal to the U.S. Supreme Court. The U.S. Supreme

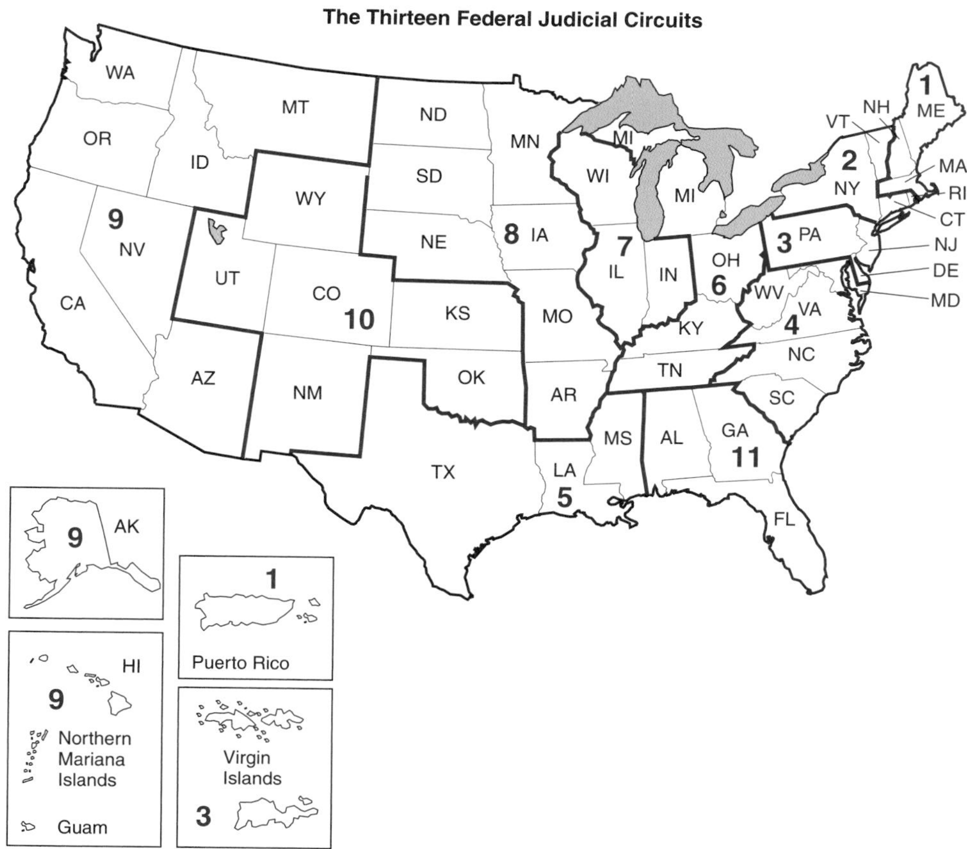

Figure 12.2 ■ The 13 federal judicial circuits. (Copyright © 2003, West Group. Reprinted with permission.)

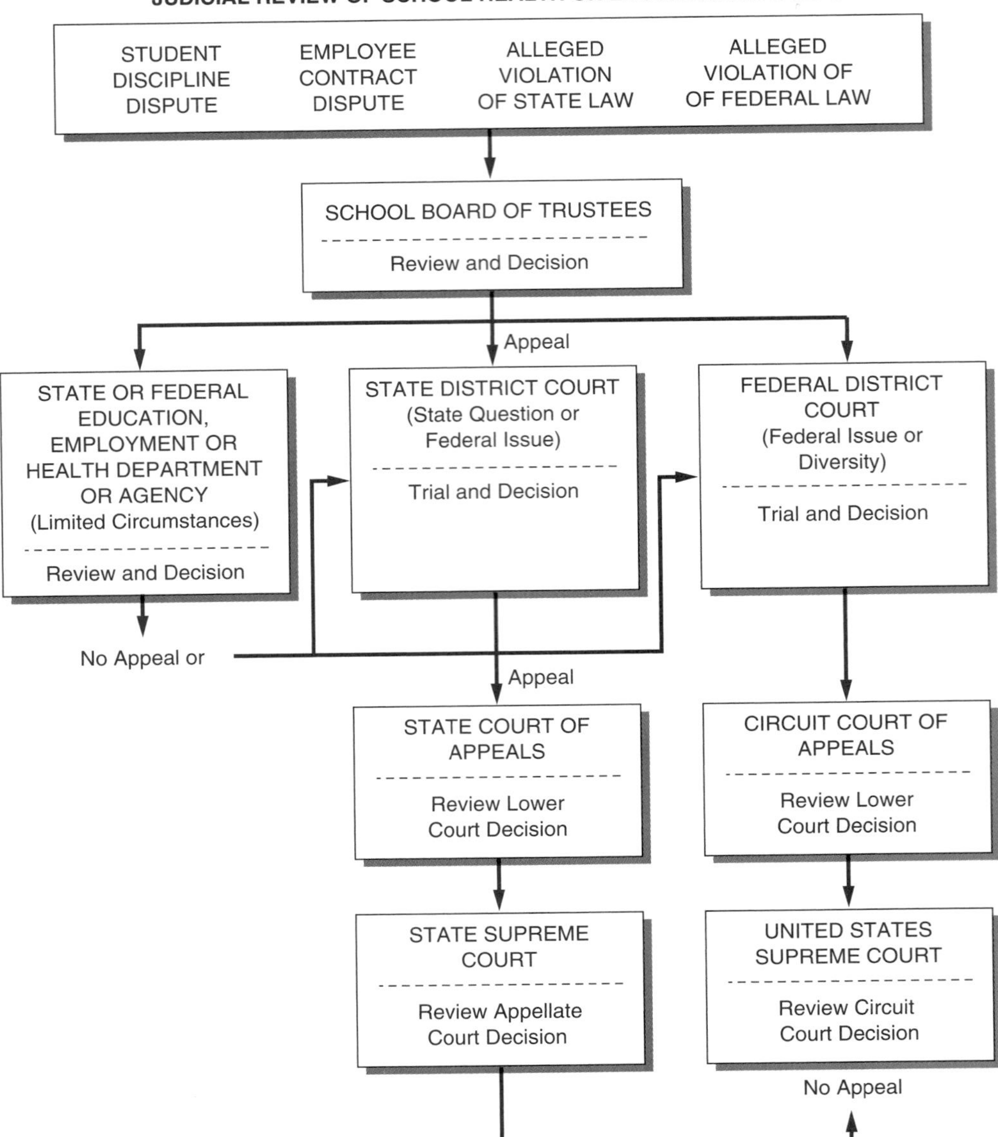

Figure 12.3 ■ Judicial review of school health or education matters.

Court's decisions are final and are the law of the land; their decisions are controlling throughout the country.

For example, in *New Jersey v. TLO*, in the original lawsuit the state of New Jersey brought delinquency charges against a student in New Jersey juvenile court after a school employee searched the student's purse and found drugs and drug paraphernalia. Despite the student's claim that the search violated her Fourth Amendment rights, the juvenile court found that the search was reasonable and determined that the student was delinquent. The student then appealed that decision to the Appellate Division of the New Jersey Superior Court. The appellate court affirmed the trial court's finding that the search of the student's purse did not violate the student's Fourth Amendment rights. The student next appealed the decision to the New Jersey Supreme Court. The state supreme court concluded that the search of the purse was unreasonable and reversed the lower courts. Finally, the state appealed the decision to the United States Supreme Court. The Supreme Court agreed to hear the case, to determine the appropriate application of a student's Fourth Amendment rights in all public schools. The Supreme Court decided that the Fourth Amendment protection from unreasonable searches and seizures applies to searches conducted by public school officials, but the Court further concluded that the search at issue in this case was reasonable. The Court's decision then became the controlling law for searches of a student's belongings by public school officials throughout the country.

Special education cases are handled differently, however, as shown in FIGURE 12.4. When a parent alleges that a school district violated his or her child's rights under the federal Individuals with Disabilities Education Act (IDEA) (see Chapter 14), the parent requests a due process hearing, which is a trial conducted by a hearing officer assigned by the state education agency. Because IDEA is a federal law, that hearing officer's decision can be appealed to federal district court, which normally reviews the due process hearing transcript and evidence, rather than conducting another trial on the same facts, and which may conduct only a limited trial on new information. After the court reaches a decision regarding whether or not the school district violated IDEA, that federal district court decision can then be appealed to the proper federal circuit court of appeals. That circuit court of appeal's decision can be appealed to the U.S. Supreme Court and the Supreme Court can decide whether or not it wants to hear and decide the case.

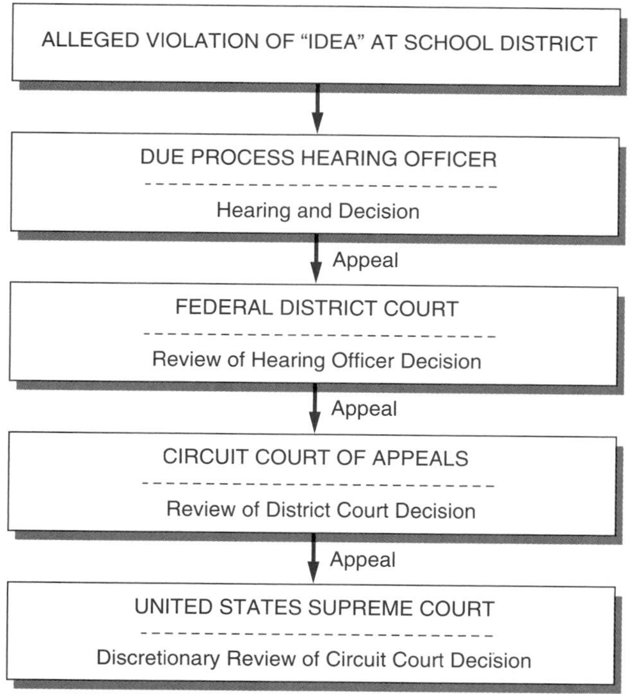

Figure 12.4 ■ Judicial review of special education dispute.

For example, in *Cedar Rapids Community School District v. Garret F.*, a parent complained that the school district was violating IDEA by failing to accept financial responsibility for all the services required by a special education student who was wheelchair-bound and ventilator dependent. The dispute was first presented to a hearing officer at an Iowa Department of Education hearing. The hearing officer concluded that IDEA required the school district to bear financial responsibility for all disputed services. The school district appealed the hearing officer's decision to the federal district court, which agreed with the hearing officer's decision. The school district next appealed the decision to the Eighth Circuit Court of Appeals, which affirmed the lower court's decision. Finally, the school district appealed the decision to the United States Supreme Court. The Supreme Court provided the final determination that the IDEA required the school district to provide the special education student with the nursing services required during school hours.

Civil and Criminal Courts

Just as there are civil and criminal laws, there are civil and criminal courts. Criminal cases are brought by law enforcement authorities when evidence of a crime is discovered or when an individual files a complaint or charge alleging criminal conduct against another person. Examples of criminal cases of concern to the school nurse may include assault, fraud, records tampering, kidnapping, child abuse, and controlled substance abuse. Criminal authorities must prove that an individual is guilty "beyond a reasonable doubt" in order for a judge or jury to find an individual guilty of a criminal law. "Beyond a reasonable doubt" is a very high standard of proof, requiring that the proven facts must establish guilt. This high standard has been implemented to increase the probability that only the truly guilty are convicted of crimes.

Civil cases are brought by individuals or organizations against others. Examples of civil cases of concern to the school nurse include personal injury cases, medical or professional malpractice cases, wrongful employment termination cases, breach of contract cases, and child custody cases. Civil law violations are normally brought to the attention of the courts through lawsuits brought by someone who claims to be an injured party. The lawsuit can be brought in state or federal court, depending on the law allegedly violated and the residency of the parties.

Civil cases typically have a much lower burden of proof than criminal cases—a preponderance of the evidence, which is merely evidence that is more convincing than the evidence offered in opposition to it. In other words, it is merely the degree of proof that establishes that something is more probable than not.

Civil and criminal cases are entirely separate from each other and involve separate court systems. The civil and criminal courts address different laws, have different standards of proof, and result in different consequences. If appropriate, both civil and criminal cases can be brought as a result of a single incident or situation, and the outcomes of the cases will not be dependent on each other. Because of the different kinds of laws and burdens of proof, it is possible for different decisions to result from a criminal case and a civil case involving the same facts and circumstances. For example, imagine that a school employee physically harmed a child, which resulted in serious injury to a child. Further, imagine that the child's parents file a civil personal injury case against the school and the employee as a result of the incident, and the district attorney files a criminal assault case against the employee. The school or the employee could be found civilly liable for monetary damages to the child to compensate him for the injuries he sustained, because the parents may be able to prove that it was more probable than not that the employee was negligent. However, that same employee could be found to be not guilty of the criminal offense of assault, based on the same conduct, because the district attorney may not be able to prove beyond a reasonable doubt that the employee had the necessary criminal intent to harm the child.

Agency Contested Cases

There is another kind of quasi-judicial decision of particular importance to school nurses: public agency reviewed and contested cases. For example, a state Nursing Examiner Board may investigate and hear disciplinary cases filed against school nurses and their licensures. Because licensure is a property right, the due process clause of the United States Constitution requires adequate due process (notice and hearing) before licensure can be removed. Typically, a nurse will be given complete and detailed notice of the allegations, and will be entitled to respond generally to those allegations. The nurse will then typically be provided a hearing, in which he or she is confronted with all witnesses and evidence, may cross-examine all witnesses, may present witnesses and evidence, and may present oral and written argument to the agency. Normally, only after due process is provided in a contested case does the agency decide whether any action should be taken against a nurse's license. (See, e.g.,, 22 Texas Administrative Code § 217.19; New York Education Law § 6510 (McKinney), a Texas regulation and a New York law that specifies the amount of due process required to revoke a nurse's license.) If the nurse fails to take advantage of the due process opportunity, revocation proceedings can continue in the nurse's absence, as a nurse learned in New York in *In re Allen*, when she declined to attend her revocation proceedings.

Grounds to initiate agency proceedings also vary by state, but may include fraud, material violations of a nurse practice act, criminal conviction, incompetency or incapacity, unethical behavior, illegal drug or alcohol use, violation of licensure probation, child abuse or neglect, failure to report child abuse or neglect, gross negligence in nursing practice, falsification of records, immoral conduct in the work environment, or violation of confidentiality, among others (225 Illinois Compiled Statutes 65/10-45; California Code of Regulations title 16, § 1442-1444.5).

Any inquiry or contested case must be taken very seriously by the school nurse. Cooperation by the school nurse is vital to the process, as is competent legal counsel. Once all facts are known and all applicable laws are assessed, the school nurse is in a much better position to determine what action is appropriate. While a full defense may be appropriate, a negotiated settlement may also be a viable option.

Many agencies and boards, including Boards of Nursing, may have a procedure in place to informally resolve a contested case, whether through mediation, arbitration, or settlement, in the interest of economy and efficiency. It is often in a school nurse's best interest to at least explore some form of alternative dispute resolution, especially when the facts are not in dispute, in order to prevent the inevitable drain of time, energy, resources, and concentration required of all parties involved in a contested case.

An example of a public agency review is the federal Equal Employment Opportunity Commission (EEOC), which hears complaints of alleged discrimination related to employment matters under the Equal Employment Opportunity Act, 42 U.S.C. § 2000e, et seq. Both parties have the opportunity to provide position statements and evidence, and must cooperate in investigations. However, because EEOC is a reviewing agency, no due process hearing is conducted. Rather, after receiving all information from all parties, the EEOC or its corresponding state agency may mediate a claim, do a full investigation, and issue a letter of findings. That letter may be accompanied by a "right to sue" letter, which then entitles the complainant to proceed by filing a lawsuit in federal district court. For employment discrimination matters, this federal agency complaint is a prerequisite to the filing of a lawsuit, a process known as "exhausting administrative remedies."

State education agencies and health departments may also conduct investigations based on complaints received from parents or students. Typically, these proceedings are more informal, as they do not result in the loss of licensure. An agency may receive a complaint and, based on the facts of the complaint, request information from the school and the school nurse. The school and the school nurse are expected to cooperate fully with the agency's investigation, providing all requested information and position statements. After receipt of that information, the agency then may decide that the complaint has no merit or may recommend that the school or the nurse take some type of corrective action.

STANDARD OF CARE

A school nurse takes many discretionary actions during the course of a school day. Most of a school nurse's work involves the exercise of judgment and discretion on a time-sensitive basis. As a result, courts typically defer to the professional judgment and discretion of the school nurse as a school employee. To a great degree, courts do not see their role as second-guessing education professionals or as serving as "super school boards." However, some lawsuits are brought against school professionals, and some of those court rulings are adverse to the school professionals. For nurses, those cases could arise in the context of physical injuries to students, the provision of health-related services to students who are disabled, failure to prevent injuries to students, the provision of healthcare instruction, and emergency care (Schwab & Gelfman, 2001). Should a lawsuit be filed, the inquiry regarding a school nurse will likely focus on whether or not that nurse provided the appropriate standard of care.

Legal Bases for Standard of Care

The standard of care by which a school nurse will be judged is derived from a variety of sources, including the federal and state constitutions, federal and state laws and regulations (including standards of practice), applicable court decisions, local policies, procedures and job descriptions. For example, a school nurse's interaction with students may not infringe upon a student's Constitutional rights, such as the Fourth Amendment's prohibition against unreasonable search or seizure. In *New Jersey v. T.L.O.*, the United States Supreme Court, in 1985, proclaimed that the Fourth Amendment's prohibition against unreasonable searches and seizures applies to a search or seizure conducted by a public school official. The Court recognized that students are entitled to some expectation of privacy, but also acknowledged the school's interest in maintaining an environment conducive to learning. To achieve the appropriate balance, the Court ruled that it is not necessary for a school official to obtain a warrant or to establish 'probable cause' (the police search standard) before conducting a search of a student's belongings; however, the school official's actions must be "reasonable in light of the circumstances," that is, the official must have "reasonable cause." For example, if a student arrives in the school nurse's office exhibiting signs of illegal drug use, it would be reasonable for the nurse to search the student's backpack or purse for drugs. But, it may not be reasonable for a nurse to search the purse or backpack of a student who comes in to obtain acetaminophen for a headache, when there is no reason to suspect a student is carrying an illegal substance.

Similarly, it may certainly be reasonable for a school nurse to view the unclothed chest of a student complaining of chest pains, after the student's privacy is protected. However, if that student was complaining of leg pains, while it may be appropriate for the school nurse to take vital signs and listen to the student's heartbeat, it would not be appropriate for the nurse to ask a student complaining of leg pain to remove her blouse.

Federal laws and regulations also establish certain responsibilities of a school district related to the appropriate standard of care for students with special needs. For example, the Individuals with Disabilities Education Act (IDEA) (originally enacted in 1970 as the Education of the Handicapped Act), was enacted to ensure that all children with disabilities receive a free appropriate public education that includes special education and related services that meet their unique needs. In addition, Section 504 of the Rehabilitation Act of 1973 prohibits discrimination against disabled students by schools that receive federal funds. Some of the responsibilities to serve students with disabilities may be assigned by the school district to the school nurse through a student's Individual Education Program (IEP) for IDEA students or a 504 Plan for Section 504 students. Chapters 9 and 14 have information on these laws and their applicability to the school setting.

A public school district's responsibility to provide a free appropriate public education to disabled students may require a school nurse to provide certain nursing services for a disabled child, such as clean intermittent catheterization, as the U.S. Supreme Court decided in *Irving Independent School District v. Tatro* in 1984. Certain nursing services, such as one-on-one nursing care, may be required under IDEA for a medically fragile, ventilator-dependent, quadriplegic child, as the U.S. Supreme Court decided in 1999 in *Cedar Rapids Community School District v. Garrett F.*

A school nurse may also be asked to provide input into determining the extent of related services necessary to allow a disabled student to benefit from special education, as well as educate the student's IEP team about a student's medical conditions, and the effect those conditions might have on his or her educational performance. The nurse may also be called upon to give input to the student's IEP team about the health challenges faced by the student and accommodations and services that might address the student's disabilities, to allow the student to benefit from special education.

State laws, including school and health laws, also define specific expectations that establish the school nurse's standard of care, as do state licensure laws and regulations. Because some laws may conflict or be subject to different interpretation, establishing the proper standard of care is not always a simple matter. For example, in *Stamps v. Jefferson County Board of Education*, special education teachers in Alabama sued the Jefferson County Board of Education because the school district, in attempting to follow IDEA, required teachers to perform duties such as direct line feedings, suctioning of tracheotomy tubes and changing of colostomy bags, which the teachers believed made them liable for criminal prosecution for the unauthorized practice of nursing. The Supreme Court of Alabama decided that the state's Board of Nursing was an indispensable party in the lawsuit, because the nursing board was the organization that would determine whether an individual was guilty of the unauthorized practice of nursing.

Licensure laws, nurse practice standards, and specific statutes addressing health issues may all impact on determining the appropriate standard of care expected of a school nurse. Nurse licensure laws are state laws, because health care is a state responsibility. As a result, there can be significant variations among states regarding the education, duties, responsibilities, expectations, and delegation authority of nurses, in general, and school nurses, in particular. Most state nursing practice standards will cover areas such as compliance with nursing practice rules, maintenance of confidentiality, application of appropriate nursing interventions for stabilization and prevention of complications, systematic approaches to individualized goal-directed care, clarification of unclear or contraindicated orders and treatments, prevention of communicable disease exposure, administration of medication, accurate record-keeping and reporting, professional development, client education, delegation of tasks, and supervision of others. For example, Texas Administrative Code Title 22, Section 217.11, provides a list of the standards for nursing practice in the state of Texas applicable to all nurses as well as standards specific to vocational nurses and registered nurses.

Case law from other court decisions may also serve as precedential guidance in determining the appropriate standard of care. Employer expectations are another source of standard of care, and may be identified in contracts, local policies, job descriptions, employee handbooks, and student handbooks. Several factors may affect the standard that is applied to a particular school nurse's actions, such as the nurse's education, experience, and current community practices. For example, an LVN with a few months' experience may not be held to the same standard of care as an RN with 15 years of school nursing experience.

Further, the specific factual situation may factor into the determination of the school nurse's appropriate standard of care. The school nurse's job responsibilities, the student's special needs, the geographical location of the nurse in relation to the students, and the nurse's caseload may all be factors. For example, a school nurse assigned to two separate schools that are 15 minutes apart by car cannot be held to the same standard of care for a medically fragile student as a school nurse assigned to monitor that one medically fragile student, and whose sole responsibility is to provide lifesaving measures to that child at any time throughout the school day.

Finally, other available resources may establish a standard of care. In *Debord v. Ferguson-Florissant School District*, the federal Court of Appeals for the Eighth Circuit ruled, in 1997, that a school nurse may rely on the *Physician's Desk Reference* to guide the nurse's decisions regarding the appropriate standard of care. In that case, the court held that, even though a student may require a higher than recommended dosage of a medication, a nurse does not act unreasonably if she refuses to administer a dosage that exceeds the maximum dosage recommended in the *Physician's Desk Reference* and the school agrees to accommodate home administration of the medication.

Therefore, it is important for a school nurse to be very familiar with the laws and regulations in the nurse's geographical location. A complete and thorough knowledge of expectations will assist the school nurse in achieving those expectations on a daily basis. A good documentation system consistently used by the nurse will provide proof that the appropriate standard of care is *met* (Schwab & Gelfman, 2001).

Determinations of Standard of Care—Negligence

In civil cases seeking money damages for personal injury (tort claims), the standard of care is based on a negligence standard. Typically, a negligence action would be brought against the nurse and the nurse's employer, and the standard of care would be examined for both the employee and the employer. The *standard of care is what a reasonably prudent person would do under the same or similar circumstances.* In a professional malpractice case, the standard of care is what an ordinary prudent professional would provide under the same or similar circumstances. The best course of action for a school nurse, therefore, is to act as an ordinary, prudent professional would act. Reasonable justification for actions taken in the best interest of student safety can reduce or eliminate liability.

Negligence, therefore, is the failure to act as a reasonably prudent person would act under the same or similar circumstances. In order to prevail in a negligence case in court, a plaintiff normally must prove that: (1) the defendant owed a legal duty to the plaintiff; (2) the defendant breached (or failed to accomplish) that duty by failing to act as a reasonable person would in the same or similar circumstances, that is, by failing to prevent foreseeable harm; (3) the defendant's breach is what caused the plaintiff's harm (called "proximate cause"); and (4) the plaintiff was injured or harmed as a result of the defendant's breach (Restatement (Second) of Torts § 281 (1965)). In a medical or nursing negligence case, then, the plaintiff must prove: (1) standard of care (duty); (2) failure to comply with the standard of care (breach of duty); (3) that failure to comply with the standard of care caused injury (proximate cause); and (4) injury (harm) (*Sullivan v. Edward Hospital*).

To prevail in a negligence case, a plaintiff must prove facts that establish all four elements of a negligence action: (1) duty, (2) breach of duty, (3) proximate cause, and (4) harm (Restatement (Second) of Torts § 281). An individual or entity cannot be held liable for negligence unless all four elements are proven. For example, it is possible for a student to sustain an injury, even though the school nurse does everything that a reasonably prudent nurse would do, such as when providing proper inhalation therapy and summoning emergency medical assistance fail to save a student undergoing a severe asthma attack. Conversely, a school nurse can breach his or her duty to perform a legal responsibility, but, if no one is harmed as a result, then the nurse is not liable for negligence. For example, a school nurse could switch the medications of two students, both of whom were taking the same dosage of Ritalin. Although the nurse erred, no harm was done. Neither scenario described above would support a negligence cause of action, because an essential element of the cause of action would be missing.

Duty

To establish a legal duty owed by a school nurse, the court could look to federal or state statutory or regulatory responsibilities, job descriptions, employment contracts, employee or student handbooks, individualized education programs, or any other document or rule that establishes the legal duty owed by the nurse. At trial, expert witnesses can also testify regarding the standards prevalent within the professional community and about nurse practice standards. In *Sullivan v. Edward Hospital*, the Illinois Supreme Court in 2004 specifically stated that a physician cannot testify as an expert witness to the appropriate standard of care expected of a nurse; only another nurse can serve as that expert witness. The Court held that the expert: (1) must be a licensed member of the same school of medicine; and (2) must be familiar with the methods, procedures, and treatments ordinarily observed by others of the same profession. Only after that foundation is established, is it then within the court's discretion to determine whether the expert is competent to testify, that is, whether the negligence allegations concern matters within the expert's knowledge and observation. Therefore, typically, another nurse will testify as an expert witness regarding the standard of care expected of a school nurse.

An injured party's status as an invitee or a trespasser can also impact the determination of whether a legal duty is owed. For example, a school nurse present at an athletic field day to render first aid may owe a legal duty to the student participants, but will not owe that same legal duty to a neighbor who wanders over to the school uninvited to see what all the excitement is about.

Establishing the existence of a legal duty or responsibility is not always a simple task. For example, in *Griffith v. New York*, an appellate court in New York in 1986, ruled that a school has a duty to exercise the same degree of care over a student at school as a reasonable parent would exercise, but that duty ceases once the student is back under the parent's authority. Therefore, the court ruled that even though a school nurse in New York City improperly denied medical attention to a student with asthma and sent her home, the school was not responsible when the student fell out of a window at home in a panicked attempt to get more air into her lungs while waiting for an ambulance.

In *Federico v. Order of Saint Benedict*, the federal Court of Appeals for the First Circuit, in 1995, ruled that a school was not subject to a heightened duty of care because it was a boarding school. The court determined that, although a school must do whatever a reasonably prudent person would do to safeguard the health of its students, the school is not responsible for guaranteeing the health of its students. Rather, the court ruled that a school's legal duty is to act reasonably in responding to a student's medical needs. In *Federico*, the court concluded that the school nurse met her legal duty when, upon notice that a student was suffering from a severe asthma attack in his room, she immediately called for emergency services and went to check on the student. Once in the student's room, the nurse attempted to administer mouth-to-mouth resuscitation, but was unsuccessful. Emergency personnel were unable to revive the student. The student's parents argued that a boarding school should be held to a higher duty of care that includes individualized standing orders in the event of an emergency. Then, according to the parents, the nurse would have been alerted and authorized to administer epinephrine immediately. Expert witnesses testified that, if the nurse had given the student an epinephrine injection as soon as she arrived in the student's room, it may have saved the student's life. However, the court concluded there was no basis for holding the boarding school to a higher standard of care and ruled that the nurse met her duty to act reasonably by calling for emergency services and attempting resuscitation.

Breach of Duty

In determining whether a breach of a legal duty occurred, a court would look to those same statutory or regulatory responsibilities, contracts, job descriptions, employee or student handbooks, and expert witness testimony about prevalent standards and nurse practice standards that established the legal duty. For example, a court would review a state's child abuse reporting laws to determine whether a school nurse who suspected child abuse breached a statutory reporting responsibility by failing to report that reasonable belief to the proper authorities.

As another example, a court could determine that a school nurse breached a duty to a student if the nurse failed to call for emergency help when a reasonable person would seek such assistance. In *Declouet v. Orleans Parish School Board*, a Louisiana state court, in 1998, determined that a school counselor was liable for a student's death, because the counselor failed to call 911 when the student had an asthma attack. Further, the court held the school board liable for failing to properly train school employees about how to properly respond to emergencies.

Similarly, in *Barth v. Board of Education*, an Illinois state court, in 1986, held the school board liable for negligence for failing to secure prompt medical attention for an injured student. In that case, the court held that the state's immunity statute did not apply because the immunity protection did not apply when the school's conduct was willful or wanton. The court concluded that the school's conduct was willful or wanton because the school's staff displayed a reckless disregard for the student's safety by ignoring the student's symptoms that clearly indicated a serious illness and did not take advantage of the fact that there was a hospital directly across the street from the school.

Causation

The causation element of negligence requires the plaintiff to show a direct link between the defendant's negligent conduct and the resulting injury. In *Mogabgab v. Orleans Parish School Board*, a Louisiana state court, in 1970, determined that the causation element was met when school coaches failed to provide prompt treatment to a football player suffering from heat stroke. The boy's parents brought a negligence claim against the football coaches, the school principal, the physical education director, and the school board. The court concluded that, under the preponderance of evidence standard, it was more likely than not that the student would have survived if the coaches had provided prompt medical attention when the heat stroke symptoms first developed, instead of waiting. However, the court also determined that negligence was established against the coaches only for their failure to act. There was no causal link between any conduct by the other defendants and the boy's death; therefore, the court declined to hold the other defendants liable.

When determining whether a school nurse's breach was the proximate cause of an individual's injury, a court will also consider any intervening cause for the injury. For example, a school nurse may breach a legal duty by failing to look at a child's arm that is painful and swelling after a playground injury. However, if the child's parent refuses to take the child to the doctor for several days after learning of the child's complaint, and the arm resets incorrectly, the child's parent's actions would be an intervening cause of the child's injuries.

Damages

When proving damages in a negligence case, a plaintiff must show some harm or injury, such as physical injury, pain and suffering, emotional distress (with its attendant physical symptoms) or an economic loss, such as medical expenses or lost wages. Without harm or injury, there is no recovery. For example, a plaintiff may be able to prove that a school nurse provided a child with another child's medication, but unless the child was harmed by that administration error, the plaintiff will not be able to recover any monetary damages from the school nurse or the nurse's employer.

Even when a plaintiff can prove harm, the amount of money the plaintiff can recover may be limited by statute. For example, in Maine, tort claims against individual employees of a government entity are limited to $10,000, as long as the employee is acting within the scope of employment, while tort claims against school districts are limited to $400,000 per occurrence (Maine Revised Statutes title 14 §§ 8104-D, 8105).

Defenses

There are a number of defenses to a negligence action. Defenses are reasons of law or fact that establish why a plaintiff should not recover damages in a lawsuit, even if the defendant was negligent and the plaintiff suffered damages. Depending on the state, defenses to negligence actions may include consent, waiver and release, assumption of the risk, statute of limitations, contributory or comparative negligence, sovereign immunity, and qualified immunity.

A consent defense arises when a plaintiff, understanding the risks, agrees to the actions later claimed to be negligent. A waiver and release defense arises when a plaintiff, with knowledge of the risks or the loss, and usually in writing, voluntarily relinquishes any right to recover damages for negligent actions which have already taken place or which may take place in the future.

Statutes of limitations are laws that determine how long after a negligent act the injured party can file a lawsuit, usually 2 to 4 years for tort actions. However, in many states, a child's age stops a statute of limitations from running. In other words, a child's time for filing a lawsuit does not usually start to run until the child becomes an adult. For example, a 10-year-old student in a state with 18 as the age of majority and a 2-year tort claims statute of limitations, may have ten years, or until the student's 20th birthday, to file suit for the personal injuries suffered, whereas an adult who is harmed by that same negligent action would be required to file a lawsuit within 2 years of the injury.

Contributory negligence is another defense to a negligence action. This defense arises when the plaintiff's own behavior was not the behavior of a reasonable person, and it, at least partially, caused the harm suffered by the plaintiff, which reduces or eliminates the defendant's liability for damages. Comparative negligence assigns blame among all negligent parties, all of whom acted unreasonably, and holds each party responsible for a share of the damages in proportion to that party's negligence. Immunity is another defense, which will be discussed in detail below.

Immunity

Sovereign or governmental immunity, in some states, protects public entities such as school districts, and employees of school districts acting in their official capacities, from tort liability, except when they consent to be sued. The concept behind sovereign immunity is that public tax money should not be spent on righting individual wrongs, but should only be spent on the public educational purposes of the school district. A number of states, however, have abandoned sovereign immunity in favor of allowing personal injury actions against public entities, within certain limits and restrictions. Qualified immunity and official immunity, in some states, protect from liability individual employees who are acting in good faith in their official capacities.

State immunity laws are generally interpreted to provide a broad scope of protection for state employees exercising discretion in the performance of official duties or responsibilities. For example, in *Cook v. Hubbard Exempted Village Board of Education*, an Ohio state court of appeals, in 1996, considered whether the state's statutory immunity provisions protected a school nurse when the nurse failed to call an ambulance after a student involved in a fight at school sustained a fractured ankle. The relevant portion of the applicable Ohio statute provides immunity from liability if "the action or failure to act by the employee involved that gave rise to the claim of liability was within the discretion of the employee . . . by virtue of the duties and responsibilities of the office or position of the employee" (Ohio Revised Code § 2744.03(A)(3)). In *Cook*, the court concluded that the decision to call or not call an ambulance involved the exercise of the school nurse's discretion, because school policy required the nurse to call an ambulance when needed. The court stated that the fact that the school nurse was not required to call an ambulance in response to every medical emergency indicated that the nurse had discretion in such matters, and so the nurse was immune from liability for the student's injuries.

Similarly, the Alabama Supreme Court, in *Nance v. Matthews* in 1993, considered the scope of that state's immunity statute, which grants immunity for discretionary acts. The school nurse was sued for negligent supervision because an aide under the nurse's supervision failed to catheterize a special education student after being directed to do so. The court noted, "in determining whether an employee makes difficult decisions and exercises discretion, the courts must focus on the process employed to arrive at the decision." The court concluded that the nurse was entitled to immunity because her role as the aide's supervisor required constant decision-making and judgment calls; therefore, her supervision of the aide was discretionary, which entitled the nurse to immunity under Alabama law.

There are also federal statutory sources for immunity that may protect a school nurse and the school district from liability. For example, the No Child Left Behind Act, a federal law, contains immunity provisions for professional employees who work in schools, and who, in their jobs or in emergencies, are called upon to maintain discipline or to insure safety (20 USC § 6731). Arguably, this new federal immunity could be applicable to school nurses, as they are regularly called upon to ensure the safety of students.

Some state and federal laws may include provisions that grant immunity to persons who act in good faith when they comply with the statutes' requirements. For example, most states have a statute that requires licensed professionals to make a report to the proper law enforcement agency if there is reasonable cause to believe a child has suffered abuse or neglect. In *Spurrell v. Block*, a Washington state appellate court, in 1985, reviewed the provisions of that state's child abuse reporting law when parents sued the school nurse for making a report to a child protective services caseworker. The parents sought damages for wrongful infliction of emotional distress, defamation, and civil rights violations. In response, the court held the school nurse had no liability because the Washington Revised Code § 26.44.030 required the nurse to make a report if she had "reasonable cause" to believe the child had suffered abuse or neglect. Further, the court cited Code Section 26.44.060, which expressly states that "any person participating in good faith in the making of a report pursuant to this chapter . . . shall in so doing be immune from any liability arising out of such reporting."

Negligence cases against school nurses are generally based on failures to meet standards of care. Schwab and Gelfman (2001) note the following "recurring themes" in successful lawsuits: (1) failure to keep abreast of nursing knowledge; (2) failure to document properly; (3) failure to recognize urgent and emergency situations; (4) failure to follow school district policy; and (5) failure to challenge administrative decisions that put students at risk. Knowledge that these are the recurring themes in prior litigation can assist current school nurses in avoiding obvious pitfalls in their professional arenas. Some strategies the school nurse might use to avoid these pitfalls are as follows:

- Attend continuing education programs.
- Read journals and articles related to current nursing practice.
- Develop and follow a documentation policy.
- Be familiar with the school district's policies adopted by the Board of Trustees.
- Be familiar with proper procedures to challenge administrative decisions if the school nurse believes it is necessary for a student's well-being.
- If the school nurse believes that a school district's policy or practice may result in an unnecessary risk to students, challenge the policy or practice before an incident arises.

CONSEQUENCES FOR VIOLATIONS OF STANDARD OF CARE

The consequences for violating a standard of care vary depending on the legal proceeding brought against the school nurse. Responsible authorities or victims may decide to bring one or more types of proceedings against a violator: civil, criminal, or administrative. Because they are different proceedings in different forums, with different standards of proof and different consequences, there is no legal prohibition against proceeding against a violator in one, two, or three different types of actions. Therefore, all three types of actions and their consequences will be reviewed here.

Civil Consequences

Civil actions are brought by those who claim, or allege, that they have been harmed by someone who breached their duty or violated a law, and who then seek compensation for the harm they suffered by filing a lawsuit in state or federal court. A judge, sometimes with the help of a jury deciding fact issues, may rule that an individual, a school, or a school district violated a standard of care by breaking the law or breaching a legal duty, which proximately caused damage to another. Once that determination is made, the consequence in a civil action is that the victim is compensated for the damages suffered.

The most common damages compensation is monetary. Damages can be compensatory or punitive. For compensatory damages, or actual damages, a judge or jury will decide what amount of money would fairly compensate an individual for the harm or loss, physical loss, that individual suffered, and nothing more. Monetary damages may compensate an individual for actual out-of-pocket education; medical, rehabilitation or living expenses; physical loss; sometimes pain and suffering; fair market value of lost property; or other documentable losses. To assist the court in determining the amount of compensatory damages owed, both parties present evidence at trial to show what each party believes is fair compensation for the harm caused. Expert witnesses, bills and receipts, long term care estimates, and "a day in the life" scenarios may be presented to the trier of fact. All the introduced evidence will be considered in making an ultimate determination of the amount of money the defendant should pay to fairly compensate the plaintiff for the damages suffered. Compensatory damages are sometimes recoverable through insurance policies.

Exemplary or punitive damages represent a monetary sum in excess of compensatory damages, which are designed to punish the defendant for his or her wrongful conduct, to make an example of the defendant, and to provide comfort to the plaintiff for mental anguish and other emotional harms. Punitive damages are designed to be amounts awarded in addition to all compensatory damages, and can sometimes far exceed the amount of compensatory damages awarded. Punitive damages are generally not recoverable under insurance policies, because they are designed to punish the violator, not the violator's insurance company.

Other damages sometimes awarded in civil matters include consequential damages, which are damages that do not flow directly from the wrong committed, but that flow from some of the consequences of the wrongful act. For example, the time that a mother must take off work, at a loss of pay, in order to care for an injured child, while not resulting directly from the wrongful act that injured the child, may be compensable as consequential damages.

A damages award by a judge or jury is generally appealable. Generally, an appealed award is not paid until all appeals are exhausted. As a result, parties sometimes agree to settle damage awards for less than the amount awarded, in order to obtain the monetary award in a timely manner and to avoid the uncertainty of the results of an appeal decision. Of course, cases can also settle prior to damage awards, to avoid the expense of litigation, to buy peace between the parties, and to avoid the uncertainty of the outcome of litigation.

A judge or jury may also determine other consequences to be appropriate in civil proceedings. For example, injunctive relief may be available. Injunctive relief typically forces an individual or organization to refrain from taking a certain action or prevents an individual or organization from stopping another who is taking some action. Injunctive relief may be temporary or permanent, a one-time time-sensitive matter, or a long-term continuing legal obligation. For example, a school nurse who does not believe that students with attention deficit hyperactivity disorder should be treated with psychotropic medication could be stopped from preventing students from receiving their prescribed Adderall. Declaratory relief could also be a consequence in a civil action. Declaratory relief, in effect, "declares" the respective rights of the parties in litigation, when those rights are uncertain or are in dispute.

Criminal Consequences

A school nurse, a staff member, or a student who violates a penal or criminal law could face criminal charges. Criminal cases normally result in either acquittals or convictions. An acquittal means that an individual defendant is determined to be not guilty of the criminal offense charged. There are no further consequences of an acquittal; the individual is free to continue on with his or her life. A conviction, on the other hand, means that an individual is found to be guilty of the criminal offense charged "beyond a reasonable doubt." In other words, the facts proven at trial establish the guilt of the defendant. The consequence of a conviction is that punishment must be assessed. In some jurisdictions, the assessment of punishment requires a separate trial regarding the level or amount of punishment to be assessed.

Criminal cases that result in a finding adverse to a defendant normally result in the imposition of one or both of the following punishments: imprisonment and fines. In very serious murder and capital crimes cases, in some states, a convicted defendant can be put to death. Sometimes, monetary restitution to a victim can also be ordered.

If imprisonment is assessed, the length of imprisonment normally depends upon the seriousness of the criminal act, whether the defendant has previously committed the same or a similar offense, and the risk of danger the defendant poses to others. The length of imprisonment can also sometimes be shortened for time served while awaiting trial or for good behavior while in prison.

Prison sentences can also be "probated," so that an individual does not have to serve time in prison or may get out of prison earlier, unless the individual commits another criminal offense that causes the probation to be revoked. Individuals on probation must normally report to an officer of the criminal justice system, at regular intervals, so that the system can determine whether or not the probationer is following all requirements of his or her probation. Conditions of probation may include such things as staying away from certain people or places, not working in certain kinds of jobs, voluntarily relinquishing a license, remaining drug-free and alcohol-free, attending rehabilitation meetings, and other corrective conditions designed to prevent the individual from committing additional criminal offenses or designed to protect certain people or property. Community service or some other community contribution can be a condition of probation or could be a separate criminal consequence ordered in a case.

Fines levied in criminal cases normally go to the entity bringing the criminal case against the defendant, which can be a state, a county, or a municipality. Sometimes, fines can be deposited in a victims' fund, designed to help crime victims. Normally, however, a fine paid by a defendant does not go to compensate the victim of the crime. Restitution to a crime victim is, therefore, sometimes assessed against the criminal defendant to aid the victim. Without such restitution to the victim from the criminal case, the victim would be forced to bring a civil lawsuit against the defendant in order to obtain monetary compensation for damages the victim suffered.

Plea bargains in the criminal context, like settlements in the civil context, are common. In a plea bargain, a defendant may plead guilty or *nolo contendere* (no contest) and may receive a somewhat reduced sentence or fine than that sought through a criminal case. A plea bargain eliminates the uncertainty and risk of a trial for both sides, and allows the government to save the cost of a potentially expensive trial.

Administrative Consequences

Administrative consequences for a school nurse who violates a standard of care normally result from two situations. In the first, an employer school or school district may decide to terminate the employment. In the second, the state agency that licenses nurses may decide to revoke or otherwise censure the nurse's licensure.

The formality of an administrative proceeding to terminate an employee's employment depends upon a number of factors. The first is whether the employer is a public or private employer. A private employer's relationship with an employee is determined by the employment contract signed between the parties, if any, and any state or federal laws that control the employment relationship. For example, a contract that states that employment is "at will" intends that either party can terminate the relationship at any time without any formality (*Galloway v. Roger Williams University*, 777 A.2d 148 (R.I. 2001)). On the other hand, a contract for a school year, which states that it can be terminated only "for good cause" and explains what constitutes "good cause," requires a determination that good cause exists by whichever party makes that decision under the terms of the contract (*Jones v. Costco Wholesale Corp.*, 34 Fed. Appx. 320 (9th Cir. 2002)). A contract may also specify appeal or review rights or compensation to be paid for early contract termination.

For a public school district, on the other hand, there is one more issue that determines the formality of an employment termination. Under the U.S. Constitution's Fourteenth Amendment, a governmental entity such as a school district may not deprive an individual of property without due process of law. In *Perry v. Sindermann*, a state university employment termination case, the U.S. Supreme Court, in 1972, stated that an individual must look to state law to determine whether a property right to continued employment exists. The court held that if a property right exists under state law, then due process must be provided before that property right is taken away by the governmental entity. At the same time it issued a decision in *Perry*, the Supreme Court also decided *Board of Regents v. Roth* and emphasized that an employee claiming a right to due process must be able to establish a claim of entitlement to continued employment; a unilateral expectation of continued employment is not sufficient to invoke due process protection. Due process is a very flexible concept, which consists of notice and a hearing. How much notice and the type of hearing that must be provided depend upon the extent of the property right to be taken away. If the property right is minimal, the due process required is minimal. If the property right is extensive, on the other hand, then the due process required is extensive.

For example, in Texas, public school district nurses are entitled to probationary and term contracts (Texas Education Code § 21.101 et seq.; 21.201 et seq.). Therefore, those contracts and their attendant rights are property rights for Texas public school nurses. The statutes spell out the amount and type of process required to terminate these contracts at the end of a school term and during a school term. To terminate a probationary contract at the end of a school term, the standard is very low—"best interests of the district" as determined by the Board of Trustees, because there is no property right to a probationary contract beyond the term of that contract. To non-renew a term contract at the end of the contract term in Texas, the Board of Trustees is limited to the list of reasons for non-renewal located in its Board policies, and the nurse is entitled to a hearing before the school district Board to determine whether the nurse's conduct constitutes a Board policy reason for nonrenewal. However, termination of a probationary or term contract *during* a contract term is the termination of a property right. Therefore, the Texas public school nurse facing a mid-year contract termination has the right to a hearing regarding whether "good cause" exists in front of an independent hearing examiner, who hears the case in a trial-type setting and makes a recommendation to the board of trustees. The Board, then, is limited in its ability to change the hearing examiner's findings of fact and conclusions of law and must decide whether or not to terminate the contract based on the hearing transcript, the hearing examiner's recommendation, and oral argument. That decision is then subject to an expedited appeal to the Texas Commissioner of Education (Texas Education Code §§ 21.101 et seq.; 21.201 et seq.; 21.251 et seq.). Clearly, the amount of due process provided expands in proportion to the extent of the property right at risk. Although each state differs, these concepts are similar for all states.

A state licensing board may also decide, on the basis of a complaint, a news item, a required report, an investigation, or some other method, to take administrative action against a school nurse's license. Again, the state agency is bound by the same constitutional due process restrictions discussed above, because nursing licensure bestows on the license-holder a property right to pursue a livelihood in nursing. Therefore, an administrative proceeding to revoke a nursing license or to take some other action against a nurse's license will normally require an extensive notice and hearing process, as described above. The nurse is given notice of the allegation and given an informal initial opportunity to respond. Then, a trial-type procedure is normally conducted, with both parties having the right to legal counsel and the nurse having the right to be confronted with the evidence and witnesses against the nurse, to cross-examine the witnesses, to present witnesses and evidence on the nurse's behalf, and to have a fair and impartial tribunal to hear the case (22 Texas Administrative Code § 217.19; New York Education Law § 6510 (McKinney)). Due process is a right that a nurse can refuse through a voluntary surrender of a license or through refusal to participate in the administrative proceedings. Refusal to participate in the nurse's own defense can result in the proceedings continuing in the nurse's absence (*In re Allen*).

Consequences of an adverse decision can include revocation of licensure or some lesser action, such as a reprimand, probation, annulment, or suspension; a fine or penalty; an injunction; recommendations/mandates for supervision or monitoring, counseling or treatment, or limitations on practice; civil or criminal penalties; a mandate for additional training or education; or required public service hours, depending upon the applicable state laws and regulations (Texas Occupations Code Chapter 301; New York Education Law § 6511 (McKinney); 225 Illinois Compiled Statutes 65/10-45). Of course, revocation or suspension of a license will result in the nurse being unable to work as a nurse (*In re Anderson*).

FINANCIAL AND LIABILITY PROTECTION AND RESPONSIBILITY

Given the potential liability and risk to a school nurse when a standard of care is violated, it is incumbent upon the nurse to ensure that adequate legal protection exists and to ensure that legal advice is received from counsel knowledgeable about the laws and regulations impacting on the education and healthcare professions.

To provide employees adequate legal protection, many employers carry professional liability insurance to protect school professionals from errors and omissions. In an insurance policy, the insurance company agrees to compensate those injured by an insured's errors or omissions, and to defend the individuals and organizations accused of wrongdoing.

It is important for the school nurse to review that insurance policy very carefully to determine how much insurance coverage is provided by the employer. Typically, coverage is limited to certain amounts for certain situations. As important as the listed coverages in the policy, are the listed "exclusions," which describe what the insurance does *not* cover. For example, typical exclusions might include intentional acts, acts taken outside the scope of employment, corporal punishment, sexual harassment or abuse, or criminal acts. Professional liability policies may or may not cover an accused professional who is facing disciplinary consequences from a licensure board, but certainly would not protect a nurse from the consequences of licensure revocation.

A school nurse who determines that there is not sufficient insurance coverage provided by the employer is well advised to purchase additional insurance coverage, either individually, through an association of nurses, if available, or through a homeowner's policy. Adequate insurance protection is essential to peace of mind and for financial protection.

Of course, the best protection against liability is an informed knowledge of the specific federal and state laws and regulations affecting school nurses, strict adherence to their terms and requirements, a systematic method of performing job functions, and a documentation system that reflects the work performed. It is essential for a school nurse to keep up to date on laws, regulations, and standards that control the nurse's practice. Prudent, careful action taken in the best interests of the students served by the nurse, with all discretionary decisions being made in the best interests of the safety of the students served, and documentation that supports those decisions, will place a school nurse in an excellent position to defend any potentially adverse action filed against the nurse.

THE SCHOOL NURSE AS A WITNESS

While this chapter has addressed a school nurse's conduct and the legal issues related to that conduct, another important legal issue can arise for the school nurse who may be peripherally involved in a legal action involving third parties. For example, the nurse may be called as a fact witness or as an expert witness in a student's personal injury case against another person, in a child custody case between parents, or in a negligence action against another nurse. The nurse may be interviewed or may be subpoenaed to testify in a deposition involving an investigation about a child or the parents of the child to whom the nurse has provided nursing services. To assist the school nurse in understanding the role she played in those matters, some peripheral issues will be addressed, including compliance with subpoenas, admissible testimony, and parental termination evidence.

Subpoena Compliance

If a school nurse is served a subpoena instructing the nurse to provide documents or to appear in court, or to appear to answer questions in a deposition, the nurse should promptly contact a school administrator and request legal counsel to guide the nurse in proper compliance with the subpoena. Valid subpoenas are legal documents, which must be carefully reviewed and followed. However, the potential exists that subpoena compliance could violate federal law, and, in some states, medical records and privacy laws.

For example, to the extent a subpoena requests the disclosure of student records maintained by a public school district, without written consent from the student's parents, a school district must first comply with the federal Family Educational Rights and Privacy Act ("FERPA") before complying with the subpoena (20 U.S.C. § 1232g(b)(2)(B)). Under FERPA, while student records may be released pursuant to a valid subpoena, the District is required to notify the student and parents of the subpoena "in advance of the compliance" (20 U.S.C. § 1232g(b)(2)(A)). The regulations implementing FERPA make it clear that the purpose of the notice to the students and/or parents is "so that the parent or eligible student may seek protective action" (34 C.F.R. § 99.31(a)(9)(ii)). Therefore, it is necessary for a school district to notify parents prior to the production of student records pursuant to a subpoena.

In some instances, a subpoena recipient may attempt to assert the Fifth Amendment privilege against self-incrimination and refuse to produce requested documents or refuse to answer questions at a court appearance. When this occurs in a federal court or a hearing before a federal agency, the person presiding over the proceeding may compel the witness to comply with the order in exchange for immunity. Then, no testimony or documents produced may be used against the witness in any subsequent action, except prosecution for perjury (18 U.S.C. § 6002).

Hearsay Statements

A school nurse may often be called on to testify about what a student said to the nurse, especially in cases involving assaults and child abuse. Generally, a trial witness is not allowed to testify at a trial about statements made to the witness by another person, although those same statements can be stated by the witness during an investigation, a student disciplinary proceeding, or during a deposition taken pursuant to discovery in a lawsuit. These statements heard by a witness are called "hearsay statements." They, generally, are not admissible in court because it is not possible for the judge or jury to assess the trustworthiness or the reliability of the person who originally made the statements. However, there are several exceptions to that general rule. For the most part, these exceptions represent situations in which the degree of trustworthiness is higher than usual.

For example, Federal Rule of Evidence 803(2) and most state evidence codes recognize an "excited utterance" exception. This exception allows witnesses to testify about statements that they heard another person make, when such statements are made in response to a "startling event." Lawmakers and courts agree that statements blurted out while a person is in an excited state are unlikely to be the result of conscious thought. Therefore, the perception is that these "off the cuff" remarks represent a person's immediate response to the startling event, rather than a contrived falsehood, because the person does not have time to reflect before responding to the event. The exception only applies if there has been a startling event, the declarant was under the influence of the event at the time the statements were made, and the statements related to the startling event. It is up to the judge to determine whether the "excited utterance" exception applies to the hearsay rule in any given trial.

A school nurse may often be one of the first people with whom a student comes in contact following an accident, a fight or some other incident of violence. In these cases, it may be common for the student to blurt out a comment to the nurse. Especially when children are involved, it is often advantageous to allow the adult listener to testify, in lieu of putting a child through the trauma of testifying in court. However, all the elements of the "excited utterance" exception must be present before a school nurse could testify as to the statements made by a student. For example, in *U.S. v. Fink*, a military court in 1991 determined that the exception did not apply when a 12-year-old female who was mentally impaired reported acts of sexual abuse by her father to the school nurse. Although the alleged acts allegedly occurred the night before the conversation with the nurse, the court noted that the time lapse was not determinative. Instead, the child's demeanor, which the school nurse described as "very calm" and "not overly emotional," but "kind of resigned," led the court to decide that the child was not in a state of excitement, but rather was more likely in a state of depression.

In response to this type of decision by courts, many states adopted child hearsay rules intended to allow the admission of a child's statements into evidence without putting the child witness through the trauma of testifying in court. However, these rules are often challenged on constitutional grounds because of the defendant's constitutional due process right to cross-examine a witness. To balance a defendant's constitutional rights and the court's interest in protecting the well-being of child witnesses, most states place some type of limitation on the admissibility of child hearsay statements. For example, some limit admissibility to statements by a child victim and exclude hearsay statements by a child witness to abuse, such as Florida Evidence Rule 90.803. Other states' rules, such as Colorado's Evidence Rule 13-25-129, allow child hearsay testimony by a child victim or a child witness, but only if the statements are corroborated by other evidence. Texas law includes child hearsay provisions in Texas Family Code Section 54.031 and in the Code of Criminal Procedure Section 38.072; both statutes provide that only the first adult to whom the child victim reveals an incident of abuse may testify as to the child's statements. Under any of these child hearsay provisions, a school nurse may be the person called upon to testify as to a student's statements. Therefore, a school nurse should take care to pay attention and listen closely to student complaints and statements and to also note their nonverbal communication.

Parental Termination Evidence

State actions involving allegations of child abuse or neglect may lead the state to seek removal of the child from the home or termination of parental rights. Generally, these actions are based upon statutory provisions that allow the state to intervene in the parent-child relationship if it is in the child's best interest. In building a case to prove a pattern of abuse or neglect, the state may call upon the school nurse to testify about any signs of physical abuse the nurse has witnessed, especially if documented over a period of time. Often, the school nurse is one of several witnesses called to identify a pattern of abuse.

In 1986, a Connecticut state appellate court found *In re Jason S.* that there was sufficient evidence to find a 7-year-old child was neglected, within the statutory definition of that term, based in part on the testimony of the child's principal, teacher and school nurse regarding physical marks each observed on the child. *In re Sandra C.*, a New York appellate court, in 2002, relied upon the testimony of a child's teachers and the school nurse to corroborate statements by the child and her siblings that their father repeatedly burned one of the older children and used excessive force in disciplining all but the two youngest children; therefore, the court upheld the family court's decision that the father was guilty of abuse.

While it is certainly an uncomfortable aspect of a school nurse's job to testify or provide information in third-party proceedings, it is vitally important for the school nurse to tell the truth and provide necessary information when required by law to do so, in the best interests of a child's safety and well-being.

CONCLUSION

No single book chapter can adequately address all of the legal issues that confront school nurses on a day-to-day basis. The best preparation for the school nurse is a basic understanding of the legal framework in place and the legal principles at work. This foundation then enables the school nurse, when confronted with a situation, to analyze and understand the legal issues related to the nurse's professional practice and the nurse's licensure, and assists the nurse in determining the proper professional response. When a school nurse's nursing practice standards, or state or federal statutes or regulations create conflicts, making the school nurse unsure of the proper action to take, the best option is to seek competent legal counsel and, ultimately, to bring the conflict to the attention of the proper legal authorities for resolution.

References

Barth v. Board of Education, 490 N.E.2d 77 (Ill. App. Ct. 1986).
Board of Regents v. Roth, 408 U.S. 564 (1972).
California Teachers' Association v. Livingston Union School District, 219 Cal.App.3d 1503 (1990).
Cedar Rapids Community School District v. Garret F., 526 U.S. 66 (1999).
Cipollone v. Liggett Group, Inc., 505 U.S. 504 (1992).
Cook v. Hubbard Exempted Village Board of Education, 688 N.E.2d 1058 (Ohio Ct. App. 1996).
Debord v. Ferguson-Florissant School District, 126 F.3d 1102 (8th Cir. 1997).
Declouet v. Orleans Parish School Board, 715 So. 2d 69 (La. Ct. App. 1998).
Doe v. Voluntown of Board of Education, 25 Conn. L. Rptr. 629 (Conn. Super. Ct. 1999).
Federico v. Order of Saint Benedict, 64 F.3d 1 (1st Cir. 1995).
Freightliner Corp. v. Myrick, 514 U.S. 280 (1995).
Galloway v. Roger Williams University, 777 A.2d 148 (R.I. 2001).
Griffith v. New York, 507 N.Y.S.2d 445 (N.Y. App. Div. 1986).
In re Allen, 259 N.Y.S. 2d 366 (N.Y. App. Div. 1965).
In re Anderson, 464 N.Y.S. 2d 868 (N.Y. App. Div. 1983).
In re Jason S., 516 A.2d 1352 (Conn. App. Ct. 1986).
In re Sandra C., 748 N.Y.S.2d 129 (N.Y. App. Div. 2002).
Irving Independent School District v. Tatro, 468 U.S. 883 (1984).
Jass v. Prudential Health Care Plan, 88 F.3d 1482 (7th Cir. 1996).
Jones v. Costco Wholesale Corp., 34 Fed. Appx. 320 (9th Cir. 2002).
Mogabgab v. Orleans Parish School Board, 239 So. 2d 456 (La. Ct. App. 1970).
New Jersey v. T.L.O., 469 U.S. 325 (1985).
Nance v. Matthews, 622 So. 2d 297 (Ala. 1993).
Perry v. Sindermann, 408 U.S. 593 (1972).
Schwab, N., & Gelfman, M.H.B. (2001). *Legal issues in school health services: A resource for school administrators, school attorneys, and school nurses*. North Branch, MN: Sunrise River Press.
Spurrell v. Block, 701 P.2d 529 (Wash. App. 1985).
Stamps v. Jefferson County Board of Education, 642 So. 2d 941 (Ala. 1994).
Sullivan v. Edward Hospital, 806 N.E.2d 645 (2004).
Uhr v. East Greenbush Central Sch. Dist., 720 N.E.2d 886 (N.Y. 1999).
U.S. v. Fink, 32 M.J. 987 (1991).
Restatement (Second) of Torts § 281 (1965).
Texas Attorney General Opinion No. GA-0178 (2004).

Constitutions
U.S. Constitution articles I, II, III.
U.S. Constitution amendments I, IV, V, X, XIV.

Statutes
Americans with Disabilities Act (1990) (ADA), 42 U.S.C. §§ 12101 et seq.
Asbestos Hazard Emergency Response Act (AHERA), 15 U.S.C. §§ 2641, et seq.
California Education Code § 45028.
California Government Code § 3543.2.
Coins and Currency, 18 USC § 331.
Counterfeiting and Forgery, 18 USC § 501.
Employee Retirement Income Security Act of 1974 (ERISA), 29 U.S.C. §§ 1001 et seq.
Equal Employment Opportunity Act of 1972, 42 U.S.C. §§ 2000e et seq.
Family and Medical Leave Act of 1993 (FMLA), 29 U.S.C. § 2611.
Family Educational Rights and Privacy Act of 1974 (FERPA), 20 U.S.C. § 1232g.
Health Insurance Portability & Accountability Act of 1996 (HIPAA), 26 U.S.C. § 294, 42 U.S.C. §§ 201, 1395b-5.
Illinois Compiled Statutes, 225 Ill. Comp. Stat. 65/10-45.
Individuals with Disabilities Education Act (IDEA), 20 U.S.C. § 1400 et seq.
Maine Revised Statutes title 14, §§ 8104-D, 8105.
Medicaid Act, 42 U.S.C. § 1396a.

New York Education Law §§ 6510, 6511 (McKinney).
No Child Left Behind Act of 2001 (NCLB), 20 U.S.C. § 301; 20 U.S.C. § 6731 et seq.
Ohio Revised Code § 2744.03(A)(3).
Rehabilitation Act (Section 504), 29 U.S.C. § 794 et seq.
Stewart B. McKinney Homeless Assistance Act, 42 USC § 11431 et seq.
Texas Code of Criminal Procedure § 38.072.
Texas Education Code §§ 21.101 et seq.; 21.201 et seq.; 21.251 et seq.; 25.002; 38.001.
Texas Family Code § 54.031.
Texas Occupations Code Chapter 301.
Washington Revised Code §§ 26.44.030, 26.44.060.
Witness Immunity, 18 U.S.C. § 6002.

Regulations

California Code of Regulations title 16, §§ 1442-1444.5.
Colorado Rule of Evidence 13-25-129.
Federal Rules of Evidence 803(2).
Family Educational Rights and Privacy Act Regulations, 34 C.F.R. § 99.31(a)(9)(ii).
Florida Rule of Evidence 90.803.
Texas Administrative Code, 22 Tex. Admin. Code §§ 217.11; 217.19.

Chapter 13

Legislation Affecting School Nurses

LYNN KELLY

Chapter Outline

INTRODUCTION

"Politics has often been described as the "art of the possible." It is politics and the political process that translate our ideas and values into public policy" (Lee & Estes, 2001, p. 181). Branches of government at the federal, state, and local levels define accepted practices and policies affecting both individual and institutional actions. When it comes to health issues, major political parties often agree on what problems exist. However, solutions to these health crises differ widely among political parties and individual legislators. Policies are shaped by individual beliefs, attitudes, and values. Lee and Estes argue that what directs healthcare policy is whether decision makers perceive health care as a "social good or as a market commodity" (p. 143). Economic factors are much more likely to influence policy when health care is viewed as a market good.

> Is it a coincidence that over the last fifteen years public health reports have emphasized personal responsibility at a time of conservative government? These are "blame the victim" approaches. It's clearly cheaper than funding *public* health. (McBeath, 1990)

Understanding the current political climate is essential for school nurses who are continually challenged to provide students the services and resources necessary for maintaining health. This chapter focuses on legislative issues of which school nurses must be aware when delivering health services to children in schools. Included are discussions regarding immunizations and control of communicable disease regulations, reporting of suspected child abuse, mandated screenings and services, and the impact of federal and state legislation on school nursing practice.

INDIVIDUAL RIGHTS AND THE LEGAL SYSTEM

"Perhaps the most important social and economic entitlement is the right to health. Considerable disagreement exists, however, whether 'health' is a meaningful, identifiable, operational, and enforceable right or whether it is merely aspirational or rhetorical" (Gostin, 2001, p. 30). In our society, decisions regarding how services will be allocated are based on the concept of justice. However, how individuals or groups make judgments regarding whether an act is just vary greatly, as do policies that claim to treat groups equally and fairly. The American Nurses Association Code of Ethics for Nurses (2001) provides sound guidance for how nurses should make judgments regarding quality and professional behavior. The Code places the needs of individuals as the factor to consider when implementing care.

Issues regarding access to care have grown as the healthcare system has evolved from a human service model to a business model that stresses cost containment measures (Galarneau, 2002). Access to health services within schools is tied directly to the economic reality of different groups vying for limited resources. If one were to apply the concept of justice, it would seem that fairness would identify children as the most vulnerable segment of the population who must be provided with the most resource access. However, providing resources to one group often involves denying another group these same resources. So again, the issue of defining justice remains gray rather than simply black and white.

Legal rights are ensured by a court of law. One might argue that individuals are also afforded rights on moral grounds. Although the Constitution does not contain language that addresses a right to health care (Schwab & Gelfman, 2001), many believe that this is a moral right held by all individuals.

Rights are often presented from the perspective of the individual. However, decisions regarding one individual's rights must be regarded in relationship to the impact that a given decision may have on others. Within the school, claims of rights are also complicated by the fact that a student may not have reached the legally mandated age to take an independent action, despite his or her desire to do so. When making decisions about a student's rights, it is helpful to remember that all share moral rights. Therefore, it is wrong to support a student or parental claim to a right that results in denial of the same right to others. When students or parents make demands based on their assumptions about rights, it is important to clarify whether what they are requesting is truly a right or whether they are seeking a special privilege. Provision of special privileges places the school or the school nurse at risk for allegations of discrimination.

EXPANDING HEALTH SERVICES THROUGH FEDERAL FUNDING

In 1997, Congress passed the Balanced Budget Act (Public Law 105-33) with the principal purpose of providing health insurance for low-income children not eligible for Medicaid. Data collected in 2002 showed that 15.5% of the population was without health insurance (Mills & Bhandari, 2003). Many of these individuals were employed in low-paying jobs. CHIP (Children's Health Insurance Program) was developed for the purpose of providing free or low-cost healthcare coverage to the children of these working poor. While Medicaid regulations are regulated at the Federal level, individual states are allowed more leeway in how their CHIP program will be constructed and implemented (Dick, Allison, & Haber, 2002).

The federal government allocated $40 billion in 2000 to be dispersed among states for their SCHIP (State Children's Health Insurance Program). States develop guidelines for enrollment qualifications, processes for reimbursement for services, and types of services covered. This plan is then submitted to the Health Care Financing Administration for approval (Nabors & Mettrick, 2001). Each state has its own eligibility rules; however, most cover children until their eighteenth birthday. Eligibility requirements are based on income and are adjusted yearly. In 2003 families were eligible for CHIP coverage if their income, for a family of four, was no more than $36,816. Recently, a number of states have approved use of SCHIP funds to help parents who are working, but at minimum wage jobs, acquire health insurance. Some states have approved the use of some SCHIP funding to help small-business employers provide health insurance for their employees.

School nurses can access enrollment qualifications for their state from the Insure Kids Now Web site (http://www.insurekidsnow.gov). A link will take the viewer to a specific state's program. The program stresses the need to identify children whose families may meet the criteria for SCHIP enrollment but who are unaware of the program. States publish posters and other informational material that can be provided to parents during school enrollment or displayed in areas where parents can access the material during visits to the school. The school nurse may also recruit community groups to help educate families about SCHIP and assist in helping families to enroll.

REQUIRING IMMUNIZATIONS FOR SCHOOL ATTENDANCE

States began enacting immunization laws in the early 1800s when Massachusetts required citizens to be immunized against smallpox. In an effort to improve low childhood immunization rates, states enacted laws requiring certain immunizations as a prerequisite for school entry. Immunizations have been responsible for a dramatic reduction in morbidity and mortality rates previously associated with certain communicable diseases. For example, during the measles epidemic of 1978, those states that strictly enforced their immunization statutes were able to reduce the incidence of the disease by 90% (Satcher, 1999). States with less stringent regulations had a much higher incidence of measles cases that year.

The recommended schedule of immunizations is reviewed and updated at least annually in compliance with guidelines set up by two organizations: the Advisory Committee on Immunization Practices (ACIP) of the U.S. Department of Health and Human Services (USDHHS), Public Health Services Centers for Disease Control and Prevention (CDC) and the Committee on Infectious Diseases of the American Academy of Pediatrics (AAP). All states require that children receive a series of immunizations. However, states do vary in their requirements. There are no federal laws that specify which schedule of vaccinations a child must receive in order to attend school. The U.S. Supreme Court has ruled that states have the right to enact and enforce individual compulsory immunization statutes (Satcher, 1999). Students who fail to meet the designated state immunization requirements can be excluded until the necessary immunizations are obtained. Some states such as Pennsylvania allow for provisional enrollment. For example, in Pennsylvania, if a student has at least one dose of each required immunization, then that student can be provisionally enrolled for 8 months to allow the family to complete the required series (Pennsylvania Department of Health, 2001).

The Immunization Action Coalition (IAC) (http://www.immunize.org), an organization that works closely with and is partly funded by the Centers for Disease Control and Prevention, provides current information about vaccine-preventable diseases. From their Web site, school nurses can access changes in state immunization laws. For example, proposed changes in Minnesota's vaccination requirements were posted on the IAC Web site (FIGURE 13.1). See TABLE 13.1 for state immunization program Web sites.

Reports regarding adverse effects experienced by children after receiving the DPT (diphtheria, pertussis, tetanus) immunization resulted in many parents questioning the safety of the vaccines (see Chapter 21). Families who believed their child had experienced a negative consequence as a result of the administered immunization sued companies manufacturing the vaccine and healthcare personnel administering the vaccine. Because of the liability concerns, some companies stopped producing vaccines, resulting in a shortage of some vaccines. To ensure adequate supplies of vaccines and also provide a way for families to register claims related to alleged injuries from vaccines, the United States Congress enacted the National Childhood Vaccine Injury Act of 1986. The act covers all childhood vaccines that currently are recommended by the Centers for Disease Control and Prevention. If parents believe that their child experienced an adverse response to a vaccine, they may file for compensation. The claim names the Secretary of Health and Human Services as the Respondent. If the case is supported, then the compensation is awarded by the government, rather than by any company or individual involved in the manufacturing or administration of the vaccine. Information related to what constitutes an injury due to a vaccine and the process for filing a claim can be found on the U.S. Department of Health and Human Services, Health Resources and Services Administration Web site (http://www.hrsa.gov/osp/vicp).

Schools that elect to provide immunizations on the school premises should develop a clear policy that is consistent with sound practice and incorporates the tenets of the National Childhood Vaccine Injury Act (National Vaccine Information Center, 2003) and the Vaccine for Children's Program (CDC, 2004). This Act requires that both the parents and older students be informed regarding the risks and benefits of receiving the immunization. It is also necessary to obtain written consent. In addition, the Vaccine Information Statement (VIS), providing information specific to each vaccine developed by the CDC, is to be reviewed with the parent(s) before the immunization is administered. The VIS for

(text continues on page 288)

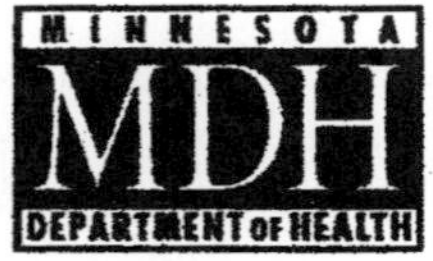

Summary of New Immunization Requirements: 2003 and 2004
(Minnesota Rules, Parts 4604.0100 to 4604.1000)

In the fall of 2003, the Minnesota Department of Health (MDH) modified the immunization requirements for children in child care, grades K-12, and students at post-secondary institutions. These changes do not alter the medical exemption or the option for parents to decline any or all vaccines due to conscientious objections.

Effective October 2003

1. Schedule: Shortens the **grace period** school-age children have to complete any immunization series from **18 to 8 months** to make it easier for school nurses to bring children into compliance in the school year.
2. Schedule: Allows vaccine doses administered **four or fewer days before the minimum age** required in law to be considered valid in order to be consistent with nationally established recommendations.
3. Immunization Documentation: Whenever child care facilities and elementary and secondary schools **communicate** with parents/guardians regarding immunization requirements, they must include information on exemption procedures. Therefore, they are required to use the Minnesota Department of Health's **official record form** or a similar document approved by the department when sending notices to parents/guardians.
4. Hib Vaccine: Clarifies the current *Haemophilus influenzae* type b **(Hib) dosage** series by requiring that one dose be given at or after 12 months of age to be consistent with clinical guidelines.
5. Hepatitis B Vaccine: Allows both the three-dose and the alternate **two-dose hepatitis B** vaccine series for 11 through 15 year olds in order to comply with the 7th grade hepatitis B requirement.
6. Suspension of Law: Gives the commissioner of health authority to suspend immunization law requirements (121A. 15 and 135A. 14) to address a **vaccine shortage or emergency situation.**

Effective September 2004

1. Varicella (Chickenpox): Requires documentation of varicella vaccine or history of disease for children age 18 months to 5 years who are enrolled in **child care,** as well as for **school-age children** entering **kindergarten** and **seventh grade.** Documentation of a history of varicella disease must include one of the following:
   (A) Signature of a provider and the date of the child's varicella illness; or
   (B) Signature of a provider and a statement that a parent's or legal guardian's description of the disease history is indicative of past varicella infection; or
   (C) Signature of a provider or a representative of a public clinic and laboratory evidence of the child's varicella immunity; or
   (D) Signature of the child's parent or legal guardian and the year the child had varicella disease. This item expires on September 1, 2010.
2. Pneumococcal: Requires documentation of pneumococcal conjugate vaccine for children enrolled in **child care** who are **between 2 and 24 months** of age. This vaccine protects against meningitis, bloodstream infections, and pneumonia. **THIS REQUIREMENT HAS BEEN TEMPORARILY SUSPENDED AS OF APRIL 2004 DUE TO A VACCINE SHORTAGE.**
3. Measles, Mumps, Rubella Vaccine: Requires children entering kindergarten to provide documentation of a second dose of vaccine each for measles, mumps, and rubella. (Minnesota currently requires and will continue to require the second dose for children in grades 7-12 until spring 2012.)

For more information and a detailed copy of the rule requirements, contact the Minnesota Department of Health Immunization Program at 612-676-5414 or immunizerule@health.state.mn.us or on the web at www.health.state.mn.us/immunize.

Figure 13.1 ■ Minnesota's vaccination requirements.

Table 13.1 ■
STATE IMMUNIZATION PROGRAM WEB SITES

STATE	WEB ADDRESS
Alabama	http://www.adph.org/immunization
Alaska	http://www.epi.hss.state.ak.us/id/immune.stm
Arizona	http://www.azdhs.gov/phs/immun/index/htm
Arkansas	http://www.healthyarkansas.com

(continued)

STATE	WEB ADDRESS
California	http://www.dhs.ca.gov/ps/dcdc/izgroup
Colorado	http://www.cdphe.state.co.us/dc/immunization/immhom.asp
Connecticut	http://www.dph.state.ct.us/BCH/infectiousdise/immuniza.htm
Delaware	http://www.state.de.us/dhss/dph/dph/immunize.html
District of Columbia (Washington)	http://dchealth.dc.gov
Florida	http://www.doh.state.fl.us/disease_ctrl/immune/index.html
Georgia	http://www.ph.dhr.state.ga.us/programs/immunization/index.shtml
Hawaii	http://www.vaxhawaii.com
Idaho	http://www2.state.id.us/dhw/immun/immun.htm
Illinois	http://www.idph.state.il.us/about/shots.htm
Indiana	http://www.in.gov/isdh/programs/immunization.htm
Iowa	http://www.idph.state.ia.us/adper/immunization.asp
Kansas	http://www.kdhe.state.ks.us/immunize/index.html
Kentucky	http://chs.state.ky.us/publichealth/index-immunization-programs.htm
Maine	http://www.maine.gov/dhs/boh/ddc/Immunization.htm
Maryland	http://www.edcp.org/html/immpg.html
Massachusetts	http://www.mass.gov/dph/cdc/epii/imm/imm.htm
Michigan	http://www.michigan.gov/immunize
Minnesota	http://www.health.state.mn.us/immunize
Mississippi	http://www.msdh.state.ms.us/msdhsite/index.cfm/14,0,71,html
Missouri	http://www.dhss.mo.gov/Immunizations/index.html
Montana	http://www.dphhs.state.mt.us/hpsd/pubheal/disease/immuniz/
Nebraska	http://www.hhs.state.ne.us/imm/immindex.htm
Nevada	http://www.health2k.state.nv.us/immune
New Hampshire	http://www.dhhs.state.nh.us/DHHS/IMMUNIZATION/default.htm
New Jersey	http://www.state.nj.us/health/cd/vpdphome.htm
New Mexico	http://www.health.state.nm.us/immunize
New York	http://www.health.state.ny.us/nysdoh/provider/disease.htm
North Carolina	http://www.immunizenc.com
North Dakota	http://www.health.state.nd.us/disease/immunization/
Ohio	http://www.odh.state.oh.us/ODHPrograms/IMMUNIZE/index.htm
Oklahoma	http://www.health.state.ok.us/program/imm
Oregon	http://www.ohd.hr.state.or.us/imm
Pennsylvania	http://www.dsf.health.state.pa.us/health/cwp/view.asp?a=178&Q=199020
Rhode Island	http://www.health.ri.gov/family/immunization/index.php
South Carolina	http://www.scdhec.net/HS/diseasecont/immunization/
South Dakota	http://www.state.sd.us/doh/disease/index.htm

(continued)

Table 13.1 ■ (Continued)

STATE	WEB ADDRESS
Tennessee	http://www2.state.tn.us/health.CEDS/immunization.htm
Texas	http://www.tdh.texas.gov/immunize
Utah	http://www.immunize-utah.org
Vermont	http://www.state.vt.us/health/hcprov.htm
Virginia	http://www.vdh.state.va.us/imm
Washington	http://www.doh.wa.gov/cfh.immunize
West Virginia	http://www.wvdhhr.org/immunizations/
Wisconsin	http://www.dhfs.state.wi.us/immunization/index.htm
Wyoming	www.immunizewyoming.com

measles, mumps, and rubella can be found in FIGURE 13.2. Copies of these documents can be obtained from the CDC's Web site, National Immunization Program (http://www.cdc.gov/nip). If the school population contains families who do not speak or read English, the law requires that the information in the document be modified in a way that ensures that the parent is providing informed consent (Schwab & Gelfman, 2001).

COMMUNICABLE DISEASE CONTROL AND REPORTING

Among the rights provided to individuals is the right to be protected from undue exposure to communicable disease. Schools are among the institutions that are assigned the responsibility of establishing policies for communicable disease control. In most school districts, the primary responsibility for identifying potential and actual cases of communicable disease falls to the school nurse. In some areas, school nurses are responsible for screening students for typical childhood infestations such as pediculosis (see Chapter 26). Nurse practice statutes in most states limit the authority to make medical diagnoses to advanced practice nurses. School nurses prepared at the baccalaureate level have physical assessment skills that provide them with the ability to identify deviations from normal findings. Therefore, in the case of a potential communicable disease, such as conjunctivitis, the child is excluded from school until a healthcare provider can diagnose the child's clinical findings as infectious or produced by another cause such as an allergy.

Each state health department publishes guidelines specifying diseases that must be reported, as well as personnel required to file reports. The process for reporting communicable diseases is similar among states. The reporting process for New York State is found in FIGURE 13.3. A copy of each state's communicable disease reporting policies and procedures can be accessed on the Centers for Disease Control and Prevention Web site (http://www.cdc.gov/mmwr) by clicking on Public Health Resources and then selecting State Health Departments. School nurses should develop collaborative relationships and maintain good communication with their local health department. When a number of cases of a particular communicable disease occur among the students in the school, the local health department can provide valuable guidance and assistance in applying school or health department policies and procedures, as well as developing guidelines for parental notification.

School policies on communicable disease management should be based on guidelines developed by health authorities. These authorities should be clearly identified in school policies on communicable diseases. Both the *Red Book* from the American Academy of Pediatrics (Committee on Infectious Diseases, 2003) and *Control of Communicable Disease Manual* published by the American Public Health Association (2004) provide clear evidence-based guidelines on which to base decisions regarding school exclusion and disease management. Written policies should reference these authorities within the text as this action provides strong support for the actions taken when a student is

(text continues on page 291)

MEASLES MUMPS & RUBELLA VACCINES

WHAT YOU NEED TO KNOW

1 Why get vaccinated?

Measles, mumps, and rubella are serious diseases.

Measles
- Measles virus causes rash, cough, runny nose, eye irritation, and fever.
- It can lead to ear infection, pneumonia, seizures (jerking and staring), brain damage, and death.

Mumps
- Mumps virus causes fever, headache, and swollen glands.
- It can lead to deafness, meningitis (infection of the brain and spinal cord covering), painful swelling of the testicles or ovaries, and, rarely, death.

Rubella (German Measles)
- Rubella virus causes rash, mild fever, and arthritis (mostly in women).
- If a woman gets rubella while she is pregnant, she could have a miscarriage or her baby could be born with serious birth defects.

You or your child could catch these diseases by being around someone who has them. They spread from person to person through the air.

Measles, mumps, and rubella (MMR) vaccine can prevent these diseases. Most children who get their MMR shots will not get these diseases. Many more children would get them if we stopped vaccinating.

2 Who should get MMR vaccine and when?

Children should get 2 doses of MMR vaccine:

✓ The first at **12-15 months of age**

✓ and the second at **4-6 years of age.**

These are the recommended ages. But children can get the second dose at any age, as long as it is at least 28 days after the first dose.

Some **adults** should also get MMR vaccine:

Generally, anyone 18 years of age or older, who was born after 1956, should get at least one dose of MMR vaccine, unless they can show that they have had either the vaccines or the diseases.

Ask your doctor or nurse for more information.

MMR vaccine may be given at the same time as other vaccines.

3 Some people should not get MMR vaccine or should wait

- People should not get MMR vaccine who have ever had a life-threatening allergic reaction to **gelatin,** the antibiotic **neomycin,** or to **a previous dose of MMR vaccine.**
- People who are moderately or severely ill at the time the shot is scheduled should usually wait until they recover before getting MMR vaccine.
- Pregnant women should wait to get MMR vaccine until after they have given birth. Women should avoid getting pregnant for 4 weeks after getting MMR vaccine.
- Some people should check with their doctor about whether they should get MMR vaccine, including anyone who:
  - Has HIV/AIDS, or another disease that affects the immune system
  - Is being treated with drugs that affect the immune system, such as steroids, for 2 weeks or longer.
  - Has any kind of cancer
  - Is taking cancer treatment with x-rays or drugs
  - Has ever had a low platelet count (a blood disorder)
- People who recently had a transfusion or were given other blood products should ask their doctor when they may get MMR vaccine.

Ask your doctor or nurse for more information.

4 What are the risks from MMR vaccine?

A vaccine, like any medicine, is capable of causing serious problems, such as severe allergic reactions. The risk of MMR vaccine causing serious harm, or death, is extremely small.

Getting MMR vaccine is much safer than getting any of these three diseases. Most people who get MMR vaccine do not have any problems with it.

Mild Problems
- Fever (up to 1 person out of 6)
- Mild rash (about 1 person out of 20)
- Swelling of glands in the cheeks or neck (rare)

If these problems occur, it is usually within 7-12 days after the shot. They occur less often after the second dose.

Moderate Problems
- Seizure (jerking or staring) caused by fever (about 1 out of 3,000 doses)
- Temporary pain and stiffness in the joints, mostly in teenage or adult women (up to 1 out of 4)
- Temporary low platelet count, which can cause a bleeding disorder (about 1 out of 30,000 doses)

Severe Problems (Very Rare)
- Serious allergic reaction (less than 1 out of a million doses)
- Several other severe problems have been known to occur after a child gets MMR vaccine. But this happens so rarely, experts cannot be sure whether they are caused by the vaccine or not. These include:
  - Deafness
  - Long-term seizures, coma, or lowered consciousness
  - Permanent brain damage

5 What if there is a moderate or severe reaction?

What should I look for?

Any unusual conditions, such as a serious allergic reaction, high fever or behavior changes. Signs of a serious allergic reaction include difficulty breathing, hoarseness or wheezing, hives, paleness, weakness, a fast heart beat or dizziness within a few minutes to a few hours after the shot. A high fever or seizure, if it occurs, would happen 1 or 2 weeks after the shot.

What should I do?
- **Call** a doctor, or get the person to a doctor right away.
- **Tell** your doctor what happened, the date and time it happened, and when the vaccination was given.
- **Ask** your doctor, nurse, or health department to report the reaction by filing a Vaccine Adverse Event Reporting System (VAERS) form.
  Or you can file this report through the VAERS web site at www.vaers.org, or by calling 1-800-822-7967.
  VAERS does not provide medical advice.

6 The National Vaccine Injury Compensation Program

In the rare event that you or your child has a serious reaction to a vaccine, a federal program has been created to help you pay for the care of those who have been harmed.

For details about the National Vaccine Injury Compensation Program, call **1-800-338-2382** or visit the program's website at www.hrsa.gov/osp/vicp

7 How can I learn more?

- Ask your doctor or nurse. They can give you the vaccine package insert or suggest other sources of information.
- Call your local or state health department's immunization program.
- Contact the Centers for Disease Control and Prevention (CDC):
  - Call **1-800-232-4636 (1-800-CDC-INFO)**
  - Visit the National Immunization Program's website at www.cdc.gov/nip

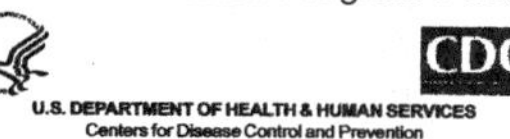

Vaccine Information Statement

MMR (1/15/03) 42 U.S.C. § 300aa-26

Figure 13.2 ■ Vaccine information statements.

NEW YORK STATE DEPARTMENT OF HEALTH
COMMUNICABLE DISEASE REPORTING REQUIREMENTS

Reporting of suspected or confirmed communicable diseases is mandated under the New York State Sanitary Code (10NYCRR 2.10). The primary responsibility for reporting rests with the physician; moreover, laboratories (PHL 2102), school nurses (10NYCRR 2.12), day care center directors, nursing homes/hospitals (10NYCRR 405.3d) and state institutions (10NYCRR 2.10a) or other locations providing health services (10NYCRR 2.12) are also required to report the diseases listed below.

- Amebiasis
- ☎ **Animal bites for which rabies prophylaxis is given**[1]
- ☎ **Anthrax**[2]
- ☎ **Arboviral infection**[3]
- Babesiosis
- ☎ **Botulism**[2]
- ☎ **Brucellosis**[2]
- Campylobacteriosis
- Chancroid
- Chlamydia trachomatis infection
- ☎ **Cholera**
- Cryptosporidiosis
- Cyclosporiasis
- ☎ **Diphtheria**
- E. coli O157:H7 infection[4]
- Ehrlichiosis
- ☎ **Encephalitis**
- ☎ **Foodborne illness**
- Giardiasis
- ☎ **Glanders**[2]
- Gonococcal infection
- Haemophilus influenzae[5] (invasive disease)
- ☎ **Hantavirus disease**
- Hemolytic uremic syndrome
- Hepatitis A
- ☎ **Hepatitis A in a food handler**
- Hepatitis B, C (specify acute or chronic)
- Pregnant hepatitis B carrier
- Hospital associated infections (as defined in section 2.2 10NYCRR)
- Influenza, laboratory-confirmed
- Legionellosis
- Listeriosis
- Lyme disease
- Lymphogranuloma venereum
- Malaria
- ☎ **Measles**
- ☎ **Melioidosis**[2]
- Meningitis
  - Aseptic or viral
  - ☎ **Haemophilus**
  - ☎ **Meningococcal**
  - Other (specify type)
- ☎ **Meningococcemia**
- ☎ **Monkeypox**
- Mumps
- Pertussis
- ☎ **Plague**[2]
- ☎ **Poliomyelitis**
- Psittacosis
- ☎ **Q Fever**[2]
- ☎ **Rabies**
- Rocky Mountain spotted fever
- ☎ **Rubella** (including congenital rubella syndrome)
- Salmonellosis
- ☎ **Severe Acute Respiratory Syndrome (SARS)**
- Shigatoxin-producing infection[4]
- Shigellosis[4]
- ☎ **Smallpox**[2]
- Staphylococcus aureus[6] (due to strains showing reduced susceptibility or resistance to vancomycin)
- ☎ **Staphylococcal enterotoxin B poisoning**[2]
- Streptococcal infection (invasive disease)[5]
  - Group A beta-hemolytic strep
  - Group B strep
  - Streptococcus pneumoniae
- ☎ **Syphilis, specify stage**[7]
- Tetanus
- Toxic shock syndrome
- Transmissable spongiform encephalopathies[8]
- Trichinosis
- ☎ **Tuberculosis current disease (specify site)**
- ☎ **Tularemia**[2]
- ☎ **Typhoid**
- Vibriosis[6]
- ☎ **Vaccinia disease**[9]
- ☎ **Viral hemorrhagic fever**[2]
- Yersiniosis

1 Local health department must be notified prior to initiating rabies prophylaxis.
2 Diseases that are possible indicators of bioterrorism.
3 Including, but not limited to, infections caused by eastern equine encephalitis virus, western equine encephalitis virus, West Nile virus, St. Louis encephalitis virus, La Crosse virus, Powassan virus, Jamestown Canyon virus, dengue and yellow fever.
4 Positive shigatoxin test results should be reported as presumptive evidence of disease.
5 Only report cases with positive cultures from blood, CSF, joint, peritoneal or pleural fluid. Do not report cases with positive cultures from skin, saliva, sputum or throat.
6 Proposed addition to list.
7 Any non-treponemal test ≥ 1:16 or any positive primary or secondary stage disease or prenatal or delivery test result regardless of titer should be reported by phone; all others may be reported by mail.
8 Including Creutzfeldt-Jakob disease. Cases should be reported directly to the New York State Department of Health Alzheimer's Disease and Other Dementias Registry at (518) 473-7817 upon suspicion of disease. In NYC, cases should also be reported to the NYCDOHMH.
9 persons with vaccinia infection due to contact transmission, and persons with the following complications from vaccination: eczema vaccinatum, erythema multiforme major or Stevens-Johnson syndrome, fetal vaccinia, generalized vaccinia, inadvertent inoculation, ocular vaccinia, post-vaccinial encephalitis or encephalomyelitis, progressive vaccinia, pyogenic infection of the infection site, and any other serious adverse events.

SPECIAL NOTES

- Diseases listed in **bold type** (☎) warrant prompt action and should be reported **immediately** to local health departments by phone followed by submission of the confidential case report form (DOH-389). In NYC use case report form 395V.
- In addition to the diseases listed above, any unusual disease (defined as a newly apparent or emerging disease or syndrome that could possibly be caused by a transmissible infectious agent or microbial toxin) is reportable.
- Outbreaks: while individual cases of some diseases (e.g., streptococcal sore throat, head lice, impetigo, scabies and pneumonia) are not reportable, a cluster or outbreak of cases of any communicable disease is a reportable event.
- **Cases of HIV infection, HIV-related illness and AIDS are reportable to:**

Division of Epidemiology
P.O. Box 2073, ESP Station
Albany, NY 12220-2073
(518) 474-4284

In New York City: New York City Department of Health and Mental Hygiene
For HIV/AIDS reporting, call:
(212) 442-3388

WHO SHOULD REPORT?

Physicians, nurses, laboratory directors, infection control practitioners, health care facilities, state institutions, schools.

WHERE SHOULD REPORT BE MADE?

Report to local health department where patient resides.

Contact Person______________________

Name/Address ______________________

____

____

Phone______________________

Fax______________________

WHEN SHOULD REPORT BE MADE?

Within 24 hours of diagnosis:

- phone diseases in bold type,
- mail case report, DOH-389, for all other diseases.
- in New York City use form 395V.

For more information on disease reporting, call your local health department or the New York State Department of Health Bureau of Communicable Disease Control at (518) 473-4439. In New York City, 1 (866) NYC-DOH1. To obtain reporting forms (DOH-389), call (518) 474-0548.

PLEASE POST THIS CONSPICUOUSLY

Revised 2/05

Figure 13.3 ■ New York State Department of Health communicable disease reporting requirements.

identified with a communicable disease or infestation.

Clear communication to families of the school's policies on communicable disease management is crucial, and it should be provided annually in writing. Information included in this communication identifies procedures for screening various communicable diseases and criteria for student exclusion and readmittance. Included in the communication to parents should be an explanation of how the student's rights to confidentiality will be ensured. When performing group screenings, procedures should include strategies to prevent other students in the class from learning of a peer's situation.

There must be consistency in the determination of student exclusion, as well as the criteria for readmission. If "special case" status is assigned to particular students exempting them from the policy, then parents of a child who was treated according to the policy can claim discrimination or harassment (Schwab & Gelfman, 2001). Students who present repeatedly at school with a communicable condition, such as ringworm, may require repeated assessment by the school nurse; when she or he determines that treatment has not been initiated, the student may be repeatedly excluded. Clear policies based on the judgment of medical authorities support the need to protect other students from unnecessary exposure to a communicable disease.

Families may request that their child be exempted from receiving immunizations either because of religious beliefs or the immunization is contraindicated owing to a medical condition. In 15 states, including California, philosophical reasons are also acceptable as requests for immunization exemption (Schwab & Gelfman, 2001). Mississippi and West Virginia are the only two states that do not have provisions in immunization guidelines for religious exemptions.

A thorough understanding of the mode of transmission of communicable diseases is necessary to develop sound policies directed at minimizing student and staff risk for acquiring a disease. These policies should also ensure that the rights to privacy and education of those infected with the disease are protected. An example of how the mode of transmission will direct policy involves the various forms of hepatitis. Hepatitis B, C, and D are transmitted via exposure to bodily fluids, particularly blood. All faculty and staff should be educated yearly on use of Standard Precautions and provided with appropriate barrier supplies. Policies that exclude students with hepatitis B or C from attending school are generally not supported by the courts, which rule that such action is discrimination, citing section 504 of the 1973 Rehabilitation Act as support. Hepatitis A and E commonly have a fecal–oral pattern of transmission. Therefore, policies to minimize transmission of hepatitis A in the school should focus on measures that limit the healthy student's access to contaminated food or water (Chin, 2002). Schools should ensure appropriate hand washing facilities, including sufficient supplies of soap and paper towels. Alcohol-based hand rubs should be available when students do not have access to soap and running water (CDC, 2002). Policies that address how food is handled by staff should clearly specify measures that prevent contamination. Schools may also develop policies that forbid students to share food.

Probably human immunodeficiency virus/acquired immunodeficiency syndrome (HIV/AIDS) raises more concern regarding communicability than any other disease. As with hepatitis B and C, HIV is transmitted primarily by direct contact with infected blood and body fluid. The American Academy of Pediatrics, Committee on Infectious Diseases states that "in the absence of blood exposure, HIV infection is not acquired through the types of contact that usually occur in school settings, including contact with saliva or tears" (AAP, 2003, p. 345). The AAP also provides specific guidelines for cleaning up spills that contain blood and other bodily fluids (see Chapter 21). These guidelines should be clearly articulated in the school policy.

In the past, many school districts included tuberculosis (TB) testing as one of the required screenings. Although the incidence of TB is increasing worldwide, the disease is found primarily in specific high-risk groups. Schools should apply the recommendations outlined by the American Academy of Pediatrics (2003) in policies related to TB testing requirements. The AAP recommends immediate testing only for students who have had contact with an individual diagnosed with TB, those with clinical findings suggestive of TB, or those immigrating from an area endemic for TB (see Chapter 21). Annual and periodic testing for TB is clearly aligned with recognized recommendations for specific groups.

Control of communicable disease requires that certain parties, such as parents of other students, be notified of a disease that is likely to be contracted by others. When it is in the best interest of the public, the court allows for release of certain personal information. Often "limited disclosure" fulfills the purpose of the notification to protect others, but also preserves the privacy of the student. For example, when a student in a class is diagnosed with scarlet fever, his or her classmates' parents can be notified of the presence of the disease without identifying the specific student who is ill. Other communicable diseases pose such a significant risk to others that states require that individuals who contract these diseases be identified and information sought related to contacts. State law determines which diseases are reportable. These may include, but are not limited to, bacterial meningitis, hepatitis, measles, sexually transmitted diseases, and tuberculosis.

CHILD ABUSE REPORTING

In 1963, the first statutes mandating reporting of child abuse were enacted. At present all states and the District of Columbia have laws requiring the reporting of child abuse. The Child Abuse Prevention and Treatment Act (CAPTA) of 1974 provides federal funds to states to implement programs that identify, treat, and prevent child abuse. States must include in their child abuse reporting laws the following: (a) the individuals who are considered mandated reporters; (b) a definition of maltreatment; (c) the procedure for reporting suspected abuse and neglect; and (d) the agencies that are designated to receive and investigate the report. It also requires that the statute provide immunity from prosecution for reporters and penalties for failure to report and false reporting. States must identify acts or omissions that are exempt from definitions of child abuse. Lastly, reporting laws must include provisions that nullify certain privileged communication rights (U.S. Department of Health and Human Services [USDHHS], 2003a). Variations exist across states in regard to who is a mandated reporter, definitions of maltreatment, and standards and procedures for reporting. Each state's statutes can be found on the National Clearinghouse on Child Abuse and Neglect Information Web site at http://www.calib.com/nccanch.

CAPTA defines a child as someone who has not attained the age of 18, and defines child abuse and neglect as "any recent act or failure to act by parent or caretaker, which results in death, serious physical or emotional harm, sexual abuse, or exploitation, or an act or failure to act which presents an imminent risk of serious harm" (National Clearinghouse on Child Abuse and Neglect Information, 2003, p. 5). The perpetrator is defined by CAPTA as a parent or caretaker. Individual states may add additional descriptors to these definitions. For example, in Oregon a child is defined as an unmarried person who is younger than 18 years of age (National Clearinghouse on Child Abuse and Neglect Information, 2003).

Mandated reporters face criminal or civil liability for failure to report suspected child abuse. Each state defines who is included as a mandated reporter, with many states including the phrase "any person but not limited to." Eighteen states include in their statutes that any person who suspects child abuse or neglect is required to report. There were 2.6 million cases of suspected abuse and neglect reported to child protective services in 2002. Of this number, 896,000 were judged to require investigation. More than half of all cases investigated were reported by professionals, with school personnel the most frequent (16.1%) source, followed by legal or law enforcement professionals (15.7%) and social service professionals (12.6%) (National Clearinghouse, 2003).

Thirty-three states include in reporting laws that the religious beliefs of the parents should be considered when assessing indications of child abuse or neglect. For example, Alaska legislation states that "there is no failure to provide medical attention to a child (as an element of the offense of criminal nonsupport) if the child is provided treatment solely by spiritual means through prayer in accordance with the tenets and practices of a recognized church or religious denomination by an accredited practitioner of the church or denomination" (Alaska Statute, 1996). However, several states mandate that children receive intervention in life-threatening situations even if in conflict with parental religious beliefs. For example, in Pennsylvania, agencies are directed to seek a court order for medical intervention (National Clearinghouse on Child Abuse and Neglect Information, 2003).

The majority of states require that oral reports be made immediately on the suspicion of child abuse or neglect. Most states require that mandated reporters then follow up with a written report. The written reports must contain the child's and parent's names, age of the child, nature and extent of the injuries, and any other pertinent information. Many states have standard forms showing injuries on figures that allow for accurate documentation seen on the child's body. The school nurse should be the individual who documents physical findings, as reporting of physical findings by someone who is not licensed to perform physical assessments might not be admissible in legal proceedings (Schwab & Gelfman, 2001).

CAPTA requires that states include provisions for immunity from prosecution for individuals who make "good faith" reports. Because good faith may be open to judicial interpretation, some states include the phrase "is presumed to be acting in good faith," which provides better protection in case of litigation (National Clearinghouse on Child Abuse and Neglect Information, 2003). Forty-six states and the District of Columbia impose penalties on mandatory reporters who knowingly fail to report. This is a misdemeanor that can result in fines and/or imprisonment. In situations in which a child dies or is seriously injured, failure to report can result in criminal penalties.

School nurses should know their state regulations associated with child abuse reporting. In some states the individual who has identified the suspicion of abuse must file the report. Other states specify that individuals identified in a supervisory role or a special team of qualified members file the report. In some school districts school nurses cannot independently file suspected abuse or neglect reports. The authority for filing may be held by an administrator. However, once the school nurse has identified a situation that requires the filing of a report, an administrator cannot make an independent determination that no report is necessary. When school personnel report to a supervisor that child abuse or neglect is suspected, the supervisor, by law, must file a report. The supervisor cannot base decisions to report the suspected abuse or neglect on his or her independent assessment of the situation or the child. It is important to note that school personnel are responsible for reporting, not investigating, suspected cases of abuse or neglect. Once the report has been filed, the state's child protective agency will gather the evidence associated with the report.

All data collected and documented by the school nurse should be clearly objective and free from multiple interpretations. School districts should have policies specifying documentation procedures and storage of records. Records concerning child abuse allegations should always be kept in the records within the child's current school. As with all personal data, these records should be stored following strict confidential procedures. Even in cases in which the investigations have not found sufficient evidence of abuse, it is important to maintain the report in the child's file in order to track any other incidences that may support future concerns of abuse or neglect.

Although photographs provide strong evidence to support abuse claims, the school nurse should be clear on state laws regarding who is legally permitted to take pictures of physical evidence. It is important to emphasize again that the school nurse's responsibility is to perform only those assessments that are necessary to raise a suspicion of child maltreatment. Taking pictures may be interpreted as an investigative function more appropriately conducted by child protective services (Schwab & Gelfman, 2001).

There may be times when child protective services are unable to arrive at the school and assess the student before the end of the day. The child's safety may be a concern if the child is sent home according to regular procedures. It is critical that school personnel never transport the child in a personal vehicle off school property. The family would then have a legal basis for the charge of kidnapping. If there is documented concern for the child's safety, then police or medical emergency transport is contacted to either take the child to the hospital or to another designated safe place.

Parental notification by school authorities or social service agencies is required for any child for whom a suspected child abuse or neglect report is filed. School policy should specify the procedure for parental notification. Parents are allowed access to review any reports that have been filed. They can also request a copy of the report. In most cases they do not have the legal right to know the name of the individual who has filed the report and this information can be eliminated from the copy provided to the parent (Schwab & Gelfman, 2001).

The Child Abuse Prevention and Treatment Act (CAPTA) requires that states follow specific guidelines for protecting the confidentiality of the family who is the focus of a child abuse investigation. The records can be made available only to:

- Individuals who are the subject of the report
- Federal, state, or local government entities, or any agent of such entities, having a need for such information in order to carry out its responsibilities under law to protect children from abuse and neglect
- Child abuse citizen review panels
- A grand jury or court, upon a finding that information in the record is necessary for the determination of an issue before the court or grand jury
- Other entities or classes of individuals statutorily authorized by the state to receive such information pursuant to a legitimate state purpose (National Clearinghouse on Child Abuse and Neglect Information, 2003, p. 12).

Individual state statutes may stipulate others who may have access to records. Professionals who are often provided such access include law enforcement officers and physicians.

LEGAL ISSUES RELATED TO MANDATED SCREENINGS

Schools provide an optimal setting for health promotion. Through a program of health screenings, school nurses are able to identify a number of conditions that have the potential for preventing students from attaining their optimal physical and mental levels. Individual states mandate the type and schedule of screening required. Many states require that schools provide screenings for vision and hearing, as well as for posture/scoliosis (see Chapter 20). Clear procedures and policies must be in place that identify the qualifications of personnel performing the screening, equipment necessary, and procedure to be followed. All forms used to document findings should be organized to be congruent with the school district's written policy. Both normal and abnormal findings are documented on student records. Forms notifying parents of the results of screenings should provide for instructions regarding necessary follow-up and communication of the results of that follow-up to the school nurse.

Parents cannot be required to allow their child to receive screenings. Neither can a school nurse force a student to participate in a screening against his or her will. To force a student to participate in a particular procedure can place the school nurse at risk for charges of assault and battery (Schwab & Gelfman, 2001). Clear documentation of the parental or student refusal of the screening in the student's health record is necessary. Parents should be notified if the parents have consented to the screening but their child refuses. Even with parental consent the student should never be forced to complete the screening.

Student rights to privacy and confidentiality during screenings must be ensured. Other students should not have access to information about a student's weight or visual acuity. During mass screenings it is important to organize the room in such a way that students in the waiting area are not able to observe the screening of their peers. Screenings that require removal of clothing, such as a physical exam or scoliosis screening, should be performed with a witness present.

When schools provide physical examinations that go beyond routine screenings, parents must be provided an explicit description of what the exam will involve and provide written consent for the exam to be performed. These exams are typically provided to students who participate in sports or in some cases to students who failed to receive a mandated physical from their family physician. Some states, including Pennsylvania, require schools to provide physical exams for students who have not received a mandated exam from a family physician. However, a school district in Pennsylvania was charged with violating the rights of eight female students whose school physical examination included assessment of external genitalia. The federal judge ruled that the girls' Fourth Amendment rights protecting against unreasonable searches were violated (Schwab & Gelfman, 2001).

It is important that parents are notified of planned screenings, as well as the results, particularly when follow-up is necessary. Individual state laws regarding the guidelines associated with abnormal findings may include parental notification, student referral, and follow-up to determine results of the referral. Although a time-consuming process, school nurses should always track the family's action regarding a report of abnormal screening findings. Even when there is no specific mandate in state law that requires follow-up, standards within nursing practice do expect follow-up with families whose child requires treatment for an abnormal finding identified during a school screening.

REGULATING STUDENT SERVICES

Although all would agree that health is tied to learning ability, current focus on educational reform has all but ignored school health services. The No Child Left Behind Act enacted into law by President George W. Bush, on January 8, 2002, amends the Elementary and Secondary Education Act (ESEA) of 1965. This act focuses on defining success in terms of student accomplishments. Millions of dollars are provided to local and state agencies to promote student learning. The Act focuses on increasing local control over educational initiatives, expanding educational options for parents, and emphasizing teaching approaches proven to produce student achievement. Nowhere in the Act's language is there a discussion of the need to ensure that students are healthy and ready to learn. This characteristic lack of attention to the health needs of students within the educational system continues to challenge the school nurse's ability to obtain the resources necessary to provide optimal health-related services to students.

The Center for Disease Control and Prevention (2005) has developed guidelines for a comprehensive school health program. However, there is no consistent provision of school health services among states. Some of this lack of clarity is explained by the fact that the major decision-making body determining health services are educators whose mission is primarily focused on academics. The fact that learning is clearly tied to a healthy mind and body has done little in some states to expand health services provided to students. State law governs the mandated health services that schools provide. However, at times, state laws may not be consistent with federal guidelines. Schwab and Gelfman (2001) provide an example of such a disparity in the Connecticut state education law that does not require schools to administer medications. Federal guidelines could rule this policy as discriminatory.

Laws mandating school health services have clearly not kept up with the changing needs of the school-age population. Nurse-to-student ratios established almost 50 years ago do not reflect the needs of an increasing population of students with complex physical, psychological, and social needs. School nurses are in a perfect position to help to inform families and legislators of the needs to revise state health mandates to better meet the needs of the current population of students.

REGULATING SCHOOL NURSE EDUCATION

Controversies surrounding the preparation of nurses for practice have been present since 1964 when the American Nurses Association (ANA) produced a statement that entry into practice should be at the baccalaureate level (ANA, 1965). Almost 40 years later, nurses take the same licensing exam and receive the RN license whether they complete a hospital diploma program, or an associate or baccalaureate degree. As a result, it is not surprising that wide differences exist in the preparation that individual states require for school nurses.

Professional organizations support the baccalaureate degree as the minimal requirement for school nursing practice (American Nurses Association, 2001; National Association of School Nurses, 2002). In addition, further preparation in the area of school nursing is also recognized as essential (see Chapter 5). Acquiring certification in the area of school nursing provides additional evidence of achieving the specialized knowledge and skills necessary for practice within the school. However, certification is not required to practice school nursing in all states. Certification can be obtained through completion of the educational preparation required by a state, which then issues a certificate similar to teachers, or by national certification. The National Board for Certification of School Nurses offers a standardized exam that, when passed, provides national certification. This standardized exam is required by some states for school nurse certification.

School nurse responsibilities also differ widely among states. Few states require the student-to-nurse ratio of 750:1 that is recommended by the National Association of School Nurses (NASN) as well as other organizations (NASN, 2004). As late as 2002, Delaware, District of Columbia, and Vermont were the only three states that required a student-to-nurse ratio of 750:1 or better. School nurses in a number of states, including Washington, have supported legislation supporting the 750:1 ratio. Although the legislators in Washington supported more school nurses, they cited budgetary problems tied to increasing school nurse ratios. During 2005 a bill was created to continue to study the issue of school nurse/student ratios in Washington. Alabama, Arkansas, Louisiana, Minnesota, Pennsylvania, Tennessee, and West Virginia also specify a specific student-to-nurse ratio. However, each ratio is above the recommended 750:1. The remaining states have no mandated student-to-nurse ratio. Data collected by the CDC in the latest Social Health Policies and Programs Study highlight the difference in school nurse qualifications required among states, as well as school nurse responsibilities (CDC, 2001).

School nurses are advised to consult their state school nurse association for information on the status of changes in school nurse-to-student ratios, as many states are examining this issue and proposing reducing ratios to those more consistent with the recommendation advocated by NASN.

School nursing, as a specialty within professional nursing, requires additional educational preparation. However, there are no consistent preparation requirements across states. In some states, such as New Jersey, the focus is on preparing the nurse to teach, while in other states, such as Pennsylvania, school nurses cannot teach in the classroom without additional teacher certification. Baccalaureate degree programs prepare school nurses for caring for clients within the community. A focus within community health curricula on case management, communicable disease management, and community and family assessment provides the school nurse with a sound foundation for practicing in the school setting. States that require school nurse certification specify competencies that the school nurse should possess at the program completion. These also differ among states. Lack of consensus related to basic and advanced preparation for school nursing practice limits a clear role definition.

APPLYING LAWS TO RECORD KEEPING AND COMMUNICATION RELATED TO STUDENTS

"Management of student health records is one of the most challenging responsibilities of school nurses. These responsibilities, usually shared with school district administrators, include the generation, maintenance, protection, disclosure, and destruction of students' school health records" (NASN, 2004). Federal, state, and local laws address guidelines regarding student records within schools. However, inconsistencies often exist in guidelines outlined among these sources. Adding to the confusion for school nurses is how health room and student health records are defined in relation to the laws regulating educational records. States differ in how they classify aspects of a student's record; student health information in some states is classified as part of the health record and access to information contained in the record is limited to healthcare professionals. If, however, all student records are considered educational records, then access to health-related information would be less restricted.

States vary in their regulations regarding retention of student records. School policies must be in line with state and federal guidelines and should include length of time specific records are maintained in the school, as well as which records can be destroyed at the end of the year.

Family Educational Rights and Privacy Act (FERPA)

Federally mandated regulation of school records began in 1974 with the enactment of the Family Educational Rights and Privacy Act (FERPA), also called the Buckley Amendment. This Act gives parents the right to access their child's educational records and protects the release of personally identifiable student information to others, including student health information. FERPA defines records as "any information recorded in any way, including but not limited to, handwriting, print, computer, media, audio or videotape, microfilm, and microfiche" (National Task Force on Confidential Student Health Information, 2000, p. 8). Any information on a student within a school is considered an educational record; therefore "FERPA governs all student health records maintained by school employees or by contracted employees who provide "school health services"...[especially] services directed to supporting students' participation and progress in school. These services are generally considered health promotion, health maintenance, and "related" or "support" services that enable students, especially those with special healthcare needs, to attend school, maintain (or improve) their health status during the school day, progress toward independence in self-care in the school setting, and achieve educational success" (NASN, 2004).

Some individual states (Washington and Massachusetts) and some school districts exempt the nursing record from inclusion in educational records when applying FERPA regulations. While records of health screenings and immunization status are considered part of the educational record, records of student health room visits, individualized health plans, and records of medication administration are typically viewed as health records (Schwab & Gelfman, 2001).

Certain types of information can be released without parental approval. FERPA uses the term "Directory Information" for this form of student data and defines it as:

> Information contained in an educational record of a student, which would not generally be considered harmful or an invasion of privacy if disclosed. It includes, but is not limited to the student's name, address, telephone listing, date and place of birth, major field of study, participation in officially recognized activities and sports, weight and height of members of athletic teams, date of attendances, degrees and awards received and the most recent previous educational agency or institution attended. (Schwab & Gelfman, 2001, p. 382)

Schools are required to notify parents that they have the option to request that their child's information not be included in any publications of directory information. Also, school districts may also place restrictions on what they want to consider directory information and may choose not to release student information that is included in FERPA guidelines.

FERPA guidelines specify that decisions regarding where student records are kept should be based on the necessary frequency of access, as well as the sensitivity of the information that is contained in the record. School districts are encouraged to classify student information into the following categories:

Class A: Academic information such as grade transcripts and attendance information and educational records, including IEPs for students with special education needs.

Class B: Temporary records that are usually discarded at the end of the school year or sooner.

Class C: Sensitive records, such as child abuse reports, nursing records, medical and psychiatric reports, hospital records, psychological test results, and counseling records (National Task Force on Confidential Student Health Information, 2000, p. 35).

There may be some concern regarding the classification of IEPs in the Class A category. However, for each category, access is limited to those with "legitimate educational interest." Within the FERPA regulations is the requirement that school districts define "legitimate educational interest." Therefore, protection of particular information within student records can be ensured with careful stipulation of the district's determination of who is considered to have legitimate educational interest.

Class C records are the most restricted, allowing access only to those professionals whose educational background makes these records relevant. If other professionals in the school require information contained in class C records, then this information should be communicated to the individual rather than providing open access to the student's record. "Ideally, access should be strictly limited to licensed health professionals who originate the records because they can best interpret their meaning" (National Task Force on Confidential Student Health Information, 2000, p. 36).

Increasingly, part or all of student records, including health records, are being stored on computer files. Safeguards need to be implemented to ensure the same level of security for electronic data that is in place for paper records. Records stored on computer files require protection from unauthorized access by implementing measures that limit access, require placement of the computer in a secure site, and establish a record-keeping procedure related to who has accessed files. Homeland security requirements often contradict FERPA by mandating that hard copy lists be kept of students with special needs. The school nurse should discuss school and district protocols at the beginning of each school year to ensure compliance.

Prompt transfer of school records when students leave one school and enter another is necessary in order to ensure that the new school has what is needed to plan the child's educational program. Parental consent, under the FERPA guidelines, is not necessary when transferring school records to the student's new school. However, it is recommended that schools have in place clear policies regarding transfer of student records. Included should be notification of parents that their child's records will be transferred to the new school. Some state laws do not allow medical records in the school record that are from a source outside of the school to be released. Examples of such records include those from a hospitalization or family physician. Special consideration should be taken when sending health records through the mail, including labeling the envelope confidential and addressing it specifically to the school nurse. When it is necessary to fax health information, it is important that the cover sheet also state that the data are confidential. Timing the faxing of health information should be such that the school nurse is able to immediately receive it rather than allowing the record to sit on the fax machine for unauthorized persons to see.

"FERPA does not require school district personnel to be trained in confidentiality requirements, nor does it impose consequences on school employees for non-permitted disclosures. Rather, it provides that, if a school district violates the requirements of FERPA, the district may by sanctioned through the loss of federal financial assistance" (NASN, 2004).

Health Insurance Portability and Accountability Act (HIPAA)

Concern over the confidentiality of health records transmitted electronically resulted in the creation of the Health Insurance Portability and Accountability Act first published in 2000 and amended in 2002. The Act went into effect April 14, 2001. The Act instituted national requirements for ensuring the privacy of all identifiable data related to an individual's health status. Regulations within the Act place restrictions and procedures on health information that is produced or retained electronically by healthcare providers. Also included are regulations regarding health-related data collected by health plans and healthcare clearinghouses (USDHHS, 2002). In general, "student records in schools and school districts that receive federal funding are generally not subject to HIPAA privacy provisions" (NASN, 2004).

HIPAA was intended to ensure that personal medical information is shared responsibly and to protect client confidentiality. It was not intended to interrupt necessary communication between healthcare providers. Those who provide health care are considered to be 'covered entities' according to HIPAA. When a patient or their family gives personal health information to a covered entity, that information is then considered to be "Protected Health Information" or PHI (Selekman, 2004). In most cases, permission is required of the parents before PHI is released.

The Preamble to HIPAA specifically excludes schools as 'covered entities,' as they are already covered by FERPA; however, many school nurses have experienced difficulty communicating with other healthcare providers regarding students in their care. This was never the intent of HIPAA. The question is how much information can be shared outside of the office or clinic where children and adolescents receive their care. Information should be shared on a "need to know" basis and follows "minimum necessary" standards. PHI can be shared for the purposes of treatment. Therefore, healthcare providers should not feel restricted to share necessary information with the school nurse regarding specific treatments, including medications, or other interventions when a question arises about a specific student.

Consulting with another healthcare provider

about a patient is within the HIPAA Privacy Rule's definition of "treatment" and, therefore, is permissible. In addition, a healthcare provider (or other protected entity) is expressly permitted to disclose "protected health information about an individual to a healthcare provider for that provider's treatment of the individual" (USDHHS, 2003b). This consultation includes the healthcare provider and the school nurse.

"School-based health centers administered by covered entities and, in most instances, school-based healthcare providers employed by an agency other than a school district and who engage in certain electronic transactions, are subject to HIPAA. Schools and school health professionals whose records are covered by FERPA and who engage in certain electronic transactions (such as Medicaid billing) are likely covered by the HIPAA Transaction Rule but not the HIPAA Privacy Rule" (NASN, 2004).

When comparing the two laws, "the fundamental ethical and legal principles underlying FERPA and HIPAA are the same. FERPA protects student information in education records, while HIPAA protects individually identifiable health information, in any form, that is used or disclosed by a covered entity. HIPAA privacy requirements, which are more detailed and directive than FERPA privacy requirements, provide useful reference standards for school district policy, procedures, and practices related to the protection and disclosure of student health information" (NASN, 2004). In addition, violation of HIPAA can result in criminal and monetary penalties. Guidelines for communication regarding the health of students should place emphasis on the functional symptoms and their implications related to the student's ability to participate in the learning environment in a state of health; it does not require the sharing of the diagnosis.

ACCESSING STATE AND FEDERAL LAWS

Laws that govern behavior of individuals in the United States can have a federal or a state source. The U.S. Constitution serves as the foundation for Federal law, as does each state's constitution (see Chapter 12). Both federal and state constitutions define three branches of government with different functions. The legislative branch makes the laws, the executive branch administers the laws, and the judicial branch is charged with the responsibility for interpreting laws (Schwab & Gelfman, 2001). Three types of laws govern at the federal, state, and local level: statutory, administrative, and case law. Statutory laws state whether something is required or prohibited. Many of the laws discussed in this chapter, including FERPA and child abuse reporting, are examples of statutory law, as are nurse practice acts that define the legal scope of practice within a given state. Within the nurse practice acts, nurses are required to perform certain duties. These acts can also include behaviors that are prohibited to be performed by nurses. For example, in most states, nurses without an advanced degree and state approval are prohibited from prescribing medications. A state's legislative body enacts specific regulations that define the scope of professional nursing practice. Departments of Education, both at the federal and state levels, apply statutory law to requirements for regulations related to health-related services provided to students. Statutory law regulates state-mandated requirements regarding immunizations for school attendance and scheduled health screenings.

While statutory law defines what must, what can, or what cannot be done in a given situation, administrative law defines who will interpret and enforce or regulate the law. Various agencies, including State Boards of Nursing, are charged with the task of enforcing statutory laws. While a board of nursing may apply professional nursing standards to hearings for nurses, they cannot change the way the scope of practice is defined within the law. Only the state legislature holds authority to change laws. Rulings by State Boards of Nursing, however, can revoke a nurse's license if they determine that the nurse's behavior did not meet an accepted standard as defined within the state's nurse practice act.

The last form of law, case law, involves courts of law in which lawsuits brought by one individual or group against another are heard and judged. Various statutes and regulations are applied to the case to make a determination of the legality of the action that is the focus of the court case.

Laws at the local, state, and federal levels influence school nursing practice. Therefore it is important for school nurses to be knowledgeable regarding the current legal status of such laws. School nurses can keep updated on the legislative issues in their state by becoming familiar with where such information is communicated. At the federal level, laws can be accessed on a number of Web sites depending on the nature of the topic. TABLE 13.2 lists Web sites for obtaining information on common legal issues pertinent to school nurses.

Professional organizations are another valuable resource for knowledge related to legislative issues. The National Association of School Nurses (http://www.nasn.org) frequently includes on their Web site current discussions of legal actions that have an impact on school nurses. An example was

Table 13.2 ■
ACCESSING LEGISLATIVE INFORMATION ON THE WORLD WIDE WEB

1. The Library of Congress—Thomas (http://thomas.loc.gov) A service of the Library of Congress that provides legislative information from the House of Representatives and the Senate. Information on proceedings for the current day is updated every 15 minutes.
2. Children's Health Insurance Programs (http://www.insurekidsnow.gov). This purpose of CHIP is to provide free or low-cost healthcare coverage to low-income children not eligible for Medicaid. The viewer is able to link onto a specific State for enrollment guidelines.
3. National Association of School Nurses (http://www.nasn.org). Click on Legislative News for current issues relevant to school nurses. Also from this site you can click on State organizations for legislative action within the state.
4. FIRSTGOV (http://www.firstgov.org). This site is the official gateway to all Federal, State, and Local agencies. From this site you can access just about any governmental agency. There are vast numbers of links, including those that connect the individual to each state's governor's e-mail.
5. E-Gov (http://www.whitehouse.gov/omb/egov). The E-Government Act 2002 (public law 107-347) was signed into law by President Bush in February, 2002 for the purpose of expanding access and use of governmental resources via the Internet. Individuals can file most governmental forms on this site and conduct other governmental business.
6. Centers For Disease Control (http://www.cdc.gov/nip). This is for the National Immunization Program. Information on this site provides the current childhood immunization recommendations, National Childhood Vaccine Injury Act, Vaccine Information Statement, as well as links to many other sites providing information on legislative issues affecting school-age children.
7. The Immunization Action Coalition (http://www.immunize.org). This is an organization that works closely with and is partly funded by the Centers for Disease Control. From their Web site school nurses can access information on changes in state immunization laws.
8. National Clearinghouse on Child Abuse and Neglect Information (http://nccanch.acf.hhs.gov). This site provides extensive information on both state and federal child abuse regulations. Each state's child abuse statutes can be found on this site.

the focus on the reauthorization of the IDEA legislation in which school nurse services would be included in the legislative language of the Related Services Personnel Section. School nurses were provided a thorough explanation of the legislation as well as how the outcome would influence school nursing. Lastly, within the "action needed" section, suggestions were given for topics to include in communication with legislators.

Some of the state affiliates of NASN provide extensive information on the current status of legislation in their state. One of the best examples is the California School Nurses Organization (CSNO) (http://www.csno.org). On their Web site is a document stating their current legislative priorities. Those outlined for the 2004–2005 legislative cycle included restriction of the sale of certain foods and beverages in the school and regulations regarding specialized healthcare procedures performed by unlicensed school personnel. In addition, there is a continuously updated Bill status report. Each Bill is described in detail with the position taken by CSNO identified, as well as the last action taken on the Bill. The CSNO is a model for how an organization can provide its members with important legislative information impacting on practice.

On the South Carolina Association of School Nurses Web site (http://www.scasn.org), there is a description of the proposed Diabetes Mellitus School Care Act that describes guidelines for training school personnel in diabetes care. The organization clearly outlined their rationale for opposition to the Bill.

CONCLUSION

This chapter focused on how legislation, on both the state and federal levels, impacts on school children and therefore on school nursing practice. Schools are more and more viewed as an ideal setting for providing expanded services beyond those traditionally tied to education. It is often said that a child must be healthy to learn. It is obvious that the school nurse is central to fulfilling the mission of promoting healthy outcomes for children. Political factors continually impact on all aspects of society and on every individual. Keeping current on the laws and regulations that guide school nursing practice can be a daunting task, but one that ensures maintaining professional standards and providing a high standard of care to the nation's children and adolescents.

References

Alaska Statute. (1996). *Religious Exemption to Criminal Child Abuse and Neglect*, Ala. Code 13A-16-6.

American Nurses Association (ANA). (2001). *Code for nurses with interpretive statements*. Washington, DC: American Nurses Association.

American Nurses Association (ANA). (1965). American Nurses Association first position on education for nursing. *American Journal of Nursing, 65*,106–107.

Chin, J. (2002). *Control of communicable disease manual*. Washington, DC: American Public Health Association.

Centers for Disease Control and Prevention (CDC). (2001). SHPPS 2000. *Journal of School Health, 7*(1), 1–98.

Centers for Disease Control and Prevention (CDC). (2002). *Healthy handwashing fact sheet. Retrieved March 25, 2005 from http://www.cdc.gov/od/oc/media/pressrel/fs/021025.htm*

Centers for Disease Control and Prevention (CDC). (2004). *National Immunization Program: Vaccines for children program*. Retrieved August, 2005 from http:www.cdc.gov/nip/vfc/default.htm

Centers for Disease Control and Prevention (CDC). (2005). *Comprehensive school health*. Washington, DC: National Center for Chronic Disease Prevention and Control.

Committee on Infectious Diseases (2002). *Red book 2002: Report of the Committee on Infectious Diseases* (26th ed.). Evanston, IL: American Academy of Pediatrics.

Dick, A. W., Allison, R. A., & Haber, S. G. (2002). Consequences of states policies for SCHIP Disenrollment. *Health Care Financing Review, 23*(3), 65–88.

Family Educational Rights and Privacy Act, 20 U.S.C.A. 1232g, regulations at 34 C.F.R.

Galarneau, C. A. (2002). Healthcare as a community good: Many dimensions, many communities, many views of justice. *The Hastings Center Report, 32*(5), 33–40.

Gostin, L. O. (2001). The human right to health: A right to the "highest attainable standard of health." *The Hastings Center Report, 31*(2), 29–30.

Lee, P. R., & Estes, C. L. (2001). *The nation's health*. Sudbury, MA: Jones and Bartlett.

McBeath, W. H. (1990). *Opening remarks, annual meeting of the American Public Health Association*. New York, October, 1, 1990.

Mills, R. J., & Bhandari, S. (2003). *Health insurance coverage in the United States: 2002*. Washington, DC: U.S. Census Bureau.

Nabors, L. A., & Mettrick, J. E. (2001). Incorporating expanded school mental health programs In State Children's Health Insurance Program plans. *The Journal of School Health, 71*(2), 73–76.

National Association of School Nurses (NASN). (2004). *Position statement: Caseload assignments*. Retrieved August, 2005 from http://nasn.org/positions/2004pscaseload.htm

National Association of School Nurses (NASN). (2002). *Position statement: Education, licensure and certification of school nurses*. Retrieved October 2005 from http://nasn.org/position/education.htm

National Association of School Nurses (NASN). (2004). *Issue brief: School health nurse's role in education. Privacy standards for student health records*. Retrieved April 2005 from http://www.nasn.org

National Clearinghouse on Child Abuse and Neglect Information (2003). *Child abuse and neglect state statutes elements*. Washington, DC: Department of Health and Human Services.

National Task Force on Confidential Student Health Information. (2000). *Guidelines for protecting confidential student health information*. Kent, OH: American School Health Association.

National Vaccine Information Center (2003). *National Childhood Vaccine Injury Act*. Retrieved August, 2005 from http://www.909shot.com

Pennsylvania Department of Health. (2001). *Procedure manual: School immunizations*. Harrisburg, PA.

Satcher, D. (1999). *Statement before the U.S. House of Representatives Committee on Government Reform*. Washington, DC, August 3, 1999.

Schwab, N. C., & Gelfman, H. B. (2001). *Legal issues in school health services*. North Branch, MN: Sunrise River Press.

Schwab, N. C., Panettieri, M. J., & Bergen, M. D. (1998). *Guidelines for school nursing documentation: Standards, issues and models*. Scarborough, ME: NASN.

Selekman, J. (March, 2004). The pediatrician, HIPAA, and the school nurse. What's AAP, doc? *The Delaware Chapter of the American Academy of Pediatrics Newsletter*, 2–3.

U.S. Department of Health and Human Services (USDHHS). (2002). *Final modification to the HIPAA Privacy Rule. Retrieved March 25, 2005 from* http://www.hhs.gov/ocr/hipaa/finalreg.html

U.S. Department of Health and Human Services (USDHHS). (2003a). *The Child Abuse and Treatment Act, including Adoption Opportunities and the Abandoned Infants Assistance Act, as amended by the Keeping Children and Families Safe Act of 2003*. Retrieved March 10, 2005 from http://www.hhs.gov/Programs/cb/laws/capta03/index.htm

U.S. Department of Health and Human Services (USDHHS). (2003b). *Questions and answers*. HIPAA Web site of the Office for Civil Rights. Retrieved August 2005 from http://www.hhs.gov/ocr/hipaa/

Chapter 14

Federal Laws Protecting Children and Youth with Disabilities

ELIZABETH K. GREGORY

Chapter Outline

INTRODUCTION

This chapter provides a history of U.S. federal laws, regulations, and court decisions related to students and staff with chronic conditions. It focuses on the Individuals with Disabilities Education Improvement Act (IDEA, 2004), the Americans with Disabilities Act (1990), and Section 504 of the Vocational Rehabilitation Act (1973). These laws provide educational opportunities, protection, and support for students in both special education and regular education who have special needs because of their disabilities.

There are many categories of students with special needs under the disabilities umbrella (Box 14.1), yet those listed do not cover all those with chronic conditions who do not require special education or additional educational services. Chapter 27 goes into great detail regarding various terminologies used when discussing this population as well as descriptions of many of the chronic conditions and their impact on the student. School districts have guidelines they must follow to serve students with disabilities. Many of these guidelines are based on federal laws.

FEDERAL LAWS ADDRESSING EDUCATION FOR CHILDREN WITH DISABILITIES: THE INDIVIDUALS WITH DISABILITIES EDUCATION IMPROVEMENT ACT

The Tenth Amendment to the United States Constitution (1791) states "powers not delegated to the United States by the Constitution, nor prohibited

Box 14.1 ■ ■ ■

DISABILITY CLASSIFICATIONS

Individuals protected under IDEA include those children who, after evaluation, are found to have mental retardation, a hearing impairment including deafness, a speech or language impairment, a visual impairment including blindness, serious emotional disturbance, an orthopedic impairment, autism, traumatic brain injury, and other health impairment, a specific learning disability, deaf-blindness, or multiple disabilities, and who, by reason thereof, need special education and related services (IDEA Regulations, 1999, 300.7 (a) (1).

Complete definitions of each disability term are located in IDEA Regulations, 1999, 300.7 (c).

by it to the states, are reserved to the states respectively, or to the people." Education has remained with state and local governments throughout the history of the United States. Certain activities, such as printing money and making treaties, are restricted to the federal government. States regulate many laws and services for residents of their states; education and nursing practice are two that relate to this chapter. How did the federal government, then, become involved in education?

Initially, every state provided free education, but only to some residents. The ability of a child with a disability to attend school depended on the interest of the state in which a child resided, the nature of the child's disability, and the parents' determination to provide their child with an education. Prior to 1975 more than half of the children with disabilities did not receive an education in the public schools. Many were excluded from school or misclassified, and therefore did not receive an appropriate education. Still others were sent to schools far from home in order to receive an education (Gelfman & Schwab, 2000; Gould, 2002; Reauthorization of IDEA, 2002). Public pressure and a growing awareness of the needs of individuals with disabilities led to enactment of many laws to protect their right to an education. Box 14.2 lists historic and current federal laws that support education and related services for students with disabilities. School nurses and school health services personnel are part of the education team serving these students and considered under *related services*.

Box 14.2 ■ ■ ■

FEDERAL STATUTES (LAWS) PROMOTING EDUCATION IN UNDERSERVED AREAS AND SPECIAL EDUCATION FOR CHILDREN WITH HANDICAPPING CONDITIONS

The United States Congress began enacting laws supporting special education in the 1960s. For state or local education agencies to continue to receive federal commodities or grants, the entity must comply with federal laws. Ensuring federal and state oversight of local education districts to ensure compliance was part of the rules for each statute.

1965—The Elementary and Secondary Education Act of 1965 (PL 89-10) was one of the first federal commitments to improve education for all. Congress authorized funds to support school-based programs for educationally disadvantaged children from low-income families. This law included the statutory basis upon which early special education legislation was drafted (Goodman, 2003).

1965—The Elementary and Secondary Education Amendment of 1965 (PL 89-313) became law a few months later and Congress authorized the first state-level grant program specifically to help states educate children with handicaps.

1966—The Elementary and Secondary Education Amendment of 1966 (PL 89-750) permitted school districts to apply for grants to help educate handicapped children, even though their state did not apply. The first federal education agencies, the Bureau of Education of the Handicapped (BEH) and the National Advisory Board (now the National Council on Disability), began to supervise compliance (Summarized at http://ahowell.usc.edu, 1998).

1970—The Elementary and Secondary Education Act (ESEA) Amendments of 1970, PL 91-230 introduced Part B, the Education of the Handicapped Act (EHA) (Goodman, 2003).

1974—The Education Amendments of 1974 (PL 93-230) was the first law to mention a provision for a *free, appropriate public education (FAPE)* for all children ages 5 to 18 regardless of handicap (Summarized at http://ahowell.usc.edu, 1998).

1975—The Education for All Handicapped Children Act of 1975 (EHA) (PL 94-142) was the landmark legislation that required all school districts receiving federal funds to provide a free, appropriate public education (FAPE) to all children 5 to 18 years of age regardless of the handicapping condition. This statute also stated that all related services necessary for a child to learn must be included.

1983—The Education of the Handicapped Amendments of 1983 (PL 98-199) provided federal funding to states that would develop parent training and information centers (PIC) so parents would learn more about their children's disabilities, their children's rights under EHA (1975), and how best to help their child learn. It also provided financial incentives to states to establish early intervention and early childhood education programs and demonstration projects for school-to-work and/or adult living transition programs.

1986—The Handicapped Children's Protection Act of 1986 (PL 99-372) permitted parents or guardians to be reimbursed for reasonable legal costs incurred when disputing special education and related services for their child with a school district, if the parents won the petition. The law requires parents and lawyers to discuss the cost of the legal council and the particulars of the case prior to beginning legal action.

1986—The Education for All Handicapped Children Amendments of 1986 (PL 99-457), also known as the Early Intervention Amendments, offered special funding incentives for states that would make a free, appropriate public education (FAPE) available through early intervention programs for infants and toddlers with handicaps and early childhood schooling for all preschool children, 3 to 5 years of age, with developmental delays (summarized at http://ahowell.usc.edu, 1998).

1988—The Technology-Related Assistance for Individuals with Disabilities Act of 1988 (PL 100-409), also known as "The Tech Act," assists states to develop comprehensive programs using the special equipment or assistive devices needed to support handicapped students and their learning needs. When IEP teams identify something that may enable a student to achieve the IEP objectives, it must be provided. This includes equipment, training, and services for the item for staff and parents.

1990—Individuals with Disabilities Education Act of 1990 (PL 101-476) (hereafter IDEA 1990) updated existing legislation. IDEA (1990) combined the concepts in the prior legislations [the Education for All Handicapped Children Acts of 1975 (PL 94-142); 1975 (PL 89-313); 1976 (PL 89-750); and 1983 (PL 98-199)], judicial decisions, and issues parents and educators had brought to the Department of Education. IDEA (1990) has also been known as the "Person first" law since the wording of the statute recognized the child first and the disability second; terms such as the asthmatic or handicapped student became the child with asthma or the student with a handicap. IDEA (1990) goals were to ensure that all children with disabilities had available to them a FAPE in the least restrictive environment (LRE). It also defined the rights of parents in the special education process.

1991—The Individuals with Disabilities Education Amendment Act of 1991 (PL 101-119) IDEA (1991) amended IDEA (1990) to mandate early intervention programs for children with developmental delays from birth to 5 years of age as a requirement for a state to continue to receive federal funds and commodities. States were to target children from at-risk or underserved groups, including families with low-income, and those who were from rural, minority, and other underserved populations for special education services.

1994—Improving America's Schools Act of 1994 (PL 103-382, also called the Amendment to the Elementary and Secondary Education Act of 1965), provided funds to address educating homeless children and youth. While educational opportunity for children who are disadvantaged had improved, further financial incentives were appropriated to ensure "that a high-quality education for all individuals and a fair and equal opportunity to obtain that education are a societal good, are a moral imperative, and improve the life of every individual, because the quality of our individual lives ultimately depends on the quality of the lives of others" (Improving America's Schools Act of 1994, Title 1, Sec. 1001).

1994—Goal 2000: Educate America Act of 1994 (PL 103-227) provided a framework of eight goals to assist states to reform educational programs for the next century. These included ensuring that students enter school ready to learn and that they demonstrate competence; that teachers receive continuing professional development; and that schools are free of drugs, alcohol, violence, and

(Continued on the following page)

Box 14.2 ■ ■ ■

FEDERAL STATUTES (LAWS) PROMOTING EDUCATION IN UNDERSERVED AREAS AND SPECIAL EDUCATION FOR CHILDREN WITH HANDICAPPING CONDITIONS *(Continued)*

firearms so that the environment is appropriate for learning to occur and that schools work with parents in partnerships.

1997—The Individuals with Disabilities Education Act Amendments of 1997 (PL 105-17) [hereafter IDEA (1997)] updated IDEA (1990) by including new Supreme Court decisions and comments from parents and educators. Congress authorized a complete revision of the IDEA Regulations (1999). It took 2 years to complete and must be updated every 5 years.

2001—No Child Left Behind Act of 2001 (PL107-110) (hereafter NCLB) is another landmark education reform bill. It reauthorized the Elementary and Secondary Education Act (1965), first enacted to assist children in underserved areas to receive a quality education. NCLB (2001) requires schools to demonstrate accountability; providing a quality education by using testing standards to measure student achievement; and requiring teachers to be credentialed for the courses they teach. Teachers and their administrators are accountable to parents for student success. Parents have the right to know how their local school measures against other schools in the district and may request a transfer if their children's school is 'low performing' (Walsh, 2003).

2004—Assistive Technology Act (H.R. 4278) was signed into law in October 2004. It revised the Assistance Technology Act of 1998 by continuing guaranteed funding through 2010 for students in need. The law will provide block grants to states with the stipulation that 60% to 70% of the money goes to direct service for students. It includes a provision for universal design principles that will be usable by people with the widest possible range of functional capabilities (CEC, 2004).

2004—IDEA (Individuals with Disabilities Improvement Act of 2004, PL 108-446). Signed December 2004 and implemented in July, 2005. Most revisions are to Part B, Assistance for Education of All Children with Disabilities (CEC, 2004).

Congress was also interested in equalizing educational opportunities for children living in rural or low socioeconomic areas of the country. Over time the federal government began providing states with some support for education, usually in the form of grants or commodities. In the 1960s Congress began awarding grants to states to encourage extra educational efforts for rural or underserved areas and for children with handicapping conditions. For a state or local education agency to continue to receive federal dollars or commodities for education, it had to comply with federal laws. Federal and state oversights to ensure compliance are part of the regulations for each law. By 1975, Congress required states that wanted to continue to receive federal grants or subsidies to provide educational opportunities and the necessary related services to all handicapped children (Education for All Handicapped Children Act, 1975). The purpose of this law (Box 14.3) was to provide children with disabilities an education tailored to their needs and abilities.

Box 14.3 ■ ■ ■

PURPOSE OF THE EDUCATION OF ALL HANDICAPPED CHILDREN ACT OF 1975 (PL 94-142)

It is the purpose of this Act to assure that all handicapped children have available to them... a free appropriate public education which emphasizes special education and related services designed to meet their unique needs, to assure that the rights of handicapped children and their parents or guardians are protected, to assist States and localities to provide for the education of all handicapped children, and to assess and assure the effectiveness of efforts to educate handicapped children.

(The Education of All Handicapped Children Act, 1975).

In the years following the Education for All Handicapped Children Act (1975), some students with handicapping conditions were provided access to an education, but students with profound physical disabilities or multiple healthcare needs, when enrolled, were centralized at one school in a district or assigned residential placement, rather than being served at their home school (Gelfman & Schwab, 2000). These arrangements did not provide all students an education in the *least restrictive environment* (LRE) as required by law.

Between 1975 and 1990, Congress amended the Education for All Handicapped Children Act (1975) several times to extend the age for children with handicaps who were entitled to services from birth through 21 years of age and to support training for parents of these children. In 1990 Congress approved the Individuals with Disabilities Education Act (hereafter IDEA [1990]). IDEA incorporated all prior special education laws and Supreme Court decisions.

The definitions of special education and related services did not change, but the term "handicapped child" became "a student with a disability." IDEA (1990) added the additional diagnoses of autism and traumatic brain injury as conditions eligible for special education services, an option to apply for grants to support services to infants and toddlers, and two additional related services that must be included in a student's Individualized Education Program (IEP)—assistive technology and transition services. The IEP is discussed later in this chapter.

IDEA was amended in 1997. It continued to affirm the basic principles of the Education for All Handicapped Children Act (1975), but required updating to include changes brought about by more Supreme Court decisions and concerns expressed by parents and educators.

IDEA (1997) is not a static law. As the services needed by students with disabilities change and technology introduces new services, updates are required. Congress included a plan to update IDEA Regulations every 5 years. IDEA Regulations (1999) has four parts: Part A, General Provisions; Part B, Grants to States; Part C, Infants and Toddlers Programs; and Part D, Support Programs. The Office of Special Education and Rehabilitative Services (OSERS) at the U.S. Department of Education held a series of public forums from 2002 to 2003 to solicit comments on the newest reauthorization of IDEA.

IDEA (1997) requires every school district that receives any federal money to provide special education services to eligible students. To qualify, a student must have a full and individual evaluation to determine if the student has a disability as defined under IDEA and because of that disability, needs special education and/or related services [IDEA Regulations, 1999, Sec. 300.7(a)(2)(ii)]. The evaluation must be sufficiently comprehensive so that all the student's special education and related services needs are identified [IDEA Regulation, 1999, Sec. 300.532(h)], including hearing, vision, and social and emotional status. The evaluation by trained and knowledgeable personnel must assess a child's actual abilities if sensory, motor, or language impairment is present (Goodman, 2003). If the evaluation shows that the student does, indeed, have a disability and that, because of that disability, he or she needs special education and related services, then he or she meets the criteria for access to special education and related services.

An appropriate evaluation enables a school team to discuss the impact of the child's disability on educational performance, identify his or her needs, and develop an appropriate educational program for the student (Eichman, 2003). In addition, team members must be aware of federal civil rights, special education laws, and Office of Civil Rights (OCR) opinions and meet their criteria. IDEA (1997) also mandates that students have the right to:

1. Assistance with educational needs that result from the disability
2. Advance appropriately toward attaining their annual goals
3. Be involved and progress in the general curriculum (i.e., the curriculum used by non-disabled students)
4. Participate in extracurricular and other nonacademic activities with other children with disabilities and non-disabled children [IDEA Regulations, 1999, Sec. 300.347(a)(3)].

Parents may request an independent evaluation if they can show that all avenues or evaluations were not used to determine their child's particular learning disability (Eichman, 2003). In one case, a parent arranged for an independent educational evaluation (IEE) following an IEP (Individualized Education Program) team's decision that a 15-year-old student was ineligible for special education as learning disabled (LD). Parents sought and received reimbursement for the IEE because the district's evaluation was insufficient in scope. The assessment did not include social/emotional/adaptive behavior assessments or process testing, although the district's assessment plan did list these areas of evaluation, and no observations of the student's behavior by anyone other than her teachers were reported. Observation of a student's behavior by professional personnel is a regulation for the evaluation of an LD (IDEA Regulations, 1999, 300.542). In addition, the health assessment was also inadequate, as it was based entirely on a review of school health records (Eichman, 2003).

Although Congress approved funding to states for the excess cost of educating students in special education at 40% in 1975, the reality is that the extra financial support has been only between 7% and 15% (Reauthorization of IDEA, 2002; Katsiyannis & Yell, 1999; Walsh, 2003). While Congress often proposes an increase in the government's contribution to districts for special education costs, the U.S. Department of Education does not always receive these funds (Walsh, 2003; What Congress is thinking, 2000).

Infants and children with disabilities are served through Early Childhood Intervention (ECI) programs. These programs require school districts to identify and provide assistance for infants and toddlers up to age 3 who have disabilities and their families (Education of All Handicapped Children Amendments, 1986; IDEA Regulations, 1999). In an ECI program, healthcare practitioners, such as dieticians, nurses, occupational and physical therapists, as well as speech language pathologists, social workers, and teachers, provide assessment and intervention services to the child and parent in the home or at a central location. Practitioners evaluate for deficits or delays in physical, cognitive, communication, social or emotional, or adaptive development or delays in multiple areas (IDEA Regulations, 1999).

Teams in these programs prepare an Individualized Family Service Plan (IFSP) for infants and young children with disabilities. All children with disabilities may be enrolled in early childhood education classes in the public schools at the age of 3; a child need not have been in an infant/toddler program to enter school at 3 years of age.

The No Child Left Behind Act (NCLB) (2001) reauthorized the Elementary and Secondary Education Act (1965), which was the first statute that addressed underserved populations. NCLB provides grants to states for disadvantaged children. The introduction to NCLB (2001) includes a report from the National Assessment of Educational Progress for the year 2000 that states that only 34% of fourth-grade students can read at a proficient level. While scores of the highest performing students have improved over the years, those of the lower performing students continue to decline. The NCLB (2001) goal is for all schools to accomplish high achievement for all children. States must ensure strong accountability for providing a quality education as measured by student achievement on standardized tests (Walsh, 2003). All teachers must be certified for the classes they teach and administrators are accountable to parents for student success. In some states, this certification requirement includes school nurses as well. Most of the funding for the initial (2003–2004) school year was earmarked for Title I: Improving the Academic Achievement of Disadvantaged Children (*Section 504 Compliance Book*, 2003).

The NCLB (2001) requirements include having qualified teachers and paraprofessionals in each classroom and ensuring that all students achieve at grade level. Almost every student is expected to take standardized tests or an alternative assessment. Modifications in testing for students with disabilities should be limited to those few students who cannot be tested by alternate assessment (*Section 504 Compliance Book*, 2003).

Approximately six and a half million children ages 3 to 21 were enrolled in special education during the 2001–2002 school year (National Center for Education Statistics, 2004). The number of additional students with chronic conditions who need accommodations under IDEA and the other laws is unknown, but is assumed to be significant.

The President's Commission on Excellence in Special Education Transition Task Force Hearing (Gould, 2002) presented problems among states with compliance to federal guidelines for students in special education. These included the fact that regulations were stipulated from multiple federal agencies; there was a lack of awareness among families of children in special education or with special needs regarding the laws and their rights; and problems existed with retention of students in special education. These difficulties contribute to the fact that many students do not complete their education or transition to another program (Gould, 2002). Approximately one in thirteen students, or 500,000 students in special education, did not complete their education or continue in another program (Gould, 2002).

In 1998, 75% of students in regular education classes completed their high school education and earned a diploma. Although this is a dismal reality, only 27% of students in special education who were eligible to graduate with a diploma did so. States reported graduation rates for students with disabilities ranging from 7% to 81% (Gould, 2002). The wide variance among the states indicates a problem in providing a *free, appropriate public education* (FAPE) for every student with a disability.

Supreme Court Rulings for Children with Disabilities that Impact on School Health Services

Many court cases followed the enactment of these laws as parents and school districts sought interpretation and clarification of special education laws. As federal laws first encouraged, then required, special education, parents and state and local education departments did not always agree on the required services. Parents were seeking the best educational opportunity for their children and districts were determined to provide required services, but no more.

Disagreements between parents and IEP teams (multidisciplinary teams) or the school district on required services are presented at due process hearings at the district level, before state Department of Education hearing officers, and in the courts. Both sides present their arguments for or against a program or service according to their interpretation of the law, and a judge or a group of judges makes a decision.

Judicial rulings provide precedent. A precedent is a previous judicial decision taken as a rule when dealing with subsequent, similar cases. The ruling may modify, disagree with, or strengthen the law being tested. When a parent requests a due process hearing in a district, the decision affects only that child and that district. An appeal to a state department of education hearing officer or to a state court becomes a precedent for similar cases in school districts in that state. Federal Court rulings impact every school district in each state in that court's jurisdiction; a Supreme Court ruling becomes a precedent for every school in the United States.

The Rowley decision (The Board of Education, 1982) identified the Supreme Court's definition of related services. Amy, an 8-year-old student with a hearing impairment, was enrolled in a regular education class and doing well. The parents requested that an interpreter for the deaf be provided for Amy to assist her in school. The school district refused because Amy was doing well in school. A lower court determined that Amy should have an interpreter. The district appealed to the Supreme Court. The Court agreed that Amy did not need an interpreter. Amy's educational program complied with the substantive requirements of FAPE (free and appropriate public education) since she performed better than the average child in her class (The Board of Education, 1982). The Court concluded that Amy's IEP offered an education equal to that provided her nonhandicapped classmates.

Based on this decision, school districts now determine the need for related services for a student using the "Rowley test." This is an important definition of what constitutes a required related service. The Justices' ruling limited related services to those things necessary for the student to learn. Significant court rulings that further define school health services for a child with a disability include the cases of Tatro (Irving Independent, 1984) and Garret F. (Cedar Rapids, 1999). Background information on these two cases is provided in BOXES 14.4 and 14.5.

Amber Tatro (Irving Independent, 1984), an 8-year-old student with spina bifida, attended special education classes in Irving ISD (Texas). The district had prepared an IEP that included speech and physical and occupational therapies, but they refused to provide clean intermittent catheterization because the district considered it a medical service.

The Supreme Court cited U.S. Department of Education regulations defining related services to include school health services [Education of the Handicapped Amendments of 1983, Sec. 300.24(b)(12)]. The Court determined the definition of medical services did exclude physicians' services as such, but that did not relate to nursing services (Irving Independent, 1984). The Supreme Court established these criteria to determine required services, sometimes called the "bright-line test" or the two-step test. A related service must be provided if it will assist the student to benefit from special education and the service does not have to be performed by a physician (Cedar Rapids, 1999; Irving Independent, 1984; NASN, 2001a).

A sub-case in Tatro (Irving Independent, 1984) was a request by the parents that the district pay legal fees incurred over the 4-year legal contest. Section 504 of the Rehabilitation Act (1973) allows for recovery of attorney's fees. They claimed discrimination by a program that receives federal funds under Section 504 of the Vocational Rehabilitation Act of 1973. The Texas District Court awarded compensatory damages and attorney fees to the parents. The Justices did not agree with the District Court's judgment for attorney fees under Section 504 of the Rehabilitation Act (1973), since the case was decided under the Education of the Handicapped Children Act (1975). Two years later, Congress passed the Handicapped Children's Protection Act (1986), which allowed parents or guardians to be reimbursed for reasonable legal costs if they prevail.

Families continued to demand services for their children with special needs. Following the Tatro decision (Irving Independent, 1984), a number of

Box 14.4

IRVING INDEPENDENT SCHOOL DISTRICT V. TATRO

Irving Independent School District V. Tatro Et Ux., Individually and as Next Friends of Tatro, a Minor Certiorari to the United States Court of Appeals for the Fifth Circuit No. 83-558. (Irving Independent, 1984).

Eight-year-old Amber Tatro, a child with spinal bifida, had been enrolled in special education classes since she was 3 years of age. Amber has orthopedic problems, speech impairment, and a neurogenic bladder. To prevent kidney damage, Amber required clean intermittent catheterization (CIC) every 3 to 4 hours. The district had prepared an IEP for the student that included speech and physical and occupational therapies. The parents cited the Education of All Handicapped Children Act (1975), arguing that CIC is an included related service under the statutory definition.

The Tatros could not resolve the issue of CIC through district or state due process hearings or litigation (Tatro v. Texas, 625 F.2d 557 CA5, 1980). The Texas District Court ruled in favor of the school district, holding that CIC was a medical service and, therefore, not required. The family appealed to the U.S. Court of Appeals for the Fifth Circuit (Tatro v. Texas, 1983) and that court determined that CIC was a related service, not a medical service, and thus, had to be provided by the school because the service was necessary for Amber to attend school.

Irving ISD then appealed to the U.S. Supreme Court (Irving Independent, 1984) and lost their case. The Supreme Court ruled that CIC services were not subject to exclusion as a medical service because the service did not need to be provided by a physician; indeed it is "a simple procedure that can be performed in a few minutes by a layperson with less than an hour's training" (Irving Independent, 1984, p. 2.).

Box 14.5

CEDAR RAPIDS COMMUNITY SCHOOL DISTRICT V. GARRET F. AND CHARLENE F

Garret Frey, paralyzed in a motorcycle accident when he was 4 years old, was ventilator dependent. Garret required ventilator supervision, tracheotomy supervision and suctioning, repositioning every hour, assistance with eating, catheterization, and assessments for respiratory distress and autonomic hyperreflexia. [Autonomic hyperreflexia is an uncontrolled visceral reaction to anxiety or a full bladder. Blood pressure increases, heart rate increases, and flushing and sweating may occur (Cedar Rapids, 1999, footnote 3)].

Garret successfully participated in a regular education class with assistance. He used a motorized wheelchair operated with a straw and a computer that responds to head movements (Cedar Rapids, 1999; Katsiyannis & Yell, 1999). During his early school years, Garret's family provided for his physical care during the school day through relatives or a licensed practical nurse (LPN) whose fee was paid by medical insurance.

The district had always assigned a teaching assistant to Garret and at one time the assistant was an LPN. Since the Iowa State Board of Nurse Examiners allows registered nurses to delegate client care to an LPN, the school nurse supervised Garret's care at minimal additional expense to the district. By middle school the family requested the district provide a nurse for Garret and the district refused. The family brought their request to a state hearing officer, an Administrative Law Judge (ALJ) at the Iowa State Department of Education. The ALJ determined that the district had to provide all the services the parent requested based on the Tatro bright-line test (Irving Independent, 1984), state law, and IDEA (1990) including provisions for nursing services for the student. The ALJ concluded that the district cared for other students with needs similar to Garret, except for ventilator dependency. While Garret needed a greater amount of complicated healthcare services than other students in special education, none were medical procedures that could be provided only by a physician.

The district challenged the decision of the federal court and the Court of Appeals (Cedar Rapids Community School District v. Garret F., 1997). That Court agreed with the ALJ, so the school district then appealed to the Supreme Court to hear the case on the basis that continuous one-on-one nursing service as a medical service was excluded under IDEA (1990).

courts ruled that the definition of medical services should go beyond the provider to consider complexity, cost, and burden of services to a school. That is, when health services were extremely expensive and complex, they were medical services and therefore not the responsibility of the school district. Courts in several states held different opinions on the scope of allowable school health services and medical services (Cedar Rapids, 1999; Macomb v. Joshua, 1989).

The question presented in Cedar Rapids Community School District v. Garret F. and Charlene F. (1999) was whether the definition of related services requires a public school district to provide a ventilator-dependent student with nursing services during school hours (Box 14.5). The Supreme Court decision required the district to pay for complex healthcare services when a medically fragile student needs them to be able to learn. This decision affirmed the rights of students with complex medical problems to a free, appropriate education in the least restrictive environment (Gelfman & Schwab, 2000). "This landmark decision solidifies and reaffirms the central role that school nurses play in the delivery of school health services under the IDEA . . ." (NASN, 2001).

The Justices maintained that the IDEA (1990) definition of related services, the Court decision in Tatro (Irving Independent, 1984), and the overall statutory scheme support the decision of the lower courts in this case (Cedar Rapids, 1999). The decision was based on law, not on the district's broad concerns for the financial burden of providing school health services to one student. The Court did acknowledge that the school district may have had legitimate concerns about the financial burden of providing the services Garret needed and the limit of existing staff; however, cost cannot be considered in determining a required service and this issue was outside the Court's authority (Cedar Rapids, 1999).

The Individualized Education Program (IEP)

IDEA Regulations (1999) define special education as specially designed instruction to meet the unique needs of a student with a disability. Every student in need of special education must have an *Individualized Education Program* (IEP). When a student with disabilities requires special services or assistive technology to access an education, the student's IEP must include a specific statement of such, including the nature and amount of such services [IDEA Regulations, 1999, Sec. 300.346 (a)(3)]. In addition, the plan must include specific goals to assist the student to learn; any related services the student might need; long-range vocational goals by age 14; and a transition to work/continuing education plan by age 16. The plan must specify when a service will begin, its frequency, where it will take place, and the duration [IDEA Regulations, 1999, Sec 300.347(a)(6)]. Box 14.6 presents an overview of a district's requirements under IDEA (1997).

Box 14.6 ■ ■ ■

DISTRICT REQUIREMENTS UNDER IDEA (1997)

Highlights of IDEA (1997) requirements for a school district include:

- Identifying all children with disabilities, birth through 21
- Providing a free, appropriate education in the least restrictive environment
- Monitoring by a state agency
- Defining members of the IEP team—school personnel and parents
- Evaluating a student with a multidisciplinary team of professionals knowledgeable in the area of a student's disability. An evaluation must include all areas of a student's unique needs
- Preparing IEPs that address the specialized needs of each student including long-range vocational goals
- Providing for at least an annual review of the IEP
- Notifying parents of their rights to:
  - –Approve evaluation and placement
  - –Participate as a member of the IEP team
  - –Access all records on their child
  - –Provide written consent for evaluation, placement, and re-evaluation
  - –Request an independent evaluation (Approval by the district is not automatic.)
- Developing mediation guidelines between parents and the school district
- Developing disciplinary procedures for students with disabilities and the relationship of a behavior to a disability (Gelfman, 2001; IDEA Regulations, 1999)

The district must provide assistive technology at no cost to parents [IDEA Regulations, 1999, Sec. 300.1 and 300.17 (a)(1) and (2)]. For example, an amplification system may be considered assistive technology under IDEA's definition when the IEP team determines that a child with a disability requires aided hearing and specifies such. If a student has difficulty mastering a goal, the IEP team must meet to review, evaluate, and revise it. Besides the need to provide required services for a student to learn, the district must include a plan to support a student on field trips and extracurricular activities.

For students 14 years of age and older, vocational or higher education goals must be included as part of their IEP and a transition plan needs to be provided for them. The purpose of the plan is to facilitate the transition of students from public school to college or vocational rehabilitation services and to define the financial responsibilities of each agency (IDEA, 1997). The state education agency oversees and coordinates a student's transition plan from school to vocational rehabilitation services, so this part of the IEP must include the procedures for coordinating activities between the designated state agency and the school personnel responsible for the public education of students with disabilities.

Individualized Education Program (IEP) Team

The Individualized Education Program (IEP) team, sometimes called a special education team or multidisciplinary team, includes professional school personnel, the parents or guardians, and at times the student. The team leaders must be knowledgeable about IDEA Regulations and other laws, such as the Americans with Disabilities Act (1990) and Section 504 of the Rehabilitation Act (1973), and services available within the district and community. Team members, including parents, must agree to the plan. Any risks to the student and/or training for personnel must be evaluated before determining an appropriate placement and intervention. Team members develop strategies to help the student learn. These are based on a student's test results, professional testing and evaluation, and a student's disabilities. Educational goals and related services necessary for the student to achieve these goals are recorded in the IEP. Health service needs for students that assist them and allow them to benefit from their educational program should be part of the plan (Cedar Rapids, 1999; IDEA, 2004; Irving Independent, 1984).

Parents are members of the IEP team. They need to be encouraged to speak out for their child. The family of a student dependent on nursing care in order to access a free, appropriate education needs to be sure the health care will be administered by properly educated and licensed individuals. If nursing services are required for students to maintain or improve their health status, the district must include such services, and as with other related services, it must be delivered by a qualified individual [IDEA, 2004, 612(14)(B)].

School Health Services as Part of the IEP Team

The Preface for IDEA (1997) proposes that the makeup of the IEP team include other individuals who have knowledge regarding the student. Related services personnel should be at a meeting when their particular specialty service will be discussed or at the request of the parents or the school (Gelfman, 2001). School health services described as related services in IDEA (1997) are "services provided by a qualified school nurse or other qualified person" (IDEA Regulations, 1999). The Supreme Court justices wrote, "As we noted in Tatro, the IDEA requires schools to hire specially trained personnel to meet disabled students' needs" (Cedar Rapids, 1999, footnote 8).

The role of the school nurse in school health services is an integral part of the school support team (Box 14.7). When a student requires a health service, the school nurse should be a member of the IEP team. However, it would be beneficial for the school nurse to be present for most IEP meetings or have access to the plans, as he or she will most probably interact with the identified student during the academic year during a health-related visit, a required screening, or in a class the school nurse is teaching.

Students must be at their optimum level of wellness in order to take full advantage of their educational opportunities. It is important to check state policy, as some states provide related services only for students receiving special education (Gelfman, 2001). IDEA (2004) states that "special education and related services..., based on peer reviewed research to the extent practical, to be provided a child, or on behalf of the child, and a statement of the program modification or supports for school personnel that will be provided for the child..." [IDEA, 2004, Sec. 614(d)(i)(A)(IV)].

Most often, the school nurse is the only school professional who can interpret medical records for the team; evaluate a student's specialized healthcare needs required as related services for the student to benefit from the educational program; and plan for the student's healthcare needs. School nurses and administrators will share a leadership role in fulfilling district obligations to students with complex health needs. The nurse or health services administrator is also responsible for designing the service delivery system, that is, framework, model,

Box 14.7 ■ ■ ■

THE ROLE OF THE SCHOOL NURSE AS PART OF THE IEP TEAM

The school nurse is prepared to:

- Assist in identifying children who may need special educational or health-related services.
- Assess the identified child's functional and physical health status, in collaboration with the child, parent(s)/guardian(s) and health-care providers.
- Develop individualized health and emergency care plans.
- Assist the team in developing an Individual Educational Plan (IEP) that provides for the required health needs of the child, which enables the student to participate in his/her educational program.
- Assist the parent(s) and child to identify and utilize community resources.
- Assist the parent(s) and teachers to identify and remove health related barriers to learning.
- Provide in-service training for teachers and staff regarding the individual health needs of the child.
- Provide and/or supervise unlicensed assistive personnel to provide specialized health-care services in the school setting.
- Evaluate the effectiveness of the health related components of the IEP with the child, parent(s), and other team members, and makes revisions to the plan as needed.
- Participate in the identification and evaluation of students who may be eligible for services under IDEA. Through shared responsibility with other team members, the professional school nurse assists in the planning and implementation of Individual Education Programs or Individual Family Service Plans as needed.
- Develop student goals and objectives and nursing protocols to meet student specific health needs during a school day, monitors student progress, and initiates an IEP reassessment when indicated.
- Serve as the team liaison to the medical community (NASN, 2002).

staffing patterns, and maintaining compliance with state nurse practice acts regarding delegation of nursing tasks (Schwab & Pohlman, 2002).

Nursing administrators and school nurses must be aware of specific state nursing board rules governing invasive procedures and delegation. Supreme Court decisions in Tatro (Irving Independent, 1984) and Garret (Cedar Rapids, 1999) did not address nursing services from the parameters of any state's nursing licensing board. Nurse licensing board rules vary from state to state. IDEA Regulations (1999) state that professional personnel serving special education students must meet the entry level requirements that are based on the highest requirements of the state applicable to the profession, and unlicensed assistive personnel need to be appropriately trained and supervised, in accordance with state law, regulations, or written policy (IDEA Regulations, 1999, Sec. 300.136). State agency guidelines that address school health services for special healthcare needs may include staffing requirements, infection control, medication administration, nursing procedures, classroom modifications, transportation, and policies (Porter, Haynie, Bierle, Caldwell, & Palfrey, 1997).

School health services may include interpretation of medical records, assessment of the student's symptoms, interventions, health appraisals, health education, a listening ear, the use of an assistive health device to compensate for the reduction or loss of a body function, case management, and advocacy. Students with special needs may require medication administration, chronic disease management, intermittent catheterization, tracheostomy care and suctioning, gastrostomy care and feedings, skin assessment, positioning, or equipment monitoring. They may have ventilators, central lines, or mobility devices that may require intermittent intervention.

The blanket mandate that all services a student needs in order to access an education are to be covered as long as a physician is not the provider is challenging to school districts, especially in light of shrinking budgets. Budget limitations and staffing plans are also part of the IEP team's discussions. The school nurse administrator or the school nurse should be prepared to offer suggestions. For example, if two students who require full-time nursing care can be transported together and educated in the same or adjoining classrooms, then only one nurse would be required to provide services to both students. The costs for specialized care must be weighed against the cost of residential placement; for example, a student with a psychiatric disorder requiring one-on-one services will be served in the home school at far less expense to a district than in a residential placement (Gelfman & Schwab, 2000).

The National Dissemination Center for Children with Disabilities (NICHCY, 2004), formerly titled the National Information Center for Children and Youth with Disabilities, provides information about special education services to parents and educators (see Chapter 27).

Districts may also explore the option of contracting school health services from the private sector. Such an option has already been adopted by many school districts when providing counseling or psychotherapy to students in special education (Katsiyannis & Yell, 1999). Some laws that fund medical care for children with disabilities are noted in Box 14.8.

A school district can assume all financial costs for healthcare services or look for other options. If a student is on Medicaid, the school nurse may bill for nursing services. "Depending on individual state Medicaid provisions, health services included in a Medicaid-eligible student's IEP are generally reimbursable to a school district if they participate in the Medicaid billing program" (Gelfman & Schwab, 2000, p. 56) (see Chapter 44).

District personnel cannot ask parents to use private insurance benefits toward the cost of school care if doing so would decrease the child's lifetime benefits under the insurance plan, if there is a deductible involved or if the insurance premium would increase (Shook v. Gaston County Board of Education, 1989). Parents cannot be required to provide the essential services a child needs to access an education (IDEA Regulations, 1999, Sec. 300.13). Indeed, since Garret (Cedar Rapids, 1999), insurance companies have exercised a government exclusion clause for services provided by a governmental agency (Gelfman & Schwab, 2000).

Box 14.8 ■■■

LAWS THAT FUND MEDICAL CARE FOR CHILDREN WITH DISABILITIES

1988—The Catastrophic Coverage Act (PL 100-360) permits "states to obtain limited funds for IEP-related services and for early intervention/family support services as defined in the individualized family service plan (IFSP)" (summarized at ahowell.usc.edu, 1998).

1989—Medicare Amendments (PL 101-239) "expands Medicaid's Early and Periodic Screening, Diagnosis, and Treatment (EPSDT) and allows Medicaid funds for "medically necessary" treatment without regard to the limits on a state's Medicaid plan" (summarized at ahowell.usc.edu, 1998).

The Student with Medically Complex Problems

IDEA (1997) has had a great impact on educational systems, including school health services. School personnel are faced with legal, ethical, and moral dilemmas as they try to meet the purpose of the law and the health and safety needs of students with disabilities. While students with chronic health problems may need direct or indirect professional nursing services, a small percentage of students with disabilities, identified as medically fragile, medically complex, or technology-dependent, require a great deal of support including constant monitoring. These students probably survived catastrophic physical events that required intensive and prolonged healthcare management. Their educational needs were secondary to survival. Students may have missed blocks of time from school or their cognitive ability may have been compromised. Learning potential may also be hampered by fatigue, lethargy, short attention span, and limited mobility (DePaepe, Garrison-Kane, & Doelling, 2004).

The issue of educating students with medically complex problems has evolved over many years through court decisions and amendments to federal laws. Several Supreme Court decisions on related services for healthcare needs define the role of school health services. Students with a medically complex health status usually have chronic conditions that require specialized health care, often because they are dependent on a ventilator, tracheostomy, supplemental oxygen, or nutritional supplements; they may have congestive heart problems or need apnea monitoring or kidney dialysis. Each medical condition presents its own unique set of characteristics that must be addressed before students can benefit from their educational experience (see Chapter 27). Since Garret (Cedar Rapids, 1999), IDEA requires "school districts to provide nursing services when such support services are necessary for students to access and benefit from their education program" (NASN, 2001, p. 1).

It is beneficial to all parties when the school nurse and administrator are aware of the needs of a student with medically complex needs prior to enrollment. Schools are allowed to postpone admission of a student for up to 10 days in order to prepare for the student (Gelfman, 2001). Before a student with healthcare needs arrives at school, the school nurse needs to speak to the parents and request access to the healthcare professionals responsible for the care of the child. If a student is transferring from another school, contact the caregivers at that school. When a student will be coming from a hospital or institutional setting, ask the parents to request all pertinent records for your review and use. A home visit may be in order. School nurses must be able to clearly describe a student's needs and existing laws that regulate health care and the credentials of the persons who may safely provide the care. Gelfman and Schwab (2000) identify the role of school health services for the student with healthcare needs to include:

- Developing policies that support a safe, school environment;
- Developing district school health services procedures;
- Preparing clear lines of decision making for the level of health care required by a medically complex student;
- Collaborating with administrators in hiring and assigning responsibilities to staff; and
- Training and supervising auxiliary personnel, if indicated (Gelfman & Schwab, 2000).

The IHP for a student with complex healthcare needs should include treatments or assessments with a focus on the level of care to be provided by school personnel on the service delivery team (Schwab & Pohlman, 2002). The school nurse will be responsible for ensuring that the staff is comfortable with and prepared to safely perform all procedures necessary for the student. Written guidelines for each treatment plan should be provided to each trainee, including a check off list of steps to follow and a skill sheet for training. Skill sheets should be signed, dated, and reviewed according to district or state protocols.

School nurses and parents are not the only people concerned with the level of care for a student. Special education college professors voice concern that those studying to be teachers do not get adequate training to serve students diagnosed with a variety of physical and health impairments. They consider special education students to be at risk when educators are not prepared to meet specialized healthcare needs for students. The Council for Exceptional Children (CEC) preservice preparation program standards for beginning special education teachers includes specific knowledge and skills that special educators need to acquire (DePaepe, Garrison-Kane, & Doelling, 2002). In one situation, a Florida appeals court ruled that paraprofessionals should not be expected to perform specialized procedures, even if the paraprofessional was trained and supervised by a registered nurse (Citation in the Courts, 2000).

The school nurse may be caught in an ethical dilemma trying to follow district policies or parent wishes when deciding which school personnel will be allowed to perform treatments and care of the students with invasive or noninvasive procedures. IDEA Regulations (1999) include a provision encouraging states to set standards for paraprofessionals who work with students in special education and related services (Schwab & Gelfman, 2001, p. 3; Weiss, n.d.). IDEA describes related services paraprofessionals as individuals who are appropriately trained and supervised [Sec. 612(14)(B)(iii)]. It is important to remind school administrators that the rules of the nurse practice act are to protect the public from unqualified or unlawful nursing, not to protect a nurse from liability (Schwab, Hootman, Gelfman, Gregory, & Pohlman, 2001). There are books describing specialized healthcare procedures, such as *Children and youth assisted by medical technology in educational settings: Guidelines for care* by Porter et al. (1997). In addition, home health agencies or children's hospitals may share the procedure guidelines they use to train parents. NASN publications Web site (http://www.nasn.org) has a vast array of resources. With these varied resources, the school nurse may find answers to specific delegation issues within his or her practice following what is required by the state nurse practice act.

The student with medically complex needs may have additional special needs not requiring nursing care, but still related to his or her healthcare needs. In situations as this, the school nurse may be requested to coordinate the care and support needed by this student. For example, a student with limited mobility and limited respiratory function may require a battery-operated wheelchair and a battery-powered ventilator in order to attend school. In addition to the health-related needs, the school nurse may be responsible to oversee the operation of the motorized wheelchair and ventilator. The school nurse will need to consult with the parents, the healthcare practitioner, a respiratory therapist, and perhaps a physical therapist to determine a plan of care. Questions that need to be addressed include what written plans are in place to provide training for the school health services staff, school support staff, and bus monitors, so everyone will know what to do if there is a battery failure. Everyone involved with the care of a student with special needs must know where the back-up generator is for the ventilator, in case of a battery failure. The teacher and classroom aide must know how to evacuate a student in an emergency. The emergency evacuation plans should be located in an easily identified place and reviewed with staff throughout the school year.

Questions, such as what to do if needed machinery is left on the bus, must be addressed.

FEDERAL LAWS PROTECTING ALL INDIVIDUALS WITH DISABILITIES: THE AMERICANS WITH DISABILITIES ACT AND SECTION 504 OF THE REHABILITATION ACT

If, after evaluation, a student does not qualify for special education services, the IEP team must consider whether or not the student may qualify for special services under Section 504 of the Rehabilitation Act of 1973 and/or the Americans with Disabilities Act (ADA) (1990) (Eggert, 2001). The Office of Civil Rights (OCR) in the U.S. Department of Education enforces Section 504 and ADA with regard to education. OCR interprets Section 504 and ADA requirements identically (Wrigley, 2002). Federal laws that protect all individuals are listed in Box 14.9.

In cases in which a student, after evaluation, is not in need of special education services, but, for example, is diagnosed as having attention deficit hyperactivity disorder (ADHD), the student may still be eligible for special services under Section 504 of the Rehabilitation Act of 1973 (1973). ADHD is one of the most frequent conditions identified as *other health impairment* (OHI) (see Chapter 30). Students with ADHD may qualify as disabled under other health impaired (OHI), learning disabled, or emotionally disturbed (IDEA, 1997), because ADHD may result in limited alertness (Eggert, 2001).

More than 254,000 students were classified as OHI in 1999–2000 (DePaepe et al., 2002). That number represents a 351% increase from 1990. Other health impairments are defined as:

> having limited strength, vitality or alertness, including a heightened alertness to environmental stimuli, that results in limited alert-

Box 14.9 ■ ■ ■

FEDERAL LAWS PROTECTING ALL INDIVIDUALS

1964—The Civil Rights Act of 1964 PL 88-352, based on the 14th Amendment, made it unlawful to discriminate against persons. Title VI of the civil rights act prohibits discrimination in federally funded programs. Discrimination occurs when the civil rights of an individual are denied or interfered with because of their membership in a particular group or class.

1973—Section 504 of the Vocational Rehabilitation Act of 1973 PL 93-112 (hereafter Section 504) is an anti-discrimination statute that protects persons with disabilities. This includes regular and special education students. The handicapped person is defined as one who:

1. Has a mental or physical impairment that substantially limits one or more major life activities,
2. Has a record of such impairment, or
3. Is regarded as having such impairment (Sec. 504 C).

1983—Vocational Rehabilitation Act of 1983 (PL 98-199). Revised and expanded the Vocational Rehabilitation Act of 1973.

1984—The Carl E. Perkins Vocational Act of 1984 (PL 98-524) assured individuals with special needs equal access to vocational education assistance with recruitment, training, and placement. It was amended in 1990 (PL 101-392).

1990—Americans with Disabilities Act of 1990 (PL 101-336) (hereafter ADA) ensures civil rights protections to individuals with disabilities and makes it illegal to discriminate on the basis of physical or mental disabilities in the areas of employment, public services, transportation, public accommodations, and telecommunications. ADA is an extension of two previous laws: The Civil Rights Act of 1964, barring discrimination on the basis of gender, race, religion and national origin and the Vocational Rehabilitation Act of 1973, barring discrimination in federally funded programs.

1992—Rehabilitation Act Amendments of 1992 (PL 102-569) revised and expanded the Vocational Rehabilitation Act of 1973 (PL 93-112) to ensure that an individual's wishes, strengths, resources, interests, and concerns are considered during the rehabilitation process, especially in the individualized written rehabilitation plan (IWRP). This law provides for personal assistance, transition, and supported employment services for individuals with more severe disabilities (summarized from www.ahowell.usc.edu, 1998).

ness with respect to the educational environment, that (i) is due to chronic or acute health problems such as asthma, attention deficit disorder or attention deficit hyperactivity disorder, diabetes, epilepsy, a heart condition, hemophilia, lead poisoning, leukemia, nephritis, rheumatic fever, and sickle cell anemia; and (ii) adversely affects a child's educational performance. (IDEA Rules and Regulations, 300.7(c)(9))

Section 504 of the Vocational Rehabilitation Act (1973) (Section 504) is an antidiscrimination statute that prohibits discrimination against qualified person with disabilities in federally funded programs and activities. The Vocational Rehabilitation Act (1973) provides vocational rehabilitation training or assistance in college to individuals in need, so they may gain employment. The OCR regards learning as a major life activity (Wrigley, 2002). Section 504 states that "No otherwise qualified individual with handicaps . . . shall solely by reason of his or her handicap, be excluded from the participation in, be denied the benefits of, or be subjected to discrimination under any program or activity receiving Federal financial assistance" (Section 504 of the Vocational Rehabilitation Act of 1973, abbreviated by Wrigley, 2002). The law was amended in 1978 to include all programs and activities conducted by federal agencies and the U.S. Postal Service and again in 1987 to codify the Supreme Court's decision that persons with AIDS and tuberculosis are also protected (*Section 504 Compliance Book*, 2003).

Section 504 protections are for any individual with a disability. A student does not have to fit into a disability category to receive services under Section 504. Regular and special education students with disabilities that affect learning are included in Section 504 services. For example, ADHD is not a listed disability under IDEA (1997), although in some cases a student with ADHD may fit into an IDEA (1997) category because of existing comorbidity. Under Section 504, the issue is simply whether the ADHD substantially limits the child's ability to learn (Wrigley, 2002). Some of the rulings related to the Civil Rights of students with special needs are listed in Box 14.10.

Schools, usually via a 504 team, must identify eligible students and notify parents and students of their rights. This team must include the parents and individuals who have the knowledge and relevant information to determine both the student's eligibility for accommodations as well as the accommodations that are necessary (Moses, Gilchrest, & Schwab, 2005). Students with conditions or disabilities that affect learning, such as dyslexia, ADHD, asthma, orthopedic impairments, emotional illness, and others, may qualify, if learning is substantially affected. The National Council on Disability reported that parents and educators continue to

Box 14.10 ■ ■ ■

THE U.S. DEPARTMENT OF EDUCATION'S OFFICE OF CIVIL RIGHTS (OCR) RULINGS FOR STUDENTS

The U.S. Department of Education's Office of Civil Rights (OCR) rulings for students so they may have a free and public education (FAPE) in the least restrictive environment (LRE) under IDEA (1997) and Section 504 include:

1. Physical site: All programs must be accessible to a student with disabilities, even if some parts of a school may not be.
2. Program: Education should be in the most integrated setting appropriate, preferably the regular education classroom. Section 504 defines a FAPE as regular or special education and related aids and services that are designed to meet individual educational needs of students with disabilities as adequately as the needs of nondisabled students are met.
3. Eligibility: Under IDEA and 504, the student must be provided with a comprehensive, individualized evaluation and periodic reevaluations and a written plan. For IDEA a special education student must have an IEP. A student protected by Section 504 does not need an IEP. Most important is that Section 504 requires students who have a disability, but are not in special education, to receive services in order to fully participate in the school program.
4. Students with disabilities but not in special education must receive assistive technology if needed to reach their full potential. Some health related assistive technology devices that have been ruled as necessary include:
   - Classroom hearing assistive device,
   - Closed caption decoder for a student with a hearing impairment while viewing videotapes, and
   - Tutorial software and a laptop for a student with narcolepsy (Wrigley, 2002).

complain about the lack of services for children with disabilities served in regular classrooms (Reauthorization of IDEA, 2002).

While IDEA Regulations (1999) refer to special education and related services, Section 504 refers to *accommodating* a student by the use of supplementary aids or services in regular education (*Section 504 Compliance Book*, 2003). School districts are required to:

- Identify and notify qualified, disabled students of their rights
- Evaluate students to determine eligibility
- Meet the needs of eligible disabled students as adequately as the needs of nondisabled students in all programs
- Provide a free, appropriate education
- Provide the parents of each eligible student with the required procedural safeguards (*Section 504 Compliance Book*, 2003; Vocational Rehabilitation Act, 1973).

A student evaluation in Section 504 may not mean testing. Information on a student may be gathered from a variety of sources, including aptitude and achievement tests, teachers' reports, discipline referrals, health information, parent information, and students' grades. Student placement by the IEP team or the 504 team usually refers to the regular education classroom with individually planned accommodation (*Getting to know Section 504 . . .*, n.d.).

The school nurse may play a vital role in identifying and evaluating students who may be eligible for services under Section 504. What accommodations might a student with a chronic health problem, such as asthma or diabetes, need? Accommodations may include a rest period in the school health office, permission to use the bathroom at any time without permission, or special writing implements. Specialized areas of assessment and implementation may include, but are not limited to, the following:

- Assessment of student health status through communication with the parents and health-care providers
- Consultation with the classroom teacher and guidance counselor on medical issues related to the student
- Development of student goals and objectives and nursing protocols to meet student specific health needs during a school day
- Monitoring student progress, and initiation of a new accommodation plan, when indicated
- Serving as the team liaison to the medical community
- Maintaining open communication with the family on the health status of the student

"Students who qualify for special education services under the IDEA Act will automatically qualify as a handicapped person under Section 504, and...such students' individualized education plans (IEPs) will almost always satisfy the requirements for an accommodation plan" (Moses et al., 2005, p. 49). While an IEP will usually include everything that might be included in a 504 plan (see Chapter 9), occasionally a student has more than one problem where one condition is addressed in an IEP and the other requires a 504 plan.

The Americans with Disabilities Act (ADA) (PL 101-336, 1990) ensures civil rights protections to individuals with disabilities. The ADA defines a person with a disability as one who has impairments that substantially limit major life activities such as seeing, hearing, speaking, walking, breathing, performing manual tasks, learning, caring for oneself, and working (ADA, 1990). The Act makes it illegal to discriminate on the basis of physical or mental disabilities in the areas of employment, public services, transportation, public accommodations, and telecommunications. Individuals with a record of a disability, such as a person who has recovered from cancer or mental illness, would be protected from discrimination. ADA (1990) also protects individuals who are regarded as having a substantially limiting impairment, even though the impairment may not impact on their ability to work or study. For example, an individual who is disfigured after facial burns is protected from being denied employment because an employer might fear negative reactions from customers.

THE SCHOOL NURSE'S ROLE

The role of the school nurse is to maintain or improve optimum health of all students so they can participate in their educational program. The specialty of school nursing has a foundation in general nursing practice and these nursing skills and services are utilized in school health services for students with special needs. Supreme Court rulings specify that school districts must provide a particular health service as a related service when it is necessary for a student to attend school, as long as it is a procedure that can be performed by a school nurse or other qualified person (Cedar Rapids, 1999; Irving Independent, 1984; Weiss, n.d.).

Because students with chronic and special healthcare needs have unique health considerations, individualized nursing assessment, planning, and intervention are critical to identifying appropriate placement and service decisions and must be included in an Individualized Healthcare Plan (IHP) (NASN, 2002). Nursing diagnoses must be client specific and current. Student-centered goals for maintaining or improving health and all treatment plans need to be written. The nurse will usually need to contact the parent and healthcare providers in order to develop an appropriate plan, but records from a prior school may be available and current. School nurses should use the IEP team meeting as an opportunity to educate other team members on the special health service needs of a student and the value to the student when the Individualized Healthcare Plan (IHP) and emergency action plan are incorporated into the IEP.

Some students may also need an emergency plan for situations such as an emergency evacuation or a power outage that "includes specific information about the child's medical condition, current and emergency medications, and appropriate emergency intervention" (NASN, 1998). (See Chapter 9 for more information on IHPs.)

When school nurses are not invited to participate on the IEP team, nurses need to assert their role as advocate for the health of the students. The school nurse needs to know and have an impact on all decisions approved by the IEP team because a student in special education will come to the health office for care. When school nurses are not included in IEP team meetings, they should discuss each student's perceived needs with the parents, administrator, and IEP team leader to explain how the student's diagnosis or healthcare needs may require school nurse intervention.

The nurse may need written treatment plans approved by the ordering physician and a request to provide the service from the parent. This requirement may vary among states, so it is important to be aware of the regulations for physicians' orders in state nurse practice acts.

Skills necessary for a student to access an education may range from the simple, such as providing a clean, safe place for the student to perform self-catheterization, to the complex, such as providing treatments to a student who is ventilator dependent. The school nurse may need to seek knowledge and skills training in order to care for a particular student. This is a personnel, not an IEP team matter, that the nurse must discuss with his or her supervisor (Schwab & Pohlman, 2002). That knowledge or skill training may come from the student's physician or case manager as well as from the family and community agencies. Advanced practice nurses in specialty clinics are an ideal resource for information on skills and updates on treatments. The Supreme Court determined in Garret (Cedar Rapids, 1999) that school health services provided by a qualified school nurse or other qualified person are considered to be related services under IDEA (1997), regardless of whether these services require a nurse for one-half hour per week or one-on-one throughout the school day. This ruling has not been challenged.

Children enrolled or awaiting testing for early childhood education class at a school provide new challenges for a school nurse. The reality may be that a 3-year-old child is admitted to an early childhood class by an IEP team before the nurse evaluates the child. The child needs to be screened and a health history obtained, whether the child is awaiting testing or is currently enrolled. The school nurse will have to assess the student as soon as possible. It may take more than one visit to complete screening for a young child. Should a child enter an early childhood program before vision and hearing testing and a health history are completed, the nurse needs to remind the IEP team privately of these requirements before admitting a child to a special education program. The school team would be out of compliance with federal and state evaluation guidelines [IDEA Regulation, 1999, Section 300.532(g)].

Communication

Parents see the nurse as a qualified professional who helps their child. They may ask the school nurse for advice and counsel about special education services for their child. Nurses, by nature, want to help, but there are many legal implications to advising about special education services. The school nurse is the authority on nursing care. When the questions are about school health service delivery, refer to district guidelines and the director of school health services for answers. While the school nurse is not expected to know everything about a student's health problem or remediation to promote health, the nurse should have resources available.

A topic that parents may have concerns about and solicit a school nurse's opinion or support could be the benefits of an independent evaluation for their child. When the questions are out of the realm of health care, defer to the experts. As a member of the IEP Team, unless the school nurse is fully versed in the intricacies of special education laws and school board policy, when parents ask about a child's educational program, the nurse should refer them to the child's teacher, counselor, a school administrator, or the district special education department. Those educational professionals will be better versed in district, state, and federal guidelines for special education.

Discipline as Part of IDEA (1997) and Section 504

IDEA Regulations (1999) provide explicit provisions for disciplining students with disabilities. These provisions are intended to protect the rights of children with disabilities and their parents, while at the same time addressing the concerns of school administrators and teachers regarding school safety and order. The provisions are also intended to help schools respond appropriately to a student's behavior and promote the use of behavioral interventions to prevent troubling behavior from recurring. As part of the IEP team, the school nurse will be involved in discussions about discipline measures for students. Should a student exhibit unacceptable behavior at school, positive behavioral interventions must be addressed in the IEP. Positive behavioral interventions (see Chapter 38) and supports involve a comprehensive set of strategies aimed at providing a student with a disability an improved lifestyle that includes reductions in problem behaviors, changes in social relationships, an expansion of prosocial skills, and an increase in school and community inclusion (Fox, Vaughn, Dunlap, & Bucy, 1997).

School personnel, the student, or the student's parents may need to discuss differences with the district special education specialist or the 504 specialist when parties do not agree. The school or district special education or the 504 specialists will have legal information about discipline that they can share with the parent.

Section 504 offers protection for students with behavior problems similar to IDEA (1997). When a student begins to exhibit behavior problems, the district should first attempt to address the problem by determining whether the placement is appropriate or whether additional services are needed (Wrigley, 2002). Students with disabilities are not protected from suspension or expulsion for the following infractions:

- "Violate a school rule or code of conduct that is subject to disciplinary action
- Carry a weapon to (or possess a weapon at) school or a school function
- Knowingly possess or use illegal drugs or sell or solicit the sale of a controlled substance while at school or a school function
- Are substantially likely to injure themselves or others, if left in their current educational placement" (IDEA Regulations, 1999, Sec. 300.520–529).

The school nurse should not be in the role of disciplinarian, but should follow the behavior plan as a team member while always being an advocate for all students. The school nurse will want to be sure that the student's healthcare needs are considered when an intervention plan is developed and carried out. The nurse should be an advocate for the student concerning the positive or negative effects of an intervention. The nurse may be a daily participant in the care of students with behavioral problems, especially if they receive daily medication or specialized treatments. The nurse is often well acquainted with these students and their families and will need to follow a student's behavioral intervention plan as the need arises. The school nurse must assess if the behavior the student is exhibiting is consistent with the student's past behaviors, or whether it might be a symptom of disease, distress, or medication. If parents voice a concern to the school nurse, or if the school nurse has concerns about the appropriateness of disciplinary actions, a meeting of the IEP team can be called to address the student's need for positive behavioral interventions.

CONCLUSION

Special education and educational accommodations have evolved over many years through the diligent work of students, parents, educators, and the federal government. These expectations, coupled with the financial constraints every school faces, are still a dilemma today. Whereas 30 years ago only one fifth of all children and adolescents with disabilities in the United States were being educated, at present almost every child with disabilities attends school (Gould, 2002). There is still much work to be done on the national, state, and local levels to provide an adequate education for all students. Many of the terms used in the laws are confusing to the public and to health professionals. A synopsis of terms is provided in Box 14.11.

Advocacy groups and school nurse leaders have paved the way for the still-evolving inclusion of the registered nurse and school health services for students with disabilities. The issue of qualifications for individuals providing health care is an ongoing debate. It is important to consider current school healthcare practices for all students as well as the increase in the numbers of children with disabilities

Box 14.11 ■■■

DEFINITIONS OF TERMS IN SPECIAL EDUCATION STATUTES

Free appropriate public education (FAPE) is provided at public expense, under public supervision and direction, and without charge. It meets the standards of the state agency and includes preschool, elementary and secondary school education that is provided in conformity with the IEP [IDEA, 1997, Sec. 614(d)].

Individualized Educational Program (IEP) is a written statement for each child within a district that includes the nature of the student's educational needs, the services to be provided, and specific goals for the student. The IEP must be developed, reviewed, and revised in accordance with this section [IDEA, 1997, Sec. 614(d)(1)(A)].

Least restrictive environment (LRE)—each public agency shall ensure that to the maximum extent appropriate, children with disabilities, including children in public or private institutions or other care facilities, are educated with children who are non-disabled; and that special classes, separate schooling or other removal of children with disabilities from the regular educational environment occurs only when the nature or severity of the disability is such that education in regular classes with the use of supplementary aids and services cannot be achieved satisfactorily [IDEA Regulations, 1999, Sec 300.550(b)].

Related services—those specialized services necessary for a child to access and progress in their education program. Covered items include "transportation and such developmental, corrective, and other supportive services as are required to assist a child with a disability to benefit from special education" [IDEA Regulations (1999), Sec. 300.24(a)].

Special education—specially designed instruction, at no cost to parents, to meet the unique needs of a child with a disability [IDEA Regulations, 1999, Sec. 300.26(a)].

School health services—services provided by a qualified school nurse or other qualified person [IDEA Regulations, 1999, Sec. 300.24(b)(12)].

and complex healthcare needs in regular and special education classes. Will the number of school nurses increase to adequately care for this population? Every school nurse needs to understand the past, work in the present, prepare for the future, and always advocate for the child and parent.

References

Amendment to the Elementary and Secondary Education Act of 1965, PL 103-384. (1994). Retrieved January 16, 2004 from http://www.ed.gov/legislation/ESEA/toc.html

American Academy of Pediatrics (AAP), Committee on Pediatric Emergency Medicine. (2000). *Emergency preparedness for children with special health care needs. Pediatrics, 104*(4). Retrieved January 10, 2004 from http://www.pediatrics.org/cgi/content/full/104/e53

Americans with Disabilities Act (ADA) of 1990, PL 101-336; USCA 12101 (West 1993); 2,104 Stat. 328 (1991). Retrieved March 18, 2003 from http://www.unc.edu/-ahowell/exceplaw.html

Assistive Technology Act (H.R. 4278). (2004). Retrieved on November 3, 2004 from http://www.cec.sped.org/pp/legislative_update/modules/news/article.php?storyid=84

Bill of Rights. (1791). Retrieved March 12, 2004 from http://lcweb2.loc.gov/const/bor.html

Carl E. Perkins Vocational Act of 1984, PL 98-524. (1984). Retrieved March 18, 2003 from http://www.unc.edu/-ahowell/exceplaw.html

Catastrophic Coverage Act, PL 100-360. (1988). Retrieved March 18, 2003 from http://www.unc.edu/-ahowell/exceplaw.html

Cedar Rapids Community School District v. Garret F, 119 S.Ct. 992, 29 IDELR 966 (U.S. 199). (1999). Retrieved February 12, 2003 from http://supct.law.cornell.edu/supct/html/96-1793.ZS.html

Citation in the Courts . . . (2000). Court finds catheterization not 'expected work' for paraprofessionals. *Health & Health Care in Schools, 1*(10), 1.

Civil Rights Act of 1964, PL 88-352. (1964). Retrieved January 16, 2004 from the Legal Information Institute at http://www.law.cornell.edu/topics/civil_rights.html

Definition of a Child with a Disability. IDEA. (1997). (20 U.S.C. 1401(3)(A) and (B); 1401(26)).

DePaepe, P., Garrison-Kane, L., & Doelling, J. (2002). Supporting students with health needs in schools: An overview of selected health conditions. *Exceptional Children, 35*(1), 1–22.

Detsel v. Auburn Enlarged City School District Board of Education, 820 E2d 587 (2nd Cir. 1987). January 16, 2004 from http://www.ed.gov/legislation/ESEA/toc.html

Education of All Handicapped Children Act of 1975, PL 94-142. (1975). Retrieved August, 2005 from http://asclepius.com/angel/special.html

Education Amendments of 1974, PL 93-280. (1974). Retrieved March 18, 2003 from http://www.unc.edu/-ahowell/exceplaw.html

Education of the Handicapped Act Amendments, PL 98-199. (1983) Retrieved August, 2005 from http://www.unc.edu/~ahowell/exceplaw.html

Education of the Handicapped Act Amendments of 1986, PL 99-457. (1986). Retrieved August 2005 from http://www.nichy.org/pubs/outprint/nd/5txt.htm Introduction.

Eggert, D. (2001). *Special education law update*. Presentation to Nashua School District on April 14 2001. Retrieved March 20, 2003 from: http://www.wadleighlaw.com/Articles/School/special_education_update.htm

Elementary and Secondary Education Act of 1965, PL 89-10. (1965). Retrieved March 20, 2003 from http://www.ed.gov/legislation/ESEA/toc.html

Eichman, S. (2003). Ascertaining the Adequacy, Scope, and Utility of District Evaluations University of Northern Iowa. *Exceptional Children, 69*(2), 227–247.

Fox, L., Vaughn, B., Dunlap, G., Bucy, M. (1997). Parent–professional partnership in behavioral support: A qualitative analysis of one family's experience. *Journal of the Association for Persons with Severe Handicaps, 22*(4), 198–207.

Gelfman, M. H. B. (2001). Special Education Law. In N. C. Schwab & M. H. B. Gelfman (Eds.), *Legal issues in school health services, a resources for school administrators, school attorneys, school nurses* (pp. 373–397). North Branch, MN: Sunrise River Press.

Gelfman, M. H., & Schwab, N. (2000). School health services after Cedar Rapids Independent School District v. Garret F. *Journal of School Nursing, 16*(4), 54–59.

Getting to know Section 504 of the Rehabilitation Act of 1973: A guide for parents. (n.d.). [Brochure]. Sugar Land, TX: Ft. Bend Independent School District.

GOALS 2000: Educate America Act (PL 103-227). (1994). Retrieved March 18, 2003 from http://222.unc.edu/-ahowell/exceplaw.html

Goodman, S. (2003). *What's reauthorization all about? NICHCY's IDEA News* (March 2003). pp. 1–6. Retrieved April 10, 2004 from http://www.nichcy.org

Gould, M. (2002). *Written remarks of Martin Gould submitted for the record to the President's Commission on Excellence in Special Education, Transition Task Force Hearing, April 30, 2002*. Retrieved March 18, 2003 from http://www.ncd.gov/newsroom/testimony/gould_04-30-02.html

Handicapped Children's Protection Act of 1986, PL 99-372. (1986). Retrieved March 18, 2003 from http://www.unc.edu/-ahowell/exceplaw.html

Individuals with Disabilities Education Act (IDEA), PL 101-476. (1990). *Also called the Education for All Handicapped Children Act Amendments of 1990*. Retrieved March 18, 2003 from http://www.unc.edu/-ahowell/exceplaw.html

Individuals with Disabilities Act (IDEA). (1991). *Individuals with Disabilities Education Act Amendments, PL 101-119*. Retrieved April 5, 2003 from http://www.ed.gov/offices/OSERS/IDEA/index.html

Individuals with Disabilities Education Act (IDEA) Amendments. (1997). PL 105-17, (1997). 20 U.S.C. Chapter 33, Sections 1400–1485, 1997. Retrieved March 18, 2003 from http://www.unc.edu/-ahowell/exceplaw.html

Individuals with Disabilities Act (IDEA) Regulations. (1999). Code of Federal Regulations: Title 34; Education; Part 300–399; 20 U.S.C. 1401 (3) (B); *Federal Register, 64*(48), 12406-1267. Retrieved April 5, 2003 from http://www.ed.gov/offices/OSERS/IDEA/index.html

Individuals with Disabilities Act (IDEA). (2004). Individuals with Disabilities Education Improvement Act of 2004, PL 108-446. 118Srat.2647. Retrieved December 2004 from http://www.cec.sped.org/pp/legislative_update

Improving America's Schools Act, PL 103-382. (1994). Retrieved September 2, 2004 from http://www.ed.gov/legislation/ESEA/toc.html

Irving Independent School District v. Tatro Et Ux., Individually and as Next Friends of Tatro, a Minor Certiorari to the United States Court of Appeals for the Fifth Circuit No. 83-558. (1984). (short title—Irving Independent School District v. Tatro, 468 U.S. 883, EHLR 555:511) Retrieved January 2003 from http://caselaw.lp.findlaw.com/ scripts/getcase.pl?navby=search&court=US&case=/us/468/883.html

Katsiyannis, A., & Yell, M.I. (1999). The Supreme Court and school health services: Cedar Rapids v. Garret F. *Exceptional Children, 66*(3), 317–326.

Macomb County Intermediate School District v. Joshua S., 715 E Supp. 824 (E. D. Mich. 1989). Retrieved January 16, 2004 from http://www.ed.gov/legislation/ESEA/toc.html

Moses, M., Gilchrest, C., & Schwab, N. (2005). Section 504 of the Rehabilitation Act: Determining eligibility and implications for school districts. *The Journal of School Nursing, 21*(1), 48–58.

National Association of School Nurses (NASN). (1998). *Position statement: Emergency care plans for students with special health care needs*. Retrieved September 1, 2004 from http://nasn.org/positions/emer_care.htm

National Association of School Nurses (NASN). (2001). *Issue brief: Impact of Cedar Rapids Community School District vs. Garret F. on school nursing services*. Scarborough, ME: Author.

National Association of School Nurses (NASN). (2002). *Issue brief: School health nursing services role in health care: School nurses and the Individuals with Disabilities Education Act (IDEA)*. Scarborough, ME: Author.

National Center for Education Statistics. (2004). *Digest of Educational Statistics, 2003*. Retrieved December, 2004 from http://necs.ed.gov/programs/digest/d03/tables/dt054.asp

National Dissemination Center for Children with Disabilities (NICHCY). (2004). Retrieved September 2, 2004 from www.nichcy.org

No Child Left Behind Act (NCLB), PL107-110. (2001). Retrieved August, 2005 from *http://www.ed.gov/policy/elsec/leg/esea02/index.html*

Porter, S., Haynie, M., Bierle, T., Caldwell, T., & Palfrey, J. (1997). *Children and youth assisted by medical technology in educational settings: Guidelines for care*. Baltimore: Paul H. Brookes.

Reauthorization of IDEA. (2002). *Federal Register. April 3, 2002, 67 (64), pp. 15830–15834. National Council on Disability. Retrieved March 5, 2004 from http://frwebgate.access.gpo.gov/cgi-bin/getdoc.cgi?dbname=2002_register&docid=fr03ap02-81*

Schwab, N. C., Hootman, J., Gelfman, M. H. B., Gregory, E. K., & Pohlman, K. J. (2001). School nursing practice: Professional performance issues. In N. C. Schwab & M. H. B. Gelfman (Eds.), *Legal issues in school health services, a resources for school administrators, school attorneys, school nurses. (pp. 123–166)*. North Branch, MN: Sunrise River Press.

Schwab, N. C., & Pohlman, K. J. (2002). Legal and ethical issues: Questions and answers. *Journal of School Nursing, 18*(5), 301–305.

Section 504 compliance book. (2003). Washington, DC: Thompson Publishing Group.

Section 504 of the Vocational Rehabilitation Act of 1973. (1973). Retrieved March 18, 2003 from http://www.unc.edu/~ahowell/exceplaw.html

Shook v. Gaston County Board of Education. (1989). 882 F.2d 119, EHLR 441:561 (4th Cir.). Retrieved January

16, 2003 from http://supct.law.cornell.edu/supct/html/961793.ZO.html

The Board of Education of the Hendrick Hudson Central School District, Westchester County, et al., Petitioners v. Amy Rowley, by her parents, Rowley et al. Respondent (1982). No. 80-1002 U.S. S. Ct, 1982. Retrieved January 16, 2004 from http://www.ed.gov/legislation/ESEA/toc.html

Vocational Rehabilitation Act of 1973, PL 93-112. (1973). Retrieved March 18, 2003 from http://www.unc.edu/-ahowell/exceplaw.html

Walsh, J. (2003). A look at the no child left behind act: Two years later. *Legal Digest, 19*(9), 1–3.

Weiss, J. (n.d.). *Providing safe health care: The role of education support professionals*. Washington, DC: National Education Association Office of Support Personnel and the National Center for Innovation.

What Congress is thinking. (2000). Health and Health Care in Schools, 1(10), 1.

Wrightslaw Web page. (2004). *Updates on discussions on IDEA Reauthorization of 2004*. Retrieved November 4, 2004 from http://www.wrightslaw.com/news/idea2002.htm

Wrigley, J. (2002). *Section 504 and students with disabilities: An overview*. Retrieved February 2, 2003 from http://www.oradvocacy.org/pubs/sec504overview.htm

PART IV

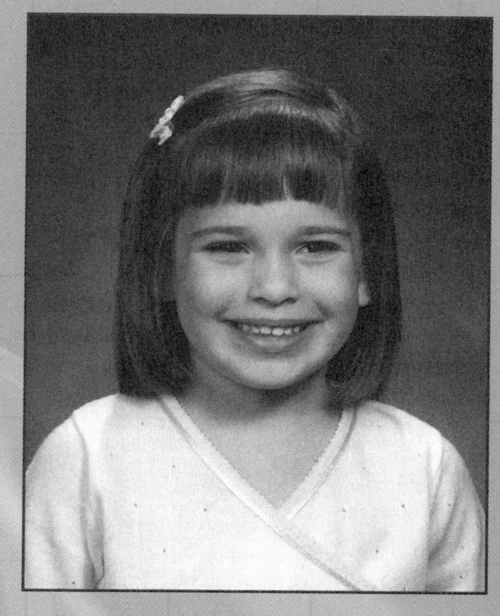

The Well Child: Preschool, School Age, and Adolescent

Chapter 15

The Demographics of Children and Adolescents

KATHY RILEY-LAWLESS

Chapter Outline

INTRODUCTION

The demographics of children and adolescents provide descriptive information to school nurses about the populations they serve. Population numbers and trends, family-centered statistics, and health-related information present school nurses with information that may influence their practice and assist in future planning. Through use of and understanding of these demographics, nurses promote both health and school success in children and adolescents.

POPULATION OF CHILDREN AND ADOLESCENTS

According to the 2000 population survey, there are a total of 80,473,265 children and adolescents in the United States. This accounts for 28.6% of the total U.S. population (U.S. Census Bureau, 2000). Table 15.1 lists the breakdown by age. However, it should be recognized that this number may not account for those children who are homeless, living in shelters and group homes, and or who are non-citizens.

By excluding the approximately 11,416,676 infants and children younger than 3 years, that leaves approximately 69 million American children considered to be school age. Of these, between 56 and 58 million are enrolled in preschool, elementary, and high school.

The racial and ethnic composition of children younger than 18 years of age is shown in Table 15.2. The percentage of white non-Hispanic children has declined steadily over the past two decades and this decline is expected to continue. While the percentage

The author thanks Dyane Bunnell, MSN, RN for her assistance in collecting data for this chapter.

Table 15.1 ■

POPULATION OF CHILDREN AND ADOLESCENTS BY AGE

Younger than age 5	19,175,798
5–9	20,549,505
10–14	20,528,072
15–19	20,219,890

Source: U.S. Census Bureau (2000).

of the black, non-Hispanic population has stayed relatively the same, the percentage of the Hispanic population has doubled in that same period of time and is projected to increase further.

It is estimated that 53,167,000 children are enrolled in American elementary and secondary schools. Of these, 47,223,000 attend public and parochial schools and 5,944,000 attend private school. This chapter does not address the needs of those children who are home schooled or not otherwise in the formal educational system.

FAMILY STRUCTURE

Families and the environments in which they live influence all aspects of a child's development. Family environment characteristics such as family structure, economic status, and use of professional health services influence children's health status, health behaviors, and school achievement. Knowledge of these family influences enables the school nurse to foster child health and ultimately school achievement (see Chapter 17).

Table 15.2 ■

PERCENTAGE OF CHILDREN AND ADOLESCENTS BY RACE

White non-Hispanic	64%
Black non-Hispanic	15%
Hispanic	16%
Asian/Pacific Islander	4%
American Indian/Alaska Native	1%

Source: http://ChildStats.gov (n.d.).

Although a majority of children are living with two parents, there is increasing diversity of family structure and composition. Children today are being cared for by single parents, mixed-race families, foreign-born parents, gay and lesbian parents, kinship families comprised of relatives, adoptive families, and foster families. Family structure influences child health and has a dramatic impact on family economics and use of health professional services (see Chapter 17).

Sixty-eight percent of children live with two parents, 23% live with their mothers, and 5% live with their fathers (Federal Interagency Forum on Children and Family Statistics, 2004); 4% live with neither parent. More white and Hispanic children live with two parents than do black children ages 5 to 17. Because of the stabilization of both divorce rates and the number of unmarried women giving birth, little change is predicted in these numbers (Annie E. Casey Foundation, 2004).

For children living with one or both parents, characteristics of the family have the potential to affect child health, health behaviors, and school achievement. For example, the number of interracial families is growing. According to the 2000 population survey, almost 7 million Americans, including 2.8 million children younger than 8 years of age, identify themselves as more than one race (U.S. Census Bureau, 2000). This blending of cultures influences the family environment and ultimately child development and school achievement (see Chapter 18).

The number of families with a foreign-born parent is also increasing. Twenty percent of children have at least one foreign-born parent (Federal Interagency Forum, 2004). Within these families, children may or may not be foreign born. Children with a foreign-born parent have challenging economic and educational needs. Between 30% and 45% of foreign-born parents lack a high school diploma and more than 70% speak a language other than English in the home (Federal Interagency Forum, 2004). Many children with a foreign-born parent will need additional resources at school.

The number of families with lesbian and gay parents is receiving increasing attention. Although the actual number of families is not known, the U.S. Census identified 301,026 households headed by a male householder and a male partner, and 293,365 households headed by a female householder and a female partner (Kurdek, 2004; Proctor & Dalaker, 2003). The number of same-sex households has grown significantly in Connecticut, Delaware, Illinois, Indiana, Louisiana, Massachusetts, Montana, Nebraska, Nevada, and Vermont. One third of lesbian households and one fifth of gay male households include children (Proctor & Dalaker, 2003). It is estimated that 6 to 14 million children have a gay or lesbian parent through a previous marriage, donor insemination, or adoption. Most states do not deny custody or visitation based on sexual orientation and 22 states allow gay and lesbian couples to adopt children. Since the literature on this development is relatively new, little has been studied regarding this family structure.

Children also become a part of a family through kinship care, adoption, and foster care. Often these children come from challenging economic situations and may have complicated health needs. Each situation presents a challenge to the school nurse.

Grandparents are a part of the family structure of 5.6 million children (Urban Institute, n.d.). More children younger than 6 years of age than older children live with a grandparent. This family structure is more common in black and Hispanic families than in white families. The majority of children (65%) have at least one parent living with them although most live in the grandparent's house. When only one grandparent is present, it is most often the grandmother. Other children live in kinship care arrangements with relatives such as aunts, uncles, or siblings without the presence of a parent.

The number of children adopted into families is difficult to estimate. Although statistics are available for public welfare system and international adoptions, no reporting mechanism is in place for private adoptions. In 2001, there were 50,000 adoptions from the public welfare system and 19,237 international adoptions (Child Welfare League of America, n.d.). Adoption policies vary in foreign countries. In 2003, more children were adopted from China, followed by Russia, Guatemala, Korea, Kazakhstan, Ukraine, and India (Travel.State.gov, 2004).

When comparing adoptions from the U.S. public welfare system and international adoptions, there were no gender differences except for those adoptions from China in which 96% were girls (Child Welfare League of America, n.d.). There was an age difference; children adopted within the United States were older. Only 2% of U.S. adoptions involved children younger than 1 year of age compared to 44% of international adoptions, while 24% of U.S. adoptions involved children older than 9 years of age compared to 5% of international adoptions (Child Welfare League of America, n.d.).

TABLE 15.3 lists the percentage of children within the U.S. public welfare system waiting to be adopted and adopted by race. There were more black children waiting to be adopted and more white children adopted in 2001. Sixty-seven percent were adopted by a married couple, 30% by a single woman, 2% by a single man, and 1% by an unmarried couple

Table 15.3 ■
PERCENTAGE OF CHILDREN BY RACE/ETHNICITY IN THE U.S. PUBLIC WELFARE SYSTEM

	WAITING TO BE ADOPTED (%)	ADOPTED (%)
American Indian/Alaskan Native non-Hispanic	2	1
Asian/Pacific Islander non-Hispanic	1	1
Black non-Hispanic	43	35
Hispanic	13	16
White non-Hispanic	34	38
Unknown/unable to determine	5	5
Two or more races non-Hispanic	2	3

Source: U.S. Department of Health and Human Services (2003).

Table 15.4 ■

PERCENTAGE OF CHILDREN IN FOSTER CARE BY PLACEMENT

Foster family home (non-relative)	48
Relative foster home	24
Group home or institution	18
Preadoptive homes	4
Other placement types	6

Source: Annie E. Casey Foundation (2004).

(USDHHD, 2003). It is not uncommon for adopted children to have additional educational and healthcare needs, as they may have received substandard care, have been born to mothers whose pregnancies were complicated by drug or alcohol use, or have special healthcare needs.

There are more than half a million children in foster care. On average, 290,000 children enter and 263,000 exit foster care each year (U.S. Department of Health and Human Services [USDHHS], 2003). Table 15.4 lists the type of foster care placement. The median age is 10.6 years. Males comprise 52% of the children and females 48%. The race and ethnic composition of children in foster care are presented in Table 15.5. The outcome for black children is less favorable, as they are more likely to be in foster care longer, placed in residential or group care, and least likely to be reunified with family.

Of the children who exited foster care, 57% were reunited with their families, 18% were adopted, 13% went to live with a relative or guardian, 7% were emancipated (considered to be an adult and allowed to live independently), and 5% had other outcomes (Annie E. Casey Foundation, 2004). Outcomes of children exiting foster care are now being assessed. It appears that children reunited with parents reenter foster care at higher rates than children who exit for kinship care, adoption, or legal guardianship (USDHHS, 2002).

Table 15.5 ■

PERCENTAGE OF CHILDREN IN FOSTER CARE BY RACE AND ETHNICITY

Black/non-Hispanic	38
White/non-Hispanic	37
Hispanic	17
Other races/ethnic origins	8

Source: Annie E. Casey Foundation (2004).

A majority of the children who have been or are in foster care have challenging healthcare and educational needs. The children may have health or mental health problems resulting from abuse or neglect. They are often behind educationally and require special education (Annie E. Casey Foundation, 2004).

In summary, family structure has a powerful influence on child development. It influences the health of family members, their health beliefs and practices, and the educational success of the children. Increasing diversity among family structures presents many challenges for the school nurse. Changes in family composition, parent characteristics, and family culture influence the child. Sensitivity to family structure is needed in regard to parent and grandparent days, parent gift making, holiday celebrations, dietary habits, and health beliefs and practices.

FAMILY ECONOMICS

Income influences the health of all family members. For the poor, it is a negative influence; research shows that there is a higher incidence of disease and death among families with a low income (Loveland-Cherry & Bomar, 2004). In the child health literature, the percentage of children living in poverty is the most widely used indicator of child well-being. For children, direct links have been identified between poverty and undesirable outcomes related to health and education (Annie E. Casey Foundation, 2004). Only 64% of children in the lowest quartile of income distribution graduate high school compared to 92% of children in the highest quartile (Annie E. Casey Foundation, 2004). This section examines family economics as represented by poverty, healthcare coverage, and use of preventative healthcare services.

Poverty

The official poverty measure consists of a series of income guidelines based on family size and composition. The guidelines, revised each year, are used to determine financial eligibility for certain federal programs such as Head Start and the National School

Table 15.6 ■

CHILDREN IN LOW-INCOME WORKING FAMILIES BY GEOGRAPHICAL REGION

REGION	NO. OF CHILDREN	PERCENTAGE OF CHILDREN
Northeast	1,567,000	15
Midwest	1,927,000	19
South	3,786,000	37
West	2,883,000	28

Source: Annie E. Casey Foundation (2004).

Lunch Program. The 2005 poverty guideline for a family of one adult and two children would be $16,090 for the contiguous 48 states, $20,110 if the family was living in Alaska, and $18,510 if the family was living in Hawaii (USDHHS, 2005). Based on these income thresholds, poverty rates for children fell dramatically during the mid- to late-1990s but increased slightly each year. In 2003, 17.6% or nearly 13 million children under the age of 18 lived in poverty (Institute for Research on Poverty, n.d.).

While the poverty rate was declining, there was an increase in the number of working poor families. As a result of the economic boon of the 1990s, many parents were able to secure employment for at least part of the year. Because of this, between 1976 and 2002 the number of children living in poor families, with income from earnings but no income from public assistance, increased from 4.4 million to 7.3 million (Annie E. Casey Foundation, 2004). Parental employment does not necessarily mean a family can move above the poverty line or that the job includes benefits such as health insurance. Table 15.6 lists the geographical location of working low-income families. Interestingly, 32% of the families live in the suburbs, 30% in cities, and 23% in rural areas; 15% did not identify their residential status (Annie E. Casey Foundation, 2004).

In 2002, 30% of children lived in families with incomes below $30,000 and 17% of children lived in poverty (National Center for Health Statistics, 2004). While the percentage of children living in poverty was not statistically different from 1976, children are still more likely to be living in poverty than working-age adults or older Americans (National Center for Health Statistics, 2004). To put this in perspective, an average of 750 children were added to the poverty population each day from 2000 through 2002 (Annie E. Casey Foundation, 2004). Eighteen percent of children lived in families labeled as "food insecure" by the USDA while more than half a million children lived in households classified as "food insecure with child hunger" (Annie E. Casey Foundation, 2004).

Poverty rates differ by race/ethnicity. Across all age groups, a higher percentage of Hispanic and black persons are poor. Percentages for children by race/ethnicity are listed in Table 15.7. The percentage of Hispanic and black children is more than double the percentage of white children.

Family structure has a dramatic impact on family economics. For the majority of children who live in two parent families, most had at least one (97%) and often two (62%) parents in the work force. Thus, it is not surprising that only 9% of families with two parents live in poverty. In contrast, about 40% of children living in female-headed households live in

Table 15.7 ■

PERCENTAGE OF CHILDREN LIVING IN FAMILIES BELOW THE POVERTY LEVEL BY RACE/ETHNICITY

White only	13.1
Black or African American only	32.1
Asian only	11.4
Hispanic or Latino	28.2

Source: National Center for Health Statistics (2004).

Table 15.8 ■

PERCENTAGE OF CHILDREN UNDER 18 YEARS OF AGE IN FEMALE-HEADED HOUSEHOLDS LIVING IN POVERTY BY RACE/ETHNICITY

White only	34.7
Black or African American only	47.5
Asian only	29.8
Hispanic or Latino	47.9

Source: National Center For Health Statistics (2004).

poverty (ChildStat.gov, n.d.). TABLE 15.8 lists poverty percentages by race/ethnicity. It should be noted that two thirds of female-headed households do not receive child support or alimony payments (Annie E. Casey Foundation, 2004).

Many children with foreign-born parents live in poverty (Maternal and Child Health Bureau, 2002). This has been linked to lack of education and language difficulties. Children living with grandparents also face economic hardships whether a parent is present or not. When the parent is present, 15% of the children live in poverty. When a parent is not present, the percentage doubles to 30% (Urban Institute, n.d.).

HEALTHCARE COVERAGE

In 2002, 8.5 million children and adolescents did not have health insurance (Mills & Bhandari, 2003). However, more children have health insurance now than a decade ago. An increase in the number of children covered by a parent's private employer-based insurance and the introduction and implementation of the State Children's Health Insurance Program (SCHIP) contributed to this increase. Using federal monies, SCHIP helps provide coverage to 8.4 million children who would otherwise be uninsured. In 2000, Virginia had the smallest percentage of children with SCHIP coverage (8.7%) and Vermont had the highest percentage at 37%. The national state average was 20.6% (Maternal and Child Health Bureau, 2002). Three quarters of children who are uninsured are eligible for this program but are uninsured because of lack of parental knowledge and complicated enrollment procedures (Holahan, Dubay, & Kenney, 2003).

Race/ethnicity, poverty and family structure all combine to influence health insurance status. Hispanic persons and non-Hispanic black persons were more likely to lack health insurance than non Hispanic white persons. Access to health insurance coverage through employment is lowest for Hispanic persons (National Center for Health Statistics, 2004). Families with incomes near or below the poverty level were three times more likely to be without health insurance as compared to families with incomes twice the poverty level or higher (National Center for Health Statistics, 2004). In relation to family structure, more children in families with one parent (19%) were not covered by health insurance than children in two-parent families (11.4%) (Maternal and Child Health Bureau, 2002). Children living with a foreign-born parent or a grandparent were at the greatest risk for being uninsured.

Use of Preventive Healthcare Services

One of the responsibilities of a family is to promote and maintain health as well as prevent disease in family members. One of the ways to accomplish this is through the use of professional health services (Loveland-Cherry & Bomar, 2004). These preventive health services include but are not limited to preventive healthcare visits, immunizations, and dental care. Together they promote child health and subsequently school success.

Twenty-three percent of children and adolescents, 3 to 17 years of age, do not have an annual well-child visit (Yu et al., 2002). The statistics of who does and does not receive preventive health care are interesting. More children with public insurance (85%) then with private (76%) or no insurance (68%) have preventive visits. This may be related to SCHIP that provides coverage of preventive healthcare visits. Younger children were more likely than older children to have preventive care; across all age groups, Hispanic children were the least likely to access these services (TABLE 15.9). Children and adolescents who do not have preventive healthcare visits are denied health screenings, confidential time with a healthcare provider, as well as counseling on risk behaviors that can have detrimental effects on their health. This increases the responsibilities of the school nurse.

Immunization status is another indicator of family use of preventive health services. One quarter (25%) of young children, less than 3 years of age, have not received the recommended doses of five key vaccines (4 DTaP, 3 polio, 1 MMR, 3 Hib, 3 hepatitis B) (The Commonwealth Fund, 2004). (See Chapter 21.)

Table 15.9 ■

PERCENTAGE OF CHILDREN AND ADOLESCENTS WITHOUT A PREVENTIVE HEALTHCARE VISIT IN THE PAST YEAR BY AGE AND RACE/ETHNICITY

	WHITE	BLACK	HISPANIC
Younger than age 4	5.6	5.6	9.5
Ages 5–9	10.7	13.3	20.8
Ages 10–14	13.8	20.4	26.0
Ages 15–17	13.7	17.7	28.2

Source: Maternal and Child Health Bureau (2002).

Nationally, the percentage of children without the vaccines ranged from 14% in Massachusetts to 37% in Colorado.

Immunization status varies by race/ethnicity, poverty level, and urban area. Poor, minority, and urban young children are less likely to be fully immunized. More white (80%) than Hispanic (76%) and black children (71%) were fully immunized. The gap narrowed between white and Hispanic children but widened between white and Black children. A gap in having received the full complement of vaccines remains between children living below the poverty level (76%) and children at or above the poverty level (83%) and between children living in urban (75%) versus suburban areas (80%) (The Commonwealth Fund, 2004).

Among children ages 2 to 17 years, 26% had not received dental care during the past year. Again, this varied by race/ethnicity, poverty level, and type of insurance. Minority children, children in families with lower income, and those with public or no insurance are less likely to receive regular dental care (National Center for Health Statistics, 2004).

In summary, as a result of family characteristics, children are presenting to schools with challenging health and educational needs. Effective care requires knowledge and understanding of the family environment and the resulting influences on all aspects of the child's development, health, and potential for success in school; it also requires that these health-related services be available to the school population. School nurses are in an ideal position to assess the effects of family, family economic status, and family use of preventive services on the student's health. In all areas, poverty emerges as one of the largest negative influences on child development. Many families do not participate in available government programs (Table 15.10). School nurses can use this knowledge and their advocacy role to support families and guide them toward available programs.

Table 15.10 ■

PERCENTAGE OF CHILDREN FROM LOW-INCOME FAMILIES PARTICIPATING IN GOVERNMENT ASSISTANCE PROGRAMS

Food stamps	23
Free or reduced-cost school meal	58
At least one child covered by public insurance (Medicare, Medicaid, or SCHIP)	42
Social Security Insurance (SSI)	3
Public or subsidized housing	12
Energy assistance	8
WIC	21

Source: Annie E. Casey Foundation (2004).

CHILDREN IN THE SCHOOL SETTING

Outside of the home, school is where children and adolescents spend most of their time. Characteristics of the school affect not only the child but the nurse as well. Within the United States, school type, size, location, and policies impact on the child's potential for success and the role of the school nurse.

Preschool

Preschools help prepare young children for school or provide child care for working parents. Programs may be center based, such as daycare centers, nursery schools, Head Start programs, or other early childhood centers. Almost 8 million children ages 3 to 5 years old attend preschool, reflecting a 20% increase over the early 1990s. Preprimary enrollment (nursery and kindergarten) grew significantly (20%) between 1991 and 2001. The percentage of children attending is influenced by the child's age, race/ethnicity, poverty level, and maternal education. More 5-year-olds (73%) than 4-year-olds (66%) or 3-year-olds (43%) attend preschool. More black (63%) and white (59%) than Hispanic (36%) children attend. Children living at the poverty level and above are more likely to attend than children living below the poverty level. The more educated the mother, the more likely the child is to attend preschool. Seventy percent of children with mothers who attended college versus 38% of children with mothers who did not graduate high school attend preschool (National Center for Education Statistics, 2002a).

Prekindergarten

In an effort directed at preparing more children for school, about one third of elementary schools are now offering prekindergarten programs. The programs tend to be offered in city public elementary schools with enrollments greater than 700 students. Of the 822,000 children attending prekindergarten, 61% were eligible for free or reduced-cost lunch. In schools with low levels of children living in poverty, 4% were black, 8% were Hispanic, and 81% were white. In schools with high levels of children living in poverty, 22% of the children were white, 36% were black, and 39% were Hispanic (National Center for Education Statistics, 2002b).

Elementary and Secondary Schools

Student enrollment in both public and private schools has been increasing. Between 1995 and 2000, enrollment increased 4% in public elementary schools, 8% in public secondary schools, and 5% in both private elementary and secondary schools. The largest increases have been in Arizona, Colorado, Florida, New Jersey, and Nevada. It is predicted that enrollments will total between 53.5 and 53.9 million children through 2012. During this time, enrollment is expected to rise by 9% in the West and 1% in the South, and decrease by 4% in the Midwest and 5% in the Northeast (National Center for Education Statistics, 2002c).

As of 2000, 53,167,000 children are enrolled in American elementary and secondary schools. Of these, 47,223,000 attend public and parochial schools and 5,944,000 attend private school. Total enrollment for grades prekindergarten through grade 8 is 38,387,000 or 71.4% of students. Total enrollment for grades 9 through 12 is 14,780,000 or 28.6% of students. TABLE 15.11 lists the number of schools by grade level. The category "other" includes special education programs, alternative schools, and schools not classified by grade level. New subcategories of schools are becoming increasing popular. In 2002, there were 1,736 magnet schools and 2,348 charter schools. Magnet and charter schools are usually part of the public school system. Students attend them by choice rather than by neighborhood assignment. TABLE 15.12 lists private schools by type. The average public elementary school enrollment is 477 students and the average secondary school enrollment is 795.

The race/ethnicity of students varies dramatically by school type. The overall percentage of enrollment by race/ethnicity in public schools is 61.2% white, 17.2% black, 16.3% Hispanic, 4.1% Asian/Pacific Islander, and 1.2% American Indian/Alaskan Native. Thus, 39% of students are members of a minority group, up from 17% in the 1970s. This

Table 15.11 ■
TOTAL NUMBER OF SCHOOLS BY GRADE LEVEL

	PUBLIC	PRIVATE
Total	92,012	27,223
Elementary	64,131	16,530
Secondary	22,365	2,538
Combined	4,042	8,155
Other	1,474	

Source: National Center for Education Statistics (2002c).

Table 15.12 ■
NUMBER OF PRIVATE SCHOOLS

	ELEMENTARY	SECONDARY	COMBINED
Catholic	6,707	1,114	282
Other religious	6,843	718	5,672
Non-sectarian	2,981	707	2,201

Source: National Center for Education Statistics (2002c).

increase is largely attributable to increasing numbers of Hispanic students. There are more minority students in public schools in the West and South. In contrast, almost half of private schools have fewer than 10% minority students (National Center for Educational Statistics, 2002c).

Larger percentages of black and Hispanic students attend schools with high poverty levels. Eligibility for the free or reduced-cost lunch program provides a proxy measure for poverty. Overall, 40% of fourth-graders were eligible for free or reduced-cost lunch programs in 2003. More black and Hispanic students participated in these programs. The states with the largest number of students eligible for free or reduced meals are California (2.9 million), Texas (1.9 million), and New York (1.2 million) (Hoffman, 2003).

In addition to students, there are a total of 3,343,000 teachers in these schools. The majority (2, 953,000) teach in public schools while 390,000 work in private schools. Teacher/pupil ratios range from 1:15 to 1:30. Approximately 50,000 guidance counselors and staff work in high schools. Guidance counselor/student ratios range from 1:250 to 1:300. In addition, there is a large number of support staff working in schools. School nurses often serve as a resource to these adults in addition to their roles related to students.

CHILDREN WITH SPECIAL HEALTHCARE NEEDS

Special consideration must be given to families in which there is a child with special healthcare needs (CSHCN). Inconsistency in the definition of a CSHCN has led to confusion as to the actual number of children. In 1995, the definition was revised to identify CSHCN based on who requires health and related services beyond that generally required by a child (see Chapter 27). It also includes children who are at risk for a chronic physical, developmental, behavioral, or emotional condition that requires services (McPherson et al., 1998).

In 2000, the Maternal and Child Health Bureau and the National Center for Health Statistics conducted a telephone survey to determine the number of children with special healthcare needs and the impact on the family. The survey found that 12.8% of children younger than the age of 18 had special healthcare needs. It did not include children and adolescents at risk for developing special needs.

Prevalence was higher for 12- to 17-year-old adolescents (15.8%) as compared to 6- to 11-year-olds (14.6%) and children age 5 and younger (7.8%) (Allen, 2004; Van Dyck, 2003). Table 15.13 lists the services that the students required.

Access to coordinated, comprehensive care was a concern of many families. Regardless of type of

Table 15.13 ■
PERCENTAGE OF SERVICES REQUIRED BY CSHCN

Prescriptive medicines	74.3
Elevated service use (more frequent visits/needs)	45.6
Emotional/behavioral developmental services	28.7
Limitation in activities	21.3
Specialized therapies	17.4

Source: Allen (2004).

insurance, many families felt that their child had unmet healthcare needs. Many families also had financial concerns related to insurance that did not cover the child's healthcare needs and the need to cut back or stop work.

CSHCN are more likely to be absent from school because of healthcare provider visits, illness, and hospitalization. While at school they may require procedures such as catheterizations or tube feedings. The school nurse often serves as the link between the child and family and teachers. More information on this population is provided in Chapter 27.

STUDENTS RECEIVING SCHOOL SERVICES UNDER IDEA

Within the population of school children is an increasing number of children receiving services under the Individuals with Disabilities Education Act (IDEA). This legislation mandates that children with disabilities who are having trouble learning as a result of the disability receive a free appropriate public education in the least restrictive environment (see Chapters 14 and 27). The categories of disabilities include autism, deafness, hearing impairment, mental retardation, multiple disabilities, orthopedic impairment, serious emotional disturbance, specific learning disabilities, speech or language impairment, traumatic brain injury, visual impairment, and other health impairment. The category "other health conditions" includes any health condition that may limit strength and/or cause problems with learning. Some children require the support of services such as speech or occupational therapy while others require nursing care and health-related interventions.

Infants and Toddlers

The number of infants and toddlers with disabilities receiving services under the Individual with Disabilities Education Act (see Chapter 14) has increased 40% from 1994 to 2000. Of the 230,853 children receiving services, 18% are between birth and 1 year of age, 33% are between 1 and 2 years of age, and half are 2 to 3 years old. More than 60% of the children are white, 17% are black, and another 17% are Hispanic (U.S. Department of Education, 2002). Most services are provided in the home or as part of specific programs for young children with developmental delay or disabilities. While school nurses have minimal contact with infants and toddlers requiring special education, the increasing number of young children receiving services warns of the potential of increasing numbers of school-age children requiring services.

Preschoolers

Almost 600,000 preschool children ages 3 to 5 receive services under IDEA. TABLE 15.14 lists the race/ethnicity of preschoolers receiving those services. As with infants and toddlers, the number of children has increased since the early 1990s. Forty-four percent more 3-year-olds, 37% more 4-year-olds, and 22% more 5-year-olds received services in the 2000–2001 school year as in the 1992–1993 school year. Children received services for speech or language impairments (55%), development delay (25%), mental retardation (4%), specific learning disability (3%), and autism (2%) (U.S. Department of Education, 2002). Services were provided in a number of settings, including early childhood centers, special education centers, homes, residential facilities, and schools.

School-Age Children

Between 5 and 6 million Americans ages 6 through 21 years receive special education services. TABLE 15.15 lists the race/ethnicity of school-age children receiving services. The number of those receiving services has increased 19% for children 6 to 11 years old and 40% for children 12 to 17 years old in the 2000–2001 school year as compared to the 1992–1993 school year. For ages 6 to 11 years, specific learning disability was the largest category, followed by speech or language impairment, mental retardation, and emotional disturbance. For children and adolescents ages 12 to 17 years, specific learning disability was the most common, followed by mental retardation, emotional disturbances, and speech or language impairment.

Missing from the data collected on students served under IDEA and lost in the revised definition

Table 15.14 ■

PERCENTAGE OF PRESCHOOLERS WITH DISABILITIES BY RACE/ETHNICITY RECEIVING SERVICES UNDER IDEA

White	67.4
Hispanic	13.9
Black	14.8
Asian American/Pacific Islander	2.1
American Indian/Alaska Native	1.2

Source: U.S. Department of Education (2002).

Table 15.15 ■

PERCENTAGE OF 6- TO 21-YEAR-OLDS WITH DISABILITIES BY RACE/ETHNICITY SERVED UNDER IDEA

White	62.3
Black	19.8
Hispanic	14.5
Asian/Pacific Islander	1.9
American Islander/Native American	1.5

Source: U.S. Department of Education (2002).

of children with special healthcare needs is the nursing care that the students require. Under this program, children with complex medical needs are being educated in school settings. The dramatic increase in the number of students of all ages participating in school-based programs has implications for school nurses. Data as to numbers of children who are technology-dependent and/or require treatments such as tracheostomy care, tube feedings, catheterizations, and insulin injections are not available.

SELECTED DEMOGRAPHICS

School nurses must be knowledgeable about a variety of healthcare conditions, current treatments, and a wide scope of issues. Many are addressed in other chapters in this book. However, when addressing the demographics of children and adolescents, attention needs to be focused on child and teen death, child maltreatment, and school violence. School nurses are in a position to provide education to help prevent child and teen deaths, detect and address the after effects of child maltreatment, and provide both care and support to students and staff post victimization.

Child and Adolescent Death

Child death rates have declined. In 2001, there were approximately 33 deaths per day among children ages 1 to 14 or 22 deaths/100,000 children; this is down from 26 deaths per 100,000 children in 1996. The leading causes of death for children 1 to 4 years are listed in TABLE 15.16. The leading causes of death for children 5 to 14 years old are listed in TABLE 15.17. By state, rates improved in 44 states and were worse in five states including Alaska, Delaware, Kentucky, New Hampshire, and Oklahoma (Annie E. Casey Foundation, 2004). Childhood mortality rates were lowest in Connecticut and New Jersey and highest in Mississippi. Rates improved across all race/ethnic groups but remained higher for black and American Indian/ Alaskan Native chil-

Table 15.16 ■

LEADING CAUSES OF DEATH IN CHILDREN 1 TO 4 YEARS OF AGE PER 100,000 CHILDREN

Unintentional injury	11.7
Congenital malformations	3.1
Malignant neoplasms	2.6
Homicide	2.1
Diseases of the heart	1.1
Pneumonia and influenza	0.6
Septicemia	0.6

Source: National Center for Health Statistics (2004).

Table 15.17 ■

LEADING CAUSES OF DEATH IN CHILDREN 5 TO 14 YEARS OF AGE PER 100,000 CHILDREN

Unintentional injury	7.3
Malignant neoplasms	2.6
Congenital malformations	1.0
Homicide	0.9
Suicide	0.7
Diseases of the heart	0.6
Chronic lower respiratory disease	0.3

Source: National Center for Health Statistics (2004).

dren and for children living in poverty. As a result of advances in medical care and decreases in deaths from motor vehicle accidents, the rate is predicted to continue to decline. However, it should be noted that more than half the deaths from motor vehicle accidents are the result of children not wearing seat belts (Federal Interagency Forum, 2003).

Teen death rates are determined based on the number of accidents, homicides, and suicides. Together, these three account for 75% of all teen deaths. The teen death rate has declined. In 2001, there were 50 deaths per 100,000 teens as compared to 60 deaths per 100,000 children in 1996. Rates improved across all race/ethnic groups but are still higher for black and American Indian teens (TABLE 15.18). Teen deaths decreased 1% from accidents, 34% from homicides, and 11% from suicides. Rates among states varied widely from a low of 10 deaths/100,000 teens in New Jersey to 126 deaths/100,000 teens in the District of Columbia. Nationally, on an average day, there were 18 accidental deaths of teens, 5 homicides, and 4 suicides, with motor vehicle accidents being the leading cause of death. Sadly, most of these teen deaths were preventable (Annie E. Casey Foundation, 2004).

Secondary school students engage in many behaviors that contribute to unintentional injuries and possibly death (see Chapter 40). Many of these behaviors impact on the number of motor vehicle accidents. These accidents are a leading cause of death and disability in teenagers. For example, 18.2% of students had rarely or never worn a seat belt. Sixty-two percent of students who had ridden a bicycle in the preceding 12 months had rarely or never worn a helmet. Thirty percent had ridden in a car or other vehicle one or more times with a driver who had been drinking. Twelve percent had driven a car or other vehicle after drinking (Centers for Disease Control and Prevention, 2004). Many states now use graduated driving licenses to combat the effects of lack of driving experience and the prevalence of these risk behaviors.

Table 15.18 ■

DEATH RATE BASED ON ACCIDENTS, HOMICIDES, AND SUICIDES IN ADOLESCENTS 15 TO 19 YEARS OF AGE BY RACE/ETHNICITY PER 100,000

Total	50
White	48
African American	63
Asian/Pacific Islander	28
American Indian	92
Latino	47

Source: Annie E. Casey Foundation (2004).

Child Maltreatment

In 2000, state protective agencies received reports from community professionals, family, friends, relatives, and neighbors alleging maltreatment of approximately 3 million children (Maternal and Child Health Bureau, 2002). TABLE 15.19 lists types of child abuse. Some children suffered more than one type of maltreatment (see Chapter 39). In a majority of cases (79%), one or both parents were involved in the abuse. Incidence and death related to abuse and neglect are highest among children age 3 and younger.

The role of school nurses in reporting suspected cases of child maltreatment has long been recognized (see Chapter 13). Receiving less attention is the role of school nurses in dealing with the effects of child maltreatment. Maltreatment has long-term mental, physical, and behavioral effects on child development. Studies show that children who were maltreated at young ages receive lower ratings from teachers on cognitive, social, and emotional functioning (The Commonwealth Fund, 2004). (See Chapter 39.)

School Violence

The percentage of students victimized at school decreased from 10% in 1996 to 6% in 2001 (DeVoe et al., 2003). The percentage of students reporting

Table 15.19 ■

PERCENTAGE OF CHILD ABUSE BY TYPE

Neglect	63
Physical abuse	19
Sexual abuse	10
Psychological maltreatment	8
Other forms of maltreatment	17

Source: Maternal and Child Health Bureau (2002).

Table 15.20 ■

STUDENT VICTIMIZATION RATES PER 1,000 STUDENTS BY SCHOOL GRADE

	TOTAL	THEFT	VIOLENT CRIME
Elementary	40	28	12
Middle/junior high	78	46	33
High school	78	47	31

Source: DeVoe et al. (2003).

being the victim of theft fell from 7% to 4% and violent victimization at school fell from 3% to 2%. TABLE 15.20 lists student victimization by school grade. Violent crime includes rape, sexual assault, robbery, aggravated assault, and simple assault. Twenty percent of all public schools experienced one or more serious violent crimes. Forty-six percent of all public schools reported property crimes or thefts. Victimization was more likely to occur in larger secondary schools. At least 89% of schools with 1,000 or more students experienced a violent incident compared to 61% of schools with fewer than 300 students (deVoe et al., 2003) (see Chapter 39).

Even though the number of students who are victims is decreasing, students are still more afraid of being attacked when they are at school then when they are not. Attention needs to be focused on student behaviors that contribute to violence in the school setting. Counseling and interventions continue to be needed (Chapter 39).

The Youth Risk Behavior Surveillance System (YRBSS) monitors risk factors nationally in students in grades 9 to 12 attending public and private schools. Many of these risk factors are behaviors that support school violence. TABLES 15.21 AND 15.22 list the percentage of male and female high school students engaging in violence-related risk behaviors by race/ethnicity for 2003. The risk behaviors of carrying a weapon, carrying a gun, and being involved in a fight were all higher in males. Almost 30% of students had property stolen at school during the preceding 12 months. In addition, in 2001, 8% of students reported that they had been bullied at school in the preceding 6 months.

Between 1997 and 2001, teachers were the victims of approximately 1.3 million nonfatal crimes in

Table 15.21 ■

PERCENTAGE MALE HIGH SCHOOL STUDENT VIOLENCE-RELATED RISK BEHAVIORS BY RACE/ETHNICITY

	WHITE	BLACK	HISPANIC
Carried a weapon	27.1	24.9	24.3
Carried a gun	10.0	10.6	8.2
Involved in a fight	38.4	45.6	42.6
Had property stolen or damaged	30.6	33.9	37.0
Did not go to school	3.3	7.9	8.9

Source: Centers for Disease Control and Prevention (2004).

Table 15.22 ■

PERCENTAGE OF FEMALE HIGH SCHOOL STUDENT VIOLENCE-RELATED RISK BEHAVIORS BY RACE/ETHNICITY

	WHITE	BLACK	HISPANIC
Carried a weapon	5.5	9.8	8.5
Carried a gun	1.5	1.4	2.6
Involved in a fight	22.1	34.0	29.5
Property stolen	25.6	27.0	27.6
Did not go to school	2.9	9.0	10.0

Source: Centers for Disease Control and Prevention (2004).

schools including 817,000 thefts and 473,000 violent crimes (rape or sexual assault, robbery, and aggravated and simple assault). The majority of victims were high school teachers in urban areas. Nine percent of all elementary and secondary school teachers were threatened by a student and 4% were physically attacked (DeVoe et al., 2003).

In response to violence in schools, both public and private schools have instituted a number of safety measures. TABLE 15.23 lists security measures in public schools. TABLE 15.24 lists security measures in private schools. In public and private schools, the larger the school the more security measures were employed. However, type of security measure

Table 15.23 ■

PERCENTAGE OF SECURITY MEASURES IN PUBLIC SCHOOLS

	ELEMENTARY	SECONDARY	COMBINED
Require visitor sign-in	96.9	96.4	93.4
Daily metal detector checks	0.8	3.1	8.5
Random metal detector checks	5.0	13.9	18.9
Closed lunch	94.4	77.3	82.0
Drug sweeps	10.0	49.3	40.0
Daily presence of police/security	14.6	48.1	28.6
Video surveillance	10.9	25.5	19.7
Violence prevention program	59.2	59.1	61.1

Source: National Center for Education Statistics (2002c).

Table 15.24 ■
PERCENTAGE OF SECURITY MEASURES IN PRIVATE SCHOOLS

	ELEMENTARY	SECONDARY	COMBINED
Require visitor sign in	80.7	80.7	80.7
Daily metal detector checks	0.3	0	1.1
Random metal detector checks	0.2	3.5	1.0
Closed lunch	94.0	84.7	88.9
Drug sweeps	1.3	18.8	7.3
Daily presence of police/security	2.6	15.9	5.7
Video surveillance	7.8	13.1	7.2
Violence prevention program	24.6	31.0	19.1

Source: National Center for Education Statistics (2002c).

varied by location. For example, drug sweeps were more common in rural schools as compared to the presence of police or security in city schools.

Adolescents are more likely to be victims outside of school. Even though rates have decreased, 51.6/1,000 of adolescents ages 12 to 15 and 53/1000 adolescents ages 16 to 19 were victims (Child Trends Data Bank, n.d.). Race/ethnicity and gender did not affect the likelihood of being victimized but did influence the type of violence encountered.

Victimization rates are important to the school nurse. Adolescents who have been violently victimized are more likely to have physical and mental health concerns, substance abuse problems, and difficulties in their academic work (Wordes & Nunez, 2002).

Gay, Lesbian, Bisexual, and Transgender Identity

Secondary school is a time of sexuality development. An area receiving much needed attention is gay, lesbian, bisexual, and transgender identity among high school students. No clear data are available on the number of gay, lesbian, and bisexual adolescents. It is thought that an increasing number of adolescents are declaring a gay, lesbian, or bisexual identity (Graber & Archibald, 2001). Studies of the coming out process reveal disclosure more to friends than family and mothers rather than fathers (Krudek, 2004).

Significant to school nurses is the finding that gay, lesbian, and bisexual adolescents feel not only the regular adolescent stressors, but also additional stressors related to their sexuality. Many feel different, lack family support, and are often targets of abuse. They are at risk for school problems, as well as running away, prostitution, drug and alcohol abuse, and suicide attempts (Russell, Seif, & Truong, 2001; Savin-Williams, 2001). Negative reactions at school include social isolation, rejection, and verbal and physical abuse (Rivers & D'Augelli, 2001). It is not surprising that many gay, lesbian, and bisexual students do not feel safe at school (see Chapter 47).

Gay, lesbian, and bisexual adolescents have a greater incidence of sexually transmitted diseases and HIV. Forty percent of the HIV infections reported in 2000 were among adolescent males. More than 60% of these new cases were the result of male-to-male transmissions.

Black adolescent males were 1.7 times more likely to report HIV infection than white adolescent males, and 9.3 times more likely than Hispanic adolescent males. In comparison, 38% of adolescent females acquired HIV from heterosexual contact and 5% from intravenous drug use. Black adolescent females were 3.7 times more likely to report HIV infection than white adolescent females and 13.5 times more likely than Hispanic adolescent females. TABLE 15.25 lists race/ethnicity of the 5,536 adoles-

Table 15.25 ■

HIV CASES DIAGNOSED IN 1981–2000 BY GENDER AND RACE/ETHNICITY FOR AGES 13 TO 19

	MALES	FEMALES	
White, non-Hispanic	814	628	
Black, non-Hispanic	1,442	2,330	
Hispanic	150	172	
American Indian/Alaskan Native	17	21	
Asian Pacific Islander	9	7	
Total	2,388	3,148	5,536

Source: Maternal and Child Health Bureau (2002).

cents diagnosed with HIV between 1981 and 2000 (Maternal and Child Health Bureau, 2002).

THE IMPACT OF DEMOGRAPHICS ON SCHOOL NURSES

There are approximately 45,000 school nurses employed in the United States (American Federation of Teachers, n.d.). The national ratio of school nurses to students is 1:1,155 students. The actual ratio varies widely by school district, type of school, and educational level. In many districts, nurses cover more than one school while in other districts there is no school nurse. Thus, in many districts the ratio is greater than 1:2000.

Professional and governmental organizations, such as the National Association of School Nurses, the American School Health Association, and the Centers for Disease Control and Prevention recommend one nurse for every 750 students in general education. This ratio is also supported by the Healthy People 2010 objectives. Currently decisions regarding the role and responsibilities of the school nurse are made on the state and local school district level.

With the increasing numbers of students with special healthcare needs, students requiring medications or procedures during the school day and students with unmet healthcare needs, there are not enough school nurses to meet the needs of the millions of children and adolescents in schools. Many feel that federal legislation is needed to mandate that a school nurse be present during school hours. In response, the American Federation of Teachers has launched the "Every Child Needs A School Nurse" campaign.

Because of the lack of a school nurse, many districts have developed policies that permit others to assume some of the school nurse's responsibilities. For example, it is not uncommon for teachers, secretaries, coaches, aides, and sometimes even parents to dispense medication. Yet, the role of the school nurse involves so much more than the dispensing of medications or completion of procedures. Who assumes responsibility for all the other dimensions of the school nurse's role and what happens to the school children who lack the contact and expertise with a school nurse? Who addresses the issues specific to each level of education?

Elementary school nurses may be the ones to diagnose a previously undetected chronic condition, support the mainstreaming of a child with disabilities, and provide education to promote health and prevent disease. Using his or her expertise, the nurse is in a position to help counteract the detrimental effects of poverty.

The majority of elementary school students undergo a transition from elementary school to a middle school or junior high school. Although the number of such schools is mixed in with the total number of elementary school, an estimated 88% of public school students make this transition (National Middle School Association, n.d.). This is a challenging time for students as physically their bodies begin to change, socially they have a new peer group, and educationally they have exposure to more teachers and increased work demands. It is a complicated time to begin redefining roles and responsibilities. Decision-making becomes important and at-risk behaviors may start to emerge. Statistics regarding risk behaviors within this population are desperately needed. The school nurse is in a position to support this transition and influence student outcomes.

Secondary school nurses may be the ones to address the special needs, educational issues, and risk behaviors of the older student. Chapters on Athlete Health (24), Violence (39), Mental Health Needs (34), High-Risk Behaviors (40), Pregnancy (41), and STDs (42) provide more information on these issues. Success in high school is vital to the well being of the adolescent as they move into adulthood.

CONCLUSION

Examination of the demographics of children and adolescents reveals important information for school nurses. Family structure, family economics, and use of preventive healthcare services interact to exert powerful influences on the health of children and their potential for success. Changes in these influences are altering the culture and language of schools and presenting challenges for school personnel. Striving to meet these challenges presents opportunities to enhance the school environment. Changes in school populations, characteristics of schools, and characteristics of the students in the schools also offer challenges. School size and safety are of primary concern. As students with chronic conditions survive once-fatal conditions, the nature of school nursing services has changed significantly. Children with special needs, whether physical, psychosocial, or cultural, will continue to force school nurses to make adaptations in policies, protocols, and the care provided. The goal is to enhance the health of students and support their educational success. Understanding of student and school demographics enables school nurses to accomplish these goals.

References

Allen, P. (2004). Children with special health care needs: National survey of prevalence and health care needs. *Pediatric Nursing, 30* (4), 307–313.

American Federation of Teachers. (n.d.). *Every child needs a school nurse*. Retrieved December 8, 2004, from http://www.aft.org/topics/school-nurses/

Annie E. Casey Foundation. (2004). *Kids count data book*. United States: Author.

Centers for Disease Control and Prevention. (2004). Surveillance summaries. MMWR, 53 (No. SS-2).

Child Trends Data Bank. (n.d.). *Violent crime victimization*. Retrieved October 9, 2004 from http:// www. childtrendsdatabank.org/indicators/ 71ViolentVictimization.cfm

Child Welfare League of America. (n.d.). *International adoption: Trends and issues*. Retrieved October 17, 2004 from http://ndas.cwla.org/include/text/ IssueBrief_International_Adoption_Final.pdf

ChildStats.gov. (n.d.) Racial and ethnic composition. *America's Children 2002*. Retrieved October 29, 2004 from http://childstats.gov/ac2002/indicators.asp? IID=10&id=2

DeVoe, J. F. Peter, K., Kaufman, P., Ruddy, S. A., Miller, A. K., Planty, M., Snyder, T. D., & Rand, M. R. (2003). Indicators of school crime and safety. *Education Statistics Quarterly, 5* (4). Retrieved December 1, 2004 from http://nces.ed.gov/programs/quarterly/vol_5/ 5_4/3_6.asp

Federal Interagency Forum on Child and Family Statistics. (2004). *America's children in brief: Key indicators of well-being, 2004*. Washington, DC: U.S. Government Printing Office.

Graber, J. A., & Archibald, A. A. (2001). Psychosocial change at puberty and beyond: Understanding adolescent sexuality and sexual orientation. In A. R. D'Augelli & C. J. Patterson (Eds.), *Lesbian, gay, and bisexual identities and youth: Psychological perspectives* (pp. 3–26). New York: Oxford University Press.

Hoffman, L. (2003). *Overview of public elementary and secondary schools and districts: School year 2001–02. Education Statistics Quarterly, 5*(2). Retrieved December 15, 2004 from http://nces.ed.gov/programs/ quarterly/vol_5/5_2/q3_5.asp

Holahan, J., Dubay, L., & Kenney, G. M. 2003. Which children are still uninsured and why. *Future Child, 13*(1), 55–57.

Institute for Research on Poverty. (n.d.). *Who was poor in 2003?* Retrieved March 7, 2005 from http://irp.wisc.edu/ faqs/faq3.htm

Kurdek, L. A. (2004). Gay men and lesbians: The family context. In M. Coleman & L. H. Ganong (Eds.), *Handbook of contemporary families: Considering the past, contemplating the future* (pp. 96–115). Thousand Oaks, CA: Sage.

Loveland-Cherry, C. J., & Bomar, P. J. (2004). Family Health Promotion and Health Protection. In P. J. Bomar (Ed.), *Promoting health in families: Applying family research theory to nursing practice* (pp. 61–89). Philadelphia: Saunders.

Maternal and Child Health Bureau. (2002). *Child health USA 2002*. Retrieved November 1, 2004 from http:// mchb.hrsa.gov/chusa02/

McPherson, M., Arango, P., Fox, H., Lauver, C., McManus, M., Newacheck, P. W., Perrin, J. M., Shonkoff, J. P., & Strickland, B. (1998). A new definition of children with special health care needs. *Pediatrics, 102*(1), 137–140.

Mills, R., & Bhandari, S. (2003). *U.S. Census Bureau: Current population reports, P60–223: Health insurance coverage in the United States: 2002*. Retrieved November 29, 2004 from http://www.census.gov/prod/ 2003pubs/p60223.pdf

National Center for Education Statistics (NCES). (2002a). *Participation in education: Preprimary education*. Retrieved December 15, 2004 from http://nces.ed.gov// programs/coe/2002/section1/indicator01.asp

National Center for Education Statistics (NCES). (2002b). *Participation in education: Prekindergarten in U.S. public schools*. Retrieved December 15, 2004 from http://nces.ed.gov//programs/coe/2004/section1/indicator02.asp

National Center for Education Statistics (NCES). (2002c). Elementary and secondary education in *Digest of education statistics, 2002* (Chap. 2). Retrieved December 15, 2004 from http://nces.ed.gov/pubs2003/2003060b.pdf

National Center for Health Statistics (NCHS). (2004). *Health, United States, 2004 with chartbook on trends in the health of Americans*. Retrieved November 23, 2004, from http://www.cdc.gov/nchs/data/hus/hus04.pdf

National Middle School Association (n.d.). *Supporting students in their transition to middle school*. Retrieved December 2005 from http://www.nmsa.org/news/transition.html

Proctor, B. D., & Dalaker, J. (2003). *U.S. Census Bureau: Current population reports, P60–222: Poverty in the United States: 2002*. Retrieved November 29, 2004 from http://www.census.gov/prod/2003pubs/p60–222.pdf

Rivers, I., & D'Augelli, A. R. (2001). The victimization of lesbian, gay, and bisexual youths. In A. R. D'Augelli & C. J. Patterson (Eds.), *Lesbian, gay, and bisexual identities and youth: Psychological perspectives* (pp. 199–223). New York: Oxford University Press.

Russell, S. T., Seif, H., & Truong, N. L. (2001). School outcomes of sexual minority youth in the United States: Evidence from a national study. *Journal of Adolescence, 24*(1), 111–127.

Savin-Williams, R. C. (2001). Suicide attempts among sexual-minority youths: Population and measurement issues. *Journal of Consulting and Clinical Psychology, 69*(6), 983–991.

The Commonwealth Fund, Child Trends, and Center for Childhealth Research. (2004). *Early childhood development in social context: A chartbook*. Retrieved November 16, 2004 from http://www.cmwf.org/usr_doc/chartbook_quick_download.pdf

Travel.State.Gov. (2004). *Immigrant visas issued to orphans coming to the U.S*. Retrieved October 17, 2004 from http://www.travel.state.gov/family/adoption_resourses_02.html.

Urban Institute. (n.d.). *Children in kinship care*. Retrieved October 31, 2004 from http://www.urban.org/url.cfm?ID=900661

U.S. Census Bureau. (2000). DP-1. *Profiles of general demographic characteristics: 2000*. Retrieved October 26, 2004 from http://www.census.gov/prod/census2000/dp1/2kh00.pdf

U.S. Department of Education (USDOE). (2002). Student characteristics. In Twenty-fourth annual report to Congress on implementation of the IDEA (Chap. 2). Retrieved December 15, 2004 from http://www.ed.gov/about/reports/annual/osep/2002/section-ii.doc

U.S. Department of Health and Human Services (USDHHS), Administration for Children and Families. (2002). *Child welfare outcomes: 2000: Annual report to Congress*. Washington DC: U.S. Government Printing Office.

U.S. Department of Health and Human Services (USDHHS), Administration for Children and Families. (2003). *The AFCARS report*. Retrieved November 16, 2004 from http: //www.acf.dhhs.gov/programs/cb/publications/afcars/report8.html

U.S. Department of Health and Human Services (USDHHS). (2005). *The 2005 HHS poverty guidelines*. Retrieved March 7, 2005 from http://aspe.hhs.gov/poverty/05poverty.shtml

Van Dyck, P. C. (2003). *The national survey of children with special health care needs*. DataSpeak, Health Resources and Service Administration Maternal and Child Health Bureau.

Wordes, M., & Numez, M. (2002). *Our vulnerable teenagers: Their victimization, its consequences, and directions for prevention and intervention*. Retrieved December 8, 2004 from http://www.ncvc.org/ncvc/AGP.net/Components/documentViewer/Download.aspxnz?DocumentID=32558

Yu, S. M., Bellamy, H. A., Kogan, M. D., Dunbar, J. L., Schwall, R. H., & Schuster, M. A. (2002). Factors that influence receipt of recommended preventative pediatric health and dental care. *Pediatrics, 110*(6), E73. Retrieved November 21, 2004 from http://www.medscape.com

Chapter 16

Growth and Development: Preschool through Adolescence

ELIZABETH MATTEY

Chapter Outline

INTRODUCTION

Growth and development are the hallmark features of childhood and adolescence. The school nurse sees large numbers of students in the well setting of the school environment and thus is an ideal healthcare provider to promote normal and identify potential alterations in growth and development. The traditional age groups covered by school nursing are those in kindergarten through 12th grade, or 5 through 18 years of age. As more children ages 3 to 5 attend preschool programs, school nurses are also providing services to this age group. Therefore, this chapter focuses on the normal cognitive, psychosocial, moral, and physical growth and development of children and adolescents, ages 3 through 18.

Growth and development encompasses many parameters. *Growth* refers only to an increase in size of an organ or structure. It is change that can be measured, such as height and weight. *Development* is the maturation of a body or system; it involves the process of acquiring new abilities and skills. The development of language, the ability to process a thought and reach a logical conclusion, and the ability to form social relationships are all part of development. Growth and development are affected by genetics and the environment. Health and nutritional status also have a significant impact, as do community expectations. School nurses need to understand their specific population, the families that make up the population, and the expectations within the community. Cultural, racial, and socioeconomic backgrounds each have their own set of growth and developmental norms.

School nurses will need to use their knowledge of normal growth and development in interactions with students. For example, a ninth-grade student may be much smaller than his or her classmates but a review of the student's growth and development might indicate that he or she is within normal limits. A younger child might not understand humor and abstract ideas and may misinterpret cues and instructions from adults. Health teaching may not be effective when a child does not understand cause-and-effect relationships. By understanding the growth and development of a student, school nurses can plan their interactions and interventions most effectively.

PHYSIOLOGICAL GROWTH

Height and Weight

Children physically grow at different rates. The preschool and school-age years can be considered periods of slow, steady growth, compared to the very rapid growth that occurs during adolescence. This has implications for developmental expectations, nutritional needs, and physiological changes.

Growth charts were revised in 2000 by the U.S. Centers for Disease Control and Prevention (CDC) to more accurately reflect the growth of children and adolescents (CDC, 2002a, 2005a). These charts (Figures 16.1 and 16.2) are available online at http://www.cdc.gov/growthcharts/. Preschool children, ages 3 to 5, grow an average of 1.5 inches per year and their weight increases approximately 2 pounds per year. Boys and girls from age 6 until puberty grow in height approximately 2 to 3 inches per year. By age 6, boys and girls average 45 inches and weigh 45 pounds.

Girls gain 6 to 8 pounds per year until puberty begins, at which time 4 pounds per year can be expected as she begins a fast growth spurt and begins sexual development. Boys average a weight gain of 4 to 6 pounds per year during the elementary years; around age 10, their growth rate increases to add 10 to 12 pounds per year (CDC, 2002a).

Children will generally follow their own curve on the growth scale. If a child is identified in the 45th percentile, he or she will likely remain in that percentile during periods of growth. Children should be referred to their healthcare provider if the school nurse notes a significant change in either the height or weight percentile from the student's normal pattern, if they grow less than 5 cm per year, or if there is more than a 10% change based on successive measurements (Williams, McCarthy, Bragadottir, & Reed, 2002). An abnormal growth pattern may be the only sign of a growth disorder that may also affect multiple body systems. For example, children with genetic growth disorders such as Marfan syndrome, in which they are very tall, can also have cardiovascular defects, ocular abnormalities, and dental crowding. Children with Turner syndrome are short in stature and may also have learning difficulties (Williams et al., 2002). Early recognition and treatment are essential for both their physical health and their school success. *Healthy People 2010* suggests that special attention be given to children from low-income families because 8% of low-income children younger than the age of 5 experience growth delay (U.S. Department of Health and Human Services [USDHHS], 2001b).

Delayed growth can be caused by illness or malnutrition; once the problem is resolved, the child can usually "catch-up" to peers, depending on the severity of the problem (Haywood & Getchell, 2001). As students get older, they may be more sensitive about being too tall or too short. For some with short stature, growth hormone therapy may be considered. Treatment may be considered for the psychosocial issues related to short stature as well as to increase height (Hull & Harvey, 2003). Some students with short stature have been shown to have an immature self-concept and academic deficits and tend to repeat a grade more often than their taller peers even though they have a normal IQ (Hull & Harvey, 2003; Williams et al., 2002). Those treated with growth hormone therapy have shown positive responses and improvement in behavior; final adult height ranges from minimal increases to increases of 4 to 6 cm (Finkelstein et al., 2002; Willhaus, 1999) (Box 16.1).

Most school nurses will care for at least one child with a growth disorder every year (Williams et al., 2002). Nurses will need to educate staff and

(text continues on page 347)

Box 16.1 ■ ■ ■

GROWTH HORMONE THERAPY MAY BENEFIT CHILDREN WHO HAVE:

- Idiopathic short stature (below 10th percentile)
- Turner syndrome
- Chronic renal failure
- Achondroplasia/hypochondroplasia
- Prader-Willi syndrome
- Growth hormone deficiency
- Noonan's syndrome

(Adapted from Finkelstein et al., 2002; Hull & Harvey, 2003)

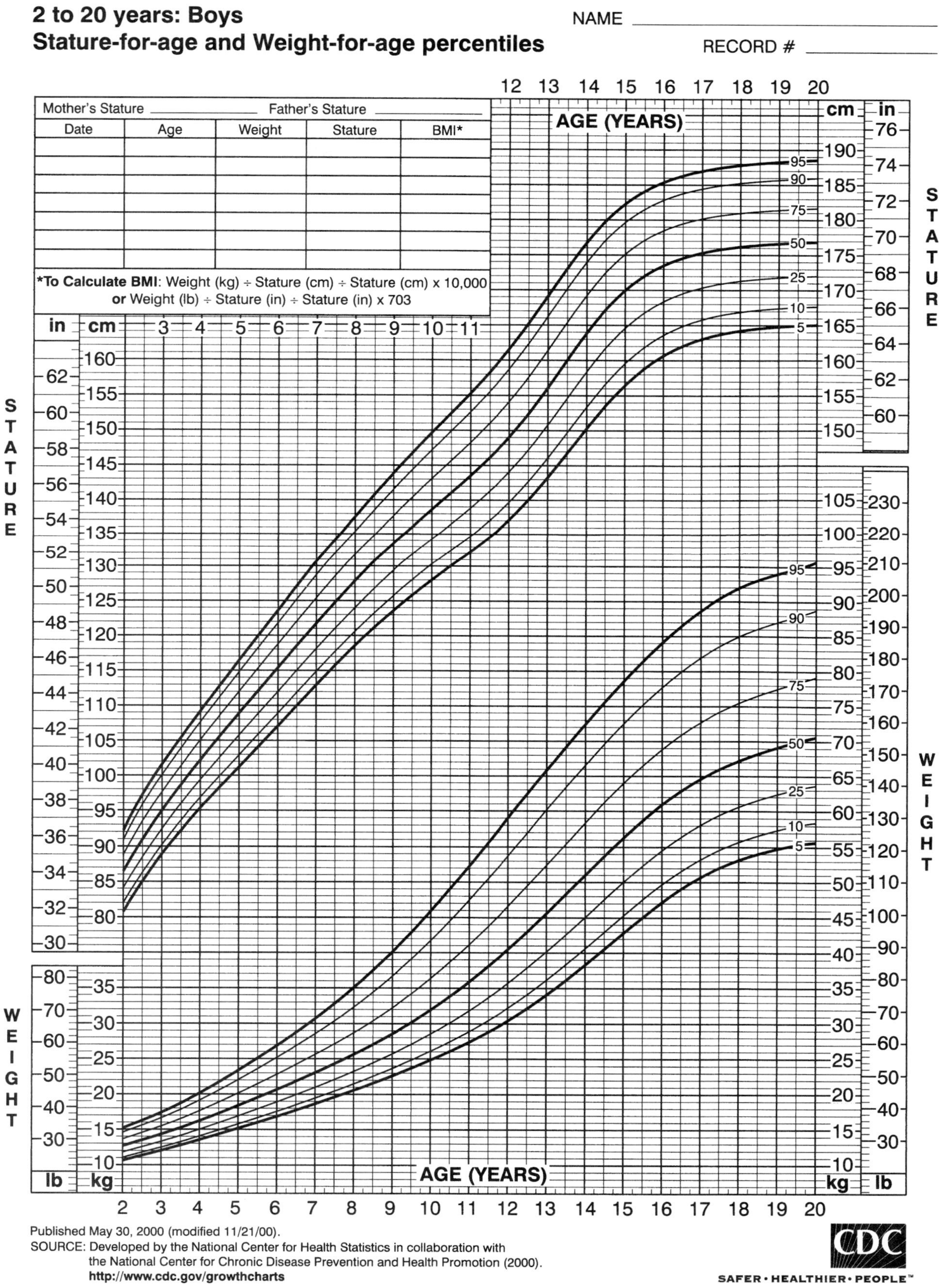

2 to 20 years: Boys
Stature-for-age and Weight-for-age percentiles

NAME ______________________

RECORD # __________

Date	Age	Weight	Stature	BMI*

Mother's Stature ____________ Father's Stature ____________

***To Calculate BMI**: Weight (kg) ÷ Stature (cm) ÷ Stature (cm) x 10,000
or Weight (lb) ÷ Stature (in) ÷ Stature (in) x 703

AGE (YEARS)

STATURE

WEIGHT

Published May 30, 2000 (modified 11/21/00).
SOURCE: Developed by the National Center for Health Statistics in collaboration with the National Center for Chronic Disease Prevention and Health Promotion (2000).
http://www.cdc.gov/growthcharts

CDC
SAFER • HEALTHIER • PEOPLE™

Figure 16.1 Growth chart for boys.

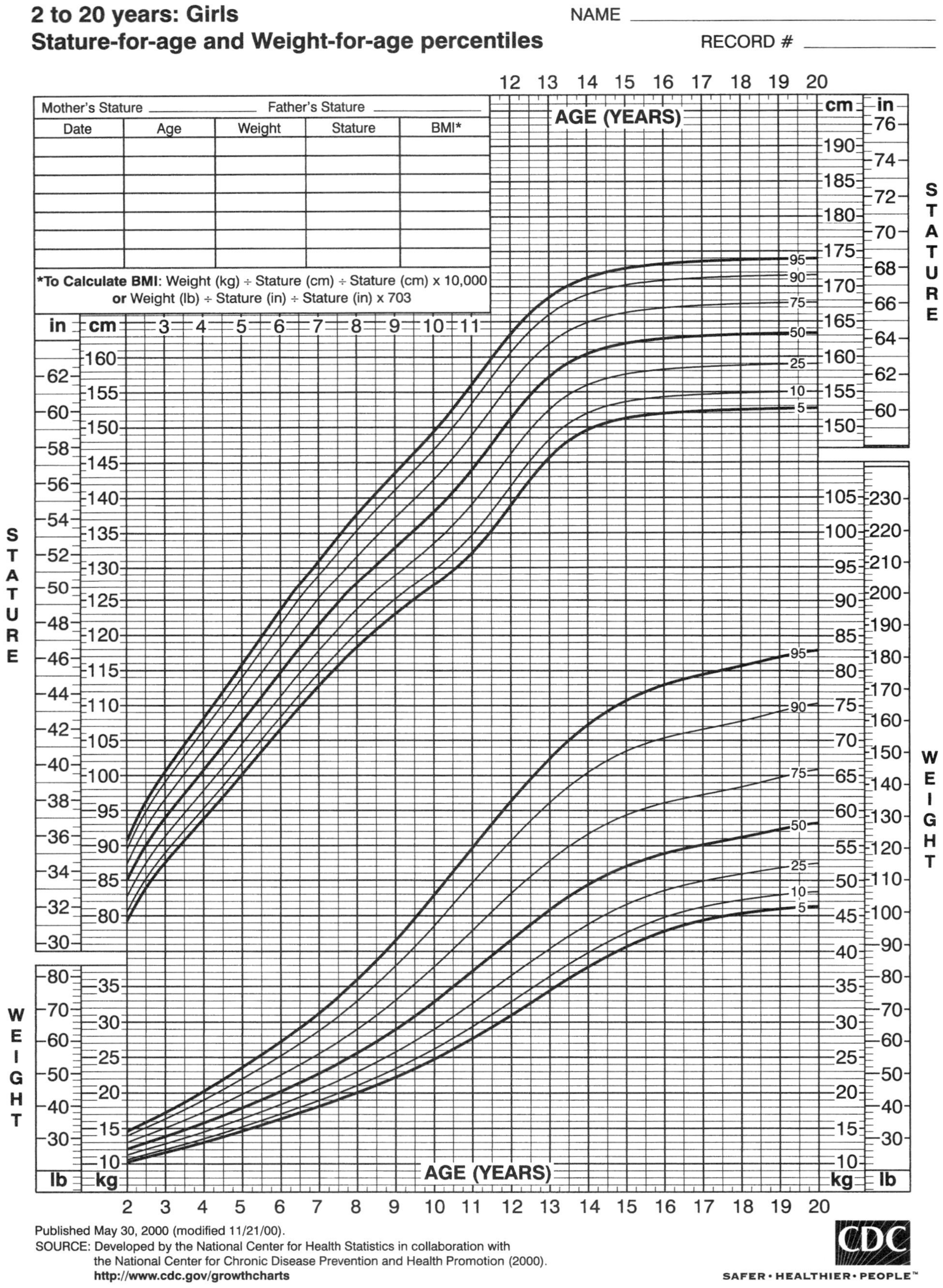
2 to 20 years: Girls
Stature-for-age and Weight-for-age percentiles
NAME
RECORD #
Mother's Stature
Father's Stature
Date
Age
Weight
Stature
BMI*
*To Calculate BMI: Weight (kg) ÷ Stature (cm) ÷ Stature (cm) x 10,000
or Weight (lb) ÷ Stature (in) ÷ Stature (in) x 703
AGE (YEARS)
STATURE
WEIGHT
in
cm
kg
lb
95
90
75
50
25
10
5
Published May 30, 2000 (modified 11/21/00).
SOURCE: Developed by the National Center for Health Statistics in collaboration with
the National Center for Chronic Disease Prevention and Health Promotion (2000).
http://www.cdc.gov/growthcharts
CDC
SAFER • HEALTHIER • PEOPLE™

Figure 16.2 ■ Growth chart for girls.

prepare to manage the additional health issues that accompany a growth disorder, including self-esteem issues, peer relationships, and injury prevention. Parents who are also short in stature may be more sensitive to information concerning the height of their child. Short-statured parents may or may not be receptive to information based on their own life experience. It is always best to be prepared with facts and documentation when offering information to parents. Information can then be shared in a nonjudgmental, caring manner.

Childhood obesity has become a national epidemic (Denehy, 2003). Chapter 36 covers this topic in depth. Youth who are overweight have an increased risk of chronic diseases in adulthood such as heart disease and type 2 diabetes. Obese or overweight students may also experience high blood pressure or glucose intolerance, diseases previously considered to be adult onset. In addition, they may suffer from psychosocial issues during childhood and adolescence including negative self-esteem, social discrimination, and learning problems (CDC, 2003).

The Centers for Disease Control and Prevention (CDC, 2002a) now recommends the use of body mass index (BMI) to determine obesity. Body mass index can be plotted for children after age 2 (FIGURES 16.3 and 16.4). To calculate BMI, the child's weight is divided by the square of his height [BMI= (weight/height^2)]. The results are then charted on the corresponding growth chart (see Chapter 36 for information on obesity and Chapter 20 for screening information and calculation of the BMI).

Communicating to parents that their child may be over- or underweight should be handled in a sensitive manner. Parents may also have a weight issue. A nonjudgmental, factual approach works best in providing education and suggesting interventions. The CDC height, weight, and BMI charts can offer solid documentation to a parent of standardized norms. A parent may still react negatively, but a calm demeanor may help communicate the information. Allow the parent to take the written documentation home to digest later in a less stressful environment. Some nurses may choose to mail the information home to parents. It is important to follow up through personal contact if at all possible. The school nurse should be prepared to offer information about healthy diet and exercise as well as a referral for the child to be evaluated by the healthcare provider to rule out a medical cause for the condition.

Bone Growth

Ossification of bone, or the conversion of cartilage to bone, occurs from before birth through childhood and adolescence with peak bone mass occurring in early adulthood (Neinstein, 2002). Linear skeletal growth occurs at the epiphysial plates at the end of long bones. The epiphysial plate has many cell layers and the blood supplies nutrients to form new cell layers that then ossify to produce new bone (Haywood & Getchell, 2001). In a complex process, cartilage cells at the epiphyses are replaced by osteoblasts which deposit calcium. Phosphate and vitamin D help to promote mineralization and the formation of developing bone. Calcium intake during childhood and adolescence is extremely important in providing adequate bone density in adulthood (Mourad, 1998).

Bones grow in diameter by addition of new tissue layers under the periosteum. Throughout the life span, old bone is replaced by new bone. During adolescence, the growth plate disappears and the epiphysis and metaphysis fuse. At this point, growth is completed. Children generate new bone faster than the older bone is absorbed, thus skeletal mass increases. Skeletal age can be determined by X-ray film; it is used to determine the proportion of total growth that has been completed. The left hand and wrist bone are most commonly used to determine skeletal age because the wrist bones (carpals) ossify in a particular order. The X-ray film is then compared to an assessment atlas based on the child's chronological age and his or her skeletal age. It can help the healthcare provider determine whether children with short stature will continue to grow and catch up to their expected height percentile

(text continues on page 350)

Box 16.2 ■ ■ ■

PROMOTING BONE HEALTH

Powerful Bones, Powerful Girls™ is a social marketing campaign to promote bone health among adolescent girls. For more information visit their Web site: http://www.cdc.gov/powerfulbones/parents/toolbox/toolbox.html

Box 16.3 ■ ■ ■

Osgood-Schlatter disease (aseptic necrosis of the tibial tuberosity) is an irritation of the traction epiphysis where the patellar tendon attaches to the shin, causing pain with knee flexion. Treatment often involves rest of the knee.

2 to 20 years: Boys
Body mass index-for-age percentiles

NAME ____________________

RECORD # ____________

Date	Age	Weight	Stature	BMI*	Comments

***To Calculate BMI**: Weight (kg) ÷ Stature (cm) ÷ Stature (cm) x 10,000
or Weight (lb) ÷ Stature (in) ÷ Stature (in) x 703

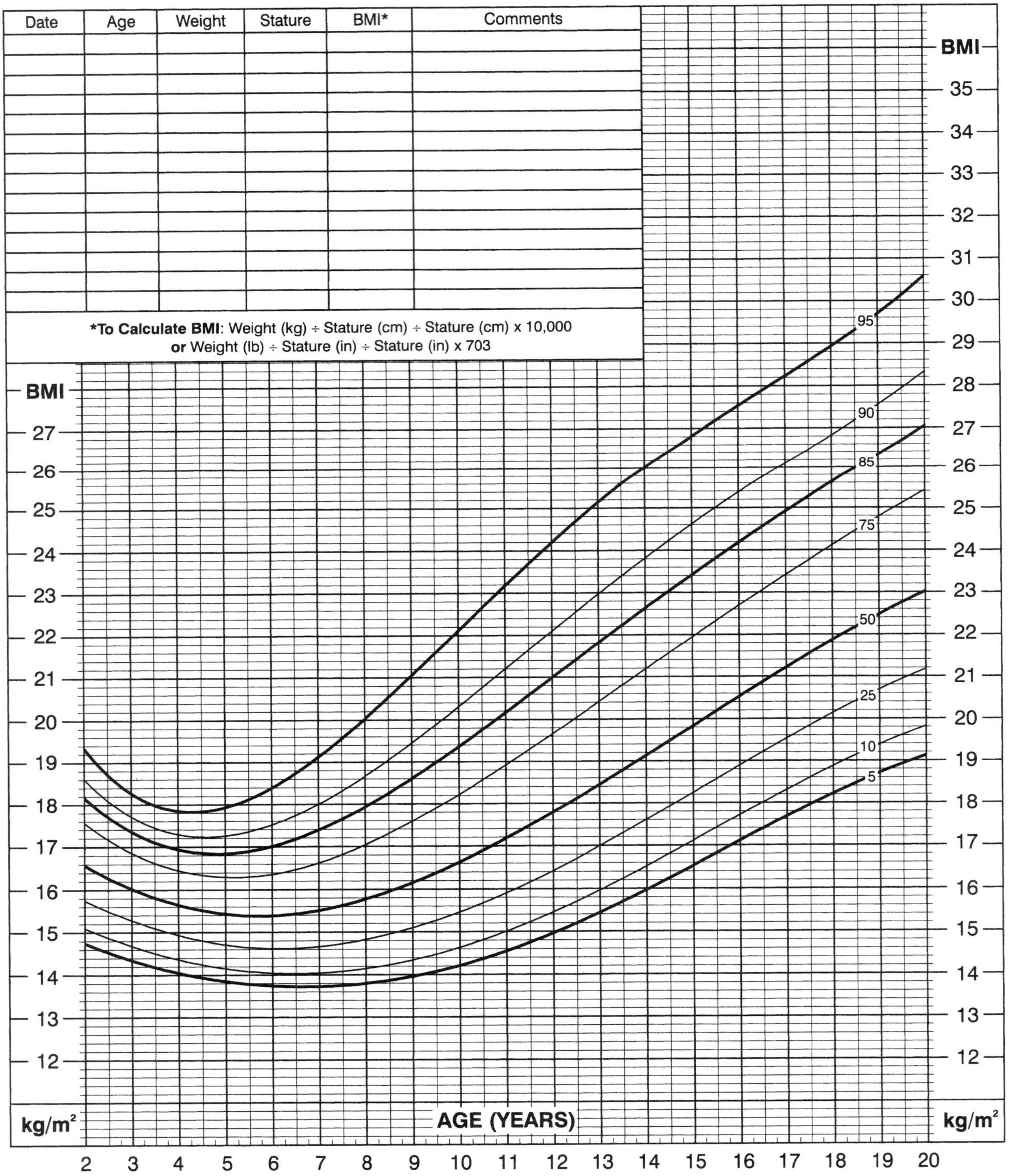

BMI

35
34
33
32
31
30
29
28
27
26
25
24
23
22
21
20
19
18
17
16
15
14
13
12

95
90
85
75
50
25
10
5

kg/m²

AGE (YEARS)

2 3 4 5 6 7 8 9 10 11 12 13 14 15 16 17 18 19 20

Published May 30, 2000 (modified 10/16/00).
SOURCE: Developed by the National Center for Health Statistics in collaboration with the National Center for Chronic Disease Prevention and Health Promotion (2000).
http://www.cdc.gov/growthcharts

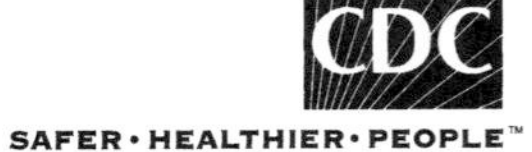

Figure 16.3 ■ Male body mass index.

2 to 20 years: Girls
Body mass index-for-age percentiles

NAME 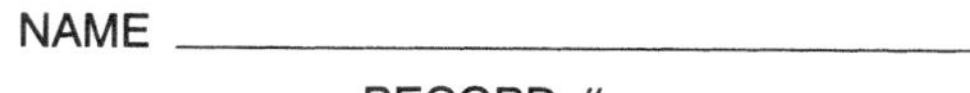

RECORD #

Date	Age	Weight	Stature	BMI*	Comments

***To Calculate BMI**: Weight (kg) ÷ Stature (cm) ÷ Stature (cm) x 10,000
or Weight (lb) ÷ Stature (in) ÷ Stature (in) x 703

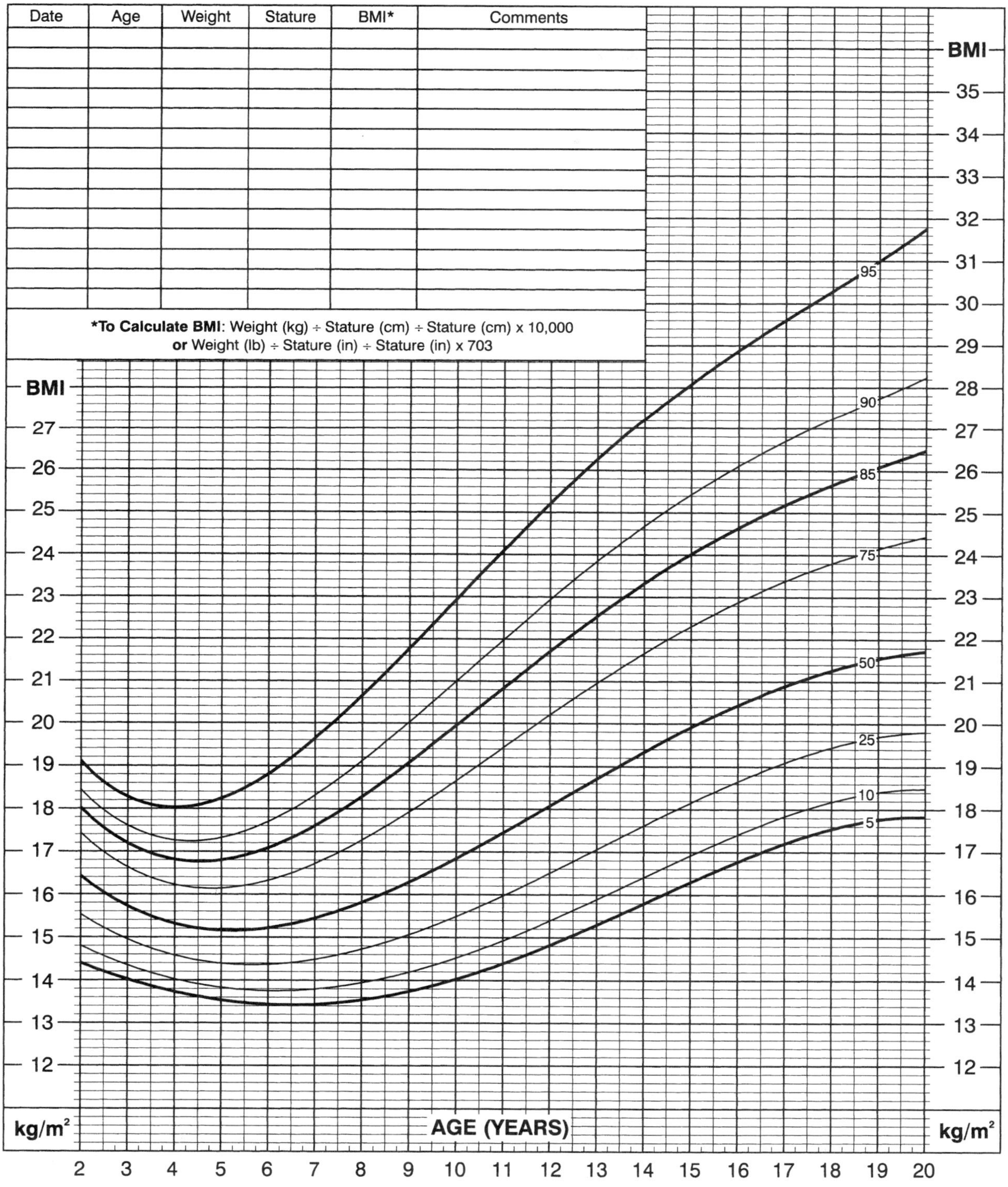

BMI
35
34
33
32
31
30
29
28
27
26
25
24
23
22
21
20
19
18
17
16
15
14
13
12
kg/m²

95
90
85
75
50
25
10
5

AGE (YEARS)

2 3 4 5 6 7 8 9 10 11 12 13 14 15 16 17 18 19 20

Published May 30, 2000 (modified 10/16/00).
SOURCE: Developed by the National Center for Health Statistics in collaboration with the National Center for Chronic Disease Prevention and Health Promotion (2000).
http://www.cdc.gov/growthcharts

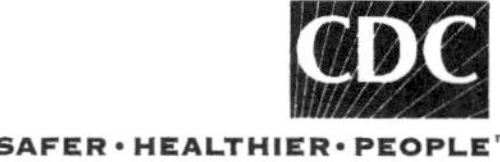

Figure 16.4 ■ Female body mass index.

even though their chronological age height is below expected percentiles (Germak, 2002; Haywood & Getchell, 2001). Bone age can also examine those who grow too fast too early.

Growing bones are flexible and highly porous. Thus, the younger child's bones can absorb a great deal of energy and not sustain a fracture (Bowden, Dickey, & Greenberg, 1998). The bones of children can bend slightly and heal quickly. Although the bones are more flexible, children can suffer fractures of the growth plate or epiphysial plate. Growth plate fractures may affect the future growth of the bone if the fracture interrupts the integrity of the epiphysial plate (D'Ambra & Jack, 1999). It is extremely important that these injuries are adequately assessed and treated so that bone deformity does not occur.

Muscle Growth

Muscles grow in length and width to accommodate the growing bones. Muscles grow naturally by the addition of sarcomeres, which make up the muscle cells and the muscle fiber. The muscle is composed of bundles of fiber (Haywood & Getchell, 2001). The more activity the muscles are subjected to during growth, the greater the diameter and thus the larger the muscle.

Muscle mass in childhood is similar for boys and girls. A marked difference in muscle mass between boys and girls begins at puberty due to the influence of androgens. Girls generally add muscle mass up until age 13 with 45% of their body weight due to muscle mass. Boys will continue to add muscle mass until approximately age 17, and 54% of their body weight is due to muscle mass (Haywood & Getchell, 2001).

Dentition

Most preschool children have all of their primary teeth. The U.S. Department of Health and Human Services (USDHHS, 2001a) recommends that dental services begin at approximately 12 months of age, or shortly after the primary teeth begin to erupt. Preschool children can brush their own teeth with some assistance. Dental health lessons help to reinforce the importance of dental hygiene with the preschool child. Some preschool programs make brushing teeth part of the morning ritual. Regular preventive dental care should be continued during the school years with biannual check-ups and cleaning.

Traumatic dental injury, even of deciduous teeth, should always be referred to a dentist, as trauma to the underlying permanent tooth may require evaluation when the deciduous tooth is injured. Avulsion of a permanent tooth is a dental emergency if the tooth is to be saved (see Chapter 24).

Most children do not start losing primary teeth until they have reached school age. The permanent teeth develop in the jaw beneath the primary teeth. The roots of the primary teeth gradually are absorbed and eventually the crown is all that is left which then becomes loose and falls out allowing the permanent teeth to erupt. As the child grows, the jaw also grows to allow room for larger permanent teeth. Eruption of the permanent teeth generally follows a sequential pattern (Figure 16.5). During the school-age years, the central and lateral incisors erupt, followed by the second and third cuspids, then the first and second molars.

The second molars erupt around age 12 to 13, whereas the wisdom teeth, or third molars, may not erupt until the student has graduated (between ages 17 and 21). Because the jaw does not reach its

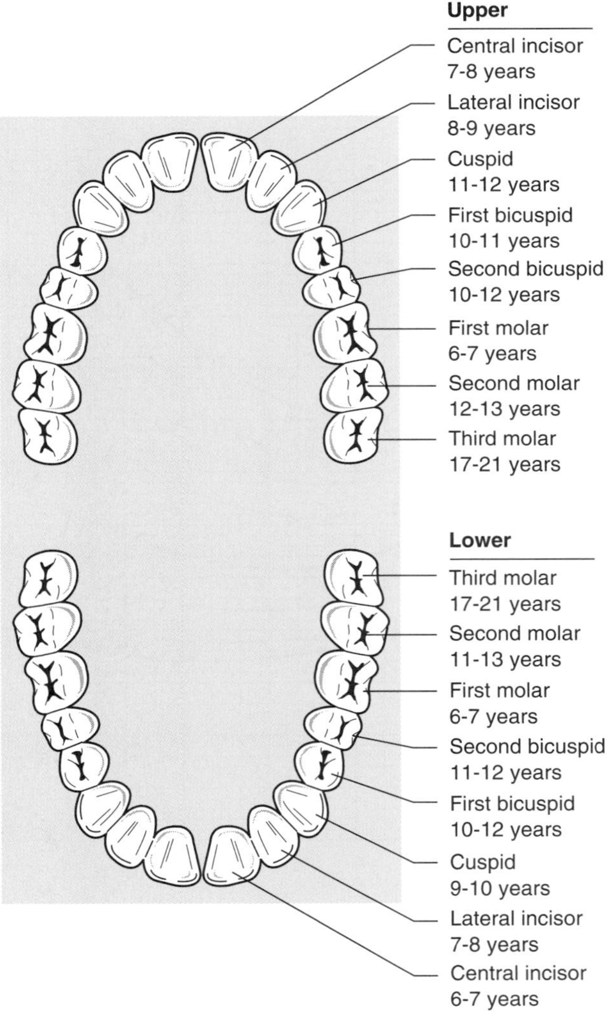

Figure 16.5 ■ Eruption of permanent secondary teeth.

full size until the end of adolescence, early eruption of the wisdom teeth may cause pain and discomfort. This may result in the third molars having to be removed. In addition, during the adolescent years and while the jaw continues to develop, many students have orthodontic work done, including the use of dental braces to realign teeth.

Losing the first tooth occurs generally during kindergarten or first grade; this is an important event for a child. Across cultures, it is heralded with fanfare. The "tooth fairy" is an American tradition and when a tooth is left under a pillow, it is replaced with money. In Europe, a mouse takes the tooth away and the child is left with assurances that the tooth will be replaced by another tooth (Austrian, 2002). Children need to know that losing deciduous teeth is a normal part of development. Primary teeth may not fall out naturally. If the erupting permanent tooth is visible, a visit to the dentist may be necessary to remove the primary tooth to allow the permanent tooth room to erupt.

Students who lose a tooth in school are often sent to the school nurse, perhaps because of the small amount of bleeding that may occur. School nurses often keep a collection of special containers so that the student can safely take the tooth home to show family members. Losing the first tooth can lead to a teachable moment and give the nurse the opportunity to discuss brushing and dental hygiene.

Dental caries are the most common disease of childhood, occurring five times more frequently than asthma in the 5- to 17-year-old age group (CDC, 2005b). Regular dental visits and proper brushing and flossing can prevent the formation of dental caries. However, for many children and adolescents, dental care is not available. It has been shown that children from some racial and ethnic minority groups and children from low socioeconomic areas have more untreated oral disease than the general population (CDC, 2005b). Students may present to the school nurse with poor dental hygiene or possibly a large painful cavity.

Proper dental hygiene is essential for the development and maintenance of good oral health. School nurses can teach students about brushing and flossing. If school nurses continue to deliver the message to children, they will take the message home and teach the parents. Prevention is still the best treatment in dental health. Contact local organizations to donate toothbrushes for distribution to children. Look in the community for dentists who will accept Medicaid clients or ask local dentists to adopt your school for children in need. The month of February has been designated Dental Health Month by the American Dental Association. School nurses can take advantage of numerous opportunities during this time to incorporate lessons into the school day. Invite a local dentist or dental hygienist to the school to speak to students. Information should be provided to children as well as parents. The American Dental Association has classroom ideas and resources available on its Web site, http://www.ada.org.

Multiple situations occurring during childhood can affect the developing teeth. Areas with high fluoride content in the water can cause mottling or white or brownish discolorations in the teeth. Malnutrition, illness, and trauma can also affect developing teeth causing hypocalcification or hypoplasia. Hypocalcification is seen as white opaque patches on the tooth and hypoplasia occurs as areas of pitting or the absence of enamel. Local trauma to primary incisors can affect the formation of permanent incisors, so trauma even to primary teeth should be referred to the dentist for evaluation. Repeated or prolonged antibiotic therapy with tetracycline before age 7 can cause brownish-yellow discoloration of the teeth (Johnsen & Tinanoff, 2000) and chronic Dilantin use for control of seizures can cause the gums to grow over the teeth (gingival hyperplasia).

Box 16.4 ■ ■ ■

WEB SITES FOR DENTAL HEALTH INFORMATION

http://www.ada.org American Dental Association
http://www.adha.org American Dental Hygienists Association
http://www.bmcc.org/Headstart/Dental Dental health lessons

Commercial Sites

http://www.colgateoralcare.com Colgate
http://www.cresthealthysmiles.com Crest

PHYSIOLOGICAL CHANGES

Metabolism

Metabolism refers to all physical and chemical changes in the body. The basal metabolic rate (BMR) is the minimum energy expenditure of the body at rest. It is affected by many different factors including age, sex, height, weight, exercise, hormones, and stress (Berne & Levy, 1998). Children and adolescents

Box 16.5 ■■■

THE STUDENT ATHLETE

Flavored sports drinks help to increase the amount of fluid a student athlete consumes and allows for better hydration than just drinking water. Water has been shown to replace only half of the fluids lost during exercise.

(National Athletic Trainers Association, 2003)

have higher metabolic rates than adults in order to produce energy for growth. During periods of exercise or illness, the basic metabolic rate increases even more. For each centigrade increase of body temperature, the BMR will increase approximately 10% (Curran & Barness, 2000). During sleep the metabolic rate decreases (Berne & Levy, 1998).

With an increased metabolic rate, caloric and fluid intake must increase to maintain adequate body function. For example, physical activity during hot weather, whether related to sports or marching band practice, requires an increased intake of fluids to maintain adequate hydration and body function due to the influence of exercise and the environment on metabolic rate. The student with a fever should be encouraged to drink fluids to help maintain hydration because of the increased demands of the body. The presence of fever is an indication that a student should not participate in sports and physical activity. The increased body temperature puts the student at increased risk of developing a heat-related illness (Binkley, Beckett, Casa, Kleiner, & Plummer, 2002; Coyle, 2000).

School nurses are often asked about excessive heat or extreme cold when deciding to send children outside for recess, hold field days, or continue with some other athletic event. Because children have a higher metabolic rate than adults, they produce more heat during exercise but do not transfer the heat generated from the muscles to the skin for cooling as well as adults (Coyle, 2000; Steen & Bernhardt, 2000). Sweating is the primary method of cooling the body temperature and children younger than 14 years of age do not sweat as much as adults. Less circulating blood volume in children is even more dramatic when sweating lowers blood volume (Coyle, 2000).

In extreme temperatures, exercise can cause heat-related illness in children. Experts advise the best measurement to determine whether it is safe to exercise in heat is a wet-bulb globe temperature. This is an index based on the measurement of air temperature, evaporative cooling, and radiation, although this is generally not available to the school nurse. School guidelines should be developed. For example, if an activity lasts more than 30 minutes, exercise in 90°F air temperature at 20% humidity approaches the dangerous zone. A critical zone would be humidity at 40% and the temperature at 90°F (Coyle, 2000). (See heat-related injuries in Chapter 24.) It might be prudent on extremely hot days to shorten the length of physical activity to lessen the risk of heat injury. Vepraskas (2002) adapted the Heat Index Chart in Figure 16.6 based on the National Weather Service Heat Index chart. Additional information is provided in Box 16.7.

Fluid replacement is important, and drinking from a cup allows more fluid intake than drinking from the water fountain (Coyle, 2000). Children on certain medications, such as anticholinergic drugs, diuretics, certain antibiotics, and antihistamines,

Box 16.6 ■■■

Recess during school is often scheduled around lunchtime. Not only is this the hottest part of the day, but also sun exposure is at its highest. Students should be protected from harmful sunrays by using sunscreen with an SPF greater than 15. In a recent study, adolescents were found to be exposed to enough ultraviolet radiation during the course of a normal school day to cause sunburn (American Academy of Dermatology, 2002). Encourage parents to include sunscreen as part of the daily routine. School nurses can educate students on the importance of sunscreen in protecting the skin from the short- and long-term consequences of sun exposure.

Box 16.7 ■■■

TO EXERCISE OR NOT TO EXERCISE. THAT IS THE QUESTION.

Heat index and wind chill can be calculated on the National Weather Service Web site http://www.crh.noaa.gov/lsx/calc.php

The National Athletic Trainers Association Heat Illness Consensus statement. http://www.nata.org/publicinformation/files/heatillnessconsensusstatement.pdf

Temperature (F)	Relative Humidity (%) 90.0	80.0	70.0	60.0	50.0	40.0	30.0	20.0	10.0	
75	79.7	76.7	75.8	74.8	73.9	72.9	72.0	71.1	70.1	Green Zone Below 80
80	88.2	85.9	84.2	82.8	81.6	80.4	79.0	77.4	76.1	
85	101.4	97.0	93.3	90.3	87.7	85.5	83.5	81.6	79.6	
90	119.3	112.0	105.8	100.5	96.1	92.3	89.2	86.5	84.2	Yellow Zone 80 to 100
95	141.8	131.1	121.7	113.6	106.7	100.9	96.1	92.2	89.2	
100	168.7	154.0	140.9	129.5	119.6	111.2	104.2	98.7	94.4	
105	200.0	180.7	163.4	148.1	134.7	123.2	113.6	105.8	100.0	Red Zone Above 100
110	235.6	211.2	189.1	169.4	151.9	136.8	124.1	113.7	105.8	

Green Zone : Outdoor conditions ideal.
Yellow Zone: Heat exhaustion possible with prolonged exposure & activity
Red Zone: Heat cramps & exhaustion likely with prolonged exposure. Heatstroke possible. Limit or cancel outdoor rehearsals.

Figure 16.6 ■ Heat index chart. (Reprinted with permission from Vepraskas, C. [2002].)

are more sensitive to heat and sun exposure and these children will need special accommodations (Coyle, 2000). Students who are taking antipsychotic medications such as Seroquel (U.S. Food and Drug Administration [FDA], 2004), Abilify, or Risperdal, or antiepileptic medications such as Topamax (FDA, 2003) should exercise caution when participating in activities that may expose them to excessive heat.

Children are also more affected by extreme cold temperatures, although more injuries are associated with heat than with cold. The larger skin surface to body-mass ratio and less subcutaneous fat in children make them more susceptible to cold than adults (Coyle, 2000). During exercise in cold weather, a child's higher metabolic rate allows him or her to stay warmer. Not all children run around and stay warm during recess, and it is harder for a child to stay warm at rest. Guidelines are fairly liberal when gauging temperature, wind chill, and the risk of freezing exposed flesh. There is increased risk of freezing exposed flesh when the air temperature is 10°F and the wind chill factor is –25°F. However, frostnip, severe chilling without freezing can occur on the nose, ears, face, and fingers (Coyle, 2000e). Again, common sense should prevail and children should have adequate clothing to protect themselves from cold exposure, including hat and gloves.

Nutritional Needs

Nutrition is a major component in promoting growth and health and in preventing disease. Research shows that good nutrition lowers the risk for developing heart disease, stroke, diabetes, some types of cancer, and osteoporosis (USHHS & USDA, 2005). Lack of adequate nutrition also affects the immune response to fight disease and is linked to lowered ability to concentrate and limited overall learning potential (Center on Hunger and Poverty, 1998).

School nurses will be the first to identify a hungry child who cannot concentrate or pay attention in class. The importance of a nutritious breakfast every morning is widely recognized, yet many students come to school without breakfast. Many schools have federal breakfast programs, and all efforts should be made to ensure that children eat before school. A stomach pain at 10:00 in the morning may be related to hunger and may be relieved by a nutritious snack.

As stated earlier, physical growth will catch up if nutritional needs are met at a later date, but lack of nutrition may be an indicator of other familial problems that may require intervention. The child may suffer from a lack of parental supervision, chaotic and unsafe living conditions, or extreme poverty. At the other end of the spectrum, sedentary activities, such as television viewing and computer and video games, and excess calorie intake con-

Box 16.8 ■ ■ ■

School nurses often keep nutritious snacks on hand to help students who may have missed breakfast. It is important to find out why the student is not eating breakfast. The nurse may intervene and enroll the student in a breakfast program, or talk to the parents about nutrition at home.

tribute to the increasing obesity problem among youth.

Intake affects multiple systems and body functions. Eating large amounts of sweetened foods is linked to tooth decay (Nemours Foundation, 2001a). It is not, however, linked to hyperactivity. Large amounts of soda may replace milk in a child's diet and therefore the student may not get sufficient amounts of calcium. Sweetened foods and soda are also high in calories, contributing to the obesity problem. Drinks high in caffeine such as cola, root beer, coffee, or tea can create additional concerns. Caffeine is a stimulant and can interfere with a student's sleep patterns. It has also been linked to nervousness, irritability, and headaches, all of which will interfere with learning (National Association of School Nurses [NASN], 2002).

Preschool and school-age children enjoy helping to prepare meals and are beginning to make snack choices. This is an ideal time to include nutrition education to help children make wise food choices, including portion size. A play area with plastic food items to make pretend meals and pretend grocery shopping can help to guide a child to make good food choices. Children can also participate in real cooking experiences. Three-year-old children can spread soft spreads, knead and shape yeast dough, pour liquids, and mix other ingredients. Four-year-old children can peel eggs or oranges and 5-year-old children can measure ingredients.

Adolescence is a time of significant growth, and good nutrition is essential to attain optimal health and meet metabolic demands. However, there are multiple demands on students' time that interfere with healthy eating. While some students make wise choices, far too many subsist on snack foods and foods high in sugar with little or no nutritional value. Teens participate in sports and have after school jobs leading to irregular schedules, so prepared family meals may be uncommon. In the rush to get out of bed and to school on time, breakfast may be an afterthought, or given no thought until the hunger pains occur at midmorning.

Most adolescent females require about 1,800 to 2,400 calories a day and adolescent boys require between 2,200 and 3,200 calories per day (U.S. Department of Agriculture, 2005). A variety of food choices is important and should be stressed with emphasis on limiting foods high in sugar and fat. Students can also be taught to be wise consumers and read nutrition labels on food choices.

Teens who participate in strenuous athletic activities will require more calories. Frequent nutritious snacks will help to supply the energy and nutrition needed. The school nurse may suggest that athletes eat a nutritious snack after school before they engage in the athletic activity.

Students will benefit when the school nurse communicates regularly with the cafeteria staff or food vendor about student nutrition. Vending machines create controversy in schools over the nutritious value of snacks and drink versus the income derived from sales. It may be difficult to offer only fruit and healthy foods in the snack line, but if the goal is to have teens eating with nutrition in mind, efforts should be made to support that goal.

Adolescent athletes are prime targets for nutrition education (see Chapter 24 on athlete health). They need to understand that good nutritional habits will boost their performance. Establishing a link between performance and good nutrition may encourage the athlete to exercise good eating habits. If possible, all sport teams should receive information on good nutrition at the start of each season. A follow-up session during mid-season may be helpful.

Quick weight gain or weight loss of the adolescent athlete should be discouraged. Wrestlers who are trying to make a certain weight class may crash diet or try to "sweat-out" water to make the weight. This is a dangerous practice, as evidenced by the deaths of three college athletes in 1997. The National Collegiate Athletic Association (NCAA) took steps to eliminate any weight control practices that would risk the health of the participant (NCAA, 2001). The National Federation of State High School Associations took steps to require each state association to develop and use a weight-control program to prevent severe weight reduction by 2004 (Perriello, 2001).

Female athletes may exhibit signs of eating disorders such as anorexia nervosa or bulimia. The Female Athlete Triad (see Chapter 24) is a pattern of disordered eating, amenorrhea and osteoporosis (Donaldson, 2003; Kazis & Iglesias, 2003; Sherman & Thompson, 2004). Multiple orthopedic fractures or secondary amenorrhea should be red flags for the school nurse to refer the female athlete for a more complete assessment. Sports such as gymnastics, dance, or running, in which a lean physique is encouraged, put athletes at risk for developing this triad. The athlete herself may strive for an unnatural weight loss and control eating by restricting intake, or exhibit patterns of binging and purging.

Student athletes should focus on eating the proper diet so they can get the most out of their training and be at peak performance on game day. An athlete should eat a full meal 2 to 3 hours prior to an event, which includes complex carbohydrates and limits excessive fat and protein. A well-balanced meal after the event should include protein and fat (Nemours, 2005). Athletes who participate in day-long activities should have high-energy nutritious snacks to eat during the day to maintain adequate energy and nutrition. Fluid intake is essential during periods of exertion and care should be taken to ensure adequate hydration. If an athlete is adequately hydrated, the urine will be clear.

A balanced diet is needed with a variety of food choices, as no one single food supplies the necessary nutrients. TABLE 16.1 offers guidelines for calorie intake for the school-age child and adolescent.

If the diet is adequate, vitamin and mineral intake is most likely adequate. Poor eating habits, eating disorders, or unhealthy weight loss are examples of situations that may cause a vitamin defi-

Table 16.1 ■
FOOD GROUPS

FOOD GROUP	MODERATELY ACTIVE CHILDREN AGES 4-8 (1,400-1,600) CALORIES	MODERATELY ACTIVE FEMALES AGES 9-13 (1,600-2,000 CALORIES) AGES 14-18 (2,000 CALORIES)	MODERATELY ACTIVE MALES AGES 9-13 (1,800-2,200 CALORIES) AGES 14-18 (2,400-2,800 CALORIES)	WHAT IS A SERVING	IMPORTANT BECAUSE THEY SUPPLY:
Bread, cereal, rice, and pasta group (whole grains recommended)	6 servings per day	6–8 servings per day	6–11 servings per day	• 1 slice of bread • 1 cup cold cereal • 1/2 cup cooked rice, hot cereal or pasta	Body fuel in the way of complex carbohydrates; Vitamin B-complex (folate); Bulk to help eliminate waste
Vegetable	3–4 servings per day	4–5 servings per day	5–7 servings per day	• 1 serving • 1 cup raw leafy vegetables • 1/2 cup other cooked vegetables • 3/4 cup vegetable juice	Vitamins A and C Potassium Folate
Fruit	3 servings per day	3-4 servings per day	3-5 servings per day	• 1 medium apple • 1/2 cup cooked or canned fruit • 3/4 cup fruit juice	Vitamins A and C Potassium Fiber to help with elimination

(continued)

Table 16.1 ■ *(Continued)*

FOOD GROUP	MODERATELY ACTIVE CHILDREN AGES 4-8 (1,400-1,600) CALORIES	MODERATELY ACTIVE FEMALES AGES 9-13 (1,600-2,000 CALORIES) AGES 14-18 (2,000 CALORIES)	MODERATELY ACTIVE MALES AGES 9-13 (1,800-2,200 CALORIES) AGES 14-18 (2,400-2,800 CALORIES)	WHAT IS A SERVING	IMPORTANT BECAUSE THEY SUPPLY:
Low-fat or fat-free dairy foods	2 or 3 servings per day	2 or 3 servings per day	3 servings per day	• 1 cup milk or yogurt (reduced or fat free) • 1 ½ ounces of cheese (reduced or fat free)	Vitamins A and D Calcium Protein
Meat, poultry, fish, nuts seeds legumes	1–2 servings per day	1–2 servings per day	1–2 servings per day	• 3 ounces of cooked lean meat, poultry or fish • ½ cup cooked dry beans • ⅓ cup nuts • ½ oz. seeds	Protein Iron and zinc Vitamin B complex
Fats and oils	sparingly < 30% of total calories	sparingly < 30% of total calories	sparingly < 30% of total calories	• 1 tsp. vegetable oil • 1 tsp. soft margarine	

Source: Adapted from Health and Human Services and U.S. Department of Agriculture (2005).

ciency (Peel, 2002). Vegetarian diets are generally healthy; however, consultation with a dietician or healthcare provider may be necessary to ensure that all the nutritional requirements are being met. TABLE 16.2 describes the different vegetarian diets.

Vital Signs

Temperature

The normal body temperature for children and adolescents is between 97.5° and 98.6°F when measured orally. The body temperature may fluctuate based on the time of day, exercise, excessive clothing, or environmental temperature (Bowden et al., 1998; Huether & Leo, 2002). Oral electronic thermometers can give an estimate of body temperature and are generally accepted as accurate measures (Dinu, 2003). The ear-based temperature readings with an infrared sensor reliably measure the temperature in the ear canal. Both methods may be affected by environmental factors. It must be noted that some ear-based thermometers commonly used in schools do not measure tympanic temperature and should not be referred to as tympanic thermometers. Other methods, such as axillary measurements with electronic thermometers and the thermographs (plastic strip thermometers), have

Table 16.2 ■
VEGETARIAN DIETS

TYPE OF DIET	FOOD CHOICES	SUPPLEMENTS THAT MAY BE NEEDED
Semivegetarians	• Milk products • Limited seafood • Poultry No red meat	Increased risk for iron and zinc deficiencies
Lactovegetarians	• Milk products No eggs, meat, fish or poultry	Increased risk for iron and zinc deficiencies
Ovolactovegetarians	• Milk products • Eggs No meat, fish or poultry	Increased risk for iron and zinc deficiencies
Ovovegetarians	• Eggs No milk, meat, fish or poultry	Riboflavin Vitamins D and B_{12} Increased risk for iron and zinc deficiencies
Vegans	• Vegetable food only No foods of animal origin	Riboflavin Vitamins D and B_{12} Increased risk for iron and zinc deficiencies

Source: Adapted from Neinstein, L. & Schack, L. (2002).

been found to underestimate body temperature. The thermographs have also given false elevated temperature readings due to the influence of air temperature (Dinu, 2003).

There is concern about the mercury in glass thermometers, should the thermometer break. The cumulative effects of mercury getting into the environment and the ease and availability of electronic thermometers make mercury thermometers unnecessary and they should not be used (Goldman & Shannon, 2001). If glass thermometers are still being used, a policy approved by public health should be in place in the event of breakage regarding the cleanup and removal of the mercury (DiCarlo, Ruck, & Marcus, 2002). Contact the local public health officials to determine how to dispose of the broken thermometer and the mercury. The area of the breakage is considered contaminated and must be cleaned promptly using special gloves, mercury-absorbing powder, and a special container for disposal of the mercury.

Blood Pressure in Children

Screening for blood pressure in children has not routinely been undertaken in the schools. Although hypertension has been associated with increased morbidity in adulthood, children were previously not thought to be at risk for high blood pressure. The Fourth Report on the Diagnosis, Evaluation and Treatment of High Blood Pressure in Children and Adolescents (National High Blood Pressure Education Program Working Group on High Blood Pressure in Children and Adolescents, 2004) found that hypertension in children and adolescents occurs commonly and can be detected at a young age. Furthermore, there is a strong association between hypertension and obesity. Approximately 30% of overweight children are hypertensive. In adolescence, the incidence of hypertension increases as BMI increases.

Guidelines now exist for the diagnosis and treatment of hypertension in children. Lifestyle changes that focus on prevention of excess weight, regular physical activity, and appropriate nutrition have had success in the treatment of hypertension in adults and are now thought to benefit children who have been diagnosed with hypertension. In addition, children identified at risk of developing hypertension can be taught appropriate lifestyle changes and management to prevent long-term health consequences (Vessey et al., 2001).

One study indicates that blood pressure screening in schools is warranted but cautions that more formalized study is needed before a definitive decision is made to include blood pressure as part of routine screening in school (Vessey et al., 2001). If students are screened and identified as having high blood pressure or being at risk for it, health education from the school nurse concerning diet and exercise can be initiated. Interventions started at a young age for high-risk individuals can prevent future complications in adulthood. School nurses can and do promote wellness, which includes regular physical activity and maintaining a healthy weight and proper nutrition. Health promotion activities and targeted education can and should be initiated for all students whether or not they have been identified with hypertension.

When measuring blood pressure, care must be taken to choose the appropriate cuff size. Blood pressure should be taken in the upper right arm. The right arm is preferred for consistency and comparison to standard tables. To choose the appropriate cuff size, the width of the bladder in the cuff should be approximately 40% of the arm circumference midway between the olecranon and the acromion. The cuff should cover approximately two thirds of the upper arm and the cuff bladder should cover 80% to 100% of the arm circumference. Younger school-aged students will need a pediatric size cuff. Most adolescents will need an adult cuff size and large adolescents may need to have blood pressure taken with an extra large cuff. A cuff that is too small will give false high readings (Turman & Mahan, 2002). It is recommended that blood pressure be taken by auscultation and not by an automated device. Calibration and a lack of standards for these machines make auscultation the better choice (National High Blood Pressure Education Program, 2004).

Students should sit for 3 to 5 minutes in a quiet environment before the blood pressure is measured. The systolic measurement should be recorded when the first Kortokoff sound is heard. The diastolic measurement should be recorded at the disappearance of the Kortokoff sound for both children and adolescents or at the fifth Kortokoff sound (NHBPEPWGHBPCA, 2004). Blood pressure tables now consider age and body size when determining normal or high blood pressure. Students with a blood pressure measurement exceeding the 95th percentile for either the systolic or diastolic readings should be referred for evaluation and treatment. If a student is symptomatic with a marginal blood pressure reading, an immediate referral should be made to the primary care provider (PCP) (Thede & Iverson, 1999). Tables 16.3 and 16.4 provide a quick reference of blood pressure readings for the 50th percentile based on age in the 50th percentile of height. It is to be used only as a guide. The complete tables can be found in The Fourth Report on the Diagnosis, Evaluation and Treatment of High Blood Pressure in Children and Adolescents. (National High Blood Pressure Education Program Working Group on High Blood Pressure in Children and Adolescents, 2004.) A quick estimate can be predicted using the formulas in Box 16.9.

Often, initial identification of elevated blood pressure may be made by the Primary Care Provider (PCP) and the school nurse will be asked to collaborate with the PCP to monitor blood pressure on a regular basis. These repeated office visits provide an opportune time to educate students about proper diet and exercise and to reinforce the education provided by the PCP.

Risk factors such as family history cannot be

Table 16.3 ■

BLOOD PRESSURE READINGS IN THE 50TH PERCENTILE FOR GIRLS BY AGE IN THE 50TH HEIGHT PERCENTILE

AGE	SYSTOLIC/DIASTOLIC READINGS IN THE 50TH PERCENTILE
4	91/52
6	94/56
7	96/57
8	98/58
9	100/59
10	100/60
11	102/61
12	104/62
13	106/63
14	107/64
15	109/65
16	110/66
17	110/66

Source: Adapted from The Fourth Report on the Diagnosis, Evaluation and Treatment of High Blood Pressure in Children and Adolescents

Table 16.4 ■

BLOOD PRESSURE READINGS IN THE 50TH PERCENTILE FOR BOYS BY AGE IN THE 50TH HEIGHT PERCENTILE

AGE	SYSTOLIC/DIASTOLIC READINGS IN THE 50TH PERCENTILE
4	93/50
6	96/55
7	97/57
8	99/59
9	100/60
10	102/61
11	104/61
12	106/62
13	108/62
14	111/63
15	113/64
16	116/64
17	118/67

Source: Adapted from The Fourth Report on the Diagnosis, Evaluation and Treatment of High Blood Pressure in Children and Adolescents (National High Blood Pressure Education Program Working Group on High Blood Pressure in Children and Adolescents) (2004).

changed, but exercise and physical activity can be stressed as a method of controlling blood pressure by preventing obesity. Diets high in salt and caffeine have been linked to hypertension, as well as other behaviors such as smoking. Certain drugs, such as amphetamines and cocaine, can also increase blood pressure (Turman & Mahan, 2002). All of this information can be discussed during the brief period it takes to measure blood pressure.

Box 16.9 ■■■

A quick estimate for the average blood pressure in children can be determined using this formula for children ages 8 to 18:

Systolic pressure:
(2 × age in years) + 83

Diastolic pressure:
Age in years + 52

(Hockenberry, 2003)

Heart Rate

Heart rate slows as children grow older (Table 16.5). The heart rate in children should be recorded for a full minute to more accurately assess the rate and rhythm. Students may have a normal change in heart rhythm during respiration. The nurse can ask the student to hold his breath to evaluate the heart rhythm if she is concerned about an irregular rhythm.

Peripheral pulses can be used as a measure of heart rate in school-aged children and adolescents. The radial pulse is the most frequently used and the most convenient. Rhythm, rate, and amplitude

Table 16.5 ■

HEART RATES AT REST

AGE	LOWER LIMITS OF NORMAL		AVERAGE		UPPER LIMITS OF NORMAL	
4	80		100		120	
6	75		100		115	
8	70		90		110	
10	70		90		110	
	Girls	Boys	Girls	Boys	Girls	Boys
12	70	65	90	85	110	105
14	65	60	85	80	105	100
16	60	55	80	75	100	95
18	55	50	75	70	95	90

Source: Reprinted from Behrman, Kliegman, & Jenson (2000), with permission from Elsevier, Inc.

should be recorded. Normal amplitude is recorded as 2+. One note of interest is that the dorsalis pedis pulse can be found in different locations on the dorsum of the foot and is absent in 15% of normal individuals (Thede & Iverson, 1999).

Respiration

Normal respiration should be regular, smooth, and effortless (Table 16.6). School-age children have a ratio of inspiratory time to expiratory time of 1:2. The trachea should be at midline. The transverse measurement of the chest is proportional to the anterior posterior measurement with a ratio of 2:1 (Synoground & Thiele, 2000). Students with chronic respiratory conditions, such as asthma and cystic fibrosis, may have a barrel-shaped chest as a result of air trapping.

Sleep

Adequate sleep and rest are necessary for restoration and growth. Non-rapid eye movement (NREM) sleep has four stages and the child and adolescent will progress to stage 4 sleep within 20 to 30 minutes. In stage 4, respirations are slow and deep, heart rate slows, and temperature drops. Blood pressure also drops. In this deep stage of sleep, if the child is awakened, he or she may experience confusion and disorientation. Rapid-eye movement sleep (REM) follows the NREM stages. Dreams will occur during the REM stage of sleep and last between 10 and 30 minutes. Nightmares occur during NREM stage 3 and night terrors occur during the NREM stage 4 (Huether & Leo, 2002). Children will then start a new sleep cycle moving into the NREM sleep stages again. Each cycle lasts approximately 90 minutes. Bedwetting can occur at any stage of the sleep cycle (Scott & Dalton, 2000).

Preschool children need about 12 hours of sleep per night. Three-year old children may still need a nap during the day, but by age 4, most children have outgrown that need. Preschool-age children do not always sleep through the night and may experience periods of nighttime awakening.

Preschool children may not stay dry through the night. This is not considered enuresis until after age 5; even then, 15% to 25% of 5-year-old children wet the bed (Thiedke, 2003). The school nurse may be asked to talk with parents to ensure that the child is bathing before coming to school if he is still bedwetting to avoid unpleasant odors.

Secondary nocturnal enuresis occurs between the ages of 5 and 8 years. Primary nocturnal enuresis occurs in a child who has never been dry at night. Several factors may contribute to nocturnal enuresis. Children whose parents also had a history of nocturnal enuresis have been shown to have almost a 65% to 85% chance of developing nocturnal enuresis (Thiedke, 2003). Some believe that affected children sleep soundly and do not awaken with the urge to void. Others believe that children with enuresis have a smaller bladder capacity than those who do not wet the bed or have insufficient anti-diuretic hormone interfering with the kidney's ability to concentrate urine (Hockenberry, 2003; Thiedke, 2003). Transient environmental stressors may also cause secondary nocturnal enuresis and the behavior generally will be short lived once the stressors are reduced. Children should always be referred to their healthcare provider for a urinalysis and physical examination to rule out an organic cause (Scott & Dalton, 2000).

Several treatment programs exist to help with enuresis. These include:

- Bladder training to stretch the bladder by encouraging the child to hold urine after the urge to void appears.

Table 16.6 ■ NORMAL RESPIRATORY RATES

AGE	BREATHS PER MINUTE
4	23–30
6	21–26
8	20–26
10	20–26
12	18–22
14	18–22
16	16–20
18	12–20

Source: Reprinted from Bowden, Dickey, & Greenberg, (1998) with permission from Elsevier.

Box 16.10 ■ ■ ■

Drinking warm milk prior to bedtime to help a child sleep may not just be an old wive's tale. Milk contains the amino acid tryptophan, which synthesizes serotonin. It is thought that serotonin may be the neurotransmitter of the sleep-producing center in the brain and enhance sleep.

(Campbell, Reece, & Mitchell, 1999)

- A nighttime bell or buzzer alarm that awakens the child when the bed is wet. This method has been shown to be the most effective when treating nocturnal enuresis.
- Medication can also be used to help control bedwetting, but is not recommended for children younger than 6 years of age. Studies have shown that the relapse rate after the discontinuation of drug therapy is high so other methods may be preferable (Thiedke, 2003).
- Decrease nighttime fluids and avoid caffeine.

Punishment should never be used to control bedwetting, although the child should be encouraged to help with changing the sheets when wet (Nemours Foundation, 2001b). Parents can be reassured that nocturnal enuresis diminishes as the child gets older.

Children 10 to 12 years of age can get by on 9 to 10 hours of sleep (Thiedke, 2001). Sleep patterns may be an important assessment piece for the school nurse. Children who chronically do not get enough sleep may be irritable and have difficulty concentrating in the classroom, which impacts on learning. The school nurse may need to investigate sleep patterns of the child at home. The school nurse may assist the parents with strategies to ensure the child is getting adequate sleep. These may include finding a quiet place to sleep, bedtime rituals to establish a sleep routine, and enforced quiet time.

Sleep requirements vary in the adolescent population. Teens need between five and seven sleep cycles per night, that is, cycles of non-rapid-eye-movement (NREM) and rapid-eye-movement (REM) sleep. As each cycle lasts 90 minutes, teens may require between 7.5 and 9.5 hours of uninterrupted sleep. Lack of adequate sleep or interrupted sleep cycles can cause a disturbance of behavior and mood (Paolicchi, Pakalnis, & Joseph, 2002) as well as multiple visits to the school nurse's office with vague complaints such as headaches or body aches. Insomnia affects 10% to 20% of adolescents and may be due, in part, to alterations in regular sleep patterns (Behrman et al., 2000).

Daytime sleepiness is common in adolescents. Delayed sleep phase syndrome (DSPS) may be one possibility. In this case, the adolescent has difficulty falling asleep at night, but once he or she does fall asleep, he or she then has difficulty awakening in the morning (Paolicchi et al., 2002). Another cause may be the fact that the student has a paying job that requires working late hours. Late night school work and socializing with friends may also cause late sleep onset. Several clinicians advocate for a later starting time for high school students based on the adolescent's body clock. A later school starting time would allow students the extra hour to sleep.

Some teens have their sleep interrupted because of painful leg cramps they get in the middle of the night. These are common during adolescence and occur at transitions between sleep–wake cycles (Paolicchi et al., 2002). Stretching the cramped muscle at the time of the cramp can provide immediate relief.

DEVELOPMENT

Achievement of developmental tasks at specific ages or stages has always been the gauge by which "normal" development is measured. These are divided into motor development, cognitive and language development, and psychosocial and moral development.

Motor Development

The development of purposeful movement takes place over time. Gross motor development refers to the development of movement using large muscle groups and fine motor refers to small muscle groups; both mature as the child grows and gets stronger. The school environment is often a setting where professionals, other than parents, can observe a child over a period of time. It is important for the school nurse to be cognizant of the motor skills expected of various age groups. Early identification of possible delays can help access services to help the student reach his or her potential.

Balance is important in the overall synthesis of motor coordination and helps with spatial awareness. Balance is well established by the time a child reaches school age. A 3-year-old preschool child is a proficient walker and the speed and rhythm of his walk improves through childhood. Throwing, running, and combination movements such as a hop, skip, and a jump will continue to be developed through school age (Feldman, 2004; Haywood & Getchell, 2001). Young children can throw a ball but an adolescent is able to coordinate the shoulder, the leg, and the arm to put his body behind the force of the throw.

The 3-year-old should be able to jump off a step 12 inches high with both feet and can walk on a balance beam. He or she should be able to hop on one foot and ride a tricycle. By age 4, a child can walk down steps using alternate feet. After age 8, children should be able to move a limb without looking. Sixty percent of children have achieved a mature kicking pattern by age 8 (Gomez, 2000). Most children by age 9 do not make mistakes in body awareness, such as overreaching for a glass. Children up to age 12 are still developing directionality or spatial location; for example, the child may have difficulty when told to throw the ball to the right of the line (Haywood & Getchell, 2001). During the period of rapid growth in adolescence, the teen may become more awkward than he had been previously due to rapidly growing extremities. The young adolescent may underestimate the length of his arms or legs and appear awkward or gangly in movements. He or she may be clumsy when performing certain activities or misjudge the height of a step based on changing leg length and trip or fall.

Fine motor skills also continue to develop throughout childhood. By age 3, the child can undo clothes when going to the bathroom and can copy a circle with a pencil and use scissors; by age 4, he or she can copy a cross and should be able to draw a man in three parts (Lissauer & Clayden, 1997). A 4-year-old child can lace his or her shoes and by age 6 can tie his or her shoes, although this skill often occurs later because of the prevalence of Velcro fasteners on shoes.

The refinement of skills continues throughout school age. Writing and typing skills improve. Children may play a musical instrument, paint, or build models. Between ages 6 and 8, the speed with which messages are relayed to the muscles is significantly increased because of an increased production of myelin in the brain allowing fine motor skills to improve (Feldman, 2004). The child's increasing ability to concentrate and focus on a task for prolonged periods also helps fine muscle development.

Children who may appear clumsy or uncoordinated or are not achieving the milestones expected should be referred to the healthcare provider for evaluation. School nurses can also help to identify types of motor activities that are appropriate for children. They can observe students in both structured classroom settings and unstructured settings, such as recess.

School nurses are often called upon to help evaluate playground safety and to make recommendations for equipment that is both safe and promotes development. Hopscotch on the playground during elementary years will help develop motor coordination. A low-to-the-ground balance beam will help a child refine balance and spatial awareness. Climbing can help a child develop body awareness and increase upper body strength; however, children younger than 4 years of age should not play on climbing apparatus (Agnvall, 2000). Climbing apparatus for the school age child should be no higher than 7 feet. Ground cover on playgrounds should be at least 12 inches deep with materials such as wood chips, bark mulch, wood fibers, sand, or shredded tires in any area where falling is a possibility (National Safety Council, 2002; Nemours Foundation, 2002). Playground equipment is designed and made for two age groups: children ages 2 to 5 and children ages 5 to 12. Younger children should not play on equipment designed for older children. These Web sites offer further information and guidelines for playgrounds: http://www.nsc.org (National Safety Council) and http://www.uni.edu/playground/home.htm (National Program for Playground Safety).

In farming communities, children may be performing tasks while working on the family farm that may exceed the motor development of the child. The school nurse can help parents understand motor development and what tasks are safe for the school-age child or adolescent to perform. For example, children 7 to 9 years of age have slower reaction times than older children. This may increase the risk of injury around equipment with moving parts (National Children's Center for Rural and Agricultural Health and Safety, 1999). A good resource for school nurses and parents can be found at http://research.marshfieldclinic.org/children/Resources/default.htm.

Cognitive Development

Piaget examined the development of intelligence and cognitive thinking, and the reasons why children have certain beliefs and opinions (Beard, 1969). He described operational thinking as the way a child uses mental activity to reach a logical conclusion. He used the terms *equilibrium, assimilation, accommodation,* and *organization* to describe how a child interprets, adapts, and modifies his thinking into new and more complex abilities. Piaget described stages (CHART 1) to explain how a child develops and improves his operational thinking, with each stage representing the way a developing child looks at the world (Gardner, 1999). Piaget said that each stage is a building block on the previous stage and the sequence does not vary; however, different children of the same age may be at different stages in the sequence.

The preschool child, described by Piaget as ages 2 to 7, is in the stage of *preoperational thought*, having moved on from the sensorimotor stage. Preschool children look at what is happening around them as it relates to what they see or hear. They have not developed the ability to think logically. They view events from their own perspective and cannot take another view; thus, they are egocentric. Preschool children see what is presented at the moment; their perception of an object or an event is limited to what is seen, heard, or felt.

(text continues on page 364)

Chart 1 ■

MAJOR THEORIES OF DEVELOPMENT IN THE SCHOOL - AGE CHILD AND ADOLESCENT

AGE IN YEARS	COGNITIVE (PIAGET)	PSYCHOSOCIAL (ERIKSON)	MORAL (KOHLBERG)	IMPLICATIONS FOR THE SCHOOL NURSE
Preschool and Kindergarten Ages 2–7	**Preoperational Thought** The preschool child is an egocentric thinker. The child believes others see things exactly as they do. Children do not see the whole picture and generally think about one object at a time. Magical thinking is present.	**Initiative vs. Guilt** Children ages 3–6 are becoming more interactive with environment and are learning how to start action, thus initiative. Conflict comes when the child feels guilty about actions.	**Preconventional Level** Most concerned with needs of self.	Play is important during the preschool and early school years. Children learn about their environment and their place by acting out different roles, such as Doctor's Office, or grocery shopping play.
School Age 6/7 years–12 years	**Concrete Operations** Children build ideas one at a time. Concepts may change if the child is presented with different facts. Children begin to understand that matter can exist in different forms. They can classify objects, and understand reversibility.	**Industry vs. Inferiority** Children learn how to do things and make things. The child produces a product at home or school and hopefully receives positive feedback to build self-esteem. Child enjoys the positive feedback from doing something well.	**Conventional Level** Children are aware of the rules and follows rules to be viewed as a good person. Authority figures, such as parents, teachers and healthcare providers are important. Structure and framework are important and rules maintain the social order.	Health education is very effective during this time. Children want to be good and do what is right. Information to build a good foundation for health behaviors is important. Children value health lessons and can take the message home to parents. Visual aids such as models of the body can help to explain pain and other health issues.
Adolescent Age 12 and older	**Formal Operations** Adolescents can think about concepts in the abstract, although some may always think concretely. They understand past, present and future. They can envision consequences of actions and identify alternative outcomes. They enjoy debating issues and examining different ideas.	**Identity vs. Role Confusion** The changing body and the separation from parents help adolescents figure out where they belong. They search for their own identity and may experience some confusion in the process. Peers are very important.	**Postconventional Level** Adolescents follow the rules and laws of society for the good of all. They understand that some laws may need to be changed to benefit the society as a whole.	High-risk behavior can result from teens trying to fit in with peers, or find their own identity. Health behaviors may not be valued even though cognitively adolescents understand the outcomes of poor choices. Many teens choose to participate in pro-social activities such as the anti-tobacco movement.

Preschool children tend to be more fearful than school-age children because they cannot always separate the imagined or fantasy from the adult real world; they engage in magical thinking (Hockenberry, 2003; Kail, 2004). They also believe that everyone else sees exactly what they see (Gleitman, Fridlund, & Reisberg, 1998).

As the preschool child and kindergartener reach the end of the preoperational period, they enter the stage of *concrete operational thinking*, the ability to understand concepts in the concrete form; this stage encompasses ages from 7 to 11 to 12 years (Miller, 2004). Piaget concluded that early school-age children build ideas one at a time and are unable to keep more than one idea at a time; thus ideas will change when presented with different facts. Objects may take on a different view depending on the surroundings. These children are still egocentric in their thinking but are beginning to think logically. Children in concrete operations understand cause-and-effect, the concept of time and numbers, and where pieces fit into other pieces, as with puzzles. They understand the concepts of conservation of matter and reversibility.

They can understand events and consequences and thus make changes based on the expected results. They are able to categorize and classify objects and begin to serialize, arranging objects in categories and in order. By age 8, students using these skills can be involved in simple science experiments.

This is the age when they learn to read, write, and work with numbers. However, school age children can benefit from introducing new concepts using the various intelligences described by Gardner (1999). For example, a narrative or story may be valuable as a way to introduce a subject. The narrative helps provide the base and overall context of the subject and will provide a framework that helps a child relate to lessons taught. Multiple approaches can help to retain what is taught, such as music and rhymes.

Formal operations usually occur between the ages of 12 and 15. These adolescents can deal with the past, present, and future; they develop abstract thinking and an increased ability to analyze, synthesize, reason, and form logical conclusions. They understand scientific reasoning and benefit from talking about different attitudes and opinions (Piaget, 1961). Early adolescent teens, however, may fluctuate between concrete operations and formal operational thought. As they develop in this stage, adolescents become more confident in their ability to hypothesize and predict results and reflect on the results. Thinking becomes more flexible and input from various sources can be considered and applied (Austrian, 2002). Adolescents can generate different possibilities from certain situations and can begin to anticipate potential consequences of actions. Not all adolescents achieve formal operational thought and many continue to think in a concrete manner (Brown, 2002).

Box 16.11 ■ ■ ■

Children ages 8 or 9 may show an interest in comic books (Pillitteri, 1999). There are many health education comic books directed at this age group and it may be helpful to have them available in the school nurse's office for children to read.

Health teaching can be quite effective during this time. Adolescents want facts and explanations. They can identify different alternatives or outcomes based on choices and situations. However, their cognitive awareness does not guarantee that they will act on this knowledge. It is well known that adolescents make inappropriate choices, even though they are cognitively aware of the facts.

Inherent in understanding cause-and-effect and how things work is an interest in how the body works and stays healthy. Health teaching can be more effective if visual, hands-on models are available for children in all stages of development. Teachable moments can help a child connect his actions with an outcome.

While Piaget explained the stages and development of cognitive thinking, other theorists have offered additional observations. Vygotsky focused on how culture influences the development of cognitive learning. He claimed that social-mediated activity shapes cognitive growth. This involves observation of others, dialogue with elders and with other experienced members of society, and the lived experience within a culture (Shaffer, 1999). Therefore, new skills that are mastered are a function of the lived culture and a result of actively participating in culturally relevant tasks.

Gardner developed the concept of multiple intelligences (Kail, 2004). He thought that Piaget's cognitive theory favored the development of logical–mathematical thinking and did not explore different cognitive strengths. He describes "Nine Intelligences" that develop over time and can be used as *entry points* to develop cognitive strengths (Gardner, 1999; Kail, 2004). These include:

- *Linguistic* intelligence—the gift of language (a strong area for writers and poets)
- *Logical–mathematical* intelligence—strength

in problem solving (a strong area for scientists and mathematicians)

- *Spatial* intelligence—cognitive awareness of spatial relationships (strong for sailors, artists, and engineers)
- *Musical* intelligence—the ability to play an instrument, sing, and create music
- *Body–kinesthetic* intelligence—using the body to solve problems or perform (strong among dancers, professional athletes, and craftspeople)
- *Naturalist* intelligence—the ability to distinguish between different kinds of animals and different kinds of plants
- *Interpersonal* intelligence—the ability to work with people (strong for salespeople, teachers, and politicians)
- *Intrapersonal* intelligence—understanding and using one's own emotions and feelings to guide behavior
- *Existential* intelligence—ability to consider the purpose of life and death (Gardner, 1999).

Children may show strength in one or several areas. Children should be given an opportunity to explore and develop all of their intellectual strengths through a multitude of opportunities. Music education, physical education, and art education as well as traditional cognitive lessons are important in the overall development of the child (Gardner, 1999).

Children also learn through social contacts, whether directly or indirectly. The person, the environment, and behavior make up the triad of relationships that shapes the child (Merrell, 2003). Behavior that is rewarded will be repeated.

Language Development

Language development reflects cognitive development and is a sign of intelligence. Several theories exist describing the development of language, one of which is the Interactionist Perspective Theory. This describes language development as a result of a complex relationship between biological growth, cognitive development, and the changing linguistic environment of the child (Shaffer, 1999). Language development is important because it is the primary method of communication among people.

Preschool children master language at a rapid rate, forming sentences and developing social conversation. They can speak in sentences and begin to use adjectives in speech. They often ask questions about "who," "what," and "how". By age 4, most adults should be able to understand a child's speech (Lissauer & Clayton, 1997; Shaffer, 1999). They may have difficulty with pronouns and with pronunciation of certain words. As the child develops cognitively, they learn to adjust their language to the situation. For example, a preschool child can adjust his language when talking to a 2-year-old, as opposed to more formal speech when talking to an adult.

Language or speech disorders are frequently identified during early childhood education. A child may have older siblings and a language delay in "the baby" may go unnoticed. Once the child arrives at school, his lack of language development may become obvious in his interactions with others. Language concerns may be either expressive or receptive. A child may have difficulty expressing what he wants to say, even though his actual speaking skills are adequate. Conversely, a child may have difficulty comprehending language. Language and speech delay may be due to a hearing loss, inadequate stimulation in the home environment, or another developmental delay. If a language or speech delay is suspected, the child should be referred to a speech therapist for more thorough diagnosis and treatment (Lissauer & Clayton, 1997).

By age 6, most children have a vocabulary of between 8,000 and 14,000 words (Feldman, 2004). Children ages 6 to 8 can make inferences based on spoken communication and understand more than what was actually said (Shaffer, 1999). School age youth can communicate in code, tell jokes, and communicate nonverbally. They can speak in future tense and use nouns, plurals, and possessives. By 10 to 12 years of age, students can use formal versus informal speech and can change patterns depending on the audience, for example parents versus peers. Students can also understand the multiple meanings of words.

Difficulty pronouncing certain sounds such as j, v, th, ch, and sh may be noticeable (Feldman, 2004). Generally speech therapy is not required for common errors if the difficulty clears by second grade (Pillitteri, 1999). If there is a concern, the child can be further evaluated by a speech and language pathologist.

Communicating in the Health Office

It is often difficult to determine why a child has arrived at the health office. If the student is shy and has had a bad experience with clinicians, he or she may be reluctant to tell the nurse what is hurting. Other children may feel intimidated by the nurse without the support of a parent.

Deciphering the reason for a health room visit may take creativity and time. A nurse may keep dolls in her office to help children talk about an injury. It is always best to let a child explain what is

Box 16.12 ■■■

It is important for the school nurse to visit the classroom in the primary grades to familiarize the students with the school nurse and her role in the school. The school nurse should be seen as a helper and healthcare provider, health educator, and a valuable resource. The school nurse's office should be seen as a "safety zone."

happening; however, that may not always happen. A picture of different feelings such as "Happy," "Sad," "Angry," and "Afraid" may be helpful allowing the child to point to how they are feeling; the nurse can ask the child to "point to where it hurts." Pain rating scales may help to determine the severity of pain in a child. Several visual pain-rating scales are available for pediatric use.

Psychosocial Development

Erikson described certain challenges over the life span that individuals must address in order to develop a healthy personality and function in society. He called these challenges the "Eight Stages of Man" (Erikson, 1968) and they describe psychosocial development throughout life (Chart 1).

The preschool and kindergarten years are the stage of *initiative vs. guilt* as described by Erikson. The child is beginning to develop a conscience as he or she experiences self-observation and self-guidance and thus may feel guilty when his actions or thoughts cause conflict (Erikson, 1968; Shaffer, 1999). Preschoolers play with other children. It is at this stage that children recognize there is a difference in the sexes (Erikson, 1968). The child will imitate adult roles in play as he begins to learn about his adult role in the world, such as playing "family" or "doctor." The school nurse may want to provide the early childhood classroom with health-related equipment to foster imaginative play. Invite the class to come visit in the nurse's office to describe the role of the school nurse. This early role-play can help children see the school nurse as a helper and lessen future anxiety.

Three- to five-year-olds entering school for the first time may experience some separation anxiety when they realize that their parent or caregiver is planning to leave them in a new place with many different people. A visit to the new school prior to the start of school may help to familiarize the child with the new environment. The school can help by having the same staff member meet the child each day and escort him or her into the classroom. It may be necessary for the parent to remain in the classroom for a period of time to help the child adjust, but the time can be shorter each day. Good-byes should not be prolonged, but the parent should not "slip-away" either. Routines are important to the preschool child and decrease anxiety.

School-age children enter the stage of *industry versus inferiority*, where they have a need to accomplish and make things and become industrious. Projects that allow the child to succeed, such as papers, pictures, projects, and recitals, help to build self-confidence and thus encourage industry. Positive recognition of accomplishments provides feedback to the child and helps to establish a sense of purpose and productivity, in turn promoting positive self-esteem. Failure at these tasks and criticisms by those around him or her can lead to feelings of inferiority. This inferiority has a direct impact on the child's self-esteem and the child may feel unable to accomplish tasks. Repeated failures and negative feedback may cause the child to quit trying.

Musical talents may be encouraged or physical movements may be useful to help master skills. A student skilled in interpersonal relationships may be given roles that allow his talent to receive recognition. The school nurse may need to help a child find success when the school nurse's office becomes an outlet or respite from a stressful academic situation.

Adolescence brings on the stage of *identity versus role confusion*. The adolescent body is growing, maturing and changing and they are concerned with how others see them. Peer groups and cliques become important as adolescents try to figure out where they belong and look to others to provide feedback. Acceptance by peers provides a sense of self worth. Indeed most activity during this stage revolves around activities with peers.

Teenagers can be quite cruel to those they perceive as different from themselves. This searching for identity can lead to some role confusion as teens examine different values and norms. Thus the current fads of tattoos and body piercing are the adolescent's way of "fitting in" and belonging to a group. Late adolescents enter the stage of *intimacy versus isolation*. After learning one's identity, the person is ready to share his identity with others. Thus the search for a significant other begins.

Moral Development

Kohlberg (1981) examined the moral development of an individual and identified stages of moral development (Chart 1). A major criticism of Kohlberg's theory was that he only studied males; thus, gender differences were not accounted for (Austrian, 2002).

The **Preconventional Level** has two stages and identifies the most basic and primitive of moral development. During stage 1, right and wrong are understood but are judged by who has the power, that is, parents. Avoidance of punishment is of most importance; thus it is called the Punishment and Obedience Orientation. Stage 2, The Instrumental Relativist Orientation, examines fairness, equal sharing, and reciprocity. Thus, children can work in groups and be expected to cooperate with each other. This stage begins around the age of 4, and children can be expected to accept differences in other children, whether they are cultural, racial, or socioeconomic.

They conform to the rules imposed by others and respond to labels such as good or bad. Cultural and familial attitudes are understood by preschool children; thus many biases and prejudices are learned at this time (Feldman, 2004). Care must be taken to expose children to different cultures as a way of learning about differences in others at an early age.

At the **Conventional Level**, good behavior is judged by what is generally acceptable by the majority. Rule following and respect for authority are of primary importance. Certain behavior is expected in order to maintain the social order, such as obeying the law. Most of society functions at this level. Early and middle adolescence function at the conventional level, where it is important to obey the rules and follow the laws set by society.

As they enter school, children are exposed to authority figures other than their parents, and usually believe what they say as "law." By age 10, fairness is important and children consider cooperation and the respect of others when deciding on rules to follow. After age 10, the needs of a group help determine the rules and children follow the rules to please others and be part of the group.

Children enjoy helping others because this is "nice behavior"; they enjoy the recognition and praise received for being "nice." This stage is complicated by cultural differences of what is "right" and "nice." Therefore, schools must stipulate the rules of the school. For example, bullying must be defined and bullying behaviors must be identified (see Chapter 39 on violence).

The teen has a sense of justice but tends to see issues in black and white. The adolescent looks to peers for moral approval rather than to family. This is an ideal time for students to become involved in activities to influence legislation to change laws.

The **Postconventional, Autonomous, or Principled Level** recognizes the moral code of individuals apart from the rules of society. The values are followed because the individual believes in the rightness of the principles. At this level, one recognizes that laws can be changed if they can be shown to benefit the whole of society. Adolescents can be expected to follow this adult standard. By late adolescence postconventional moral values develop and they are able to look at the laws and rules as they affect society. The older adolescent considers whether the rules fit his own inner principles and values.

Studies show that the development of moral codes in females is based on interpersonal relationships. The emphasis on nurturing and caring that is encouraged in females influences their moral decisions and thus may be different than those identified in males (Austrian, 2002). Gilligan asserts that females base their moral decisions on caring whereas males base their moral decisions on the principles of justice as described by Kohlberg (Austrian, 2002).

INFLUENCES ON DEVELOPMENT: DEVELOPMENTAL THEORIES

Expert school nurses know they cannot work with a student in isolation of his or her parents and family. Family systems theory views the family as a system that continually interacts with its environment. Each family member affects other family members. The family is viewed as adaptable and can respond to positive and negative feedback. An open family system accepts feedback and information from outside the family; this allows the family to use resources within the community and accept new information and opportunities. A closed family system is more reluctant to accept information from outside sources. The student's family is discussed in Chapter 17.

Bronfenbrenner (1979) criticized other theorists such as Piaget and Erikson because they studied the child in isolation. He argued that the child is part of his lived experiences, his cultural experiences, and the expectations of the family. He described the external systems affecting the family and thus the child. These include the parents' workplace, the parents' social networks, and the influence of the community on the family. He defined the microsystem as the immediate setting and the mesosystem as the connection to the child's immediate microsystem such as school, family, day care, and church. The exosystem is the community not directly connected to the child, such as neighbors, friends of the family, the workplace, and community services. The macrosystem is the broad ideology of the culture and laws of the child's culture or social class (Shaffer, 1999).

Bronfenbrenner (1986) suggested that the family's occupational status, education, family income, role within the community, and geographical mobility, as well as the influence of television influence family development. Families that experience changes in normal expected life events, such as loss of a job, frequent moving, or something as positive as lottery winnings will have an effect on the development of the child.

Social support is helpful to relieve stress. It is beneficial to identify who is available to support the family in times of stress. Some children are being raised by grandparents; they need to have a support system as well. Community support, family support, and cultural practices all influence what will be available for the child. The expert school nurse recognizes the wealth of resources within the community for the student and initiates appropriate referrals.

Low socioeconomic status has been associated with poor nutrition, lack of immunization, and increased illness and injury. Children living in poverty are more likely to have difficulty in school (Federal Interagency Forum on Child and Family Statistics, 2002; Feldman, 2004). On the other hand, a child living in wealth may have difficulty forming trusting relationships (Hockenberry, 2003). Thus the influence of socioeconomic status can be quite important in the development of the child.

Payne (1998) offers a framework to understand children living in poverty. Each class, whether the status is poverty, middle class, or wealth, has a set of hidden rules. An assumption cannot be made that those living in poverty understand the hidden rules of middle class, just as those in middle class do not know the rules of poverty. For example, in poverty the quantity of food is important, whereas in middle class the quality of the food is important. Those living in poverty consider money as something that is to be spent and shared with others, but in middle class, money is to be managed. In wealth, money is to be conserved and invested. In poverty, personality and people are important whereas in middle class possessions are considered important. In wealth, one-of-a-kind items and pedigrees are important (Payne, 1998).

The school nurse will benefit from understanding the rules of the different classes represented in her school. A child from poverty may laugh when being disciplined. This is considered a way of "saving face" and the child may need to be taught more appropriate responses (Payne, 1998). A family with limited financial resources may rely on public transportation if they do not own a car. If the school nurse refers a sick child to the healthcare provider, she may need to determine if transportation is available. An appointment that requires two bus changes with a sick child may not be easy for a single parent with other small children to bring along. It may be helpful to write sequential instructions when giving healthcare instructions to a parent. However, in poverty, the importance of the sequence may not be valued (Payne, 1998).

The school nurse can be a valuable resource for a family living in poverty. Children living in generational poverty (poverty that lasts over two generations) are taught that people and relationships are very important. Children are more likely to comply with requests by a person they trust (Payne, 1998). Developing a trusting relationship with the students and families may allow the school nurse to make a difference in their health care.

DEVELOPMENTAL ISSUES FOR SPECIFIC AGE GROUPS

The Preschool Child, Ages 3 to 5

Introduction to Early Childhood Education

Increasing numbers of children are enrolled in early childhood programs. During the past 30 years, attendance at early childhood preschool programs has increased 45% (Federal Interagency Forum on Child and Family Statistics, 2002). Head Start, a 1965 federal program, was introduced to narrow the achievement gap of children from low-income families and improve their readiness for kindergarten. In 1968, children with disabilities were accepted into Head Start programs. This was followed by the *Individuals with Disabilities Education Act* (Chapter 14), which mandated that public schools offer special education services to eligible 3- to 5-year-old children with disabilities. Federal programs such as these have encouraged the creation of quality preschool programs. Furthermore, families have frequently looked to preschool programs as an alternative to day care when both parents work. As more and more of these programs become available, school nurses will be called upon to provide services to this age group.

Quality early childhood programs can benefit from access to a school nurse. Early childhood screening, control of communicable diseases, care of acute or chronic illnesses, injury prevention, and parent education are just a few of the services a school nurse can provide in this setting.

Several screening tools are available to help determine school readiness and other important milestones of development (Table 16.7). The most well known is the Denver II Developmental Screening Test. This can be used on children from birth to age 6 and takes approximately 30 minutes to administer. It screens for social interaction, fine and gross motor ability and language ability. The Battelle Developmental Inventory Screening Test can test children ages 6 months to 8 years of age. It can be given in approximately 30 minutes and tests gross and fine motor skills, expressive and receptive language, cognitive skills, and personal and adaptive skills (McCabe, 1997; Pulcini, 1997). These screening tests identify the child who may need further evaluation.

Table 16.7 ■
SKILLS OF THE PRESCHOOL CHILD

AGE	FINE MOTOR	GROSS MOTOR	LANGUAGE AND COMMUNICATION	SELF-HELP	PLAY
>3	• Copies a circle • String large beads • Cuts with scissors • Can put pegs in pegboard	• Hops on one foot • Jumps from a height of 12 inches • Rides a tricycle • Walks on balance beam	• Sentences with three or four words • Understands biggest/smallest • Follows two-step commands	• Dresses with some assistance • Know which shoe goes on which foot • Washes hands • Brushes teeth with help	• Role play becomes important and children experiment with adult roles. • Begin to take turns • Can usually play cooperatively with other children
4	• Draws three-part person	• Walks down steps alternating feet • Walks backwards • Good kicking motion	• Asks, who, what when, why often • Uses five- or six-word sentences • Can communicate effectively	• Dresses self • Brushes teeth • Laces shoes • Buckles belt	• Children become aware of different genders. • Proud of accomplishments
5	• Uses pencil • Draws seven-part person • Colors in the lines	• Skips • Throws and catches a ball • Jumps rope • Can balance on one foot with eyes closed	• Can communicate feelings • Can participate in a conversation	• Covers mouth and nose when coughing or sneezing • Ties shoes	• Can play table games • Understands rules

Source: Adapted from Battelle Developmental Inventory (1988). Allen, TX: LINC, Associates, Inc.; Brigance, A. (1991). Inventory of Early Development; Birth to Seven Years. N. Billerica, MA: Curriculum Associates; Lemay, D., Griffin, P. & Sanford, A. (N.D.) Learning Accomplishment Profile (LAP). Chapel Hill Training-Outreach Project.

It is helpful for the school nurse to be familiar with the screening tests used in his or her school community. School nurses may participate in Individualized Education Program meetings and other multidisciplinary team meetings, and will benefit from knowledge of the abilities of the child and the skills being assessed by the various tools.

School nurses need to be sensitive to the parent whose child may have a developmental delay or a learning disability. The diagnostic period can be stressful and school nurses may need to reinforce information being provided by the healthcare provider. Although parents may suspect that their child is different or slower than other children, having this confirmed by school officials is often upsetting to a parent.

Toilet Training

Most children entering preschool are toilet trained. However, the school nurse may choose to keep an extra set of clothing on hand for times of accidental incontinence. Most children will train themselves if given the chance, but for those who arrive at school and are not toilet trained, the school nurse may be asked to provide guidance. If a child is not toilet trained by age 5, the child should be referred to the HCP for evaluation (Arnold, 1997).

A private area close to the classroom should be made available to help a child become toilet trained while at school. A toilet low to the ground or a potty chair should be available so the child can use it with minimal help from adults. Never punish or demean a child for accidents. In a school setting, hygiene and asepsis are essential, especially if staff are asked to change diapers. Good hand-washing for staff and students is necessary when helping a child learn to use the toilet. The use of underpants is considered a badge of success, especially those designed with the child's favorite characters. Parents should be encouraged to leave an extra set of clothing in the student's cubby in case of accidents. Be sure that wet or soiled clothes are bagged to avoid contamination with other student materials.

Classroom teachers should ensure that toileting is included in the class schedule every 2 hours. They must be alert for signs of urination or defecation and usher the child quickly to the toilet. If the child does not show an interest in learning to use the toilet at school, a schedule can be developed. The child can be escorted to the toilet every hour and placed on the toilet for 5 minutes. Attempts and successes should be rewarded with praise and positive reinforcement. Several books about using the potty are available and these can be shared with preschool students.

The School-Age Child, Ages 6 to 12

Head and Neck Changes

The school-age years reflect the continuing development of the immune system. Lymphatic tissue grows until about 9 years of age; excess tonsillar and adenoid tissue may be mistaken for enlargement during an upper respiratory illness during this time and may even interfere with hearing. Once the tissue recedes normally, hearing returns to normal (Pillitteri, 1999). In addition, the frontal sinuses develop around age 6 and thus students may experience sinus headaches.

Skills and Play of the School-Age Child

The beginning school-age child is interested in simple board games, cards, music, water, and clay; action games such as tag and hide and seek are popular. Children like to pretend play and will imitate adult behavior. They may play in groups, but the groups are loosely organized. Children are becoming more industrious and may start to take things apart just to put them back together again. They enjoy collecting and sorting items, whether they be cards or stickers. They then trade with their peers.

As the child masters skills of reading and writing, books and pads of paper can occupy a child. As the child develops, games with rules become more important. Group play allows the child to learn cooperation from others and the rules help form the structure for the games. Social rules are incorporated into play. Winning is important and although they have an awareness of rules, children may cheat at games to win. Informal clubs and organized group activities become more prevalent (Taylor, Menarcheck-Fetkovich, & Day, 2000). See TABLE 16.8 for the skills the school-age child would be expected to accomplish.

School-age children spend much of their day in school and friends become very important. A sense of belonging develops as they begin to take part in group activities. Peer group activities help the child to develop interpersonal interactions, self-concept, and sex-role behavior (Selekman & Saunders, 1996). Best friends are important at age 8 and children may have a first "best friend" as well as a second "best friend."

During the school-age years, music lessons, swimming lessons, scouts, sports groups, and other

(text continues on page 372)

Table 16.8 ■

SKILLS OF THE SCHOOL - AGE CHILD

AGE	FINE MOTOR	GROSS MOTOR	LANGUAGE	PLAY
6	Should easily tie shoelaces. Can cut and paste, draw a person with good detail and print	Can jump, skip, and hop. Can walk a straight line and can ride a two-wheeled bicycle. Becoming skilled at throwing a ball.	Talk in full sentences and their use of grammar becomes more correct.	Imaginative play is present.
7	Can write and wants writing to be perfect. Can read regular size type. Between ages 6 and 12, students typing skills improve with computer use.	Can jump with coordination to play hopscotch and skip rope. Can play games with balls.	Can tell time in hours and knows the months of year. Begins to use complex passive sentences and constructs conditional sentences.	Gender differences in games begin to surface; for example, boys may be interested in a game of catch while girls may be more interested in hopscotch. Will need more props with play. May develop an interest in collecting items such as baseball cards, dolls, and coins.
8	Learns to read and use script writing. Can use a hand tool such as a screwdriver	Can adjust body position to successfully catch a ball. Can crouch on tiptoes and can put right or left foot forward on command.		Likes to ride bicycles and participate in organized sports. Likes to sort and catalogue items
9	Writing looks more mature. Continues to refine skills	Can balance on one leg with eyes closed and can catch a ball with one hand.	Inferences in language are understood.	Likes to play rough and are more interested in the play than perfecting skills. Music lessons for children are common and talent becomes evident. Children like to take lessons with other children and school music programs are important.

(continued)

Table 16.8 ■ *(Continued)*

AGE	FINE MOTOR	GROSS MOTOR	LANGUAGE	PLAY
10	Eye-hand coordination is sufficient for children to become quite proficient in computer games and handheld computer games.		Begins use of formal and informal speech and can change patterns depending on audience. Can understand the multiple meanings of words. Can comprehend approximately 40,000 words.	Continues to improve at organized sports. Rules are important and clubs with social order may be present, such as those with officers. Building toys
11				Growth spurts may make body awareness more difficult; thus some children may not participate in sports. Time with friends is spent talking. Like to listen and dance to popular music.
12			Sense of humor develops	Organized sports are important.

Source: Adapted from Haywood & Getchell (2001); Pillitteri (1999); and Shaffer (1999).

organized activities introduce children to multiple aspects of life as well as build skills and encourage group activities. Schools often promote and may even provide these activities after school hours. The school nurse can often recommend these activities to students, especially those who need companionship and building self-esteem. Groups such as scouts or the Police Athletic League or local community centers may be available.

Daily activity should be encouraged. Fewer than half of students are able to meet the requirements of standard fitness tests (Kail, 2004). Children age 6 and older can begin to participate in organized sports; however, the emphasis should be on having fun and trying different sports. Children between ages 6 and 10 may have difficulty handling the stress of intense competition or the disappointment of loss or failure, so winning should not be the most important goal. Learning skills and teamwork should be encouraged at this level (Denehy, 2002).

Children who cannot physically handle the demands of the sport may feel discouraged when they fail and thus not make further attempts. The development of balance, coordination, and reaction time improves with age; therefore, beginning ball sports such as T-ball or soccer should be encouraged. They still have a shorter attention span and are not adept at making quick decisions. Also, their ability to anticipate the projection and direction of a ball may make them appear uncoordinated, but this does improve with age.

Improved skills and increasing memory skills that help to remember patterns and plays for sports enhance their success and enjoyment. Sports participation can incorporate physical skill-building activities and appropriate socialization, as well as anger management and problem-solving skills. The importance of developing these skills should be stressed over the need to win at this age level (Patel, Pratt, & Greydanus, 2002)

The emphasis on daily physical exercise and the link to obesity indicates that all children should be encouraged to participate in physical activity. Sport activities should be developmentally appropriate for

Box 16.13 ■■■

Sports activities for children ages 6 to 9

- Dance
- Hopscotch
- Soccer
- T-Ball
- Baseball
- Kickball
- Karate
- Swimming
- Gymnastics
- Hiking

Sports activities for children ages 10 to 12

- Ball sports
  - Baseball
  - Softball
  - Football
  - Soccer
  - Kickball
  - Tennis
- Field hockey or ice hockey
- Biking
- Inline skating
- Skateboarding
- Wrestling
- Lacrosse
- Dance
- Gymnastics
- Hiking
- Running (not distance)
- Swimming

the child to allow for success in the activity. If the child is successful, it is likely that he will continue to enjoy the sport. In addition, the positive feedback achieved from participation will enhance self-esteem.

Developing Sexuality and a Sexual Identity

From a young age, boys and girls learn sexual identity. Sexuality develops over time and school-age children have a curiosity about sex. In fact, they may engage in some form of sex play. Generally this should not be alarming and is most likely temporary (Hockenberry, 2003). The school nurse may, however, be asked to talk with the young child who is masturbating or otherwise acting out sexually in class. A frank non-judgmental discussion with the child about appropriate behavior in public may be all that is necessary. In addition, the nurse should assess whether a medical problem or problems at home may be causing the behavior.

Healthy sexuality can be supported by giving accurate information, correct terminology and reassurance that sexuality is part of normal growth and development (Hockenberry, 2003). Sex education in the early school-age years should include factual information using correct terminology. It should be treated as a normal part of growth and development and can be incorporated into a unit on Family Life or a study of animals.

Some children do begin to sexually mature during elementary school; therefore it is important to introduce body changes and sex education in the grade school curriculum. There are several programs available to teach normal sexual development during the middle school years. Many of these programs are available for bilingual children. The

Box 16.14 ■■■

TEACHING SEXUAL DEVELOPMENT

Resources for the school nurse:
It's a Girl Thing®
It's a Guy Thing®
http://www.kotex.com/na/talk/educators/edukitinfo.asp
Kotex Lifetime Learning Systems, Inc., P.O. Box 638, Deavan, WI 53115-9909

Always: http://www.always.com.
Also has a Web site for mothers and daughters.

Midol Parent and Teacher Guide: http://www.midol.com/ParentTeacherGuide/index.asp
Also has resources and reading suggestions

Puberty information for boys and girls:
American Academy of Pediatrics Fact Sheet

school nurse and the health education teacher should consider informing parents and administration about the content of the reproduction or sexuality curriculum. The school nurse may be called on to explain menarche for the 7- or 8-year-old who develops early. Simple, factual information should be the hallmark of instruction given to the younger child.

The Pediatric Endocrine Society issued new recommendations in 2003 to determine when pubertal development is precocious. Precocious puberty should be considered in boys younger than age 9, and in African-American girls younger than age 6 and Caucasian girls younger than age 7 who show signs of early development (Midyett, Moore, & Jacobson, 2003). Therefore, signs of pubertal development in 7- and 8-year-old girls should be considered normal and benign. School nurses in elementary, middle, and high schools should keep a supply of feminine products available for the young girl who may start her menstrual cycle at school.

Puberty

Puberty is the stage when secondary sexual characteristics develop. In males, the hypothalamus produces gonadotropin-releasing hormone (GnRH) that signals the anterior pituitary gland to release the gonadotropins, luteinizing hormone (LH) and follicle-stimulating hormone (FSH) (Berne & Levy, 1998). LH causes testicular enlargement and development of Leydig's cells in the testes that produce testosterone. FSH stimulates the development of the seminiferous tubules of the testes, leading to spermatogenesis and fertility. Enlargement of the testicles signals the start of puberty. See Table 16.9 for a complete view of the chemical changes during puberty.

Spermarche, the onset of sperm emission, is an early pubertal event in boys. It occurs at approximately 13.4 years of age and generally occurs prior to pubic hair development and prior to the peak growth spurt (Neinstein & Kaufman, 2002). Nocturnal emissions, frequently referred to as "wet-dreams," are common during puberty and are sometimes misinterpreted as "wetting the bed." Approximately one third of boys will have some breast growth and tenderness due to the influence of the hormone estradiol, although, as their testosterone level increases, this breast growth stops (Berne & Levy, 1998).

The appearance of breast buds is the first sign of puberty in girls (Tanner, 1962). In females, as in males, the hypothalamus produces gonadotropin-releasing hormone (GnRH) that signals the anterior pituitary to release gonadotropins, luteinizing hormone (LH) and follicle-stimulating hormone (FSH). The effects of these hormones in girls start the development of secondary sexual characteristics: FSH stimulates ovarian development and estrogen production while estrogen influences the development of secondary sex characteristics (see Table 16.9).

Table 16.9 ■
CHEMICAL CHANGES DURING PUBERTY

HORMONE	SEX	CHANGES	ACTIONS
Gonadotropin (released by the anterior pituitary)			
FSH (follicle-stimulating hormone; stimulated by gonadotropin releasing hormone)	Females	Growth of ovarian follicles Production of estrogens	Estradiols stimulate the development of internal and external genitalia and breasts and increase body fat. Estradiols trigger LH production at mid cycle which causes maturation and release of an ovum. Estradiols at low levels encourage linear growth and at high levels increases the rate of epiphysial fusion.

(continued)

HORMONE	SEX	CHANGES	ACTIONS
FSH (stimulated by gonadotropin-releasing hormone)	Males	Makes cells receptive to testosterone	Testosterone stimulates spermatogenesis Development of the seminiferous tubules in testes
LH (luteinizing hormone; stimulated by gonadotropin-releasing hormone)	Females	Initiates ovulation Formation of the corpus luteum Production of progesterone	Progesterone along with estrogen regulate the menstrual cycle and stimulate breast development.
LH (stimulated by gonadotropin releasing hormone)	Males	Promotes maturation of testicles and increased size Development of Leydig's cells in testes which lead to the production of testosterone Promotes production of small amount of estrogen	Testosterone increases linear growth and rate of epiphysial fusion. It increases muscle mass and bone density. Testosterone stimulates development of internal and external sexual characteristics and increases libido. It increases the size of the larynx which deepens the voice. It stimulates sebaceous glands to secrete oil. Estradiol increases the rate of epiphysial fusion and increases bone mineral density.
Adrenal androgens (the sex steroids) are produced by adrenal glands.			
DHA (dehydroepiandrosterone) DHEAS (dehydroepiandrosterone sulfate)	Male	Testosterone released	Axillary and pubic hair growth although influence in puberty is much less than for gonadotropins.
DHA (dehydroepiandrosterone) DHEAS (dehydroepiandrosterone sulfate)	Female	Testosterone, estrogen and progesterone released	Axillary and pubic hair growth and an increase in female libido

Source: Adapted from Berne & Levy (1998); Hockenberry (2003); & Neinstein & Kaufman (2002).

Menarche, the onset of menses, occurs on average at 12 years of age. It occurs approximately 3 years after the start of the growth spurt and 1 year after the peak height velocity. Growth after menarche is minimal and breast development ends shortly after the start of menses. Culture, race, economic status, heredity, and nutrition all influence the age of menarche. Menstrual cycles will become increasingly more regular 5 to 7 years after menarche (Gordon & Neinstein, 2002).

Tanner (1962) described this sexual development of the adolescent in stages. The average boy

Stage 1 Pre-adolescent testes, scrotum and penis are same size and proportion as in early childhood. No pubic hair

Stage 2 Enlargement of scrotum and testes. Scrotum skin redness and changes in texture. Sparse growth of long, downy hair, straight or slightly curly, appears at base of penis.

Stage 3 Enlargement of penis, mainly in length. Testes and scrotum continue to enlarge. Darker, coarser and more curled pubic hair.

Stage 4 Increased size of penis with growth in breadth and development of glands. Increase darkening of scrotal skin. Pubic hair now resembles adult, but there is less surface area covered by hair. Axillary hair generally appears 2 years after appearance of pubic hair. Facial hair begins to grow at the same time as axillary hair. Testosterone influences the deepening of the voice due to increased size of larynx, which coincides with the penis nearing complete growth.

Stage 5 Adult genitalia in size and shape.

Figure 16.7 ■ Description of male development.

takes about 2 years to develop from stage 2 to stage 4 and an additional 2 years to progress to stage 5 (description in FIGURE 16.7 and picture in FIGURE 16.8).

Females progress through similar stages according to Tanner (see description in FIGURE 16.9, a breast development picture in FIGURE 16.10, and a pubic development picture in FIGURE 16.11).

Other characteristics occur during adolescence. Girls develop a widening of the hips and boys develop broadening shoulders. Facial characteristics become more adult-like as the lips protrude and the nose and jaw become more prominent (Shaffer, 1999).

During puberty, the sweat glands will increase their activity and axillary sweating begins to appear at about the time of axillary hair growth. As apocrine sweat glands and sebaceous glands become more active, body odor and acne become an issue for the adolescent. Sweating can set up the environment for tinea to grow in the groin or foot. This is an ideal time to promote good body hygiene and the use of deodorant with the rationales for their need. It is not uncommon for younger students to be unaware of body odor as they begin pubertal changes.

School nurses must be sensitive to various culture differences in regard to hygiene. Certain societies do not bathe as frequently as practiced by most Americans. In one study, Saudi girls did not shower during their menstrual cycle (Moawed, 2001). Women in Jordan reported bathing just once a week (Mahasneh, 2001). Refugees from countries where running water is scarce may be reluctant to use such a valuable resource for bathing. Poverty may influence whether a teen has access to a shower or

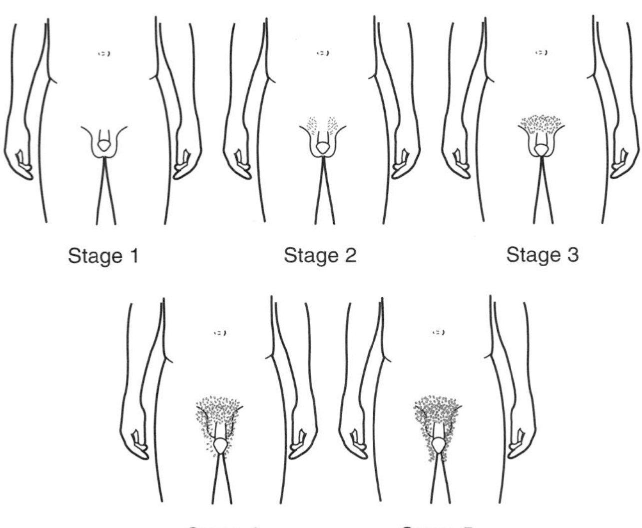

Figure 16.8 ■ Picture of male development. (Illustration: Valerie Probst)

Stage 1 Pre-adolescent: elevation of papilla only. No pubic hair.

Stage 2 Breast buds: slight elevation of breast. Enlargement of the diameter of the areolar. Sparse growth of downy pubic hair.

Stage 3 Further enlargement and elevation of breast and areola. Darker, coarser and more curled pubic hair.

Stage 4 Projection of areola and papilla to form secondary mound above the level of breast. Pubic hair now resembles adult type, but surface area not as large.

Stage 5 Mature stage: projection of papilla only. Adult pubic hair.

Figure 16.9 ■ Description of female development.

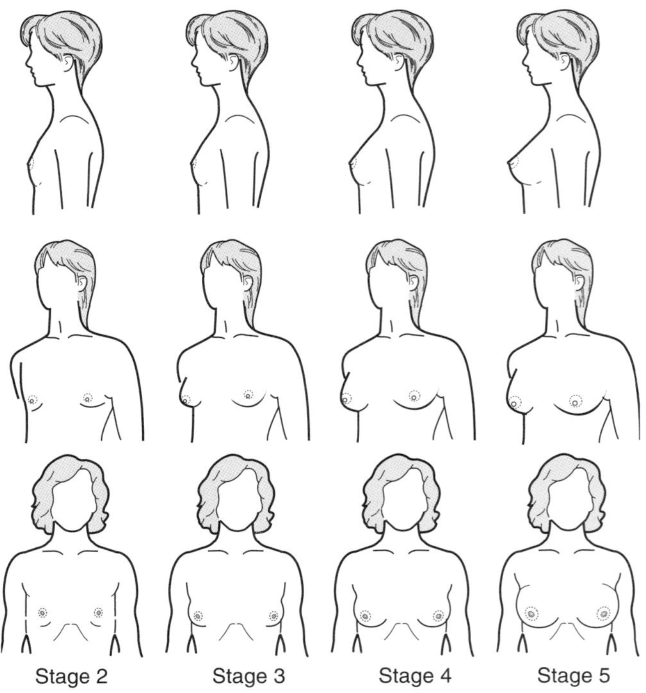

Figure 16.10 ■ Female breast development. (Illustration: Valerie Probst)

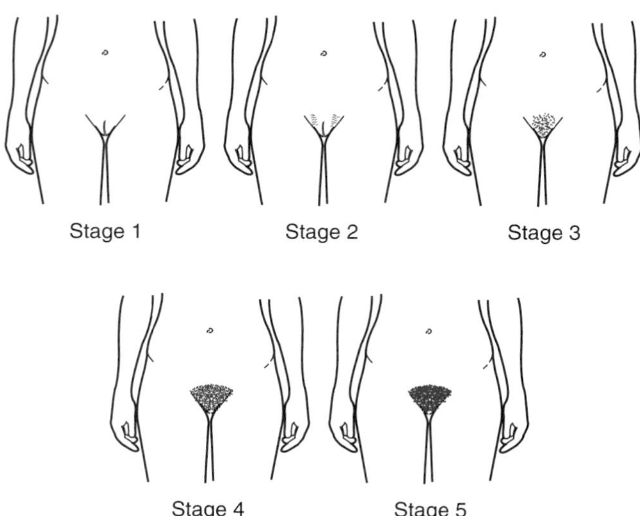

Figure 16.11 ■ Female pubic development. (Illustration: Valerie Probst)

bath. The school nurse may need to intervene to help the adolescent assimilate into the adolescent culture. The teen may be unaware of the effect he or she is having on others and it is up to the school nurse to educate the teen on accepted hygiene.

An increase in the production of sebum by the sebaceous follicles of the skin in response to increased hormone levels during puberty causes acne. Acne is an inflammation of the sebaceous glands and hair follicles of the skin with papules and pustules (see Chapter 25). Stress and genetic factors have also been shown to influence the development of acne. Despite beliefs by some parents, food choices have not been shown to be a significant link in the development of acne (Bechtel, 2002).

Washing the face at least twice daily helps to wash off excess oil and help to prevent acne eruptions. Acne that may cause scars or causes disturbance in body image can be treated by the healthcare provider using a variety of methods, either topically or systemically.

The Adolescent, Ages 12 to 18

Adolescence is a time of rapid physiological and psychological changes. These changes can occur in a nonsequential pattern. Although the biological changes are related to hormones and occur sequentially, the psychosocial and cognitive changes may not occur when expected.

Physical Growth and Development

The key hormone responsible for growth is growth hormone (GH). Growth hormone levels rise during puberty stimulating the peak years of physical growth and are also linked to the stage of puberty. During non-rapid-eye movement sleep, stage IV, growth hormone (GH) is released (Huether & Leo, 1998; Kail, 2004). The increase of the hormones testosterone and estradiol stimulates linear growth, increases bone density and increases the rate of epiphysial fusion. The end of growth occurs when the epiphysial plates close and bone growth stops.

Skeletal growth peaks during the adolescent growth spurt, accounting for 20% of the final adult height (Neinstein & Kaufman, 2002). The formation of skeletal bone mass during puberty is extremely important, as this is the time when an individual establishes peak bone mass. This bone mass has significant implications on the loss of bone mass that occurs throughout adulthood (Neinstein & Kaufman, 2002).

Girls start their growth spurt earlier than boys and once a girl reaches puberty, her growth will slow to 1 inch per year, gradually leveling off at approximately 15 years of age. Girls generally will stop growing 2 to 2 1/2 years after menarche (Hockenberry, 2003). This is important when screening for scoliosis since no further changes will occur after growth stops. Boys begin their maximum growth beginning around age 14 and continue through puberty until approximately age 18. Boys at age 17 still average a weight gain of 6 pounds per year (CDC, 2002a). Adolescent boys who mature late tend to be taller than early maturers because the period of growth will be longer (Haywood & Getchell, 2001).

At adolescence, muscle mass in boys increases rapidly and accounts for 54% of body weight. Boys may experience a spurt of increased strength during adolescence while girls have a steady increase in strength before leveling off (Haywood & Getchell, 2001). The percentage of body fat decreases in adolescent males and increases in females. During puberty, a female in stage 1 of the Tanner scale has 15.7% body fat. By the development of stage 4, the average female will have 26.7% body fat. Menarche can occur with about 17% body fat, but in order to maintain menstruation, 22% body fat is needed (Gordon & Neinstein, 2002). Boys on the other hand during stage 1 have 14.3% body fat and during stage 2 decreases to 11.2% body fat. The level remains stable for boys during stages 3, 4, and 5 (Neinstein & Kaufman, 2002). Scientific explanations for changes that are occurring will help the teen understand that the changes that he or she is experiencing are universal and normal.

Biopsychosocial Development

The different hormonal changes that occur influence growth and development during adolescence. Although these changes occur to almost all adolescents, there is a wide variation among individuals, based on sex or racial and ethnic groups (Neinstein, 2002). Recent studies on normal teen brain development indicate that the brain continues to change well past the teen years. Magnetic resonance imagining has shown that the brain develops in stages, from back to front. The prefrontal cortex, which is the area of the brain used in planning, priority setting, organizing thoughts, and recognizing consequences, is the last area to develop. Thus risk-taking behavior may be explained by this delayed brain development. In addition, the hormonal influence on the brain may be the reason that teens seek thrills and intense excitement (Wallis, 2004).

Adolescence has been divided into three stages. Early adolescence occurs between ages 10 and 13, the middle school years; middle adolescence occurs between ages 14 and 17, or the high school years; and late adolescence extends from age 17 to age 20, after high school. These categories help to define the behaviors more succinctly, but teens may fluctuate between the early, middle, and late behaviors of adolescence.

Early adolescence is characterized by concrete thinking; therefore, when thinking about the consequences of their actions, early adolescents look at the immediate rather than long term consequences. They may be more rebellious as they test their independence from the family. They may be confused about their changing role from child to adolescent and may lack confidence and self-esteem. Peers are extremely important, for the early adolescent looks to their friends to determine normal behavior. Pubertal changes usually occur during early adolescence.

Middle adolescence is characterized by more abstract thinking and the long-term consequences of their behavior are considered. Dating and interest in sexual experimentation are common in middle adolescence; thus, prevention of sexually transmitted diseases (STDs) and pregnancy become important topics for the school nurse to discuss with students. Teens seek increasing independence from the family and value their privacy. Late adolescence marks the transition into adulthood, with increasing responsibility and making independent choices. These adolescents leave home for college or jobs and often establish relationships with a significant other.

Teens must adapt to a changing body image and they must experience the separation and struggle for independence as they change their social relationships. Adolescents become much more independent, and spend more time with friends than family. As the adolescent seeks independence, the separation from the parents may create tension in family relationships; however, major conflicts between parents and teens are not normal (Radzik, Sherer, & Neinstein, 2002).

During this time, teens will increasingly learn how to interact in an adult world. For some, it may be hard to live up to the expectations of parents and teachers. Four main tasks should be achieved during adolescence:

1. Accepting a changing body image with a mature and positive self image
2. Establishing independence and separating from parents
3. Making a career decision
4. Developing a mature sexuality (Brown, 2002)

Issues that arise during adolescence require assurance of confidentiality based on local laws. Inform teens about what information cannot remain confidential. Listening is an invaluable tool in a sometimes hurried world. A simple request for ice for an injury may uncover a multitude of physical and emotional needs of an adolescent. The key is to take the time to listen in a nonthreatening, nonjudgmental environment.

As an emerging adult, health behavior and practices often are more valued when the adolescent takes part in the decision-making process. If teens see the school nurse as an advocate for their needs, a beneficial partnership can develop. Teens will respect the knowledge and the care and concern with which it is delivered. Nurses need to be prepared to offer accurate and up-to-date healthcare information.

Sexuality

Early adolescent teens often fantasize about the opposite sex, but little activity is usually initiated. The early adolescent female may daydream of the perfect love interest. Crushes are common. Boys experiment sexually through masturbation (Hockenberry, 2003). However, young adolescents may misperceive "love interests" as extremely significant.

It is likely that early adolescents are confused as a result of the messages conveyed in films and television, which offer unrealistic expectations and information. Consider that children and teens spend more time in front of a television than in the classroom. The education that occurs in the media is often misleading and promotes high-risk behaviors. Music videos often portray women as sex objects and television shows suggest that everyone is sexually active. Advertising media use sexual messages to sell their products (Kilbourne, 1999).

During middle adolescence, teens still spend time with peer groups, but now may look to members of the opposite sex for companionship. Intense feelings of infatuation and "love" may be short lived but no less real to the adolescent. The break-up of a relationship is quite traumatic for the adolescent and the teen may benefit from formal or informal counseling.

Teens start to date and sexual experimentation may begin. Data from the 2001 Youth Risk Behavior Survey (CDC, 2002b) indicate that 34.4% of 9th graders and 40.8% of 10th graders have had sexual intercourse. Education can be the key in combating the influence of the media, dispelling myths, offering facts and reassuring teens.

Issues of sexual orientation arise during adolescence. Approximately 15% of adolescents report they are attracted to members of the same sex. This may be related to experimentation and exploration of one's sexuality during adolescence. One source notes that 5% of all teens indicate that they are homosexual (Kail, 2004). Bakker & Cavender (2003) dispute these numbers saying it is difficult to determine prevalence due to the large number of students who question their sexuality and who may be transgendered or bisexual. Nonetheless these students are at risk for STDs, depression and other risky behaviors. The school nurse will need to be aware of mental and physical health issues that may affect these students and offer appropriate support and guidance.

CONCLUSION

This chapter gives the school nurse an overview of the growth and development of the preschool and school-age child and the adolescent. Each student is different and individualized approaches based on the specific growth and developmental pattern of the individual student are necessary. The educational process and the health of each child are closely linked. School nurses may need to advocate for the student and ensure that arrangements are made to accommodate each child's differences.

References

Agnvall, E. (2000). *Is your child's playground safe? National Safety Council Family Safety & Health Playground Safety*. Retrieved March 29, 2005 from http://www.nsc.org/pubs/fsh/archive/spr00/playgrnd.htm

Arnold, D. (1997). Common parenting concerns. In Fox, J. (Ed.). *Primary health care of children* (pp. 276–300). St. Louis: C. V. Mosby.

Austrian, S. (2002). *Developmental theories through the life cycle*. New York: Columbia University Press.

Bakker, L., & Cavender, A. (2003). Promoting culturally competent care for gay youth. *Journal of School Nursing*, 19(2). 65–72.

Beard, R. (1969). *An outline of Piaget's developmental psychology for students and teachers*. New York: Basic Books.

Bechtel, M. (2002). Dermatology. In C. Holland-Hall & R. Brown (Eds.), *Adolescent medicine secrets* (pp. 67–72). Philadelphia: Hanley & Belfus.

Behrman, R., Kliegman, R., & Jenson, R. (2000). *Nelson textbook of pediatrics* (16th ed.). Philadelphia: W. B. Saunders.

Berne, R., & Levy, M. (1998). *Physiology* (4th ed.). St. Louis: C. V. Mosby.

Binkley, H., Beckett, J., Casa, D., Kleiner, D., & Plummer, P. (2002). National Athletic Trainers's Association Position Statement: Exertional heat illnesses. *Journal of Athletic Training, 37*(3), 329–343.

Bowden, V., Dickey, S., & Greenberg, C. (1998). *Children and their families*. Philadelphia: W. B. Saunders.

Bronfenbrenner, U. (1979). *The ecology of human development*. Cambridge, MA: Harvard University Press.

Bronfenbrenner, U. (1986) Ecology of the family as a context for human development: research perspectives. *Developmental Psychology, 22*(6), 723–742.

Brown, R. (2002). Adolescent growth and development. In C. Holland-Hall & R. Brown, (Eds.), *Adolescent medicine secrets* (pp. 21–28). Philadelphia: Hanley & Belfus.

Centers for Disease Control and Prevention (CDC). (2002a). *CDC growth charts, United States*. Retrieved June 3, 2003 from http://www.cdc.gov/growthcharts

Centers for Disease Control and Prevention (CDC). (2002b). Youth Risk Behavior Surveillance—United States, 2001. *MMWR, 51*(No. SS-4), June 28, 2002.

Centers for Disease Control and Prevention (CDC). (2003). *Overweight children and adolescents: Recommendations to screen, assess and manage*. Retrieved April 16, 2004 from http://www.cdc.gov/nccdphp/dnpa/growthcharts/training/modules/module3/text/module3print.pdf

Centers for Disease Control and Prevention (CDC). (2005a). *CDC growth charts: United States*. Retrieved March 29, 2005 from http://www.cdc.gov/nchs/about/major/nhanes/growthcharts/background.htm

Centers for Disease Control and Prevention (CDC). (2005b). *Preventing chronic diseases: Investing wisely in health*. Retrieved March 6, 2005 from http://www.cdc.gov/OralHealth/factsheets/dental_caries.htm

Center on Hunger and Poverty. (1998). *Childhood hunger, childhood obesity: An examination of the paradox*. Retrieved February 29, 2004 from http://nutrition.tufts.edu/pdf/publications/hunger/hunger_and_obesity.pdf

Coyle, J. (2000). Thermoregulation. In J. Sullivan & S. Anderson (Eds.), *Care of the young athlete* (pp. 65–80). Rosemont, IL: American Academy of Orthopaedic Surgeons and American Academy of Pediatrics.

Curran, J., & Barness, L. (2000). Nutrition. In R. Behrman, R. Kliegman, J. Jenson (Eds.), *Nelson textbook of pediatrics* (16th ed., pp. 138–149). Philadelphia: W. B. Saunders.

D'Ambra, P., & Jack, J. (1999). Musculo-Skeletal. In Bradley, B. (Ed.), *Nursing assessment of school age youth*. Scarborough, ME: National Association of School Nurses.

Denehy, J. (2002). Promoting the Health of Student Athletes. *Journal of School Nursing, 18*(6), 309–312.

Denehy, J. (2003). The health effects of soft drinks. *Journal of School Nursing, 19*(2), 63–64.

DiCarlo, M., Ruck, B., & Marcus, S. (2002). How should a fever mercury thermometer be disposed of? A survey of those likely to be asked. *Pediatrics, 109*(5), 71.

Dinu, B. (2003). Route of temperature measurement in children. In M. Hockenberry, (Ed.), *Wong's nursing care of infants and children* (7th ed., pp. 180–181). St Louis: C. V. Mosby.

Donaldson, M. (2003). The female athlete triad. A growing health concern. *Orthopedic Nursing, 22*(5), 322–324.

Erickson, E. (1968). The human life cycle. In S. Schlein (Ed.) (1987), *A way of looking at things: Selected papers from 1930 to 1980* (pp. 595–610). New York: W. W. Norton.

Federal Interagency Forum on Child and Family Statistics. (2002). *America's children: Key national indicators of well-being, 2002*. Federal Interagency Forum on Child and Family Statistics, Washington, DC: U.S. Government Printing Office.

Feldman, R. (2004). *Child development* (3rd ed.). Upper Saddle River, NJ: Pearson Prentice-Hall.

Finkelstein, B., Imperiale, T., Speroff, T., Marrero, U., Radcliffe, D., & Cuttler, L. (2002). Effect of growth hormone therapy on height in children with idiopathic short stature: A meta-analysis. *Archives of Pediatric Adolescent Medicine, 156*(9), 946–947.

Gardner, H. (1999). *The disciplined mind*. New York: Simon & Schuster.

Germak, J. (2002). Endocrinology. In C. Holland-Hall & R. Brown (Eds.), *Adolescent medicine secrets* (pp. 73–91). Philadelphia: Hanley & Belfus.

Gleitman, H., Fridlund, A., & Reisberg, D. (1998). *Psychology* (5th ed.). New York: W. W. Norton.

Goldman, L., & Shannon, M. (2001). Technical report: Mercury in the environment: Implications for pediatricians. *Pediatrics, 108* (1), 197–205.

Gomez, J. (2000). Growth and Maturation. In J. Sullivan & S. Anderson, (Eds.), *Care of the young athlete* (pp. 25–32). Rosemont, IL: American Academy of Orthopaedic Surgeons and American Academy of Pediatrics.

Gordon, C., & Neinstein, L. (2002). Normal Menstrual Physiology. In Neinstein, L. (Ed.), *Adolescent health care: A practical guide* (4th ed., pp. 947–951). Philadelphia: Lippincott, Williams & Wilkins.

Haywood, K., & Getchell, N. (2001). *Life span motor development* (3rd ed.) St. Louis: Human Kinetics.

Hockenberry, M. (2003). *Wong's nursing care of infants and children* (7th ed.). St. Louis: C. V. Mosby.

Huether, S., & Leo, J. (2002). Pain, temperature regulation, sleep, and sensory function. In K. McCance & S. Huether (Eds.), *Pathophysiology: The biologic basis for disease in adults and children* (4th ed., pp. 401–437). St. Louis: C. V. Mosby.

Hull, K., & Harvey, S. (2003). Growth hormone therapy and quality of life: possibilities, pitfalls and mechanisms. *Journal of Endocrinology*, 179, 311–333.

Johnsen, D., & Tinanoff, N. (2000). The oral cavity. In R. Behrman, R. Kliegman, & J. Jenson (Eds.), *Nelson textbook of pediatrics* (16th ed., pp. 1108–1121). Philadelphia: W. B. Saunders.

Kail, R. (2004). *Children and their development* (3rd ed.). Upper Saddle River, NJ: Pearson Prentice-Hall.

Kazis, K., & Iglesias, E. (2003). The female athlete triad. *Adolescent Medicine, 14*(1), 87–95.

Kilbourne, J. (1999). *Can't buy my love*. New York: Simon & Schuster.

Kohlberg, L. (1981). *The philosophy of moral development*. San Francisco: Harper & Row.

Lemay, D., Griffin, P., & Sanford, A. (N.D.) Learning accomplishment profile (LAP). Chapel Hill Training-Outreach Project.

Lissauer, T., & Clayden, G. (1997). *Illustrated textbook of paediatrics*. London: C. V. Mosby.

Mahasneh, S. (2001). Health perceptions and health behaviours of poor urban Jordanian women. *Journal of Advanced Nursing, 36*(1), 58–68.

McCabe, M., (1997). Developmental Assessment. In J. Fox (Ed.). *Primary health care of children* (pp. 144–147). St. Louis: C. V. Mosby.

Merrell, K. (2003). *Behavioral, social, and emotional assessment of children and adolescents*. Mahwah, NJ: Lawrence Erlbaum Associates.

Midyett, L. K., Moore, W., & Jacobson, J. (2003). Are pubertal changes in girls before age 8 benign? *Pediatrics, 111* (1), 47–51.

Miller, S. (2004). Piagetian Research. In L. Nadelman (Ed.), *Research manual in child development* (2nd ed., pp. 111–123). Mahwah, NJ: Lawrence Erlbaum Associates.

Moawed, S. (2001). Indigenous practices of Saudi girls in Riyadh during their menstrual period. *Journal of East Mediterranean Health,* 7, 197–203.

Mourad, L. (1998). Structure and function of the musculoskeletal system. In K. McCance & S. Huether, (Eds.), *Pathophysiology* (3rd ed., pp. 1405–1434). St. Louis: C. V. Mosby.

National Association of School Nurses (NASN). (2002). *Position statement: Soft drinks and candy in the school setting*. Retrieved May 17, 2003 from http://nasn.org/positions/softdrinks.htm

National Athletic Trainers Association. (2003). *Inter-Association Task Force on Exertional Heat Illnesses consensus statement*. Retrieved March, 29, 2005 from http://www.nata.org/publicinformation/files/heatillness-consensusstatement.pdf

National Children's Center for Rural and Agricultural Health and Safety, (1999). *North American Guidelines for Children's Agricultural Tasks*. Retrieved March 29, 2005 from http://research.marshfieldhclinic.org/children/Resources/default.htm

National Collegiate Athletic Association. (2001). *Wrestling with weight loss: The NCAA Wrestling weight management policy*. Retrieved May 23, 2003 from http;//www.ncaa.org.

National Safety Council. (2002). *Fact Sheet Library: Playground safety*. Retrieved June 3, 2003 from http://www.nsc.org/library/facts/plgrdgen.htm

National High Blood Pressure Program Working Group on High Blood Pressure in Children and Adolescents. (2004). The Fourth Report on the Diagnosis, Evaluation, and Treatment of High Blood Pressure in Children and Adolescents. *Pediatrics, 114*(2), 555–576.

National High Blood Pressure Education Program Working Group on High Blood Pressure in Children and Adolescents. (2004). The Fourth Report on the Diagnosis, Evaluation, and Treatment of High Blood Pressure in Children and Adolescents. *Pediatrics, 114*(2), 555–576. Retrieved March 8, 2005 from http://pediatrics.aappublications.org/cgi/content/full/114/2/S2/555

Neinstein, L. (2002). *Adolescent health care: A practical guide* (4th ed.). Philadelphia: Lippincott, Williams & Wilkins.

Neinstein, L., & Kaufman, F. (2002). Normal physical growth and development. In Neinstein, L. (Ed.), *Adolescent health care: A practical guide* (4th ed., pp. 3–51). Philadelphia: Lippincott, Williams & Wilkins.

Neinstein, L., & Schack, L. (2002). Nutrition. In L. Neinstein (Ed.). *Adolescent health care: A practical guide* (4th ed., pp. 170–185). Philadelphia: Lippincott, Williams & Wilkins.

Nemours Foundation. (2001a). *Caffeine, sugar, fat, and your child*. Retrieved January 19, 2004 from http://www.kidshealth.org/parent/nutrition_fit/nutrition/caffeine.html

Nemours Foundation. (2001b). *What parents need to know about bedwetting*. Retrieved June 3, 2003 from http://www.kidshealth.org./PageManager.jsp?dn=KidsHealth&lic1&ps=107&cat_id=190&article_set=22116

Nemours Foundation. (2002). *Playground safety*. Retrieved June 3, 2003 from http://www.kidshealth.org/PageManager.jsp?dn=KidsHealth&lic=1&ps=107&cat_id=152&article_set=22032

Nemours Foundation. (2005). Do you know how to feed your child athlete? Retrieved July 6, 2006 from http://www.kidshealth.org/parents/nutrition_fit/fitness/feed_child_athlete.html

Paolicchi, J., Pakalnis, A., & Joseph, S. (2002). Neurology. In C. Holland-Hall & R. Brown (Eds.), *Adolescent medicine secrets* (pp. 131–137). Philadelphia: Hanley & Belfus.

Patel, D., Pratt, H., & Greydanus, D. (2002). Pediatric neurodevelopment and sports participation: When are children ready to play sports? *Pediatric Clinics of North America, 49*, 505–531.

Payne, R. (1998). *A framework for understanding poverty*. Highlands, TX:RFT Publishing.

Peel, L. (2002). Nutrition. In C. Holland-Hall & R. Brown (Eds.), *Adolescent medicine secrets* (pp. 35–42). Philadelphia: Hanley & Belfus.

Perriello, V. (2001). Aiming for healthy weight in wrestlers and other athletes. *Contemporary Pediatrics, 18*(9), 55–74. Retrieved March 29, 2005 from http://www.nfhs.org/staticcontent/PDFs/k9a055.pdf

Piaget, J. (1961). *The growth of logical thinking from childhood to adolescence*. New York: Basic Books.

Pillitteri, A. (1999). *Child health nursing: Care of the child and family*. Philadelphia: Lippincott, Williams & Wilkins.

Pulcini, J. (1997). Assessing school readiness. In J. Fox (Ed.), *Primary health care of children* (pp. 263–275). St. Louis: C. V. Mosby.

Radzik, M., Sherer, S., & Neinstein, L. (2002). Psychosocial development in normal adolescents. In L. Neinstein (Ed.), *Adolescent health care: A practical guide* (4th ed., pp. 52–58). Philadelphia: Lippincott, Williams & Wilkins.

Scott, C., & Dalton, R. (2000). Vegetative disorders. In R. Behrman, R. Kliegman, & J. Jenson (Eds.), *Nelson textbook of pediatrics* (16th ed., pp. 72–75). Philadelphia: W. B. Saunders.

Selekman, J., & Saunders, A. (1996). *Pediatric nursing*. Springhouse, PA: Springhouse Corporation.

Shaffer, D. (1999). *Developmental psychology: Childhood and adolescence* (5th ed.). Pacific Grove: Brooks/Cole.

Sherman, R., & Thompson, R. (2004). The female athlete triad. *Journal of School Nursing, 20*(4), 197–202.

Steen, S., & Bernhardt, D. (2000). Nutrition and weight control. In J. Sullivan & S. Anderson (Eds.), *Care of the young athlete* (pp. 81–94). Rosemont, IL: American Academy of Orthopaedic Surgeons and American Academy of Pediatrics.

Synoground, G., & Thiele, J. (2000). Respiratory Function. In Bradley, B. (Ed.), *Nursing assessment of school age youth*. Scarborough, ME: National Association of School Nurses.

Tanner, J. M. (1962). *Growth at adolescence* (2nd ed.). Oxford: Blackwell.

Taylor, K., Menarchek-Fetkovich, M., & Day, C. (2000). The play history interview. In K. Gitlin-Weiner, A., Sandgrund, & C. Schaefer (Eds.), *Play diagnosis and assessment* (2nd ed., pp. 114–138). New York: John Wiley & Sons.

Thede, J., & Iverson, C. (1999). Cardiovascular health. In Bradley, B. (Ed.), *Nursing assessment of school age youth*. Scarborough, ME: National Association of School Nurses.

Thiedke, C. (2001). Sleep disorders and sleep problems in childhood. *American Family Physician, 63*(2), 277–284.

Thiedke, C. (2003). Nocturnal enuresis. *American Family Physician, 67*(7), 1499–1506.

Turman, M., & Mahan, J., (2002). Renal system. In C. Holland-Hall & R. Brown(Eds.), *Adolescent medicine secrets* (pp. 139–146). Philadelphia: Hanley & Belfus.

U.S. Department of Agriculture. (2005). New 2005 Food Pyramid Information. Accessed October 2005 from http://www.ring.com/health/food/food.htm

U.S. Department of Health and Human Services (USDHHS). (2001a). National Center for Education in Maternal and Child Health Bureau. *Trends in children's oral health*. Washington, DC: Author

U.S. Department of Health and Human Services (USDHHS). (2001b). *Healthy People 2010*. Retrieved February 29, 2004 from http://www.healthypeople.gov

U.S. Department of Health and Human Services (USDHHS) & U.S. Department of Agriculture (USDA). (2005). *Dietary guidelines for Americans, 2005*. Retrieved March 29, 2005 from http://www.health.gov/dietaryguidelines/dga2005/document/

U.S. Food and Drug Administration (FDA). (2004). *Seroquel*. Retrieved April 2, 2004 from http://www.fda.vob/cder/foi/label/2004/20639se1-017,016_seroquel_lbl.pdf. U.S. Food and Drug Administration (FDA). (2003). *Topamax. Retrieved April 2, 2004 from http://www.fda.gov/medwatch/SAFETY/2003/tpamax.pdf.*

Vepraskas, C. (2002). Beat the heat: Managing heat and hydration in marching band. *Journal of School Nursing, 18* (4). 237–243.

Vessey, J., Ben-Or, K., Mebane, D., Krapac, N., Cobb, N., Poltrack, M., Shack, L., Terrell, L., & Wilson, S. (2001). Evaluating the value of screening for hypertension: An evidence-based approach. *Journal of School Nursing, 17* (1). 44–49.

Wallis, C. (2004, May 10). What makes teens tick. *Time*, 56–65.

Willhaus, J. (1999). Growth hormone therapy and children with idiopathic short stature: A viable option? *Pediatric Nursing, 25* (6), 662–665.

Williams, J., McCarthy, A., Bragadottir, H., & Reed, D. (2002). School nurses'experiences, concerns, and knowledge of growth disorders in children: Development of a monograph. *Journal of School Nursing, 18*(1), 25–32.

Chapter 17

The Student's Family

ELIZABETH DIETZ ■ DARYL CANHAM

Chapter Outline

INTRODUCTION

The school nurse constantly interacts with families to provide comprehensive health care in the school setting. Changing family constellations and roles can be quite challenging for the school nurse and other health professionals in providing effective care. Challenges can include many factors outside of the normal healthcare delivery model, such as legal issues regarding custodianship and privacy issues with respect to information sharing. Dealing with "family" can also be an issue for faculty and staff related to parent conferences and sending notes home to parents or guardians.

Yet, "families are the most central and enduring influence in children's lives...The health and well-being of children are inextricably linked to their parents' physical, emotional and social health, social circumstances, and child-rearing practices" (American Academy of Pediatrics [AAP], 2003, p. 1541). This chapter explores the various family constellations from which students come.

DEFINITION OF FAMILY

The definition of family has changed over time and varies based on one's frame of reference and values. A broad definition of family is "two or more persons who are joined together by bonds of sharing and emotional closeness and who identify themselves as being part of a family" (Friedman, Bowden, & Jones, 2003). This definition provides the healthcare provider with a comprehensive concept of family and is especially applicable to the school setting, which encompasses a variety of family structures. Because this text focuses on school health, only those definitions that include children are addressed in this chapter.

FAMILY THEORIES

Family theories provide a framework for school nurses to assess and evaluate family interactions, functions, and structures. Family nursing theories evolved from combining nursing, social science, and family therapy theories to develop a set of integrated models. Several models have been developed. Family Systems Theory (Kerr & Bowen, 1988) views the family as a whole system that continually interacts with its members and the environment. A change for one member results in change in another. Forces outside the family, such as the school system, can influence the family system. Dysfunction of the family is considered to be the result of the type of interaction and not caused by any one person. "Chronic anxiety is the underlying basis for dysfunction" (Hanson, Kaakinen, & Friedman, 1998, p.91). This model is most helpful in exploring parent–child relationships.

Family Stress Theory is useful in examining family stressors and strengths as well as resources in adaptation and restoring family stability (Boss, 2002). Because stress is inherent in all families, even positive stress will affect the family. Some stress is expected, such as having a child dressed, fed, and ready for the school bus in the morning; other stress is cumulative or unexpected. This model applies primary, secondary, and tertiary preventive approaches and is helpful for any family situation where stress occurs, such as divorce, illness, two working parents, and teenage behaviors.

Family Development Theory is also a useful approach in studying family patterns, the dynamic nature of the family, and how change occurs in the family. In this dynamic theory, eight stages of the family life cycle are identified. Each stage has a list of developmental tasks that need to be accomplished. As one changes stages, disequilibrium occurs, requiring adaptation. Stage 3 involves families with preschoolers. Socialization of children begins as early as 1 month of age in interactions with parents and other siblings; however, socialization becomes more dynamic in the preschool years as children separate from parents in order to attend preschool. Stage 4 involves families with elementary-age children. During this stage, children develop friends outside the family unit. Parents must adjust to the influence of peers and the school on their child. Stage 5 involves families with teenagers. At this time, adolescents are developing autonomy and responsibility as they mature and emancipate themselves (Friedman, Bowden, & Jones, 2003). Parents and other significant adults maintain the relationship with the teenager by listening with respect and clearly stating parental counsel. Parents are also focusing on their careers and their relationships. Knowledge of these developmental stages in families is helpful for those planning parent programs; it offers guidance in providing parents with anticipatory guidance for each developmental stage.

School nurses can use one or more of these models as guides in working with families to assess problems and plan appropriate interventions. There are other theories that may be better suited for particular populations, but the advantage of using family theory is the ability to describe the family unit and how the family responds to the changes and stressors that occur.

FAMILY FUNCTIONS AND STRUCTURE

Kaakinen, Hanson, and Birenbaum (2003) identified six different family functions: (1) financial survival; (2) reproduction; (3) protection; (4) passing along the culture; (5) education and socialization; and (6) conferring status in society. If the family is unable to maintain any of these functions, family instability results.

The classic American fairy tale shows the family constellation as an idealistic, static never changing female mother, male father, two children of either sex, "nice" house, white picket fence, dog and/or cat, living in the sweet village or town with multiple family generations and all members living in close proximity. Holidays and vacations are spent together in this idyllic picture enhanced by the warmth of "comfort" foods. The main problem is that it is a fairy tale and not a picture of real life. The truth is that the concept of family is a constantly morphing perception. In the twenty-first century, there is no "typical" picture of a family.

Family constellations are changing throughout the United States. Social and sexual rules are changing, resulting in a great diversity of family constellations. Only 69% of children live in a two-parent family and 26% live with only one parent (AAP, 2003); 15% of households include blended families, with at least one step-parent, step-sibling, or half sibling. Unmarried couples of the same or different genders are rearing children, as well as unmarried single parents. In 2000, 33.2% of births were to unmarried women (AAP, 2003). Grandparents, most commonly grandmothers, are rearing their grandchildren and other relatives. Families are fluid networks, with members coming and going depending on social situations, financial needs, and availability.

The biologic family is the family into which the child is born. The term "source family," or the family that legally and pragmatically functions as the biological family, even if the child was born to another, has frequently replaced this term.

Friedman et al. (2003) delineate traditional and nontraditional family structures. This list is not inclusive and other authors have defined additional structures. The traditional structures include nuclear (a married heterosexual couple with children, including adoptive children), single parent (previously married), extended families (includes at least three generations), and blended families (two single parents with children marry, resulting in step-parents and stepsiblings). Nontraditional family structures include single parent (never married) with children, unmarried couples with children (cohabitating couples, common law marriage, gay/lesbian couple), foster families, augmented families (nuclear or single parent family with unrelated persons living in the household), grandparents raising grandchildren, and communal households (usually composed of unrelated individuals and couples with children where all members share responsibility for daily living tasks, including child care and child rearing).

Birth rates, in general, are declining or static for much of the population, allowing parents more freedom from child-rearing duties. Many women with children have entered the work force because of the necessity of dual parent incomes, the freedom to choose as a result of the women's movement, and more opportunities available because of increased education for women. There are also those who have chosen to remain single and to have children using donated sperm and in vitro fertilization. International adoptions are commonplace today, adding new complexities, including health, language, and culture. Examples include adopting children who are chronic carriers of hepatitis B or who have been exposed to tuberculosis. Families often attempt to learn the cultural practices of the child's original heritage. Some families have to learn to care for different skin or hair textures than those with which they are familiar. Incidents of life sometimes cause great alterations in families, such as serious illness or death of members, divorce, new marriage, and families breaking up due to finances (Doherty & Beaton, 2000). These all pose challenges for the school nurse in order to best serve students.

New members added through birth, adoption, marriage, or cohabitation that add other children with their particular needs and expectations also impact families. All of these changes in the family dynamics cause multiple alterations but many cope without complications.

THE "POTENTIALLY AT-RISK" CHILD

The changes in family constellations and altered support systems can leave children "at risk" in a variety of situations. These situations include children who are "latchkey" (see definition below), homeless, in the foster care system, members of recent immigrant families, adopted, experiencing the separation or divorce of parents, incarcerated, or being raised by grandparents. The school and the school nurse can be a resource and a support for these students as well as their families.

"Latchkey" Children

The term "latchkey" refers to children who spend unsupervised time at home, usually before or after school. The majority of the literature addressing this problem was written in the late 1980s. The 1990s saw an increase in after-school programs and community programs to alleviate the risks of children spending time at home alone without adult supervision. Recent studies have documented the use of public libraries as an alternative to children returning home after school; in this format, children spend time in the library until a parent or caregiver can pick them up. Other schools have "after-care" programs that offer crafts or sports in a supervised setting in the school until parents can pick up their children.

Safety is the major concern for latchkey children; they need information regarding who to contact in case of emergency, how to treat minor injuries, how to avoid dangerous situations, and how to access resources by telephone. Some communities have developed intervention programs to address the needs of "latchkey" children, or guidelines for working parents to assess the appropriateness of their children staying home alone and to prepare their children for self-care. The school nurse can be instrumental in providing information to parents and children that will provide a safer environment.

Children Who Are Homeless

Families are the fastest growing segment of the homeless population (Freidman et al., 2003). Healthcare problems and needs of homeless families include inadequate immunization status, poor nutritional status, and limited access to healthcare. The impact of homelessness affects all family members. The parents experience depression and chronic health problems more frequently than the general population (Freidman et al., 2003). The children also experience more acute and chronic illnesses, and are more prone to develop tuberculosis, asthma, anemia, gastrointestinal problems, chronic otitis media, and lice infestations (Freidman et al., 2003). Homeless children also have more developmental, behavioral, and emotional problems than their peers (Morris & Strong, 2004). There are also adolescents who have left home voluntarily or involuntarily;

some have been physically, sexually, or emotionally abused, and some are angry that their parents will not allow them to engage in particular behaviors. It is estimated that almost 8% of teenagers have spent at least one night "on the streets, in a shelter, in some public place, such as a train station or park, or with a stranger" (Monsen, 2003, p. 137). When including the number of "runaways," the number could approach 2 million young people without a home. Those living on the street are at increased risk of substance abuse (used by 71% of street youth), sexual activity (often used to buy food or drugs), crime, and physical abuse. They are at risk for depression as well as sexually transmitted diseases. Rew, Taylor-Seehafer, Thomas, and Yockey (2001 as cited in Monsen, 2003) questioned 15- to 22-year-olds who were homeless and found that "having someone who cared about them was important to their respondents, both in their family lives and at school. Resilience was correlated positively with having hope and correlated negatively with loneliness, high-risk behaviors (attitudes about suicide and being prone to suicide), and social connectedness" (p. 138).

The school nurse can intervene with the family that is homeless to facilitate access to health care through public health, especially related to completion of immunizations. In addition, referrals to nutrition resources, such as the Women's, Infants, and Children federal health program (WIC) and assisting children of homeless families to access free school lunch programs can help to increase the nutritional status of students. These students also often perform below grade level academically, and may need in-school assistance to boost their achievement (Morris & Butt, 2003). The child or adolescent who is homeless is also exposed to environmental hazards, violence, and substance abuse. Banouli (1996) identified this combination of health problems, environmental dangers, and stress as the "homeless child syndrome."

Children who are homeless need to be provided with tools to enhance their self-care. Rew (2003) found that her study population of homeless adolescents demonstrated a social process of self-care within the high-risk environment of homelessness. Supporting this population in the areas of self-awareness, use of resources, and maintaining health are interventions appropriate for school nurses. The school nurse might be the students' only resource for assessment and referrals to medical care.

Because hospitalizations are more frequent and behavioral problems are prevalent, school attendance may be sporadic and school performance suffers as a result. The school nurse should focus on preventive and follow-up care and treat acute/immediate problems. This population would benefit from access to or provision of physical exams, behavioral and developmental assessments, nutritional support, screening tests, and immunizations within the school setting (Banouli, 1996). The school nurse is in a prime position to facilitate all of these interventions and assist the homeless student to achieve a higher level of health. The manner in which the school staff and the school nurse respond to the needs of students experiencing homelessness will have a profound effect on how those children approach school and how successful they are (Hindman & Mincemeyer, 2004).

Children in Foster Care

"Foster care refers to the substitution of some alternative parent, parents, or institutional provider for the source parents of a child who has been removed from the source home as a result of maltreatment" (Ellis, Dulmus, & Wodarski, 2003, p. 101). Foster care has increased greatly in the last 20 years, and currently there are record numbers of children in foster care (Lindsey, 2001). There are 550,000 children in the foster care system in the United States (Rubin et al., 2004). Some of this care is provided in single-family homes, while others are group homes; the goal is to provide a safe, stable living environment that resembles a family setting. Foster care can be short term (less than a week), long term, or permanent.

There are concerns regarding the quality of care and the provision of health care for children in foster care. There is an increased incidence of chronic conditions and mental health problems in those children and adolescents who had multiple foster home placements than if they had episodic foster care placement (Rubin et al., 2004; Schneiderman, 2004). The literature documents that many foster children experience depression, poor self-esteem, anxiety, and separation trauma. They may tend to distrust adults and have inappropriate social skills (Ellis et al., 2003).

Chernoff, Combs-Orme, Risley-Curtiss, and Heisler (1994) identified the health problems of children entering the foster care system. They found that more than 90% of the children examined had an abnormality in at least one body system. They also found that a significant percentage of the children failed vision and hearing screenings (25% failed vision and 15% failed hearing). Heights and weights were below the norms for age, and they also exhibited abnormal results (23%) on developmental screenings. Although this study was completed 10 years ago, it indicates that this population has many healthcare needs.

"Frequent change of placements, poor caregivers, and incomplete health records made continuity of care difficulty" (Schneiderman, 2004, p. 344). School nurses can provide support for children in foster care who are in the school setting by assessing for health problems and referring for supportive services and counseling, if needed. In addition, facilitating screenings and screening follow-ups are critical to this population.

Immigrant Children

Immigrant children include those who are legal and illegal (undocumented), refugees, and international adoptees. Challenges for immigrants can result in unsatisfactory health care and decreased family health status. Challenges include adjustment to new social rules, maintaining family cohesion, maintaining their own cultural practices, and accessing health care (Kaakinen et al., 2003). Because of the cost of health care, immigrants may avoid routine health care, not seek preventative care, and only utilize emergency departments and health clinics for episodic care.

The school nurse can play a vital role in linking these families to appropriate health care. The school nurse is in a position to understand the cultural implications of accessing and receiving health care (see Chapter 18). Immigrant children are at risk due to possible inadequate immunization levels and possible undiagnosed pre-existing conditions. Priority interventions for this population include thorough screenings, updating of immunizations, thorough physical evaluation, and mental health assessments.

Children Who Are Adopted

Children are adopted at all ages and from all around the world. The first requirement is that the birth parents terminate their legal rights and responsibilities as parents. This is a legal proceeding and occurs when (1) the birth family does not want custody of the child, (2) the birth family is unable or incapable of caring for the child, (3) the birth family cannot be located for an extended period of time, (4) the birth family is deceased, or (5) "no suitable kinship arrangement can be made in which custody can be arranged without TPR" (terminating parental rights) (Ellis et al., 2003, p. 169). Although these factors do not guarantee that adoption will occur, they allow the legal system to begin the process.

In some jurisdictions, adolescents may refuse to be adopted. For these youth and those who are difficult to place, they may be in foster care or be wards of the state. It is possible that students are eligible for or in the process of being adopted during the school year. They may need assistance in bonding with their new families and may not know or remember the needed information to answer staff questions, such as home address and phone number or where the parent works. Their adoption may result in their entering the school mid-year.

The school nurse can be a significant source of support for these students and can encourage staff to help them become involved with peers. Multiple books have been written for children on the topic of being adopted and loved; these can be read in classes and available in the library. The school nurse and perhaps the counseling staff should communicate directly with the parents who have adopted children to provide support and a connection with the school.

Students adopted from other countries, whether as infants or older children, may have additional concerns, such as for those of immigrant children above. More than 21,000 infants were adopted from outside the United States in 2003, many from Asia and Eastern Europe (Monsen, 2004). While some are well cared for and have minimal adjustment problems, others may have been abused or neglected in their orphanage. Some have tuberculosis, syphilis, parasites, and human immunodeficiency virus disease and some are developmentally delayed. Some younger than the age of 6 may display self-stimulating behaviors, such as persistent rocking, self-injury, or feeding problems (Monsen, 2004). Consistency in the care provided and emotional support are essential in promoting a successful transition.

Children Experiencing the Separation or Divorce of Their Parents

More than one million children and adolescents experience the separation or divorce of their parents each year in the United States. "Approximately 50% of first marriages and 60% of second marriages end in divorce" (Cohen, 2002, p. 1019). While tension from parental conflict may have caused the divorce, stress levels continue after the one spouse has moved out of the house. Children and adolescents feel a sense of loss, especially on holidays or special school events. Students may become aware of changes in their routines, parental work schedules, and financial status. They endure the stress of perhaps "living in two homes," with varied schedules and needing to keep duplicate supplies at each home. Teachers are acutely aware of the behavior changes in some students when they were with one parent over the weekend and now have returned to the other parent's home.

Half of all children "show a symptomatic response during the first year after their parents divorce" (Cohen, 2002, p. 1019). Preschoolers may blame themselves for the breakup; they may cling to one parent, fearing that they will also be abandoned, or they may experience sleep problems or acting-out behavior. School-age youth and adolescents may be sad, moody, or aggressive, and may feel rejected by the absent parent. Their schoolwork may suffer and they may act out and engage in high-risk behaviors. Psychosomatic complaints are also common, such as stomachache or migraine headaches.

All children and adolescents need to understand that (1) they are loved, (2) they are not the cause of the divorce, and (3) they are not alone. Some school nurses have developed support groups for children whose parents are divorced. Parent conference can help identify the legal and practical issues, especially related to any accommodations needed by the student. Conferences can be initiated by the family, the faculty, the counseling staff, or the school nurse.

Students Who Are Incarcerated

Research literature relating to health problems of this population is limited. However, Shelton (2000) studied the health needs of young offenders in the care of state juvenile justice systems. It was found that 45% had some medical condition, 53% had a history of abuse, and 36% had been injured but 12% had not received treatment for injuries. Although 86% of the youth in the study reported they were healthy, the health indicators did not support their self-reports. When working with this population, it is important to remember that although they see themselves as healthy, there may be several underlying health problems. They may also have engaged in high-risk behaviors leading to sexually transmitted diseases, HIV, drug abuse, and so forth.

Violence, both family and community, are components of the incarcerated child's life. All of the socio-cultural and psychological, as well as physical risk factors of violence are present. The school nurse functions in a collaborative role with many other resources in providing care to this population and assuring a smooth transition back into the school setting or an alternative arrangement.

Children Living in Grandparent-Headed Households

In the past two decades, increasing numbers of grandparents have been assuming the parenting role as a result of multiple family issues. These include teen pregnancy, death, divorce, substance abuse, incarceration, abandonment, AIDS, and child abuse (Nolan, 1999). About one in 20 children, or 1.4 million children, are raised in a household without a parent present. Ten percent of grandparents are raising their grandchildren and 4 million children live in a grandparent-headed household. "African-Americans are more likely to raise their grandchildren because of parent-absent circumstances…and have twice the odds of becoming caregivers to their grandchildren" (Kataoka-Yahiro, Ceria, & Caulfield, 2004, p. 315).

The grandparent functioning in the parent role may need assistance with child development information, financial support, and educational resources, as well as assistance with emotional, medical, and legal issues. Grandparents caring for a child or children may need support from the community. The school and school nurse are major contacts for the grandparent. There are multi-levels of health care required in this family structure. The grandparents need information about immunizations, well child health care, and treatment for acute and chronic childhood illnesses that has changed from when they raised their children. In addition, the grandparent may have chronic conditions themselves that require treatment and may limit their ability to provide adequate child care. The school nurse can assist the "grandparent" family with linkages to healthcare providers and other community resources.

IMPACT ON THE SCHOOL NURSE

Nursing education has always promoted family-centered care. All pediatric nurses recognize the importance of family to the child's growth and development and the importance of good communication between the school and the family. Parent contact information kept in the health office should include who to call and their relationship to the student. It should be known by the school who the legal guardian is for the student and if there are any restraining orders preventing one of the parents from making contact with their child.

When interacting with parents, it may be helpful for the school nurse to know (1) who is involved in the student's care, (2) who lives in the home, (3) whom the parents can rely on for their emotional support, (4) if the biological parents are not in the home, where are they and what are their parenting responsibilities, if any, and (5) if the family is "at risk," do they need to be connected with community resources for health care (such as accessing immunizations), financial support (such as accessing free lunch programs), and childcare after school (such as Boys' and Girls' Clubs or Police Athletic League).

Resources such as Help Directors printed by the United Way and manuals and directories from the Public Health Department as well as local health-care agencies or HMOs can provide additional information for parents and guardians.

CONCLUSION

School nurses utilize components of family assessment to assess and implement health care for students identified with health needs. The school nurse can provide health information, health promotion, health protection, and illness prevention at the primary prevention level. When problems occur, school nurses can obtain needed assistance for families to deal more effectively with a student's health problems. The school nurse plays an integral role in facilitating family interactions with health and social systems regardless of the family structure. The school nurse must remain sensitive to the changing dynamics of the students' families and of the school environment in general. Evolving sociological, cultural, and economic conditions must be constantly considered in the school setting.

References

American Academy of Pediatrics (AAP). (2003). Family pediatrics: Report of the Task Force on the Family. *Pediatrics, 111*(6), 1539–1571.

Banouli, J. (1996). *Homelessness in America*. Phoenix: Onyx.

Boss, P. (2002). *Family stress management*. Thousand Oaks, CA: Sage.

Chernoff, R., Combs-Orme, T., Risley-Curtiss, C. & Heisler, A. (1994). Assessing the health status of children entering foster care. *Pediatrics, 93*(4), 594–601.

Cohen, G. and the Committee on Psychosocial Aspects of Child and Family Health. (2002). Helping children and families deal with divorce and separation. *Pediatrics, 110*(6), 1019–1022.

Doherty, W. J., & Beaton, J. M. (2000). Family therapists, community, and civic renewal. *Family Process, 39*, 149–161.

Ellis, R., Dulmus, C., & Wodarski, J. (2003). *Essentials of child welfare*. Hoboken, NJ: John Wiley & Sons.

Freidman, M., Bowden, V., & Jones, E. (2003). *Family nursing: Research, theory, & Practice* (5th ed.). Upper Saddle River, NJ: Prentice Hall.

Hanson, S., Kaakinen, J., & Friedman, M. (1998). Theoretical approaches to family nursing. In M. Friedman (Eds.), *Family nursing: Research, theory, & practice* (pp. 75–98). Stamford, CT: Appleton & Lange.

Hindman, J., & Mincemeyer, J. (Fall, 2004). *School nurses: It's not just bandages anymore. Project Hope Virginia. Information Brief No. 3: Children who are homeless.* Retrieved April, 2005 from http://www.wm.edu/hope.

Kaakinen, J., Hanson, S., & Birenbaum, L. (2003). Family development and family nursing assessment. In M. Stanhope & J. Lancaster. *Community and public health nursing* (pp. 563–591). St. Louis: C. V. Mosby.

Kataoka-Yahiro, M., Ceria, C., & Caulfield, R. (2004). Grandparent caregiving role in ethnically diverse families. *Journal of Pediatric Nursing, 19*(5), 315–328.

Kerr, M., & Bowen, M. (1988). *Family evaluation*. New York: W. W. Norton.

Linsdey, E. W. (2001). Foster family characteristics and behavioral and emotional problems of foster children. *Family Relations*, 50(1), 19–22.

Monsen, R. (2004). Adopting children. *Journal of Pediatric Nursing, 19*(3), 214–215.

Monsen, R. (2003). Sheltering children. *Journal of Pediatric Nursing, 18*(2), 137–138.

Morris, R., & Butt, R. (2003). Parents' perspectives on homelessness and its effects on the educational development of their children. *Journal of School Nursing, 19*(1), 43–50.

Morris, R., & Strong, L. (2004). The impact of homelessness on the health of families. *The Journal of School Nursing, 20*(4), 221–227.

Nolan, J. (1999) *Grandparents as parents again*. Ohio State University Extension, Senior Series. Retrieved November 21, 2003 from http://www.ag.ohio-state.edu/~seniors.

Rew, L. (2003). A theory of taking care of oneself grounded in experiences of homeless youth. *Nursing Research, 52*(4), 234–241.

Rubin, D., Alessandrini, E., Feudtner, C., Mandell, D., Localio, A. R., & Hadley, R. (2004). Placement stability and mental health costs for children in foster care. *Pediatrics, 113*(5), 1336–1341.

Schneiderman, J. (2004). The health of children in foster care. *The Journal of School Nursing, 20*(6), 343–351.

Shelton, D. (2000). Health status of young offenders and their families. *Journal of Nursing Scholarship, 32*(2), 173–178.

Wright, L., & Leahey, M. (2000). *Nurses and families: A guide to family assessment and intervention* (3rd ed). Philadelphia: F. A. Davis.

Chapter 18

Cultural Competence in Professional School Nursing Practice

DONNA J. MAZYCK ▪ MARIA RIVERA (KLEIN)-MATZA

Chapter Outline

INTRODUCTION

The United States has experienced a growing shift in its cultural demographics that requires changes in the manner in which healthcare professionals and healthcare organizations provide care for clients. Schools in the United States reflect the changing cultural landscape, and school nurses have the opportunity to expand their scope of practice by adding to their knowledge and understanding of various population groups. The purpose of this chapter is to define culture and cultural competency in relationship to health outcomes in school-aged children, and to describe the methods school nurses can use to bridge communication among educational systems, healthcare systems, and children and their families. School nurses who work with children and families of diverse cultures need to understand the complex social, political, and economic forces that shape people's lives in order to promote health in a community; they must also render care that is sensitive to the different needs of diverse groups.

When discussing cultural issues, one cannot generalize to all individuals of a certain culture. Culture is a *process* and changes over time. Thus a third-generation Vietnamese-American or Cuban-American would have distinctly different values, attitudes, and health practices than a first-generation or a newly arrived immigrant.

School nurses may have not received professional development on cultural competence, especially as it relates to children and their families. In an effort to better assist students and families, school nurses must learn about the factors that influence them. The models and frameworks of cultural competency developed by Leininger, Purnell, and Giger and Davidhizar will provide organizational structure for this process.

Racial and ethnic groups may view health care and healthcare professionals from a perspective based on their previous experience and knowledge. School nurses who are aware of these views may provide health care more appropriately and respectfully. School nurses also must examine their personal cultural beliefs and identify potential prejudice or stereotypical triggers and thoughts. Being culturally competent corresponds well with the holistic approach to nursing.

DEMOGRAPHICS

Schools are among the most culturally diverse environments in the United States. In 1972 the student population in public schools was 79% white, non-Hispanic; 14% black; 6% Hispanic; and 1% Asian, Pacific Islander, and other races. In 1999, it was 64% white, non-Hispanic; 16% black; 15% Hispanic, Asian, and Pacific Islander; and 5% other races in public schools (U.S. Department of Commerce [USDC], 2001). In 2000, 39% of public school students were classified as minorities (U.S. Department of Education [USDOE], 2003). Census figures show the Hispanic population reached about 37 million as of January 2004, making Hispanics the nation's largest minority.

Of the 57 million children and adolescents enrolled in school, "20% had at least one foreign-born parent, including 5% who are themselves foreign-born" (USDC, 2001). During the past 20 years, the number of young people 5 to 24 years of age who speak a language other than English at home or who speak English with difficulty has increased from 6.3 million to 13.7 million and from 2.2 million to 4.5 million, respectively (USDOE, 2003).

School nurses are not as diverse a group as the students to whom they deliver school health services. Approximately 12% of registered nurses with current licenses in the United States are African-American, Asian, Hispanic, or American Indian/Alaskan Native (Spratley et al., 2000).

HEALTH DISPARITIES

The history of the United States is replete with examples of gross discrimination against various racial and ethnic groups, including Native Americans, enslaved Africans, and immigrants landing on Ellis Island in New York City. This discrimination extended to the healthcare arena. Huff and Kline (1999) noted that "cultural differences can and do present major barriers to effective health care intervention" (p. 6). Discrimination in society continues, as evidenced by the diminished quality of health care received by minority and ethnic populations compared to Caucasian populations in the United States (Institute of Medicine, 2002).

One goal of *Healthy People 2010* is to eliminate healthcare disparities in the United States, including differences that occur by gender, race or ethnicity, education or income, disability, geographical location, or sexual orientation (U.S. Department of Health and Human Services [USDHHS], 2000). Students and their families reflect the health beliefs, values, and customs of the community from which they come. "Likewise, community health is profoundly affected by the collective beliefs, attitudes, and behaviors of everyone who lives in the community" (USDHHS, 2000). "Healthy People 2010 is firmly dedicated to the principle that every person in every community across the Nation deserves equal access to comprehensive, culturally competent, community-based health care systems that are committed to serving the needs of the individual and promoting community health" (USDHHS, 2000).

Clients' access and response to healthcare services is greatly influenced by their cultural and ethnic backgrounds (New Hampshire Department of Health and Human Services, 2002). On an individual and organizational level, healthcare professionals must intentionally reduce barriers to healthcare services.

The differences in the cultural backgrounds of the school nurse, the parent/guardian, and the student can present challenges in the delivery of school health services. In the *Scope and standards of professional school nursing practice*, one of the measurement criteria for the professional performance standard on ethics is "the school nurse delivers care in a nonjudgmental and nondiscriminatory manner that is sensitive to student diversity in the school community" (NASN & ANA, 2001, p. 21). It is therefore the responsibility of the school nurse to find a way to deliver school health services in a culturally competent manner.

Multiple factors impact on providing culturally competent care. The presence of language barriers requires an understanding on the part of the school nurse of the process in learning a second language. The presence of an interpreter who is trained in medical terminology helps bridge the communication gap as the student learns English. Attention to the family's ethnic and religious practices allows the school nurse to gain knowledge about potential reasons behind the practices and beliefs of students (Gambol & Gambol, 2002). Awareness of the students' previous experiences, such as witnesses to and survivors of war crimes, will alert school nurses to the potential of somatic and emotional health problems in students who are immigrants (Gambol & Gambol, 2002). The school nurse may work with an interdisciplinary team representing the school and community in order to assist the student and family with their multiple healthcare needs.

UNDERSTANDING CULTURAL TERMS

Culture

Many terms are involved in understanding the concept of cultural competence, the first of which is defining the concept of culture. Culture is a learned behavior; and all behavior is influenced by culture. Multiple theories and models have been developed to explain culture. Each defines culture within the context of their theory. Some of the more popular definitions of culture are as follows.

- Culture is a "totality of socially transmitted behavioral patterns, arts, beliefs, values, customs, *lifeways*, and all other products of human work and thought characteristics of a population of people that guide their worldview and decision making" (Purnell & Paulanka, 2003, p. 3).
- Culture is a "metacommunication system" wherein not only the spoken words have meaning, but everything else as well (Spector, 2004, p. 9).
- "Culture is a system of symbols that is shared, learned, and passed on through generations of a social group. Culture mediates between human beings and chaos; it influences what people perceive and guides people's interactions with each other. It is a process rather than a static entity and it changes over time" (Lipson, 1996, p. 1).
- "Culture is the values, beliefs, norms, and practices of a particular group that are learned and shared and that guide thinking, decisions, and actions in a patterned way" (Leininger & McFarland, 2002, p. 83).
- "Culture is a patterned behavioral response that develops over time as a result of imprinting the mind through social and religious structures and intellectual and artistic manifestations.... passed down from one generation to the next" (Giger & Davidhizar, 2004, p. 3)

Culture guides the interactions individuals have with one another, including with healthcare providers. The common universal thread in examining culture is the idea that values and beliefs are passed from generation to generation.

Cultural Diversity/Ethnicity/Race

The multiple cultures, races, religions, income levels, ethnicity, and languages are what contribute to the cultural variety in society. Cultural diversity includes age, race, gender, ethnicity, religion, sexual orientation, socioeconomic status, and education, as well as health and emotional challenges. Ethnicity and race are separate entities that are often confused. Race refers to the biological factors of blood type, skin color, and bone structure, while ethnicity refers to the identity of members of a group based on shared social and cultural traditions (Davidhizer, Havens, & Bechtel, 1999).

Cultural diversity is related not only to racial and ethnic groups. When a particular group has a pattern of beliefs, values, and actions that they share, one may view them as a cultural group. For example, groups of students who are athletes or involved in creative arts represent a cultural group. Men in nursing are another group. It is beneficial to learn basic information about the different culture groups represented in the school and community. One way in which school nurses can learn about the beliefs and values of the groups is by asking members from these groups to explain their culture to them. School nurses may informally explore details of the cultures of students and families during routine interactions. Collaborations with other school staff may provide opportunities for the school community to learn about various cultures in more formal arrangements, such as Parent–Teacher–Student Organization (PTSO) presentations and school staff meetings. School nurses may also seek this information in structured, formal ways such as through postgraduate or continuing education formats. Cultural inquiry is a rich field for school nursing research.

Cultural Competence versus Cultural Sensitivity

Cultural sensitivity refers to a person's attitudes toward a culture or ethnic background different from one's own but not saying things that would be offensive to members of those other groups (Purnell & Paulanka, 2003). However, cultural sensitivity is only a beginning step towards cultural competence. Cultural competence in health care is the process of understanding and respecting the cultural values and practices of clients. According to Purnell and Paulanka (2003), cultural competence incorporates:

- Developing an awareness of one's own existence, sensations, thoughts, and environment without letting it have an undue influence on those from other backgrounds.
- Demonstrating knowledge and understanding of the client's culture, health-related needs, and meanings of health and illness.
- Accepting and respecting cultural differences.
- Not assuming that the healthcare provider's beliefs and values are the same as the client's.
- Resisting judgmental attitudes such as "different is not as good."
- Being open to cultural encounters.
- Adapting care to be congruent with the client's culture. Cultural competence is a conscious process and not necessarily linear.

Cultural competence is a fundamental human right. Various aspects of cultural competency include the clients' views about health and health care, family relationships, language (including communication styles), and religion. One does not attain cultural competence; rather one increasingly grows in knowledge and skills in this area. Cultural competence is not a static process.

Knowledge about particular people groups is helpful in the process of developing cultural competence. Ethnic groups and religious groups may have views that will influence how they receive healthcare services. Learning basic information about the groups will enable the school nurse to consider those points of view while interacting with students and family members. Other people groups may have beliefs and practices that require some additional knowledge by school nurses, such as students who have immigrated as refugees from war-torn nations or students who are deaf.

Acculturation

Acculturation reflects a modification in one's culture resulting from association with members of another culture (Purnell & Paulanka, 2003). When immigrants or refugees settle in a new country, they experience new cultural customs. Some immigrants and refugees choose acculturation as a means of adapting to their surroundings by continuing to maintain their own culture while embracing some aspects of the dominant culture. Acculturation usually reflects a minority group adopting habits and language patterns of the dominant group; it can also be a reciprocal process. For example, immigrant adolescents who begin wearing styles of clothes similar to those of their classmates rather than their country of origin demonstrate one aspect of acculturation. In a reciprocal process, a Caucasian child living in a primarily Latino community may begin to incorporate Spanish into his or her conversations with neighborhood friends.

Assimilation

Many newcomers to a foreign land ultimately assimilate to the new culture. According to Purnell and Paulanka (2003), to assimilate is "to gradually adopt and incorporate the characteristics of the prevailing culture" (p. 351). Assimilation may be evidenced by changes in language preference, adoption of common attitudes and values, and loss of separate political or ethnic identification. An example of this can be seen when families no longer practice the traditions of their country of origin, such as national holidays, or no longer speak their native language.

Ethnocentrism

Assuming that one's thoughts, actions, and beliefs are the only correct thoughts, actions, and beliefs is called ethnocentrism (Purnell & Paulanka, 2003). School nurses must examine their view of the cultures represented by students and staff in their efforts to consciously move toward culturally competent care. The school nurse's personal culture may directly affect how he or she responds to students of differing cultures. There may be a desire on the part of healthcare providers and school staff to have the students assimilate when, in fact, they do not want to. The following examples illustrate ways in which a school nurse's culture may affect responses to clients:

- The school nurse who believes in Western medicine and is not accepting of the cultural practice of coining to respond to fever and attempts to discourage this practice.
- A school nurse may consider fasting during the day inappropriate for a young student, although it is practiced within some religions, for example, Islam during Ramadan. The assumptions by the school nurses about the ways of "people groups" are often based on their limited experiences.

Ethnocentrism may keep healthcare professionals from becoming aware that their views may be causing misunderstandings with groups that are different from their culture. In addition, healthcare professionals must learn not to judge a different culture by their own cultural values. School nurses can sometimes recognize their assumptions about "people groups" by noting their reactions in encounters with students and family members. Rather than deny the reactions, one can recognize them and accept that the assumptions exist. Only with self-awareness can a conscious decision to alter those assumptions be made.

NATIONALLY RECOMMENDED STANDARDS

The National Association of School Nurses (NASN) supports cultural competence and promotes provision of "age appropriate, culturally, and ethically sensitive care" (NASN & ANA, 2001, p. 11). Standard V (Ethics) of the Standards of Professional Performance of School Nursing Practice includes the following:

- "The school nurse delivers care in a manner that promotes and preserves student and family autonomy, dignity, and rights."
- "The school nurse delivers care in a nonjudgmental and nondiscriminatory manner that is sensitive to student diversity in the school community" (NASN & ANA, 2001, p. 21).

The National Council for Accreditation of Teacher Education developed six standards that "prepare educators to work effectively" in preschool through grade 12 schools (National Council for Accreditation of Teacher Education, 2002, p. 10). One standard focuses on diversity in curriculum and on experiences of working with colleagues and students. In helping all students learn, school personnel are encouraged to consider student ethnicity, race, gender, language, and geographical origins (National Council for Accreditation of Teacher Education, 2002). States vary on requirements for staff development and other course work in topics on cultural competence for educators.

The Office of Minority Health of the U.S. Department of Health and Human Services (2001) has developed *National Standards for Culturally and Linguistically Appropriate Services in Health Care (CLAS)* (Box 18.1). The first three standards concern culturally competent care. Standards four through seven deal with the use of appropriate language and the final seven standards define organizational supports necessary. These standards address healthcare organizations and indicate a growing concern for culturally competent care in health care.

Box 18.1 ■ ■ ■

NATIONAL STANDARDS FOR CULTURALLY AND LINGUISTICALLY APPROPRIATE SERVICES IN HEALTH CARE

HEALTHCARE ORGANIZATIONS:

1. Should ensure that patients/consumers receive from all staff members effective, understandable, and respectful care that is provided in a manner compatible with their cultural health beliefs and practices and preferred language.
2. Should implement strategies to recruit, retain, and promote at all levels of the organization a diverse staff and leadership that are representative of the demographic characteristics of the service area.
3. Should ensure that staff at all levels and across all disciplines receive ongoing education and training in culturally and linguistically appropriate service delivery.
4. Must offer and provide language assistance services, including bilingual staff and interpreter services, at no cost to each patient/consumer with limited English proficiency at all points of contact, in a timely manner during all hours of operation.
5. Must provide to patients/consumers in their preferred language both verbal offers and written notices informing them of their right to receive language assistance services.
6. Must ensure the competence of language assistance provided to limited English proficient patients/consumers by interpreters and bilingual staff. Family and friends should not be used to provide interpretation services (except on request of the patient/consumer).
7. Must make available easily understood patient-related materials and post signage in the languages of the commonly encountered groups and/or groups represented in the service area.

(Continued on the following page)

Box 18.1 ■■■

NATIONAL STANDARDS FOR CULTURALLY AND LINGUISTICALLY APPROPRIATE SERVICES IN HEALTH CARE *(Continued)*

8. Should develop, implement, and promote a written strategic plan that outlines clear goals, policies, operational plans, and management accountability/oversight mechanisms to provide culturally and linguistically appropriate services.
9. Should conduct initial and ongoing organizational self-assessments of CLAS-related activities and are encouraged to integrate cultural and linguistic competence-related measures into their internal audits, performance improvement programs, patient satisfaction assessments, and outcomes-based evaluations.
10. Should ensure that data on the individual patient's/consumer's race, ethnicity, and spoken and written language are collected in health records, integrated into the organization's management information systems, and periodically updated.
11. Should maintain a current demographic cultural, and epidemiological profile of the community as well as a needs assessment to accurately plan for and implement services that respond to the cultural and linguistic characteristics of the service area.
12. Should develop participatory, collaborative partnerships with communities and utilize a variety of formal and informal mechanisms to facilitate community and patient/consumer involvement in designing and implementing CLAS-related activities.
13. Should ensure that conflict and grievance resolution processes are culturally and linguistically sensitive and capable of identifying, preventing, and resolving cross-cultural conflicts or complaints by patient/consumers.
14. Are encouraged to regularly make available to the public information about their progress and successful innovations in implementing the CLAS standards and to provide public notice in their communities about the availability of this information.

In the first standard, culturally competent care by healthcare professionals considers the health-related beliefs, values, and health disparities of the particular cultural group. The second standard recommends diversity in staff and leadership. When healthcare organizations recruit, retain, and promote staff on all levels who reflect the diversity of the community, they are promoting culturally competent care. The third standard moves from cultural diversity reflected among staff to a commitment to continuing education and training in culturally competent health services delivery. Cultural competence is a process that requires ongoing training and growing knowledge.

The CLAS standards set forth a commitment to culturally competent communication with clients and for healthcare organizations to make prompt self-assessments concerning their culturally and linguistically appropriate services. If clients cannot comprehend what is being communicated in healthcare delivery via verbal and written methods, there is minimal chance for adherence to treatment, getting families to complete needed health-related paperwork, or follow through with referrals. All of these principles directly relate to the care and interactions provided by the school nurse.

THEORIES AND MODELS OF CULTURE

A variety of theories and models are available for teaching concepts about cultural diversity. All have some relevance to school nursing practice and it is up to the school nurse to determine which work best in their practice setting. Leninger's Transcultural Model was developed in the 1970s and set the stage for the focus on culturally sensitive health care. Leininger wanted nurses to focus on "promoting and maintaining the cultural care needs of human beings" (Leininger & McFarland, 2002, p. 3). Leininger (1999) coined the term "transcultural nursing" in the mid-1950s to reflect "a new and potentially relevant discipline with a unique body of knowledge to help nurses provide culturally competent care" (p. 187). As a psychiatric clinical nurse specialist in pediatrics and a nurse anthropologist, Leininger noted the difficulty in working with children and parents of various cultures. She identified that "culture was the critical and major missing dimension of care" (Leininger & McFarland, 2002, p. 21).

In 1968, Leininger established the Committee on Nursing and Anthropology within the Medical Anthropology Council and by 1975, she had developed the world's first masters of nursing and doctorate in transcultural nursing (Leininger &

McFarland, 2002). The Organization of the National Transcultural Nursing Society was established in 1974. This Society began a certification program for transcultural care nurses in 1988, and in 1989 awarded certification to nurses who met the program's requirements (Leininger & McFarland, 2002).

Transcultural Nursing and the Culture Care Theory: Leininger

The definition of transcultural care nursing focuses on the primary element of caring. "Transcultural nursing has been defined as a formal area of study and practice focused on comparative human-care (caring) differences and similarities of the beliefs, values, and patterned lifeways of cultures to provide culturally congruent, meaningful, and beneficial health care to people" (Leininger & McFarland, 2002, pp. 5–6).

Transcultural nursing focuses on the comparison of differences and similarities of various cultures (Leininger & McFarland, 2002). Nurses developing cultural competence must be aware of these differences and similarities in order to render respectful care to students, staff, and families.

Leininger's culture care theory, also referred to as Culture Care Diversity and Universality (Leininger & McFarland, 2002), incorporates concepts from anthropology, including the five basic interactional phenomena, which are:

1. Culture encounter or contact refers to a situation in which a person from one culture meets or briefly interacts with a person from another culture.
2. Enculturation is the process by which one learns to take on or live by *all* aspects of a particular culture with its specific values, beliefs, and practices.
3. Acculturation refers to the process by which an individual or group from Culture A learns how to take on *many* (but not all) values, behaviors, norms, and lifeways of Culture B.
4. Socialization refers to the social process whereby an individual or group from a particular culture learns how to function within the larger society (or country).
5. Assimilation refers to the way an individual or group from one culture very selectively and usually intentionally selects certain features of another culture without necessarily taking on many or all attributes of lifeways that would declare one to be acculturated (Leininger & McFarland, 2002, pp. 55–56).

The culture care theory begins with the premise that nursing is a caring profession. It then acknowledges that "care diversities (differences) and universalities (commonalties) existed among and between cultures in the world" (Leininger & McFarland, 2002, p. 78). Culture care theory promotes "three major care actions and decisions to arrive at culturally congruent care for the general health and well-being of clients or to help them face death or disabilities:

- Culture care preservation or maintenance—assists in the preservation or retention of care values of a client's particular culture that help maintain well-being or recovery from illness." School nurses demonstrate culture care preservation when they acknowledge and encourage a cultural practice that will enhance the well-being of a student, such as advocating for a Muslim student to wear her hijab (headcovering) in a school that prohibits head coverings in the building.
- "Culture care accommodation or negotiation—assists in adaptation and negotiation with clients of a particular culture in identifying beneficial health outcomes." The school nurse exhibits this care action when accommodating a Vietnamese family's practice of coin rubbing while negotiating with them to also give their child the medication prescribed by the healthcare provider.
- "Culture care repatterning or restructuring—assists with modification of clients healthcare patterns to new and beneficial ones while respecting their cultural values and beliefs" (Leininger & McFarland, 2002, p. 78). School nurses assist with culture care restructuring when assisting a student and family to begin visiting the primary care provider for routine maintenance visits for chronic health needs rather than utilizing the emergency room exclusively only after a crisis occurs.

Models for cultural competence in nursing and other health professions have emerged from the culture care theory (Figure 18.1).

Transcultural Assessment Model: Giger and Davidhizar

The Giger and Davidhizar Transcultural Assessment Model was developed in 1988 and provides a more eclectic approach. This framework provides a systematic approach that can be helpful in developing skills for providing culturally competent care.

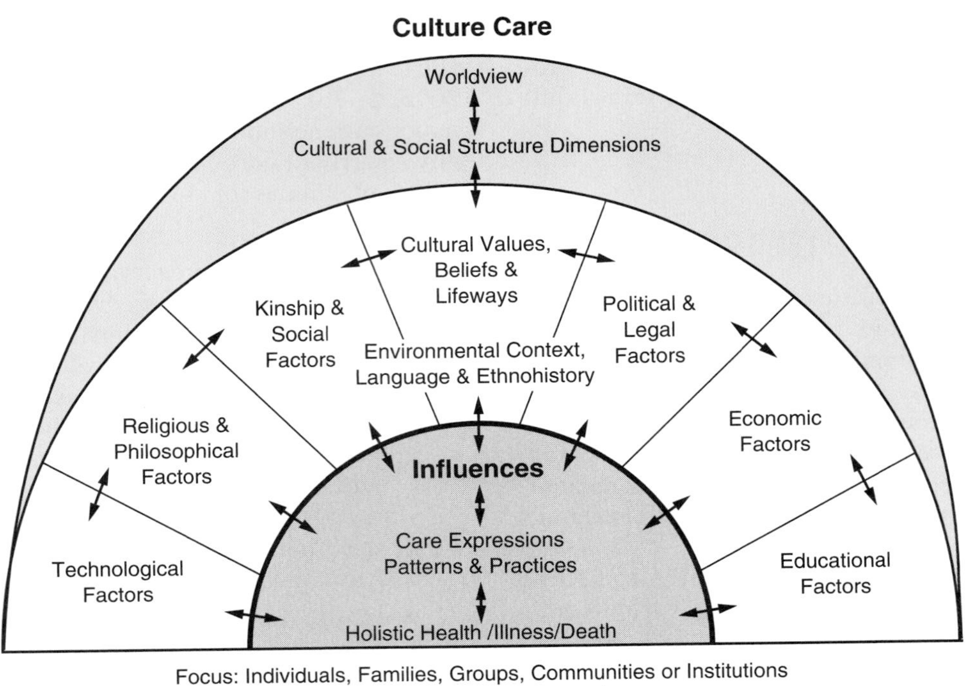

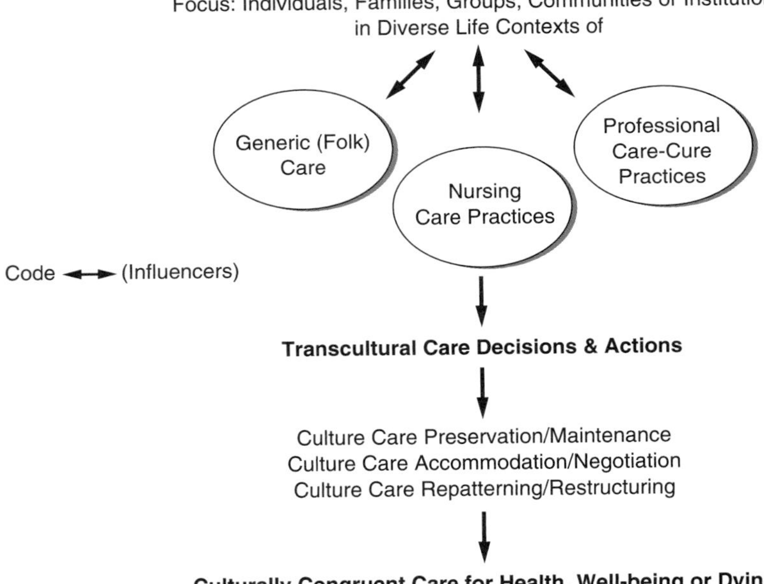

Figure 18.1 ■ Leininger's sunrise enabler.

The model emphasizes six cultural phenomena that make each individual unique: communication, space, social organization, time, environmental control, and biological variation (2004). These phenomena provide a framework for patient assessment and a basis from which culturally sensitive care can be designed. The work of Giger and Davidhizar builds on the seminal work of Leninger and other nurses as well as experts in space phenomena, communication, and anthropology (Giger & Davidhizar, 2002).

Communication incorporates all human interactions and behaviors, both verbal and nonverbal. This is "the means by which culture is transmitted and preserved" (Giger & Davidhizar, 2002, p. 185). *Space* is the distance individuals maintain between themselves when they interact. It is divided into intimate, personal, social and consultative, and public zones. *Social organization* refers to the family structure and organization. This includes the roles that family members play as well as their religious values and beliefs. *Time* refers to time orientation and one's view of past and future. *Environmental control* involves one's ability "to control nature and to plan and direct factors in the environment that affect them" (p. 185). *Biological variations* imply that there are innate differences among cultural groups, including genetic factors and conditions to which they are more susceptible.

Giger and Davidhizar's (2004) model is broad enough in scope to be recognized for applicability by many other healthcare professionals, and has been used for analysis of current trends in multiculturalism in health care. This is quickly producing a way for staff across disciplines to understand cultural diversity and learn culturally competent care. The Giger and Davidhizar model is a clear and effective tool to use in the assessment of students' and other clients' cultural care needs in the school health environment.

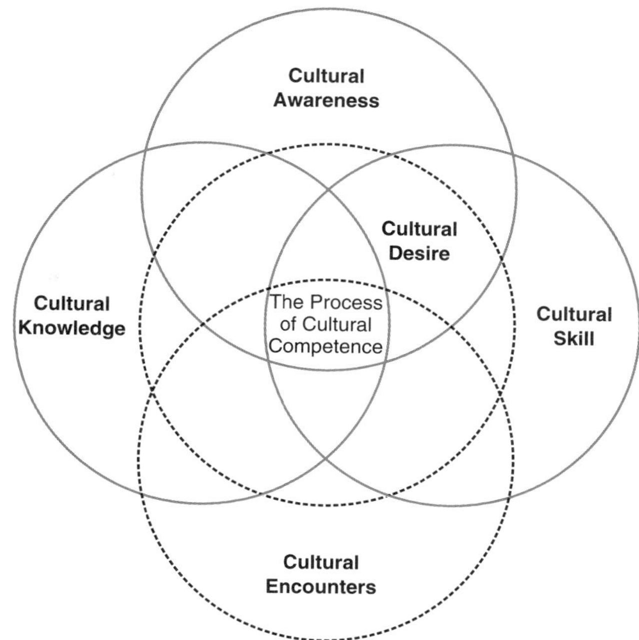

Figure 18.2 ■ Conceptual model of cultural competence. (From Campinha-Bacote [2002] Reprinted with permission from Transcultural C.A.R.E Associates.)

A Model for Cultural Competence in the Delivery of Healthcare Services: Campinha-Bacote

Campinha-Bacote (2002a) developed a conceptual model of cultural competence to assist nurses in their journey toward rendering culturally competent care. According to Campinha-Bacote, cultural competency is a goal one works toward rather than a place of arrival. Healthcare professionals must continually seek a higher level of cultural competence.

The model includes five interdependent constructs (Figure 18.2):

1. *Cultural awareness* refers to the healthcare professional's self-assessment regarding one's own culture and the biases and prejudices one has about those who are different.
2. *Cultural knowledge* refers to the knowledge sought and gained by healthcare professionals as they seek information on and understanding of the cultures of clients.
3. *Cultural skill* refers to the healthcare provider's ability to complete cultural assessments in a culturally sensitive manner. It also involves accomplishing culturally informed physical assessments on clients.
4. *Cultural encounter* refers to the healthcare professional's intentional pursuit of interactions with multiple members of diverse cultural backgrounds to refine one's beliefs about cultural groups. It may require the use of an interpreter in order to facilitate this process.
5. "Cultural desire" requires a motivation of the healthcare professional to "want to, rather than have to, engage in the process of becoming culturally aware, culturally knowledgeable, culturally skillful, and familiar with cultural encounters" (p. 182). The inward desire and motivation for cultural competence is reflected in an outward manifestation of genuine caring as the healthcare professional works with clients of various cultures (Campinha-Bacote, 2002a).

In this model, one's attitude and willingness are key in becoming more culturally competent. Cultural desire is a beginning point for the other constructs of this model.

Campinha-Bacote (2002b) also developed a self-administered tool for measuring the level of cultural competence of healthcare professionals: the Inventory to Assess the Process of Cultural Competence among Healthcare Professionals (IAPCC). This instrument works best if used to measure effectiveness of cultural competence training that teaches the five constructs developed by Campinha-Bacote. The instrument can be obtained from the Transcultural C.A.R.E. Associates at http://www.transcultural-care.net.

An informal assessment of cultural competency is reflected in the mnemonic "ASKED" (Box 18.2).

Box 18.2 ■ ■ ■

"ASKED"

A wareness: Are you aware of your biases and prejudices toward other cultural groups?

S kill: Do you know how to conduct a cultural assessment?

K nowledge: Are you knowledgeable about the world views of different cultural groups?

E ncounters: Do you seek out face-to-face interactions with individuals who are different from you?

D esire: Do you really "want to" become culturally competent?

Campinha-Bacote (2002)

Answering these questions posed in the mnemonic is a reasonable starting point for school nurses who choose to embark on a journey toward cultural competence.

Box 18.3 ■ ■ ■

THE TWELVE DOMAINS OF CULTURE

1. Overview, inhabited localities, and topography
2. Communication
3. Family roles and organization
4. Workforce issues
5. Biocultural ecology
6. High-risk health behaviors
7. Nutrition
8. Pregnancy and childbearing practices
9. Death rituals
10. Spirituality
11. Healthcare practices
12. Healthcare practitioners

(Purnell & Paulanka, 2003, p. 11)

Purnell's Model for Cultural Competence

Purnell presented another model of cultural competence that focuses on cultural domains as they affect the global society, community, family, and the individual person (Purnell & Paulanka, 2003). The Purnell Model (Box 18.3) displays the cultural domains that are necessary for cultural assessments.

Each of these domains provides a framework by which healthcare professionals can track the thoroughness of their cultural assessments. For example:

- *Inhabited localities and topography* refer to the family's reason for migration, educational status, economic factors, heritage of the "people group," and an overview of the part of the world from which they originate.
- *Communication* involves more than spoken language; nonverbal expressions and preferred greeting approaches are explored with clients.
- *Family roles and organization* require identifying the head of household, gender roles, priorities, and acceptable and forbidden behaviors for children and adolescents.
- *Workforce issues* focus on cultural considerations when working with the specific group in the workplace, as well as issues affected by immigration.
- *Biocultural ecology* deals with skin color, responses to medications, and health conditions more common to the cultural group.
- *High-risk behaviors* identifies common high-risk behaviors in the specific "people group," and explores their healthcare practices.
- *Nutrition* encompasses the foods the members of a cultural group eat and the importance of food and therapeutic nutritional practices of the cultural group.
- *Pregnancy and childbearing practices* include cultural views about pregnancy, as well as acceptable and forbidden behaviors on a continuum from pregnancy to postpartum care.
- *Death rituals* of specific groups identify responses to death and grief and burial practices.
- *Spirituality* identifies the influence of religion, the meaning of life, and the impact of spiritual beliefs on healthcare practices.

- *Healthcare practices* include exploration of the cultural health beliefs, traditions, and responses to health and illness.
- *Healthcare practitioners* includes knowledge of the acceptance of healthcare practitioners in the culture and the interface with other practitioners, for example, folk and religious healers (Purnell & Paulanka, 2003).

IMPLICATIONS FOR SCHOOL NURSES

Conducting cultural assessments of the students and their families provides valuable information for school nurses as they plan for student healthcare needs, especially related to healthcare practices and communication. These practices or special needs should be added to any health plans or parent information cards in the nurse's office. Asking students and their families about aspects of their culture is one way to gain knowledge about them and to communicate respect and acceptance of their practices.

Communication, both verbal and nonverbal, often reflects cultural differences and the need for cultural competence. Awareness of difficulties with English will determine if interpreters are needed to assist with student, family, and school nurse communication. The use of students as primary translators for their families is not recommended because of the possibility of reversing the parental position as well as issues of confidentiality.

Communication helps to build trust between school nurses and families; this trust can become essential in hearing the families' needs and accessing appropriate resources for them. Students and families of various cultures are more likely to perceive the genuineness of the school nurse's desire to provide health care when the nurse incorporates knowledge of the individual and cultural group to which the individual belongs.

Understanding nonverbal communication assists the school nurse in approaching students and families and interpreting the interaction. For example, some individuals from Asian countries avoid direct eye contact with authority figures out of respect (Taylor & Willies-Jacobo, 2003). Another nonverbal communication in which cultural differences may become apparent is touch. In the United States, handshake greetings are common in business settings. However, for devout Muslims and Orthodox Jews, public touching between genders is not generally acceptable (Purnell & Paulanka, 2003). The school nurse who is aware of this can make necessary modifications in this form of greeting in order to show cultural sensitivity to a parent coming into the school for a meeting.

Other implications of cultural practices may be the young student from Vietnam who presents with an unusual bruising. The school nurse needs to ask questions as to whether the mother used a coin-rubbing practice in her attempt to cure the child's cold. The school nurse can also advocate for students who are Moslem, Orthodox Jewish, or Amish whose cultures require them to wear long sleeves and who are then "unable" to change to short tops for gym class. Posters displayed in the school should reflect the cultures represented therein. This is also true for any videos that are used in teaching the students.

It is important to keep in mind that as one learns more about the specific cultures represented in the school, particular students may not fit all the general cultural aspects of their culture. Development of trusting and respectful relationships with the students and their families is a priority. This helps the school nurse to be more effective in the role of student advocate. Learning about the individual is as essential as learning about the cultural group to which the person belongs.

In addition to students and their families, cultural competence in school nursing extends to interactions with the school staff. School staff may also represent various cultural groups. The school nurse can model and promote cultural competence throughout the entire school community.

Increasing one's awareness, knowledge, and skills to provide culturally competent care requires planning. The components of action planning include identifying current cultural issues, planning for the culturally diverse student body, and evaluating the cultural competence of school staff. Cultural competence is a life-long pursuit, and the school nurse can increase awareness, knowledge, and skills through formal and informal methods. Exploring various models of culturally competent care can assist the school nurse in choosing an approach to follow. A haphazard approach to providing culturally competent care may leave gaps in meeting the student's healthcare needs.

SELECTED CULTURAL GROUPS

Additional information regarding selected groups has been included in this chapter. The selected groups are African-Americans, American Indians and Alaskan Natives, Asians and Pacific Islanders, and Hispanic immigrants. These are some of the more common cultures represented in American schools.

African-American

The term African-American refers to a diverse group of people including those whose ancestors originated from the continent of Africa and more recent immigrants from African nations and other areas of the world. In the 2000 U.S. Census, "the South had the largest Black population, as well as the highest proportion of Blacks in its total population" (McKinnon, 2003, p. 2). It is important to distinguish between recent immigrants from Africa and African-Americans whose families have lived in the United States for multiple generations. Recent immigrants from Africa represent numerous cultures, and they maintain many cultural distinctions. African-Americans who have been living in this country for many generations are generally acculturated and assimilated into American culture. Conducting a thorough cultural assessment of individual African-Americans will unveil the nuances of specific cultural distinctions.

Some groups of African-Americans are more relaxed about time; they are less concerned about arriving hours late for an appointment than the fact that they arrived. "Therefore, flexibility in timing appointments may be necessary for African Americans who have a circular sense of time rather than the dominant culture's linear sense of time" (Glanville, 2003, p. 42). Parenting reflects belief in a firm parenting style. Parents expect respect and obedience from their children; when they are old enough, youth are encouraged to work as part of their family responsibility (Glanville, 2003).

Some African-Americans may employ folk healers, faith healers, and alternative medicine practices to manage illnesses. School nurses should attempt to understand their health beliefs and, if appropriate, incorporate them into the child's care. For example, if a child's family believes that prayer will help his asthma, the school nurse's awareness of this information may lead to discussions on how both traditional medicine and the faith of the family can work together to bring the desired results. Respect is a significant value in the African-American culture. This can be demonstrated by addressing adults with their last name and title.

Developing a collaborative relationship with the student and family may aid in gaining accurate information. An example of this is seen when limited funds affect how the child uses medication. For example, if dollars are limited, stretching the longevity of an asthma medication (e.g., by skipping doses when the child appears to be well) may be the way the parent attempts to solve the financial problem rather than using the medication as ordered. The school nurse can assist the family in understanding the chronic nature of asthma and the need for ongoing medication and obtaining financial assistance for prescriptions.

If the school nurse is working with recent immigrants from African nations, remember that each nation has its own culture and sometimes will include multiple cultures. Self-study and asking the student and family to instruct you will add to your knowledge of the nation. In addition, this lets the family know that you care and respect their heritage.

African-Americans experience health disparities in many areas, including an increase in cancer rates, cardiovascular disease, human immunodeficiency virus/acquired immunodeficiency syndrome (HIV/AIDS), and diabetes compared with the white population. They make up the vast majority of those with sickle cell disease. There is a higher rate of poor outcomes with teen pregnancies; "furthermore, the teenage mother is expected to assume primary responsibility for her child" (Glanville, 2003, p. 43). Johnston, O'Malley, and Bachman (2002) reported lower rates of illicit drug use in African-American secondary school students compared to illicit drug use by white secondary school students.

American Indian and Alaska Native

American Indian and Alaska Native refer to "people having origins in any of the original peoples of North or South America (including Central America), and who maintain tribal affiliation or community attachment" (Oqunwole, 2002, p. 2). Many different tribes comprise this group; therefore school nurses will need to learn about specific tribal groups in order to deliver culturally competent care. The United States Bureau of Indian Affairs has information on the tribes on their Web site at http://www.doi.gov/bureau-indian-affairs.html.

Health challenges in the American Indian and Alaska Native cultural groups of children and youth are primarily the result of physical trauma from motor vehicle accidents, drowning, fire, firearms, and suicide; rates for these injuries are two times higher than for other racial and ethnic groups in the United States (Centers for Disease Control and Prevention, 2003). Alcohol use and fetal alcohol syndrome are also more common in American Indian and Alaska native groups.

Discovering the lifeways of the tribal groups can assist the school nurse in developing culturally relevant health services to students, families, and communities. American Indians and Alaskan Natives believe in balancing mind, soul, and body, as well as living in harmony with nature (Still & Hodgins, 2003). School nurses can express awareness of the use of traditional healing for illnesses. In Navajo tribes, children may have the freedom to determine if they will comply with a medication regimen (Still & Hodgins, 2003). Understanding this privilege may assist the school nurse in explaining the purpose and value of the medication regimen, in addition to discussing alternative effective treatments.

Asian and Pacific Islander

This cultural group actually consists of various subgroups, including Japanese, Chinese, Indian, Korean, Philippino, Cambodian, Laotian, Thai, and Vietnamese. Reeves and Bennett define Asian as "people having origins in any of the original peoples of the Far East, Southeast Asia, or the Indian subcontinent" (2003, p. 1). Pacific Islander refers to those with origins in Hawaii, Guam, Samoa, and the Pacific Islands. The Asian population in the United States is a mixture of groups that have been in the United States for generations (e.g., Japanese and Chinese) and those who have arrived in recent decades, in many cases fleeing wars or political unrest in their native lands (e.g., Cambodian and Vietnamese).

As school nurses work with students from Asian groups, specific information about the culture and the history of the particular family's immigration will guide the services accessed for the student. Understanding the reason for migration and immigration, the customs of the land they left, and medical and mental health concerns related to refugee status will assist the school nurse in planning for the care of students (Hoxie, 1999). Gambol and Gambol (2002) provided suggestions on communicating effectively with this population, particularly when the student or family has limited English-speaking skills; they suggested tips for speaking, listening, and asking questions (Box 18.4).

Cambodian

Gambol and Gambol (2002) noted common challenges in children from Southeast Asia whose families have immigrated to the United States. Health challenges include a tendency toward parasitic infections, hepatitis A and B, tuberculosis, as well as symptoms related to stress. Many immigrants from Cambodia experienced torture, malnutrition, and poverty, causing deep physical, spiritual, and psychological wounds (Tellep, Chim, Murphy, & Cureton, 2001). Some refugee children suffered brain damage and small stature resulting from prolonged malnutrition (Tellep et al., 2001). Post-

Box 18.4 ■■■

TIPS FOR IMPROVING COMMUNICATION WITH IMMIGRANT CHILDREN

When speaking:

- Speak at a slow pace; show objects, draw pictures, and act out meanings.
- Simplify messages and focus the student's attention.
- Use short, simple sentence structures (subject-verb-object).
- Choose your words carefully. Use common words and names rather than pronouns.
- Pause after phrases and sentences; the child will need time to attach meaning to message.
- Do not talk louder than necessary; it sounds angry and does not increase comprehension.
- Repeat cheerfully; use the same simple words, sentence structures, and gestures.

When listening:

- Demonstrate support for attempts to communicate. Give feedback, nods, encouragement, and praise.
- Give the child your complete attention and put forth your best effort at attempting to understand communication. Demonstrate your patience through body language.
- Offer several interpretations to check meaning of communication.
- Encourage children to draw or act out meaning if communication fails.
- If someone is translating for the child, speak directly to the child.
- Correction of errors will cause anxiety and diminish efforts to speak. Give indirect rather than direct correction. The child says, "My mom sick. He no eat." Respond with, "Oh, your mom is sick. She is not eating. Tell your mom to drink lots of water." Pantomime drinking water as you speak.

(Continued on the following page)

Box 18.4 ■■■

TIPS FOR IMPROVING COMMUNICATION WITH IMMIGRANT CHILDREN *(Continued)*

Tailor oral questions:

- Ask children to point to items, words, or locations.
- Ask simple questions that can be answered with yes or no. Instead of asking, "Where does it hurt?" try "Does your stomach hurt?" while pointing to the child's stomach or "Does your head hurt?" while pointing to the head.
- Ask questions that may be answered in a single word or phrase; embed the answer in an either–or question. This way, the child only needs to identify the answer rather than recall it. "Did you throw up [pantomime throwing up] last night [pantomime sleeping] or did you throw up [pantomime again] this morning?" [pantomime waking]
- Accept one-word responses; supply the complete sentence in your acknowledgment. You ask, "What should you do if you feel sick?" The student responds, "Water." You acknowledge "Yes. Very good. You need to drink lots of water."
- Break complex sentences into components. Instead of asking, "Did you ever have tuberculosis when you lived in Vietnam?" Try, "When you were little [point to child and put hand out to express height of the younger child] did you have a bad cough? [Pantomime bad coughing]?" "Did you live in Vietnam [point to map] when you had a bad cough [pantomime again]?"
- Allow plenty of wait time. A child learning English as a second language may understand your question but will need extra thinking time (at least 15-20 seconds) to frame his or her answer verbally.

(Gambol & Gambol, 2002)

traumatic stress disorder, anxiety, and depression are common in this population (Tellep et al., 2001).

Tellep et al. (2001) studied the responses of school nurses and Cambodian liaisons as they worked together to provide healthcare services to children of Cambodian refugees. School nurses appreciated the multifaceted roles of the Cambodian liaisons in their cross-cultural teams. Some recommendations for nursing practice included, "individualize care based on family's background and refugee history, suspend assumptions and worldview, look beyond the behavior to understand the underlying dynamic, incorporate spiritual healing practices and the temple into delivery of health services, and provide support to parents and elders" (Tellep et al., 2001, p. 272).

Hispanic/Latino

The term Hispanic refers to an ethnic entity that is composed of multiple subgroups, the largest being Mexican-Americans, Puerto Ricans, and Cubans (USDOE, 2003). The word "Latino" can be used synonymously with Hispanic; there are regional and individual preferences in the use of these terms. When the school nurse encounters one of the subgroups of Hispanics, the specific cultural ways of that student and family cannot be generalized from one group to another. Two thirds of Hispanics currently residing in the United States were born in the United States; Hispanic children and adolescents younger than 18 years of age represent 16% of the total population (USDOE, 2003).

The health of Hispanic children is affected by the lack of health insurance; in 2000, 25% of Hispanic children and adolescents younger than 18 years of age did not have health insurance (USDOE, 2003). Some of the reasons for the lack of health insurance are inadequate finances, limited knowledge of available services, and the undocumented status of immigrant parents.

The level of acculturation in Hispanic populations depends on the history of immigration, socioeconomic status, and the family's longevity in America. The Hispanic worldview generally includes a sense of fatalism or resignation that emerges from religious beliefs that there is little one can do about "fate" (Lassetter & Baldwin, 2004). They live for today and often are not concerned about "tomorrow." This may result in an apparent lack of concern related to the need for immunizations. In their view, sickness and pain may be God's will for them, and therefore need to be endured (Zoucha & Purnell, 2003).

Respect and formality characterize communication, both verbal and nonverbal. Direct eye contact and direct confrontation are not encouraged. Children are cherished and elders are respected. The father or oldest male maintains decision-making authority. Women can be both idealized and oppressed. The school nurse's awareness of gender roles in the culture can help foster understanding with a mother of a student who says she cannot make a decision regarding the nurse's request until she speaks with her husband.

Health beliefs of some Hispanics include the use of folk healers (*curanderos*) to achieve good health. Illness results from an imbalance between the person and the environment (Zoucha & Purnell, 2003). School nurses who want to provide culturally competent care must learn about the Hispanic concepts of health and illness. For example, *mal de ojo*, or evil eye, is the belief that someone with strong eyes who looks at a child could cause illness; a cure is sometimes a seed-like charm the child wears (Taylor & Willies-Jacobo, 2003).

Mexican Immigrants

Cowell, McNaughton, and Ailey (2000) developed a Mexican-American problem-solving (MAPS) school nursing intervention designed to advance the mental health, family functioning, children's health conceptions, and self-esteem of immigrants (mothers and children). While conducting focus groups, Mexican mothers shared some of the stresses that accompanied their relocation from Mexico, for example, the higher cost of living that forced mothers into the workplace, differences in child discipline, increased availability of drugs and alcohol, and domestic violence (Cowell et al., 2000). An interesting finding was the preference of the mothers for home visits rather than group activities. There was also an increased incidence of depression in mothers and their children (Cowell et al., 2000). "Affective support, health information, and decisional control...were successful strategies" for school nurses working with these mothers and children (Cowell et al., 2000, p. 38).

SUBCULTURES WITHIN STUDENT GROUPS

Childhood has a culture that is specific to the age group. However, within the student body, there are subcultures about which the school nurse should be informed. These may be smaller student groups who are like-minded or share a common problem. Leininger and McFarland (2002) define subculture as "closely related to culture, but refers to subgroups who deviate in certain ways from a dominant culture in values, beliefs, norms, moral codes, and ways of living with some distinctive features that characterize their unique lifeways" (p. 47). These subculture groups are rarely hidden.

With inclusion guiding the composition of schools, many students who may have been educated in a special school are now in the comprehensive schools. For example, if more than two or three students in the school are deaf, they are potentially a subculture; the larger deaf community certainly sees themselves as having a separate culture. Athletes in specific sport groupings, for example, soccer players, football team, and cheerleaders, are another subculture. Students who excel in computer work, musicians, teen parents, teens who are gay and lesbian, gothic-interested students, gangs, and other groups may be seen as a subculture. These subcultures do, in fact, have a culture in which they function. Getting to know the life ways of the groups provides school nurses with valuable information for collaborating with the student on health issues. Culturally respectful health services emerge when the school nurse moves toward cultural competence.

If the subcultures promote destructive behaviors, knowledge about their ways and genuine caring for that group may promote trusting relationships between the school nurse and group members. From the platform of a trusting relationship, school nurses may have the opportunity to promote healthy behaviors and redirect their energies.

In some situations, subcultures may have unique health concerns, for example, gay and lesbian students and students with chronic conditions. Acknowledgment of subcultures is a first step in learning about them in order to deliver culturally competent care.

Barriers are attributable to lack of knowledge, misinterpretation of cues to affect, or a clash between value systems. Silence and the word "yes" can lead to numerous misunderstandings. Neither necessarily signifies agreement. Silence can mean I do not agree, but I am too polite to disagree with authority. "Yes" can mean I am listening but I do not agree. "Yes" can mean I do not understand what you are telling me but I am going to respect your authority (Gropper, 1996). For example, a recent immigrant student may have learned that being respectful to an adult means saying *yes* even when you neither understand nor agree with what has been spoken to you.

CONCLUSION

North American cultural values and non-Western cultures tend to clash. Every culture tends to assume that other people's cultures are more similar to their own than is actually true. A lack of awareness of some aspects of our own cultures exists, so that many basic assumptions are not questioned. For example, many middle-class Americans believe in self-actualization. This is not the case for many cultures. Direct verbal communication is highly esteemed in American culture but is a sign of rudeness in many other cultures, where people rely heavily on multichannel systems in which body posture and indirect phrasing have primacy over words.

The school nurse is in an ideal position to assess for cultural beliefs and practices and to incorporate these into any health-centered encounters. It is important to be aware that not all persons show respect, handle time and space, interpret behaviors and gestures, or prioritize values in the same way. One way that school nurses can develop skills in cultural awareness and competency is to identify students of different cultures and backgrounds. By utilizing the cultural frameworks and theoretical models, nurses can analyze the meaning behind the behavior. Health education and health promotion interventions can be created that will respect the values and cultural nuances of each cultural group. Practical interventions will be the result of understanding the differences.

School nurses need creativity, caring, and clinical competence in order to grow in cultural competence. The journey begins with the first step. Self-assessments and cultural assessments are available to enable the school nurse in this pursuit. "Cultural competence means nurses modify and adapt their care to meet the cultural needs of each client, but modifications alone may not be sufficient if that care is not documented and communicated to clients and other providers" (Clark et al., 2000, p. 203). Box 18.5 contains a self-assessment that school nurses can complete.

School nurses are role models to staff and students. As school nurses grow in cultural competence, school staff and students may be open to examining their cultural ways and learning about other cultures. Cross-cultural teams are ideal because they reflect cultural competence in supporting student success.

Remember that cultural competency is a process, not a static state. The process begins with a self-assessment, knowing one's cultural viewpoint. Begin and enjoy the journey.

Box 18.5 ■■■

CULTURAL DIVERSITY TEST

QUESTIONS FOR COMMUNICATION AND CULTURAL DIVERSITY	ANSWERS
1. Native language explanations and understandings can be more accurate.	
2. All cultures favor directness in communication.	
3. Demonstration of emotion is culturally influenced.	
4. All gestures mean the same thing in all cultures.	
5. Discussing personal matters outside the family is seen as embarrassing by many cultures	
6. It's generally best to be reserved and formal initially.	
7. Making a human-to-human connection and building rapport is an essential first step in relationship building.	
QUESTIONS FOR CULTURALLY COMPETENT CARE	
1. It is not necessary to involve understanding & respect of the patient's cultural values, beliefs, and practices.	
2. Factors that may differ from patient to patient include ethnic, religious, and occupational factors.	
3. Pay no attention to body language, facial expressions, and other behavioral cues.	
4. Smiles and laughter may indicate discomfort or embarrassment.	

QUESTIONS FOR COMMUNICATION AND CULTURAL DIVERSITY	ANSWERS
5. Avoid making judgments about the patient's beliefs and practices.	
6. In the Middle East, it is normal for people to stand close enough to feel each other's breath on their faces.	
7. A handshake is generally accepted as a standard greeting in business, yet the kind of handshake differs.	
8. It is not important to consider religious rules when dealing with patients.	
9. Do not assume that a particular patient fits the general cultural descriptions of his or her culture.	
10. Spend time cultivating relationships by getting to know patients & co-workers and by establishing comfort before jumping into the task at hand.	

ANSWERS TO CULTURAL DIVERSITY TEST

Communication and Cultural Diversity	Culturally Competent Care
1. True	1. False
2. False	2. True
3. True	3. False
4. False	4. True
5. True	5. True
6. True	6. True
7. True	7. True
	8. False
	9. True
	10. True

(Courtesy: http://www.HospitalSoup.com. All About Hospitals, Medical Jobs, & Healthcare. http://www.hospitalsoup.com/cultural_competency/culturaldiversity.asp.)

Resources

Diversity Rx is sponsored by The National Conference of State Legislatures, Resources for Cross Cultural Health Care, and Henry J. Kaiser Family Foundation Web site:
http://www.diversityRx.org

National Center for Cultural Competence. Georgetown University Center for Child and Human Development (also known as Georgetown University Child Development Center)
3307 M Street, NW, Suite 401, Washington, DC 20007-3935
Tel: 800/788-2066 or 202/687-5387
Fax: 202/687-8899
cultural@georgetown.edu
http://www.georgetown.edu/research/gucdc/nccc/index/html.

National Center for Cultural Healing
http://www.culturalhealing

Office of Minority Health
http://www.cdc.gov/omh

Office of Minority and Women's Health
http://www.cdc.gov/hcidod/omwh

School Health*Culture Zone.
http://courses.international.edu/bc680/nmcgahn

Transcultural C.A.R.E. Associates
http://www.transculturalcare.net/trancultural_care_home_page.htm

The Transcultural Nursing Society.
http://www.tcns.org

Transcultural Nursing. Assessment and bookstore available.
http://www.culturediversity.org

References

American Nurses Association (ANA). (1991). *Position Statement: Cultural diversity in nursing practice.* Council on Cultural Diversity in Nursing Practice, Congress of Nursing Practice. Washington, DC: ANA.

Campinha-Bacote, J. (1999). A model and instrument for addressing cultural competence in healthcare. *Journal of Nursing Education, 38*(5), 203–207.

Campinha-Bacote, J. (2002a). The process of cultural competence in the delivery of healthcare services: A culturally competent model of care. *Journal of Transcultural Nursing, 13*(3), 181–184.

Campinha-Bacote, J. (2002b). *The process of cultural competence in the delivery of healthcare services: A culturally competent model of care*. Retrieved December 31, 2002 from http://www.transculturalcare.net

Centers for Disease Control and Prevention (CDC). (2003). Injury mortality among American Indian and Alaska Native children and youth—United States 1989–1998. *MMWR, 52*, 697–701.

Clark, L., Zuk, J., & Baramee, J. (2000). A literary approach to teaching cultural competence. *Journal of Transcultural Nursing, 11*(3), 199–203.

Cowell, J. M., McNaughton, D. B., & Ailey, S. (2000). Development and evaluation of a Mexican immigrant family support program. *Journal of School Nursing, 16*(5), 32–39.

Davidhizer, R., Havens, R., & Bechtel, G. (1999) Assessing culturally diverse pediatric clients. *Pediatric Nursing, 25*(4), 371–376.

Gambol, P., & Gambol, M. (2002). Vulnerability in the Asian or Pacific Islander immigrant child. *Journal of School Nursing, 18*(6), 314–321.

Giger, J., & Davidhizar, R. (2002). The Giger and Davidhizar transcultural assessment model. *Journal of Transcultural Nursing, 13*(3), 185–188.

Giger, J., & Davidhizar, R. (2004). *Transcultural nursing: Assessment and intervention*. St. Louis: C. V. Mosby.

Glanville, C. (2003). People of African American Heritage. In L. Purnell and B. Paulanka (Eds.), *Transcultural health care* (pp. 40–53). Philadelphia: F. A. Davis.

Gropper, R. C. (1996). *Culture and the clinical encounter*. Yarmouth, ME: Intercultural Press.

Hoxie, A. (1999). Immigrant and refugee students: Legal, health, and cultural considerations. In M. Arnold & C. Silkworth (Eds.), *The school nurse's source book of individualized healthcare plans: Issues and applications in school nursing practice* (pp. 89–105). North Branch, MN: Sunrise River Press.

Huff, R. M., & Kline, M. V. (1999). *Promoting health in multicultural populations: A* handbook for practitioners. Thousand Oaks, CA: Sage Publications.

Institute of Medicine. (2002). *Unequal treatment: What healthcare providers need to know about racial and ethnic disparities in healthcare*. Washington, DC: National Academy Press.

Johnston, L., O'Malley, P. M., & Bachman, J. G. (2002). *Monitoring the future national results on adolescent drug use: Overview of key findings 2001*. (NIH Publication No. 02-5105). Bethesda, MD: National Institute on Drug Abuse.

Jones, M. E., Kubelka, S., & Bond, M. L. (2001). Acculturaltion status, birth outcomes, and family planning compliance among Hispanic teens. *Journal of School Nursing, 17*(2), 83–89.

Lassetter, J., & Baldwin, J. (2004). Health care barriers for Latino children and provision of culturally competent care. *Journal of Pediatric Nursing, 19*(3), 184–192.

Leininger, M., & McFarland, M. R. (2002). *Transcultural nursing: Concepts, theories, research, and practice* (3rd ed.). New York: McGraw-Hill.

Leininger, M. M. (1999). Response to the commentaries on defining transcultural nursing. *Journal of Transcultural Nursing, 10*(3), 187.

Lipson, J. (1996). Culturally competent nursing care. In J. Lipson, S. Dibble, & P. Minarik. *Culture and nursing care: A pocket guide*. San Francisco: UCSF Nursing Press.

McKinnon, J. (2003). *The black population in the United States: March 2002*. Current Population Reports. U.S. Census Bureau. Washington, DC: U.S. Department of Commerce.

National Association of School Nurses (NASN) & American Nurses Association ANA). (2001) *Scope and standards of professional school nursing practice*. Washington, DC: American Nurses Publishing.

National Council for Accreditation of Teacher Education (2002). *Professional standards for the accreditation of schools, colleges, and departments of education*. Washington, DC: Author.

New hampshire department of health and human services (2002). *Diversity plan: cultural competency—"a way of life."* New Hampshire: author.

Ogunwole, S. (2002). *The American Indian and Alaska Native population*. U.S. Census Bureau. Washington, DC: U.S. Department of Commerce.

Purnell, L. D., & Paulanka, B. J. (2003). *Transcultural health care: A culturally competent approach* (2nd ed.). Philadelphia: F. A. Davis.

Reeves, T., & Bennett, C. (2003). *The Asian and Pacific Islander population in the United States: March 2002*. Current Population Reports. U.S. Census Bureau. Washington, DC: U.S. Department of Commerce.

Spector, R. (2004). *Cultural diversity in health and illness*. Stamford, CT: Appleton & Lange.

Spratley, E., Johnson, A., Sochalski, J., Fritz, M., & Spencer, W. (2000). *The registered nurse population: Findings from the national sample survey of registered nurses*. Washington, DC: U.S. Department of Health and Human Services, Health Resource and Service Administration, Bureau of Health Professions.

Still, O., & Hodgins, D. (2003). Navajo Indians. In L. Purnell & B. Paulanka (Eds.), *Transcultural health care* (pp. 279–293). Philadelphia: F. A. Davis.

Taylor, L., & Willies-Jacobo, L. (2003). The culturally competent pediatrician: Respecting ethnicity in your practice. *Contemporary Pediatrics, 20*(6), 83–105.

Tellep, T. L., Chim, M., Murphy, S., & Cureton, V. Y. (2001). Great suffering, great compassion: A transcultural opportunity for school nurses caring for Cambodian refugee children. *Journal of Transcultural Care, 12*(4), 261–274.

U.S. Department of Commerce (USDC), Bureau of the Census. (2001). *School enrollment in the United States: Social and economic characteristics of students*. Washington, DC: Author.

U.S. Department of Education (USDOE), National Center for Education Statistics (2003). *Status and trends in the education of Hispanics* (NCES 2003-008).Washington, DC: 2003.

U.S. Department of Health and Human Services (USDHHS). (2000). *Healthy People 2010: Understanding and improving health* (2nd ed.). Washington, DC: U.S. Government Printing Office.

U.S. Department of Health and Human Services (USDHHS), Office of Minority Health (2001). *National standards for culturally and linguistically appropriate services in health care*. Rockville, MD: IQ Solutions, Inc.

Zoucha, R., & Purnell, L. (2003). People of Mexican Heritage. In L. Purnell & B. Paulanka (Eds.)., *Transcultural health care* (pp. 264–278). Phildelphia: F. A. Davis.

Chapter 19

Collaboration with the Community

RUTH ELLEN LUEHR ▪ JANICE SELEKMAN

Chapter Outline

INTRODUCTION: INVOLVEMENT WITH THE COMMUNITY

The school is a community within a community; in addition, the community is within the school. Caring for children and youth in schools can be successful only when considered from the context of the community from which the students come and in which the school is located. Understanding the social context of students recognizes the importance of family, peers, community, and the school as influences that support development and social and educational achievement. This chapter is designed to describe the role of the school nurse as a collaborator with the community in promoting the health of children and youth in schools.

Because school attendance is a nearly universal experience, every parent, community service provider, business person, and resident often feel he or she can speak with some authority on what schools could or should be like. Everyone has an opinion about what needs improvement, how it "used to be," and a story about his or her best or worst school experience. And everyone takes pride in and ownership of the local school when things go well.

According to the U.S. Centers for Disease Control and Prevention (CDC), from 20% to 75% of a community have links to the schools (Bogden, 2003). They may have children or grandchildren in the schools, they may live near or have businesses near the school property, they may be employed by or provide services to the school, or they may pay taxes that keep the schools running. Schools may provide services to the community through evening programs related to parenting young children or adolescents, or classes in tax preparation, quilting, computer literacy, and recreation programs.

In the Community Schools Movement, the school is the very hub of the community, offering everything for families from primary health care, dental services, and mental health services to social services for job training and placement, English literacy classes, housing assistance, and emergency food and clothing (Dryfoos & Magure, 2002). In other cases, the school is a distinctly separate entity from the community, where the school day program makes little effort to involve parents, has few links to community resources, or few or no programs or services available to community members.

Sometimes community members/parents want a high level of control over what is taught, not only to their own children but also to everyone else's children. Examples include what textbooks or library books are recommended and available. Others want to be informed when sensitive content is taught so that they have the option of withdrawing their children from those classes. State government also makes mandates, initiated by both the schools and the community at large, regarding school curricula and content that must be taught, such as information on human immunodeficiency virus (HIV), screenings and assessments to be conducted and services to be provided, including the extent of nursing services in school (with the hope that they mandate for a school nurse in every building).

Schools want to be known as a safe place in the community for students to learn and play. Many have special protections, such as being labeled "drug-free zones," where the penalties for drug use are higher than for other areas of the community; many school zones also have reduced speed limits for drivers.

Given these examples where the school is greatly influenced by the community and vice versa, it is clear that the role of the school nurse goes beyond the boundaries of the school property to meet the health-related needs of the students and their families. Collaboration with the community incorporates the African proverb of "It takes a village to raise a child."

WHO MAKES UP THE COMMUNITY?

The community in which a school resides is a microcosm of society. It is usually part of a school district directed by the state education agency, usually the Department of Education. Therefore, school boards and governmental agencies determine the policies and resources available to a school.

Integral to the school nurse's role is the medical community, including healthcare providers, clinics, available health-related services, and allied health providers, including emergency medical response agencies. In addition, there are the state and federal programs that fund these programs and services, including Medicaid and third-party insurance companies.

The community thrives on its businesses and industry. Equally important are the social components to any community. These may include special interest groups, service organizations, such as Kiwanis or Lions Clubs, and religious organizations. Police and fire resources are essential to the security of a community. Youth organizations, such as scouts, Girl's Clubs, Police Athletic Leagues, and Little League, provide for additional growth experiences beyond school hours. The availability of higher education in a community not only provides for the possibility of a concrete goal following graduation, but also may be a resource for collaboration and provide opportunities for mentoring. The media in the community, whether by radio, newspaper, television, or billboards, can assist schools in transmitting messages. In addition to these, there is a retired population with a wealth of experiences whose services are rarely tapped. All of these are ripe for collaboration with the school, especially related to its mission of supporting the health of students, staff, and family members.

COLLABORATION: THE CONCEPT

Collaboration is the process of working together to achieve common goals that cannot be reached as efficiently by individuals or agencies acting singly. Considering the wide range of numbers of students and staff for whom school nurses are responsible, it is imperative that school nurses work with others, especially when they share common goals related to student health and education. Many public and private healthcare providers and service agencies dedicated to health in the community have analogous goals, and collaboration may be more cost efficient and result in more efficient use of manpower. Having multiple groups working together may make the limited services in a community more accessible and more acceptable.

Building collaborative partnerships takes time, commitment, and good communication. These partnerships can improve the efficiency in and effectiveness of services, pool resources when budgets are tight, and allow for sharing of strategies to improve professional practice and services to students. Sometimes, working together in an interdisciplinary team is required. Collaboration is often required in order to qualify for large research or service grants from private and public funding agencies; oversight agencies mandate collaborative partnerships to increase accountability and reduce duplication of services.

Collaboration occurs on several levels. It starts with *communication*, during which the players come to the table and talk, listen, and network. Astute listening skills are key. Individuals with common interests decide how to share resources and ideas and to benefit from being together. The second level is *cooperation*, in which people and agencies share work but have their own identities. An example would be two groups sharing a workshop day, announcing it on one brochure but with a separate time slot for each group's presentation.

The third level is *coordination*, in which the focus is on doing tasks together with each partner remaining distinct yet enhanced by the relationship. In *collaboration*, the final level, work is integrated and the specific contributions of individual agencies are not identified. Although each contributes unique resources, the resources cannot function without those of the partner agency. This process does not require an equal distribution of resources or responsibilities. Some partners may contribute more personnel time or in-kind services (space, transportation, food, printing, contacting staff, or parents), while others provide their expertise.

Collaborating is an essential aspect of school nursing practice and is specified in the Scope and Standards of School Nursing Practice (NASN & ANA, 2001) as Standard VI, which focuses on collaboration. It states, "The school nurse collaborates with the student, family, school staff, community, and other providers in providing student care" (p. 21). The measurement criteria are shown in TABLE 19.1.

The measurement criteria for collaboration are the minimum expectations that the public can expect when accessing school nursing services. This means that the school nurse is expected to consider the need for, the resources to, and the partners in collaboration when providing care to students. In terms of the nursing process, collaboration is often necessary when assessing students or the school community. For example, the decision to screen adolescents for depression or suicide risk may require support from parents and awareness and support from school faculty; data gathering or analysis assistance may come from community mental health agencies, school counselors, or school psychologists; and agreement on criteria for assessment and referral may come from public and private providers. Following through with the steps of the nursing process and planning with each of these groups will be needed to determine appropriate and congruent interventions for students by the family, school, and community. Without collaboration, the school nurse would not be able to adequately meet the mental health needs of these students and find the needed supports for them in the community.

Table 19.1 ■

MEASUREMENT CRITERIA FOR STANDARD VI. COLLABORATION

1. The school nurse communicates verbally and in writing with the student, family, school staff, community, and other providers regarding client care and nursing's role in the provision of care.
2. The school nurse collaborates with the student, family, school staff, community, and other providers in the formulation of overall goals, time lines, the plan of care, and decisions related to care and the delivery of services.
3. The school nurse assists individual students in developing appropriate skills to advocate for themselves based on age and developmental level.
4. The school nurse consults with and utilizes the expertise of other providers for client care, as needed.
5. The school nurse makes referrals, including provisions for continuity of care, as needed.

Source: National Association of School Nurses & American Nurses Association (2001, p. 21).

The National Parent–Teachers Association (2004) also recognizes the importance of collaborating with the community. They have a national standard that states "Community resources are used to strengthen schools, families, and student learning" (National PTA, 2004). Their rationale for this standard is shown in BOX 19.1.

Many who engage in collaborative partnerships find them worthwhile and rewarding. They provide a source of affiliation (feeling included in another aspect of the community), collegiality with others interested in the same mission, and a sense of working together so that the responsibility is shared and thus, more can be accomplished. Kaye's (2001) six R's of participation (TABLE 19.2) echo these benefits and can serve as a useful guide when participating in collaborative efforts.

Box 19.1 ■■■

NATIONAL PTA STANDARD VI

When schools and communities work together, both are strengthened in synergistic ways and make gains that outpace what either entity could accomplish on its own:

- Families access community resources more easily.
- Businesses connect education programs with the realities of the workplace.
- Seniors contribute wisdom and gain a greater sense of purpose; and ultimately,
- Students serve and learn beyond their school involvement.

(National Standards: VI. Collaborating with the Community, National PTA, 2004. http://www.pta.org)

Working in integrated partnerships takes time, growing pains, a history of testing out working styles, the establishment of trust among its members (people and organizations), and gained confidence of the community. The inevitable push–pull of power struggles, unpredictable short-term funding streams, unavailable broadly focused long-term funding streams, and the dynamics of a changing school and community are factors that cause partnerships to transition among the four levels (communicate, cooperate, coordinate, and collaborate) for given sub-projects and over time (Benson, Roehlkepartain, & Sesma, 2004).

Table 19.2 ■

SIX R'S OF PARTICIPATION

Members:

1. Need to be *Recognized* publicly for their coalition efforts.
2. Must have clear expectations of the *Role* or roles they play in the coalition.
3. Should be *Respected* for the diversity they represent according to their culture, ethnicity, race, and educational level (as examples).
4. Should be *Rewarded* for their contributions.
5. Should develop meaningful *Relationships* with other members and leaders.
6. Should expect that their efforts will lead to measurable *Results*.

Source: Kaye (2001).

LINKING HEALTH AND LEARNING: A FRAMEWORK FOR COMMUNITY OUTREACH

A connection has consistently been made between health and learning. For students to grow, develop, and be successful academically, they must be ready to learn and be present and participating in their optimal state of health. The school nurse plays an important role in ensuring that students are healthy and ready to learn. Learning includes synthesizing knowledge; acquiring and refining intellectual, interactive, and physical skills; and making sense of social interactions and the environment. The characteristics that are essential for learning are that the student is (1) ready to learn, (2) willing and able, and (3) present and participating. The following questions can be asked by the school nurse; all have implications for nursing interventions.

1. *Ready to learn.* Are the students' basic needs met: sleep/rest, nutrition, having clothes to wear? Are students free of physical or mental health problems and sensory limitations (e.g., vision or hearing problems)? Are students free of chemical substances?
2. *Willing and able.* Are students motivated and engaged? Do they value learning and value school? Do students have the ability or capacity to learn? Are they free from interference, such as interruptions (e.g., seizures), distractions (e.g., attention-deficit/hyperactivity disorder [ADHD]), or being disturbed (e.g., stressed, worried or anxious about peers or family members)?
3. *Present and participating.* Are students attending school and classes regularly? When students are out of class seeking assistance for any reason, do they return promptly and re-focus on learning? Are students paying attention, meaningfully involved, and contributing? (Adelman & Taylor, 2003; Costante, 2002).

A student's readiness and ability to learn is affected by *academic achievement/school success, health/social behaviors*, and *school connectedness*. Their impact extends beyond the school setting. Academic success is reflected in good grades, recognition for effort and improvement, and a sense of contributing. These result in pride in one's work. The more successful a student is in school, the more he or she will like school, have better attendance, and feel like he or she belongs. The more educated a person is, the less likely he or she is to engage in health risk behaviors. The converse also holds: If a student feels like a failure at school, he or she is more likely to engage in health risk behaviors and the more likely his or her attendance suffers; their school connectedness declines. While the school nurse is not directly responsible for academic achievement, he or she can certainly identify students whose self-esteem is low and who need external measures of recognition (Luehr, 2004).

Health and social issues are clearly within the domain of school nursing practice. The CDC identified six risk behaviors in children and adolescents that lead to the highest morbidity and mortality in adults: poor nutrition; sedentary lifestyle; tobacco use; alcohol and other drug use; early and unprotected sexual activity (leading to HIV/sexually transmitted infections (STIs), unintended pregnancy), and internal and external injury. Although the behaviors are manifest in adulthood, the foundation for these behaviors occurs during the school years and should be addressed by the school nurse. These behaviors contribute to the adult health problems of heart disease, cancer, infectious diseases, and injury. In addition, social problems, such as violence and other antisocial behaviors, directly affect student learning—from limiting attendance, to reducing attention and feeling invested in school, to interfering with planning and having dreams for the future. These variables are so interconnected that one researcher said, "The number one goal of public health should be to assist schools and parents in getting youth to graduate from high school. The higher the level of education, the lower the health risk factors" (Kahn, 2000).

Research links school connectedness to increased graduation rates, decreased violence, and decreased substance abuse (McNeely, Nonnemaker, & Blum, 2002; MDE, 2003). Students who have a sense of attachment to their school are more likely to be motivated learners. How the school climate is perceived by students affects their success in school. Do adults care about them? Do teachers invite their ideas and participation? Are classrooms well managed and students given clear directions? These factors are also reflected in whether students feel welcomed in the health office, whether they are recognized by name, afforded privacy, and treated with respect when seeking health care.

The school nurse can identify multiple collaborative partners to support these positive factors to promote health and thus success in learning. The three primary areas for support are the school learning environment, the family/parents, and the community. The school learning environment can contribute to students' basic safety and learning needs when the following three characteristics are present in the school environment: safe and caring, academically stimulating, and adaptable to student learning styles and inclusive. The school nurse can assess these characteristics by asking the following questions:

1. *Safe and caring*: Is the school an emotionally safe and physically safe place to be for the student, staff, and parents? Is conflict addressed—first among staff, between staff and students, among students, and between staff and parents? Do students have access to the basics—things that relate to basic human dignity such as hot water/soap in bathrooms; clean and attractive space, not crowded so there is enough space to "breathe," good air quality, good food choices, physical activity, and time between classes? Do the students count? Are they acknowledged, recognized, and known? At a minimum, are there smiles and eye contact from adults in hallways? Are students respected? Is there a response plan in place that assures management of crises and protection from harm?
2. *Academically stimulating*: Does the school place a high value on learning? Is learning celebrated and has as high a priority as other school functions (such as discipline and athletics). Are the studies meaningful and relevant? Are students' work and accomplishments displayed, honored, and celebrated?
3. *Adaptable to student learning styles, responsive, and inclusive*. Is a positive, stimulating, flexible yet predictable learning environment established and sustained? Do students consistently feel connected and involved and therefore committed (Luehr, 2004)?

The figure of the climate continuum (Box 19.2) illustrates what can happen when the learning environment is positive versus when it is negative. The school nurse is in a unique position to assess the impact of the learning environment when students present with various health concerns.

Supports by the family take into account the value that parents, siblings, and other family members have related to learning and how they express that value. Do they regularly read to their children, ask about specific learning activities, check

Box 19.2 ■■■

CLIMATE CONTINUUM

Intimidation *Isolation/Rejection* *Opportunities/Support* *School Success/Productivity* *Personal/Social Self-Determination*

ASHA, Jan/Feb 2003.

homework, communicate with teachers, and attend special events? Are parents involved in their own learning (modeling lifelong learning)? Are parents able to separate their own experiences and needs from those of their children?

Supports by the community also reflect the value that is placed on education. Are community members involved in student learning by volunteering, providing funds, or providing program materials and staff? Does law enforcement attend to "minor" problems such as truancy and tobacco or alcohol use? Do merchants and service providers invest in education by posting notices of school academic as well as drama, music, and athletic activities? Do they support the academic and health components of the school program? Do they post signs saying youth are welcome in their establishment after school hours? Does the community provide recognition to teachers and other school staff (Luehr, 2004)?

The Education and Development Center (2003) has compiled a list of action steps and rationales to promote family and community involvement in school health (Table 19.3). School nurses should examine each of these steps to determine what can be done in their schools to promote this involvement.

The Comprehensive Prevention Model for Schools

Recognizing the importance of having a supportive environment in order to build the linkages between health and learning, the school nurse can use the *Comprehensive Prevention Model for Schools* from Minnesota (Minnesota Department of Education) (Box 19.3) to build partnerships and to explain to other school staff the value of collaboration in preventing health and learning problems before they interfere with the student's ability to be successful. There are four components of the model: policy and procedures, curriculum and instruction, student services, and parent and family involvement. All

Table 19.3 ■

COMMUNITY INVESTS IN EDUCATION

ACTION STEPS FOR IMPLEMENTING FAMILY AND COMMUNITY INVOLVEMENT IN SCHOOL HEALTH
With the enactment of the No Child Left Behind legislation, family and community partnerships with schools have become central. • Supportive families and social support within communities contribute to students' success. • When children feel valued they are more likely to develop healthy skills, avoid risky behaviors and remain in school. • When parents are involved, students achieve more, regardless of socioeconomic status, ethnic/racial background, or the parents' education level. • The more extensive the parent involvement, the higher the student achievement. • Negative student behaviors, such as alcohol and substance abuse, violence, and antisocial behavior decrease as parent involvement increases. • Students are less likely to succeed when communities are economically deprived, disorganized, and lack opportunities for employment or youth involvement; when families do not set clear expectations, monitor children's behavior, or model appropriate behaviors; and when schools present a negative climate and do not involve students and their families.

Source: EDC, Health is Academic - Action Steps (2003).

Box 19.3 ■■■

COMPREHENSIVE PREVENTION MODEL FOR SCHOOLS

COMPONENTS		ENGAGE SCHOOL AND COMMUNITY PARTNERS	ASSESS. PLAN AND IMPLEMENT	PROVIDE STAFF DEVELOPMENT	EVALUATE
Policy and Procedures	Youth Involvement and Advocacy				
Curriculum and Instruction					
Student Services					
Family and Parent Involvement					

Minnesota Department of Education, 2004

rely on community involvement. The value of this model is that it can guide the school nurse working with the school health team to include the coordinated strategies in order to have a well supported, organized, and meaningful program with measurable outcomes.

Policies and procedures are the standards of behavior set by the school. In families, youth groups, and many community programs these "policies" are known as rules or behavior expectations. A goal is a consistent approach that clearly articulates rules, reinforces positive behavior, and has meaningful sanctions for illegal and harmful behavior. School policies and procedures related to health promotion and the learning environment need to be in concert with the community or county ordinances and state laws and clearly articulated to and supported by staff, students, and the community. School nurses have a responsibility to review all relevant policies, make sure they are implemented, and initiate plans for revision or policy development when needed.

Health curriculum and instruction are primarily the role of classroom teachers, with a focus on enhancing personal, family, and community health as outlined in the National Health Education Standards (American Association for Health Education, 2005) (TABLE 19.4). Student services team members and community agency partners are involved in planning, co-teaching, and providing resource materials for the classroom and referral to credible community sources. To ensure support and reinforcement of student learning, parents need to be included via student assignments, parenting suggestions and culturally relevant resources. Peer education and school-wide initiatives support classroom health education but are no substitute. In addition to classroom health education, students need to have basic social skills and refusal skills reinforced early and often by teachers, coaches, student services staff, and family members. As outlined in Chapter 7 on the role of the school nurse as an educator, the school nurse can be active in health promotion in the classroom, in the health office, school-wide, and with families in the community.

Providing **student services** requires school nurses, counselors, social workers, psychologists, and antidrug health coordinators to work together. This team reinforces the classroom-taught decision-making and behavior skills with vulnerable students on a one-to-one basis, directs peer helper/leader programs, works with students identified as

Table 19.4 ■

PROPOSED REVISION OF THE NATIONAL HEALTH EDUCATION STANDARDS

1. Students will comprehend concepts that enhance personal, family, and community health.
2. Students will demonstrate the ability to apply health literacy skills to enhance personal, family, and community health.
3. Students will demonstrate the ability to apply self-management skills to enhance personal, family, and community health.
4. Students will analyze the influence of family, peers, culture, media, technology, and other factors on healthy behaviors.
5. Students will demonstrate the ability to use interpersonal communication to enhance personal, family, and community health.
6. Students will demonstrate the ability to use decision-making and goal-setting skills to engage in health-advancing behaviors.
7. Students will demonstrate the ability to advocate for personal, family, and community health.

Source: American Association for Health Education (2005).

having behaviors of concern, and provides intervention services or refers students to public and private providers, assists in policy development and implementation, and communicates with parents and family members. The National Guidelines for Student Services (Adelman & Taylor, 2003) summarizes this coordinated teamwork as focusing on academic success, addressing barriers, and providing specialized student and family assistance and support. In addition to providing direct health services to students, the school nurse must provide comprehensive coordinated services that reach beyond the school walls and involve the family and community in order to promote health.

Family and parent involvement incorporates parent representatives and feedback on policy development and review committees and curriculum selection and program development committees, having health and school connectedness on the agenda of the parent–teacher association and encouraging parents to volunteer at school. Involvement also includes the daily emphasis by parents on academic success and positive health behaviors and skills with their children. Being role models and encouraging pro-social behaviors also pertains to adults in the community who are in contact with youth, such as employers, youth program leaders, faith community leaders, coaches and staff, and those in parks and recreation programs, to name a few. The school nurse can be instrumental in identifying individuals who need to be involved in offering support and guidance for parents with evidence-based information and by maintaining open lines of communication with parents and community partners.

Youth development is a strand that is integral to each of the above components. Engaging youth in planning policy, curriculum, and student services makes the programs current and relevant. While each component is essential to linking health and learning, the model also includes strategies, or coordinating processes to systematically determine that all aspects are considered. These strategies have much in common with the decision-making process inherent in the School Nursing Standards of Care (NASN & ANA, 2001) (Table 19.1). The coordinating strategies to promote this comprehensive prevention model for schools include engaging partners, systematically identifying needs, planning and implementing programs or solutions, evaluation, and staff development.

Engaging school and community partners is essential in gaining buy-in from school staff and community partners. This begins with building an awareness of health and learning issues and their connections, and enlisting support for changing policies and programs. The intent is to have consistency among school, home, and community approaches and to connect them so that scarce school and community resources, including ideas, materials, and people, are shared.

Assessing, planning, and implementing steps include a systematic review of the needs of the students. It means looking at what is in place and what is working and building connections among program elements so that key concepts and youth skills are reinforced. It also means setting realistic timelines with tasks shared by school and community partners. An essential aspect of this strategy is effective and repeated communication.

In the planning phase, the school nurse can help determine the measures that will be periodically reviewed to see if progress is being made (process and outcome measures) and set intervals to provide the relevant documentation. Systematically monitoring what is being done and the outcomes helps link the results to improvement in academics. A plan needs to be in place regarding the sharing of results. Celebrating the small steps and recognizing the impact on student health and learning are essential to building a collaborative partnership for health promotion. School nurses, students, families, staff, and community partners need regular reinforcement to help maintain momentum and enthusiasm.

Staff development that includes administrators, teachers, and student services staff can make the connections between policy and setting social norms, between health and learning, and between the school and the family's roles. When there is inconsistency between the classroom messages and policy and what happens at home, students are skeptical. For example, youth learn that tobacco use impacts on cognition (neurological effects), yet the school policy of no-tobacco-use may not be enforced because it requires increased staff involvement and consistent discipline; parents say that smoking is bad yet they might send their adolescent to the store to buy cigarettes for them. Youth may be buying cigarettes for themselves because the community is not enforcing the laws on youth purchasing tobacco.

One connection that can easily be made is that the decision-making steps learned by students in their health education class can be posted in the health services and school counseling offices, in the community pediatric clinic, and on parents' refrigerators at home. Then the steps can be recalled when students bring up their real-life situations. This strategy enhances the school–home link, educates parents, and provides reinforcing messages to students and the community. The National Staff Development Standards provide a foundation for designing ways over time to influence school programming and approaches (NSDC, 2002). The school nurse can refer to these standards when contributing suggestions for staff development programs or when implementing them.

COLLABORATORS: SCHOOL NURSES

School nurses are in an optimal position to serve as school–community collaborators because of their breadth of knowledge of wellness and illness, human development, behavior, social systems, and learning theory. No one else in the school has this breadth of knowledge. This knowledge base applies to individuals, peer groups, families and groups, the school community, and the community-at-large. School nurses have skills as problem solvers and communicators. These skills are demonstrated in the school nurse's roles as educator and advocate who speaks for children and youth, not the system. School nurses articulate the problems and needs based on professional knowledge, research, clinical experience, and the perspective of others. School nurses can see future possibilities and envision a plan to see it succeed. As mediators, with astute communication skills and having nonjudgmental interpersonal skills, school nurses help others with differing points of view be acknowledged and heard. School nurses have the skills to understand individual, group, and community dynamics, goals, motivations, and perspectives and draw on these to inform, engage, involve, and invest families and the community in partnerships with the schools.

Nursing cannot do it alone; there are too many students with needs and not enough school nurses. However, school nurses can take a leadership role in the collaborative process, for leadership is part of every baccalaureate nursing program. Working with different families and different programs in the school and community, school nurses are called on to implement all of the standards of care and many of the standards of professional performance in working with partners. This is most clearly identified in the standard on collaboration (Table 19.1) which specifies the expectation that the school nurse will collaborate with students, staff, families, and healthcare providers in providing care. The measurement criteria for this standard include communication, consultation, making referrals, and providing for continuity of care. Under this broad framework of collaboration, the school nurse uses many skills to promote healthy partnerships.

School nurses, especially those who are newer to the specialty, need to use the expertise of their colleagues to expand their repertoire of creative approaches and community contacts. *State school nurse consultants* are an invaluable resource for the school nurse. These registered professional nurses are employed by state departments of education or state departments of health and have statewide responsibilities related to the practice of school nursing and the provision of school health services. Although their job descriptions vary, they provide leadership, advocacy staff development, and technical assistance; they also influence public policy related to school health.

Consultants typically have a broad background in the principles and practices of school nursing, public health, adult learning, administration, and comprehensive school health programs. They must also understand program and project development, including a strong understanding of evaluation and data analysis. Consultants have a complete understanding of the state's nurse practice act to address the ever-increasing complexity of student health situations in an education setting. They may be able to identify funding sources or other agencies interested in a similar project as the school nurse. This makes them ideal for consultation and collaboration.

The remaining sections of this chapter describe collaboration with multiple groups followed by a description of the role of the school nurse as collaborator with the family, healthcare providers, school staff, and the community. While collaboration with students is essential, it is assumed that all school nurse actions begin and end with the student. Standards of care direct school nurses in gathering data, identifying needs, formulating plans, implementing care, and determining its value. Each of these steps requires active student involvement. Where student collaboration is not obvious in the collaborative partnership discussed, specific guidelines will be addressed.

COLLABORATION WITH FAMILIES

Nursing has at its core the view of a client in the context of his or her family and community. Nursing recognizes significant others as partners in health; likewise, school nurses recognize parents or other adult care providers as partners in education. Although some in the school may not share this philosophy of working closely with parents and significant others, the school nurse is in a unique position to offer ideas and resources for connecting parents to the classrooms and vice versa.

Recognizing the diversity in families is important. The term "parent" is often used to designate the adult care provider in the family. This may or may not be a biological or adoptive parent. In some families, it is a step-parent, grandparent, aunt or uncle, adult sibling, foster parent or court-appointed guardian (see Chapter 17). In some cases, an adolescent is an emancipated minor and makes his or her own healthcare decisions as well as decisions for her children. It may be the religious leader who guides a student. In rare cases, the most significant stable adult in an adolescent's life is his or her employer.

Parents' own educational experiences, their attitudes toward education, and their involvement in their children's learning have been identified as having a potential impact on their child's learning. Several key ideas have been recognized in research studies: parental styles, attitudes, and involvement. Authoritative parenting (not autocratic) benefits children's academic success, their acquisition of positive lifetime health attitudes and behaviors, and their connectedness to school and community. As noted previously, these positively impact on academic success.

Parents' attitudes toward learning have at least as much influence on student attitudes and behaviors toward learning as parent actions regarding learning. Parents' attitudes and expectations about youth health behaviors have as much impact toward students' acquisition of positive health behaviors as parents' own health behaviors. Lastly, parent involvement in education is less about showing up at school and being leaders in the parent–teacher organizations (although schools have a difficult time functioning without parent volunteers being part of daily in-school activities) and is more about making learning at home a priority (establishing a routine time and place for children to do homework undistracted, reading regularly to children) and feeling comfortable communicating with the children's teachers. From the child's perspective, "showing up" at special events is the main job of parents (Partnerships for Family Involvement in Education, 1998; Simpson, 2001).

DeBord (2001) has outlined the following four reasons why parents should be involved: (1) Students do better in school; (2) parents become empowered; (3) teacher morale improves; and (4) communities grow stronger. School nurses can use this information to encourage parental participation and involvement in school activities. In addition, partnerships with parents can be enhanced when the school nurse recognizes the strengths and contributions that families make to the learning environment.

Although these guides serve to remind us of basic principles of interacting with community members, the National Standards for Parent/Family Involvement (National PTA, 2003) offers a framework for describing how schools can engage parents and family members in the major acitivities of schools (TABLE 19.5). The Standards are consistent with other literature supporting family collaboration.

In simple or complex referrals, the family also has responsibility; however, the family's capacity depends on the family's physical and mental health, its stability in terms of place of residence and who is in the family, and workplace stability. The family's past experiences with education play an important role in their problem-solving approaches related to school issues—whether the parent(s) liked school, had a good or bad school experience, had their education interrupted, or had positive or negative school experiences with other children. In addition, their past experiences with health care, mental health counseling, or chemical use treatment, social services, or law enforcement all affect the family's ability to cope with a health-related problem, see a possible resolution, seek services, and focus on what

Table 19.5 ■
NATIONAL STANDARDS FOR PARENT/FAMILY INVOLVEMENT

I. **Communicating:** Communication between home and school is regular, two-way and meaningful.
II. **Parenting:** Parenting skills are promoted and supported.
III. **Student Learning:** Parents play an integral role in assisting student learning.
IV. **Volunteering:** Parents are welcome in the school, and their support and assistance are sought.
V. **School Decision Making and Advocacy:** Parents are full partners in the decisions that affect children and families.
VI. **Collaborating with Community:** Community resources are used to strengthen schools, families and student learning.

Source: National PTA (2003).

will improve the child's education (Mostert, 1998). Therefore, the community providers to which families are referred should be welcoming, able to meet cultural needs, practical in terms of matching the families' ability and tolerance to the treatment regimen recommended, accessible, and acceptable. If the community resource provides feedback to the school saying the student or family is noncompliant, the provider has not heard what the family sees as the problem and the plan does not meet what the family knows or has been convinced will resolve the problem (White, 2001).

COLLABORATION WITH THE HEALTHCARE COMMUNITY

The school nurse collaborates with healthcare providers in a variety of ways, including making referrals, providing follow-up care, and in serving on school and community-based committees to promote health and learning. In addition, many schools are fortunate to have school-based health centers. The school nurse is the link between the school and the community in order to provide comprehensive services to the students.

Referral

A referral is more than sending a student to a healthcare provider or clinic for medical care. The intuitive and subtle assessment, negotiation, and communication skills used by the school nurse in decision-making are complex. Referral is a component of the nursing process whereby, after a nursing assessment has been conducted and nursing diagnosis made, the school nurse reaches a conclusion, and communicates the conclusion to the student and his or her parent or guardian to identify options for accessing the community healthcare system. For example, it may be apparent that the student is experiencing an acute health problem or an exacerbation of a known chronic health problem; therefore further examination and diagnosis are necessary to rule out problems or to identify and treat the medical condition.

The following key areas can be used by the school nurse when considering the need for a referral:

- In most situations, the parent or guardian will need to be contacted if care is to be provided beyond that provided by the school. The school nurse must know which exceptions do not require parental permission, especially related to child abuse, public health issues, and reproductive services.
- Outline the presenting problem for the student and parent or guardian and check to see if they concur with the health history findings and signs and symptoms. It may be necessary to provide education at this point.
- Elicit past practices (e.g., clinic use) and satisfaction with those services (e.g, Were they able to get the medications and did they work? Did they use medications as prescribed? If they didn't follow recommendations, why? What home-based practices have they tried and were they successful?)
- Determine student and family resources and resourcefulness as related to the immediacy of the problem (e.g., neither parent nor emergency contacts can be reached; parents get off work; there are no evening clinic hours; student usually carries medicine but forgot it, but his brother is carrying his medicine which is the same prescription; a school-based health center opens in an hour but parent has not signed permission for the student to receive services there).
- Determine whether or not services are accessible and acceptable. Consider distance,

transportation, culture and language, cost of care, and wait time at the clinic (e.g., parent has to take a taxi to school to pick up their child at school, to get to the health clinic and then to get back home but has limited finances; family newly immigrated to the United States and the town's clinic does not have translators).

- Inform the parent or guardian of school policies regarding attendance (e.g., students with a temperature of 100.5°F in the morning are to go home; acute transmitted diseases, such as streptococcal infection, are to be treated for 24 hours with antibiotics prior to return to school; attendance is strongly encouraged on days when the state academic tests are given, otherwise the school is penalized; after 10 days of absence in a quarter the student must drop the class and receive no credit).
- Weigh exposure of the ill student to others and vice versa. (Does this student need to be removed from the school environment because they are a risk to other students, or might infections of other students put this student at risk?)
- Determine whether the school nurse needs to contact the care provider instead of the parent or in addition to the parent to confer on the nature of the problem, ramifications for the student's education, school policy, and so forth. Obtain permission from the parent to do so according to federal and state data practices requirements and school policy and procedures. Follow appropriate guidelines in obtaining signed consent from the parent.
- Anticipate whether follow-up treatment, education, or other problem-solving may need to occur at school (e.g., administering antibiotics that cannot be given during off-school hours at home; revising the asthma action plan due to a change in the frequency of recurring symptoms; educating parents, the student and staff regarding a new insulin pump; contacting local ambulance drivers regarding the expectation by parents that they would provide epinephrine in an emergency).

Follow-up for Continuity of Care

If the student and parent promptly get medical care and treatment and comply with the medical recommendations and school procedures (i.e., treat with antibiotics for 24 hours before returning to school; temperature normal for 24 hours prior to returning to school; daily medication given at school only if it cannot be scheduled to be given at home; signed physician order and parent permission to give medication during school hours or before/after school at school-age childcare), a subsequent aspect of healthcare provider collaboration is following up to confirm that the plan was appropriate and worked.

The school nurse needs to determine that the problem has resolved or is resolving and that there are no untoward effects (i.e., medication allergy, secondary infection, insulin level instability due to dehydration from stomach flu, parent's workplace docked pay due to absence for the medical appointment, food for the family was a priority and there was not enough money to pay for medication; term paper is late and student's grade is affected).

The school nurse can increase student awareness of health and illness, its impact on learning and daily life, the process of seeking care and treatment, the assets of early intervention, and competence in self-care. The National Health Education Standards (American Association for Health Education, 2005) (Table 19.5) offer a valuable framework for increasing knowledge, cognitive skills, and behavioral skills in students. The student's personal experience "brings to life" the theory outlined in the Standards and is a valuable learning experience. Students are more likely to connect the classroom-taught information and skills and be able to generalize the lessons learned when the school nurse facilitates guided reflection about the healthcare experience.

The school nurse should monitor over time to ensure that the problem does not recur, the chronic condition has stabilized, a new regimen of medications is understood by the student and staff, and no adjustments in the education program are needed (i.e., absences counted as "excused," the student not being penalized, due date of a paper delayed by 1 or 2 days, snack/lunch and recess time switched because of changes in insulin type and dosage). The monitoring for an acute health problem may be within the time period the student is taking an antibiotic and then 2 weeks later. For a chronic health problem, the monitoring may need to occur daily for 5 days, every 2 weeks, and then monthly, depending on the severity of the problem.

Follow-up also includes communication with the classroom teachers and student services team to note changes that may show a recurrence of a health concern or related problems that would cause an interference in the student's education (i.e., student who has a distance vision limitation has stopped wearing his glasses after a recent name-calling incident on the playground). Communication with the family, permission to share pertinent information with school staff, and obtaining written consent for being able to contact the healthcare provider are essential components of collaboration with other healthcare providers.

School-Based Health Centers

School-based health centers (SBHC) (sometimes called school-based wellness centers) are part of the community that is within the school. They started 35 years ago in elementary schools as a way to provide services to those who could not afford or access health care. They now exist in more than 1,300 schools in the United States, and are available to anyone (with parental consent), with the majority (41%) being in high schools (American Academy of Pediatrics, 2004; Swider & Valukas, 2004).

SBHCs are freestanding entities located in the school or in a portable unit on school property. No two centers are the same; the services they provide are varied and are specific to the population. A list of some of the services that may be provided is shown in TABLE 19.6. SBHCs are managed by a variety of entities. They may be operated and staffed by local hospitals, public health departments, departments of education, school systems, university medical or nursing schools, youth agencies, or community agencies. Some are open to students for a few hours a week, some for the entire time that school is in session, and some have hours during evenings and weekends.

Some in the community are opposed to SBHCs, fearing that their use by their children usurps parental authority. The services that receive the most opposition relate to reproductive health care. Yet, one of the first SBHCs to provide pregnancy prevention services was able to demonstrate a 50% reduction in the birth rates among teens in 7 years (Button & Rienzo, 2002). In fact, SBHCs "that offer comprehensive family-planning services and condom distribution—delay the initiation of sexual intercourse, upgrade the quality of contraceptive use, and lower pregnancy rates" (Button & Rienzo, 2002, p. 12); they increase the use of condoms among adolescents who are already sexually active but they do *not* increase the incidence of sexual activity among students. Despite these statistics, many SBHCs are prohibited from providing reproductive health services.

Other benefits of SBHCs are that they allow students to receive acute care services in school rather than missing a day of school or causing parents to miss time from work to take their child to see a healthcare provider. One study demonstrated a decrease in absence rates by 50% for those screened and referred for mental health services (Geierstanger, Amaral, Mansour, & Walters, 2004). It decreases the waiting time and travel inconveniences for health care. In general, research has demonstrated "a direct link between SBHCs and academic performance that can be widely generalized" (Geierstanger et al., 2004, p. 350).

There can be a significant amount of collaboration between the school nurse and the school-based health center. While there may be overlap in the services provided, good communication can decrease any conflict and perhaps increase the cost efficiency of both. The school nurse is responsible for the day-to-day health of *all* students while they are in the school. State laws and district policies mandate some of the screenings, stipulations, and interventions that must be done for all students, such as required immunizations and vision screening.

The SBHC is a referral source for the school nurse for students who require services beyond those of the school nurse and who have permission

Table 19.6 ■

SELECTED SERVICES THAT MAY BE PROVIDED BY SCHOOL-BASED HEALTH CENTERS

- Physical examinations for school entry and sports participation
- Diagnosis and management of acute illness
- Maintenance and monitoring of chronic health conditions
- Limited laboratory services
- Dental screening
- Pregnancy testing
- Diagnosis and management of sexually transmitted diseases
- Reproductive health counseling
- Mental health counseling (individual or group)
- Crisis intervention
- Diagnosis and interventions for students with learning or behavior problems
- Nutrition counseling
- Substance abuse counseling
- Tobacco cessation programs
- Social services (assistance with assuring that families have food, clothing, shelter and are free of abuse)
- Wellness programs

from their parents to use the center. The National Association of School Nurses, along with other agencies committed to the health of those in the schools (2001), issued a joint statement on the partnership between the school nurse and the SBHC. It acknowledges that they share the mission of protecting and advancing the health of school-age children and that by working together, they can "increase compliance with treatment plans, facilitate access to needed health and mental health care, monitor outcomes of care, uniformly document care, collect data about health needs and outcomes of care, and provide case management." They must communicate with each other, within the bounds of HIPAA.

Just as the school nurse must collaborate with the community, so must the school-based health center. Many have community advisory boards and develop partnerships with the healthcare community to access services for students and funding for the center, as this is a major concern in the survival of these programs (Swider & Valukas, 2004). NASN (2001) recommends that the school nurse be part of the team that develops the SBHC and facilitates access for students to use the services provided. In addition, the SBHC should include the school nurse as part of their advisory team and that, in partnership, they:

- Develop a shared case management structure to track outcomes of care and share workload
- Coordinate nursing and treatment compliance care plans for clients who require follow-up care
- Work together to document services that will allow data collection to study outcomes of care, cost-effectiveness of care and other key data needed to identify outcomes using an evidence-based system of care
- Develop policies and systems that ensure the quality and confidentiality of care received by students
- Jointly plan and implement health promotion and disease prevention programs to improve health outcomes for all members of the school community
- Within parameters of confidentiality, notify school staff of students with acute or chronic health needs who may require health counseling and/or health education and accommodations during the school day (NASN, 2001).

SBHCs have been successful in meeting the needs of students that could have resulted in barriers to learning. They are supported by the American Academy of Pediatrics, although they are not intended to replace the primary care provider or the medical home for the student. They are, however, an excellent avenue of collaboration for the school nurse. There have been recent reports of pediatric healthcare providers who have informed their clients that if students use the SBHC, they may not also be clients in that pediatrician's practice. This mandate often has a financial basis, but may be addressed by providing the healthcare provider with the above positive statistics of the SBHC and reminding them of their advocacy role for students and their families.

COLLABORATION WITH COLLEAGUES WITHIN THE SCHOOL

A student services team or student assistance team is a multidisciplinary team consisting of the partnering student services disciplines: teachers, school social worker, school psychologist, school counselor, antidrug health specialist, and the school nurse. Depending on the resources in the school and community and the nature of student concerns, the school administrator may join the team, as well as various special education specialists and in-school family advocates if such a service exists. In the broadest use of the model, any concern of teachers could be referred to the team, including learning problems, attention or attendance problems, family troubles reported by a student, conflict between an educator and a student, health problems (not episodic care, or well-managed chronic health conditions), chemical use, death of a student or close friend of a student, or other mental health concerns.

A multidisciplinary team that collaborates in school is important because educators are well prepared to identify when there is a sudden change in a student or even when the change is subtle over time. In the Student Assistance Model, this "behavior of concern" is anything a teacher can see that has changed in a student, or has heard the student say, such as not being as prepared in class, having a change of affect, separating from peers, lack of participation, and changing expectations. Change might also be noticed by sports coaches or Boy Scout leaders who might notify the school nurse.

The student assistance team can observe the student and decide who should best assess the student to identify the problem. The team can then "brainstorm" possible interventions. The team leader for that student's problems might be the person best able to assist the student to resolve or cope with the problem, whether it be a learning problem, a problem with peers, rejection by the opposite sex, family disruption (whether by moving or divorce), bullying in the school, or a health-related concern.

The premise is that educators and other school personnel are well prepared to identify "behaviors of concern." In so doing, the integrity of the process is important; problems referred must be addressed in some way. The knowledge and astute awareness of the teaching staff are essential. Transient or minor issues are not referred and teachers can first try a number of strategies to engage the distracted or disagreeable student. The expertise of the student services team is critical. It provides a broad breadth of experience and access to resources, and together, they are authorized to work creatively with families, the school, and the community to mediate or resolve problems. The assessment, referral, intervention and after-care model also require willing and competence of the educators to function as a collaborating team and a clear structure or process for communication and action (Mostert, 1998).

TABLE 19.7 outlines the strategies to promote health and learning in school accompanied by the collaborative impact that occurs. The school nurse can be the staff or team member described in these interactions.

This model differs from those in which the special education process is handled by one school team, the chemical-use–student-assistance-process by another, discipline handled singly by the dean or principal, and health concerns case managed only by the school nurse.

Table 19.7 ■

STUDENT ASSISTANCE TEAM PROCESS: PROBLEM IDENTIFICATION, REFERRAL, AND FOLLOW-UP

EDUCATORS' ACTIONS	SYSTEM INTERACTIONS
a. Staff aware of growth and development, deviations from the norm, and the impact of problems on learning. b. Staff observe and name "behaviors of concern" in a student and inform the student services team. Concerns may also come to health services or student services team from the student, a peer, a parent, or a community member. c. Staff discuss behavior with student using the "See it, say it" approach* .	1. Responsive school environment: Staff have permission to "see" problems and an obligation to respond. 2. Staff development sessions to increase awareness of "behaviors of concern," signs and symptoms of problems and how to "see it, say it" with students. 3. System in place to "hear" staff concerns, to "intake" concerns from students themselves, peers, parents/family, or community members.
* See it, say it approach: The educator may interact directly with the student, saying, "I am concerned (or express another feeling). I see ____ (state observations, not judgments). I will listen to what you think is going on.______. I want ____ (expectation) (see nurse, tell parent, consult counselor). I will assist you by ______."	
d. Student services team identifies a case manager. e. Case manager observes student with the staff/teacher, collects relevant information. Use the "see it, say it" approach. f. Case manager may return to the student services team, asking another team member with more expertise to take the next steps; or may proceed.	4. Student assistance team works in conjunction with a special education team to differentiate the nature of the problem. 5. Policies in place for sharing information, observing students. 6. Respect and trust among student services team members, acknowledging each others' expertise, connections with families, community linkages, and so forth.

(continued)

Table 19.7 ■ *(Continued)*

EDUCATORS' ACTIONS

g. Parent, student, and case manager explore options: what has/has not worked in the past, accessible and acceptable sources for care and support, follow-up steps. Options include modifying home or school environment, interventions at school or assessment/intervention from non-school sources, and so forth.
h. Contact made with the student/family to check (1) understanding of the problem and its impact on learning, (2) readiness and capacity to act, (3) whether or not the plan is realistic and perceived as helpful, (4) barriers to action steps, (5) changes that would alter the plan, (6) other options, and (7) a realistic timeline.
i. Case manager reports to the reporting staff that follow-up is occurring and a timeline for possible changes/resolutions, but is not likely to report what steps are being taken.
j. If treatment/therapy or other interventions are provided, the student is supported through the duration. Modifications in the school schedule, class assignments, etc. are supported.
k. On conclusion of the intervention, the student is supported in the transition to school and/or the routine education plan.
l. Periodically, the student and/or family are contacted to ensure there is not recurrence of the original problems or that the sustained changes in the education plan, school environment, or home continue to be manageable and helpful.

SYSTEM INTERACTIONS

7. Policy and practice of engaging parents early and often in identifying and resolving issues.
8. Student services personnel are cross-trained in gathering relevant information: health status, health behaviors, social interactions, community connections, family factors, learning processes and obstacles.
9. Student service team regularly reviews student interviewing and brief intervention skills to share strategies and keep current with developing practices.
10. A broad range of current in-school and community resources are identified, contacted, and are known to provide useful services to students/families.
11. Policies are clear regarding in-school referrals (e.g., for special education assessment) and out-of-school referrals including issues of transportation, payment or reimbursement (if appropriate), and whether the referral is a recommendation or a requirement.
12. Cultural, language, economic, and other barriers are acknowledged and school personnel readily work with student/family to mediate the obstacles.
13. Procedures are in place; gain written consent to release information to or request it from non-school provider(s). Other data practices and confidentiality requirements are respected and followed.
    ** Feedback system in place to acknowledge the first observations by staff, to verify that action is being taken. Privacy is maintained. Feedback may be necessary at several points during an assessment, referral and follow-up process.
14. Staff development sessions discuss the principles of confidentiality and data privacy.
15. Policies and practices support short term modifications in education plans, advocacy and monitoring of progress.
16. Policies and practices support staff and student time and energy necessary to make transitions.
17. Supports are in place to track and contact students over time and from one school year to the next as needed.

Sources: Minnesota Prevention Resource Center (2002); NASN & ANA (2001); Schwab & Gelfman (2001); Svendsen, Luehr, & Helke (2003).

When school nurses and the other student services disciplines work together, teams are more likely to see the students as children and youth with roles, work, relationships and involvement in many activities that are separate from schools. Because it is teachers' expertise to provide the environment, resources, and experiences for student learning, they focus on what students bring to the classroom. Teachers need to anticipate that students are "ready to learn, willing and able, present and participating" (Linking Health and Learning Model described earlier in the chapter). The school nurse and other student services team members can be the bridge to the family and community as they know of, understand, and make efficient use of family and community resources. The work of the students is learning, growing, and developing. The work of the student service team mirrors that of an occupational health program: to assist the student coming to "work" fully prepared and returning to work with a minimum of interruption and at the best capacity possible.

Depending on the collaborative relationships with key community members (and having the legal agreements that permit sharing of student information), the student assistance team may include public health and social services representatives. In the model of a Community School, full service is available at the school site for students and family members from collaborative partners. The goal is seamless services, but a great deal of weaving of services and partnership agreements need to be in place for the services to work and work well (Dryfoos & Magure, 2002).

COLLABORATION WITH YOUTH

Because all school–community collaborations focus on students, it is essential that students are involved in providing advice and in decision-making. As is often said by inclusive educators, "It's not about them without them." This type of positive connection between youth and adults "is associated with a decrease in risk behaviors, stronger communication skills and leadership experience, increased status and stature in the community, and improved competencies and self-esteem" (U.S. Department of Health and Human Services [USDHHS], 2005). Programs benefit from fresh, new ideas and new perspectives as well as relevant information about the needs and interests of youth. This increases the program's credibility.

According to the National Clearinghouse on Families and Youth (USDHHS, 2001), youth development occurs within the context of the family and the community. It relies on the mentoring of caring adults to foster motivation, connectedness, and competence. Youth involvement in school–community collaborations can be facilitated by including the principles of representation, equality, input, and leadership opportunities.

When youth are invited to have a voice at the advisory or decision-making table, they should be invited at least in pairs or triads. A single youth may not have the nerve to speak in front of an adult group or may have the nerve, but not the perspective to represent more than a single point of view. Each young person also needs a meeting tutor to orient the student to the context, process, and content of the discussion. The leader of the group informs all members of the collaborative that this sharing is not only permissible but expected during the meeting. Periodically through the meeting, the leader should ask the youth for their input. The intent is to be supportive and inclusionary, not pejorative.

When collaboration involves multiple partners, there should be equal representation from the student body as for each of the collaborating partners. If programs or concerns discussed involve multiple age groups, then all should be represented. Older youth can even participate in preparing the agenda for meetings, presenting information, and leading discussions, all with the assistance of an adult mentor. At the conclusion to each meeting is a check-in with all present on whether or not: (1) tasks were prepared and agenda items of a meeting jointly were equally presented by youth and adults; (2) adults and student listened respectfully to each others' ideas, (3) adults and students provided input and correction to each other when there was an imbalance of power, and (4) the follow-up tasks were equally assigned to adults and youth. The successes need to be named and celebrated and suggestions for improvement made.

In many ways, this shared-responsibility approach can be more challenging for the adults in the school and community than for youth. It takes more time, but builds capacity in youth and adults and can have benefits that extend to other school functions and the community. In the long run, the actions taken by the collaborative may have a greater impact due to the direct and indirect involvement of energetic students, their family members, and others with whom they interact (Box 19.4).

Youth input can be essential in collaborative efforts. This input does not need to come just from student delegates to the committee, but can come from student government, student clubs, or representatives from specific classes. For example, if the financing of health services in schools is the issue being tackled, discussion of insurance benefits and

Box 19.4 ■ ■ ■

YOUTH DEVELOPMENT OUTCOMES

The youth development approach is predicated on the understanding that all young people need support, guidance, and opportunities during adolescence, a time of rapid growth and change. With this support, they can develop self-assurance in the four areas that are key to creating a happy, healthy, and successful life:

A sense of competence: being able to do something well

A sense of usefulness: having something to contribute

A sense of belonging: being part of a community

A sense of power: having control over one's future

(U.S. Department of Health and Human Services, National Clearinghouse on Families and Youth.[2005]. *Youth development.* Retrieved April 2005 from http://www.ncfy.com/youthdev/p.htm)

reimbursement rates may not be of interest to youth. But hearing from youth on why they do or do not use school-based services would be critical. The challenge would be to clarify the reason for seeking youth input and then, in fact, using that input.

Youth-led, adult directed initiatives are often more complicated. The issues, messages, and logistics need to be negotiated delicately between the youth and adults involved; the funders; and the established local, state, and national organizations. For example, while there is an adult–youth generational gap in the understanding and appreciation of media and technology use and influence, advertisers of youth products are savvy. The clever, continuing promotion of tobacco use "to adults," as stated by the tobacco industry, continues to have direct appeal to youth who want to be adult-like. When the prevention field wants to emulate those media strategies to sway social norms, the goal is to have youth lead the way in defining the message and messenger. Yet, which youth are to lead: the trendsetters, mainstream, disenfranchised, "older" high school youth, or "younger" junior high or freshmen youth? When trendsetters define edgy messages, do they work for the mainstreamers, the majority of whom do not and will never use tobacco yet want to be "on the edge," too? Do the edgy messages irritate the boring adult funders? Do messages that use sophisticated humor and sarcasm leave behind the younger adolescents who developmentally are not ready, do not "get it", and feel left out? Younger adolescents may gravitate to the "scary" and gory messages, yet there is clear evidence that this has intrigue but no impact on behavior formation or behavior change. The balance is in adults providing timely and relevant guidelines and direction in the politics of limited funds and the long-term vision, and still have the youth be directors and the visible leaders of initiatives.

Youth development is an approach that views youth as having an important voice regarding the programs and services that affect them. Youth need to be seen as resources with strengths and abilities to develop within their own community.

COLLABORATION WITH THE COMMUNITY

School nurses cannot be effective if they limit their scope of practice to the school building. Students have needs that require community involvement, and often community assistance. In addition, school nurses who handle large numbers of students may need volunteer assistance from the community in order to complete all required activities and to develop and carry out health-promotion and disease-prevention programs. Examples of community resources follow.

Businesses

Businesses have a variety of resources that they can bring to the table in collaborative efforts. One pizza company donated coupons for free pizzas to a school district to be given to students who read a certain number of books. Another encouraged their employees to volunteer to read to students or help them with homework. Still others rebuilt playgrounds and spruced up school buildings. While these activities focus more on the academic mission and physical plant, school nurses can engage businesses to assist in health-related initiatives. One company donated billboard space for an antismoking message developed by high school students. Another funded the printing of posters to encourage adolescents to make wiser choices and to take care of their bodies.

Some businesses may provide money to fund motivational speakers for students or health-related books for the library. One paid for the development of a walking track in the back yard of an elementary school. Still others have bought supplies that were needed by the school nurse for the health office.

Grandparents

Grandparents or other senior citizens in the community often have the time, the experience, and the patience to assist students in the school setting. It benefits them, by making them feel useful. It may be helpful for young students who need special attention or assistance in focusing on their work. School nurses may use their services as extra pairs of hands, such as during mass screenings in the school or to assist with students who need technical assistance, such as sitting with a student who needs tube feedings.

Government Agencies

Multiple local and state government agencies are available to assist the school nurse. Many, such as the Division on Mental Retardation, can provide in-service programs for staff, suggest resources for the school nurse, and assist in working with families. Public Health is an essential collaborative agency, both for their mandates and guidelines related to communicable disease control and the guidance they can provide to the school nurse related to questions. Child Protective Services are usually the resource for suspected child abuse or for domestic abuse that may be occurring in the home. Vocational Rehabilitation agencies can assist in explaining the laws, recommending accommodations, and assisting in developing transition plans for adolescents on the Individual Education Programs.

Social service agencies often work closely with school nurses, especially for students who are in foster care, homeless, or impoverished. They may be the collaborators to assist with students who are truant from school or those who are new immigrants and trying to assimilate cultures. The Social Security offices may provide information related to those who qualify for their services and support.

Police and Fire Companies

Police and fire companies often provide fire and gun safety programs in the schools. They provide security in many high schools and may offer assistance related to drug and alcohol education. Police can assist in reinforcing that businesses not sell cigarettes or alcohol to students; they also can ensure bike and car safety and assist with programs that promote these health-promoting behaviors.

Ambulance companies must work closely with schools. When the school nurse knows that there are students in the school who are prone to anaphylaxis, these emergency response companies must be alerted that they must carry epinephrine and oxygen. If students are on portable ventilators, emergency care providers must be informed and prepared for emergencies involving these students.

Transportation Companies

Many schools provide bus transportation from the students' neighborhoods to the school and back. Bus drivers must receive the same in-service programs that school staff receives. They must know how to handle blood and body secretions, what to do if a student has a seizure or an allergic attack, and how to communicate with students who are hearing impaired, should they have students with these needs. At the same time, they may identify problems they observe on the bus or at the bus stop, such as bullying, inappropriate outer clothing for the weather, or unsafe behavior on the bus. These can then be incorporated into intervention programs within the school that include the bus drivers. Public transportation groups also need to communicate with and collaborate to ensure that services are cost effective for students and that students are well behaved when using those services.

Schools of Nursing

A wonderful collaborative avenue involves schools of nursing in the area. Nursing programs are always looking for clinical placement for their students. This allows the school nurse to function in the role of mentor and teacher. Often student nurses need to engage in a community project related to their pediatrics or community health courses. This allows the school nurse to initiate health-related programs that might need to be developed. Developing health fairs, doing screening for nonmandated health needs, developing posters that send a message, and presenting educational programs in the classroom are all projects that can be accomplished with the assistance of nursing students and their faculty. Graduate students in nursing programs might assist in writing grants to fund health-related initiatives.

Service Organizations

Many school nurses have a strong relationship with service organizations in the community. The Lions Club is well known for its assistance in assisting school nurses obtain glasses for students who have visual difficulties and cannot afford them. The American Lung Association has state agencies that will provide multiple resources to teach staff and students about asthma, smoking, and air pollution. They provide inservice education to school nurses to ensure that they use proper technique in monitoring peak flow and in assisting students in using their inhalers or nebulizers. Organizations that focus on individuals with blindness, deafness, mental retardation, cerebral palsy, and so forth provide information on the use and care of equipment that may be used in the school setting for individuals with these conditions, as well as materials that will help them learn or assist in their accommodation to the school setting.

The School Nurse as a Resource to the Community

Most of this chapter has focused on the nurse as someone who looks to the community to assist in promoting the health mission of the school. However, the nurse may be viewed by the community as an expert on health issues and someone who can be approached with questions. Many school nurses can relate stories of individuals who walked into the school from the community to ask a health-related question or to seek medical assistance. School nurses are asked to speak to service organizations about the healthcare needs of students or to assist the local community center with health-related programs. The school nurse may also be asked to be a member of a board of directors or an advisory committee for any number of service organizations in the community.

STRATEGIES TO PROMOTE COMMUNITY COLLABORATION

School and Community Assessment

Collaboration with the school system and referral to other healthcare providers and community services requires that the school nurse knows the community and its resources. This knowledge is based on a thorough and systematic assessment of community demographics, values, and resources.

Community and school assessment serves a number of purposes that help the school nurse:

- Learn the landscape of the community: its resources for work, play, and worship; places to get goods and services; its methods of providing protection and response to needs; how things get done; and who is in charge.
- Broadly determine the assets and needs of the community.
- Determine the community's readiness for change.
- Identify, for a specific initiative and for a specific population, the current programs and activities and gaps in communication, knowledge, or services.
- Establish an inventory of what exists or a measurement of how well the programs and activities meet a standard or a goal.

The assessment could take several forms: a focus on the school's emergency preparedness and its connection with community resources; a review of the chronic health problems of students and utilization of services for care, education, and support; a focus on a specific health condition, such as asthma; assessment of the community's awareness of and beliefs regarding mental health and mental illness; community resources available in a new prevention initiative to assist teachers or to reach parents through the schools; readiness of educators to take on another prevention initiative (i.e., obesity or mental health screening); and the school's policies regarding health risk behaviors or antisocial behaviors compared to neighboring schools, community ordinances, and parents' rules. The Surgeon General's 2000 report outlined ways in which schools and communities can link together to promote health (Table 19.8). However, these linkages will not be successful without first establishing an understanding of the community through appropriate assessment tools and methodologies.

Assessment tools are helpful in three ways. They serve as instruments to gather baseline data so that changes made in programs or services can be documented and the impact on the population can

Table 19.8 ■

SCHOOL–COMMUNITY CONNECTIONS: SURGEON GENERAL

School programs can connect to comprehensive community programs in these ways:

- Complementary messages for youth and adults
- Highlight positive health behaviors as the majority behavior
- Note dangers of risky behaviors; provide alternatives
- Use multiple non-preachy voices
- Use grassroots advocacy and community tie-ins
- Youth empowerment and involvement

Source: Reducing Tobacco Use: A Report of the Surgeon General (2000).

be measured over time. They facilitate communication among partners (school, family, and community) regarding their various roles and the potential for coordinated approaches and strengthen the development of strong interdependent networks. Community sectors may include public health, social services, law enforcement, advocacy groups and voluntary service organizations, employers of youth, youth recreation sites, religious communities, and other involved community members. Assessment tools also drive planning efforts to increase consistency, reduce gaps, and make change in programs to better meet the needs of the population. They can be used to anticipate and be able to take advantage of new resources and utilize new community partnerships.

Methodologies for community assessment vary greatly and are determined by the goal of the assessment. Examples include paper–pencil survey of parents in the school; stand-on-the-corner interviewer with one opinion question; a search of records (i.e., mission statements of agencies, written school board policies); computer online questionnaire; a yes–no survey of spectators at a school ballgame or attendees at parent–teacher conferences; and meeting with community agencies where they each bring their annual plans and compare targeted groups, strategies, and timelines. These and other approaches may be used as a cluster of strategies for gaining information.

Sometimes governing bodies such as the school board or a planning committee request that a school or community needs assessment be conducted, especially prior to initiating new programs. In some cases, the community itself or a local public health department may initiate the assessment, to which the school should provide input regarding the questions to be asked. While a staff member could collect reams of data, compile and summarize it, the outcomes are often more productive when a wide variety of people are involved in seeing and hearing about resources, processes, gaps, needs, and innovations. A large committee can be divided into subgroups that conduct the assessment on one aspect either that they know little about (naïve) or in which they are highly invested (experts already). Both need to guard against jumping to conclusions, either from too little information or from a predetermined point of view. Findings are summarized in small groups and then shared with the larger group.

Getting a large sector of the community involved is critical, especially if major changes are expected to result. It is important to publicize the assessment effort and to have open lines of communication via several methods (drop-in, telephone, write, e-mail, meetings, focus groups, community forums, on-line-chat-lines, etc.). Surveys or polls provide responses to the questions plus some additional comments.

Even with an open-door policy, some people are reluctant to contribute their ideas. One method to broaden the base of awareness and input is the structured grapevine. At the conclusion of every meeting, the group decides what one or two things were accomplished (and need to be celebrated) and on what question they need new ideas. Every meeting participant then contacts three to five others to share the accomplishments and to elicit ideas. The three to five others are people not assigned to the committee, but have an important relationship with the informer. Messages pass quickly through the informal networks. Each of the three to five contacts on the "first tier" are then to reach three to five others and so on. The first tier contacts have a timeline for relaying information back to the meeting participant. Everyone knows what is going on and no one is surprised at the decisions. This process promotes community identification with the process and the plan, as they can "hear" their own contributions in the messages that fly back and forth. When community members on the second or third tier get a message from two or three sources, they are at the intersection of important social networks and become key informants.

It is essential that students in the school also be part of a community assessment, for their input is vital to the process and the outcomes. Youth may be the instigators, having identified a specific problem or need (i.e., there is no place to skateboard) and wanting a plan of action. They can also, with training, be the interviewers, both for their peers and for key people in the school, home, and community. Data collected by others should be shared with them. Youth can compile data; write computer programs to synthesize the data; summarize the findings; identify an innovative action plan; and present a plan to educators, parent advocates, and community coalitions. Youth groups from different schools within the same school district or from community to community may want to compare findings for consistency of programs and for new ideas for school and community-based activities.

There are a number of structured tools for review and planning of school health and prevention programs, such as school climate inventories, school and community assets, and so forth. CDC's School Health Index is an extensive tool that guides teams of educators through the review and scoring of the eight components of the Coordinated School Health Program and is focused on physical activity, nutrition and preventing tobacco use (see http://www.cdc.

gov/healthyyouth/). Whatever tool or approach is used, it should be well planned and articulate with the purpose of the assessment.

Planning the Assessment

There are many processes for assessment and planning but all follow very similar steps. The first is to have a plan for the assessment (steps 1 to 3) and then a plan for the planning, evaluation and reinvesting phases (steps 4 to 9). The following steps outline a systematic approach to planning and implementing a community assessment.

1. Establish **who** will be involved in each phase of assessment and planning. As has been outlined, many players need to be connected for a comprehensive approach. Gaining the investment and support of school, parents, and community key leaders is important.
2. Determine **what** will be assessed within a realistic goal.
3. Determine **how** the assessment will be done. Select the method that best fits the goal or topic and one that fits with the timeline for when the findings are expected. Key-informant interviews of community leaders take much longer than surveys of parents attending the "author's tea" event to read the books their children have written. If using guidelines against which a program will be measured, the responses can be numeric on a Likert-type scale (i.e., 0—Does not exist, 3—Polices in place but not used consistently, 5—Procedure in place and used by all staff consistently). Additional information can then be gathered that provides evidence (such as school board policies or school building procedures, brochures, etc.), and any clarifying comments that identify gaps, barriers, or ways to improve the particular item being assessed.
4. Establish a plan to **synthesize data** in order to determine how data will be reviewed, summarized, and reported.
5. **Set priorities** based on availability of resources and the purpose of the assessment. Consider opportunities for change. Find the weaknesses and determine what actions could be taken to improve the situation. Consider the strengths and see what additions or changes can be made to make the assessment even stronger. This is the time to select the priority components for action, and then write actions or strategies as recommendations. For each recommendation, consider the variables that could impact success, such as commitment, feasibility, cost, or time.
6. **Set goals, action steps, resources needed, and timeline**. Clearly state the goals and objectives of the program improvement plan. Describe the specific steps that need to be taken to ensure successful completion of each stated goal. Outline the resources needed to ensure successful completion of this task, such as time, funding, people, materials, technical assistance, and expertise. Determine when and how the progress will be checked.
7. **Measure progress** by describing the process measures or steps that have been taken. At that time, outline the expected and unexpected outcomes.
8. **Communicate** how the summary of information and the priority(ies) will be communicated to those involved, including the school, families, and community members.
9. **Anticipate the next steps.** Once the evaluation is done, for those goals that were accomplished, what needs to be in place to ensure continued success? What goals and actions need to be continued? Priorities were set at the beginning of the project in the assessment phase. Determine if the next priority areas are still pertinent. Analyze what has changed (i.e., the key people involved, the team or network of people involved, community support) that will affect future steps. Then determine the steps needed to renew the investment and plan for continued work and determine the steps needed to increase investment and involvement for new work.

Community Assessment Approaches

The following paragraphs describe four different community assessment approaches.

Sight Seeing in Your Own Community

Once a week for 4 weeks, walk, take public transportation, or drive from the school in a different direction for 2 miles. The task is to see the resources the community provides. Look for indicators of basic needs, such as safety, access to goods and services (food, clothing, medical services, social services), transportation, recreation for all ages, libraries, arts, cultural and spiritual centers, and open space. Observe who is in the community, including their ages, race, and ethnicity. What types of employment are available? Is the community stable or fluid? What needs of the community are not being met? The hazards can be noted as well as gaps in services. A variation of this "tour" is to ride the school bus to the end of the line once a week for 4 weeks in four different directions. Students of different ages could act as travel guides.

This informative community assessment is a useful orientation to the community for new school staff. Two or three new staff could journey together. The joint observers would share and analyze their findings and present their "travel log" to other staff. It would be useful for experienced educators, too, to travel their routine route "wearing a new pair of glasses." The best results come from different disciplines or roles within a school sharing the "trip."

Key to the City—Key Informant, That Is

People who know the "lay of the land" have a way of watching the comings and goings in a community; they know how it operates and how it has changed over time. They know the nooks and crannies that are either a haven or a danger. It is well known that, at school, key informants are the building engineer or lead custodian and the school secretary. In the community, this person is not likely to be the elected official or head of the medical clinic, but the "beat cop," the community bus driver, or the matriarch or grandmother in a housing complex. It may be the parents of students who have figured out how to navigate the social service system to get their children's needs met. The approach is not to pepper key informant with questions, but to provide open-ended comments from which they can launch into sharing their perspective and wisdom. For example, "That old school building on the corner has seen children and families come and go year after year. [pause, pause, pause] It is hard for someone like me, new to the school, to know whether or not things have changed...." The first statement is likely to elicit a response—and the second can be used to nudge informants, if necessary. They may comment on the changing needs of students, education standards, instructional methods, or school climate; or about demographics of the families in the community (stable or mobile). In a second conversation, the school nurse could ask more specific questions on how new families get services or what needs to happen at school to make it a more inviting place for parent involvement. To compare and contrast, a follow-up conversation regarding the structure and processes in the community with the formal operators (the law enforcement head, the city manager, a county administrator, etc.) is helpful.

Birdseye View

A more formal approach to community assessment includes a wide range of information about the infrastructure of a community (roads and bridges, transportation, water supply, electrical and gas supply, emergency services, revenue resources and expenditures, communication vehicles, weather, public schools and public services) and the population (age, race, family structure, income, and mobility). Much of the information is readily available on existing databases, through county offices and through the internet. City and county officials have long-range plans that would provide a broad perspective on community needs. Public health agencies write periodical plans based on a complex assessment of the age of the population, health status, health needs, health services, and the effectiveness of protection measures. Social services and law enforcement have similar planning processes.

What use are these data sources and plans to the school nurse? Suppose that the focus is on the kindergarten children entering school for the first time. Is the foundation being laid at school and by parents going to serve the children well in 10 years when they enter high school? What will the community be like so that schools and families can begin early to equip them with relevant knowledge and skills? The school nurse and other student services staff are members of the educational team specially prepared to view children in the context of their families and communities and can bring this information to school program planning.

Back to the Basics

Although community perspectives are important, equally important to consider are some strategies to assess school programs. The framework of Linking Health and Learning and the Comprehensive Prevention Model for Schools discussed previously provide direction to discovering the current status of programming and to planning for better coordination and integration. Best used for one issue at a time, mapping the extent to which the six health risk behaviors identified by the CDC would provide a solid foundation for planning. For example, are there students who are obese who are having difficulty being present and participating fully? Are their academics suffering or are they becoming disconnected from school? Is the school climate interfering (name-calling, long lunch lines, and a short time to eat and digest food; snack and pop/soda machines present)? Is information being sent home to parents? In the community, are schools the only place for children and youth to gather? Using the grid, educators can review the four components of policy, curriculum/instruction, student services, and family involvement. Community connections in each of the four components can then be examined for consistency, overlaps, and gaps.

SET PRIORITIES FOR SCHOOL NURSING

Given the many features of school programs that connect to the health of students, what areas are integrally connected to school nursing and school health services? In what order should the school nurse tackle community assessments and school action plans, and build collaborative partnerships? First, consider the plan that ensures an immediate response to life-threatening emergencies and provides for the safety of individuals as well as the population of children and adults in the school. Then proceed to responses to episodic illness, managing chronic illnesses, reducing behavior problems, and then on to health promotion. While many would like to first focus on health promotion and health education, the plans need to be in place for crisis interventions first.

School nurses who work in a large school system and are affiliated with public health agencies or healthcare settings, most likely can be assured that crisis response plans are in place. But they need to understand the steps, roles, referrals, and resources of their own school(s). As many schools are experiencing high turnover in staff every few years, new staff may not have had staff development on the strategies at the school.

The school nurse has to consider whether, at each response level, the needs of individual students are being addressed and if a school-wide plan should also be in place. Then the question is, Who are the potential partners in a school-community assessment? When meeting with key community leaders, such as emergency medical personnel and law enforcement staff, remember these people can be key informants and provide information on many fronts, such as the perception of the school's education program and/or its readiness to respond to emergencies. TABLE 19.9 outlines the problems that may be encountered in schools and the need for collaboration in developing plans to address these problems.

Table 19.9 ■
PLANS FOR RESPONDING AT DIFFERENT LEVELS OF NEED

PLAN FOR RESPONDING	INDIVIDUAL LEVEL	SCHOOL-WIDE LEVEL	PARTNERS
Emergencies—crisis response plan	Major injury Health crisis If a student with an IHP or IEP, check for an Emergency Plan.	Fire, flood, air quality, threats, endangerment Check evacuation plans for students with Emergency Plans and special needs.	EMT, police, fire, hospital Providers of public safety protection. Public Health if there is a biological, chemical, or infectious agent.
Episodic illness or minor injury—need standard protocols	Individual assessment, intervention and/or referral	If in epidemic proportions, consult public health	Physician/other healthcare provider. Public Health if it is a reportable disease.
Chronic condition including mental illness or chemical use—need protocols	See the IHP Work with Student Assistance Team	Assess contributing factors, if any. (ex., air quality—asthma)	Physician/other healthcare provider. Counselor/therapist. Law enforcement regarding illegal substances

(continued)

PLAN FOR RESPONDING	INDIVIDUAL LEVEL	SCHOOL-WIDE LEVEL	PARTNERS
Health risk behaviors—violence—Student Assistance Team	Individual assessment intervention and/or referral	Address negative social norms	Healthcare provider Public Health Social Services Youth-Serving Agencies
Sensory problems (vision and hearing) that affect learning; consult spec. ed. Health education/promotion and creating social norms.	Individual assessment intervention and/or referral Individual ed. for vulnerable students to reinforce skills.	Screening program, Assess for other factors—noise Classroom—improve skills School-wide address norms	Healthcare provider Public Health Healthcare providers Media Youth-Serving agencies
Social norms that support student learning and schools	Individual ed. for vulnerable students to reinforce skills		Healthcare providers Public Health Social Service Youth-Serving Agencies

Sources: Adapted from several sources including DOE (2003).

Much like the actions steps described in the section on community assessment, collaboratives begin with identifying who are the existing partners and natural/logical partners. Adelman and Taylor (1998) outlined eight dimensions to consider: (1) Who initiates the collaborative (school or community) or does it emerge out of an existing partnership? (2) Is it a formal or informal arrangement? (3) Is the focus on programs or services or is systemic change the goal? (4) What is the scope: a few programs or a comprehensive effort? (5) Is the potential impact for a few families or is it broad to all who need services? (6) Who owns and governs the programs and services? (7) Is the program located in the school or is it community-based and school-linked? and (8) What degree of cohesiveness exists—unconnected to coordinated to integrated? TABLE 19.10 presents a way of looking at the phases of working in a partnership.

Table 19.10 ■
PHASES OF WORKING IN PARTNERSHIPS

Create the vision.	Working together does not mean it has to be for the same reasons. For example, if public health agencies want to improve the immunity of preschoolers and the schools want to improve attendance in the first days of kindergarten, both share the vision of getting children immunized before schools start in September.
Determine the structure, roles, resources and ways to resolve conflict.	A lot of energy can be put into defining structure and roles. If mired in the logistics, the real question may not be who is supposed to do what, but whether or not the vision is clear and people have buy-in. It may be that there has not been enough time and experience to build relationships and trust. Get consensus on and rehearse the way conflicts will be handled long before conflicts emerge.

(continued)

Table 19.10 ■ *(Continued)*

Make promises.	People need to feel the energy that something positive and important is going to happen.
Keep changes small and attractive.	Who will be asked to make changes? Who is going to be affected by the changes? Are both parties included in the discussion and planning?
Plan for success.	Review proposed changes in terms of their:
	Relative advantage—Will the improvement at least match or exceed the hassle?
	Compatibility—Do the changes fit with the rest of the program? Do the changes work, personality wise, with those making changes?
	Complexity—If it can't be understood or looks too hard, it can't be done.
	Trial-ability—Will small steps work vs. leaping in all at once?
	Observe-ability—Will we or anyone else see anything happening for all the time and effort we are putting in?
Manage the work; recognize shared and unique contributions.	Keep track of tasks and how things are progressing.
	Celebrate each step of the way and name each person and their contributions via written (newsletter, awards) and verbal messages. Surprise acknowledgments are rewarding, too.
Keep track; make change based on data.	Count as you go along—because outcome change takes a long time. For example, if program participation is one step toward the vision, count people who show up, call, respond to e-mails, who read the flier and do activities with their children, who comment 2 weeks later. Don't drop a program because the number of people who attended was low.
Reward and celebrate continuous improvement.	Check on every aspect of the initiative—are the meetings getting better; are more people hearing about the change; is the newsletter getting crisper, do new people know how to post things to the web, as someone new volunteered because the group looks like they are getting something done?

Sources: Adapted from Ray (2002); Steckler et al. (1992); Winer (1994).

CONCLUSION

In summary, linking health and learning involves the interactive factors of personal student characteristics, family supports, and community supports. The comprehensive prevention model engages parents and communities in the components of school programming that need to be coordinated. In the role of collaborator, the school nurse connects with parents to support the health, growth, development, and student's academic success. Multiple considerations need to be included in referral decisions. The nursing process is mirrored in the community assessment process which guides the school nurse in a systematic, comprehensive, and accountable approach to the role of school nurse as collaborator with students, the school, healthcare providers, family, and the community.

In the words of Ferber, Pittman, and Marshall (2002):

Children and youth grow up in families and communities, not programs.
Problem-free is not fully prepared.
Fully prepared is not necessarily fully engaged.
Academic competence, while critical, is not enough.
Children and youth need services, supports and opportunities.
Investments begin early and must be sustained.

References

Adelman, H., & Taylor, L. (1999). *School–community partnership: A guide. Los Angeles, CA: University of California at Los Angeles, Center for Mental Health in Schools.*

American Academy of Pediatrics (AAP). (2004). *School health: Policy & practice*. Elk Grove, IL: Author.

American Association for Health Education. (2005). *National health education standards (proposed)* . Retrieved April 2005 from http://www.aahperd.org/aahe/template.cfm

Benson, P., Roehlkepartan, E., & Sesma, A. (2004). Tapping the power of community: The potential of asset building to strengthen substance abuse prevention efforts. *Search Institute Insights and Evidence*, *2*(1). Accessed October 2005 from www.search-institute.org/research/Insights/

Bogden, J. (January, 2003). *How schools work and how to work with schools. A primer for professionals who serve children and youth*. Alexandria, VA: National Association of State Boards of Education.

Button, J., & Rienzo, B. (2002). *The politics of youth, sex, and health care in American schools*. New York: The Haworth Press.

Costante, C. (January, 2002). Healthy learners, The link between health and student achievement. *American School Board Journal*, 1–3. Retrieved October 2004 from http://www.nsba.org

DeBord, K. (2001). *Redefining parent involvement: Parents making a difference in their child's lives*. Electronic handout used in conjunction with a live interactive telephone conference. North Carolina State University Extension Programs. Dec. 11, 2001. Retrieved October 14, 2002 from http://www.cyfernet.org/training/parenthandout.html.

Dryfoos, J., & Magure, S. (2002). *Inside full-service community schools*. Thousand Oaks, CA: Sage.

Education Development Center (EDC). (2003). *Health is academic: Action steps*. Newton, MA: Author. Retrieved May 2003 from http://www2.edc.org/makinghealthacademic/Concept/actions_family.asp

Ferber, T., & Pittman, K., with Marshall, T. (2002). *State youth policy: Helping all youth to grow up fully prepared and fully engaged*. Takoma Park, MD: The Forum for Youth Investment. Retrieved August 2005 from http://www.forumforyouthinvestment.org/issues/focus.htm

Geierstanger, S., Amaral, G., Mansour, M., & Walters, S. (2004). School-based health centers and academic performance: Research, challenges, and recommendations. *Journal of School Health, 74*(9), 347–352.

Kahn, J. (2000). *Keynote presentation: Effective youth programs and their elements*. Community Health Services Statewide Conference, Cragun's Resort, Brainerd, September 15, 2000. Fore related information, see http://www.allaboutyouth.umn.edu

Kaye, G. (2001). Grassroots involvement. *American Journal of Community Psychiatry, 29*(2), 269–275.

Luehr, R. E. (2004). *Linking health and learning*. Roseville, MN: Minnesota Department of Education, Safe and Healthy Learners Section.

McNeely, C., Nonnemaker, J., & Blum, R. (2002). Promoting school connectedness: Evidence from the National Longitudinal Study of Adolescent Health. *Journal of School Health, 72*(4), 138–146.

Minnesota Department of Education (MDE), formerly the Department of Children, Families and Learning (CFL), Learner Support Services). (2003). *Six briefs: Minnesota Student Survey 2001: Tobacco use associated with alcohol and other drug use, academic success, school connectedness, mental health, violence and other antisocial behaviors, parents as partners*. Roseville, MN: Author.

Minnesota Department of Education (MDE), Safe and Healthy Learners Team. (2004). *Comprehensive prevention model for schools*. Roseville, MN: Author.

Minnesota Prevention Resource Center (MPRC). (2002). *See it, say it*. Moundsview, MN: Author. http://www.emprc.org/index.html. (Minnesota Institute of Public Health (http://www.miph.org), the Midwest Center for Applied Prevention Technology.

Mostert, M. (1998). *Interprofessional collaboration in schools*. Boston: Allyn and Bacon.

National Association of School Nurses (NASN). (2001). Position Statement. *The role of the school nurse in school based health centers*. Retrieved January 8, 2005 from http://www.nasn.org/positions/schoolbased.htm

National Association of School Nurses (NASN) and the American Nurses Association (ANA). (2001). *Scope and standards of professional school nursing practice*. Scarborough, ME: National Association of School Nurses.

National Association of School Nurses (NASN) and other agencies. (2004). *Joint statement on the school nurse/school-based health center partnership*. Retrieved January 8, 2005 from http://www.nasn.org/statements/schoolbasedjoint.htm

National Parent–Teacher Association (National PTA). (2003). *National standards for parent/family involvement programs*. Chicago, IL: Author. Retrieved April 2005 from http://www.pta.org/parentnvolvement/standards

National Staff Development Council (NSDC). (2002). *NSDC standards for staff development*. Retrieved January 2005 from http://www.nsdc.org/standards/index.cfm

Novak, J. (2000). Community health nurse in the school. In M. Stanhope & J. Lancaster (Eds.), *Community and public health nursing* (pp. 908–940). St. Louis: C. V. Mosby.

Partnerships for Family Involvement in Education (PFIE). (1998). *Join together for kids! How communities can support family involvement for kids*. Washington, DC: Department of Education.

Ray, K. (2002). *The nimble collaboration: Fine tuning your collaboration for lasting success*. Saint Paul, MN: Amherst H. Wilder Foundation.

Schwab, N., & Gelfman, M. (2001). *Legal issues in school health services*. North Branch, MN: Sunrise River Press.

Simpson, A. R. (2001). *Raising teens: A synthesis of research and a foundation for action*. Boston: Center for Health Communication, Harvard School of Public Health.

Steckler, A., Goodman, R., McLeroy, K., Davis, S., & Koch, G. (1992). Measuring the diffusion of innovative health promotion programs. *American Journal of Health Promotion, 6* (3), 214–224.

Surgeon General. (2000). *Surgeon general's report*. Atlanta, GA: U.S. Department of Health and Human Services, Centers for Disease Control and Prevention.

Svendsen, R., Luehr, R., & Helke, L. (2003). *Student assistance model for tobacco use intervention*. Moundsview, MN: Minnesota Institute for Public Health.

Swider, S., & Valukas, A. (2004). Options for sustaining school-based health centers. *Journal of School Health, 74* (4), 115–118.

U.S. Department of Education (USDOE). (2003). *Practical information on crisis planning: A guide for schools and communities*. Washington, DC: Author. http://www.ed.gov/emergencyplan.

U.S. Department of Health and Human Services (USDHHS), National Clearinghouse on Families and Youth. (2005). *Youth development*. Retrieved April 2005 from http://www./ncfy.com/youthdev/p.htm

White, B. (Summer 2001). How to make a successful referral. *Student Assistance Journal*, pp. 14–18.

Winer, R. (1994). *Collaboration handbook: Creating, sustaining and enjoying the journey*. Saint Paul, MN: Amherst H. Wilder Foundation.

Chapter 20

Health Promotion

JANICE SELEKMAN

Chapter Outline

INTRODUCTION

From its inception, health promotion and disease prevention have been at the foundation of school nursing practice. This focus stems from the public health perspective that was the impetus for hiring the first school nurse, Lina Rogers; her role was to decrease communicable disease, improve health, and improve school attendance. The National Association of School Nurses (NASN) states the following in their *Scope and Standards of Professional School Nursing Practice*: "School nurses…utilize a public health focus in their practice…Programs and health services are offered – with the goal of prevention – to individual students as well as to the entire school community" (NASN & ANA, 2001, p. 3).

The Public Health model reflects the health continuum with wellness at one end of the continuum and illness at the other. The goal is to have individuals function at their greatest level of wellness and to improve the health of society as a whole. Therefore, the focus on the wellness end becomes that of promoting health and preventing disease. These goals are explained by using the three levels of prevention: primary, secondary, and tertiary, developed by Leavell and Clark in 1965 based on the way disease evolves over time, as well as the components of health promotion.

LEVELS OF HEALTH PROMOTION AND DISEASE PREVENTION

The definition of primary prevention has changed since it was first conceived with a focus on disease prevention. It now extends to the promotion of health. Health promotion involves activities that are designed to promote the overall health of the population. It extends far beyond just preventing disease; it aims to maximize human potential and well-being and promote self-responsibility for health. Promoting health should lead to a decrease in disease and changing patterns of behavior with positive healthy results. Examples of interventions for health promotion include healthy eating, maintaining personal hygiene and dental care, being physically active, stimulating the mind, keeping safe, and getting enough rest.

Secondary prevention includes those interventions that detect disease or alterations in health and development early in their occurrence, ideally before signs and symptoms are apparent or at the very earliest signs of a problem. "Emphasis is on resolving health problems and preventing serious consequences" (Clark, 2003, p. 7). Nursing has always promoted the benefits of early detection and the fact that early intervention results in much more positive outcomes than delayed intervention. Early case finding in infectious disease can prevent the spread to others.

A major component of secondary prevention by the school nurse includes all of the screening programs performed to detect problems such as hearing and vision deficits; postural problems; alterations in height, weight, or blood pressure; the presence of pediculosis; exposure to tuberculosis; dental problems; and mental health concerns. Encouraging staff to have Pap smears to detect cervical cancer and to perform breast or testicular self-exams are examples of secondary prevention. Screening both students and staff for tuberculosis using the purified protein derivative (PPD) is also an example of secondary prevention. Other examples include promoting annual physicals, especially for staff and older students, promoting annual dental check-ups, and promoting ways to decrease stress.

Screening is a labor-intensive, preliminary process to sort out those who may have the problem from those who may not. "A screening test is not a diagnostic test" (Clark, 2003, p. 146). Screening may be a way to identify students who are at high risk for a particular condition. In screening, some sort of a tool or test is used, usually for those without obvious symptoms, for the purpose of identifying if they may be having a problem. It is an assessment but not a definitive tool; positive findings form the basis for a referral for further assessment and diagnostic testing to evaluate whether the problem actually exists. Screening is used for large population groups; its aim is to provide early detection and interventions for a more favorable prognosis. Screening also assists a school or district to understand the existence or the extent of a particular problem in its district, such as obesity or hypertension.

Screening tools must have reliability and validity. Reliability refers to consistency in getting the same results each time and place a tool is used and for any given person on whom it is used. Validity indicates that the test measures what it says it does and correctly classifies participants. It includes that the tool is sensitive to accurately identify those with the condition and specific enough to exclude those who do not have the condition. In addition, some tools are more reliable at specific ages or developmental stages; therefore screenings may occur too early or late to be at the optimal time for a particular student. The Denver Developmental Screening Tool is an example of a tool that loses its validity after children reach the age of 6 years.

Many tools need to be calibrated on a schedule recommended by the manufacturer in order to assure reliability. For example, the pure tone audiometer should be calibrated annually to current standards. Effective screening tools and programs should also be cost effective, easy to administer to large groups, and acceptable to the school population. "This means that the test should not be overly painful, embarrassing, or anxiety provoking" (Clark, 2003, p. 337).

Tertiary prevention includes interventions initiated with those who have already been diagnosed with a disease or condition. Its aim is to interrupt the progression of the condition in order to decrease the amount of morbidity or complications that are possible or to treat the complications to prevent them from worsening. It is also aimed at preventing a condition from recurring or exacerbating (Clark, 2003). Having educational programs to empower students with asthma to identify their triggers or having support groups to boost the morale of those with attention deficit hyperactivity disorder (ADHD) are examples of tertiary prevention. This chapter focuses on primary prevention, including health promotion, and secondary prevention with a focus on screening. Information on immunizations is provided in Chapter 21.

HEALTH PROMOTION INTERVENTIONS

School nurses frequently use their role as educator to relay the messages of how to stay healthy and prevent illness and disability. They may teach a structured class in a classroom or arrange an assembly for a grade or for the entire school. These challenge the nurse to plan, develop, implement, and evaluate the lesson or program. The principles used in developing a lesson plan or a program as well as the principles of teaching are discussed in Chapter 7. Health promotion and motivational posters hanging throughout the school and especially in the health office can provide reinforcement of ways to promote health. Role modeling regarding exercise and nutritional intake are other ways to promote health indirectly. Finally, assuring that school policies promote health is essential and affords the school nurse with an opportunity to provide education to the public as well as to school staff.

Many schools rely on the income generated from vending machines (see Chapter 47). Often, these machines dispense soda and snack items that have a high fat, sodium, or sugar content with little nutritional value. Consumption of large quantities of snacks and soda are in opposition to teaching good nutrition and may contribute to the national epidemic of obesity in children and adolescents. School budget constraints may also have impacted on students' access to physical education. In addition, many schools have fund-raising projects that promote students selling candy or other snack foods. Policies to curtail or change these activities can emphasize the school district's support for health promotion.

Youth risk behavior surveys can provide data to the school regarding the high-risk behaviors in which students engage. Health promotion programs in the school setting should target those identified risk behaviors to enhance the safety of students and to prevent future problems. These might include bike safety programs if it is found that students are not wearing bike helmets; seat belt or car restraint programs if it is found that students are not wearing seat belts or are not properly restrained; or an emphasis on hand-washing during outbreaks of respiratory illness.

Primary prevention includes interventions that alter susceptibility, reduce exposure, and prevent disease from developing. It usually is directed toward those who may be susceptible to a condition or disease but have no apparent pathology (McKeown & Weinrich, 2002). It includes health promotion/health protection activities within primary prevention. Examples of primary prevention include:

- Helping preteens avoid high-risk behaviors
- Providing immunizations, including annual protection against influenza
- Providing education on or condom distribution to promote barrier protection against disease and pregnancy
- Promoting the use of seat belts or bicycle helmets
- Teaching proper ways to brush one's teeth
- Providing teen parenting classes on how to handle the challenges of providing for an infant's needs
- Providing anticipatory guidance to parents regarding the next stage of development their child is entering
- Promoting environmental measures or public policies to protect the environment (i.e., prohibiting smoking in school buildings, assuring minimum standards for water and air quality, and protection against occupational hazards)

SCREENING INTERVENTIONS

Screening mandates or guidelines may be written into state law or they might be determined by the school district. Regardless of mandate, the school nurse may identify a need to screen a student or to recommend that a student be screened for a particular condition based on symptoms displayed in the school setting. Therefore, it is important for the school nurse to understand the principles of the various screening modalities. Some states mandate that school nurses be certified in their screening techniques; this chapter is not meant to replace those mandates. It is essential for the school nurse to know which students are to be screened each year; the protocols that are to be followed for notification of students, parents, and staff; and the dates by which screening is to be completed.

Preparing Parents, Personnel, and Students

Parents should be notified that the screening is required, when it will be done, and how the results will be communicated to them. Some districts also require parent/guardian permission; if this is the case, the amount of time needed to prepare for the screening is significantly increased.

Teachers and support staff also need to be prepared for the screening and the process needs to ensure minimal class disruption. Teachers and staff appreciate ample notification to schedule work and lesson plans around the screening. They are likely to be more cooperative if they understand the purpose and value of screenings. For example, a brief note to the staff describing the obesity epidemic, potential complications that arise from being overweight as a child or adolescent, and how these can impact school performance will help to increase understanding of the importance of screening for body mass index during the growth screening. They also need to know how many students to send and at what intervals.

Preparation of students should include short presentations or written explanations, depending on the grade level, to help them understand the importance of the screening, especially how it impacts on their education; their preparation should include the concept of a "range of normal," how everyone's body is different, and how growth changes at different ages. The extent to which this preparation is conducted is dependent on the school nurse's resources. Ideally, some of the discussion can take place as part of a health lesson.

If volunteers or assistive personnel are used to help with the screening process, they must be trained; they must demonstrate accurate techniques in the various screening processes and must have had training in FERPA (Family Educational Rights and Privacy Act; see Chapter 13), to ensure confidentiality of student information. Some districts require volunteers to sign a "memo of understanding" that addresses their role and their pledge of confidentiality. One governmental resource is HRSA's (Health Resources and Services Administration) Maternal and Child Health Bureau's training modules, which are online interactive modules that provide instruction on measuring and weighing techniques. They can be accessed at: http://www.cdc.gov/nccdphp/dnpa/growthcharts/training/modules/module1/text/mainmodules.htm. Ensure that all materials are in place and that they are age-appropriate and developmentally appropriate. Interpretation of the screening results is the responsibility of the school nurse and should not be delegated to volunteer help.

Height Measurement

Growth and development parameters are assessed to ensure that students are attaining expected levels. Growth, by definition, just means an increase in size. Therefore, growth implies height and weight. Accurate assessment of growth is dependent on accurate measurements. Growth charts were revised in 2000 by the Centers for Disease Control and Prevention to reflect norms of white, black, and Mexican-American children (Kuczmarski, Ogden, Grummer-Strawn et al., 2000). They can be downloaded from the CDC Web site: http://www.cdc.gov/growthcharts/

In evaluating the results that will be plotted on the charts, it is more important to identify those who cross over percentiles than those who are consistently in one percentile over time, even if it is always the 5th percentile, as these may represent cultural norms. Crossing over multiple percentiles in a short amount of time warrants further assessment, as this is not a normal occurrence. There is no evidence that children in one percentile are healthier than those in another (Chumlea & Guo, 2004).

It is essential that a quality stadiometer be used for height measures. One type is permanently fixed to the wall; the second type is portable. Ideally, the stadiometer should be permanently installed with the use of a level. An appropriate stadiometer requires a vertical ruled board or bar with a horizontal headpiece that can be brought into contact with the most superior part of a student's head. The base of the stadiometer should be a wide and stable platform on a firm, uncarpeted floor.

Accurate measurement of stature requires the use of a calibrated, vertical stadiometer with a movable headpiece, perpendicular to the vertical backboard. If a stadiometer is not available, the school nurse can tack wooden yardsticks to the wall and use something light, such as a Plexiglas bookend that is fixed at a 90-degree angle. The stadiometer should be able to measure to 0.1 cm or 1/8-inch increments and should be easy to read.

The student should stand on the footplate of the stadiometer without shoes. The student is positioned with his or her back to the backboard, heels close together, legs straight, arms at sides, shoulders relaxed, head looking straight ahead. There are four contact points between the body and the stadiometer: the head, upper back, buttocks, and heels. Ask the student to inhale deeply and to stand fully erect without altering the position of the heels. Make sure that the heels do not rise off the footplate. Lower the perpendicular headpiece snugly to the crown of the head with sufficient pressure to compress the hair. Hair ornaments, buns, braids, and so forth must be removed to obtain an accurate measurement. To ensure an accurate reading, the nurse's eyes should be parallel with the headpiece. Record height to the nearest 1 cm or 1/4 inch.

Height attachments on beam balance scales should never be used to measure height. They produce inaccurate readings because as the student steps on the weighing platform, it naturally sinks from the weight of the child. It is also often unsteady, and the headpiece is too narrow, often floppy, and rather pointed and sharp, which could result in an injury to a child and an inaccurate reading.

Weight Measurement

Recommended scales for weighing students are either a quality beam balance or electronic scale that can be easily calibrated. The scale should weigh children in 100-gram or 1/4-pound increments and have a large enough platform to support the student being weighed. The scale should be able to be "zeroed." Beam balance scales usually have "screw type" apparatus for immobilizing the zeroing weight. The scale should be calibrated on a regular basis according to manufacturer instructions.

Box 20.1 ■ ■ ■

SCALE CHECKLIST

- Private location
- High-quality beam balance or electronic digital
- Weights in 0.1 kg (100 g) or $^1/_4$-lb increments
- Weight can be "locked" in.
- Weight is read at "eye level" of measurer.
- Stable weighing platform
- Can be easily "zeroed."
- Can be calibrated.
- No wheels on scale.
- Hand post attached to base of scale.
- No stature device attached.

(Adapted from: HRSA Maternal and Child Health Bureau Growth Chart Training Module at http://depts.washington.edu/growth)

Standard weights should be available to calibrate the scale (Box 20.1).

Bathroom scales are spring balance scales and should not be used to weigh students. The spring counterbalance loses accuracy over time. Many spring balance scales cannot be read accurately to less than one-half pound, and the reading is often difficult to note exactly, since the dial is on the floor rather than at eye level.

Privacy is not an option, but rather an expectation for weighing students and recording information. Weight measures should not be announced for others to hear. The results are treated as confidential health information, although this does not prohibit the school nurse from informing the individual student of his or her results.

Students are weighed wearing only lightweight clothing. All shoes should be removed, without exception. All extra layers of clothing should be removed so the student is wearing just one top garment when weighed. Pants or skirts are not removed in a school screening setting. Screenings conducted during warm seasons will lessen the possibilities of multiple layered and heavy clothing compromising accuracy. Screenings conducted in collaboration with physical education classes may allow for students to be in lighter gym attire of t-shirts and shorts.

The student should stand in the center of the scale platform. Weight is recorded to the nearest 0.1 kg or $^1/_4$ pound. Once measurements are recorded, note their consistency with the student's measurement from previous screenings. Height and weight should fall at approximately the same percentile range with each screening. A significant percentile change should be rechecked for errors in measuring, recording, or graphing.

Body Mass Index Measurement

Once an accurate height and weight have been obtained, the Body Mass Index (BMI) can be determined. The difference of an inch or more in height, or weight that is off by several pounds, may cause a student to be mislabeled. BMI is a commonly accepted index for classifying adiposity. Although it does not directly measure body fatness, BMI parallels changes obtained by direct measures of body fat, such as underwater weighing. BMI can be considered a proxy for measures of body fat (see Chapter 36 on obesity). BMI is the result of a mathematical calculation and can be determined with the algebraic formula using either metric or English measurements. It is calculated by dividing a person's weight in kilograms by the square of the person's height in meters.

BMI for children is gender specific and based on age, and is best represented as a percentile measurement rather than an index number. A fixed BMI cutoff is used for older adolescents and adults (i.e., adult BMI $\geq$ 30 is considered obese). However, a child's BMI changes substantially as he or she gets older. After about 1 year of age, BMI-for-age begins to decline and continues falling during the preschool years until it reaches a minimum around 4 to 6 years of age. After 4 to 6 years, BMI-for-age begins a gradual increase through adolescence. The rebound or increase in BMI that occurs after it reaches its lowest point is referred to as "adiposity rebound" (Kuczmarski et al., 2000).

BMI-for-age charts can be used with children and adolescents ages 2 to 20 years. Standardized in structions for measuring height and weight and BMI can be found on the CDC web site http://www.cdc.gov/growthcharts. (See Figures 16.3 and 16.4 for BMI charts for children and adolescents.) To determine the BMI value, the height and weight for age can be plotted on the CDC tables. These tables cross list height and weight measures in both metric and English, and do not require any mathematical calculations. BMI wheels may also be used; height and weight measurements can be aligned on the wheel. These wheels are inexpensive and can be purchased through most school nurse supply catalogs. CDC also provides an online calculator that can be used to calculate BMI: (http://www.cdc.gov/nccdphp/dnpa/growthcharts/bmi_tools.htm) by entering the height and weight measurements.

Once the BMI is determined, the student's age and gender are used to select the appropriate growth chart (BMI-for-age). There are separate growth charts for girls and boys. Find the student's age on the horizontal axis and the BMI value on the vertical axis to determine the BMI-for-age percentile (Kuczmarski et al., 2000). The score can then be interpreted (see Chapter 36 on obesity).

Growth is a fundamental characteristic of childhood and adolescence. A series of measures over time are valuable in illustrating a child's pattern of growth. Growth in children and adolescents is as unique as the individual child. Increases in height and weight are expected to different degrees at different ages. Deviations from the student's normal growth pattern may be early warning signs of some intrinsic illness/disease process or environmental insult. These deviations warrant referral.

Results should be reported to the family in a meaningful format. Avoid complicated graphs without clear explanation. Information should be sent home in a way that ensures privacy. While one school nurse sent results of student's height, weight, and BMI to the parents, another was reprimanded by her principal for doing so and told that this action was not permitted. It is strongly recommended that the school nurse work with the principal to develop a mechanism to share this information with parents.

Vision Screening

Vision is the process of the brain interpreting and then giving meaning to what is seen; the lens and the cornea refract or bend light rays to form a clear image. Tears are needed to flush the eyes and prevent infection. Vision is one of the last senses to mature. While hearing is present at birth, vision develops over the first 6 years of life (Proctor, 2005). Children with vision impairment are not usually aware of their deficit and therefore do not complain. Seeing things as blurred or distorted may just be interpreted as "normal" for them. This puts the onus of responsibility on the school nurse to identify these students so that measures can be taken early to stem the morbidity that can result, especially as it impacts on their ability to learn. Without intervention, there may be permanent vision loss, learning disabilities, emotional and behavioral problems, and school failure.

Many states require vision screening on entry into the school system. There may also be mandates to rescreen at specified intervals, such as kindergarten and grades 2, 4, 7, and 9, and prior to driver education classes, as well as all students being referred for special education. In other settings, the student is referred to the school nurse by the teacher because the student is squinting, missing material on the board, holding materials close to the eyes, having difficulty reading, covering or closing one eye, or blinking or rubbing the eyes a great deal. Students who visit the school nurse for frequent headaches, dizziness, and blurred vision would be other candidates for vision screening. The goal is to detect vision problems early, refer the student for visual correction, and allow the student with the resulting increased visual acuity to enhance his or her educational success.

Vision screening is a fairly quick and inexpensive way to identify potential eye problems among the school-age population. Vision is evaluated on its acuity, refraction, eye health, visual efficiency, and ability to process the information received. Acuity is the ability of the eye to see clearly near (10 to 13 inches—as in reading a book) and at a distance (>10 feet—as in reading a chalkboard). Refractive errors occur in 15% of children and account for half of the eye defects identified. They include defects in the way light enters the eye and hits the retina. Examples are visual acuity and astigmatism. Since vision problems increase with age, there is a need for screening throughout the school years (Ferebee, 2004). Refractive errors are treated with corrective lenses. Common vision defects are listed in Box 20.2.

Box 20.2 ■■■

VISION DEFECTS

Myopia—Nearsightedness; inability to focus on distant objects

Amblyopia—Decreased visual acuity in one eye; called "lazy eye." Often caused by strabismus. Treatment involves patching the good eye before age six before vision development is complete.

Astigmatism—Light cannot focus clearly on the retina, often causing blurred vision

Hyperopia—Farsightedness; inability to focus on nearby objects

Strabismus—Abnormal ocular alignment; deviation of one eye from point of fixation

Other areas of the eye are also assessed. Eye muscle coordination is the ability to have both eyes focus on a single image (binocular vision). Convergence is the ability to turn the eyes toward each other to focus on a close object; accommodation is the ability to change or maintain focus at different distances. Color deficiency is a condition seen most commonly in males and involves the reduced ability to distinguish colors. General eye health can be determined by ensuring that there is sufficient tearing and an absence of redness on the sclera and conjunctiva.

On any student visit with a complaint of an eye problem, the school nurse should observe for:

- Red or crusty eyelids
- Swelling of eyelids
- Red or pink sclera
- Haziness or clouding of the eye
- Pupil size
- Alignment of the eyes
- Drooping of the lids

When planning for vision screening, assessment of far and near visual acuity, as well as color discrimination should be assessed, although the color discrimination needs to be tested only once during the child's lifetime.

The following supplies are needed:

- A Snellen E chart, HOVT chart Good-Lite Tester, Lea symbols, or Allen Picture Chart, posted at eye level for the student for the 20/20 line or a Titmus Vision Testing Machine
- A plastic occluder (or cone-shaped cup)
- A good light source (subdued lighting in the room but good lighting near the chart—ensure that all glare is eliminated from the chart surface). Nothing should be in the field of vision brighter than the chart.
- Place a line or tape on the floor exactly 20 feet from the chart (or 10 feet if the 10-foot parameters are being used); have the student stand with his or her heels on the line. If seated, the back legs of the chair should be on the mark and the chart should be eye level.

Teach the student to use the occluder by covering one eye but keeping both eyes open. If the student wears glasses, the testing should be done with the glasses on (unless they are only used for close reading). For young children, go over the symbols or pointing needed before the testing begins. Expose one symbol or letter or line at a time. Test the right eye first, then the left, and then both. Start at the 20/40 line and move down to the 20/20 line. If the student is unable to read the 20/40 line, move upward. Failure to read more than half of the symbols on a line requires moving to the line above until visual acutely level is established. Usually, reading the majority of symbols on a line is considered passing (Proctor, 2005). Stop when the student does not pass a line and record the last line read correctly. (The numerator is the distance from the chart; the denominator indicates the line read correctly.)

If the Titmus machine is used, ensure that the head is placed up against the machine. The occluder is controlled by the examiner. Remember to clean the machine between students.

Not passing is usually considered to be 20/50 or a two-line difference between the right and left eye for those in kindergarten or younger and 20/40 for other students. If assistants are used to perform the initial screening, the rescreening should be completed by the school nurse 2 to 4 weeks later. Remember that "vision screening instruments are not diagnostic tools and therefore some children with vision problems, even if they are part of a screening program, will be missed" (Ferebee, 2004, p. 10).

Near Vision Acuity

Equipment needed for near vision assessment includes either a Titmus machine, plus lens glasses, or a hand-held chart. Use the same procedure as for far vision.

Muscle Tests

Often referred to as the alternate cover test or the cover/uncover test, these test eye alignment. Using the occluder and something handheld on which the student can focus (a sticker on the finger, a finger puppet, a penlight), hold the object 14 inches from the student and instruct him or her to look at the object. Cover one eye and observe the opposite eye; reverse the eye covered. The eye should not move. You can go back and forth between the eyes multiple times to check for movement. Do the same for a distant small object at 10 to 20 feet away. Move the occluder quickly between eyes without touching the student's face. Move objects to all four quadrants in an "H" pattern and then move the objects toward the nose. Observe for strabismus, nystagmus, diplopia, convergence, and smoothness of movement.

In some schools, depth perception is also measured. Using polarized glasses, have students look at the picture of a fly on a test plate that is held 16 inches away and ask them to pinch the wings between the thumb and forefinger. The child's fingers should remain above the picture; if the student pinches the surface of the test plate, he or she may fail. Make sure there is no glare on the test plate. There are other pictures and panels and the test comes with a scoring card.

Color discrimination is assessed using the Ishihara Color Test Plates or the Hardy-Rand Rittler Pseudoisochromatic Plates. Students are asked to read the numbers or trace shapes with their finger or to identify numbers or shapes. Color vision deficits cannot be corrected and may be in varying degrees. Interventions may include teaching the young students to read the colors on crayons. Blue may be easier to read than black. Vocational counseling suggesting avoidance of professions requiring color acuity may be appropriate for the older student.

NASN has published an outstanding comprehensive document on vision screening and the school nurse. Proctor's text (2005), *To See or Not to See*, provides the school nurse with all of the guidelines necessary to carry out a screening program as well as the knowledge base needed to understand vision and alterations in visual function.

Hearing Screening

Good hearing is essential to language development, and language development is essential for learning. Hearing loss contributes to educational delay and social isolation. Contrary to vision, hearing is mature at birth. Sound is caused by vibrations that travel through the air, tissue, and fluid of the ear and stimulates nerve endings of the cochlea that communicate to the brain, where it is recognized and interpreted. If sound is conducted through the bone to the cochlea, such as with a cochlear implant, it is interpreted but not "heard."

Sound is measured in decibels (loudness). Normal conversational speech is 50 to 70 decibels (NASN, 1998). For comparison, a refrigerator is approximately 40 decibels, a child screaming is 90 decibels, and a jet taking off is 130 decibels. In addition to loudness, sound has pitch, or high and low sounds. This is measured in Hertz, or the frequency/number of cycles per second of pure tone. Low tone would be 250 Hertz as in the sound of a bullfrog; high tone would be 4000 Hertz as in the sound of a whistling teakettle. The threshold is the softest level at which a person can hear the frequencies.

Degrees and types of hearing loss are discussed in Chapter 27 (children with chronic conditions). Hearing can be affected by occlusion in the ear, such as by earwax, a perforated tympanic membrane, auditory nerve damage from loud noise or infection, an accumulation of fluid in the middle ear, or swollen adenoids. Therefore, there are multiple reasons why a student may not "'pass" the hearing screening. For some students, rescreening may be scheduled after the cold or allergy season has passed or after removal of cerumen. Conductive hearing loss occurs due to problems in the outer or middle ear; sensorineural hearing loss refers to nerve damage in the inner ear.

While school nurses perform many of the hearing screenings across the country, some states have hearing and speech therapists administering the screening. For the testing to be accurate, a soundproof area is preferred; if this is unavailable, a quiet area free from ambient noises (i.e., ringing phones, flushing toilets, hall traffic, music rooms, gymnasiums, or playgrounds) should be used. Rooms with acoustical tile, drapes on the windows, carpeting, and solid core doors help to eliminate extraneous noise. The room should be big enough for a table to hold the equipment and two chairs for the student and the examiner. An electrical outlet is also needed.

Audiometers are used to test hearing. They can measure both decibels (dB) and Hertz (Hz). The audiometer is plugged into an outlet and may need to warm up for 15 to 20 minutes. It can then be left on for the entire screening period. The examiner should test that sound is coming from both earpieces. The student's chair should face away from the machine so that the student cannot view the examiner pushing the buttons. Students should be instructed to raise their hand when they hear the noise. It doesn't matter which hand they raise.

For the headset to fit correctly, students should not have on earrings, headbands, glasses, or hair in front of their ear. Center and adjust the headset so that the microphone is lined up with the student's ear canal. In most sets, the red earpiece goes on the right ear. Set the decibel level according to state or district guidelines. Twenty decibels is usually the accepted screening level; if the environment has a fair amount of extraneous noise, the intensity level can be raised to 25dB. If the student cannot hear the tone at that level, raise the decibels until hearing occurs and record these. These students will be referred for further evaluation. The frequencies usually tested are 1,000, 2,000, and 4,000 Hz. Failure to respond at the recommended screening level at any frequency in either ear constitutes a failure and should be retested in 2 to 4 weeks.

Tones are pressed for 2 to 4 seconds. Because students may get into a rhythmic pattern of raising their hands, vary the pattern of presentation, that is, do two tones on one ear and one on the other, wait a longer interval between some tones, and have some follow immediately after the last. Testing for younger children can include Conditioned Play Audiometry, in which the child is instructed to complete a task, such as pointing to the picture mentioned or dropping a block in a basket when the sound is heard. A new device that can be used to test those with special needs or those who do not speak English directly measures otoacoustic emissions. These are low-level sounds generated by the outer hair cells of the cochlea in response to auditory stimuli if the person can hear. It looks somewhat like an otoscope and provides a printout of the results.

To increase reliability, annual calibrations are recommended for most hearing equipment by the manufacturers. It is recommended that the earpieces be wiped with a soft slightly damp cloth and that alcohol not be used.

Postural Screening

Postural screening was previously called orthopedic or scoliosis screening, since that is the major condition for which the screening is performed. Good posture refers to being in the standing position with a straight vertical alignment of the body from the top of the head midline over a straight spine, through the body's center, to the bottom of the feet. Good posture demonstrates equal height, left and right of the shoulders, hips, and knees. There should also be equal distance between the arms and the body. From the side, good posture is seen as an imaginary vertical line from the ear, through the shoulder, hip, knee, and ankle.

The screening process is to identify students who have physical findings that suggest postural deviation (Ryberg, 2004). Because there is insufficient evidence to support or refute the screening process to identify spinal curvatures, 17 states no longer mandate or recommend these assessments for all students. Spinal deformities are classified by their magnitude (the degree of the curve), the location on the spine (cervical, thoracic, or lumbar), the direction (right or left convexity or anterior or posterior), and the etiology (idiopathic, neuromuscular, or congenital).

Normally, "the cervical and lumbar spine are lordotic (curving forward or anterior) while the thoracic spine and sacrum are kyphotic (curving backward or posterior)" (Ryberg, 2004, p. 7). The most common deviations are kyphosis, lordosis, and scoliosis. Kyphosis presents as a rounded back, often resembling the "dowager hump" seen in osteoporosis of the elderly. It is an abnormal fixed posterior convexity of a segment of the spine (usually seen in the thoracic spine). It is a structural problem and may be due to trauma, congenital conditions, certain diseases, or secondary to surgical treatment of spinal tumors. Lordosis, also referred to as "sway back," is an abnormal exaggerated anterior convexity of a segment of the spine (usually seen in the lumbar spine). It is normal in the young toddler who is learning to walk, but may result later as a result of obesity, pregnancy, or certain neuromuscular disorders

Scoliosis is a lateral curvature of the spine greater than 10 degrees with or without a compensatory rotational component; the curve goes from side to side (Ryberg, 2004). Scoliosis occurs most commonly around the onset of puberty and the growth spurt, between the ages of 10 and 16. It occurs in 2% in 4% of the population, with a higher incidence in females than in males (4:1); females also often have a larger degree of curve. Scoliosis can also be caused by congenital anomalies and neuromuscular conditions such as muscular dystrophy and cerebral palsy. Usually the cause is unknown.

For about 20% of individuals with scoliosis, the curve continues to progress, although this is more common in females. "Girls with severe curves prior to onset of menses have a higher rate of curve progression and should be monitored closely" (Ryberg, 2004, p. 8). The most common type is a right mid-thoracic curve that curves around the heart.

Scoliosis can be functional or structural. Functional scoliosis is usually a function of an incorrect relationship between body parts; it can be due to a leg length discrepancy, poor posture, or a rapid growth spurt. Structural scoliosis is due to a fixed vertebral change.

Preparation for postural screening will result in a smoother process and greater student acceptance. Because students are often sensitive about exposing their bodies during the ages when screening normally occurs, students need to be informed about how the spine develops, why screening is necessary, and how it will be done. It should be stressed that privacy will be provided. Some school nurses recommend that students wear bathing suits under their clothes for that day so that their backs can be exposed and others recommend that dress codes be suspended for the day so that students can wear loose t-shirts. Others use physical education class as the time for the assessment, as the students are often in gym attire.

Screen males and females separately. Students should be allowed into the testing area only one at a time to preserve privacy. "Some school nurses suggest that there be a contrasting backdrop behind the student so that when the examiner is viewing the student's back, it is easier to see the contour of the back" (Ryberg, 2004, p. 15). The process takes about 30 seconds per student. The procedure for postural screening is described in Table 20.1.

Parents should be informed of the findings. Form letters are available through NASN or the school district may already have forms or standard wording to use.

Table 20.1 ■

PROCEDURE FOR POSTURAL SCREENING

STEPS	OBSERVATION
1. Ask the student to place his or her toes on a piece of tape that is on the floor. Instruct the student to stand erect with feet slightly apart, weight evenly distributed, hands hanging at sides, looking forward.	Observe from the front, side and back: • *Is the head midline?* • *Are the shoulders at equal heights?* • *Is space between arms and body the same?* • *Are the hips (waist) at equal heights?* • *Are the knees at equal heights?* • *Is there exaggerated roundness of upper back?* • *Is there exaggerated arch in lower back?* • *Is one shoulder blade higher than the other?* • *Does the spine appear to curve?*
2. While standing behind the student, have the student put hands together (as if diving) and bend forward at the waist. Ensure that the student's feet are 2 to 3 inches apart and knees are straight. The student's back should be horizontal to the floor. (This is called the Adams Forward Bend Test.)	• *Is one scapula higher than the other?* • *Is there a prominence or bulge on one side of the back?* • *Are the hip levels uneven?* • *Is there a curvature of the spine?** • *[View from side] Are there spinal humps?*
3. Have the student walk away from you a few steps and then turn and walk back.	• *Is there asymmetry of movement on walking?* • *Do the knees come together and the ankles are abducted? (genu valgum—knock-kneed)* • *Do the knees abduct when the feet are together? (genu varum—bow-legged)*

*Some measure the curvature or degree of rotation using a scoliometer. It can be placed directly across the student's back where the irregularity is most prominent. The "0" should be directly over the top ridge of the spine. Do not press down on the device; any reading >5 to 7 degrees should be rescreened or referred. A 5-degree angle of trunk rotation will result in a referral rate of approximately 12%. Referral might also be made if there is asymmetry in 2 or more areas of visual assessment.

Depending on school policy, referral is made or rescreening is scheduled in 3 to 6 months if there is a 5- to 7-degree angle of trunk rotation. (This corresponds to an approximately 20-degree curve.) While up to 12% of the student body may need rescreening, only 1% to 2% will require treatment. An X-ray film can determine the degree of curvature (referred to as the Cobb angle) and the degree of skeletal maturation. These factors will determine the treatment selection. Usually bracing is the initial treatment for moderate curvature above 25 degrees. There are different types of braces, but all are fitted to the student and are worn 23 hours a day over a t-shirt but under one's clothes. The school nurse can assist in ensuring compliance and should contact the parents if skin irritation is noted.

For angles greater than 40 degrees or for progression that continues after bone growth has finished, surgery with spinal fusion and insertion of rods and screws to stabilize the spine may be performed. Progression of untreated scoliosis can result in respiratory problems, spinal cord compression causing weakness or paralysis, persistent pain, or heart problems caused by an asymmetrical rib cage.

Screening for Exposure to Tuberculosis

Tuberculosis (TB) has been around for thousands of years and is caused by *Mycobacterium tuberculosis*. The incidence has decreased since 1992, but not in all states; however, there were still almost 15,000 cases in the United States in 2003 (CDC, 2004). Foreign-born individuals accounted for more than half of the cases, especially those from Mexico, Philippines, Vietnam, India, and China. TB is a communicable disease spread primarily by airborne particles expelled by someone with the disease. The particles can remain suspended in the air for several hours (USDHHS, 2000).

Although some of the tubercle bacilli are phagocytized by macrophages, others multiply within the alveolar macrophages. When the macrophages die, the bacilli can spread through the lymph channels and the blood stream to distant sites, in which TB can develop (i.e., the brain, kidneys, or bone). The body usually contains the infection. Although individuals in this group do not have the disease and cannot spread the infection, they do have circulating antibodies. "About 10% of infected persons will develop TB disease at some time in life" (USDHHS, 2000, p. 5) with half of these developing TB within the first year or two after exposure (USDHHS, p. 5).

TB is classified on a scale from 0 to 5 (TABLE 20.2). Screening for TB is accomplished using the Mantoux tuberculin skin test, in which 0.1 ml of purified protein derivative (PPD) tuberculin containing 5 tuberculin units is injected intradermally into the forearm to produce a wheal 6 mm to 10 mm in diameter. The reaction is read 48 to 72 hours after administration. This timing is crucial. A reaction that is seen in the first 48 hours is probably that of the neutrophils and macrophages responding to attack the foreign product, as they would any foreign antigen. This reaction only supports that the individual's immune system is working and not that he or she has had any contact with TB. At 48 hours post-administration, the specific antibodies to TB, if they are present, will attack at the administration site causing the reaction.

When reading the results, only the area of induration, which is the hardened raised palpable area, is measured. Even if a large area of the forearm is red and inflamed, but flat, it is not considered a positive reaction. "The diameter of the indurated area should be measured across the forearm (perpendicular to the long axis)" (USDHHS, 2000, p. 29). If no induration is present, record a zero (0 mm) as the results rather than using the word "negative." The results are interpreted according to TABLE 20.3.

False positives and negatives are possible; therefore, be careful in providing an interpretation to students and their parents. Some providers prefer to use a two-step method, in which the individual receives a PPD twice. The first injection is thought to boost the immune response; if it is negative, a second injection (1 to 3 weeks later) is given and the second one is the one recorded (USDHHS, 2000).

Table 20.2 ■
CLASSIFICATION OF TB

CLASS	DEGREE OF TB EXPOSURE/INFECTION	INTERPRETATION
Class 0	No TB exposure	Negative PPD
Class 1	TB exposure; no infection	Negative PPD
Class 2	TB infection; no disease	Positive PPD; no clinical, radiographic, or bacteriological evidence of active TB
Class 3	Clinically active TB	Positive PPD; TB cultured; positive X-ray
Class 4	TB NOT clinically active	Positive PPD; history of TB or abnormal but stable X-ray with negative bacteriological studies; no clinical signs of disease
Class 5	TB suspected	Diagnosis pending

Source: U.S. Department of Health and Human Services (2000).

Table 20.3 ■
INTERPRETATION OF THE TUBERCULIN REACTIONS

DEGREE OF INDURATION	SPECIFIC POPULATIONS
≥5 mm is classified as *positive* in	HIV-positive persons Recent contacts of TB cases Persons with radiographic results consistent with old healed TB Persons with suspected TB Persons who are immunosuppressed
≥10 mm is classified as *positive* in	Recent arrivals from high-prevalence countries Those with concomitant medical conditions Injection drug users Residents/employees of high-risk areas Children < 4 years of age Students exposed to adults in high risk categories
≥15 mm is classified as *positive* in	Anyone 4 years of age or older with no known risk factor for TB

Source: Adapted from Pediatric Tuberculosis Collaborative Group (2004).

Recent national policy change recommendations have been adopted by many school districts that now recommend the Mantoux tuberculin test be used *only* for those who are at high risk for contracting TB (Pediatric Tuberculosis Collaborative Group, 2004). This risk is determined by administering the TB Risk-Assessment Questionnaire to the parent. The four key questions are:

1. Was your child born outside the United States? If yes, where was the child born? (Children born in Africa, Asia, Latin America, or Eastern Europe should receive the Mantoux.)
2. Has your child traveled outside the United States? If yes, where has he or she traveled, for how long, and where did he or she stay? (If the child stayed for 1 week or longer in the above areas, he or she should receive the Mantoux.)
3. Has your child been exposed to anyone with TB disease? If yes, ask if the person had TB disease or TB infection, when the exposure occurred, and the nature of the contact. If confirmed that the child has been exposed, the child should receive the Mantoux.
4. Does your child have close contact with a person who has a positive TB skin test? (If yes, see question 3 for follow-up questions.)

Additional questions, based on local epidemiology, might be:

1. Does your child spend time with anyone who has been in jail or a shelter, uses illegal drugs, or has HIV?
2. Has your child consumed raw milk or unpasteurized cheese?
3. Does your child have a household member who was born outside the United States?
4. Does your child have a household member who has traveled outside the United States?

Adolescents can be asked these questions directly. Any "yes" response is considered a positive risk factor and is an indication for administration of the Mantoux tuberculin test to the student. This change in protocol is supported by the American Academy of Pediatrics and the Centers for Disease Control and Prevention (Froehlich et al., 2001; Pediatric Tuberculosis Collaborative Group, 2004).

Other Possible Screening Options

1. *Lead screening* is important in both secondary and tertiary prevention. Lead is neurotoxic and can harm the developing nervous system of children; it also can damage the hematopoietic and renal systems (Meyer et al., 2003). While no safe lead level at which no harmful effects occur has been determined, the goal is to eliminate blood lead levels above 10 micrograms per deciliter. Some states require screening for lead levels prior to enrollment in pre-

school or kindergarten. This testing of venous blood is usually completed by the primary care provider (if capillary blood is used, two positive readings 12 weeks apart are needed) (Meyer et al., 2003).

High lead levels have a direct impact on one's ability to learn. Blood levels of lead of 10 micrograms per deciliter produce a 7.4 point drop in IQ (Canfield et al., 2003).

The number of affected children has been decreasing, but 74,887 children had values ≥10 in 2001 (Meyer et al., 2003). It is estimated that one in every 50 U.S. children has lead levels above this level. One in ten have levels of at least 5 micrograms per deciliter. Sources of lead include the paint in houses built before 1946; the prevalence is considerably higher in children from low-income families (16.4%) compared to those of middle- (4.1%) and high (0.9%) -income families (Meyer et al., 2003). It should be remembered that lead exposure can occur in older children (and adults) because of exposure to lead in batteries, ceramics, and some traditional folk remedies (CDC, 2005).

2. *Developmental assessment* can identify whether a student's physical development is within normal limits. In addition to growth parameters, attainment of physical and social developmental tasks can be assessed formally or informally. Speech patterns, social interactions, level of fear, as well as cognitive ability are often assessed informally by school faculty, who may express their concern to the school nurse. The school nurse can then observe the student or even speak to the student to determine if assessment is needed by other members of the healthcare or coordinated school health team (see Chapter 16).

3. *Dental screening*. Some school districts have dentists or dental hygienists who come in and provide dental screening for students, especially for those unable to obtain dental services. The school nurse can also screen for oral health. Some school nurses have written grants to fund the services of these healthcare providers to promote primary and secondary prevention.

4. *Scalp screening.* Many school nurses engage in scalp screening for pediculosis, tinea capitis, and general hair hygiene. Information on pediculosis is in Chapter 26 and tinea capitis is covered in Chapter 25.

CONCLUSION

Screening is an essential role of the school nurse. Some schools are able to do many of these screenings in one session, thereby saving time and administrative work and decreasing class interruption. By keeping students in their optimal state of health and by identifying problems early and referring for appropriate interventions, students will be ready to benefit more from the educational setting and reach their optimal potential.

References

Canfield, R., Henderson, C., Cory-Slechta, D., Cox, C., Jusko, T., & Lanphear, B. (2003). Intellectual impairment in children with blood lead concentrations below 10 μg [micrograms] per deciliter. *The New England Journal of Medicine, 348*(16), 1517–1526.

Centers for Disease Control and Prevention (CDC). (2004). Trends in tuberculosis—United States, 1998–2003. *Morbidity and Mortality Weekly Report, 53*(10), 209–214.

Centers for Disease Control and Prevention (CDC). (2005). Lead poisoning associated with use of Litargirio—Rhode Island, 2003. *Morbidity and Mortality Weekly Report, 54*(9), 227–229.

Chumlea, W., & Guo, S. (2004). Physical growth and development. In P. Samour, K. Helm, & C. Lang (Eds.), *Handbook of pediatric nutrition* (pp. 3–15). Boston: Jones & Bartlett.

Clark, M. (2003). *Community health nursing: Caring for populations*. Upper Saddle River, NJ: Prentice-Hall.

Ferebee, A. (2004). *Childhood vision: Public challenges and opportunities: A policy brief*. Washington, DC: The Center for Health and Health Care in Schools.

Froehlich, H., Ackerson, L., Morozumi, P. & the Pediatric Tuberculosis Study Group. (2001). *Targeting testing of children for tuberculosis: Validation of a risk assessment questionnaire. Pediatrics, 107*(4), Retrieved August 2005 from http://www.pediatrics.org/cgi/content/full/107/4/e54

Kuczmarski, R., Ogden, C., Grummer-Strawn, L., Flegal, K., Guo, S., Wei, R., Mei, Z., Curtin, L., Roche, A., & Johnson, C. (2000). CDC Growth Charts: United States. *Advance Data, 314*, 1–27. (U.S. Department of Health and Human Services).

Leavell, H., & Clark, E. (1965). *Preventive medicine for the doctor in his community: An epidemiological approach*. New York: McGraw-Hill.

McKeown, R., & Weinrich, S. (2002). Epidemiological applications in community health nursing. In M. Stanhope & J. Lancaster (Eds.), *Foundations of community health nursing* (pp. 129–150). St. Louis: C. V. Mosby.

Meyer, P., Povetz, T., Dignam, T., Homa, D., Schoonover, J., & Brody, D. (2003). Surveillance for elevated blood lead levels among children—United States, 1997–2001. *Morbidity and Mortality Weekly Report, 52*(SS-10), 1–21.

National Association of School Nurses (NASN). (1998). *The ear and hearing: A guide for school nurses*. Scarborough ME: National Association of School Nurses.

National Association of School Nurses (NASN) & the American Nurses Association (ANA). (2001). *Scope and standards of professional school nursing practice*. Washington, DC: American Nurses Publishing.

Ozuah, P., Ozuah, T., Stein, R., Burton, W., & Mulvihill, M., (2001). Evaluation of a risk assessment questionnaire used to target tuberculin skin testing in children. *Journal of the American Medical Association, 285*(4), 451–453.

Pediatric Tuberculosis Collaborative Group. (2004). Targeted tuberculin skin testing and treatment of latent tuberculosis infection in children and adolescents. *Pediatrics, 114*(4 Suppl.), 1175–1201.

Proctor, S. (2005). *To see or not to see: Screening the vision of children in school*. Castle Rock, CO: National Association of School Nurses.

Ryberg, J. (2004). *Postural screening guidelines for school nurses*. Scarborough, ME: NASN.

U.S. Department of Health & Human Services (USDHHS). (2000). *Core curriculum on tuberculosis: What the clinician should know*. Atlanta: Centers for Disease Control and Prevention.

Chapter 21

Disease Prevention

JANICE SELEKMAN

Chapter Outline

INTRODUCTION

One of the primary roles of the school nurse is to prevent disease from occurring. One approach is to promote wellness both in the classroom and indirectly through school policies and practices (i.e., brushing teeth after lunch), role modeling, educational posters, and teachable moments. This approach aims to ensure that students come to school fed, rested, groomed, and emotionally healthy. Approaches to disease prevention include implementing policies and educational programs to meet immunization requirements, as well as infection control measures that must be implemented in the school. This chapter covers both of these components.

DISEASE PREVENTION

Disease prevention involves primary and secondary prevention efforts (see Chapter 20). The school nurse, in collaboration with classroom teachers, can promote many activities in school to prevent disease and to prevent its spread. These include frequent hand washing, especially after meals and after toileting, proper disposal of used tissues, and covering one's mouth and nose when coughing or sneezing (followed by washing one's hands for 15 to 20 seconds). Health information sent home to families can inform them of the amount of sleep children and adolescents need, recommend family activities and exercise, suggest ways to cognitively stimulate their children and to enhance communication, and promote proper nutrition, including suggestions for healthy lunches; it can also provide guidance on appropriate measures to take if their child is ill.

Immunizations are a significant adjunct in preventing disease. They are used as primary prevention measures for the vast majority of students. Some vaccinations are also used as secondary prevention aids, such as those that provide immediate protection to those exposed to diseases, such as tetanus, hepatitis B, and varicella. It is essential for the school nurse to have a comprehensive knowledge base regarding immunizations and the diseases they prevent.

IMMUNIZATIONS

Why Immunize?

There are multiple answers to the question of why immunizations are important. They keep students and staff healthy, prevent the morbidity that could occur as a result of disease, and prevent students from spreading disease to those who are most at risk (i.e., the elderly, infants and the immunocompromised). It also is the law (since 1980).

Protecting the public from disease is a public health issue and the Healthy People 2010 (U.S. Department of Health and Human Services [USDHHS], 2000) document includes numerous objectives that deal with increasing immunization levels (Box 21.1). The protection of society involves the concept of "herd" immunity. As more of the "herd" is protected, fewer are at risk for getting the disease, spreading it to others, and suffering the consequences of it. The consequences of the diseases cost far more than the immunizations and the programs that promote them. It must be kept in mind that just because "we" are protected, our global neighbors are not; infections can easily reemerge. Table 21.1 demonstrates the numbers of Americans affected by selected preventable diseases and when outbreaks have developed. In 2001, only 77.2% of children between 19 and 35 months of age had received their basic immunization series. Rates were especially low among children who were poor, members of a racial or ethnic minority, or lived in either inner city or rural areas (American Academy of Pediatrics [AAP], 2003a). By the 2003–2004 school year, more than 90% of children had the required immunizations on entry to school (Centers for Disease Control and Prevention [CDC], 2004a). However, states have different immunization requirements for school entry.

Box 21.1 ■■■

SELECTED HEALTHY PEOPLE 2010 OBJECTIVES RELATED TO IMMUNIZATION LEVELS

Goal: Prevent disease, disability, and death from infectious diseases, including vaccine-preventable diseases.
Objectives:

- Reduce or eliminate indigenous cases of vaccine-preventable disease.
- Eliminate (by 2010) congenital rubella syndrome; diphtheria; *Haemophilus influenzae*, type b; measles; rubella; mumps; polio; and tetanus.
- Reduce the number of cases of pertussis; hepatitis B; varicella; pneumococcal disease; hepatitis A; hepatitis C; meningococcal disease; Lyme disease; and tuberculosis.
- Maintain vaccination coverage for children in licensed day care facilities and children in kindergarten through first grade (at 95%).
- Increase the proportion of young children who receive all vaccines that have been recommended for universal administration for at least 5 years. (In 1998, it was 73%; the goal is 80%.)
- Increase the proportion of children who participate in fully operational population-based immunization registries. (In 1998, 32% of those under age 6 were enrolled; the goal is 95%.)
- Increase routine vaccination coverage levels of adolescents.
- Reduce vaccine-associated adverse effects.
- Eliminate vaccine-associated paralytic polio.
- Reduce febrile seizures caused by pertussis vaccine.

(U.S. Department of Health and Human Services, 2000)

Different Modalities of Immune Protection

Some immune protection is innate. Humans are naturally protected against certain organisms, such as the virus that causes distemper in dogs. Skin, gastric acidity, and intestinal flora are other natural barriers against disease. However, most immunity in humans is acquired either naturally or artificially and occurs during childhood. Within each of these categories, protection can occur actively or passively.

To actually have a disease is to "naturally" acquire it and to 'actively' stimulate the immune system to develop immunity against it (naturally acquired active). Having a case of measles (rubeola) results in the immune response, the typical signs and symptoms, and the resulting immune protection. However, it also puts the person at risk for the sequelae of the disease. There are only two ways to obtain

Table 21.1 ■

NUMBER OF CASES OF CONTAGIOUS DISEASES REPORTED IN THE UNITED STATES

DISEASE	1986	1989	1996	2001	2004
Diphtheria	0	2	1	2	0
Pertussis	4,162	5,611	6,467	7,580	18,957
Tetanus	61	47	45	37	26
Polio	2	0	0	0	0
Measles	6,273	17,850	488	116	37
Rubella	502	373	210	23	12
C.R.S.	11	3	2	3	0
Mumps	6,807	3,745	658	266	236
Hepatitis A	23,117	35,165	29,024	10,614	5,609
Hepatitis B	25,452	22,963	9,994	7,844	6,632
Hepatitis C	3,435	2,323	3,321	3,977	866
Meningococcal	2,481	2,595	3,176	2,333	1,254
AIDS	13,008	35,238	65,475	42,092	39,097
Pediatric AIDS			257	212	149
Gonorrhea	896,383	689,922	308,737	360,906	307,845
Syphilis	27,599	42,600	11,110	6,095	7,352
Congenital syphilis	107	243	225	497	312
Haemophilus influenzae			1,065	1,597	1,814
TB			19,096	15,492	11,178
Varicella				781,614	18,718

Source: U.S. Morbidity and Mortality Weekly Report, Volume 52 of the respective years. (Summary of Provisional Cases, 2005; Summary of Notifiable Diseases, 2002.)

protection "naturally" by the "passive" route (naturally acquired passive). Passive protection results in *no* stimulation of the immune system. It occurs during every pregnancy, when the mother naturally transfers some immune protection (immunoglobulin G) to the fetus, and again during breastfeeding, when immunoglobulins in breast milk are transferred to the child. The protection resulting from passive protection is short lived and the protection disappears by the second year of life.

Immunizations are "artificially" derived products that "actively" stimulate the immune system to provide protection (artificially acquired active). The immunity developed is usually not quite as good as, nor does it last as long as "naturally active," but the risks of sequelae are significantly reduced. These medically engineered and modified products are similar to the original organisms but may require "boosters" in order to keep the person's antibody titer at a high enough level to be protective.

"Artificially passive" immunizations are also available (artificially acquired passive). Gammaglobulin provides passive protection to those who are exposed to contagious disease and who are most at risk of its sequelae. It contains the pooled antibodies from approximately 8000 randomized U.S. volunteers to ensure consistent protection against the pathogens endemic to the U.S. population. It is given intramuscularly or intravenously, but because it is passive and does not stimulate the person's immune system, it has a half-life of only 22 days, and therefore is only effective for about a month. Individuals who are immunocompromised, such as those with human immunodeficiency virus (HIV) infection or primary immunodeficiencies, may receive gamma-globulin injections every month.

For some conditions, it is possible to provide specific "artificial passive" protection. Examples include varicella (VZIG-varicella zoster immune globulin), hepatitis B (HBIG-hepatitis B immune globulin), tetanus (Hypertet-tetanus immune globulin), and rabies (rabies immune globulin). Again, these only provide immediate protection; they do not stimulate the immune system and protection fades after a few weeks. However, the presence of these passively provided antibodies will significantly interfere with the development of sufficient titers of live attenuated vaccines (Atkinson, Pickering, Watson, & Peter, 2004).

Concept of Titers

A certain level of antibody (titer) is necessary before protection can be assured. The titer has implications for the number of doses of a vaccine, if boosters are required, when the vaccines should be given, and the spacing of the doses. A complicating factor in infancy is the presence of the maternal antibodies mentioned previously. Infants need frequent boosters to keep their titers high as the maternal antibodies fade; consequently, their immunizations are usually just months apart. It was the awareness of the drop in protective titers that resulted in the policy change requiring a second dose of MMR (measles–mumps–rubella). It is important to know what factors may interfere with the development of a protective titer. Being in the throes of an acute illness is not the optimal time to receive immunizations, as the immune system is already "busy" fighting the primary infection; consequently, the ultimate titer may be compromised.

Types of Artificially Acquired Active Vaccines

"The purpose of a vaccine is to stimulate the immune response without subjecting an individual to the risk of actual infection. An ideal vaccine would confer the same degree of immunity as natural infection" (Nossal, 2003). Vaccines may be live attenuated, inactivated, or genetically engineered. Viral and bacterial agents that cause some diseases must be modified in the laboratory by heat or chemicals, thus still retaining their ability to replicate and stimulate immunity to the specific virus. These "attenuated" live vaccines confer about 90% to 95% of the immunity as the naturally active disease would and protect for more than 20 years once an initial titer is established. Examples are the MMR, varicella, and the oral polio vaccine. The new nasal influenza spray vaccine is also a live attenuated vaccine. Live attenuated vaccines do have a slight risk of causing the disease; thus, adverse events following live attenuated vaccines are similar to a mild form of the natural illness.

Inactivated vaccines are created from a bacteria or virus grown in a lab and then killed or inactivated with heat or chemicals. They cannot cause the disease and do not replicate, so they result in a weakened response and require more boosters to maintain titers. The types of inactivated vaccines include toxoids, killed, or subunits. Toxoids, such as diphtheria and tetanus, are modified or inactivated toxins. To maintain immunity, they require boosters every 10 years. Killed vaccines include only the cell wall of the organism and provide only 70% protection. They include whole cell pertussis and the inactivated polio vaccines.

There is a significant increase in the number of vaccines now produced by recombinant DNA technology. The advantage is that the smallest unit of the pathogen that is able to develop an appropriate antibody titer will be able to be isolated, thus decreasing the body's exposure to additional unnecessary antigens and serious sequelae. These vaccines should be safer than the older vaccines. Fractional vaccines include inactivated subunits or components of the organism. Hepatitis B, acellular pertussis, and influenza vaccines are examples. Another type of inactivated subunit vaccines are the polysaccharide vaccines; examples are *Haemophilus influenzae*, meningococcal, and pneumococcal vaccines (CDC, 2000d).

Additives/Immune Adjuvants

To grow and modify the organisms and to maintain the effectiveness of the vaccines during transport and storage and enhance immunogenicity, numerous additives are included. Some are antibiotics (especially neomycin) to prevent bacterial growth. Some are products to hold the antigen in the tissue longer or slow the release into the body so that the immune system has more time to respond to the antigens; examples are aluminum hydroxide, aluminum phosphate, and mineral oil (Vogel & Hem, 2004). The mechanism of action for many of the adjuvant formulations is to cause an inflammatory reaction at the site of inoculation, in order to enhance immune function and the production of antibodies (Seder & Mascola, 2003). Some viruses are grown on chicken eggs. All additives have implications for those with anaphylactic allergic responses to these products.

One additive used as a preservative, thimerosal, is no longer added to pediatric vaccines. It had been included in vaccines since the 1930s. Its action was to kill bacteria and fungi and prevent bacterial contamination, especially in multidose containers. However, thimerisol contains mercury and there is concern regarding the neurodevelopmental effects of mercury, especially during the first 6 months of age. Therefore, on July 8, 1999, the American Academy of Pediatrics and the Public Health Service ordered the removal or reduction of thimerosal in vaccines for children (CDC, 1999a). There is no evidence to support the myth that thimerosal causes autism (Verstraeten et al., 2003); the discontinuation of thimerosal in vaccines in Denmark was actually followed by an increase in the incidence of autism (Madsen et al., 2003). It should be noted that the risks of not vaccinating far outweigh the unknown risks of mercury.

Vaccine Schedule

In the past, it was easy for every pediatric nurse to memorize the immunization schedule, which consisted of MMR (measles–mumps–rubella), DPT (diphtheria–pertussis–tetanus), and polio. Now, however, the number of new vaccines increases every few years. Therefore, every January, the American Academy of Pediatrics (AAP) and the Advisory Committee on Immunization Practices (ACIP) of the CDC publish the changes in the schedule for that year (Figure 21.1). This puts increased responsibility on school nurses to ensure that students are up to date according to the updated schedule.

The first consideration in immunizations is the spacing. The time that must elapse between vaccine doses depends on whether it is live or inactivated. *There is a 4-week minimum between live vaccine doses* (Figure 21.1). However, all vaccines can be administered at the same time (see later). If they are not, they must wait at least a month between doses. Remember that booster doses are the same serum as the original vaccine; their role is just to boost the titers.

Existing antibodies can interfere with the development of a protective titer. Because maternal antibodies to measles are the last to disappear (somewhere between 12 and 14 months), those infants immunized too early (at 12 months of age) had only 66% of the protection needed. Consequently, the time of the immunization was changed to 15 months and a booster was recommended. Similarly, if the person has received blood or any other antibody-containing product, such as gamma-globulin, these can inhibit the immune response, especially to measles and rubella vaccines, for up to 3 months. Therefore active immunization must be delayed until the passive antibodies have degraded. The same is true for receiving passive immunization with a serum immune globulin product. The passive antibody will interfere with the active production of immune production; exceptions are tetanus and hepatitis B, where both the active and passive protection can be administered at the same time (but in different sites).

Another consideration in the timing of vaccines depends on a balance between the titer and the risk for mortality and morbidity. In addition, infants and toddlers do not respond appropriately to some vaccines, and thus some are ineffective for those ages. Consequently, if an infant receives the measles vaccine at 9 months to stave off the morbidity and mortality occurring during a measles outbreak, this vaccine will not count as one of the child's shots, since the body will still have maternal antibodies.

One question occasionally asked by novice healthcare providers is this: "The student has a record of having one or two of the series as an infant and then has had nothing since; does the student need to start over?" The answer is "no." Immunizations can be continued from wherever they last ended. Barring an immunological catastrophe for the person, immunizations do not have to be repeated. A way for providers to remember this principle is the line, "The immune system never forgets a pretty face." Count all shots if they were given at the full

(text continues on page 458)

Recommended childhood and adolescent immunization schedule,[1] by vaccine and age — United States, 2005

Vaccine	Birth	1 mo	2 mos	4 mos	6 mos	12 mos	15 mos	18 mos	24 mos	4–6 yrs	11–12 yrs	13–18 yrs
Hepatitis B[2]	HepB#1	only if mother HBsAg (-)	HepB #2			HepB #3					HepB series	
Diphtheria, tetanus, pertussis[3]			DTaP	DTaP	DTaP		DTaP			DTaP	Td	Td
Haemophilus influenzae type b[4]			Hib	Hib	Hib[4]	Hib						
Inactivated poliovirus			IPV	IPV		IPV				IPV		
Measles, mumps, rubella[5]						MMR #1				MMR #2	MMR #2	
Varicella[6]							Varicella				Varicella	
Pneumococcal[7]			PCV	PCV	PCV	PCV			PCV	PPV		
Influenza[8]						Influenza (yearly)				Influenza (yearly)		
- - - - - - - Vaccines below blue line are for selected populations- - - - - - - -												
Hepatitis A[9]										Hepatitis A series		

Range of recommended ages | Catch-up immunization | Preadolescent assessment

1. This schedule indicates the recommended ages for routine administration of currently licensed childhood vaccines, as of December 1, 2004, for children aged ≤18 years. Any dose not administered at the recommended age should be administered at any subsequent visit when indicated and feasible. ▒ indicates age groups that warrant special effort to administer those vaccines not previously administered. Additional vaccines might be licensed and recommended during the year. Licensed combination vaccines may be used whenever any components of the combination are indicated and other components of the vaccine are not contraindicated. Providers should consult package inserts for detailed recommendations. Clinically significant adverse events that follow immunization should be reported to the Vaccine Adverse Event Reporting System; guidance is available at http://www.vaers.org or by telephone, 800-822-7967.

2. **Hepatitis B (HepB) vaccine.** All infants should receive the first dose of HepB vaccine soon after birth and before hospital discharge; the first dose may also be administered by age 2 months if the mother is hepatitis B surface antigen (HBsAg) negative. Only monovalent HepB may be used for the birth dose. Monovalent or combination vaccine containing HepB may be used to complete the series. Four doses of vaccine may be administered when a birth dose is administered. The second dose should be administered at least 4 weeks after the first dose, except for combination vaccines, which cannot be administered before age 6 weeks. The third dose should be administered at least 16 weeks after the first dose and at least 8 weeks after the second dose. The final dose in the vaccination series (third or fourth dose) should not be administered before age 24 weeks. ***Infants born to HBsAg-positive mothers*** should receive HepB and 0.5 mL of hepatitis B immune globulin (HBIG) at separate sites within 12 hours of birth. The second dose is recommended at age 1–2 months. The final dose in the immunization series should not be administered before age 24 weeks. These infants should be tested for HBsAg and antibody to HBsAg at age 9–15 months. ***Infants born to mothers whose HBsAg status is unknown*** should receive the first dose of the HepB series within 12 hours of birth. Maternal blood should be drawn as soon as possible to determine the mother's HBsAg status; if the HBsAg test is positive, the infant should receive HBIG as soon as possible (no later than age 1 week). The second dose is recommended at age 1–2 months. The last dose in the immunization series should not be administered before age 24 weeks.

3. **Diphtheria and tetanus toxoids and acellular pertussis (DTaP) vaccine.** The fourth dose of DTaP may be administered as early as age 12 months, provided 6 months have elapsed since the third dose and the child is unlikely to return at age 15–18 months. The final dose in the series should be administered at age ≥4 years. **Tetanus and diphtheria toxoids (Td)** is recommended at age 11–12 years if at least 5 years have elapsed since the last dose of tetanus and diphtheria toxoid-containing vaccine. Subsequent routine Td boosters are recommended every 10 years.

4. ***Haemophilus influenzae* type b (Hib) conjugate vaccine.** Three Hib conjugate vaccines are licensed for infant use. If PRP-OMP (PedvaxHIB® or ComVax® [Merck]) is administered at ages 2 and 4 months, a dose at age 6 months is not required. DTaP/Hib combination products should not be used for primary immunization in infants at ages 2, 4, or 6 months but can be used as boosters after any Hib vaccine. The final dose in the series should be administered at age ≥12 months.

5. **Measles, mumps, and rubella (MMR) vaccine.** The second dose of MMR is recommended routinely at age 4–6 years but may be administered during any visit, provided at least 4 weeks have elapsed since the first dose and both doses are administered beginning at or after age 12 months. Those who have not previously received the second dose should complete the schedule by age 11–12 years.

6. **Varicella vaccine.** Varicella vaccine is recommended at any visit at or after age 12 months for susceptible children (i.e., those who lack a reliable history of chickenpox). Susceptible persons aged ≥13 years should receive 2 doses administered at least 4 weeks apart.

7. **Pneumococcal vaccine.** The heptavalent **pneumococcal conjugate vaccine (PCV)** is recommended for all children aged 2–23 months and for certain children aged 24–59 months. The final dose in the series should be administered at age ≥12 months. **Pneumococcal polysaccharide vaccine (PPV)** is recommended in addition to PCV for certain groups at high risk. See *MMWR* 2000;49(No. RR-9).

8. **Influenza vaccine.** Influenza vaccine is recommended annually for children aged ≥6 months with certain risk factors (including, but not limited to, asthma, cardiac disease, sickle cell disease, human immunodeficiency virus [HIV], and diabetes), health-care workers, and other persons (including household members) in close contact with persons in groups at high risk (see *MMWR* 2004;53[No. RR-6]). In addition, healthy children aged 6–23 months and close contacts of healthy children aged 0–23 months are recommended to receive influenza vaccine because children in this age group are at substantially increased risk for influenza-related hospitalizations. For healthy persons aged 5–49 years, the intranasally administered, live, attenuated influenza vaccine (LAIV) is an acceptable alternative to the intramuscular trivalent inactivated influenza vaccine (TIV). See *MMWR* 2004;53(No. RR-6). Children receiving TIV should be administered a dosage appropriate for their age (0.25 mL if aged 6–35 months or 0.5 mL if aged ≥3 years). Children aged ≤8 years who are receiving influenza vaccine for the first time should receive 2 doses (separated by at least 4 weeks for TIV and at least 6 weeks for LAIV).

9. **Hepatitis A vaccine.** Hepatitis A vaccine is recommended for children and adolescents in selected states and regions and for certain groups at high risk; consult your local public health authority. Children and adolescents in these states, regions, and groups who have not been immunized against hepatitis A can begin the hepatitis A immunization series during any visit. The 2 doses in the series should be administered at least 6 months apart. See *MMWR* 1999;48(No. RR-12).

Approved by the **Advisory Committee on Immunization Practices** (http://www.cdc.gov/nip/acip), the **American Academy of Pediatrics** (http://www.aap.org), and the **American Academy of Family Physicians** (http://www.aafp.org). Additional information about vaccines, including precautions and contraindications for vaccination and vaccine shortages, is available at http://www.cdc.gov/nip or from the National Immunization Hotline, 800-232-2522 (English) or 800-232-0233 (Spanish).

Figure 21.1 ■ 2005 Immunization chart.

Catch-up immunization schedule for children and adolescents who start late or who are >1 month behind, by age group, vaccine, and dosage interval—United States, 2005

Catch-up schedule for children aged 4 months-6 years

Vaccine	Minimum age for dose 1	Minimum interval between doses			
		Dose 1 to dose 2	Dose 2 to dose 3	Dose 3 to dose 4	Dose 4 to dose 5
DTaP[1]	6 wks	4 wks	4 wks	6 mos	6 mos[1]
IPV[2]	6 wks	4 wks	4 wks	4 wks[2]	
HepB[3]	Birth	4 wks	8 wks (and 16 wks after first dose)		
MMR[4]	12 mos	4 wks[4]			
Varicella	12 mos				
Hib[5]	6 wks	4 wks: if first dose administered at age <12 mos 8 wks (as final dose): if first dose administered at age 12–14 mos No further doses needed if first dose administered at age ≥15 mos	4 wks[6]: if current age <12 mos 8 wks (as final dose)[6]: if current age ≥12 mos and second dose administered at age <15 mos No further doses needed if previous dose administered at age ≥15 mos	8 wks (as final dose): This dose only necessary for children aged 12 mos–5 yrs who received 3 doses before age 12 mos	
PCV[7]	6 wks	4 wks: if first dose administered at age <12 mos and current age <24 mos 8 wks (as final dose): if first dose administered at age ≥12 mos or current age 24–59 mos No further doses needed for healthy children if first dose administered at age ≥24 mos	4 wks: if current age <12 mos 8 wks (as final dose): if current age ≥12 mos No further doses needed for healthy children if previous dose administered at age ≥24 mos	8 wks (as final dose): This dose only necessary for children aged 12 mos–5 yrs who received 3 doses before age 12 mos	

Catch-up schedule for children aged 7-18 years

Vaccine	Minimum interval between doses		
	Dose 1 to dose 2	Dose 2 to dose 3	Dose 3 to booster dose
Td[8]	4 wks	6 mos	6 mos[8]: if first dose administered at age <12 mos and current age <11 yrs 5 yrs[8]: if first dose administered at age ≥12 mos and third dose administered at age <7 yrs and current age ≥11 yrs 10 yrs[8]: if third dose administered at age ≥7 yrs
IPV[9]	4 wks	4 wks	IPV[2,9]
HepB	4 wks	8 wks (and 16 wks after first dose)	
MMR	4 wks[4]		
Varicella[10]	4 wks		

Note: A vaccine series dose not require restarting, regardless of the time that has elapeed between doses.

1. Diphtheria and tetanus toxoids and acelluler pertussis (DTaP) vaccine. The fifth dose is not necessary if the fourth dose was administered after the fourth birthday.
2. Inactivated pollovirus (IPV) vaccine. For children who received an all-IPV or all-oral pollovirus (OPV) series, a fourth dose is not necessary if the third dose was administered at age ≥4 years. If both OPV and IPV were administered as part of a series, a total of 4 doses should be administered, regardless of the child's current age.
3. Hepatitis B (HepB) vaccine. All children and adolescents who have not been immunized against hepatitis B should begin the HepB immunization series during any visit. Providers should make special efforts to immunize children who were born in, or whose parents were born in, areas of the world where hepatitis B virus infection is moderately or highly endemic.
4. Measles, mumps, and rubelia (MMR) vaccine. The second dose of MMR is recommended routinely at age 4–6 years but may be administered earlier if dealred.
5. *Haamophilus Influenzae* type b (Hib) vaccine. Vaccine is not generally recommended for children aged ≥5 years.
6. Hib vaccine. If current age is <12 months and the first 2 doses were PRP-OMP (PedvaxHIB® or ComVax® [Merck]), the third (and final) dose should be administered at age 12–15 months and at least 8 weeks after the second dose.
7. Pneumococcal conjugats (PCV) vaccine. Vaccine is not generally recommended for children aged ≥5 years.
8. Tetanus and diphtheria toxoids (Td). For children aged 7–10 years, the interval between the third and booster dose is determined by the age when the first dose was administered. For adolescents aged 11–18 years, the interval is determined by the age when the third dose was administered.
9. IPV. Vaccine is not generally recommended for persons aged ≥18 years.
10. Varicella vaccine. Administer the 2-dose series to all susceptible adolescents aged ≥13 years.

Figure 21.1 ■ *(continued)*

dose and at the appropriate age for the vaccine. Longer-than-recommended intervals between doses do not reduce the final antibody concentrations (Atkinson et al., 2004). Thus for the student in the example above, the healthcare provider should administer all vaccines that are age appropriate.

If the student has no record and the guardian cannot remember if anything was given before, some professionals are concerned about giving "too much vaccine too often." In general, there is little danger to repeating immunizations. There may be an increased rate of local or systemic reactions if it is too frequent, because of the antigen–antibody complexes. This is most common in tetanus vaccines that are given too frequently; an arthus formation occurs at the site of the injection where the antibodies attack the incoming antigen in the vaccine as it enters the body causing a serious localized area of inflammation, possibly even leading to necrosis at the site of injection.

How Many Shots Can Be Given at the Same Time?

The answer to this question is an easy one and based on repeated studies. *Children can receive as many vaccines simultaneously as are age appropriate*. The vaccines can *not* be mixed into one syringe and the contents of each syringe must be administered in a different site. There are reports of four nurses all injecting vaccine into a child at the same time and reports of those who give one right after the other in different sites (with different needles) (Atkinson et al., 2004). Regardless of the approach, good titers are reported and the rates of adverse reactions are similar to those observed when the vaccines are administered separately (Offit et al., 2002). Most of the literature addresses the problem from the perspective of the trauma to the child, but there is no long-term study that demonstrates negative emotional sequelae. The bottom line is that children entering the school system who do not have their full complement of immunizations can get the first dose of everything they need at the same visit.

Which Doses of Immunizations Count Toward Meeting School Criteria?

There are five "rights" that are important for the school nurse to consider in evaluating immunization information to determine if the student has met school entry mandates: Were the immunizations given at the right age, right dose, right interval, right route, and right site? The age of administration is essential because of the fact that immunity does not occur if immunized too early. Pneumococcal vaccine is not effective in children younger than age 2. Measles vaccine will only produce a limited titer if the child is younger than the age of 12 months. However, during an epidemic, measles vaccine can be administered to the infant younger than age 1, but it will *not* count toward the two doses required for school entry.

The right dose means the full dose. Divided doses do not work and do not count. The right interval is one that is especially important for school nurses. For doses that are too close together, the latter dose does not count. While state laws differ, there is usually a 4-day grace period. If it is 5 days or more short of the 4 weeks, the student needs to wait 4 weeks and then have the dose repeated (Figure 21.1).

The last two "rights" are more difficult to document. The vaccine needs to be given by the right route, whether intramuscularly or subcutaneously. The right site ensures that vaccines are given into the right tissue. Therefore, hepatitis B vaccine given in the gluteus should be repeated, since it is going into fat.

With the increased number of vaccines for protection against the same organism, it should be noted that vaccines are not identical in the antigen content among manufacturers. However, available data indicate that infants who receive sequential doses of different HiB conjugate, HBV, and hepatitis A vaccines produce a satisfactory antibody response after a complete primary series. All brands of HiB conjugate, hepatitis B, and hepatitis A vaccines are interchangeable within their respective series. If different brands of HiB conjugate vaccine are administered, a total of three doses is considered adequate for the primary series among infants. However, any brand can be used for the booster. Less data are available for the DaPT. In one study, 1 or 2 doses of Tripedia followed by Infanrix for the rest is comparable to three doses of Tripedia. Vaccination should not be deferred because the brand used for the previous dose is not available or is unknown.

The school nurses can accept only written dated records as evidence of vaccination. The only exception is for the pneumococcal vaccine where a verbal OK is sufficient. If there are no records, consider the student to be susceptible and require that documentation of all age-appropriate vaccines be provided. This may require the student to be revaccinated. The alternative is serological testing to measure the titers; however, this is an expensive proposition.

DISEASES AGAINST WHICH VACCINES ARE EFFECTIVE AND THE VACCINES TO PREVENT THEM

Diphtheria

Diphtheria is caused by bacteria that proliferate in the respiratory tract and multiply on dead tissue in the throat, producing an exotoxin and exudate consisting of a tough fibrous membrane (pseudomembrane) across the respiratory tract at the back of the throat; this results in a mechanical airway obstruction and respiratory distress. The disease is more serious in infants and can cause renal, cardiac, and peripheral central nervous system (CNS) damage; however, it can affect individuals of any age.

While the incidence is very low in the United States, Russia reported an outbreak in 1990 of more than 400 cases in a home for children who were mentally retarded and unimmunized; forty-one deaths resulted. Diphtheria peaked in 1921 in the United States when there were almost 207,000 cases reported. Before immunizations, diphtheria was one of the most common causes of death in school-age children. Immunization has been highly effective in keeping the current annual incidence in the single digits. The full dose of diphtheria, noted by the capital "D," is part of all doses given to children younger than the age of 6. Each dose contains 10 to 12 flocculating units (Lf) of diphtheria toxoid. After that time, as the risk of the sequelae of diphtheria decreases, all subsequent boosters have a smaller dose of diphtheria, noted by the lower case "d"; each dose only contains less than 2 Lf of diphtheria toxoid (Wharton & Vitek, 2004).

Tetanus—Lockjaw

Tetanus is caused by anaerobic, spore-forming bacteria that produce an exotoxin; it can occur in soil, house dust, and animal feces. The bacteria enter through the skin and travels to the axons of the nerves, causing voluntary muscle contraction, muscular rigidity, and painful paroxysmal seizures. It starts with trismus (lockjaw) and difficulty in swallowing and can cause laryngospasm, respiratory distress, intramuscular hemorrhage, and death. One school nurse who had the disease described it as very painful; "it was like having a seizure where all of your muscles are pulling in every direction at the same time—and being awake experiencing it."

The incidence of tetanus peaked in 1923, when there were 1560 deaths in the United States. Since 1980, the annual numbers have been less than 100, with the disease affecting adults (91%) more than children (9%), with a mortality rate of 18% (Pascual, McGinley, Zanardi, Cortese, & Murphy, 2003). Therefore, protection is needed throughout life. Keep in mind that full immunization protection does not guarantee that the person will not get tetanus. Six percent of the cases between 1998 and 2000 had three or more doses of tetanus vaccine before contracting the disease (Pascual et al., 2003).

To help in the prevention of tetanus, the onus of responsibility is on the school nurse to assess the wound, clean it thoroughly, and make a referral if the student or staff is in need of tetanus antibodies. Contaminated wounds are those in contact with dirt, feces, or saliva, deep wounds, and wounds with necrotic tissue. Adolescents should be informed that the process of body piercing and applying tattoos may also be sources of tetanus if sterility is not maintained. This is a wonderful opportunity to make sure that students are up to date with their tetanus booster.

The general guidelines for recommended care are given in Table 21.2. It should be noted that "administration of extra doses of tetanus toxoid-containing vaccines earlier than the recommended intervals can increase the risk of hypersensitivity reactions" (AAP, 1999, p. 1066).

Table 21.2 ■

CRITERIA FOR EVALUATING WOUNDS FOR PROTECTION AGAINST TETANUS

- If (1) the wound is clean and (2) the person completed the primary series and (3) received a booster against tetanus *less than* 10 years ago, no treatment is needed other than cleaning the wound.
- If (1) the wound is contaminated and (2) the person completed the primary series and (3) immunization against tetanus is *more than* 5 years old, Tetanus toxoid (Td; the active vaccine) is recommended.
- If (1) the wound is contaminated and (2) there was either an incomplete series of immunizations or there is no record of immunizations, the person should receive *both* Tetanus toxoid (Td) *and* Tetanus Immune Globulin. (If the wound is clean, only Td needs to be given)

Source: CDC (2002f).

Pertussis—Whooping Cough

Pertussis is caused by a bacterium that proliferates in the respiratory tract. It is highly contagious, is transmitted person to person by aerosolized respiratory droplets or direct contact with secretions, and has an incubation period of 6 to 20 days (CDC, 2003a). It results in a spasmodic or paroxysmal cough where the person coughs repeatedly without taking a breath between coughs. At the end of the series of coughs, there is a prolonged inspiratory whoop. The spasms may result in vomiting after the coughing episode, anoxia, cyanosis, and possibly a loss of consciousness. The cough can last for weeks. The sequelae of pertussis infection include seizures (1.6%), encephalopathy (0.1%) (possibly resulting in mental retardation or stroke), pneumonia (11%), and death; it is especially dangerous for infants (Salmaso, 2003).

Outbreaks of pertussis continue to occur throughout the United States, with almost 19,000 cases reported in 2004, especially in infants who have not yet completed their initial series (29%) (CDC, 2002d, 2005). All age groups are affected, but only 20% of cases are over the age of 20. Effective immunization with whole cell pertussis, noted by a capital "P," resulted in the lowest incidence of 1,010 in 1976; it has slowly increased since that time. In 1996, an acellular pertussis was licensed, noted as "aP." It is reported to be less reactive and cause fewer serious side effects, but recently, the efficacy of some of the brands have been called into question (Plotkin, 2003). After the age of 6, the potential side effects from the traditional whole cell vaccine was considered to be of higher risk than the risk of getting the disease and suffering the side effects of that; therefore, immunization schedules do not include the pertussis vaccine after that age. "However, the availability of the acellular vaccines has opened the possibility of further vaccination in adolescents and adults" (Salmaso, 2003, p. 216).

DTaP Vaccine

The DTaP (diphtheria and tetanus toxoids and acellular pertussis) is almost always given as a combination vaccine. It is recommended (intramuscularly) at 2, 4, and 6 months with boosters between 15 and 18 months and again between 4 and 6 years (Figure 21.1). That means children should have five doses before they enter first grade. The fifth dose is not necessary if the fourth dose was given after the fourth birthday (AAP, 2003b). Daptacel (Adventis Pasteur) was approved in 2002 and requires only four doses (2, 4, 6, and 17 to 20 months) (CDC, 2002a).

If the student is entering school with no immunizations or an incomplete series, the pertussis component is *not* given after the seventh birthday. After age 7, the tetanus toxoid with the adult dose of diphtheria (Td) is given. If the child has an active neurological condition, such as active seizures, the pertussis component will probably not be given and the child younger than age 7 will receive a DT.

Three acellular pertussis vaccines are available in the United States: Infanrix (GlaxoSmithKline), Tripedia (Aventis Pasteur), and Daptacel (Adventis Pasteur, Ltd.). Many children experience side effects from this vaccine, but few of them are considered major. For the whole cell pertussis vaccines, which are no longer used in the United States, 40% developed fever, 30% developed localized redness and swelling, and a small percentage developed persistent crying for 3 or more hours, seizures, and hypotonic–hyporesponsive episodes (Salmaso, 2003). With the acellular pertussis vaccine, fever, irritability, injection site pain, somnolence, and loss of appetite were the most common side effects seen. The side effects do increase with successive doses of the acellular pertussis, especially swelling of the injected limb (Rennels et al., 2000). To be considered a side effect of the vaccine, symptoms must appear within 72 hours of the vaccination.

While it is recommended that the same vaccine be used throughout the series, research does demonstrate that Infanrix and Tripedia can be interchanged without impacting on the development of titers and safety (Greenberg et al., 2002). Only one vaccine—TriHIBit (Aventis Pasteur) (DTaP and PRP-T Hib [Hib conjugated to tetanus])—is FDA approved for mixing Hib and DTaP in the same syringe. This should not be used for the primary vaccination series, but can be used for the Hib/DTaP booster at 15 to 18 months.

Rubeola—Measles

Rubeola is caused by a respiratory tract virus. It is one of the most contagious of the communicable diseases, with an incubation period of 7 to 18 days. It starts with fever, a rasping cough, conjunctivitis, and coryza and proceeds to a red, pruritic maculopapular rash, Koplik's spots on the buccal mucosa, and photophobia. There is a high risk of consequences of this infection, including bacterial superinfections, such as pneumonia, otitis media, and encephalitis (1:1,000), often with permanent brain damage and mental retardation, subacute sclerosing panencephalitis, and death (1 to 2:1,000) (CDC, 1998).

Rubeola is differentiated from rubella by lay terms such as the "red measles," the "10-day measles," and the "sick measles." The incidence of measles has dropped precipitously since the initiation of the required MMR booster dose, yet 30% of the U.S. cases are internationally imported (CDC, 2002c). In 2000, 63% of the cases were in infants, children, and adolescents. During an outbreak of measles, infants between the ages of 6 months and 1 year may be vaccinated against measles within 72 hours of exposure, but this dose will not count toward their two required doses (CDC, 1998).

Rubella—German Measles

Rubella is also caused by a virus in the respiratory tract. It starts with subauricular (behind the ear) and suboccipital (back of the neck) lymphadenopathy and proceeds to a pink maculopapular rash; however, 20% to 50% of infected persons are asymptomatic (CDC, 2001d). Individuals who contract this disease are not very ill or uncomfortable. While there are reports of serious side effects for some, including transient arthralgia and arthritis (especially for adults), idiopathic thrombocytopenic purpura (1:3,000), and encephalitis (1:6,000), the greatest danger of contracting rubella is to the fetus of a pregnant female (CDC, 1998).

Congenital rubella syndrome (CRS) results when mothers contract rubella, primarily in the first trimester; the child can be born with growth retardation, mental retardation, cataracts, deafness, and cardiac anomalies. Since 86% of rubella cases are now seen in adults, especially those who are foreign born, it becomes more important to protect children and thereby prevent them from carrying the disease home to their child-bearing mothers (CDC, 2001a).

One dose of the MMR will probably provide protection against Rubella (within 21 to 28 days of the vaccination), although two doses are needed to provide protection against measles (CDC, 2001a).

Parotitis—Mumps

Parotitis is caused by a virus that infects the respiratory tract and usually causes swelling of the parotid glands and painful swallowing; 15% to 20% are asymptomatic and another 50% have nonspecific respiratory symptoms. The possible consequences of this infection include aseptic meningitis, orchitis, and epididymitis in older males, nerve deafness, and encephalitis; the encephalitis can result in seizures, paralysis, and hydrocephalus (CDC, 1998).

MMR Vaccine (Measles, Mumps, Rubella)

Two subcutaneously administered doses of the MMR (Merck) are recommended: at 12 to 15 months and then again between 4 and 6 years of age. However, the second dose can be given at any age, as long as it is at least 28 days after the first dose. The use of licensed combination vaccines is preferred over separate injections of their equivalent component vaccines. These live attenuated virus vaccines are now referred to as "further attenuated" and cause fewer side effects (CDC, 1998).

The measles and mumps vaccine are produced in chick embryo cell cultures; the rubella vaccine is grown in human diploid cell culture (CDC, 1998). Contraindications to the MMR include an anaphylactic reaction to gelatin or neomycin and persons with severe immunodeficiency from any cause. "Allergy to egg is not a contraindication" (CDC, 2001a, p. 16). Those with mild immunosuppression may be vaccinated. Women of child-bearing age who receive the vaccine are advised to avoid pregnancy for 28 days following the vaccine, although no cases of CRS have been identified to have occurred as a result of the vaccine (CDC, 2001c).

Side effects of the vaccine occur in 5% to 15% of individuals after approximately 7 days. They include fever, rash, and swollen glands. Arthralgia is commonly seen in 25% of adolescents and adults. Rare side effects include febrile seizures (1:100,000), encephalitis (1:1 million), and thrombocytopenia (1:30,000). To be considered a side effect of the vaccine, symptoms must occur within 15 days of the immunization.

The appropriate storage of this vaccine is essential to ensure that the vaccine will provide protection against the disease. *Light will inactivate the vaccine viruses. Once reconstituted, the vaccine must be protected from light, must be refrigerated but not frozen, and must be discarded if not used within 8 hours* (CDC, 1998).

There are a number of concerns and myths regarding the MMR vaccine. The vaccine does not exacerbate tuberculosis. It may temporarily suppress tuberculin reactivity and cause a PPD to read negative when it is in reality positive for up to 1 month. Therefore, TB testing should be done on the same day as measles vaccine is given; otherwise one should wait at least 4 to 6 weeks to do the testing (CDC, 1998). There is also no association between the MMR and inflammatory bowel disease. Likewise, there is no association between MMR vaccine and the development of autism. Multiple studies indicate that the risk for autism is the same in countries where the MMR is given during the second year of life and those where the MMR is delayed until after age 3 (DeStefano, Bhasin, Thompson, Yeargin-Allsopp, & Boyle, 2004).

Haemophilus influenzae, Type b—Hib

Haemophilus influenza is caused by a bacterium; there are six different types (a to f), of which b is the most dangerous. It was the leading cause of serious invasive bacterial disease in children under the age of 5 years until the 1980s, causing most of the bacterial meningitis, epiglottitis, sepsis, and cellulitis seen in that age group and the morbidity and mortality that resulted. It was especially common in daycare centers and is transmitted through respiratory droplets. It colonizes in the nasopharynx of 2% to 4% of normal children, most of whom do not become ill, but they can spread Hib to susceptible hosts. It is not transmitted on dry surfaces. The signs and symptoms depend on the presenting infection. In the 1980s, it had an associated mortality rate of 3% to 7% and a morbidity rate of 25% to 35% (i.e., deafness, mental retardation, ataxia) (Meissner & Pickering, 2002). Hib vaccine has significantly decreased the incidence of diseases caused by Hib.

Hib Vaccine

The initial Hib vaccines were not effective in children younger than the age of 2 years, when most were contracting the disease. In 1988, the new Hib vaccines were generated, made more effective by conjugating them to a nontoxic form of another organism, such as the meningococcal, diphtheria, or tetanus proteins. There is no antibody response to these latter products and these conjugates do not substitute for the regular immunization schedule for these products. Infants have received this vaccine since 1991, and the incidence of disease has declined by more than 99% (CDC, 2002e).

Three or four doses (depending on the manufacturer) are administered intramuscularly before the age of 15 months and vaccination is not recommended for those older than 5 years of age. Three Hib vaccines are licensed for infants; PedvaxHIB (Merck) and ComVax require only three doses (2, 4, and 12 to 15 months); HibTITER (Wyeth) requires an additional dose at 6 months. It should be remembered, however, that the vaccine protects only against type b, and not the other strains of *Haemophilus influenzae* (CDC, 2002e). ComVax is a combination vaccine and also includes the immunization for hepatitis B. TriHIBit is a combination of Hib vaccine and DTaP vaccine and can be given **only** for the 15- to 18-month dose

Hib vaccines have very few side effects. Irritability, drowsiness, anorexia, fever, diarrhea, and vomiting may be seen in addition to redness and swelling at the site of the injection. There is no foundation to the myth that Hib vaccine results in diabetes.

Poliomyelitis

Polio affected 20,000 people each year in the United States until the advent of immunization in the 1950s. Now only a handful of cases occur each year, most of which were transmitted by those receiving the live oral polio vaccine. Yet, it still exists around the world, mostly in Africa, India, and a few third world countries; the Dominican Republic had an outbreak in 2000–2001 during which 19 people were paralyzed and 2 died. Polio is caused by an enterovirus that spreads via the fecal–oral route; it can be spread person to person or transmitted by indirect contact with contaminated saliva, feces, sewage, or water. It replicates in the gastrointestinal (GI) tract and then enters the blood and spreads to the central nervous system. The virus multiplies in the motor neurons of the anterior horn and brain stem and causes destruction and paralysis. Symptoms initially include a stiff neck and muscle pains, followed by nerve damage and asymmetrical flaccid paralysis, but without sensory deficits. Although some muscle function returns, some degree of flaccid paralysis often remains. However, 30 to 40 years after the initial attack, many are developing post-polio syndrome, which presents with exacerbation of existing muscle weakness and results in the development of new areas of muscle pain and weakness.

There are three different serotypes of the poliovirus (1, 2, and 3). The initial vaccine was the Salk vaccine, which was an inactivated poliovirus. The Sabin oral polio vaccine was developed to protect against all three types plus the wild poliovirus, which was last seen in the United States in 1979 (CDC, 2000a). While the oral vaccine was very effective and did not require an injection, it posed a risk to those who received it and those who cared for them, as it moved through the GI system and was excreted in the stool. If the child or the caretaker was immunosuppressed, there was a chance that the polio could affect him or her. This was referred to as vaccine-associated paralytic poliomyelitis (VAPP). Between 1980 and 1998, 144 of the 152 cases in the United States were due to VAPP. Because of this and because the wild poliovirus was no longer present in the United States, the immunization requirements changed back to the inactivated polio vaccine in 2000. The oral polio vaccine is no longer available in the United States.

Polio Vaccine

The current vaccine, IPOL (Aventis Pasteur), is a trivalent enhanced inactivated (killed) Salk polio vaccine. It requires three doses during the first 18 months and then a booster before age 6, with the result being that 99% to 100% of children develop protective antibodies to all three types (CDC, 2000a). This is a safe vaccine with minimal side effects. An allergic reaction to the vaccine components (neomycin, streptomycin, polymyxin B) and fever are possible but rare.

Varicella—Chickenpox

Getting chickenpox used to be one of the rights of passage through childhood. Before the advent of vaccination, 4 million cases occurred each year in the United States. Although generally considered benign, the disease resulted in 11,000 hospitalizations and 100 deaths each year (CDC, 2003f). Since immunization became available, there has been a 78% decrease in the incidence of the disease, or people experience a milder form. However, as more children are immunized, varicella will become a disease of adults, in whom the risk of complications is 10 to 20 times higher than for children (AAP, 2000).

Chickenpox is caused by the varicella herpes zoster virus that is transmitted by respiratory droplets; it is highly contagious. It is diagnosed by a vesicular, pruritic rash, with each vesicle surrounded by a reddened area that begins on the trunk and progresses proximodistally. Lesions can be found in all stages simultaneously (macular rash, vesicle, scab). *Any students with papular or vesicular lesions should be excluded from school immediately. When the lesions are all crusted over, the student is no longer contagious and may return to class, as the scabs are not infectious.* Those infected are contagious from 2 days before the appearance of a rash to 6 days after; therefore, those whose rash appears during school hours have been infectious for at least 48 hours. The care at home is symptomatic focusing on measures to decrease the itch and prevent secondary infections from scratching (keep nails short; pat, don't rub; and use calamine lotion, cool oatmeal baths, antihistamines, and light loose-fitting clothes). While the incubation period is 21 days, those exposed are not at risk until day 7. An immunocompromised student and his or her family must be notified so that the student can receive passive protection of varicella antibodies.

The sequelae of the disease include bacterial superinfections, especially group A streptococcal disease, pneumonia, ataxia, encephalitis, and years later, shingles. *Aspirin should be avoided during this viral infection, since it is highly associated with the development of Reye Syndrome, which is an acute encephalopathy with cerebral cortex swelling but without inflammation.* It is accompanied by impaired liver function and hyperammonemia and is associated with an extremely high mortality and morbidity rate.

One of the interesting facts about varicella infections is that there is the possibility that they may recur in 4.5% to 13.3% of individuals, which may be due to the failure of a previously healthy individual to mount an effective antibody titer to it; this tendency may run in families (Hall et al., 2002).

Varicella Vaccine

Verivax (Merck) is a live attenuated vaccine for varicella, approved in 1995. The vaccine contains gelatin and neomycin, so those with anaphylactoid reactions to these products should not receive the vaccine. It is also contraindicated in those individuals who have a cellular immunodeficient condition or are receiving immunosuppressants. Similarly to the MMR, varicella vaccine is not given until after the first birthday. At this time, only one dose is recommended for children; however, for those older than the age of 13 years, two doses are recommended, given at least 4 weeks apart.

The vaccine is 97% effective in preventing moderate to severe disease (defined as having fewer than 50 lesions) and 85% effective in preventing all forms of varicella. Side effects from the vaccine include fever, a varicella-like rash within 2 weeks of the vaccination, and localized discomfort at the injection site. *The vaccine should be frozen and protected from light. It can then be kept in a refrigerator for up to 72 hours, but then it must be discarded. Since it must be reconstituted with specific diluent, once reconstituted, it must be used within 30 minutes or else it must be discarded.* Postexposure immunization with Varicella Zoster Immune Globulin (VZIG) is 90% effective in preventing varicella if given within 3 days of contact (AAP, 2000).

There is the possibility of breakthrough disease, which is a varicella-like rash that occurs more than 42 days after vaccination for varicella. The condition is almost always mild with a low-grade fever and fewer than 50 lesions present; it lasts 2 to 3 days. One hypothesis for this occurrence is decreased potency of the vaccine resulting from improper storage (Watson & Levin, 2004).

Hepatitis

Hepatitis, or inflammation of the liver, can be caused by many agents, such as drugs (acetaminophen, methotrexate, anabolic steroids), ionizing radiation, autoimmune processes, bacteria, alcohol, and viruses (Selekman, 1999). There are six types of viral hepatitis: A, B, C, D, E, and G. Types A, B, and C are the most common.

The liver has multiple functions. When inflammation occurs in response to viral invasion, there is resulting damage to liver cells; blockage of the bile ducts, resulting in increased bilirubin in the blood (causing jaundice and dark urine) and decreased bilirubin in the GI tract (causing clay-colored stools); and liver enlargement (causing abdominal pain). Liver function is compromised as the liver fails, resulting in bleeding tendencies (due to decreased prothrombin and decreased vitamin K absorption); decreased detoxification of drugs and poisons; and altered metabolism of fats, carbohydrates, proteins, and sugar. Most children with viral hepatitis do not demonstrate the overt symptomatology that would help make a diagnosis. Yet, as a result of poor hygiene practices, they may easily pass the disease on to adults who may be more severely impacted by it.

Hepatitis A

More than 8,700 cases of hepatitis A, previously called infectious hepatitis, were reported in the United States in 2002, with the highest rates being in the 5- to 14-year-old group and 15% occurring in day care centers. This is a stark reduction from the 30,000 cases per year in the 1980s. Up to 26% of current cases occurred in household or sexual contacts (CDC, 2003b). In 2004, the number of cases decreased to just over 5,600 (Table 21.1). However, it is believed that the numbers of those affected by hepatitis A before the advent of hepatitis A vaccine exceeded 270,000 each year, primarily because half of children affected, and 70% of those younger than age 6, have no symptoms (Armstrong & Bell, 2002; CDC, 1999b).

This highly infectious virus is spread by the fecal–oral route and is usually self-limiting. After ingestion, it multiplies in the liver and is then excreted in the bile and then through the stool. Consequently, *poor handwashing after toileting or after changing diapers puts one at risk of transmitting the virus to others directly or through food being prepared. It can transfer from an inanimate object to a person's hands up to 3 hours after being placed on the object and can be inactivated by boiling or heating to more than 185 degrees F for 1 minute or disinfecting surfaces with household bleach* (CDC, 1999b). The incubation period is from 15 to 50 days. Once the individual is infected, the period of infectivity lasts for 2 weeks before symptoms appear and for a week after jaundice develops (CDC, 1999b). Symptoms last for weeks.

Students with hepatitis A need to stay home until the symptoms disappear. It should be noted that "*children and infants can shed HAV [Hepatitis A Virus] for longer periods than adults, up to several months after the onset of clinical illness*" (CDC, 1999b, p. 3). This has implications for school nurses who work with the youngest children and change diapers. Those exposed can receive serum immunoglobulin within 2 weeks of exposure. When the children return to school, they should have specific orders regarding any limitations that should be initiated in physical education and recess activities. They may be more fatigued and have special dietary needs.

Hepatitis A Vaccine

Hepatitis A vaccine is not recommended as part of the routine immunization schedule, although some states and counties do require it for entry into day care and kindergarten. It is recommended only for those with certain risk factors, such as hemophilia or chronic liver disease, and for those who live in communities where the annual incidence is twice the average annual rate.

Two inactivated viral vaccines are available to protect against hepatitis A: Havrix (GlaxoSmithKline) and Vaqta (Merck). The first vaccine was licensed in 1996. Two doses are administered intramuscularly in the deltoid muscle at least 6 months apart (AAP, 2003b), although the first dose cannot be given until after the age of 2. They are safe vaccines with side effects of injection site soreness and headache. It should be noted that both vaccines have a pediatric version, as the dosages are different for children and adults. A combined hepatitis A and B vaccine is available for both children and adults. In some states, efforts to immunize preschoolers and children entering kindergarten have greatly decreased the number of cases seen in younger children.

Hepatitis B

Hepatitis B was previously called serum hepatitis and is much more serious than hepatitis A. It is spread through all body secretions, including blood, saliva, tears, semen, vaginal secretions, and urine. Therefore, *human bites, sharing toothbrushes, tattooing and body piercing, sexual intercourse, intravenous drug use, and even exposure to cuts and scrapes during contact sports place a student at high risk of transmission*. The majority of those affected are asymptomatic; "only 20% are overtly ill and 30% have a subclinical course that resembles influenza" (Selekman, 1999, p. 544). Children are at much higher risk than adolescents and adults of having the acute disease progress to a chronic infection (30% to 90%), which can lead to cirrhosis, liver cancer, and death (CDC, 2003b). Since the advent of mandatory immunization, the incidence of hepatitis B has decreased significantly, yet 7,000 cases still occur each year, with many more people who are carriers. The CDC (2002b) estimates that 1.2 million Americans have chronic HBV and 4,000 to 5,000 deaths each year are caused by HBV-related liver diseases.

The *hepatitis B virus* (HBV) is a hardy virus that *can remain on surfaces for weeks*. It is not killed by cleaning agents available in most schools; "it is inactivated by glutaraldehyde, formalin, urea, and gastric secretions; therefore, it is not orally spread unless there are tears in the mouth" (Selekman, 1999, p. 544). It can be *spread by direct or indirect contact with eyes, mouth, or broken or inflamed skin*. Following contact by a nonimmunized individual, hepatitis B immunoglobulin and the first of the three-shot series of hepatitis B immunization are given within 24 hours of exposure.

Hepatitis B Vaccine

Introduced more than 20 years ago, this vaccine has resulted in a significant decrease in the incidence and morbidity associated with HBV. Two vaccines are available: Engerix-B (GlaxoSmithKline), which requires three doses for individuals of all ages, and Recombivax HB (Merck), which requires three doses for infants but only two doses for those immunized after age 11. The vaccines are safe and have mild side effects, such as injection site soreness, fever, and fatigue; however, they are contraindicated in those who are allergic to yeast. There is no truth to the myth that HBV vaccine results in demyelinating neurological disorders.

As more infants are routinely immunized, more children will enter the school system protected. However, *it is important to immunize adolescents prior to their engagement in high-risk behaviors common to their age group. It is also important to ensure that school staff are immunized against hepatitis B, especially coaches of sports teams, special education teachers, preschool teachers, physical education teachers, maintenance/cleaning staff, first aid administrators (first responders) and, of course, school nurses.*

Hepatitis C

Prior to 1989, hepatitis C was known as non-A non-B hepatitis. There are at least 6 different genotypes and 90 different subtypes of hepatitis C (Selekman, 1999). Some discussion has centered on whether hepatitis C is actually two viruses, one being *hepatitis G* (Neff & Schiff, 1999). Hepatitis C is now recognized as the most common cause of parenterally transmitted hepatitis. It can be transmitted through blood and blood products (including clotting factors), intravenous drug use, contaminated multiple-dose medication vials, hemodialysis, and organ transplantation. It can also occur as a result of body piercing and tattooing. Although only 20% to 30% of those infected have symptoms of acute hepatitis, almost 60% of those infected as adolescents will develop chronic disease (CDC, 2003b). The possible sequelae for this group include chronic liver disease, cirrhosis, and liver cancer. Hepatitis C is the leading reason for liver transplants and kills approximately 10,000 Americans annually. No vaccine against hepatitis C is available. The incubation period is 6 to 7 weeks. Once symptoms occur, patients may be put on a variety of interferons (CDC, 2003b). However, they may carry the virus for the rest of their lives.

Those with hepatitis C should not share toothbrushes, razors, or other personal care items because of the chance that they may have blood on them. The disease is not transmitted by casual contact.

Hepatitis D

Hepatitis D (HDV) was formerly called delta hepatitis. This virus cannot exist alone; the patient must also have hepatitis B. Five percent of patients with HBV also have HDV and this results in symptoms that are more serious than those seen with HBV alone (Borkowsky & Krugman, 1998); there is also a greater risk of serious sequelae. Because it cannot exist alone, prevention of hepatitis B with the appropriate vaccine will also prevent hepatitis D.

Hepatitis E

This type of hepatitis was previously called enteric or epidemic non-A, non-B hepatitis. It is most similar to hepatitis A in its symptoms and mode of transmission (fecal–oral route), especially from impure drinking water, and the fact that it is also self-limiting and does not usually result in chronic liver disease. It does have a high mortality rate among pregnant women who contract the disease. No vaccine is available yet for this type of hepatitis.

Pneumococcal Disease

Since the success of the Hib vaccine, pneumococcal disease has become the most common cause of vaccine-preventable death in the United States. Each year, it causes 700 cases of meningitis, 17,000 cases of bloodstream infections, 71,000 cases of pneumococcal pneumonia, and 5 million ear infections, all in children younger than the age of 5. It has an increased incidence in day care settings and among African Americans and American Indians. It is increasingly becoming antibiotic resistant.

Streptococcus pneumoniae, also known as *Pneumococcus*, is an encapsulated, gram-positive polysaccharide with 90 different serotypes identified. Approximately 25% of these serotypes cause 90% of pneumococcal disease. Seven of the serotypes account for 80% of invasive disease in the United

States in children younger than 6 years of age: 4, 6B, 9V, 14, 18C, 19F, and 23F (CDC, 2000b). The bacteria are carried in the nose and throat of healthy people and spread from person to person. The very young, the elderly, and those with chronic conditions are most at risk of having difficulty fighting the organism, should it invade.

Pneumococcal Vaccine

The conjugated vaccines (Pneumovax [PPV23-Merck] and Pnu-imune (Wyeth-Ayerst) are 23-valent vaccines and are better for adults. The seven-valent pneumococcal vaccine, Prevnar (PCV7)(Wyeth Lederle), is better for children. To be effective in children younger than age 2, it is conjugated to another product. Common side effects include redness, tenderness, and swelling at the injection site; low-grade fever; and irritability or drowsiness. Adverse events from the vaccine include decreased movement in the injected extremity with injection site swelling and allergic reactions to vaccine products.

The ACIP recommends this vaccine for all children younger than age 2 and for children younger than age 5 with high-risk conditions, including asplenia, sickle cell disease, human immunodeficiency virus (HIV), chronic illness, a cerebrospinal fluid leak, a cochlear implant, and immunocompromised status. Asthma is not considered a high-risk condition for pneumococcal vaccine.

If the first dose is started between 2 and 6 months of age, three doses 2 months apart and a fourth dose at age 12 to 15 months are recommended. If the first dose is started between 7 and 11 months, two doses 2 months apart and a booster at age 12 to 15 months is recommended. If the first dose is given after the first birthday but before the second, two doses are given at least 2 months apart. For healthy children between 24 and 59 months who have an incomplete series, it might be beneficial to consider one dose, at least 2 months after the last dose; however, those who are high risk and between the ages of 2 and 5 years should have three doses, with at least 2 months between each dose (CDC, 2003d). For those older than the age of 5 who are considered high risk, the 23-valent polysaccharide vaccine can be administered.

The vaccine is contraindicated for those with hypersensitivity to the DaPT and latex. It needs to be remembered that there are multiple strains of pneumococcal bacteria that are not covered by the vaccines, and therefore, the vaccine does not eradicate pneumococcal disease. The duration of protection after PCV7 is unknown.

Meningococcal Disease

There are approximately 2,000 cases of meningococcal disease each year in the United States. While the greatest incidence is in infants (11:100,000), the ratio drops from 18 months through adulthood, with an average of 1.5:100,000. An increase in incidence has been observed in college freshmen who live in dormitories, however, with a rate of 4.6:100,000. The initial signs and symptoms mimic the flu, but the disease progresses very rapidly, with death possibly occurring within 12 hours of the onset of symptoms. Symptoms of meningococcal meningitis include a severe headache, stiff neck, nausea, and vomiting. Sensitivity to light and sleepiness may also be present. Within hours, the child may develop confusion, seizures, altered consciousness, and coma (Pfister & Bleck, 2003). Purpura, a rapidly spreading purplish rash, is seen in 75% of cases. Morbidity, especially neurological disability, hearing loss, and limb loss, occurs in 11% to 25% of cases (CDC, 2000c).

There are 12 serotypes of *Neisseria meningitides* (Masignani, Pizza, & Rappuoli, 2003). However, only five of them have been associated with disease: A, B, C, Y, and W-135 (CDC, 2000c). It is *spread much like pneumococcal disease, by close contact with respiratory droplets of infected individuals. It is not spread by casual contact; therefore those in the home and anyone with whom the student worked closely, kissed, shared eating utensils or played closely enough to have contact with the discharge from the patient's nose and mouth are at risk*. The incubation period is 2 to 10 days (Heyman, 2004) and the *person infected is contagious for at least 24 hours after starting antibiotics*. For those in direct contact with an infected student or staff member, antibiotics can be administered to prevent the spread of the bacteria.

Bacterial meningitis is reportable to the state health department, which is prepared to handle all aspects of the illness, including the media releases. A protocol is usually in place related to how school contacts should be notified, the directions to give them, and the treatment recommendations.

Meningococcal Vaccine

The vaccine is not effective in infants and children younger than 2 years of age, the group with the highest incidence. The vaccine includes the subgroups A, C, Y, and W-135. It does not include the B group, which causes most of the cases in children younger than 1 year of age; but the vaccine is not effective in this young age group. It is deemed most appropriate for college freshmen, especially those living in a dormitory, and for individuals with asplenia and complement deficiency.

One vaccine against *Neisseria meningitides* is called Menomune. It is considered a safe vaccine but it does not last very long in the system. "Although the need for revaccination of older children and adults has not been determined, antibody levels rapidly decline over 2–3 years" (CDC, 2000c, p. 4). It is recommended for those who are 2 to 10 years old and for adults older than age 55 and for those who cannot access the newer vaccine. A second vaccine, Menactra, also called MCV4, was approved in 2005 for those 11 to 55 years of age. This vaccine is thought to be effective for 10 years or more (Meningococcal Vaccines, 2005; Shepard, Ortez-Sanchez, Scott, Rosenstein, & the ABCs Team, 2005). The school nurse may be asked by 12th-grade students or their parents about the pros and cons of being immunized prior to leaving for college. The current recommendation for college students is especially focused on those living in dormitories (CDC, 2000e; Meningococcal Vaccines, 2005). Parents and college students need to be informed about the dangers of meningococcal disease; the vaccine is recommended to reduce the risk of this disease.

Influenza

The incidence of influenza is higher for children than for any other age group (CDC, 2003c), although morbidity and mortality are highest in the elderly. It attacks between 15% and 42% of preschool and school-age children each year (AAP, 2004). For the 2003–2004 season, there were at least 152 influenza-associated deaths in children and adolescents (Update: Influenza Activity, 2004). Epidemics usually occur during the winter months.

Two types of influenza viruses cause epidemic disease in humans: A and B. Influenza A is divided into two subtypes: hemagglutinin (H) and neuraminidase (N). "Antibody against one influenza virus type or subtype confers limited or no protection against another" (CDC, 2003c, p. 2). Viruses frequently mutate. This antigenic drift results in the annual change in the makeup of the vaccine, which usually includes two types of A and one type of B. Thus while all of the above diseases are caused by relatively stable agents over time, the influenza viruses vary significantly from year to year.

Influenza is spread by respiratory droplet; it has a very short incubation period (1 to 4 days). "Children can be infectious for ≥ 10 days, and young children can shed virus for ≤ 6 days before their illness onset" (CDC, 2003c, p. 2). Symptoms include fever, achiness, headache, nonproductive cough, sore throat, rhinitis, otitis media, nausea, and vomiting. There appears to be considerable overlap in the symptoms of influenza and those due to severe acute respiratory syndrome (SARS). *Administration of aspirin to children with flu symptoms is contraindicated, as it is strongly correlated to Reye syndrome.*

Influenza Vaccine

Each year, the CDC attempts to project which types of influenza virus are likely to circulate throughout the United States during the next flu season. The strains that were used for the 2003–2004 season in the trivalent inactivated influenza vaccine (or their equivalents) were: A/Moscow/10/99 (H3N2)-like, A/New Caledonia/20/99 (H1N1)-like, and B/Hong Kong/330/2001-like antigens. The 2004–2005 influenza vaccine contained A/New Caledonia/20/99-like (H1N1), A/Fujian/411/2002-like (H3N2), and B/Shanghai/361/2002-like viruses (Update: Influenza Activity, 2004). The vaccine is effective for only a few months; therefore, the optimal time for administration to the school-age population is November (CDC, 2003c). Flu season often peaks in February.

Most flu vaccines are grown on hen eggs inactivated, and until 2000 still contained thimerosal. However, Fluzone (Aventis Pasteur), is thimerosal free. Fluzone is the only influenza vaccine that should be used for infants and toddlers. Targeted groups for influenza vaccine include those children and adolescents with chronic cardiopulmonary disorders, including asthma and those who are taking long-term aspirin therapy, because of the risk of contracting Reye syndrome. Fluzone should never be administered if it has been frozen, as it will lose its effectiveness. Children younger than the age of 9 who are receiving injected flu vaccine for the first time will need a second dose 1 month after the first.

A new product, FluMist (MedImmune), provides the flu vaccine via a nasal spray squirted into the nares. This trivalent live attenuated cold-adapted influenza vaccine is recommended only for *healthy* individuals who are between the ages of 5 and 49; these are not the groups with the highest mortality or morbidity. The reason for caution is because of the chance of the vaccine causing disease. It is especially contraindicated in children with asthma, as it appears to increase the incidence of asthma attacks in young children (CDC, 2003f). The nasal vaccine works by stimulating the immune system through the same route as the natural virus uses: through the nasal mucosa.

COMBINATION VACCINES

Companies that manufacture vaccines are attempting to combine multiple vaccines to decrease the number of injections given to infants. Children routinely receive as many as 20 shots by age 2 (Offit et al., 2002). DaPT as well as MMR have been combined for years in specially designed products. The polio vaccine protects against three strains or serotypes of the virus. The pneumococcal vaccines contain antigens for either 7 or 23 strains. Twinrix (GlaxoSmithKline) combines vaccines for hepatitis A and B. Only in the last decade have DaPT and Hib been combined as well as Hib and Hep B. New to the market are ProQuad (Merck) which combines MMR and varicella, and Pediatrix (GlaxoSmithKline), which includes DPTa, hepatitis B, and IPV for the 2-, 4-, and 6-month doses. The use of this latter vaccine will decrease the number of shots before age 2 to 14 or 15.

The key to combining vaccines is to ensure that the new sera produces the same level of protective titers as each of the vaccines separately. It is anticipated that future combinations will decrease the cost of administration and of storage of the vaccines and increase compliance of parents to seek protection for their children.

NEW VACCINES OR RARELY USED VACCINES

As scientific advances in genetics and technology continue to expand, it can be expected that the number of vaccines being developed will increase exponentially. Vaccines are being developed in areas outside of human health care, including agriculture and manufacturing. From the introduction of the first smallpox vaccine, it took 184 years to eradicate smallpox; technology has shortened that potential timeline considerably. Today, it takes approximately 10 years and more than $100 million dollars to develop a vaccine to meet U.S. standards (Ellis, 2002).

Vaccines against rabies, Japanese encephalitis, typhoid, yellow fever, smallpox, and anthrax have been available. Because of the threat of bioterrorism, the anthrax and smallpox vaccines have been reformulated and administered to larger numbers of first-line individuals. Smallpox was last seen in the world in 1977 and routine vaccination in the United States stopped in 1971 (CDC, 2002g); in 2003, it was proposed that the vaccine be administered again on a large scale. Because of numerous severe side effects that developed in a few individuals, especially myopericarditis, the mass immunization of first-line providers was stopped, but may be reinstated after further evaluation of the threat and the associated risks.

New vaccines in clinical trials include those against HPV to ultimately decrease the risk of cervical cancer; a herpes vaccine to prevent genital herpes simplex virus type 1 or type 2; vaccines against West Nile virus, *Staphylococcus aureus*, and Alzheimer's disease; and various vaccines against HIV. Conditions being discussed as candidates for future vaccines include many of the sexually transmitted diseases. In addition to new vaccines are new routes of immunization. Bioengineering has opened doors to the possibility of putting vaccines into foodstuffs, such as bananas, potatoes, rice, wheat, and corn (Lutwick & Abramson, 2000).

VACCINE SAFETY

The National Childhood Vaccine Injury Act was passed in 1986 and required health professionals and vaccine manufacturers to report adverse effects that occur after the administration of vaccines. The Vaccine Adverse Event Reporting System (VAERS) and the Vaccine Safety Datalink Project (VSD) were established to accept the reports so that they could be analyzed (CDC, 2003e). Parents, healthcare providers, and others can make those reports. VSD attempts to analyze the adverse events and their association with the immunizations. However, the limitation of this research is that there is no comparison made to those who have not received immunizations or for those who developed delayed-onset symptomatology. Thus VAERS reports do not establish cause and effect.

Of the 1.9 billion doses of human vaccines distributed in the United States, there were more than 128,000 reports. "The most commonly reported adverse event was fever, which appeared in 25.8% of all reports, followed by injection-site hypersensitivity (15.8%), rash (unspecified) (11.0%), injection-site edema (10.8%), and vasodilatation (10.8%)" (CDC, 2003e, p. 2). Approximately 14% of the reports were for serious adverse effects. The National Vaccine Injury Compensation Program is very specific as to what constitutes an adverse event. For example, for an anaphylactic reaction to be attributed to the DaPT, it must occur within 4 hours of the vaccine administration and the encephalopathy must occur within 72 hours. For encephalopathy to be associated with the MMR, it must occur not less than 5 days and not more than 15 days from when the vaccine was administered.

Some vaccines are developed and may be released too early. The rotavirus vaccine was approved in 1998, after having been tested on 11,000 children. However, it was pulled from the market 14 months later after it was found to cause intussusception in 1 out of every 10,000 children. Lyme disease vaccine was also associated with an increased number of side effects and in 2001 it was withdrawn from the market. The swine flu vaccine of 1994 was associated with cases of Guillain-Barré syndrome. This is not part of the current influenza vaccine. VAERS also was able to demonstrate that the side effects from the acellular pertussis vaccine were half of that of the whole cell vaccine.

According to Offit and Hackett (2003), immunizations do not cause or exacerbate allergy, asthma, or autoimmune diseases such as multiple sclerosis, type 1 diabetes mellitus, and chronic arthritis. Some vaccines may actually "prevent or modify" some of these conditions. *It is essential for school nurses to keep updated on the facts related to immunization and the myths related to safety in order to provide accurate information to parents who question their efficacy* and safety. It also needs to be remembered that there is always a very small number of children in whom the vaccines are not effective and they fail to develop the necessary titer.

The Vaccine Adverse Events Reporting System can be found at http://www.fda.gov/cber/vaers/vaers.htm. The National Vaccine Injury Compensation Program can be found at http://www.hrsa.gov/osp/vicp.

PARENTS WHO REFUSE IMMUNIZATIONS FOR THEIR CHILDREN

Informal surveys indicate that the reasons for refusal to vaccinate children are the perceived danger of the vaccine and a belief that they should be the persons responsible for determining what their child receives. They believe that their environment will protect their child from the disease or the sequelae of the disease. It is important to demonstrate that the risk of the sequelae of the disease far exceeds the risk from any adverse events from the vaccine (Diekema and the Committee on Bioethics, 2005).

All states allow medical exemptions and all but two (Mississippi and West Virginia) allow for exemptions on religious grounds. Fifteen states permit exemptions on philosophical grounds. However, it is clear that those with exemptions are much more likely to contract the contagious diseases, should an outbreak occur. In most cases, it is appropriate to formally document parents' refusal to have their child immunized. While a parent signature form is available from the American Academy of Pediatrics, most states have their own, which indicates that the parent understands the purpose, risks, and benefits of the vaccine and the consequences of the disease, including spreading it to susceptible others. Some states require that exempted students be excluded from school during an outbreak of a vaccine-preventable disease.

Federal law requires that before any vaccine is administered, the parent receive information on the benefits and potential side effects. These Vaccine Information Statements must include a description of the disease, who should get the vaccine and when, a list of the possible risks and reactions, what to do in case of a reaction, and how to learn more about the vaccine. They can be downloaded free from http://www.cdc.gov/nip/publications/VIS/default.htm.

The School Nurse Immunization Program (SNIPP) was developed by the National Association of School Nurses (2002) to provide a community-focused presentation that can be presented to parents to educate them on immunizations. It includes content on what immunizations are, vaccine safety, myths and facts, immunizations for various ages, and information on selected diseases. The National Association of School Nurses endorses the Standards for Child and Adolescent Immunization Practices by the American Academy of Pediatrics (Box 21.2).

Box 21.2 ■ ■ ■

STANDARDS FOR CHILD AND ADOLESCENT IMMUNIZATION PRACTICES

- Vaccination services are readily available.
- Vaccination services are coordinated with other healthcare services and provided in a medical home when possible.
- Barriers to vaccination are identified and minimized.
- Patient costs are minimized.
- Healthcare professionals review the vaccination and health status of patients at every encounter to determine which vaccines are indicated.
- Healthcare professionals assess for and follow only medically accepted contraindications.
- Parents/guardians and patients are educated about the benefits and risks of vaccination in a culturally appropriate manner and in easy-to-understand language.

(Continued on the following page)

Box 21.2 ■■■

STANDARDS FOR CHILD AND ADOLESCENT IMMUNIZATION PRACTICES *(Continued)*

- Healthcare professionals follow appropriate procedures for vaccine storage and handling.
- Up-to-date, written vaccination protocols are accessible at all locations where vaccines are administered.
- People who administer vaccines and staff who manage or support vaccine administration are knowledgeable and receive ongoing education.
- Healthcare professionals simultaneously administer as many indicated vaccine doses as possible.
- Vaccination records for patients are accurate, complete, and easily accessible.
- Healthcare professionals report adverse events after vaccination promptly and accurately to VAERS and are aware of a separate program, the Vaccine Injury Compensation Program.
- All personnel who have contact with patients are appropriately vaccinated.
- Systems are used to remind parents/guardians, patients, and healthcare professionals when vaccinations are due and to recall those who are overdue.
- Office or clinic-based record reviews and vaccination coverage assessments are performed annually.
- Healthcare professionals practice community-based approaches.

(National Vaccine Advisory Committee, 2003)

VACCINE REGISTRIES

"Immunization registries are confidential, population-based computerized information systems that attempt to collect vaccination data about all children within a geographic area" (CDC, 2001b, p. 3). The functions should be to monitor the immunization status of individuals and defined populations; to remind individuals that they need an immunization; and to remind practitioners to administer them (Lutwick, 2000). They would certainly be helpful to school nurses in order to track students who switch schools and districts and to more easily determine which immunizations are needed. However, as of 2002, only 43% of U.S. children under age 6 are participating in a registry (CDC, 2004b). In states where the registry is functional and available to the school nurse, obtaining information related to the students' immunization status will be much easier and result in less inconvenience for parents to provide this information to the schools.

NOTIFYING PARENTS OF A COMMUNICABLE DISEASE IN THE SCHOOL

It is often the school nurse and the principal who respond when a communicable disease is diagnosed in the school setting. In addition to immediately isolating the infected student from the rest of the school and notifying the parents, letters are often drafted that go home with the students. Whether the entire school community is notified or not is a matter of policy of the school and perhaps of the nature of the infection. Letters might just go to case contacts, the child's entire grade level, or those on the child's bus. The letter usually contains a statement of the presence of a known case of a communicable disease, how the disease is usually spread, who may be most at risk, and the action that is needed to treat or prevent the disease from spread. The school nurse can certainly assist school staff as well as students and their families to get the correct information and to fight fear with facts. Public health is often an excellent resource to provide both form letters to send to parents and assistance on what measures the school should take.

INFECTION CONTROL MEASURES

Infection control includes components as simple as handwashing and wound care to components of OSHA guidelines involving bloodborne pathogens in the school setting and preventing infection via food services.

Hand Hygiene

Nurses are well aware of the need for handwashing (now referred to as hand hygiene) between patients or students and after contact with infectious materials. In 2002, the Centers for Disease Control and Prevention Healthcare Infection Control Practices

Advisory Committee (2002h) issued guidelines for hand hygiene in healthcare settings. Their recommendations provide support for evidence-based practice that applies to the school setting.

There is agreement that when the hands are visibly soiled, they should be washed with soap and water in a sink under running water. The efficacy of hand washing depends on the type of soap used and the length of time spent actively washing the hands. *Antimicrobial soaps used for at least 30 seconds are more effective than those with plain soap used for less time. Hands should be rubbed vigorously together for at least 15 seconds* (CDC, 2002h).

For all other times, *the report supports the use of alcohol-based hand rubs as being superior to soap and water in decreasing the amount of bacteria*. Alcohol-based hand antiseptics contain isopropanol, ethanol, and/or n-propanol and are most effective when the alcohol solution contains 60% to 95% alcohol (CDC, 2002h). A study by Hammond, Ali, Fendler, Dolan, and Donovan (2000) demonstrated a 19% decrease in illness absenteeism among students in elementary schools and a 10% decrease in teacher absenteeism using the alcohol-based hand hygiene agents.

Antiseptic handwash products used in the U.S. by healthcare workers are regulated by the FDA's Division of Over-the-Counter Drug Products (CDC, 2002h). They come in the form of foam, gel, or lotion. One of the negative features of the alcohol-based preparations is drying of the skin. Therefore, many of the solutions also contain moisturizers. Other negative features include allergic contact dermatitis and the fact that the alcohol is flammable. While the alcohol-based preparations are more costly than soap, the resulting decrease cost of paying for substitutes and having a healthier student body should result in more of a cost savings.

A substantial amount of the alcohol-based preparation should be used; towelettes impregnated with the alcohol solutions have too little and their effectiveness is equal to that of soap and water. The proper way to use the alcohol handrubs is to *pour a dime-sized blob on one palm and then rub the hands together covering all surfaces of the hands and fingers until it dries, which takes about 15 seconds*.

Gloves reduce hand contamination by 70% to 80%; however, using alcohol-based handrubs should be used before and after the use of gloves for a procedure. The report also recommends other infection control measures, such as keeping fingernails less than one-quarter of an inch long and avoiding wearing artificial nails (CDC, 2002h). While this research has been demonstrated multiple times in the hospital setting, there is no research to support these practices in the school setting. Box 21.3 provides additional guidelines.

Box 21.3 ■ ■ ■

GUIDELINES FOR HAND HYGIENE

- Liquid, bar, leaflet or powdered forms of plain soap are acceptable when washing hands with a nonantimicrobial soap and water. When bar soap is used, soap racks that facilitate drainage and small bars of soap should be used.
- Multiple-use cloth towels of the hanging or roll type are not recommended for use in healthcare settings.
- Do not add soap to a partially empty soap dispenser. This practice of "topping off" dispensers can lead to bacterial contamination of soap.
- Provide healthcare workers with hand lotions or creams to minimize the occurrence of irritant contact dermatitis associated with hand antisepsis or hand washing.
- Wear gloves when contact with blood or other potentially infectious materials, mucous membranes, and nonintact skin could occur.
- No recommendation can be made regarding wearing rings in healthcare settings.

(CDC, 2002h, pp. 32–33).

Environmental Control Measures for Bloodborne Pathogens

The responsibilities of the school nurse related to environmental infection control measures vary by state and school district mandates. The Occupational Safety and Health Administration's mission is to prevent work-related injuries, illnesses, and deaths. This includes protection against occupational exposure and infection from bloodborne pathogens, specifically HIV; hepatitis B, C, and D; cytomegalovirus, and the Parvovirus B19. Occupational exposure is defined as any "reasonably anticipated skin, eye, mucous membrane or parenteral contact with blood or other potentially infectious materials that may result from the performance of an employee's duties" (U.S. Department of Labor, 2001, p. 2).

Public entities, including school districts, are exempt from the OSHA regulations. However, many states have adopted these guidelines into their Public Health regulations to be incorporated into school health policy. The policy should apply to anyone who may be exposed to infectious materials on the job. It "requires school districts to develop a written Exposure Control Plan. At a minimum, the Exposure Control Plan must include: (1) the exposure determination, (2) the procedures for evaluating the circumstances surrounding an exposure incident, and (3) the schedule and method for implementing sections of the standard covering the methods for compliance, hepatitis B vaccination, and postexposure follow-up communication of hazards to employee, and record keeping" (Champion, 1999, p. 2).

Standard Precautions (previously called Universal Precautions) are to be implemented consistently by all employees to reduce the risk of transmission of pathogens via contact. "The body fluids of all persons must be considered potentially hazardous" (Champion, 1999, p. 26). These precautions involve the use of barriers or protective measures when dealing with blood, all body fluids and excretions (except sweat), nonintact skin, and mucous membranes. In addition, there must be guidelines in place for handling body fluids in the school, the use and proper disposal of sharps, equipment cleaning, how to handle waste, and employee training. If guidelines are not in place, it is within the scope of the school nurse's role to initiate policy development.

School custodians must receive training to understand their role in protecting the health and safety of the students and staff, as well as their own. The school nurse must be aware of the guidelines in place for the cleaning of spills of hazardous materials or of bloodborne pathogens with EPA-registered disinfectants according to the manufacturer's directions. They must understand about preventing the spread of organisms with infected mops and water; trash disposal procedures; how to handle potentially infectious waste; and their role in wiping down counters and toys that may contain dangerous organisms. In addition, employees providing these services must be provided with the appropriate equipment to maintain this safety. This training is usually the responsibility of the school district; however, if the school nurse notices breaches in infection control measures in the school, he or she must initiate the change process.

If a bleach solution is made by the school nurse or other school staff (1 part bleach to 9 parts water), it must be appropriately labeled, be made daily, and kept out of the reach of students. CDC (2002h) recommends specific cleaning and disinfecting strategies for patient care areas. Depending on the school setting and the public health guidelines, consideration should be given to their recommendations regarding the cleaning of floors and table tops and the proper care of mops, cloths, and solutions. There should also be a routine protocol for cleaning the toys of young children. Mops, cloths, and solutions must be changed daily or as needed; they should be cleaned after use and allowed to dry before they are reused; and they must be changed after cleaning up large spills of blood or body substances (CDC, 2002h).

Other groups that require bloodborne pathogen and infection control training include bus drivers and cafeteria workers as well as all teachers. Potentially infectious objects or spills on the bus must be cleaned and removed appropriately, according to public health standards for that state. The high risk of transmission of organisms into food being prepared by infected hands mandates that frequent reminders about hand hygiene protocols, especially after toileting, be given to cafeteria employees. In some states, this training is the responsibility of the school nurse. Therefore, school nurses need to clarify their roles and responsibilities related to training school employees on infection control measures.

Playground safety may be another area requiring surveillance, as are the grounds used for school sports. Other areas that often have high disease exposure rates are areas for children younger than the age of 5, especially if they are not completely toilet trained; settings for children who are developmentally delayed, have special medical needs, or engage in biting behaviors; and physical education settings. Another source of environmental infection may be pets in the school, especially when the pet is allowed to roam free through the classrooms. In addition to being a vehicle for disease and a possible source of allergy, there is always a consideration of the behavior of the animal (Yamauchi, 2003).

Air quality needs to be assessed. This includes the ventilation system, the amount of moisture and mold in the building, and the presence of secondhand smoke. Water quality is another possible source of pathogens (see Chapter 47). This includes water used for drinking and in ice machines, for hand washing and for showering, and the water in swimming pools. The school environment is a component of the coordinated school health model and the school nurse is a major player in this model (see Chapter 3). The primary responsibility for air and water quality should be assigned to someone in the school or school district, but it is always the responsibility of the school nurse to identify problems or to advocate for change if a problem is identified.

CONCLUSION

"Nurses remain a school's first line of defense against contagious disease" (Harkavy, 2002, p. 37). They must be participants in the development of policy to maintain a clean environment; they must be educators to the students, staff and families; they must be advocates to assure that the concepts of cleanliness and disinfection are included in all classrooms; they must be role models to demonstrate the appropriate application of standard precautions; and they must have acute assessment skills to identify early signs of contagious disease and intervene quickly and appropriately. They must also ensure compliance of students to the immunization requirements and be aware of the concerns of parents so that they can provide current and accurate information in order to promote the highest level of health among the student body.

Resources

CDC National Immunization Information Hotline 800-232-2522

Immunization Action Coalition/Advisory Committee on Immunization Practices
http://www.immunize.org/acip

Immunization Nursing Network Provider Outreach Web Education and Resources: INNPOWER (funded by the CDC and sponsored by the American Nurses Foundation)
http://www.innpower.org

National Immunization Program
http://www.cdc.gov/nip

Vaccine Information Sheets
http://www.cdc.gov/nip/publications/VIS/visInstructions.pdf

References

American Academy of Pediatrics (AAP). (1999). Combination vaccines for childhood immunization: Recommendations of the Advisory Committee on Immunization practices (ACIP), the American Academy of Pediatrics (AAP), and the American Academy of Family Physicians (AAFP). *Pediatrics, 103*(5), 1064–1068.

American Academy of Pediatrics (AAP). (2000). Varicella vaccine update. *Pediatrics, 105*(1), 136–141.

American Academy of Pediatrics (AAP). (2003a). Increasing immunization coverage. *Pediatrics, 112*(4), 993–996.

American Academy of Pediatrics (AAP). (2003b). Recommended childhood and adolescent immunization schedule—United States, 2003. *Pediatrics, 111*(1), 212–214.

American Academy of Pediatrics (AAP). (2004). Recommendations for influenza immunization of children. *Pediatrics, 113*(5), 1441–1447.

Armstrong, G., & Bell, B. (2002). Hepatitis A virus infections in the United States: Model-based estimates and implications for childhood immunization. *Pediatrics, 109*(5), 839–845.

Atkinson, W., Pickering, L., Watson, J., & Peter, G. (2004). General immunization practices. In S. Plotkin & W. Orenstein (Eds.), *Vaccines* (pp. 91–122). Philadelphia: W. B. Saunders.

Borkowsky, W., & Krugman, S. (1998). Viral hepatitis: A, B, C, D, E, and newer hepatitis agents. In A. Katz, A. Gershon, & P. Hotez (Eds.), *Krugman's infectious diseases of children* (pp. 157–188). St. Louis: C. V. Mosby.

Centers for Disease Control and Prevention (CDC). (1998). Measles, mumps, and rubella vaccine use and strategies for elimination of measles, rubella, and congenital rubella syndrome and control of mumps. *Morbidity and Mortality Weekly Report, 47* (RR-8), 1–57.

Centers for Disease Control and Prevention (CDC). (1999a). Availability of hepatitis B vaccine that does not contain thimerosal as a preservative. *Morbidity and Mortality Weekly Report, 48*(35), 780–782.

Centers for Disease Control and Prevention (CDC). (1999b). Prevention of hepatitis A through active or passive immunization. *Morbidity and Mortality Weekly Report, 48*(RR-12), 1–37.

Centers for Disease Control and Prevention (CDC). (2000a). Poliomyelitis prevention in the United States. *Morbidity and Mortality Weekly Report, 49*(RR-5), 1–22.

Centers for Disease Control and Prevention (CDC). (2000b). Preventing pneumococcal disease among infants and young children. *Morbidity and Mortality Weekly Report, 49*(RR-9), 1–35.

Centers for Disease Control and Prevention (CDC). (2000c). Prevention and control of Meningococcal Disease. *Morbidity and Mortality Weekly Report, 49*(RR-7), 1–10.

Centers for Disease Control and Prevention (CDC). (2000d). *Epidemiology and prevention of vaccine-preventable diseases*. Washington, DC: U.S. Department of Health and Human Services. Centers for Disease Control and Prevention (CDC). (2000e). Meningococcal disease and college students. *Morbidity and Mortality Weekly Report, 49*(RR-7), 11–20.

Centers for Disease Control and Prevention (CDC). (2001a). Control and prevention of rubella: Evaluation and management of suspected outbreaks, Rubella in pregnant women, and surveillance for congenital rubella syndrome. *Morbidity and Mortality Weekly Report, 50*(RR-12), 1–21.

Centers for Disease Control and Prevention (CDC). (2001b). Progress in development of immunization registries—United States, 2000. *Morbidity and Mortality Weekly Report, 50*(1), 3–7.

Centers for Disease Control and Prevention (CDC). (2001c). Revised ACIP recommendation for avoiding pregnancy after receiving a rubella-containing vaccine. *Morbidity and Mortality Weekly Report, 50*(49), 1117.

Centers for Disease Control and Prevention (CDC). (2001d). Rubella outbreak—Arkansas, 1999. *Morbidity and Mortality Weekly Report, 50*(50), 1137–1139.

Centers for Disease Control and Prevention (CDC). (2002a). Food and Drug Administration approval of a fifth acellular pertussis vaccine for use among infants and young children—United States, 2002. *Morbidity and Mortality Weekly Report, 51*(26), 574.

Centers for Disease Control and Prevention (CDC). (2002b). Hepatitis B vaccination—United States, 1982–2002. *Morbidity and Mortality Weekly Report, 51*(25), 549–552, 563.

Centers for Disease Control and Prevention (CDC). (2002c). Measles—United States, 2000. *Morbidity and Mortality Weekly Report, 51*(6), 120–123.

Centers for Disease Control and Prevention (CDC). (2002d). Pertussis—United States, 1997–2000. *Morbidity and Mortality Weekly Report, 51*(4), 73–76.

Centers for Disease Control and Prevention (CDC). (2002e). Progress toward elimination of *Haemophilus influenza type b invasive disease among infants and children—United States, 1998–2000. Morbidity and Mortality Weekly Report, 51*(11), 234–237.

Centers for Disease Control and Prevention (CDC). (2002f). Tetanus—Puerto Rico, 2002. *Morbidity and Mortality Weekly Report, 51*(28), 613–615.

Centers for Disease Control and Prevention (CDC). (2002g). 25th Anniversary of the last case of naturally acquired smallpox. *Morbidity and Mortality Weekly Report, 51*(42), 950–951.

Centers for Disease Control and Prevention (CDC). (2002h). Immunization Registry Progress: United States, 2002. *Morbidity and Mortality Weekly Report, 51*(34), 760–762.

Centers for Disease Control and Prevention (CDC). (2003a). Pertussis outbreak among adults at an oil refinery—Illinois, August–October, 2002. *Morbidity and Mortality Weekly Report, 52*(1), 1–4.

Centers for Disease Control and Prevention (CDC). (2003b). Prevention and control of infections with hepatitis viruses in correctional settings. *Morbidity and Mortality Weekly Report, 52*(RR-1), 1–36.

Centers for Disease Control and Prevention (CDC). (2003c). Prevention and control of influenza. *Morbidity and Mortality Weekly Report, 52*(RR-8), 1–34.

Centers for Disease Control and Prevention (CDC). (2003d). Reporting invasive pneumococcal disease among vaccines. *Morbidity and Mortality Weekly Report, 52*(19), 446–447.

Centers for Disease Control and Prevention (CDC). (2003e). Surveillance for safety after immunization: Vaccine adverse event reporting system (VAERS)—United States, 1991–2001). *Morbidity and Mortality Weekly Report, 52*(SS-1), 1–24.

Centers for Disease Control and Prevention (CDC). (2003f). Using live, attenuated influenza vaccine for prevention and control of influenza. *Morbidity and Mortality Weekly Report, 52*(RR-13), 1–8.

Centers for Disease Control and Prevention (CDC). (2003g). Varicella-related deaths—United States, 2002. *Morbidity and Mortality Weekly Report, 52*(23), 545-547.

Centers for Disease Control and Prevention (CDC). (2003h). Guideline for hand hygiene in health-care settings. *Morbidity and Mortality Weekly Report, 52*(RR-16), 1–48.

Centers for Disease Control and Prevention (CDC). (2004a). Vaccination coverage among children entering school—United States, 2003–04 school year. *Morbidity and Mortality Weekly Report, 53*(44), 1041–1044.

Centers for Disease Control and Prevention (CDC), Immunization Registry Progress—United States, January–December 2002. (2004b). *Morbidity and Mortality Weekly Report, 53*(20), 431-433.

Centers for Disease Control and Prevention (CDC). (2005). Summary of provisional cases of selected notifiable diseases, United States, cumulative, week ending January 1, 2005 (52nd week). *Morbidity and Mortality Weekly Report, 53*(51, 52), 1213–1220.

Champion, C. (1999). *Occupational exposure to bloodborne pathogens*. Castle Rock, CO: National Association of School Nurses.

DeStefano, F., Bhasin, T., Thompson, W., Yeargin-Allsopp, M., & Boyle, C. (2004). Age at first measles-mumps-rubella vaccination in children with autism and school-matched control subjects: A population-based study in metropolitan Atlanta. *Pediatrics, 113*(2), 259–266.

Diekema, D., and the Committee on Bioethics. (2005). Responding to parental refusals of immunization for children. *Pediatrics, 115*(5), 1428–1431.

Ellis, R. (2002). Strategic challenges in designing and producing modern biotechnology vaccines and transforming technology. In F. Brown & I. Gust (Eds.), *Orphan vaccines: Bridging the gap* (pp. 3–11). New York: Karger.

Greenberg, D., Pickering, L., Senders, S., Bissey, J., Howard, R., Blatter, M., Reisinger, K., Pichichero, M., & Howe, B. (2002). Interchangeability of 2 diphtheria-tetanus-acellular pertussis vaccines in infancy. *Pediatrics, 109*(4), 666–672.

Hall, S., Mauphin, T., Seward, J., Jumaan, A., Peterson, C., Goldman, G., Mascola, L., & Wharton, M. (2002). Second varicella infections: Are they more common than previously thought? *Pediatrics, 109*(6), 1068–1073.

Hammond, B., Ali, Y., Fendler, E., Dolan, M., & Donovan, S. (2000). Effect of hand sanitizer use on elementary school absenteeism. *American Journal of Infection Control, 28*, 340–346.

Harkavy, L. (October, 2002). Conclusions and recommendations from the Healthy School Summit. *Supplement to The Journal of School Nursing*, 36–37.

Heymann, D. (2000). *Control of communicable diseases manual*. Washington, DC: American Public Health Association.

Lutwick, S. (2000). Pediatric vaccine compliance. *Pediatric Clinics of North America, 47*(2), 427–434.

Lutwick, L., & Abramson, J. (2000). Pediatric immunization for the future: Lyme disease vaccine and beyond. *Pediatric Clinics of North America, 47*(2), 465–479.

Madsen, K., Lauritsen, M., Pedersen, C., Thorsen, P., Plesner, A., Andersen, P., & Mortensen, P. (2003). Thimerosal and the occurrence of autism: Negative ecological evidence from Danish population-based data. *Pediatrics, 112*(3), 604–606.

Masignani, V., Pizza, M., & Rappuoli, R. (2003). Genome-based approach for a vaccine against *Neisseria meningitides*. In B. Bloom & R-H. Lambert (Eds.), *The vaccine book* (pp. 333–344). Amsterdam: Academic Press.

Meissner, H. C., & Pickering, L. (2002). Control of disease attributable to *Haemophilus influenzae type b and the National Immunization Program. Pediatrics, 110*(4), 820–822.

Meningococcal Vaccines (2005). *Vaccine information statement.* Centers for Disease Control and Prevention. Retrieved August 24, 2005 from http://www.cdc.gov/nip/publications/VIS/vis-mening.pdf

National Association of School Nurses (NASN). (2002). *Immunization information resource manual for the school nurse*. Scarborough, ME: Author.

National Vaccine Advisory Committee. (2003). Standards for child and adolescent immunization practices. *Pediatrics, 112*(4), 958–963.

Neff, G., & Schiff, E. (September, 1999). Chronic hepatitis C: Populations at risk and treatment strategies. *Hospital Medicine*, 12–20.

Nossal, G. (2003). Vaccines. In W. Paul (Ed.), *Fundamental immunology* (pp. 1319–1369). Philadelphia: Lippincott Williams & Wilkins.

Offit, P., & Hackett, C. (2003). Addressing parents' concerns: Do vaccines cause allergic or autoimmune diseases? *Pediatrics, 111*(3), 653-659.

Offit, P., Quarles, J., Gerber, M., Hackett, C., Marcuse, E., Kollman, T., Gellin, B., & Landry, S. (2002). Addressing parents' concerns: Do multiple vaccines overwhelm or weaken the infant's immune system? *Pediatrics, 109*(1), 124-129.

Pascual, R. B., McGinley, M., Zanardi, L., Cortese, M., & Murphy, T. (2003). Tetanus summary of provisional cases of selected notifiable diseases, United States, Cumulative. (2005). *Morbidity and Mortality Weekly Report, 53*(52), 1213–1220.

Pfister, H., & Bleck, T. (2003). Bacterial infections. In T. Brandt, L. Caplan, J. Dichgans, H. Diener, & C. Kennard (Eds.), *Neurological disorders: Course and treatment* (pp. 601–613). San Diego: Academic Press.

Plotkin, S. (2003). Disease states and vaccines: Selected cases. In B. Bloom & P.Lambert (Eds.), *The vaccine book* (pp. 179–209). San Diego: Academic Press.

Rennels, M., Deloria, M., Pichichero, M., Losonsky G., Englund, J., Meade, B., Anderson, E., Steinhoff, M., & Edwards K. (2000). Extensive swelling after booster doses of acellular pertussis-tetanus-diphtheria vaccines. *Pediatrics, 105*(1), http://www.pediatrics.org/cgi/content/full/105/1/e12.

Salmaso, S. (2003). Pertussis. In B. Bloom & P. Lambert (Eds.), *The vaccine book* (pp. 211– 224). San Diego: Academic Press.

Seder, R., & Mascola, J. (2003). Part A. Basic immunology of vaccine development. In B. Bloom & P. Lambert (Eds.), *The vaccine book* (pp. 51–72). Amsterdam: Academic Press.

Selekman, J. (1999). Hepatitis update. *Pediatric Nursing, 25* (5), 542–546. Summary of Notifiable Diseases—US, 2002. (2004). *Morbidity and Mortality Weekly Report,* 51 (53), 1–84.

Shepard, C., Ortega-Sanchez, I., Scott, R. D., Rosenstein, N., & the ABCs Team (2005). Cost-effectiveness of conjugate meningococcal vaccination strategies in the United States. *Pediatrics, 115*(5), 1220–1232.

Surveillance—United States, 1998–2000. *Morbidity and Mortality Weekly Report, 52* (SS-3), 1–8.

Update: Influenza activity—United States and worldwide, 2003–04 Season, and composition of the 2004–05 influenza vaccine. (2004). *Morbidity and Mortality Weekly Report, 53* (25), 547–552.

U.S. Department of Health and Human Services (USDHHS). (2000). *Healthy People 2010*. Washington, DC: Author.

U.S. Department of Labor. (2001). *Occupational safety and health standards: Bloodborne pathogens*. 29 CFR, 1910.1030. As amended at 66 FR 5325 January 18, 2001.

Verstraeten, T., Davis, R., DeStefano, F., Lieu, T., Rhodes, P., Black, S., Shinefield, H., & Chen, R. (2003). Safety of thimerosal-containing vaccines: A two-phased study of computerized Health Maintenance Organization databases. *Pediatrics, 112* (5), 1039–1048.

Vogel, F., & Hem, S. (2004). Immunologic adjuvants. In S. Plotkin & W. Orenstein (Eds.), *Vaccines* (pp. 69–79). Philadelphia: W. B. Saunders.

Watson, B., & Levin, M. (February, 2004). Varicella infection and vaccination: Where are we headed from here? *Contemporary Pediatrics* (Suppl.), 4–15.

Wharton, M., & Vitek, C. (2004). Diphtheria toxoid. In S. Plotkin & W. Orenstein (Eds.), *Vaccines* (pp. 211–228). Philadelphia: W. B. Saunders.

Yamauchi, T. (2003). Guidelines for attendees and personnel. In L. Grossman (Ed.), *Infection control in the child care center and preschool* (pp. 9–20). Philadelphia: Lippincott Williams & Wilkins.

PART V

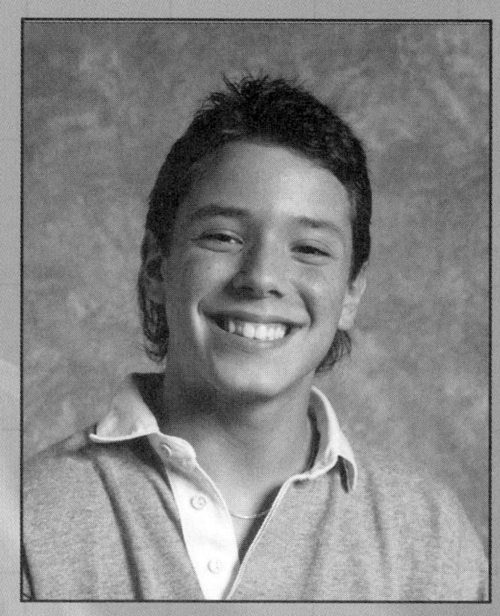

Episodic Illnesses of School Children

Chapter 22

Acute Measures for Emergent Problems

MARIE RENZI ▪ MARIANN COSBY

Chapter Outline

INTRODUCTION

The school nurse must be prepared to respond to any health-related emergency that could occur on school grounds in order to intervene in the best interest of students, staff, and school visitors. Health-related emergencies can affect a student or staff member as a result of either injury or illness, or involve large numbers of individuals in multiple casualty incidents, such as the collapse of bleachers, exposure to a toxic gas that affects multiple students and staff, or a school shooting. However, the focus of this chapter is the unexpected urgent or emergent health-related/medical emergencies of the individual student in the school setting. Mass casualty triage and treatment planning for the school setting are discussed in Chapter 10.

In an emergency, the primary objectives for the school nurse are to prevent further harm to the student, and to stabilize and expedite transport of the student to a facility where resources are available to perform a complete evaluation and provide medical treatment. After an emergency situation is identified, the school nurse is expected to complete a focused problem-based assessment of the student and to manage the condition until emergency medical services (EMS) or the parents arrive.

According to Green (2001), acute and emergency care is the area of school nursing that holds the most potential for professional liability. In numerous cases the basis of the liability was the school nurse's care of the student's injuries. Therefore it is essential that the school nurse is educated and capable of competently performing quick assessments in order to categorize or triage the severity of an illness or injury, provide initial emergency care, and determine if imminent referral to outside resources is necessary. This chapter discusses methodologies for adequate training and preparation of the school nurse to provide an appropriate response in health-related emergency situations and outlines the assessment and management of selected urgent and emergent problems.

THE SCHOOL NURSE TRAINING MANUAL

A valuable resource available to assist the school nurse in preparation and prevention of emergencies is the Managing School Emergencies Program series. The National Association of School Nurses (NASN), in collaboration with the Health Resources and Services Administration's Emergency Medical Services for Children (EMSC) program, developed a three-part modular program to prepare the school nurse to anticipate emergencies in the school setting; create plans for treating students with emergent and urgent health conditions; prepare school nurses to recognize, assess, and intervene when a student experiences an emergency condition; and introduce triage in the context of multiple casualty incidents.

The program consists of a self-study introductory module: "Preparing a Response to School Emergencies," which is followed by two didactic modules for managing school emergencies (MSE). Each of the modules is designed to be presented in a day-long format by NASN instructors, covering a variety of the more acute emergencies that occur in schools (Maloney, Doyle, Fitzgerald, Elam, & Lewis, 2002a). Although the information presented in this chapter is congruent with the NASN program, it is not meant to be a substitute for the program. It is recommended that school nurses participate in the MSE program to maximize their knowledge base and prepare for their role and response to health emergencies in schools. NASN recommends that school nurses at least complete the self-study module "Preparing a Response to School Emergencies" (Bernardo, Anderson, & Lewis, 2000). As the nurse and/or school safety team complete exercises in the self-study module, the availability of other first aid resources, such as school staff trained in first aid and basic life support, will assist with health-related emergencies. In addition, with a school plan in place (Chapter 10), school personnel will have assigned roles during emergency situations to avoid chaos and confusion and therefore provide the most appropriate and effective care.

Other courses that school nurses may want to consider to enhance their knowledge about pediatric emergencies include national programs, that is, Emergency Nurses Association's Emergency Nursing Pediatric Course, American Heart Association's Pediatric Advanced Life Support or Pediatric Basic Trauma Life Support, or other state and regional courses such as Illinois' School Nurse Emergency Care (SNEC) or Connecticut's School Nurse Emergency Medical Services for Children (SNEMSC).

THE SCHOOL NURSE'S ROLE IN EMERGENCIES

NASN defines the role of the school nurse in emergencies as follows: The school nurse must be able to: (1) distinguish emergent situations from a myriad of complaints, (2) call for the most appropriate help, (3) manage emergency care until relieved by emergency medical services (EMS) personnel, (4) communicate his or her assessment and interventions to EMS personnel, and (5) follow up with the healthcare provider and the parent or legally responsible person (Maloney et al., 2002a). If a school has an available full-time school nurse, these various activities as the first responder and manager of health-related emergency situations are feasible. However, not all schools have a full-time school nurse, and even though a school may have a nurse, the nurse may not always be on-site or readily available at the location of the emergency and should not be relied on to be the sole responder to urgent health situations in schools. Therefore, the school nurse and school building administrators should have reasonable plans for recognizing and responding to urgent and emergency healthcare problems that can reasonably be anticipated in the student population regardless of the presence of the school nurse.

As the school's healthcare expert, the school nurse's role includes involvement in the development and implementation of school emergency preparedness response plans that include planning for emergency health-related services. When planning this emergency care system, it is essential for communications to be intact among the school nurse, parents, school administration, EMS, the local emergency department, and primary care providers to ensure that optimal emergency care is available when needed in school (Abrunzo et al., 2000). The school nurse may want to consider the Coordinated School Health Program model (Chapter 3) as a part of the process so that there is collaboration and a cohesive integration of school, parent, and community in the process and approach (Knickelbein, 2004).

District policies and procedures, national and state standards, and other legal directives, such as the Education Code and the State Nurse Practice Act, should be reviewed as a guide in the development of the plan for the care of emergently ill or injured students and the requisite training of the lay staff or unlicensed assistive personnel. In addition, as an inherent aspect of the school nurse's role, it would behoove the school nurse to become keenly familiar with the job requirements and responsibilities in connection with the training of and delegation to lay staff regarding health-related emergencies, with an eye toward the concomitant legal liability and impact on licensure as a professional nurse.

It is important to realize that the school nurse will be looked to for guidance and leadership as the first responding healthcare professional when medical emergencies occur on school grounds. The nursing standard for care includes clinical assessment, diagnosis, and evidence-based interventions well beyond that of simple first aid (Hootman, Schwab, & Gelfman, 2001).

PLANNING FOR A HEALTH-RELATED EMERGENCY

Plans for a health-related emergency is a component of the more global school emergency preparedness plan. Recommendations for pediatric emergency preparedness in school were proposed in 2001 at a regional meeting of EMS providers and school nurse consultants as follows (Hohenhaus, 2001):

- Perform an emergency readiness assessment of the school; use tools developed by the Massachusetts Emergency Medical Services for Children (EMSC) program or the EMSC National Resource Center.
- Invite a group of stakeholders to participate in plan development.
- Have a school "walk through" to identify hazards.
- Create an emergency preparedness plan. Develop written procedures, policies and plans for when the nurse is available and when the nurse is not available at the school.
- Develop emergency training goals and organize staff first responder training.
- Conduct a mock emergency with the local EMS agency before an emergency occurs.
- Reevaluate the plan after all incidents occur.

Similar recommendations are contained in the NASN modules referred to earlier in the chapter.

The American Heart Association (2004) policy statement on "Response to Cardiac Arrest and Selected Life-Threatening Medical Emergencies: The Medical Emergency Response Plan for Schools" should be reviewed and considered as the school nurse and other administrative staff determine the scope of their site health-related emergency plan. The statement includes various recommendations for school preparedness including minimal staff training and elements of the plan. The American Academy of Pediatrics (2001) policy statement, "Guidelines for Emergency Medical Care in School," is another reference that should be considered and reviewed as part of the planning process. This authority recommends that the minimal training for lay staff functioning in the absence of the nurse should include first aid, basic life support, and the recognition and treatment of anaphylaxis. The National Association of Emergency Medical Technicians (NAEMT), "Guidelines for Prehospital Response to Medical Emergencies in Schools" (NAEMT, 2004), should also be reviewed as part of the planning process for recommendations regarding how to promote a seamless transfer of care from the school staff to an EMT and integrate EMS response in school emergencies.

As the plan is developed, it is essential that implications of the law for school districts and educators be considered. As addressed in Chapter 14, IDEA mandates equal rights for persons with disabilities and assures children a free and appropriate education in the least restrictive environment. In addition, Section 504 of the 1973 Rehabilitation Act mandates nondiscrimination on the basis of disability. Hence, the regular public school classroom includes an increased number of children with special healthcare needs and disabilities. Understandably, many teachers express anxiety about accepting liability for what is perceived to be a medical, rather than an educational issue, and one for which they often have received little to no education or training.

However, three of the most common school-based emergencies (breathing difficulty or asthma, seizure, and choking) can lead to life-threatening emergencies (Barrett, 2001). Further, an estimated 15% to 30% of children younger than age 18 in the United States are affected by chronic medical conditions such as asthma, diabetes, and epilepsy, which puts these children at risk for health-related emergencies while in school (Bobo, Hallenbeck, & Robinson, 2003). A delay in prompt intervention by the school nurse or other trained lay first responder personnel may exacerbate the problem or result in death.

The 1999 U.S. Supreme Court ruling on *Cedar Rapids v. Garret F.* and other recent case law rulings demonstrate that schools are responsible to provide one-on-one nursing care for students with complex medical needs and can be culpable as a result of the school's failure to provide adequate training in emergency care for its employees (Barrett, 2001; Cosby, M., 2003). Therefore, it is essential that staff training needs associated with timely access to life-saving interventions that can be rendered by lay staff who are present at the onset of the health-related emergency be evaluated and incorporated into individual school emergency response plans and the health-related emergency component.

Since unintentional injury is the leading cause of death for children and young adults, knowledge of the causes of child death and disability should also be considered in plan development (Federal Interagency Forum on Child and Family Statistics, 2005). The plan should be based, in part, on specific local community data as well as national injury data and trends.

More children die or become seriously hurt from injuries than from all childhood diseases combined. Each year, more than 21,000 children ages 1 to 19 are killed; an estimated 600,000 are hospitalized; 12 million are seen in emergency departments because of injuries; and more than 50,000 are permanently disabled. The lifetime cost of injury for 0- to 14-year-olds is estimated to be well over $13.8 billion annually (Rosenberg, 1998).

According to the Children's Safety Network (1997), 22 million children in the United States are injured each year. It is estimated that 10% to 25% of these injuries occur in and around schools. Because injuries are one of the most frequent conditions cared for by school health personnel, school districts should have policies and procedures in place to address student safety issues that support and integrate with the site-specific health-related emergency response plan.

COMPONENTS OF A HEALTH-RELATED EMERGENCY RESPONSE PLAN

Although there has been a recent surge of information and focus in the literature on school emergency response planning, the basic essential elements of the health-related emergency response plan have remained constant (Allen, Ball, & Helfer, 1998). All school plans for a health-related emergency response should minimally include the following elements:

1. Identification of a first responder who will determine if external resources will be necessary. This can be the school nurse when on-site and available, or a trained designee when the nurse is not available. This first responder determines:
   a. Appropriate on-site care and management; and/or
   b. Necessity for transport by parent/legal guardian or ambulance.
2. A protocol for calling EMS or other public safety resources that outlines criteria for when public safety resources should be summoned; and
3. A procedure for contacting a family or families in case of emergency.

Identification and Role of the First Responder

As previously discussed, the lay first responders should be identified and trained in order to respond to a health-related emergency in the absence of the school nurse or other professionally trained first responders. In addition to the identification and training components, the health-related emergency plan should address how the individual(s) renders appropriate on-site care and management of the emergency condition in the absence of the professional first responders and determine the necessity for transport by the parent/legal guardian or ambulance.

Guidelines

To accomplish this, in addition to utilizing various first-aid resources, the school health-related emergency plan should consider developing or utilizing a resource such as Ohio's "Emergency Guidelines for Schools" (Ohio Department of Public Safety, 2001) which provides emergency guidelines for "what to do in an emergency" for school staff without medical/

Box 22.1 ■■■

Emergency Guidelines can be found at http://www.ems-c.org/downloads/pdf/953OHEGS.pdf

nursing training when the school nurse is not available (see Box 22.1 for Web site address). This straightforward copy-ready color-coded resource includes algorithms for common injuries and illnesses that contain first-aid instructions, directions for on-site care and management, and recommendations of when to contact the responsible school authority or parent or legal guardian, or call EMS. Regardless of what methodology is implemented, at a minimum there should be emergency treatment guidelines for the school staff to follow should an emergency occur in the absence of the school nurse (Bernardo et al., 2000).

Guidelines that depict the management of care are also a valuable resource for the school nurse and other professional first responders and should be considered as part of the overall plan for the more frequent health-related presentations and high-risk conditions. As with the development of the school emergency preparedness plan, care guidelines can be developed within the framework of the Coordinated School Health Programs with the assistance of local school safety committees, EMS agencies, local emergency departments, and pediatricians. For example, through a collaborative effort, Illinois Emergency Medical Services for Children (2003) developed "Guidelines for the Nurse in the School Setting."

The intent of the guidelines is to provide nurses working in the school setting with a set of emergency care guidelines that can be utilized during the delivery of care to the ill or injured student. As with the guidelines for the lay first responder, these guidelines also contain algorithms for commonly encountered injuries and health-related problems of students when in school. However, in contrast, they are more comprehensive in that they contain the assessment and triage processes that the school nurse or professional first responder should utilize when determining care intervention and disposition status of the student, which are discussed later in the chapter. An example is shown in Figure 22.1. Both the Illinois and the Ohio guidelines were referenced as protocols to consider in developing a pediatric emergency preparedness plan as part of the regional conference discussed earlier (Hohenhaus, 2001).

Another resource that needs to be considered includes any other state or local guidelines for basic or specialized healthcare procedures. State school nurse consultants and state departments of education can direct the school nurse to these specific resources to ensure congruency with the district or site-specific plan.

Emergency Supplies

The availability of essential emergency supplies is an integral component of being able to render appropriate on-site care and management of the emergency condition. However, there is no nationally accepted recommended list of minimal emergency equipment or supplies for schools (Bobo et al., 2003). Variation in the recommended supply lists in the literature are primarily contingent on portability for use as a first aid kit or use for the school nurse in the health office (American Heart Association, 2004; Bernardo et al., 2000; Illinois EMS for Children, 2003; Ohio Department of Public Safety, 2001). In 2002, a national consensus group hosted by NASN, consisting of representatives from organizations and agencies having expertise in emergency care of children or school health, convened and reached consensus with regard to minimal emergency equipment and resources for schools. Although not inclusive of all equipment and resources that would be beneficial in the school setting, the minimal standard to ensure that every student has the same opportunity for effective management and stabilization of likely emergencies was established (Bobo et al., 2003; NASN, 2003). The consensus group agreed to two lists as depicted in Tables 22.1 and 22.2.

Table 22.1 reflects minimal equipment and resource required in all schools, regardless of whether the school nurse is present. Table 22.2 includes essential equipment and resources recommended in addition to the first list when a school nurse is on the premises or in close proximity all the time. Two additional optional pieces of equipment were identified to be considered for schools with the school nurse present: blood pressure cuffs in appropriate sizes (not essential but could be useful in some emergencies) and a childbirth kit (for high-risk teens). Rationale for the development of two distinct lists revolved around liability concerns including the availability of trained personnel, equipment maintenance, protocols, district policies, and state mandates.

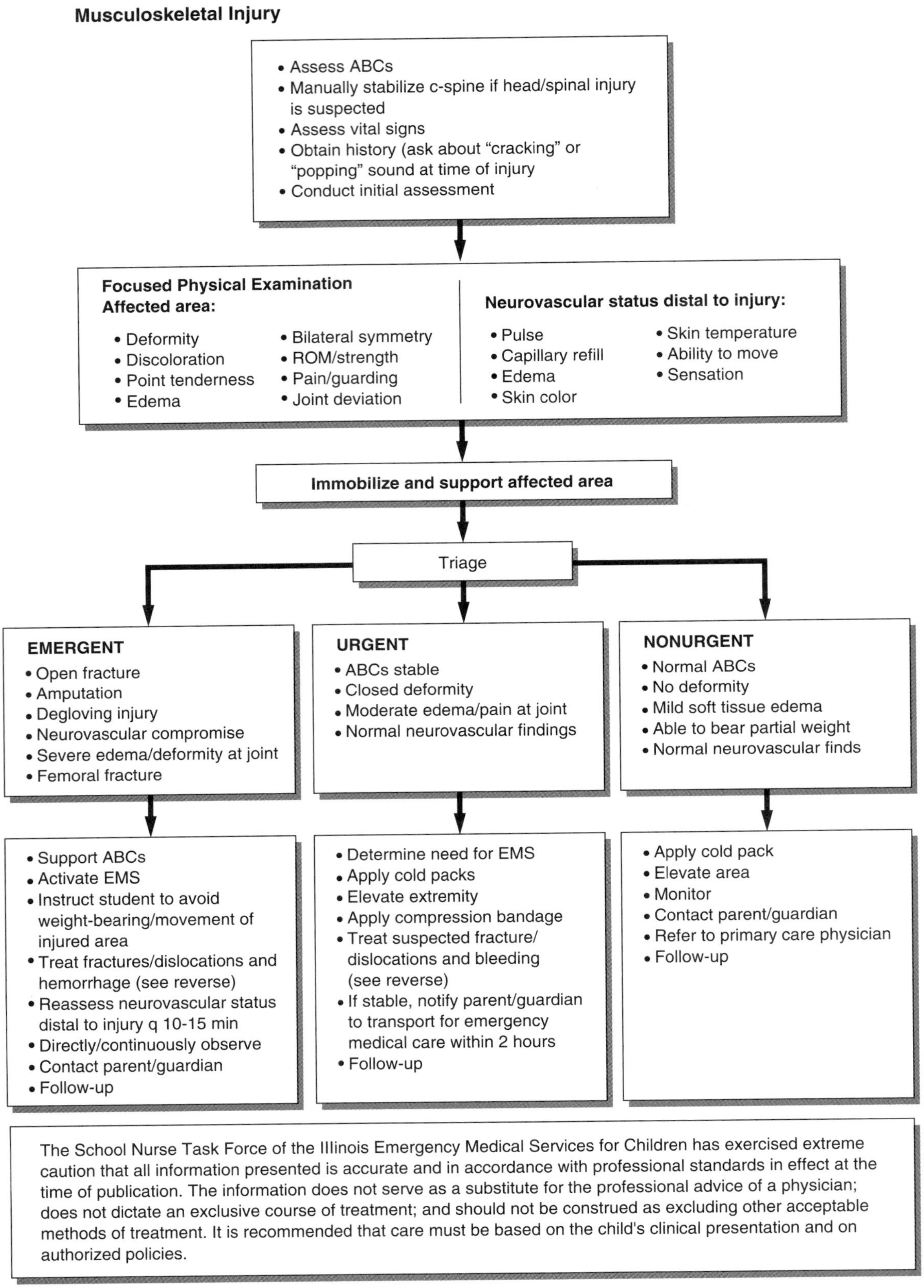

Musculoskeletal Injury

- Assess ABCs
- Manually stabilize c-spine if head/spinal injury is suspected
- Assess vital signs
- Obtain history (ask about "cracking" or "popping" sound at time of injury
- Conduct initial assessment

↓

Focused Physical Examination
Affected area:

- Deformity
- Discoloration
- Point tenderness
- Edema
- Bilateral symmetry
- ROM/strength
- Pain/guarding
- Joint deviation

Neurovascular status distal to injury:

- Pulse
- Capillary refill
- Edema
- Skin color
- Skin temperature
- Ability to move
- Sensation

↓

Immobilize and support affected area

↓

Triage

EMERGENT

- Open fracture
- Amputation
- Degloving injury
- Neurovascular compromise
- Severe edema/deformity at joint
- Femoral fracture

↓

- Support ABCs
- Activate EMS
- Instruct student to avoid weight-bearing/movement of injured area
- Treat fractures/dislocations and hemorrhage (see reverse)
- Reassess neurovascular status distal to injury q 10-15 min
- Directly/continuously observe
- Contact parent/guardian
- Follow-up

URGENT

- ABCs stable
- Closed deformity
- Moderate edema/pain at joint
- Normal neurovascular findings

↓

- Determine need for EMS
- Apply cold packs
- Elevate extremity
- Apply compression bandage
- Treat suspected fracture/ dislocations and bleeding (see reverse)
- If stable, notify parent/guardian to transport for emergency medical care within 2 hours
- Follow-up

NONURGENT

- Normal ABCs
- No deformity
- Mild soft tissue edema
- Able to bear partial weight
- Normal neurovascular finds

↓

- Apply cold pack
- Elevate area
- Monitor
- Contact parent/guardian
- Refer to primary care physician
- Follow-up

The School Nurse Task Force of the Illinois Emergency Medical Services for Children has exercised extreme caution that all information presented is accurate and in accordance with professional standards in effect at the time of publication. The information does not serve as a substitute for the professional advice of a physician; does not dictate an exclusive course of treatment; and should not be construed as excluding other acceptable methods of treatment. It is recommended that care must be based on the child's clinical presentation and on authorized policies.

Figure 22.1 ■ Musculoskeletal injury. (*Source:* Illinois EMS for Children, 2003.)

Table 22.1 ■

MINIMAL ESSENTIAL EMERGENCY EQUIPMENT AND RESOURCES FOR SCHOOLS WITHOUT A SCHOOL NURSE PRESENT

Accessible keys to locked supplies
Accessible list of phone resources
Biohazard waste bags
Blunt scissors
Clock with a second hand
CPR staff on-site when students are on the premises
Disposable blankets
Emergency cards on all staff
Emergency cards on all students
Established relationship with local EMS personnel
Ice (not cold packs)
Individual care plans for students with specialized needs
First aid tapes
Non-latex gloves
One-way resuscitation mask
Phone
Posters with CPR/Heimlich instructions
Refrigerator or cooler
Resealable plastic bags
School-wide plan for emergencies
Soap
Source of oral glucose (i.e., frosting)
Splints
Staff that have received basic first aid training
Variety of bandages and dressings
Water source/normal saline

Source: Bobo, N., Hallenbeck, P., & Robinson, J. (2003). Recommended minimal emergency equipment and resources for schools: National consensus group report. *Journal of School Nursing,* 19(3), 150–154.

Calling EMS or Other Public Safety Resources

The second element of the school plan for a health-related emergency response should include a guideline or protocol for activating EMS or directives as to when other public safety resources should be summoned and the information that should be conveyed. Protocols or guidelines as discussed earlier, and the emergency intervention guide of the Individualized Health Plan (IHP), should indicate when to activate EMS.

Table 22.2 ■

ADDITIONAL MINIMAL ESSENTIAL EMERGENCY EQUIPMENT AND RESOURCES FOR SCHOOLS WITH A SCHOOL NURSE PRESENT

C-spine immobilizer
Glucose monitoring device**
**Committee acknowledges challenges with maintenance and expense of test strips. Monitoring of machine must also be in compliance with CLIA (Clinical Laboratory Improvement Amendments)
Medications*
Albuterol
Epinephrine pen
Oxygen
*All medications should be in accordance with state laws, pharmacy, and nurse practice acts
Nebulizer
Penlight
Self-inflating resuscitation device in two sizes (500 ml and 1 liter) with appropriate sized masks to meet needs of population being served
Sharps container
Stethoscope
Suction equipment (minimal source, does not have to be electric, i.e., turkey baster)

Source: Bobo, N., Hallenbeck, P., & Robinson, J. (2003). Recommended minimal emergency equipment and resources for schools: National consensus group report. *Journal of School Nursing, 19*(3), 150–154.

Many states have 911 service to activate EMS; in other areas there are local numbers to call for emergency services. In most jurisdictions, once EMS is called, a dispatcher follows protocols to determine who responds to the school emergency. Although dependent on the local area, most responses will include an ambulance and paramedics, and may involve the fire service, police, and other public safety agencies.

It is essential that school staff stand ready to direct EMS personnel to the site of the emergency on the school grounds. School staff should provide a brief report that will be expected by the responding crew. The following key data should be included, if available:

- Name
- Gender
- Age

- Chief complaint
- Significant past medical history including allergies
- ABCD (airway, breathing, circulation, disability) assessment findings, including vital signs
- Medications
- Interventions performed
- Availability of a parent or guardian and parent contact information
- Emergency intervention plan

Although the EMS personnel will report the pertinent information to the receiving facility on their arrival, if the receiving facility is known, it is helpful to call ahead to the emergency department (ED) and make personal contact with the ED staff to facilitate communications regarding the particulars of the injury and the status of contact with the family/legal guardian.

Although the school nurse should utilize the various guidelines as previously discussed to determine when and if EMS should be summoned, the school nurse should still use professional judgment. If there is question as to the seriousness of an injury it is always better to err on the side of safety and well being for the student and transport to a medical facility that can provide diagnostic tests and deliver medical care.

Contacting the Family or Legal Guardian

The third element of the school plan for a health-related emergency response includes a mechanism to make contact with the student's family or legal guardian or emergency contact. This information is generally available on the student's health information card or form or an IHP (see Chapter 9). The card usually contains identifying data, critical parent/guardian contact information, relevant medical history information, and reference to any emergency action plan or intervention guide developed for individual students, such as the emergency care plan (ECP) or individualized emergency medical plan (IEMP). Since emergency health information will be needed for EMS and emergency care providers at the receiving healthcare facility, schools should develop a process for how health information will be shared before and during an emergency. In the event of either a health-related or school site emergency requiring building evacuation, this contact and emergency care information should be easily accessible (see Chapter 10). Equally important is development of a process by which the school nurse can ensure that this vital information is updated annually or more often as needed, to reflect both contact and health history updates and changes. As part of this process, it is essential that parents be informed of the importance of communicating major changes in health status of their child that may occur during the school year in a timely fashion to the school nurse in order for the school to better meet the child's health-related needs and emergencies that may arise.

For students with special healthcare needs (CSHCN), as an adjunct to the IHP, an Emergency Action Plan (EAP) should be developed to assist the individual who responds to a special situation or emergency involving the unique needs of the student. In collaboration with the student, family, and healthcare provider, the school nurse develops the EAP, which provides a step-by-step action plan explaining what to do for the specific student in an emergency (Seidel & Knapp, 2000). The universally accepted form, Emergency Information Form for Children with Special Needs, developed and approved in 1998 by the American College of Emergency Physicians and the American Academy of Pediatrics, should be considered a part of this process in an effort to optimize emergency care of children with special healthcare needs (AAP, 1999; AHA, 2004). (See Emergency Information Form, Figure 22.2.)

ASSESSMENT AND TRIAGE

Regardless of what precipitated the emergency and whether or not it could have been prevented, the school nurse begins evaluating a student with a health-related emergency using a systematic approach. The initial across-the-room assessment consists of observations of the student's general appearance, airway, breathing, circulation, and disability, which should take less than a minute. After securing that there are no safety hazards, the physical exam follows in two stages, beginning with a primary assessment or survey followed by the more detailed secondary assessment. The goal of the primary assessment is to provide the school nurse with a basis for identifying if a life or limb-threatening emergency exists. Using this approach, life-threatening problems can be readily treated, potentially decreasing morbidity and improving outcomes. The approach also supports a methodology for prioritizing interventions and evaluating the student's response. Experienced nurses find that they can conduct the physical assessment while simultaneously gathering information for the history, such as the chief complaint, and providing necessary interventions (Illinois EMS for Children, 2003).

While primary actions in an emergency must be directed toward care of the victim, crowd control is crucial to allow caregivers to do their work without

(text continues on page 489)

Emergency Information Form for Children With Special Needs

American College of Emergency Physicians®

American Academy of Pediatrics 

Date form completed	Revised	Initials
By Whom	Revised	Initials

Last name:

Name:	**Birth date:** **Nickname:**
Home Address:	**Home/Work Phone:**
Parent/Guardian:	**Emergency Contact Names & Relationship:**
Signature/Consent*:	
Primary Language:	**Phone Number(s):**
Physicians:	
Primary care physician:	**Emergency Phone:**
	Fax:
Current Specialty physician:	**Emergency Phone:**
Specialty:	**Fax:**
Current Specialty physician:	**Emergency Phone:**
Specialty:	**Fax:**
Anticipated Primary ED:	**Pharmacy:**
Anticipated Tertiary Care Center:	

Diagnoses/Past Procedures/Physical Exam:

1.	**Baseline physical findings:**
2.	
3.	**Baseline vital signs:**
4.	
Synopsis:	**Baseline neurological status:**

*Consent for release of this form to health care providers

Figure 22.2 ■ Emergency information form.

Last name:

Diagnoses/Past Procedures/Physical Exam continued:

Medications:	**Significant baseline ancillary findings (lab, x-ray, ECG):**
1.	
2.	
3.	
4.	**Prostheses/Appliances/Advanced Technology Devices:**
5.	
6.	

Management Data:

Allergies: Medications/Foods to be avoided	**and why:**
1.	
2.	
3.	

Procedures to be avoided	**and why:**
1.	
2.	
3.	

Immunizations (mm/yy)

Dates					
DPT					
OPV					
MMR					
HIB					

Dates					
Hep B					
Varicella					
TB status					
Other					

Antibiotic prophylaxis: Indication: Medication and dose:

Common Presenting Problems/Findings With Specific Suggested Managements

Problem	**Suggested Diagnostic Studies**	**Treatment Considerations**

Comments on child, family, or other specific medical issues:

Physician/Provider Signature: **Print Name:**

Figure 22.2 ■ *(continued)*

distraction, to protect the privacy and dignity of the injured or ill individual, and to prevent psychological trauma to bystanders. For these reasons, staff should be directed to remove bystanders and students to another location. The school nurse should direct available staff to assist with other aspects of care, such as applying pressure to a bleeding wound, reassuring the student, or communicating with the school office or EMS.

Conducting the Initial Assessment

The initial assessment consists of four components:

- Across-the-room assessment
- Scene safety assessment
- Brief physical assessment
- Brief health history

Each of these components is further explained below.

Across-the-Room Assessment

The across-the-room assessment is the nurse's first contact with the ill or injured student. The school nurse should quickly observe the student's general appearance, airway status, work of breathing, circulatory status, and disability (neurological status), focusing on the items listed in Table 22.3. The entire assessment should take less than a minute.

Table 22.3 ■
ACROSS-THE-ROOM ASSESSMENT

ASSESSMENT	OBSERVATION POINTS
General Appearance Overall impression of the student's condition. Use your intuition and experience to assess level of distress: Compared with baseline, does the student look well, ill, or seriously ill?	• Mechanism of injury • Emotional response (calm, agitated, depressed, angry, anxious) • Response to others present (irritable, apathetic) • Physical signs and symptoms (emesis, bleeding, evident pain or injury)
Airway Look for signs of patency. Facial injuries can compromise the airway; drooling or inability to talk may indicate upper airway edema from infection or anaphylaxis.	• Position (sitting upright, leaning forward, tripod position, supine) • Airway sounds (no audible sounds, stridor, signs of foreign body aspiration wheezing, coughing)
Breathing Work of breathing required for adequate ventilation.	• Rate (normal, fast or slow, apnea) • Effort (retractions, nasal flaring, difficulty speaking) • Breath odors (fruity; reminiscent of petroleum products or tobacco)
Circulation Perfusion of vital organs	• Skin color (normal, pallid, dusky, mottled, cyanotic, flushed) • Active bleeding (none, minor, moderate, profuse; controlled or uncontrolled)
Disability Awareness of environment, injury, or illness.	• Activity (talking or silent; walking or immobile; sitting or supine) • Apparent level of consciousness (alert, confused, unresponsive)

NOTE: Carry disposable gloves and a resuscitation mask at all times in case of an emergency. These items should also be available in key locations for anyone who might need them.
Source: Adapted from Illinois EMS for Children (2003). *Guidelines for the nursing in the school setting.*

Scene Safety Assessment

For incidents taking place outside the health office, the scene should be assessed to determine whether the nurse can safely approach the student. Before rendering aid, one's own safety and that of any bystanders and the student must be ensured. The school nurse should look for hazards in the form of:

- **Substances:** blood or other body fluids, noxious fumes, toxic chemicals
- **Situational dangers:** an armed perpetrator, hostages, weapons
- **Environmental dangers:** an unstable structure, fire, electrical hazards

Never place yourself in danger. If you cannot control the hazard, **do not** approach the student—call 911 or your local emergency number to activate backup assistance.

Brief Physical Assessment

A brief physical assessment supplements the across-the-room assessment with information about the student's immediate health status. The process is divided into a primary assessment or survey and a more detailed secondary assessment. The school nurse should complete this assessment in no more than a few minutes.

The primary assessment follows the ABCD format: Airway, Breathing, Circulation, and Disability, followed by the more detailed secondary assessment that continues with EFGHI: Expose/examine, Fahrenheit, Get vital signs, Head-to-toe assessment, Inspect/Isolate (TABLE 22.4). The goal of the primary assessment is to identify and treat life-threatening emergencies. The secondary assessment identifies additional problems. A full set of vital signs should be taken as part of the secondary assessment. Abnormal vital signs often indicate significant pathophysiology, physical trauma, pain, or emotional distress. During the assessment process, interventions are provided as necessary to maintain the airway, breathing, and circulation. If the student cannot maintain airway patency, adequate breathing, or adequate perfusion, EMS should be called to provide rapid transport and treatment. It should always be remembered that when performing a physical assessment, always observe body substance isolation precautions to prevent exposure to body fluids. Notify the parent or guardian as dictated by school protocols. A mnemonic helpful with the

Table 22.4 ■ PHYSICAL ASSESSMENT

Primary Assessment	Interventions
A *Airway.* Position, sounds, obstruction	Position student to maintain airway patency, using jaw thrust or chin lift as appropriate. Stabilize cervical spine if trauma is possible or mechanism of injury is unknown. Perform maneuvers for airway obstruction if indicated.
B *Breathing.* Work of breathing, adventitious sounds, rate, effort, odors, chest symmetry, drooling	Position student for maximum ventilatory ability; provide mouth-to-mask ventilation if needed.
C *Circulation.* Skin color, temperature, and moisture; capillary refill time; rate and quality of pulses; bleeding.	Initiate CPR if needed; control bleeding with pressure dressings and elevation of the affected limb.
D *Disability.* Activity level, mentation, pupil size and reactivity, emotional state. Orientation to time, place, and person. AVPU level of consciousness (see Table 22.5).	Provide reassurance; position to maintain comfort

(continued)

Secondary Assessment	Interventions
E *Expose or examine.* Open student's shirt or blouse to observe breathing; remove clothing as needed to examine injuries, rashes, bites, or stings.	Treat wounds or other findings as appropriate.
F *Fahrenheit.* Check temperature as appropriate.	Treat as necessary to maintain normothermia.
G *Get vital signs.* Obtain baseline BP, HR, RR; measure or estimate weight.	Treat as necessary.
H *Head-to-toe assessment.* Can be focused or complete, depending on the student's health status, mechanism of injury, and school policy. Inspect, palpate, and auscultate.	Perform comfort measures as indicated; for example, apply cold pack or stabilize suspected fractures. If the student's condition becomes emergent, maintain ABCs
I *Inspect and isolate.* Assess for infectious disease exposure, pediculosis, immuno-compromise.	Provide isolation measures according to public health policy and school policy.

BP, Blood pressure; HR, heart rate; RR, respiratory rate.
Source: Adapted from: ENA (2004). Initial Assessment. In *Emergency nursing pediatric course* (pp. 278–280). Des Plaines, IL: Author.

physical assessment is the AVPU mnemonic (Table 22.5) commonly used to assess level of consciousness. Establishing baseline vital signs is essential for ongoing reassessment. Normal vital signs can vary with a student's age and presenting condition (see Table 22.6).

Measuring blood pressure: In the absence of a table of normal blood pressure values, the following formula may be used to approximate the **lowest** acceptable limit for systolic blood pressure: **BP = 70 + (2 × age in years).** Do not rely solely on blood pressure to indicate the severity of the student's

Table 22.5 ■
AVPU SCALE

MEANING	ASSOCIATED FINDINGS
A Alert	The student is awake and able to speak or interact spontaneously.
V Verbal (responds to verbal stimulus)	A verbal stimulus elicits some response; for example, the student's eyes may open when you call loudly, or agitation may lessen in response to a command.
P Painful (responds to painful stimulus)	The student responds to a painful stimulus by moaning, crying, or withdrawing from pain.
U Unresponsive	The student shows no response to verbal or painful stimuli

Source: Adapted from: Dieckmann, R., Brownstein, D., & Gausche-Hill, M. (Eds.). (2000). *Pediatric education for prehospital professionals (PEPP)* (p. 47). Sudbury, MA: Jones and Bartlett.

Table 22.6 ■
NORMAL VITAL SIGNS BY AGE

AGE	RR/MIN	HR/MIN	BP
3 yr	20–30	80–120	80–110
6 yr	18–25	70–110	80–110
10 yr	15–20	60–90	90–120
15 yr	15–18	60–90	100–130
16–Adult	16–20	60–100	> 90

BP, Systolic blood pressure (mm Hg); HR, heart rate; RR, respiratory rate.

condition. Children can remain normotensive until their circulating volume has decreased by 25%, at which point decompensated shock sets in rapidly.

Gauging perfusion: A quick way to assess the adequacy of perfusion is to palpate the student's pulses. The results can be correlated with blood pressure as follows:

- If the radial pulse cannot be palpated, the systolic blood pressure is less than 80 mm Hg.
- If the femoral pulse cannot be palpated, the pressure is less than 70 mm Hg.
- If the carotid pulse cannot be palpated, the pressure is less than 60 mm Hg.

Make sure that the appropriate sized blood pressure cuff has been used (see Chapter 16).

Interpretation of findings:

- Tachycardia and tachypnea are compensatory mechanisms for shock. The heart rate and respiratory rate can also increase in the presence of fear, anxiety, fever, hypoxia, or certain medications; these elements must be factored into the evaluation.
- Hypothermia as well as certain medications can cause bradycardia.
- Combined bradycardia, slow respiration, cyanosis, and hypotension are signs of decompensated shock in a critically ill or injured child.

Brief Health History

Information gathered during the brief health history helps the school nurse form a plan of care. The school nurse may already be familiar with the student's history from information supplied by the parent/guardian, primary healthcare provider, and school staff or from previous interactions with the student. The mnemonic CIAMPEDS (pronounced *see I am peds*) from the Emergency Nursing Pediatric Course can be an aid to remembering the elements of a complete history. The components are adapted for school nurses in Table 22.7 (ENA, 2004). An alternative method for conducting the history uses the SAMPLE mnemonic shown in Table 22.8. Once the assessment is complete, it is time to assign a category that denotes the severity of the student's condition using triage.

Table 22.7 ■
CIAMPEDS ASSESSMENT

	PARAMETERS	QUESTIONS
C	*Chief complaint*	• What problem brings the student to the health office? • How long has the problem persisted? • If an injury, how and when did it occur?
I	*Immunizations, isolation*	• Are immunizations up to date? • Is isolation necessary? (pediculosis, varicella exposure, immunosuppression)
A	*Allergies*	• Does the student have any known allergies to food, medications, latex, or bee stings?

(continued)

	PARAMETERS	QUESTIONS
M	*Medications*	• Is the student using any prescription, over-the-counter, home, herbal, or cultural remedies? For what reasons? When was the last dose taken? • Did the student take any medications before coming to the health office? What was the result • Has the student used any illicit drugs?
P	*Past health history*	• Does the student have a chronic illness? (asthma, diabetes, hemophilia, seizure disorder) • Does the student have special healthcare needs? • Does the student rely on a medical device? (oxygen, tracheostomy, nebulizer, central venous line gastrostomy tube)
E	*Events preceding the problem*	• When did the problem begin? • Were there precipitating factors? • If an injury occurred, were there witnesses? What did they report?
D	*Diet/elimination*	• Is the student able to eat? • When was the last meal? • Has there been any nausea, vomiting, diarrhea? • Are bowel and bladder function normal?
S	*Symptoms associated with the problem*	• Is the student having pain, apprehension, or guarding? • What is the location, quality, and duration of the pain? • Does positioning make the pain better or worse? • What strategies make other symptoms better or worse? • What is the student's impression of his or her condition?

Source: Adapted from: ENA (2004). Initial Assessment. In *Emergency nursing pediatric course.* (pp. 51–52). Des Plaines, IL: Author.

Table 22.8 ■ SAMPLE HISTORY

MNEMONIC	HISTORY POINTS
Signs/symptoms	Ask the student to describe current symptoms, particularly pain.
Allergies	Note any allergies to medications; food; materials, such as latex; or environmental elements, such as bee stings.
Medications	List prescription and nonprescription medications the student takes regularly, including dosage regimen and time of the last dose.
Past medical history	Record information about preexisting physical or psychological disabilities. A history of previous trauma or a chronic condition is particularly relevant. Make sure immunization status, including tetanus prophylaxis, is current.
Last meal	Document when and what the student last ate or drank.
Events	Ask the student to describe events that led up to the injury.

Source: Adapted from: ENA (2004). Initial Assessment. In *Emergency nursing pediatric course.* (pp. 50). Des Plaines, IL: Author.

Assessment of Pain

A key part of the secondary assessment is the focused assessment of pain. Accurate pain assessment takes into account the age of the student, type of pain, history, and context of the pain, and parental influences. Baker and Wong describe a QUESTT approach for assessing and managing pain in children (Hockenberry, Wilson, Winkelstein, & Kline, 2003).

Q – Question the child.

U – Use pain rating scales.

E – Evaluate behavior.

S – Secure parents' involvement.

T – Take pain into account.

T – Take action.

School-age children and adolescents can give accurate ratings and descriptions of the quality of pain they are experiencing (Illinois EMSC, 2002). School nurses should use an evidence-based tool to assess a student's pain. Self-report from the student using a pain rating scale is the most accurate form of pain assessment (Franck, Greenberg, & Stevens, 2000). Quantitative assessment of pain using a reliable and valid tool is to establish a baseline so that interventions to minimize or relieve the pain through distraction or analgesics can be evaluated. TABLE 22.9 briefly describes four pain scales used to assess pain in children ages 3 to 15 years (Illinois EMS for Children, 2002).

Once pain is assessed through questioning and quantified via a pain rating scale, the nurse should evaluate the student's behavior. A student in pain may compensate by engaging in a diversionary activity such as playing or sleeping, while another child may exhibit anger and irritability when in pain (Franck et al., 2000). Physiological changes can occur as a result of acute pain and can be assessed by monitoring vital signs. Alterations in vital signs

Table 22.9 ■
PAIN SCALES

PAIN SCALES	DESCRIPTION	AGE RANGE	CONSIDERATIONS
Faces Pain Scale (Wong & Baker, 1988)	Scale consists of six cartoon faces ranging from a very happy smiling face depicting no pain to a tearful sad face depicting worst pain.	3–8 years old	Children and parents report a greater preference for the Wong and Baker model (Chambers, Giesbrecht, & Craig, et al., 1999)
	0 No hurt; 1 Hurts little bit; 2 Hurts little more; 3 Hurts even more; 4 Hurts whole lot; 5 Hurts worst		
(NRS) Numerical Rating Scale	Children rate their current pain using numbers with 0 representing the least amount of pain and 10 representing the most pain.	5–13 years old	Requires child's ability to count and have some concept of numbers and their values in relation to other numbers (Wong & Hess, 2000)
	0 1 2 3 4 5 6 7 8 9 10 — No Pain, Mild, Moderate, Severe, Worst		

(continued)

PAIN SCALES	DESCRIPTION	AGE RANGE	CONSIDERATIONS
OUCHER	Self report tool consisting of a vertical numerical scale and a photographic scale with expressions of "hurt" to "no hurt". Utilizes actual pictures of children's faces to estimate pain intensity	3–12 years old	Race-appropriate versions available. Similar to the Faces Pain Scale in that it may be more accurate for acute pain (Gregg, 1998)
Noncommunicating Children's Pain Checklist	Clinician evaluates pain based on vocal and social behaviors, facial expression, activity and physical signs.	5–15 years old	Successful across wide-range of cognitive impairments (Breau et al., 2001)

may disappear, however, when the student experiences chronic pain. Parents are often a good source of information regarding their child's pain, but parents are often not available to the school nurse.

The cause of pain should be taken into consideration when evaluating pain. An injury may cause severe pain, while a sore throat can cause pain that ranges from mild to severe. Since pain assessment is subjective, the school nurse should employ the use of a pain assessment tool to evaluate and quantify intensity.

Principles of Triage

The word *triage* comes from the French word *trier*, meaning to sort out or choose. Triage is the process of sorting and classifying individuals according to the type and urgency of their conditions and originated on World War I battlefields (ENA, 1997). The concept of triage in schools is applicable to both mass casualty situations (see Chapter 10) and to individual students as described below.

The school nurse is generally the individual responsible for determining the severity of a student's condition and deciding what interventions are necessary. While it may be easy enough to accomplish a "comprehensive triage" when a single student presents to the health office complaining of a headache and there is time to complete all the steps of the initial assessment as described previously prior to making the triage decision, the situation is more complicated when students who have sustained injuries in a fight arrive simultaneously.

Because school nursing practice is unpredictable, there may be times when there are several students as well as staff or visitors waiting in the health room for either scheduled interventions or with unexpected problems. The school nurse must also respond to episodes of acute illness or injury arising elsewhere around the facility. Consequently, the school nurse must be able to determine quickly who needs immediate interventions and who can wait. Use of the more abbreviated "spot check" or quick look triage system may be more applicable to this situation in which the school nurse obtains information and limited subjective/objective data related to the chief complaint to ensure that the most seriously ill or injured student is treated first. Hence, treatment is not based on order of arrival but rather according to the seriousness of the presenting illness or injury, placing those whose condition is most critical ahead of others. In summary, regardless of whether the presenting situation dictates a "comprehensive triage" or "spot-check triage," the process provides a systematic methodology to establish priorities of care.

In an emergency, students are initially "sorted" to determine whether their condition may threaten life, limb, or vision; then they must be reassessed and monitored on a continuing basis to detect sudden changes in their status. The school nurse may need to adjust the initial triage category based on a student's response to treatment, or a student whose condition initially appeared nonurgent may worsen abruptly, requiring immediate attention. Therefore, it is imperative for the nurse to have immediate visual access to all students waiting to be seen. The nurse must be able to physically see changes in health conditions in case there is a progression from non-urgent to urgent, or urgent to emergent.

This means that the nurse must conduct frequent reassessments of each student and arrange for ongoing monitoring and observation. Remember that it is better to over-triage than to under-triage, particularly if your intuition tells you that there is a significant underlying problem. While the school nurse may delegate tasks associated with ongoing health care, delegating tasks related to the initial assessment and triage is not recommended. Only an experienced registered nurse truly has the requisite knowledge and expertise to quickly recognize and categorize ill and injured students. Experience can also help the nurse to decide to upgrade a triage determination.

It is important for the school nurse to keep in mind that in contrast to other settings such as the emergency department where there may a significant delay from the time of the injury and presentation, the school nurse often performs the initial assessment within minutes of the injury or shortly after the onset of symptoms associated with an illness. Hence, the telltale signs and symptoms of an illness or significant injury, such as a change or altered level of consciousness, swelling, and internal bleeding, may not yet have developed. Therefore, it is important to think of what might potentially evolve as the triage decision is made. The importance of adhering to ongoing monitoring or subsequent reevaluations cannot be stressed enough.

Performing Triage

The three commonly recognized triage categories are *emergent, urgent*, and *nonurgent*. TABLE 22.10 lists triage categories and examples of problems that fall within each category.

COMPLETING THE PROCESS: INTERVENTIONS, EVALUATION, AND DISPOSITION

The triage decision is based on findings from the initial assessment and allows the school nurse to formulate a nursing diagnosis and develop the plan of care. Once the student's illness or injury has been

Table 22.10 ■
TRIAGE CATEGORIES

CATEGORY	EXAMPLES
Emergent Student requires immediate medical attention. Condition is acute and has the potential to threaten life, limb, or vision.	• Cardiopulmonary arrest • Shock (hypovolemic, cardiogenic, or distributive) • Severe respiratory distress or failure • Major burns • Cervical spine compromise • Severe medical problems, such as diabetic complications • Poisoning or overdose • Emergency childbirth • Acute seizure states • Prolonged loss of consciousness • Caustic chemical spills in the eyes
Urgent Student requires medical intervention within 2 hours. Condition is acute but not severe or life-threatening. The potential for deterioration exists if left untreated or unrecognized.	• Deformity suggesting fracture of a long bone without circulatory compromise • Lacerations in which sutures are required but bleeding is controlled and there is no significant blood loss • Moderate pain following abdominal trauma • Head injury with brief loss of consciousness • Minor burns • Persistent nausea, vomiting, or diarrhea • Avulsed tooth
Nonurgent Student may require referral for routine medical care. Minor or nonacute conditions.	• Minor abrasions or bruises • Muscle sprains and strains • Mild pain

categorized as emergent, urgent, or nonurgent, the school nurse should intervene with the most appropriate treatment or action based on approved protocols or guidelines. Evaluation of the student's response to interventions and determining whether the student's health status has improved or worsened will provide a basis for disposition, as illustrated in TABLE 22.11.

DOCUMENTATION

Assessment findings and triage category should be documented in the student's health record. List interventions and the student's response. Record the final disposition as well. Be sure relevant information is passed on to prehospital care providers so that they can include it in their report to emergency department personnel.

FOLLOW-UP

If possible, follow up any student healthcare incident with the student's primary healthcare provider, the emergency department physician, the prehospital care professionals, or the parent or guardian. Document the outcome in the student's health record and incident report, as appropriate.

STUDENTS WITH SPECIAL HEALTHCARE NEEDS

Although the pediatric assessment techniques outlined above are equally applicable to students who have special healthcare needs, the school nurse must adjust these techniques to accommodate the student's developmental age, rather than basing them on chronological age. Note also that baseline vital signs for a student with a chronic condition may be outside the range of same-age peers who do not have special needs. The school nurse may see the day-to-day variations among the school's students and is often the first to notice changes in a student's condition. With students with special healthcare needs, it is particularly important to become familiar with the student's baseline status so that changes in condition can be readily identified. Use developmentally appropriate language, gestures, and techniques when communicating with a student who has cognitive impairment or developmental

Table 22.11 ■
STUDENT DISPOSITION AFTER TREATMENT

EVALUATION	DISPOSITION*
Emergent triage category	Monitor in health office and transport to emergency care facility via ground or air EMS
Urgent triage category	Monitor in health office and transport to emergency care facility via EMS, parent/guardian, or other adult as appropriate
Non-urgent episodic illness	Monitor in health office and transport to primary healthcare provider or home, as appropriate, via parent/guardian or other adult
Insect bite or sting with **no** evidence of anaphylaxis	Monitor in health office and transport to home via parent/guardian or other adult
Minor head injury with no loss of consciousness	Return to class while you notify parent/guardian; reevaluate subsequently
Essentially well with minor illness	Return to class

*Monitoring should be performed by the school nurse.
Source: Adapted from Illinois EMS for Children (2003). *Guidelines for the nursing in the school setting.*

delay. See Figure 22.2 for the American Academy of Pediatrics' Emergency Information Form for children with special healthcare needs.

The rest of this chapter explores life-threatening emergency problems, interventions for the most serious problems, and the evaluation and follow-up as part of the school emergency medical plan.

RESPIRATORY EMERGENCIES

Etiology

Respiratory emergencies can range from mild distress to respiratory failure and arrest and the school nurse must be prepared to handle them all. Respiratory distress occurs when the work of breathing is increased. Respiratory failure is when there is an inability to maintain adequate delivery of oxygen or elimination of carbon dioxide to the tissues, which can lead to the cessation of breathing-respiratory arrest. Recognition of respiratory failure and respiratory arrest is critical, in that respiratory arrest is the precursor to cardiac arrest (Zaritsky, Nadkarni, Hickey, Schexnayder, & Berg, 2002).

Adequate respiratory function depends on oxygenation to maintain perfusion and on the elimination of carbon dioxide. Acute respiratory distress or failure usually occurs as a complication of another disease such as pneumonia, or pulmonary edema. Respiratory emergencies also occur due to airway obstructions, such as from a foreign body or from the narrowing of airways that occur in asthma or anaphylaxis (Haddad & Fontan, 2004).

Assessment

In a respiratory assessment, the nurse should start by determining if the airway is clear and if there is respiratory distress. Observe the student's position for air entry. Sitting up in a tripod position or leaning forward with the neck extended in a "sniffing" position are positions assumed with respiratory compromise. Look at the work of breathing. Is there accessory muscle use (intercostal, substernal, and supraclavicular retractions) or nasal flaring?

Inspiration is an active process and exhalation is passive. Expiration takes slightly longer than inspiration (Cosby, C., 2003). When airway passages are narrow or partially obstructed, inspiration time is relatively unchanged and expiration will be prolonged. The inspiration/expiration time ratio is then greater than 1:2.

Observe the rate, depth, and pattern of breathing. Is it deep or shallow? Is the chest expanding symmetrically? Auscultate the child's chest by placing the stethoscope at the anterior axillary line in the second intercostal space. Listen bilaterally to detect the location of abnormal breath sounds. Refer to Table 22.12 for a description of abnormal breath sounds.

Table 22.12 ■
ABNORMAL BREATH SOUNDS

TERM	CHARACTERISTICS	CAUSE
Course crackle	Discontinuous, interrupted explosive sounds	Air passing through larger airways containing fluid
Fine crackle	Discontinuous, interrupted explosive sounds, less loud and higher in pitch than course crackles	Air passing through smaller airways containing fluid
Wheeze	Continuous sounds, high pitched hissing sounds	Airway narrowed by asthma, or partially obstructed by foreign body or tumor
Rhonchus	Continuous sounds, low pitched snoring	Large upper airway obstructed by thick secretions

Source: Adapted from Hockenberry et al. (2003).

The school nurse should be alert to extremes in respiratory rate. Rate variations are obvious signs of respiratory distress and impending respiratory failure. Fast or slow rates are immediate red flags indicating a respiratory problem. In early distress, respiratory rate increases. Later it slows, as the person becomes tired and unable to compensate. A respiratory rate of greater than 60 is abnormal for any age child, just as a respiratory rate of less than 12 is abnormally slow for any age child (Dieckmann, Brownstein, & Gausche-Hill, 2000).

As respiratory distress progresses to respiratory failure, mental status changes occur due to the resulting hypoxia. Dyspnea will increase, as will the use of accessory muscles.

Interventions

If the student has a known respiratory condition that is causing the problem, such as asthma, the school nurse should give the medication prescribed by the primary care provider. Otherwise respiratory interventions include allowing the student to find a position of comfort and using basic life support skills. If distress is moderate to severe, call EMS for oxygen and advanced life support measures. If the student is not breathing or has an ineffective breathing pattern, that is, gasping, the nurse should initiate ventilations with a bag-valve-mask or mouth-to-mouth with a barrier device.

Choking

Etiology

An object or debris blocking the airway causes choking. This can occur during eating or during play when an object is placed in the mouth. Common objects that cause airway obstruction are nuts, candy, coins, hot dogs, marbles, and pieces of balloons (Nonfatal choking–related episodes among children—United States, 2001, 2002).

Assessment

If airway obstruction is due to a foreign body, there may be a sudden onset of coughing, choking, gagging, stridor, and/or shortness of breath in a previously well student. If the student can cough, cry, or speak, the airway is only partially obstructed. Try not to disturb the child and call for EMS. Prepare for the child's condition to deteriorate and be ready to perform foreign body airway obstruction maneuvers. Never perform these maneuvers on an individual with a partial obstruction (Zaritsky et al., 2002). Allow the student with a partial obstruction to attempt dislodging the foreign body through forceful coughing.

Intervention

To relieve foreign body obstruction in the unresponsive child, use the following steps:

1. Open the airway using a tongue jaw lift. Look for the object obstructing the airway. If the object is visible, remove it. Do not perform blind finger sweeps.
2. Open the airway with a head tilt-chin lift and attempt to provide rescue breaths. If the breaths are not effective, reposition the head and reattempt ventilation.
3. If the breaths are still not effective, kneel beside the victim or straddle the victim's hips and prepare to perform abdominal thrusts (Heimlich maneuver):
   a. Place the heel of one hand on the child's abdomen in the midline slightly above the navel and well below the rib cage. Place the other hand on top of the first.
   b. Press with both hands onto the abdomen with a quick inward and upward thrust. Direct each thrust upward in the midline. If necessary, perform up to five thrusts. Each thrust should be a separate and distinct movement of sufficient force to dislodge the obstruction.
4. Repeat steps 1 to 3 until the object is dislodged or the airway is patent. If the victim is still unresponsive after 1 minute activate EMS (AHA, 2001).

Asthma or Anaphylactic Reaction

Asthma is a chronic inflammatory lung disorder of the airways. Both an acute asthma reaction and a severe anaphylactic reaction can result in smooth muscle constriction of the airways, resulting in severe respiratory distress. Accurate assessment of individuals with asthma and allergy is critical to minimize complications and halt deterioration. The school nurse must recognize that students or staff with severe reactions are at risk for respiratory arrest and death. Chapter 29 on asthma and Chapter 28 on allergy discuss the etiology, assessment, and emergency interventions for these problems.

Epiglottitis

Etiology

Epiglottitis is also known as supraglottic laryngitis. Inflammation of the epiglottis and surrounding structures can rapidly occlude the airway in a matter of hours. It is always an emergent condition, usually caused by *Haemophilus influenzae*, type b (see

Chapter 21). Incidence has significantly decreased since the widespread immunization of children against *Haemophilus influenzae*, type b has occurred (Progress Towards Elimination of *Haemophilus influenzae* type b invasive disease among infants and children—United States, 1998–2000, 2002).

Assessment

The child with epiglottitis will appear ill and flushed with a high fever. The school nurse may hear stridor. The child will appear anxious with respiratory distress, and have drooling and trouble swallowing. The school nurse may observe positioning in a tripod position with the neck extended forward to keep the airway open. Do NOT attempt to visualize the back of the throat because manipulation can cause total airway obstruction (Dieckmann et al., 2000).

Intervention

When the school nurse suspects epiglottitis, keeping the child calm and quiet is a priority. EMS should be called immediately and the parents should be notified to meet the child in the emergency department. Nothing should be administered by mouth because the child may require a tracheostomy. When EMS arrives, communicate the suspected diagnosis and its implication for airway obstruction to emergency care providers so that they and whoever accompanies the child to the hospital can keep the child as calm as possible during transport. Inform EMS and the receiving hospital of the degree of respiratory distress, immunization history and suspected diagnosis.

Pneumonia

Etiology

Pneumonia is an inflammation of lung tissue, usually caused by a bacteria or virus (Hockenberry et al., 2003). The most common causative bacterial agents for children older than age 3 are *Mycoplasma pneumoniae* and *Streptococcus pneumoniae*. However, the majority of pneumonia cases are viral. Causal agents include parainfluenza, influenza, and adenovirus.

Assessment

A bacterial pneumonia is usually abrupt with a high fever, chills and a wet cough. In contrast viral pneumonia usually develops over a number of days, where the person has a cough and low-grade fever; the onset of symptoms is often associated with a recent upper respiratory infection. A student with either type of pneumonia will exhibit cough, and poor appetite, and may complain of chest pain or abdominal pain. Breath sounds may be decreased and wheezing may be present.

Intervention

If pneumonia is suspected, call the parent. For severe respiratory distress, activate EMS and call the parent. Leave the student in a position of comfort to facilitate breathing. Oral fluids may be offered if the student is not vomiting. Antipyretics such as acetaminophen or ibuprofen are indicated if a parent has authorized administration and depending on state and local rules. These medications can assist with fever management and relief of discomfort until the parent arrives. The Pneumovax® vaccine is recommended for the prevention of pneumoccocal pneumonia in children with preexisting medical conditions (Jardine, 2003).

Pneumothorax

Etiology

Pneumothorax occurs when air escapes into the pleural space of the chest. It is most likely to occur as a result of thoracic trauma. TABLE 22.13 presents the types of pneumothoraces, assessment of signs and symptoms, and interventions. Pneumothorax is a potentially life-threatening emergency. If a pneumothorax is suspected, activate EMS. The school nurse should recognize the severity of a pneumothorax and be prepared to provide supportive care until EMS arrives.

CIRCULATORY EMERGENCIES

The most common circulatory emergency that occurs in children is hypovolemic shock, although other types of shock can occur. Fluid volume deficit from nausea, vomiting, and diarrhea can occur quickly, especially in younger children. Blood loss from trauma can also quickly lead to hypovolemic shock, a life-threatening emergency.

Shock

Etiology

Shock is not a disease, but rather the end result of many different physiological events; it is a state that develops when ineffective circulation results in inadequate delivery of oxygen to the organs and tissues. As a result, vital organs are unable to function properly. There are three broad categories of shock: hypovolemic, cardiogenic, and maldistributive.

Table 22.13 ■
TYPES OF PNEUMOTHORAX

TYPE OF PNEUMOTHORAX	SIGNS AND SYMPTOMS	INTERVENTION
Open pneumothorax: An open chest wound sucking air in from the outside	• Open wound with a sucking sound • Respiratory distress • Decreased breath sounds on side with wound • Tracheal deviation • Pain	Cover the wound with an occlusive dressing, tape three of the four sides allowing air to escape, but not enter
Simple pneumothorax: Air enters the closed pleural space	• Respiratory distress • Absent breath sounds on affected side • Pain • Sometimes asymptomatic	Call parents and/or EMS depending upon severity of respiratory distress
Hemothorax: Blood enters the pleural space	• Respiratory distress • Signs of hypovolemic shock • Absence of breath sounds on affected side • Dullness on percussion of the chest	• Monitor for changes • Activate EMS
Tension pneumothorax: Air enters the pleural space and becomes trapped	• Respiratory distress • Dyspnea • Tachypnea • Decreased breath sounds on the affected side • Distended neck veins • Respiratory failure • Shock from the expanding chest volume pressing on the pulmonary vasculature	Activate EMS

Source: Adapted from Thomas, Bernardo, & Herman (2003).

Hypovolemic shock is the most common cause of shock in children; the most common cause of hypovolemic shock is loss of fluid and blood from trauma or dehydration (Zaritsky et al., 2002). The signs and symptoms of shock vary with the amount of fluid lost and the amount of time over which fluid is lost. Excessive blood loss causes decreased venous blood return to the heart and eventually a decrease in cardiac output. Tachycardia is the most common response to the fall in cardiac output (Zaritsky et al., 2002). If the volume loss is not stopped or replaced, death can occur. It is imperative that the school nurse quickly assess and intervene when shock is suspected because children decompensate very quickly.

Cardiogenic shock occurs when there is a problem with the pumping mechanism of the heart. Students with a history of a congenital heart disease or an acquired heart disease are at increased risk of developing cardiogenic shock (Thomas et al., 2003). A student with a cardiac arrhythmia or toxic drug exposure may also have cardiac dysfunction resulting in cardiogenic shock. Cardiogenic shock results in reduced cardiac output and can occur any time there is impaired heart muscle function.

Maldistributive shock occurs due to the loss of vascular tone, most often associated with sepsis, neurological injury, or anaphylaxis (Thomas et al., 2003). In sepsis and anaphylaxis, the loss of vascular tone and subsequent capillary leakage can lead to a relative hypovolemia. This means there is no true external loss of volume, but that the loss of vascular tone creates a large space in the vascular system.

The most common cause of maldistributive shock is sepsis. When left untreated, sepsis leads to circulatory shock. Cellular and immunological changes occur resulting in cell destruction, vasodilation, capillary leakage, and microemboli formation. Neurogenic shock, another type of maldistributive shock, is usually due to spinal cord injury. Vasodilation occurs due to the loss of sympathetic tone. Spinal shock most frequently occurs with total cord transection above T1. Lastly, anaphylaxis is a hypersensitive reaction to a specific allergen that causes vasodilation and capillary leakage and can result in shock (Thomas et al., 2003).

Assessment

The school nurse must recognize when a student is in shock. As the school nurse is determining what happened, she should simultaneously perform the rapid primary assessment (ABCD) (see Table 22.4) to determine if there are any life or limb-threatening injuries. Tachypnea can be an indicator of shock; however, a student who is in a compensated state of shock will breathe at a normal rate. Assess the circulatory system; remember, early signs of circulatory compromise are not only tachycardia but also include:

- Increased capillary refill time
- Decreased peripheral pulses
- Cool mottled skin
- Restless, agitated

Signs of impending circulatory collapse are:

- Change in level of consciousness
- Lethargy
- Low blood pressure
- Increased respiratory rate or respiratory failure
- Weak thready pulse

Complete a CIAMPEDS assessment (see Table 22.7).

If there is suspicion that the student is hypovolemic because of trauma, the school nurse will need to assess the mechanism of injury to determine if there was a force significant enough to cause a major injury. Students with any of the following could be considered having experienced major trauma and possibly suffering from multiple system trauma:

- Motor vehicle crash with death or serious injury to another in the car
- Motor vehicle crash with steering wheel deformity or structural incursion of more than 20 inches
- Vehicle rollover
- Fall more than 15 feet for adolescents older than 14 years of age
- Fall more than 10 feet for students or staff younger than 15 or older than 55 years old
- Pedestrian struck at more than 8 miles an hour
- Motorcycle crash victims ejected at more than 16 miles an hour
- Significant blunt trauma to head, neck, torso, or abdomen (Maloney, Fitzgerald, Elam, & Doyle, 2000)

In any of these situations, immediately direct someone to call EMS. Primary assessment always involves assessing the airway with cervical spine immobilization, breathing, circulation, and disability. The history would involve use of the CIAMPEDS mnemonic. Use all assessment data obtained to determine if the student has a potentially life-threatening condition.

If the school nurse suspects that the student is hypovolemic as a result of dehydration, then focus on assessing if there is a history of vomiting or diarrhea, or signs of diabetes or sepsis. Check mucous membranes, skin turgor, capillary refill, and vital signs, and assess if there is a history of excessive urinary output.

Diabetes is another condition that can result in dehydration and hence hypovolemic shock. Diabetic emergencies are detailed in Chapter 33. TABLE 22.14 describes physiological changes related to hypovolemic shock.

When cardiogenic shock is suspected, the focus of the assessment will be on obtaining a cardiac history. Other conditions that would cause an electrolyte imbalance and disrupt electrical conduction through the heart muscle are anorexia, bulimia, diabetes, or drug toxicity.

Maldistributive shock can be identified through assessment by determining if there is sepsis, a spinal cord injury due to trauma or previous spinal cord damage, a reaction to an allergen, or an effect from a vasodilating medication.

Intervention

School nurse interventions for shock are the same for all types of shock. Contact EMS.

Table 22.14 ■
PHYSIOLOGICAL CHANGES IN HYPOVOLEMIC SHOCK

ASSESSMENT PARAMETER	< 15% ESTIMATED BLOOD LOSS	15% TO 25% ESTIMATED BLOOD LOSS	25% TO 40% ESTIMATED BLOOD LOSS
Capillary refill	2 seconds or less	> 3 seconds	>5 seconds
Respiratory rate/work of breathing	Normal	Increased	Increased or respiratory failure
Heart rate	Normal	Increased	Increased or decreasing
Systolic blood pressure	Normal	Normal	Decreased
Sensorium	Normal	Irritable	Confused, lethargic, or unresponsive

Source: Adapted from Maloney et al. (2002).

- If spinal cord injury is a possibility, keep the head and neck stabilized and try not to move the student until EMS arrives.
- Maintain or open the airway.
- If there is no pulse or no circulation after airway and breathing are assessed then chest compressions must be initiated according to American Heart Association CPR standards for the child ages 1 to 8 or for the adult, which is considered older than age 8.
- Control any external bleeding with direct pressure; elevate the bleeding extremity
- If no spinal cord injury or head injury is suspected lay the student supine with the legs slightly elevated.
- Keep the student warm and calm.
- Document findings.

If you suspect shock due to a cardiac problem inform EMS, because they may need to give fluid boluses more slowly and monitor more closely for pulmonary edema.

Sudden Cardiac Death

Etiology

Approximately 3,000 persons between the ages of 15 and 34 experience sudden cardiac arrest each year. CDC data indicate that there has been an increase in sudden cardiac death in 15- to 34-year-olds between 1991 and 2001 (Zheng, Crosft, Giles, & Mensah, 2001). Sudden cardiac arrest is the sudden disruption of heart function caused by an abnormal heart rhythm called ventricular fibrillation or ventricular tachycardia; this frequently results in sudden cardiac death.

Assessment

If a student or staff member were to experience sudden cardiac arrest, the nurse must complete a basic life support assessment of responsiveness, airway, breathing, and circulation. Findings would indicate an unresponsive victim with a clear airway, no breathing, or gasping respirations and no palpable pulse.

Intervention

Immediate bystander CPR is indicated for sudden cardiac arrest. Ventricular fibrillation can sometimes be successfully treated with defibrillation. Automated external defibrillators (AEDs) are portable machines designed to quickly treat ventricular fibrillation. AEDs decrease the time to defibrillation in cases of sudden cardiac arrest. In response to the problem of sudden cardiac death that occurs at schools and in other public places, many areas of the country are developing Public Access Defibrillation (PAD) programs. These programs involve making defibrillation readily available through the use of AEDs in public places, including schools, and training laypersons to safely and effectively defibrillate a person with a suspected cardiac event.

The American Heart Association (AHA) has approved the use of AEDs for children ages one through eight (AHA, 2004). The American Heart Association recommends that a school medical emergency response plan include "implementation of a lay rescuer AED program in schools with an established need" (AHA, 2004).

A tertiary benefit of having an AED at school is that it will be available for use not only for children, but also by the large numbers of adults who routinely work and/or visit schools. Another benefit is the required CPR and AED training required for school staff who participate in PAD programs. The training serves to heighten awareness of the need for CPR and heart healthy lifestyles (Wolkenheim, 2000).

Sickle Cell Crisis

Etiology

The term *sickle cell disease* refers to a group of genetic disorders in which there is a predominance of hemoglobin S (see Chapter 27). Sickle cell anemia is the most severe form of sickle cell disease. Symptoms are related to anemia and vasoocclusive disease. In a student with sickle cell anemia, red blood cells are prone to taking on a sickle shape because of an amino acid substitution in their hemoglobin molecules (Thomas et al., 2003). In deoxygenated, dehydrated and acidotic states, the red blood cells take on the sickle shape and rather than flow easily through the vessels, they get stuck and impede blood flow, causing increased deoxygenation and obstruction in the microcirculation. This can lead to ischemia, infarction, and necrosis (Thomas et al., 2003).

This vasoocclusive crisis can manifest itself in a number of ways:

Acute chest syndrome—pulmonary emboli develop and the patient presents in respiratory distress and pain

Aplastic crisis—decreased RBC production

Cerebral stroke—related to sickled cells blocking blood vessels in the brain

Priapism—painful erection related to sludging of blood in the corpus cavernosum

Splenic sequestration crisis—in children younger than 5 years where the spleen pools blood leading to hypovolemic shock, anemia, and possibly death. The poor hemoglobin function and the fact that the spleen is often enlarged and non-functional puts those affected at high risk for infections.

Pain—Children with sickle cell disease may frequently experience moderate to severe pain due to ischemia and compromised circulation but without the signs and symptoms of inflammation. Pain may present as acute abdomen, arthralgias, or headache; the pain may be migratory (Hockenberry et al., 2003; Thomas et al., 2003).

Assessment

Hopefully, an IHP and an EAP (Chapter 9) have been developed for students in the school with sickle cell disease, including past incidents of vasoocclusive crisis, how they usually present, and what interventions are recommended by the family. The student may complain of joint pain, chest pain, headache, abdominal pain, nausea and/or vomiting, but without the typical signs associated with illness. Low-grade fever may be present.

Assess the ABCDs. Look for increased respiratory rate and effort and for bilateral aeration. Check capillary refill time and skin color. Use the AVPU scale to determine level of consciousness. Assess location and severity of pain. Check hydration status; ask about urinary output, and look at the mucous membranes.

Interventions

Measures for sickle cell crisis are supportive and promote oxygenation and hydration. Pain management is handled by the family, as per the healthcare provider's recommendations. If the pain is severe enough, the parents may take their child to the ER or the healthcare provider. If the student shows signs of airway compromise or neurological changes or shock, EMS should be called. Inform them that the student has sickle cell disease, so that they bring oxygen and can start an IV at the scene. If oxygen is available at the school, it should be used. Immobilize and support painful joints.

Prevention measures should also be part of the IHP. Ensure adequate hydration. Observe very closely for signs of infection and get prompt early treatment from the primary care provider. Encourage compliance with any prophylactic antibiotics. Promote compliance with immunizations. Educate the family and student regarding the importance of wearing a medical alert bracelet or carrying a card with medical information about their sickle cell disease in case of emergency, including if they normally have a very low hemoglobin.

NEUROLOGICAL EMERGENCIES

Etiology

Neurological emergencies can occur as a direct insult due to trauma or as a result of a structural abnormality of the central nervous system. Neurological compromise can be caused by alteration in cerebral blood flow, increased intracranial pressure, metabolic imbalances, infections, substance use or abuse, exposure to toxins, hypoxia, shock, stroke, and seizures.

Assessment

It is important for the school nurse to recognize the age-appropriate behavior of children and adolescents to determine if there is any alteration in neurological function. During the triage process, the school nurse determines if there is any gross alteration in motor and/or sensory function and level of consciousness using the AVPU scale. Determining the underlying cause of an abnormality will guide intervention.

The emergency assessment by the school nurse should always follow the ABCD format to determine if there is a life-threatening emergency. The AVPU scale should be used to assess neurological status. When an alteration in level of consciousness is detected, the AEIOU-TIPS mnemonic can be used to try and determine possible causes:

- A—Alcohol
- E—Epilepsy
- I—Insulin
- O—Overdose
- U—Uremia
- T—Trauma
- I—Infection
- P—Psychological
- S—Shock/stroke/syncope

(Seidel & Henderson, 1997)

The NASN Managing School Emergencies program suggests use of the mental status assessment published by the American Academy of Neurology in 1997 (Table 22.15).

Below is a list of the signs and symptoms of mental status abnormality (AAN, 1997):

- Vacant stare-confused expression
- Delayed responses

Table 22.15 ■
MENTAL STATUS ASSESSMENT

PARAMETER	ASSESSMENT
Orientation	Time, person, place and situation
Concentration	Repeat digits back in reverse order; repeat months of the year in reverse order
Memory	Names of teams playing; recall of three words and three objects (check at just after injury and five minutes later); details of a recent newsworthy event

Source: Adapted from Maloney et al. (2002b).

- Inability to focus attention
- Disoriented
- Purposeless activity
- Slurred or incoherent speech
- Gross observable uncoordinated movements
- Emotionally labile
- Memory deficits
- Repetition of phrases ("What happened?", "What happened?")

It is important to identify if there was a total loss of consciousness and whether it was a few seconds or minutes. If there was a loss of consciousness, the school nurse will activate EMS. Intervention for a neurological emergency in the school setting depends on the cause.

Traumatic Brain Injury

Etiology

Motor vehicle crashes, bicycle crashes without a helmet, falls, and sports activities are common mechanisms of brain injury in children (Thomas et al., 2003). The injury occurs at impact, when traumatic forces are applied to the brain. The brain hits the inside of the skull and contusions, fractures and diffuse axonal injury can occur. When the injured brain begins to swell, cerebral edema and increased intracranial pressure can occur. While various neurological emergencies can occur in schools, the most common cause of death among all injured children is traumatic brain injury (Thomas et al., 2003).

Assessment

After the rapid initial assessment, and intervention for abnormalities found in ABC, AVPU, and pupillary response, identify the mechanism of injury and determine if there was a total loss of consciousness and for how long. Complete a mental status assessment (see Table 22.15). Observe for pupillary changes, visual disturbances, vomiting, seizure activity, headache, weakness, or neck pain. Assess motor and sensory function by asking the student to wiggle his or her fingers and toes and ask if he or she can feel touch in each foot and each hand (Thomas et al., 2003).

Intervention

The brain and spinal cord have limited ability to regenerate after injury so immediate action must be taken to minimize long-term effects of traumatic brain injury (Thomas et al., 2003). If there was a loss of consciousness, the school nurse will activate EMS. The cervical spine is stabilized as part of the airway assessment. If there are any abnormal findings the student should be seen at the local emergency department for evaluation by a physician. Keep the student resting and continually reassess vital signs, pupils, and mental status until EMS arrives. A dressing can be applied to any open wounds and the school nurse should provide emotional support; contact the family to meet EMS at the hospital.

Spinal Cord Injury

Etiology

Spinal cord injury can occur in the cervical, thoracic, lumbar, or sacral areas. The spinal cord can be bruised, lacerated, or transected and the blood vessels supplying the cord can also be injured. The injuries occur as a consequence of hyperextension, hyperflexion, vertical compression, and rotational forces. Spinal cord injuries result most frequently from falls, diving, motor vehicle crashes, gunshot wounds, hanging, and sports activities.

Assessment

After a rapid initial assessment and determination of the mechanism of injury, assessment includes determining if there was a loss of consciousness. The student should be asked if there is any tingling or loss of sensation in any extremity. Assess for paralysis, flaccid extremities, hand grip strength, and strength of lower extremities on dorsiflexion.

Intervention

If the airway is not patent, open using the jaw thrust maneuver. Be prepared to ventilate if there is a high cervical spine injury using a bag-valve mask. Maintain stabilization to prevent further harm. Continue to monitor ABCD and call for EMS.

Seizures

Etiology

A seizure results from the abnormal discharge of cerebral electrical activity (Thomas et al., 2003) (see Chapter 37). The age of the child and the area of the brain involved influence the type of seizure that occurs. Febrile seizures are common in young children (Thomas et al., 2003). Acute seizures occur for a variety of other reasons:

- Infection
- Head trauma
- Intracranial bleeding
- Toxic exposures
- Electrolyte imbalances, hypoglycemia
- Anoxia
- Brain tumors
- Epilepsy

Status epilepticus is a continuous generalized seizure that lasts longer than 30 minutes, and/or recurrent seizures that occur without full recovery of consciousness between seizures. These children are at risk for respiratory depression and subsequent hypoxia (Thomas et al., 2003). Status epilepticus causes problems both systemically and within the brain. Systemically, the intense, prolonged muscular activity rapidly consumes tissue energy stores and leads to tissue hypoxia resulting in anaerobic metabolism and tissue breakdown (Thomas et al., 2003). Cerebrally, the increased electrical discharge increases cerebral metabolic rate that can rapidly deplete the available glucose as well as deplete the oxygen supplied to the brain. This can lead to ischemia and brain damage (Thomas et al., 2003).

Assessment

After a student experiences a seizure, the school nurse should assess what kind of seizure the child had (see Chapter 37). What time did it start and end? Describe the behavior. Was their body jerking all over, or only in one place? Does the student have a history of seizures? Did the student have an aura? Was there a head injury? Was there a toxic exposure? Was there any alcohol involved? Is there a fever or signs of an infection? After the ABCD assessment, check vital signs including temperature. The school nurse should determine the possible causes of the altered level of consciousness, as in the AEIOU-TIPS mnemonic.

Intervention

Intervention is similar regardless of cause during an active seizure. For a student who is actively seizing, the priorities are still airway, breathing, and circulation (ABC). If the seizure is due to trauma, try to maintain cervical spine stabilization. If the student begins vomiting or has oral secretions that may inhibit breathing, log roll the entire body onto one side, maintaining alignment as much as possible so that the airway remains clear of vomitus. If the student has a history of seizures or the seizure is not due to trauma, put the student in the recovery position. The main objective is to protect the student from further harm and to maintain an airway. Call EMS if the seizure is:

- The first time for the student,
- Due to trauma,
- Lasts longer than 5 minutes, or
- Different than any seizure the student has had in the past.

If incontinence accompanied the seizure, assist the student with hygiene and a change of clothing.

If the student has a history of status epilepticus, the school nurse should develop an emergency plan as part of the IHP. The nurse may wish to work with the primary care provider to get a prescription medication such as rectal diazepam or buccal midazolam to keep readily available in case the student has a prolonged seizure.

Bacterial Meningitis

Etiology

Bacterial meningitis is most often caused by *Streptococcus pneumoniae* or *Neisseria meningitides*. The incidence of cases of meningitis due to *Haemophilus influenzae* has decreased 95% since the introduction of the Hib vaccine (Selekman, 2003). It is transmitted usually from a focus of infection somewhere else in the body, such as nasal secretions. Meningococcal meningitis is the only type readily transmitted by droplet infection from nasopharyngeal secretions (CDC, 2005). This form occurs predominantly in school-age children and adolescents.

Assessment

In the early phase of meningitis, there will be a history of a "terrible" headache, fever, chills, and muscle and joint pain. The student may be extremely irritable, develop photophobia (Thomas et al., 2003), and complain of a stiff neck. Later the student will exhibit severe headache, high fever, a macular skin rash with petechiae or purpura, hypotension, slow capillary refill, respiratory distress, and an altered level of consciousness (Dieckmann et al., 2000). Be aware that these patients are at risk for seizures. This rapid change in symptoms occurs very quickly, often within a few hours.

Intervention

Because of the infectious nature of the disease, the nurse should wear personal protective equipment and should inform EMS personnel, so that protective equipment such as gloves, gowns, and masks are worn. Management of ABCDs are a priority and vital signs should be monitored until EMS arrives. Document the assessment findings and interventions. Give this information to EMS and call the emergency department to let them know ahead of time that a suspected case of meningitis is coming. Public Health must be contacted and can often be very helpful in identifying close contacts of the ill student and sending a letter home with the other students.

Syncope

Etiology

Syncope is a brief lapse in consciousness caused by cerebral hypoxia. It is usually preceded by a brief period of lightheadedness. It can be caused by a variety of factors such as, emotional stress, vagal stimulation, vascular pooling, or any sudden change in environmental temperature or body position.

Assessment

When a student presents with syncope, check vital signs, especially blood pressure and pulse, with the student lying, sitting, and standing to assess for orthostatic hypotension. Determine the onset, and if the student is able to describe what caused the syncope. Ask if there are any other symptoms and if the student is taking any medications, alcohol, or drugs. Check to see when and what the student last ate and if there are any signs of dehydration.

Check pupil size and response to light. Test hand strength bilaterally, and listen to the student's speech for clarity and articulation. Evaluate the student to see if there are any injuries associated with a fall. Check memory as described in the neurological assessment section. Check blood sugar if the student is diabetic.

Intervention

If the student feels "faint," have the student sit with the head between the knees or have the student lie down. If there are any injuries from a fall, provide first aid as needed. Assess vital signs and continue to reassess. Call the parents, and recommend consultation by the primary care provider.

ABDOMINAL EMERGENCIES

Etiology

The school nurse must be able to differentiate between a serious emergency such as appendicitis from a less serious abdominal problem, such as constipation. Stomachache can be caused by emotional distress, menstrual cramps, a cough resulting in swallowing a lot of mucus, taking antibiotics for another problem, or hunger from not getting a meal. Other causes of acute abdominal pain are listed in TABLE 22.16.

Table 22.16 ■ COMMON CAUSES OF ABDOMINAL PAIN IN CHILDREN

CHILDHOOD	ADOLESCENCE
Gastroenteritis	Ectopic pregnancy
Appendicitis	Pelvic inflammatory disease
Pancreatitis	Testicular torsion
Ulcers	Inflammatory bowel disease
Constipation	Biliary disease
Urinary tract infection	

Assessment

The pain can be assessed using the CIAMPEDS and the QUESTT mnemonics: CIAMPEDS adapted for abdominal discomfort includes:

- C—Chief complaint. Ask if the pain comes and goes or is it there all the time?
- I—Immunizations/isolation
- A—Allergies
- M—Medications: Is student taking any that upset the stomach?
- P—Past relevant medical history. Ask if the student has had this abdominal pain before. For teenage girls, ask when was the first day of the last menstrual period. Is she pregnant or could she be pregnant? Any other medical history of gastrointestinal problems?
- E—Events surrounding the incident, mechanism of injury if applicable. When did it start? Is it related to anything the student ate? Any major stressors in the student's life, like a divorce or death in the family? Does the student perceive a major problem in his or her life?
- D—Diet (intake and output). What has the student eaten? Is the student nauseous? Is there any vomiting?
- S—Signs and Symptoms—Are there any other signs and symptoms with the abdominal pain? Is there diarrhea, constipation, or fever? Is there a change in the student's activity level? (Adapted from the ENA, 2004).

Remember that if the student is not eating or drinking or if there is diarrhea and vomiting, dehydration can ensue quickly. Young children have a higher percentage of extracellular fluid and can go into shock from these fluid losses (Thomas et al., 2003).

Vital signs should be checked, especially temperature. A physical assessment of the abdomen should be performed by the school nurse, observing the shape and symmetry and assessing for any external signs of injury. Listen in all four quadrants of the abdomen for bowel sounds and have the student point to where the pain is greatest. Palpate the nonpainful areas of the abdomen first and the painful area last. Evaluate for rebound tenderness.

Intervention

Any student showing signs of shock, with an altered level of consciousness, with an abdominal mass, or showing severe signs of respiratory distress should be transported to the hospital via EMS. Any adolescent female with lower abdominal pain and who could be pregnant should go to the emergency department to rule out an ectopic pregnancy. Depending on the appearance of the young female, she may be able to wait for a parent to drive her. Anyone with severe abdominal pain (cannot walk or constantly bent over) should be evaluated by EMS and transported to the emergency department for an evaluation by a physician. If the pain persists, and a cause cannot be found, recommend that parents take the child for further evaluation. If emotional stress is determined to be the cause, consider talking to the family about seeing a psychologist or counselor for assistance. Follow up with the student, family, EMS or healthcare provider, as appropriate.

Appendicitis

Appendicitis is the most common surgical emergency that occurs in childhood. Perforation of the appendix with subsequent peritonitis can result when a diagnosis is delayed. Early diagnosis is a challenge because appendicitis can be mistaken for other illnesses.

Etiology

Appendicitis is inflammation of the appendix, a small pouch attached to the cecum, near the transition from the small intestine to the colon, on the lower right side of the abdomen. In appendicitis, the flow of mucus secretions is blocked by obstructive pressure that builds in the intestinal lumen. The resulting infection and edema can block blood flow to the area causing ischemia and infarction. Gangrene can ensue resulting in rupture of the appendix and release of toxins and bacteria into the abdominal cavity. This peritonitis can progress to sepsis, intestinal obstruction, electrolyte imbalance, and eventually shock (Hockenberry et al., 2003).

Assessment

The early signs of appendicitis are diffuse midabdominal or periumbilical pain with rebound tenderness, and pain with coughing and walking. The student's activity level will decrease and he or she will prefer to lie still for pain relief. As the appendicitis progresses, pain is localized to the right lower quadrant. The most intense pain is between the iliac crest and the umbilicus (McBurney's Point). Anorexia, nausea, and vomiting are common in the early stages (Hockenberry et al., 2003). A low-grade fever may develop. If the appendix perforates, the temperature can be expected to rise to >39°C, or >102°F, the respiratory rate increases and the abdominal pain becomes more diffuse as opposed to the earlier localized right lower quadrant pain. Often a student will report a sudden relief of pain as the appendix perforates and then an increase of a more diffuse abdominal pain (Hockenberry et al., 2003).

Using the CIAMPEDS and QUESTT mnemonics to assist with assessment, the school nurse should assess the chief complaint, vital signs, and the abdomen. Bowel sounds may be decreased on auscultation of the abdomen.

Intervention

If the school nurse suspects appendicitis, the caregiver should be called. If there is evidence of perforation, such as more diffuse abdominal pain, the school nurse may consider activating EMS. The student will require surgical intervention with perforation to avoid sepsis, shock, and potentially death. Continue to assess pain using one of the pain scales. Do not allow the student to eat or drink anything because of the possibility of surgery.

Follow-up with parents in the evening or the next day. Verify that the student was evaluated by a physician. If the student has not seen a physician, explain to the parents the potential problems if the student continues experiencing the pain characteristic of appendicitis.

GENITOURINARY EMERGENCIES

Urinary Tract Infections

Etiology

Urinary tract infections are the second most common infection seen in children, with respiratory infections being number one (Lafferty & Baird, 2001). Urinary tract infections are usually caused by bacteria, often introduced by poor hygiene or sexual activity or exacerbated by a lack of fluid intake or incomplete emptying of the bladder.

Assessment

While urinary tract infections are usually nonurgent, the presence of pain, fever, or hematuria may be signs that the problem is urgent. It is important to have the student describe the discomfort. Does it burn or sting before it comes out, while urinating, or when wiping? Is there urgency and/or frequency? Is any discharge present on the underwear or when wiping? This includes blood and mucus. Is there pain in the abdominal area or flank pain? Is the student unable to stand or walk because of the flank pain? Palpate the abdomen to assess if the bladder is distended. A urinalysis will be obtained at the care provider's site to complete the assessment.

It is important to know if the student has been diagnosed with diabetes or has other symptoms of systemic disease. A urinary tract infection can progress to a systemic infection. Students who present to the school nurse with signs of shock and/or sepsis due to infection are classified as emergent.

Intervention

There are four presenting symptoms that require urgent care by the healthcare provider:

- Unable to pass urine or can only pass a few drops (to rule out blockage of the urethra, possibly due to inflammation)
- Hematuria (to rule out hemorrhagic cystitis)
- Severe pain, especially flank pain (to rule out kidney stones)
- High fever and pain (to rule out pyelonephritis) (Schmitt, 2002).

Assuming there are no contraindications, provide clear fluids or juices high in vitamin C, but avoid caffeine and carbonated beverages "because they tend to make the urine alkaline" (Lafferty & Baird, 2001, p. 360). Medication may be prescribed to relieve the pain and burning especially on urination and to fight the infection.

Teaching young girls proper hygiene after voiding by wiping themselves front to back is key to preventing urinary tract infections. Teaching parents not to use bubble baths for young children and to avoid having children wear tight-fitting pants may also decrease the incidence. Adolescent girls who are sexually active should be taught to void and clean the perineum immediately after intercourse.

TOXICOLOGICAL EMERGENCIES

Etiology

"A poison exposure is an inappropriate contact with or use of a chemical, drug or natural toxin, by any route of exposure" (Soloway, 2003, p. 524). Poisoning means that symptoms resulted from a drug, toxin, or chemical poison exposure. Below is a list of the most common pediatric poison exposures for 6- to 19-year-olds in 2000:

- Analgesics
- Bites and envenomations
- Cleaning substances
- Cough and cold preparations
- Cosmetics and personal care products
- Plants
- Foreign bodies
- Stimulants and street drugs
- Antidepressants
- Food products and food poisoning (Litovitz et al., 2001)

Assessment

Poisonings generally enter the body through ingestion, inhalation, and cutaneous or ocular exposure. The reaction varies depending upon the agent and the quantity of substance. When a student presents to the nurse's office following exposure to a potentially toxic substance, find out what time the exposure occurred, the agent, the amount, and the route of exposure. Assess the ABCDs, use the CIAMPEDS assessment format, and check vital signs. Look for unusual odors or stains around the mouth or nose or on the clothes. Assess the skin for areas of irritation. TABLE 22.17 describes toxicological symptoms of selected toxins that the school nurse may encounter.

Intervention

For guidance on treatment of any poisoning, contact the national poison control center number 1-800-222-1222. If there are abnormal vital signs or abnormalities in ABCD, call EMS. The priority is maintaining ABCDs and identifying the toxin for EMS and the emergency department, including when, how much and any other information obtained during assessment in order to facilitate care.

While maintaining the ABCs, it is also essential to remove the student from the source of the poison or to remove any additional poisons from the student. Continuous flushing of the skin or eyes is essential if contact has been made with a poison; any contaminated clothing needs to be removed. Do not induce vomiting; however, if the student does vomit, save the vomitus in a closed container and send it with EMS (Hootman, Fratto, & Perkins, 2002). Request that another staff member contact the poison control center for guidance on management, since the nurse may be busy providing life-sustaining care to the student.

Table 22.17 ■

TOXICOLOGICAL SYMPTOMS OF SELECTED TOXINS

TOXIN	VITAL SIGNS	MENTAL STATUS	SIGNS AND SYMPTOMS
Acetaminophen	Normal	Normal	Anorexia, nausea, vomiting, right upper quadrant pain (late)
Amphetamines	Hypertension, tachycardia, fast breathing, hyperthermia	Hyperactive, agitated	Hyper alert, dilated pupils, hyperactive bowel sounds, flushed, diaphoresis
Barbiturates	Hypotension, slow breathing, hypothermia	Altered-lethargy	Slurred speech, ataxia, dysconjugate gaze, hyporeflexia
Carbon monoxide	Normal	Altered-lethargy	Headache, dizziness, nausea, vomiting, seizures
Cocaine	Hypertension, tachycardia, hyperthermia	Altered-anxiety, agitation, delirium	Paranoia, dilated pupils, tremors, diaphoresis, active bowel sounds
Cyclic antidepressants	Hypotension, tachycardia, hyperthermia	Altered-lethargy	Confusion, dizziness, dilated pupils, dry mucous membranes, flushed, seizures
Iron	Hypotension, tachycardia	Normal unless hypotensive, if hypotensive-lethargy	Abdominal pain, nausea, vomiting, diarrhea, vomiting of bright red blood, abdominal tenderness
Lead	Hypertension	Altered-lethargy	Irritability, abdominal pain, nausea, vomiting constipation, peripheral neuropathy, seizures
Opioids	Hypotension, bradycardia, slow breathing, hypothermia	Altered-lethargy	Slurred speech, ataxia, pinpoint pupils, absent bowel sounds
Organophosphates	Hypotension, bradycardia	Altered-lethargy	Salivation, lacrimation, diaphoresis, diarrhea, abdominal pain, blurred vision, vomiting, defecation, seizures
Salicylates	Hyperthermia, fast breathing	Altered-lethargic	Tinnitus, nausea, vomiting
Sedative-hypnotics	Hypotension, slow breathing, hypothermia	Altered-lethargic	Nausea, vomiting, diaphoresis, tremor, seizures

Source: Adapted from Soloway (2003).

BITES AND STINGS

While most bites and stings are relatively nonurgent and only cause minimal injury, others pose a significant risk for children. When assessing a student with a bite or envenomation, the smaller the child, the more of a health risk the poison presents. Anaphylactic reactions to bee or yellow jacket stings occur in 0.4% of children (Schmitt, 2002). Animal bites can be divided into categories of those that are wild and prone to rabies (bats, skunks, raccoon), small wild animals (rats, chipmunks, squirrels, prairie dogs, rabbits), pets (indoor animals as well as horses and other farm animals), and human bites. It should be noted that bats can transmit rabies without a detectable bite mark (Schmitt, 2002). Besides rabies, the main concern with animal bites is infection.

Assessment

Attempt to determine the type of bite the student sustained (spider, insect, snake) and the location and time of the bite. Assess the number of bites or puncture wounds, swelling, discoloration or drainage. Assess for any crush injuries or major bleeding, especially if the bite was to a major artery. Assess when the student's last tetanus shot was. TABLE 22.18 describes the pathophysiology, assessments, and interventions for deadly snake, spider, and insect bites.

Intervention

Stingers should be removed by scraping or pinching as soon as possible. Research emphasizes quick removal of the stinger without regard to the method,

Table 22.18 ■

SNAKE, SPIDER, AND INSECT BITES

TYPE OF BITE	PATHO-PHYSIOLOGY	ASSESSMENT	MANAGEMENT
Pit viper snake	Injects toxins that cause tissue necrosis hemolysis of red blood cells, and coagulation defects	Fang marks, nausea, vomiting, weakness, tachycardia, signs of shock, spontaneous bleeding, seizures, renal failure and massive pulmonary edema	Support ABCs, activate EMS, apply a constricting band 2–4 cm above the site, and a splint to the affected limb to minimize movement, keep the limb at or below the level of the heart provide information about the snake to EMS toxin.
Coral snake	Venom contains neurotoxins	Mild reaction at the site, systemic signs are delayed, but progress rapidly, nausea, vomiting, mental status changes, inability to speak and swallow, drooping of upper eyelids, visual changes, muscle paralysis	Support ABCs, activate EMS, apply a constricting band 2–4 cm above the site, and a splint to the affected limb to minimize movement, keep the limb at or below the level of the heart provide information about the snake to EMS if available.
Black widow spider	Neurotoxic venom	Mild redness and swelling, may see two tiny puncture marks, dizziness, abdominal pain, delirium, paralysis, seizures	Assess and maintain ABCDs, keep the student quiet and calm to delay absorption, cleanse with antiseptic, apply cool compress, activate EMS.

(continued)

TYPE OF BITE	PATHO-PHYSIOLOGY	ASSESSMENT	MANAGEMENT
Brown recluse spider	Neurotoxic venom	Bleb, blister at site, then purple star shaped area followed by necrotic ulceration in 7–14 days, rash, fever chills, headache, nausea, vomiting	Assess and maintain ABCDs, keep the child quiet and calm to delay absorption, cleanse with antiseptic, apply cool compress, activate EMS.
Bark scorpion	Venom contains hemolysins, endotheliolysins, and neurotoxins	Intense local pain, numbness, burning, tachycardia, increased secretions, paralysis, seizures, delirium, pulmonary edema	Assess and maintain ABCDs, keep the child quiet and calm to delay absorption, cleanse with antiseptic, apply cool compress, activate EMS
Hymenoptera (bees, wasps, yellow jackets, hornets, ants)	Venom contains histamine and allergic proteins	Small red painful area, wheal, itching and heat, systemic reaction, generalized edema, pain, nausea, vomiting, hives, shock	Remove stinger as quickly as possible to reduce the amount of venom injected (Visscher, Vetter & Camazine, 1996). Assess and maintain ABCDs, cleanse with antiseptic, apply cool compress, activate EMS as needed for systemic reaction.

Source: Adapted from Thomas et al. (2003).

as the venom sac continues to inject venom for up to 20 seconds after the sting (Visscher, Vetter, & Camazine, 1996). Methods include brushing it out gently, or scraping it with a piece of cardboard. Since speed is essential, delays in hunting for the proper removal implement should be avoided. Although pinching the stinger to pull the stinger out with the thumb and forefinger or use of tweezers may inject venom into the student, this method may be necessary to ensure removal is immediate. Wash the bite or sting with soap and water for 5 minutes (Schmitt, 2002).

If marks are small, not penetrating and the animal is known to be vaccinated for rabies, the wound should be cleansed with benzalkonium chloride (Walker, 2003). If the wound is small and the family is not seeking medical treatment, teach the caregiver to monitor the wound for any signs or symptoms of infection.

Any animal bites that occur on school property should be reported to the appropriate animal control officer. If the animal is not known to be vaccinated for rabies, the student should be evaluated in the local emergency department. The animal control officer should quarantine the animal and observe it for signs of rabies.

Human Bites

Young children may acquire bites from others in preschool, and school-age children and adolescents may bite each other during fights. Adult-sized bites may occur in abuse cases. Most human bites are superficial and heal without infection. The wound must be washed vigorously with soap and water because human bites have a greater chance of becoming infected than those of other animals (Schmitt, 2002). Apply ice to decrease pain and swelling, unless additional care is needed.

BURNS

Etiology

Burn injuries affect thousands of children each year (National SAFE KIDS Campaign, 2004). In 2003 an estimated 142,487 children newborn to 18 years of age suffered unintentional burn-related injuries in the United States (National Center for Injury Prevention and Control, 2003). More than 90% of all burn injuries are reported to be preventable. School-based burn prevention programs along with legislative and enforcement measures are effectively decreasing the number of fire injuries and deaths in the United States.

Burns are classified as:

- Thermal—from contact with hot temperatures/fire
- Electrical—from contact with alternating current, or from a lightning strike
- Chemical—from contact with an acid or alkaline chemical
- Radiation—usually from excessive exposure to ultraviolet light from the sun

Assessment

Initial assessment of a burn victim focuses on assessing if the burning process is still occurring. At the same time, assessment of the airway, breathing, and circulation should occur. The first priority is assessing the airway for any abnormal breath sounds, such as stridor or hoarseness. Then inspect the mouth, nose, and face for signs of burn injury or inhalation. When assessing breathing, auscultate the chest listening for any abnormal breath sounds. If injury is due to a flash explosion, be aware of the potential for serious inhalation injury. Assess the circulation by observing skin color, level of consciousness, capillary refill time, heart rate, rhythm, and quality. Also assess for the level of pain.

Estimate the depth of the burn (TABLE 22.19) and the total body surface area burned. Traditionally, the rule of nines charts was used to estimate body surface area burned. Be aware that the rule of nines is not accurate for young children and requires adjustment for the pediatric population (Perry, 2003). An easy method for school nurses to use for estimation the percentage of body surface area burned is that 1% of body surface area equals the size of the palm of the victim's hand. The palm size used is from student's wrist crease to beginning of the finger crease (Perry, 2003).

Intervention

Stop the burning process by extinguishing any flames; throw a blanket on the student or direct the student to stop, drop, and roll. Apply room temperature water to thermal burns for 2 to 5 minutes or until heat cannot be felt coming from the site of burn injury. Too much cooling can quickly lead to hypothermia in a severe burn (Cerepani, 2003). Remove burned clothing unless it is stuck to the burn. Quickly remove any jewelry from injured extremities, before swelling occurs and to stop the burning process. The burn wound itself has the lowest priority. Do not apply ointment or burn cream to any burn that will be assessed in the emergency department.

Table 22.19 ■
CLASSIFICATION OF BURN DEPTH

BURN DEPTH	LAYERS INVOLVED	EXAMPLES	APPEARANCE	SENSATION
Superficial (first degree)	Epidermis	Mild sunburn	Pink, red	Mild to moderate pain
Partial-thickness (second degree)	Epidermis, dermis	Mottled, pink, red, waxy areas, blisters	Moist, red, blistered	Painful, extremely sensitive to air and light touch
Full-thickness (third degree)	Epidermis, dermis, fatty tissue, can involve muscle and bone		Whitish, charred (if caused by flame) dry leathery black brown	Usually not painful unless there are areas of partial-thickness and full-thickness.

Source: Adapted from Cerepani (2003).

Management of the airway is the priority. Assist as needed with ventilations using a bag-valve mask. Continue to monitor ABCDs until EMS arrives. Measure blood pressure in an unburned extremity when assessing circulation. Cover with a sheet for warmth while waiting for EMS.

For partial thickness burns with redness, pain, swelling and blisters, determine the need to activate EMS depending on the site, total body surface area burned, and depth of the burn. Notify the parent or guardian for any partial thickness burn. If the partial thickness is greater than 15% of the total body surface area, or involving the hands feet, face or perineum, EMS should be activated; these are considered emergent burns and will need evaluation and treatment in an emergency department with possible transfer to a regional burn center. If the burn is full thickness covering 10% of the body surface area, it is considered emergent and EMS should be called (Cerepani, 2003).

If the burn is from a specific chemical consider contacting the Poison Control Center at 1-800-222-1222 for direction on management of the chemical burn. For minor, small, superficial burns, cool the burn for 2 to 5 minutes under cool running water or immerse in water. Do not use ice on a burn injury, as it will cause additional injury to tissues. Then wash the burned area with mild soap. Leave blisters intact and cover loosely with a clean dressing. The student can return to class with a small minor burn.

FOLLOW-UP

Regardless of the emergency, follow up with EMS providers and hospital staff to determine the effectiveness of your assessment and interventions in response to the emergency. Always look for ways to improve the school's response. Should protocols or guidelines be developed or changed to manage a situation like this in the future? Did the emergency plan work? Was the emergency quickly identified? Was the scene safe? Was help requested in a timely manner? Were the injuries identified? Was appropriate first aid provided? Was any information needed by the healthcare provider not available? Does the healthcare provider have any suggestions to improve emergency response?

After a school emergency, the nurse should follow up with parents and the student's healthcare provider, depending on severity of the illness or injury. There may be future back-to-school considerations for the student depending on the injury or illness. An evaluation of the assessment and management should be completed for any student that EMS transports to the hospital.

CONCLUSION

Emergency preparedness must be a priority for school nurses every day. They are often the first medical responder to any emergency at school. When the nurse is not available at the school, he or she is often still responsible for training others and developing plans for use by others serving the school in his or her absence.

References

Abrunzo, T., Gerardi, M., Dietrich, A., Lampell, M., Sanford, W. C., & Smith, D. M. (2000). The role of emergency physicians in the care of the child in school. Annals of *Emergency Medicine, 35*(2), 155–161.

Allen, K., Ball, J., & Helfer, B. (1998). Preventing and managing childhood emergencies in schools. *Journal of School Nursing, 14*(1), 20–24.

American Academy of Neurology, Quality Standards Subcommittee (AAN). (1997). Practice parameters: The management of concussion in sports. *Neurology, 48*, 581–585.

American Academy of Pediatrics (AAP). (1999). Emergency preparedness for children with special heath care needs. *Pediatrics, 104*(4), e53.

American Academy of Pediatrics (AAP). (2001). Policy statement: Guidelines for emergency medical care in school. *Pediatrics, 107*(2), 435–436.

American Heart Association (AHA). (2001). Pediatric advanced life support. *Instructor's manual*. Dallas, TX: Author.

American Heart Association (AHA). (2004). Response to cardiac arrest and selected life-threatening medical emergencies: The medical emergency response plan for schools: A statement for healthcare providers policymakers, school administrators and community leaders. *Pediatrics, 113*(1), 155–168.

Barrett, J. C. (2001). Teaching teachers about school health emergencies. *Journal of School Nursing, 17*(6), 316–322.

Bernardo, L. M., Anderson, L., & Lewis, K. (2000). *Preparing a response to emergency problems*. Castle Rock, CO: National Association of School Nurses.

Bobo, N., Hallenbeck, P., & Robinson, J. (2003). Recommended minimal emergency equipment and resources for schools: National consensus group report. *The Journal of School Nursing, 19*(3), 150–156.

Breau, L. M., Camfield, C., MacGrath P. J., Rosmos, C., & Finley, G. (2001). Measuring pain accurately in children with cognitive impairments. *Journal of Pediatrics, 138*(5), 721–727.

Centers for Disease Control and Prevention (CDC). (2005). *Meningococcal meningitis*. Retrieved February 28, 2005 from http://www.cdc.gov/ncidod/dbmd/diseaseinfo/meningococcal_g.html

Cerepani, M. J. (2003). Burn trauma. In D. O. Thomas, L. M. Bernardo, & B. Herman (Eds.), *Core curriculum for pediatric emergency nursing* (pp. 524–526). Sudbury, MA: Jones and Bartlett.

Chambers, C. T., Giesbrecht, K., Craig, K. D., Bennett, S., & Huntsman, E. (1999). A comparison of faces scales for the measurement of pediatric pain: Children's and parents' ratings. *Pain, 83*(1), 25–35.

Children's Safety Network at Education Development Center, Inc. (1997). *Injuries in the school environment: A resource guide* (2nd ed.). Newton, MA: Education Development Center Inc.

Cosby, C. (2003). Pediatric emergencies. In L. Newberry (Ed.), *Sheehy's emergency nursing principles and practice* (5th ed., pp. 719–743). St. Louis: C. V. Mosby.

Cosby, M. (2003). Supreme Court Decision: *Cedar Rapids v. Garret, F.* Impact on School Nursing and Life Care Planning, *Journal of Life Care Planning, 2*(4), 205–214.

Dieckmann, R., Brownstein, D., & Gausche-Hill, M. (Eds.). (2000). *Pediatric education for prehospital professional (PEPP)s*. Sudbury, MA: Jones and Bartlett.

Emergency Nurses Association (ENA). (1997). *Triage: Meeting the challenge* (2nd ed.). Author: Park Ridge, IL.

Emergency Nurses Association (ENA). (2004). *Emergency nursing pediatric course*. Author: Des Plaines, IL.

Federal Interagency Forum on Child and Family Statistics. (2005). *America's children: Key national indicators of well-being 2005. Child mortality*. Retrieved August 2005 from http://www.childstats.gov/americaschildren/hea7.asp

Franck, L., Greenberg, C., & Stevens, B. (2000). Acute pain in children: Pain assessment in infants and children. *Pediatric Clinics of North America, 47*(3), 487–512.

Green, M. L. (2001). The nurse in the community. In N. J. Brent (Ed.), *Nurses and the law: A guide to principles and applications* (2nd ed., pp. 396–425) Philadelphia: W. B. Saunders.

Haddad, G., & Fontan, J. (2004). Development of the respiratory system. In R. Behrman, R. Kliegman, & H. Jenson (Eds.), *Nelson textbook of pediatrics* (17th ed.). (pp. 1357–1360) Philadelphia: W. B. Saunders.

Hockenberry, M. J., Wilson, D., Winkelstein, M. L., & Kline, M. E. (2003). *Wong's nursing care of infants and children* (7th ed.). St. Louis: C. V. Mosby.

Hohenhaus, S. M. (2001). Pediatric emergency preparedness in schools: A report from the 2001 Southeastern Regional EMSC Meeting. *Journal of Emergency Nursing 27*(4), 353–356.

Hootman, J., Fratto, J., & Perkins, S. (2002). *Responding to student injury and illness*. Portland, OR: Department of School Health Services, Multnomah Education Service District.

Hootman, J., Schwab, N., & Gelfman, M. (2001). School nursing practice: Clinical performance issues. In N. Schwab & M. Gelfman (Eds.), *Legal issues in school health services* (pp. 168–169). North Branch, MN: Sunrise River Press.

Illinois EMS for Children. (2002). *Pain management in the emergency department*. Chicago: Illinois EMS for Children.

Illinois EMS for Children. (2003). *Guidelines for the nurse in the school setting*. Chicago: Illinois EMS for Children (http://www.luhs.org/depts/emsc/schl_man)

Jardine, J. (2003). Respiratory emergencies. In D. Thomas, L. Bernardo, & B. Herman (Eds.), *Core curriculum for pediatric emergency nursing*. Sudbury, MA: Jones and Bartlett.

Knickelbein, A. M. (2004). *Leadership in action: The school nurse's role in coordinated school health programs*. California School Nurses Organization, Sacramento, CA.

Lafferty, S., & Baird, M. (2001). *Tele-nurse telephone triage protocols*. Clifton Park, NY: Delmar.

Litovitz, T. L., Klein-Schwartz, W., White, S., Cobaugh, D., Youniss, J., Omslaer, A., & Benson, B. (2001). 2000 Annual Report of the American Association of Poison Control Centers Toxic Exposure Surveillance System. *American Journal of Emergency Medicine, 19*, 337–395.

Maloney, P. L., Doyle, J., Fitzgerald, S., Elam, K., & Lewis, K. D. (2002a). *Managing school emergencies I, student manual*. Castle Rock, CO: National Association of School Nurses.

Maloney, P. L., Doyle, J., Fitzgerald, S., Elam, K., & Lewis, K. D. (2002b). *Managing school emergencies II, student manual*. Castle Rock, CO: National Association of School Nurses.

Maloney, P. L., Fitzgerald, S., Elam, K., & Doyle, J. (2000). *Managing school emergencies III, student manual*. Castle Rock, CO: National Association of School Nurses.

National Association of Emergency Medical Technicians (NAEMT). (2004). *Guidelines for prehospital response to medical emergencies at schools*. Retrieved March 29, 2005 from http://emsc.naemt.org/Guidelines_Final_040826.htm

National Association of School Nurses (NASN). (2003) *Position statement preparing for school emergencies*. Scarborough, ME: National Association of School Nurses.

National Center for Injury Prevention and Control (NCIPC). (2001) *Injury prevention: Meeting the challenge*. New York: Oxford University Press.

National SAFE KIDS Campaign. (2004). *Injury facts—burn injury*. Retrieved February 28, 2005 from http://www.safekids.org/tier3_cd.cfm?folder_id=540&content_item_id=1011

National Vital Statistics System, National Center for Health Statistics and the Office of Statistics and Programming, National Center of Injury Prevention and Control. (2004). *Ten leading causes of death by age group*. Atlanta GA: Centers for Disease Control and Prevention. Retrieved February 18, 2005 from ftp://ftp.cdc.gov/pub/ncipc/10LC-2002/PDF/10lc-2002.pdf

Nonfatal choking–related episodes among children—United States, 2001 (2002). *Morbidity and Mortality Weekly Report, 51*(11), 234–237. Retrieved February 28, 2005 from http://www.cdc.gov/mmwr/preview/mmwrhtml/mm5142a1.htm

Ohio Department of Public Safety. (2001). *Emergency guidelines for schools* (2nd fed). Columbus, OH. Retrieved August 24, 2005 from http://www.ems-c.org/downloads/pdf/953OHEGS.pdf.

Perry, C. (2003). Thermal injuries. In P. A. Moloney-Harmon & S. J. Cerwinski (Eds.), *Nursing care of the pediatric trauma patient* (pp. 277–294). Philadelphia: W. B. Saunders.

Progress toward elimination of *Haemophilus influenzae* type b invasive disease among infants and children—United States, 1998–2000. (2002). *Morbidity and Mortality Weekly Report, 51* (11), 234–237. Retrieved November 12, 2003, from http://www.cdc.gov/mmwr/preview/ mmwrhtml/mm5111a4.htm

Schmitt, B. (2002). *Pediatric telephone protocols*. Elk Grove Village, IL: American Academy of Pediatrics.

Rosenberg, M. (May 5, 1998). *Statement before the Senate Committee on Labor and Human Resources on*

Unintentional Childhood Injury and Death. Retrieved February 18, 2005 from http://www.hhs.gov/asl/testify/t980505b.html

Seidel, J. S., & Henderson, D. P. (1997). *Prehospital care of pediatric emergencies*. Sudbury, MA: Jones and Bartlett.

Seidel, J. S., & Knapp, J. F. (Eds.). (2000). *Childhood emergencies in the office, hospital, and community: Organizing systems of care* (pp. 277–290). Elk Grove Village, IL: American Academy of Pediatrics.

Selekman, J. (2003). Preventing meningitis. *Pediatric Nursing, 29*(6), 467–469.

Soloway, R. A. (2003). Toxicologic emergencies. In D. O. Thomas, L. M. Bernardo, and B. Herman (Eds.), *Core curriculum for pediatric emergency nursing* (pp. 524–526). Sudbury, MA: Jones and Bartlett.

Thomas, D. O., Bernardo, L. M., & Herman, B. (Eds.). (2003). *Core curriculum for pediatric emergency nursing*. Sudbury, MA: Jones and Bartlett.

Visscher, P. K., Vetter, R. S., & Camazine, S. (1996). Removing bee stings. *Lancet, 348*, 301–302.

Walker, J. H. (2003). Bites and stings. In D. O. Thomas, L. M. Bernardo, & Herman, B. (Ed.), *Core curriculum for pediatric emergency nursing* (pp. 513–520). Sudbury, MA: Jones and Bartlett.

Wolkenheim, B. (2000). *Public access defibrillation in schools. Project ADAM*. Milwaukee, WI: Children's Hospital of Wisconsin.

Wong, D. L., & Baker, C. M. (1988). Pain in children: Comparison of assessment scales. *Pediatric Nursing, 14*, 9–17.

Zaritsky, A. L., Nadkarni, V. M., Hickey, R. W., Schexnayder, S. M., & Berg, R. A. (2002). *PALS provider manual*. Dallas, TX: American Heart Association.

Zheng, Z. J., Croft, J. B., Giles, W. H., & Mensah, G. A. (2001). Sudden cardiac death in the United States, 1989 to 1998. *Circulation, 104*(18), 2158–2163.

Chapter 23

Common Complaints

RITAMARIE JOHN ■ JEANNE KIEFNER

Chapter Outline

INTRODUCTION

The school nurse is an independent practitioner in the educational setting. A major responsibility is to create an atmosphere of safety and wellness by exercising nursing judgments and making nursing diagnoses when illnesses and physical complaints are presented. This chapter identifies many complaints that present to school health offices regardless of the age or grade of the student or whether the school is at a rural, urban, or suburban site.

The major responsibilities of the professional school nurse involve listening to the student, speaking the language of understandability, guiding parents or guardians as they make decisions with and for their students, and advocating in all areas of health promotion. The school nurse has a professional duty to maintain knowledge of and implement the standard of care that can and should be provided in the school setting.

In this unique position, the school nurse manages health policies and procedures relating to the demands presented each day. With an expertise gleaned from past nursing experiences and continuing education, the school nurse recognizes the common complaints identified by the school-age student and adolescent. To manage the daily demands of promoting and maintaining the health of students while advocating for the sick student, the school nurse collects appropriate data, documents as necessary, intervenes appropriately, and refers problems that cannot be improved with routine nursing measures. This chapter is a systematic approach to the student who presents with common complaints. The complaints are introduced by system and each complaint is handled individually except where referenced to other complaints.

Nursing documentation will include the presenting complaint, assessment, and action taken. It is important to chart the time of the arrival to the nurse's office as well as the presenting complaint. *It is assumed that the nurse will notify the parent and request an evaluation by the primary care provider where indicated. It is also assumed that a written follow-up and directions or guidance from the primary care provider will be requested by the school nurse when indicated.* Lastly, the nurse discusses student health problems with teachers within Health Insurance Portability and Accountability Act (HIPAA) and Family Education Rights and Privacy Act (FERPA) regulations only if the situation relates to class activity, student responsibility, or the environment (see Chapter 13). Following pertinent assessments, parentheses indicate the condition for which the nurse is assessing. Several tables and figures are also provided to help clarify assessment points. It is important to remember that students do not localize complaints well. It is important to evaluate above and below an area of complaint. For example, if a student complains of abdominal pain, it is possible the pain is caused by a problem in the lungs, hips, or genitalia. It is assumed that the nurse will assess the overall state of the student.

FEVER

Fever is a common presenting problem in school nursing practice. However, there is controversy regarding what temperature constitutes fever in the pediatric patient; it also depends on the method and route of taking the temperature. A rectal temperature above 100°F (Wong, Hockenberry-Eaton, Wilson, Winkelstein, & Schwartz, 2001) to 100.4°F (Behrman & Kliegman, 2002; Hay, Hayward, Levin, Sondheimer, 2003; Rudolph, Kamei, & Overby, 2002) is considered febrile, whereas oral temperatures above 99.8°F (Behrman & Kliegman, 2002) to 100.4°F (Watts, Robertson, & Thomas, 2003) would be considered febrile. Warm or cold liquid can affect the accuracy of a reading. In school nursing practice, the method of taking temperatures is usually oral, axillary, and more commonly, via the ear. Ranges for ear temperature are the same as for oral temperature, providing the nurse uses proper technique.

Physiologically, the tympanic membrane is an excellent way to measure core body temperature since both the tympanic membrane and hypothalamus in the brain share their blood supply from the internal and external carotid arteries (Childs, Harrison, & Hodkinson, 1999; Wilshaw, Beckstrand, Waid, & Schaalje, 1999). Because of the proximity of the tympanic membrane to the hypothalamus and decrease of heat loss in that site as a result of the protection afforded by the skull, the tympanic measure may be a better measurement of core temperature (Irvin, 1999; Leicke-Rude & Bloom, 1998). The tympanic membrane temperature can be calculated as either rectal or oral depending on the device used. It is important for the examiner to follow the instructions to obtain an accurate temperature. When the thermometer tip does not fit securely, the probe may measure the temperature of the ear canal, skin, or cerumen (Wilshaw et al., 1999). If the student has been out in the cold, it may be necessary for the nurse to wait for about 20 minutes before taking the student's temperature via the tympanic route. If the device is used correctly, the result of measuring temperature via the tympanic route can be rapid, sterile, convenient, and relatively risk free (Wilshaw et al., 1999).

The student may be shivering and feel cold before there is an elevation of body temperature. The main mechanisms that can raise the body temperature are:

- The hypothalamic set point in the central nervous system is raised.
- Heat production exceeds heat loss.
- A genetic defect or poisoning via anticholinergic drugs results in defective heat loss.

The control of body temperature is neurologically mediated in the preoptic area of the anterior hypothalamus (POAH). There are two locations within the POAH: one maintains normal body temperature and the second area causes a fever response. Primarily, prostaglandins act on the hypothalamus by raising the normal set point. Drugs such as acetaminophen and aspirin inhibit prostaglandin synthesis without affecting the baseline body temperature (Lorin, 2000), thus lowering the body temperature.

Fever should be differentiated from a heat illness (hyperthermia, heat stroke). Fever is a very specific response to an external pyrogen, but heat illness occurs when the body temperature is elevated despite a normal setting in the hypothalamus. Heat illness occurs when the body produces more heat than it loses as a result of extrinsic factors such as an extreme of air temperature around the body or intrinsic factors such as spinal cord or brain injury or hyperthyroidism. Use of illicit drugs that have anticholinergic actions can cause fever, as can the use of some prescription drugs, such as phenothiazines, topiramate (Topamax), and neuroleptics (FDA, 2003). The use of sympathomimetic agents such as Ecstasy in a hot environment can also cause hyperthermia (Osterhoudt, 2002).

Key History Points

School-age students can provide history to varying degrees depending on age, developmental level, verbal skills, experiences with illness, relationships with others, family experiences, and religious as well as cultural norms. There may be difficulty contacting family members who know the recent health status of the student. The following are points to consider when obtaining a history:

- Check the health records for the student's medical history and known health problems.
- Ask about excessive exercise or exercise in a hot environment.
- Look for signs and symptoms of infectious disease—associated myalgia, general malaise, and site-specific symptoms, such as cough, diarrhea, and vomiting.
- Ask about travel out of the country in the past 6 months.
- Ask about recent immunizations *(i.e., measles–mumps–rubella [MMR] vaccine may cause a fever that occurs 7 to 14 days post-administration.)*
- Ask the student about use of any illicit drugs or prescription drugs.
- Has the student voided? Is there burning or pain with urination? (*May indicate urinary tract infection, pyelonephritis.*)
- Ask about fluid intake. Is there recent change in weight, appetite, or thirst?
- Does the child have a headache or is there a history of vomiting? (*May indicate meningitis if accompanied by a stiff neck.*)

Physical Assessment

- Evaluate vital signs. Is the heart rate in proportion to the fever? Fever increases the student's metabolic rate; in fever, there is an increase of 10 pulse beats for every degree of fever and respirations increase 4 breaths per minute per degree (Lafferty & Baird, 2001).
- Assess the skin for sweating, moisture, temperature, turgor, rashes, or petechiae.
- Assess the student's behavior: is the student active, sluggish, playful, and sociable? (Words such as *listless* and *lethargic* should be avoided. A precise description of what the student is doing can demonstrate why the school nurse did or did not call 911 as part of the implementation of nursing care if the record is challenged.)
- How does the student react to stimulation?
- Does the student look ill?
- Are there any signs and symptoms of an infectious disease—lymphadenopathy, rash, pharyngitis, otitis, cough, abdominal pain, or localized area of pain?
- Are there any signs of a stiff neck? (*May indicate meningitis.*)
- Are there multiple purple spots (purpura) or petechiae? (*May indicate meningococcemia.*)

Nursing Actions

- Arrange for students to be transported to a medical facility if the student with fever is lethargic, unusually drowsy, cyanotic, has an altered level of consciousness, or has purpura.
- Notify parents once a fever is identified.
- Check school policy and nurse practice acts regarding the use of antipyretics. Many school nurses cannot dispense medications. (Antipyretics are usually not given unless the temperature is >102°F or if the student is very uncomfortable.) If they are given, and if the student is still in school, it is important to check the temperature 60 minutes later when the medication peaks to note if it was effective. Diaphoresis may occur at this time. Do not allow the student to stay in wet clothes, as this may result in chilling/shivering and an increase in body temperature. The normal dose of acetaminophen for children is 10 to 15 mg/kg per dose every 4 to 6 hours (650 mg/dose for adults); the normal dose of ibuprofen for children is 5 to 10 mg/kg per dose every 6 to 8 hours (400 mg/dose for adults) (Taketomo, Hodding, & Kraus, 2004). Do not alternate the two drugs. Do not give aspirin to children because of the risk of Reye syndrome (Schmidtt, 2002).
- Minimize the amount of clothing to improve heat loss via the skin. Keep the student comfortable and cool without causing shivering. Shivering or covering will raise the body temperature; therefore students should be encouraged not to wrap themselves in blankets or have on excessive clothing, except for comfort.
- Apply cool compresses to the forehead for comfort and to decrease the temperature.
- Offer cool fluids (ice chips, Gatorade, popsicles) to replace sweat as well as insensible loss and to cool the body, providing there are

no contraindications, that is, vomiting, head injury, spinal cord injury, or an acute abdomen.

- It should be kept in mind that fever can improve the immune response at lower temperatures except in septic patients. Fever impairs the multiplication of certain microorganisms and causes the death of certain viruses (Lorin, 2000). On the other hand, patient discomfort, oxygen consumption, carbon dioxide production, heart rate, and water loss are increased with fever and administration of antipyretics (where allowed) may be helpful.
- Despite parents' best intentions, there are occasions when the time frame for their arrival at the school dictates that the school nurse must provide comfort and make continued observations. The nurse must note notification and pick up times.
- For high fevers, anticipate the possibility of febrile seizures; if the temperature is >105°F, seek immediate care related to the high risk of sepsis (Schmidtt, 2002).

EYE PROBLEMS

Visual Complaints

Students can present to the school nurse for an eye screening after the teacher or the student has identified visual concerns. It is certainly possible for a student's vision to change during the course of the school year. It is important that both the teacher and the student recognize that the nurse can provide a screening, but a more complete assessment can be done by an eye health professional. Screening eye charts are available in most school health offices. The eye charts allow the examiner to watch the student's eyes and head posture more carefully as the student is being screened (American Academy of Pediatrics [AAP], 2003a; Simons & Kaw, 2001) (see Chapter 20.) The nurse should also observe the student in the office while the student is waiting to be seen. Having age-appropriate reading and picture books available can help the nurse observe the student's visual skills.

Key History Points

- Ask when the visual problems started.
- Is the problem sudden, gradual, or a repeated deterioration?
- Is there any history of trauma?
- Is there a history of prematurity or genetic disorders?
- What is the family history of visual problems?
- Does the student have an eye doctor?
- Did the student once wear glasses or use an eye patch?
- What were the results of previous vision screenings on the school health record?
- Does the student have any medical problems that can affect vision, such as Down syndrome, fetal alcohol syndrome, or other genetic problem?
- Does the student use any medications that may affect vision?
- Has the student recently entered puberty? Visual complaints can begin at this time since the length of the eye also changes during this period (Wright, 2003).
- When does the complaint occur? Is it more associated with close work or looking at the chalkboard?
- Does the complaint occur more often with fatigue at the end of the day?

Physical Assessment

- Look at the area around the eye for any redness, signs of trauma, or any other abnormalities.
- Evaluate the eyelids for symmetry or ptosis.
- Evaluate the pupils for symmetry, reaction to light, and accommodation by asking the student to follow an object from 18 inches away to 3 inches from his or her nose (Table 23.1).
- Look for excessive tearing or epiphora. (*May indicate glaucoma or blocked tearduct.*)
- Is the cornea clear or cloudy? (*May indicate cataracts.*)
- Evaluate the extraocular movements in the six fields of gaze using a double H or crossing.
- Evaluate for any jerking movements of the eye (*nystagmus*).
- Look at the corneal light reflex or Hirschberg test. Does the light fall into the middle of pupil or slightly nasally, or is it equal bilaterally (Figure 23.1)?
- Do a cover test (Figure 23.2). Have the student

Table 23.1 ■
PUPIL EVALUATIONS: NORMAL AND ABNORMAL FINDINGS

Evaluating pupil response	Technique • Ask patient to look in distance to maximize pupillary size • Dim the lights to maximize pupil size • Record pupil size in mm and any asymmetry or irregularity
Direct pupil response	Evaluate pupil response to pen light being shown in the eye for five seconds
Consensual pupil Xresponse	Pupil response in the other eye
Normal Variations in Pupils Anisocoria	Difference in size of pupil. If the difference is same in bright and dim lighting, then it is normal variation. If there is change in difference in the size of pupil in bright and dim lighting, then this is an abnormal finding.
Abnormal Variations in Pupils Marcus Gunn pupil or relative afferent pupillary defect	When light is shown in the affected eye, there is reduced afferent input. As a result, the pupils fail to constrict fully. Stimulation of the normal eye produces full constriction in both pupils.
Iris coloboma	Is a cat's eye or keyhole pupil because a small piece of the iris is missing
Aniridia	Lack of an iris

look at an object at a distance as well as close. Cover one eye for 5 seconds; look for movement in the uncovered eye. Then cover the other eye for 5 seconds: look for movement in the uncovered eye. Then repeat looking at the covered eye when you cover and uncover it.

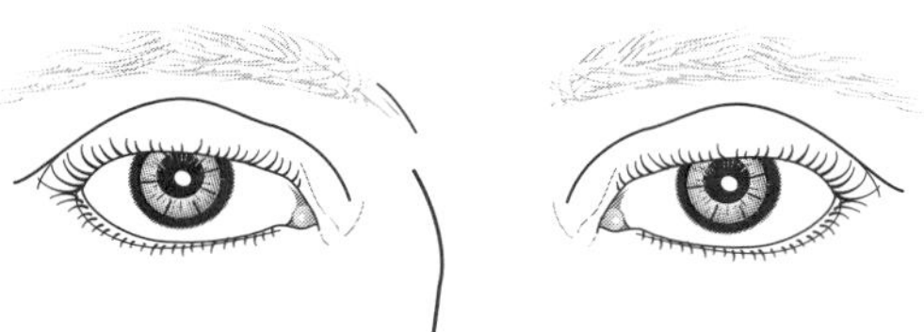

Figure 23.1 ■ Corneal light reflex. (Illustration by Traci Feldman)

- Do a vision screen using the appropriate eye chart for the student's developmental level (see Chapter 20).
  - Lea symbols, Allen picture chart, HOTV, or tumbling E may be taught to the preverbal student
  - Alphabet charts should be used on students who can read the alphabet.
  - Screen eye monocularly and binocularly. Record all three values.
  - Make sure one eye is completely occluded when testing the other eye.
- If near vision is the chief complaint, use a near vision screener (American Academy of Ophthalmology, 2002).
- Talk to the student's teacher about findings in the classroom as well as school performance.
- Evaluate for any abnormal head tilting or tor-

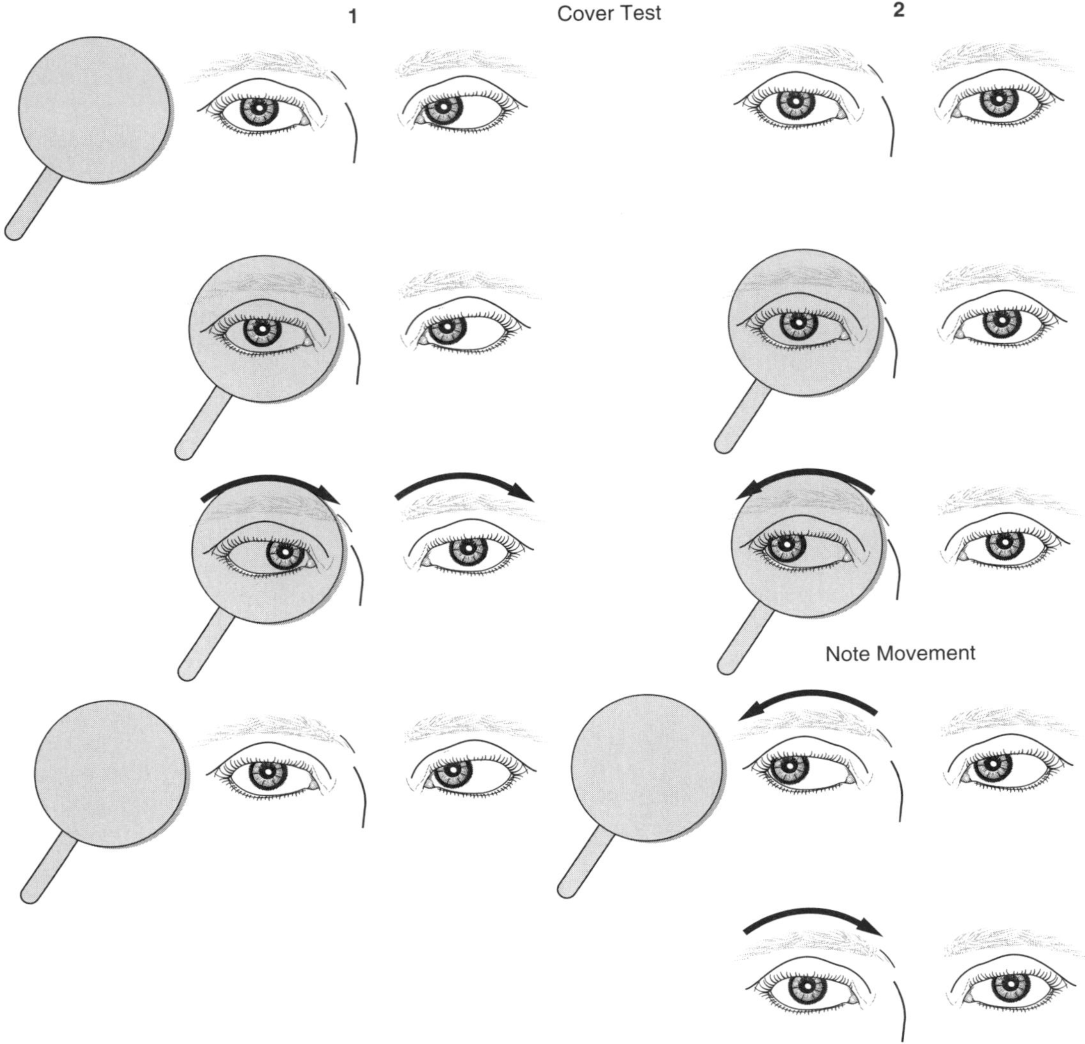

Figure 23.2 ■ Cover test. (Illustration by Traci Feldman)

ticollis when doing vision screening, which may indicate astigmatism (*abnormal lens curvature*), strabismus (*eye crossing*), or hyperopia.

- If the student is nonverbal or developmentally delayed, observe the student carefully while he colors or looks at a picture book. Can the student point to a small letter or picture on a page when asked? Put a small sticker on his hand and watch him look at it.

Nursing Actions

- Talk to the student's teacher about findings and advise preferential placement until the results of the eye exam are complete.
- Notify parent or guardian to seek evaluation by the primary care provider.
- Request a written follow-up and directions/guidance from the primary care provider.

Eye Injury/Trauma

Eye injuries presenting to the school nurse's office will need further evaluation by a primary care provider or, in some cases, a specialist. Since 20,000 to 70,000 of the 2.4 million eye injuries lead to some loss of vision, it is imperative that the initial management is correct and timely (Hoffman, 1997). Eye injury can range from corneal abrasions to globe rupture (Rhee & Pyfer, 1999). In school nursing practice, there are three likely case scenarios:

1. Clear-cut eye trauma with damage to the eyeball, or a foreign object impaled in the eye.

The plan is to activate EMS, shield the eye, and allow the student to rest. During the time you stay with the student, you may assign someone to get the health records, which should include immunization records and past vision screenings.

2. A history of eye trauma without any bleeding or obvious damage to the globe. The plan is to wait for a parent to transport the student to the primary care provider. You may have time to gather information, history, and assessment to send an appropriate referral to the primary care provider.
3. The teacher has sent a student to the school nurse reporting the student sustained a traumatic event. The student offers no complaints and has no visible signs of eye trauma. The nursing plan will include assessment and parent notification after you glean more history and complete the assessment. Normal eye anatomy is seen in FIGURE 23.3.

Key History Points

- What was the mechanism of injury (what object, solution, blunt trauma)?
- What was done after the injury?
- What are the student's symptoms? Ask specifically about visual changes such as blurring, foreign body sensation, as well as ocular pain.

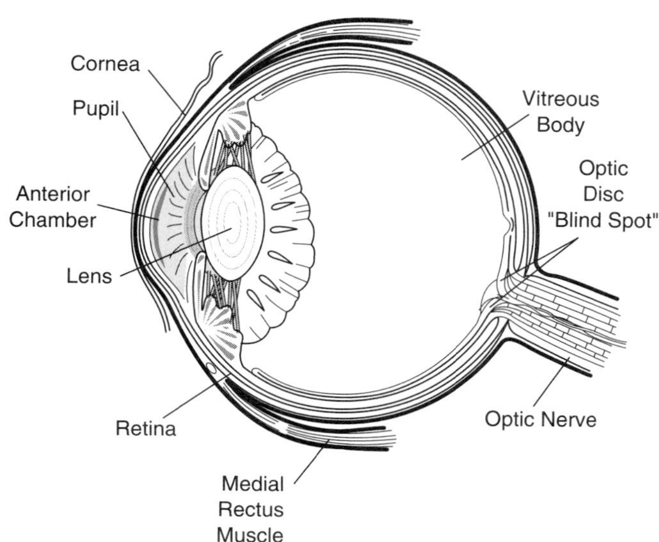

Figure 23.3 ■ Normal eye anatomy. (Illustration by Traci Feldman)

- Does it affect one eye or both?
- What is the past medical history, since certain conditions such as diabetes or immunocompromise may predispose to infection?
- What was the result of the last vision screen?
  - Does the student have any preexisting eye disorders?
  - Does the student have a contact lens in the eye at present?
- Did the student have eye protectors in use at time of injury?
- How much time elapsed between injury and presentation to the health office?
- Does the student have any drug allergies?
- When did the student last eat? (*Note for possible surgery.*)
- What was the date of the last tetanus immunization?
- Is there any ocular pain or foreign body sensation?
- Is there a history of dirt, sand, or another foreign body being thrown in the eye? (*Can indicate a corneal abrasion.*)
- Is there photophobia? (*Can indicate corneal abrasion.*)

Physical Assessment

- If there is a history of trauma, but nothing grossly abnormal is seen on initial inspection, perform an assessment as outlined below and document. Evaluate without touching the eye first to gain the student's confidence. Always look at both eyes even though the student may complain of a problem with only one eye.
- Is there a rash or any signs of trauma around the eye?
- Assess visual acuity (see Chapter 20).
- Assess the eyelids for injury or any proptosis (bulging, protrusion, or forward displacement).
- Examine the orbits by looking from in front of and above the patient.
- Look at the extraocular movements to evaluate for an orbital rim fracture.
  - Check the fourth cranial nerve function by evaluating if the student can look nasally and inward (Colyar, 2003).
  - The oculomotor or third cranial nerve can cause ptosis, lateral eye deviation, and no light or near response (Wright, 2003).

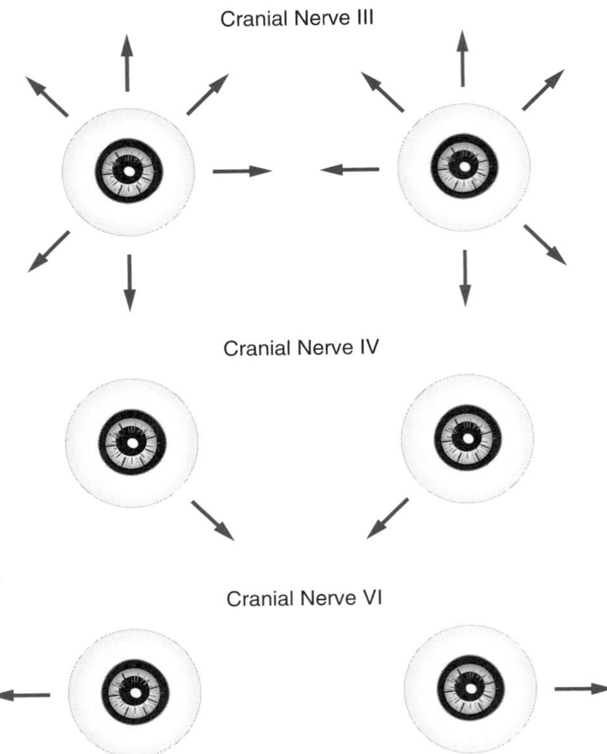

Figure 23.4 ■ Cranial nerve. (Illustration by Traci Feldman)

- Check the function of the sixth cranial nerve by testing lateral gaze (FIGURE 23.4).
- Check the lacrimal apparatus for tearing, redness, and swelling.
- Look at the sclera for subconjunctival hemorrhage, which may be associated with orbital fractures.
- Suspect orbital or eye injury if the eye is red at the limbus (the area where the iris meets the sclera) (FIGURE 23.5). This is called ciliary injection and is a sign of corneal injury in a painful eye.
- Look at the pupils for symmetry of reaction, and ability to contract to light. An irregularity in the shape of the pupil can indicate a globe rupture (Cuculino & DiMarco, 2002).
- Evaluate the pupil for blood in the anterior chamber or a hyphema (Hertle & Bacal, 1997).
- If able, check the red reflex since lack of red reflex may indicate a retinal hemorrhage.
- Examine the conjunctiva for inflammation or edema.
- Look for the presence of discharge and note color and location.

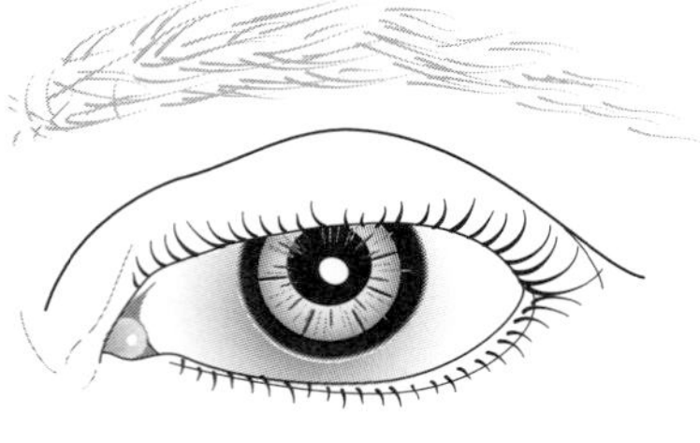

Figure 23.5 ■ Ciliary injection. (Illustration by Traci Feldman)

Nursing Actions

- For trauma, shield the eye with a cup that rests on the frontal bone above and maxillary bone below the injury. To prevent further damage, there should be no pressure on the eye. Displacement or movement of any impaled object may lead to more damage.
  - A paper cup taped over the eye is adequate if no eye shield is available. Make sure no pressure is placed on the orbits.
  - If there is a pulsatile bleed, attempt to stop the bleeding with direct pressure without further injury to the eye.
- Chemical splashes and burns are true ocular emergencies. Irrigating the eye for 20 minutes while awaiting transportation is critical. Irrigation can be accomplished with lukewarm water from a sink. The student or nurse can hold the injured eye open with one hand while flushing with the other hand. School nurses need to educate science teachers regarding initial actions to take if chemical spills occur.
- Activate EMS; transport student to the healthcare facility if the eye injury is significant (time may be crucial depending on type of injury). Stay with the student with an acute eye injury. Do a quick cephalocaudal survey for any other injury while waiting for EMS.
- Keep the student upright and quiet while awaiting transport to the healthcare facility if the student has visible hyphema or blunt trauma.
- Try to prevent further eye injury.
- Teach a class on eye health and injury prevention. Educate the teaching staff, athletic coaches, and students about the importance of wearing eye protective devices. Teachers of extracurricular activities such as art and drama also need to know this information because students may use cosmetics, paints, and dyes in play productions and art projects.

- Educate parents through presentations and newsletters about eye health and injury prevention

Red Eye

A student can have a red eye due to a simple viral or bacterial conjunctivitis (pink-eye) or there may be more serious causes for the red eye, such as iritis, glaucoma, or a hyphema following trauma (Cuculino & DiMarco, 2002; Teoh & Reynold, 2003). History and physical assessment are needed to triage the complaint effectively. Allergic conjunctivitis presents with a red eye but is frequently associated with the atopic triad of allergic rhinitis, asthma, and atopic dermatitis (Teoh & Reynold, 2003). Sometimes, a red eye can be a brief event that occurs from simply rubbing the eye. If the student looks well, has no complaints, no discharge, and normal vital signs, allow the student to lie down with the eyes closed for 20 minutes to see if the redness disappears. The most common cause of a red eye is an inflammation of the bulbar or palpebral conjunctiva. If the reason for a red eye is a bacterial or viral conjunctivitis, it is usually contagious. The American Academy of Pediatrics (AAP, 2003b) has recommended that once the appropriate therapy is started, the student can return to school (Table 23.2).

A red eye can also be the presenting complaint of a student with a systemic illness, such as Lyme disease, rheumatological disorders, and infectious disease such as pharyngoconjunctival fever, sinusitis, or herpes viral infection. In these cases, the student will have other complaints.

Table 23.2 ■

DIFFERENTIATING BACTERIAL, VIRAL, AND ALLERGIC CONJUNCTIVITIS

Bacterial conjunctivitis	Mucopurulent discharge Abrupt onset Conjunctiva erythema Normal pupil exam Burning and/or photophobia Matting of lashes
Viral conjunctivitis	Redness Gritty feeling White, stringy discharge Pain and/or photophobia May itch Preauricular adenopathy can be present Chemosis or swelling of conjunctiva
Allergic conjunctivitis	Itch is chief complaint Clear watery discharge Redness Can have swelling as well as bumpy or cobblestone appearance of palpebral conjunctiva May have associated rhinitis Gritty feeling or burning Photophobia

Source: Adapted from: Wagner, R. (2003). The child with red eye: Making the diagnosis. *Contemporary Pediatrics, 4S*, 7–11.

Key History Points

- Did anything splash in the eye—chemicals, soap, makeup?
- Does the student appear ill?
- Does the student have signs of systemic illness such as headache, nausea, diarrhea, joint pain, fever, ear pain, or sore throat (Olive-Hemker, 1999)?
- Ask about any associated history of visual loss, blurry vision, or photophobia.
- Ask when the eye became red and if it is getting worse or better.
- Is one eye or both eyes involved? Is there associated itching?
- If the eye has discharge, it is continuous or on awakening? What color is it? (Usually viral conjunctivitis does not have pus and bacterial conjunctivitis does [Schmidtt, 2002])
- Is there any history of trauma or history that indicates a foreign body?
- Does the student have any associated signs of allergy, such as allergic shiners, itchy eyes, and rhinorrhea?
- Is there any pain or tenderness around the eye? (*May indicate sinus or orbital infections or trauma.*) Is there pain in the eye? (*May indicate foreign body or corneal ulcer.*)

Physical Assessment

- Evaluate the general appearance. Is the outer lid red and swollen? (*May indicate periorbital cellulitis or ethmoiditis.*)
- Document the visual acuity in both eyes, together and alone.

- Follow the guidelines above for vision complaints and eye trauma Document any purulent discharge in the eyes.
- Look for boggy (swollen) or pale nasal mucosa (*May indicate allergies*).
- Look for grouped vesicles around the eye, which can indicate a herpes infection.
- Evaluate breath sounds for any wheezing if you think the student has allergies.

Nursing Actions

- Irrigate and cleanse eyes with warm water for 5 minutes (Schmidtt, 2002).
- Use a cool compress to relieve the itch associated with allergic conjunctivitis.
- Avoid hand to eye contact with other students while waiting for parents to pick up the student if the student has bacterial or viral conjunctivitis (AAP, 2003b).
- If the student wears contacts, he or she needs to switch to glasses until the condition is resolved.
- Work with cleaning staff if there is an outbreak of conjunctivitis within a class. Make sure the cleaning staff understands the importance of cleaning doorknobs and surfaces that children touch.
- Discuss with teachers the effectiveness of alcohol-based hand cleaners to prevent transmission of infections (Centers for Disease Control and Prevention [CDC], 2002).
- Make sure that classroom environments are free of potential allergens.
- Teach the student and parent how to clean discharge from the eye—wiping from the nasal part of the eye to outer part of the eye.
- Teach student and parent not to share towels at home and to wash hands frequently if the student has conjunctivitis to avoid passing it to siblings and guardians.
- Teach the student and his or her parents the importance of hand washing to prevent infection.
- Make sure the parent calls the primary care provider if the eye is not getting better in 48 hours or immediately if there is a change in vision.
- If antibiotic eye drops are prescribed, the student can return to school in 24 hours if pus is minimal (Schmidtt, 2002).
- When administering eye drops for bacterial conjunctivitis, "remove all dried and liquid pus from the eye with warm water and wet cotton balls. Unless this is done beforehand, the eye drops will not have a chance to work" (Schmidtt, 2002).

Tearing Eyes

Tearing from the eye may be associated with infection, intraocular pressure, a foreign body in the eye, reflex tearing secondary to dry eyes, seventh cranial nerve palsy, or abnormality of the lacrimal apparatus.

Key History Points

- Ask when the onset of the tearing occurred.
- When and where does the tearing occur?
- Is there any foreign body sensation?
- Does the student wear contact lenses?
- Are there any other signs of allergy?
- Is there any history of foreign objects thrown at or near the student?
- Is there any history of any chemical substances in the eye?
- Is there any history of medication use at home?
- Has student had this problem before?
- Does the student have a systemic illness?

Physical Assessment

- Assess the eye as outlined in the sections on visual complaints. Palpate the lacrimal sac for any mucopurulent discharge.
- Evaluate for any signs of injury or foreign body.

Nursing Actions

- Teach the student good hand washing skills.
- If there is pain, promote comfort by shielding the eye and have student rest in a darkened area.
- If a foreign body is present, see below for more details.

Eye Swelling or Periorbital Edema

Swelling around the eye can result from local or systemic problems. Sometimes the cause of the swelling is related to an obvious local reaction such as an allergic reaction, an insect bite, trauma, or infection. The area around the eye has a looseness of tissue and excess skin so the edema may be larger than expected. Systemic diseases that cause edema in various parts of the body may also cause periorbital edema. Students may not complain of any problem. However, the nurse may be the first person questioned by the parent or the teacher about this observation.

Key History Points

- Are there signs of systemic illness? (*Purulent rhinitis with redness and swelling under the eye can indicate a sinusitis or periorbital cellulitis.*)
- Are there signs of cardiac disease or renal disease, such as fatigue, exercise intolerance, or history of decreased urine output?
- Is the eye swelling bilateral or unilateral?
- Are the eyes itching or painful?
- Is the swelling noted on the inner canthus near the lachrymal apparatus?
- Is there a history of swelling following administration of drugs or food?
- Is there a history of an insect bite?
- Is there a history of trauma?
- Has the student used any face creams, makeup, or ointments around the eye?
- What does the student think the swelling is from?
- What has the student done to help with the eye swelling if it is a chronic problem?
- Does eye swelling decrease during the day and reappear the next morning? (*Dependent edema is a sign of nephrotic syndrome.*)

Physical Assessment

- Assess vital signs including blood pressure.
- Look for puffiness of the eyelids *(commonly seen in acquired hypothyroidism, nephritis, and nephrotic syndrome).*
- Note any indication of cream or makeup applied around the eye.
- Look for exophthalmos (bulging) of the eyes.
- Evaluate for an insect bite mark seen around the area of swelling.
- Note any redness associated with the swelling.
- Evaluate the student for signs of systemic illness, such as mononucleosis, which may present with puffiness of the lid, or dependent edema on other body parts later in the day (*which may indicate nephrotic syndrome*).
- Evaluate for signs of allergies—allergic shiners or nasal boggy nasal mucosa (pale, swollen nasal passages).
- Evaluate for bruising of the eyelids; if positive, evaluate for other signs of physical abuse.

Nursing Actions

- Apply cool compress to the eye.

Foreign Body in the Eyes (see p. 535)

EAR PROBLEMS

Earache

Otalgia or earache is common in pediatrics. Ear pain can arise from problems in the throat or neck, as well as the ear since the cervical nerves and cranial nerves share distribution with the ear. The causes of otalgia can be related to infection, trauma, allergy or inflammation, eustachian tube dysfunction, impacted ear wax, or rarely, tumor. Ear wax is normally sticky/waxy or flaky and ranges from light yellow to dark brown (Schmidtt, 2002).

The most common causes of ear pain are acute otitis media, otitis externa, temporomandibular joint dysfunction, ear trauma, and acute pharyngitis (Tunnessen, 1999). Based on the preceding, it is imperative to assess not only the ear but also the head and neck region to help determine the cause of the ear pain. There are no clear criteria for the diagnosis of otitis media (Matz, 2002); healthcare providers have many differing opinions. Some healthcare providers are no longer treating most cases of acute otitis media with antibiotics, as not every red ear is infected. However, a referral should still be made to the primary care provider for otalgia due to a red ear drum.

Key History Points

- Ask about any allergies.
- Are there signs of systemic illness, such as fever, cough, rhinitis, stiff neck, or headache?
- Is there buzzing, ringing, or hissing in the ears without other symptoms? Is there a muffled, crackling, or popping sound? Do the ears "feel full"?
- Are both ears affected or just one?
- Is there pain on chewing and swallowing? Is the pain different when the student is lying down or sitting up?

- Does the student have the sensation of being dizzy or feel that the room is spinning?
- How is the student's balance?
- How did the student sleep last night?
- What medications is the student using at the present time?
- Does the student have any difficulty hearing?
- Ask about the duration and severity of the pain.
- Are there any precipitating events before the onset of ear pain—trauma, infectious causes, swimming, or a history of cerumen (wax) in the ear?
- Does the student have a history of recurrent or recent ear infections and is there recent antibiotic use?
- Is there a history of recent air travel or scuba diving?
- Ask whether the student recently cleaned out the ear or put something in the ear?

Physical Assessment

- Look carefully at the pinna and the area behind the pinna.
  - Observe for any redness around the mastoid.
  - Observe for any signs of trauma.
  - If the pinna is laterally displaced and pushed forward, evaluate the mastoid bone behind the pinna for pain on pressure or redness of the bone.
  - Pain elicited when pulling gently on the pinna may suggest otitis externa or presence of a foreign object.
- Look for impacted cerumen or foreign objects as you gently place the otoscope into the ear canal.
- Be careful not to touch the ear canal with the tip of the speculum.
  - If you touch the canal, you may elicit the red reflex of the drum. This will make the drum look red. However, the landmarks will be normal.
- Observe the drum (FIGURE 23.6).
  - Observe the color and the translucency of the drum.
  - Look for any scarring of the drum. If the student has had myringotomy tubes, there will be scarring in the lower one half of the drum or a white circular device if the tubes are still in.
  - Look at the light reflex and bony landmarks. Are they in the normal position? Distortion of the bony landmarks and an abnormal light reflex with a bulging, red, and poorly mobile drum is indicative of an acute otitis media. Clear fluid behind the drum without any redness is more indicative of serous otitis media.

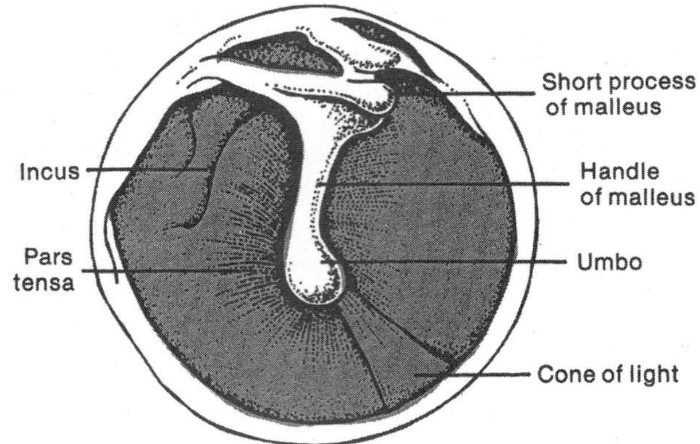

Figure 23.6 ■ Landmarks of the Tympanic Membrane (From Engel, J. (1993). Pocket Guide: Pediatric Assessment. St Louis: Mosby.)

  - Look for retraction of the drum. A retracted drum means that the bony landmark is not in the normal location.
  - Is there any drainage from the ear? Is there a foul smell to the odor?
  - Avoid putting the otoscope into the ear and then looking since it can push any foreign body into the ear canal.
- Pain can be referred from the throat and the nose. Therefore observe the entire posterior pharynx to evaluate for any signs of abscess, which may present as otalgia.
- Look into the nasal passages with a light for any foreign objects.
- Evaluate the mouth completely.
  - Assess the teeth and gums; look for signs of gum inflammation (gingivitis) and caries.
  - Assess the tongue.
  - Evaluate for any ulcers on the buccal mucosa.
  - Evaluate for tonsillar enlargement (see section on throat pain).
  - Evaluate for lymph node enlargement or neck masses.
    - Lymph nodes are considered enlarged if they are 2 cm or greater (see section on neck pain below).
    - Does the student have a tilt to the head or torticollis?

Nursing Actions

- Medicate for pain, if permitted by policy and protocol.

- Provide dry warmth to help relieve ear pain, if permitted by policy and protocol.
- Have the student lie with affected ear down.
- For swimmer's ear (external otitis) that has been diagnosed by a healthcare provider, the student may be instructed to avoid swimming until condition resolves. Parents may be advised by the healthcare provider to dilute white vinegar to half strength using water. They can then instill this solution into the child's affected ear. The child should remain on his or her side for 5 minutes, then turn over and let the vinegar solution drain. This restores normal pH and decreases swelling (Schmidtt, 2002).
- Avoid use of ear plugs, even with cotton to absorb drainage.
- Review with parents that exposure to passive smoking increases the risk of otitis media.
- Review the importance of completing the antibiotic, as prescribed, if the healthcare provider has ordered this medication.
- Encourage the parent to treat the child for pain with an appropriate dose of pain controlling medication.

Ear Discharge

Ear discharge can be due to an infectious process or cerumen. The student may have an odor from the ear due to an infection, a foreign decaying object, or skin irritation. A complaint of ear discharge is evaluated the same way as for an earache. It is important for the nurse to evaluate the complaint of ear discharge or foreign object sensation even if the nurse has previously looked in the ear. Follow the outline for earache.

Hearing Disturbances

Congenital hearing loss occurs in 1 to 3 per 1,000 students (Sokol & Hyde, 2002); any hearing loss in students can be a source of learning problems depending on the severity, duration, and time of onset (Elden & Potsic, 2002) (see Chapter 27). Mild to moderate loss in young students is easy to miss since the behavior and language problems that result are not as obvious as a marked language delay (Stockard-Pope, 2001). Therefore, the school nurse is the key person and the advocate who can make an early identification, referral, and remediation of impairments in the educational setting. Even mild hearing losses are educationally and medically significant. This section will focus on noise-related deafness.

Noise-induced hearing loss may occur due to the exposure of students to loud noise either through aircraft, firearms, lawn equipment, personal listening devices such as CD players with headphones, or a referee's whistle (Niskar et al., 2001). The hearing loss is likely to be at the range from 3,000 to 6,000 Hz (see Chapter 20). A recent study of American students showed that 12.5% of American students 6 to 19 years of age have audiograms that show noise-induced hearing loss (Niskar et al., 2001). Noise-induced hearing loss can occur after chronic exposure to sounds that are not as loud and therefore may not be as obvious to the student.

Cerumen or foreign bodies can cause hearing impairment. Evaluation of the ear should be done as suggested earlier. Sudden hearing loss can follow trauma or problems with circulation. Hypersensitivity to sound or hyperacousia may also be a complaint that brings the student to the health office. These students may complain that the classroom is too loud and may complain of a headache.

Key History Points

- Ask about noise exposure in school, play, or work exposure.
- How loud does the student keep his or her personal listening device?
- Has the student ever worn hearing devices?
- Is there a family history of hearing loss?
- Is there a history of ear infections?
- Does the student have ear pain or any upper respiratory tract infection at the present time?
- How does the student clean his ears?
- Does the student insert foreign bodies into the canal?

Physical Assessment

- Follow instructions for earache in the previous section.
- Complete a hearing screening and compare to past results
- Observe and assess student in a classroom setting.
  - Look at:
    - Changes in achievement level.
    - Frequent requests to repeat questions.
    - Irrelevant answers to questions.
    - Tilting head toward the speaker.
    - Quality of speech is changing.
    - Changes in attention level.
    - Tendency to isolate self, to become increasingly passive, easily tired, or fatigued.

Nursing Actions

- Educate students, especially adolescents, about how noises and personal listening devices can affect ability to hear.
- Instruct students to avoid the highest setting on stereos and personal listening devices.
- Talk about sources of loud noise at home, school, and work and how noises can be avoided.
- Students should be protected from sounds that are painful or annoying. Instruct them to move away from loud noise as well as not to stand by speakers in a concert. Students should understand that music delivered by ear phones should be at an audible but not loud level. Do not yell into a student's ear.
- Initiate measures to decrease noise in the school, such as in the gymnasium, machinery (lawn equipment outside of school windows), or the drums in band. Ensure that those who sit near or use the drums are given earplugs. Avoid close contact with intercom speakers.

Ear Trauma

School-age students who present with ear trauma can have damage to both the middle ear and the inner ear. These students may present to the school health office after falling or being hit by another student. If there is no obvious bleeding or ear discharge, the school nurse can evaluate the injury for triage. Bleeding into the cartilage of the auricle may require medical assessment and should be referred for possible drainage of the hematoma.

Key History Points

- What is the mechanism of injury?
- Is there associated dizziness or vertigo, which can be associated with a labyrinthitis (inflammation of the inner ear) or concussion.
- Is there any hearing loss? (*Can result from discontinuity of the ossicles or temporal bone fracture.*)
- Is there any otorrhea or rhinorrhea?
- Does the student complain of headache or earache?

Physical Assessment

- Evaluate vital signs including pain using a pain scale that is age appropriate.
- Evaluate the auricle for any signs of bleeding or clear drainage; look in front of and behind the ear. Note: If the drainage is clear, it may be cerebrospinal fluid (CSF).
- Gently palpate the skull bones for any pain or crepitus.
- Evaluate the ear canal and drum looking for any possible bruising or hematoma in the canal or drum.
- Is there are sign of facial nerve injury indicated by an asymmetrical smile?
- Does the student have mastoid ecchymosis (*Battle's sign*)?
- Look for raccoon eyes or hematomas around the eye.
- Look for bleeding behind the drum.

Nursing Actions

- Keep the student comfortable.
- Apply a cool compress, if permitted by protocol.
- If drainage is clear, cover it and call parent to take child to a primary care provider.
- If the student is bleeding, place gauze over ear and position with affected ear down.

Foreign Object in the Ear (see p. 535)

NASAL PROBLEMS

Nasal Congestion

Nasal congestion is a common presenting complaint to the school nurse's office since both allergic rhinitis and upper respiratory infections can present with rhinitis and nasal congestion. Nasal allergies affect 8% to 12% of the population and seasonal allergies are common in the school-age population (Lai & Tom, 2001) (see Chapter 28).

Key History Points

- Ask about the nasal discharge—note the character, amount, odor, duration, and whether or not it is bilateral.
- Ask about any associated symptoms such as headache, muscle aches, sore throat, and GI complaints.
- Ask whether there is seasonality to the nasal congestion.
  - Students who are allergic to trees will complain of nasal congestion in the early spring; those who are allergic to certain grasses tend to complain in late May or June; and those with ragweed allergy will

complain more in August and September (American College of Asthma, Allergies, and Immunology, 2003).

- Ask about the frequency of nasal discharge.
- Is the congestion associated with nighttime snoring?
- How does the student blow his nose?
- Is there a history of epistaxis?
- Is sneezing present?
- Is there increased burning and/or tearing of eyes?
- Has the student been rubbing the eyes?
- Has the student been exposed to cold air causing a temporary rhinorrhea?

Physical Assessment

- Have the student tilt his head back slightly.
  - You may be able to partially view both the inferior and middle turbinates.
- Check the outside of the nose—palpate the soft tissue and ridge of the nose; there should be no masses and the septum should be midline.
- Look at each nare separately using the otoscope light. Look though the glass of the otoscope and examine the external nare without putting anything into the nose.
  - The turbinates should be the same size on each side.
    - A rounded elongated mass projecting into the nasal cavity may indicate a nasal polyp or a foreign body. Foreign bodies may sometimes be only partially seen. If the color seems different, it may indicate a foreign body, such as pencil erasers.
    - Crusting over the anterior part of the nasal septum in Kiesselbach's plexus is the area where bleeding is most likely to occur.
    - If one turbinate is very narrow and the other is very large, it can indicate a deviated septum.
  - Assess the mucous membranes; nasal mucous membranes are a deeper color than buccal mucous membranes.
    - Boggy, pale with bluish-tinged turbinates indicate allergies.
    - Bright, red mucus membranes with purulent discharge indicate an infection.

Nursing Actions

- Remind the student not to forcibly blow the nose.
- Promote fluids, rest, and humidification of the air.
- If the student has medication for allergies or infection, develop a plan with the student and his family for medicine compliance; avoid triggers.
- With the staff, inspect and evaluate the classroom environment by identifying irritating substances and triggers (e.g., pets, stuffed toys, feather pillows, markers, open windows, plants, etc.). Educate the teaching, administrative, and custodial staff about avoidance of allergic triggers in the school environment.
- If the student is eligible for an air conditioner because of severe nasal allergies and asthma, educate the parent about the procedure for 504 accommodations within the school and participate in the development of the plan (see Chapters 9, 14, and 28). Section 504 allows students who have a chronic condition not covered under the Individuals with Disabilities Education Act to receive services for conditions to allow their educational needs to be met (Jackson Allen & Vessey, 2004).
- Suggest that a supply of medications be kept at school in compliance with the healthcare provider's prescriptions and parent's directions for emergency use.

Epistaxis

Epistaxis is bleeding from the nose and is common in students. Most nosebleeds in students are from the anterior part of the nose. Most epistaxis relates to minor trauma including picking, forceful blowing, exposure to dry air, or rubbing the nose (Gluckman, Barricella, & Quraishi, 2002). Students who have nosebleeds may also have allergies, have a foreign body in the nose, live in a home or a classroom with low humidity, or have an infection. Banging or hitting the nose in a fall or in contact sport may cause bleeding. Vascular malformations of the nose are rare causes of nasal bleeding. Usually, students with bleeding disorders or liver disease have other problems such as bruising easily, history of prolonged bleeding following a cut, or excessive menstrual bleeding. Hypertension is also the cause of rare cases of nosebleeds.

Key History Points

- When and how often does the student have nosebleeds?
- Is there a history of trauma, which includes picking nose, rubbing, scratching, or falling?
- Is there an associated upper respiratory tract infection?

- Does the student have allergies?
- Is there any substance abuse using the nasal route?
- If the student is a pubertal female, ask about menstrual history since bleeding disorders or acute hematological problems can present with prolonged or excessive bleeding with menses.
- Is there any family history of bleeding disorders?
- Is there a history of tarry or black stool not associated with iron administration?

Physical Assessment

- Stop the bleeding before doing any assessment by applying continuous pressure with the thumb and forefinger at the anterior nares.
- Assess vital signs, including blood pressure, especially when nasal bleeding does not stop after 10 minutes of pressure.
- Inspect the nose as outlined above, specifically looking for crusting or scabbing in the nasal septum at Kiesselbach's plexus (FIGURE 23.7).
- Assess the posterior pharynx to evaluate for a persistent dripping of blood, indicating a posterior bleed (Gluckman et al., 2002).
- Perform a general inspection of skin on arms and legs for petechiae or bruises.

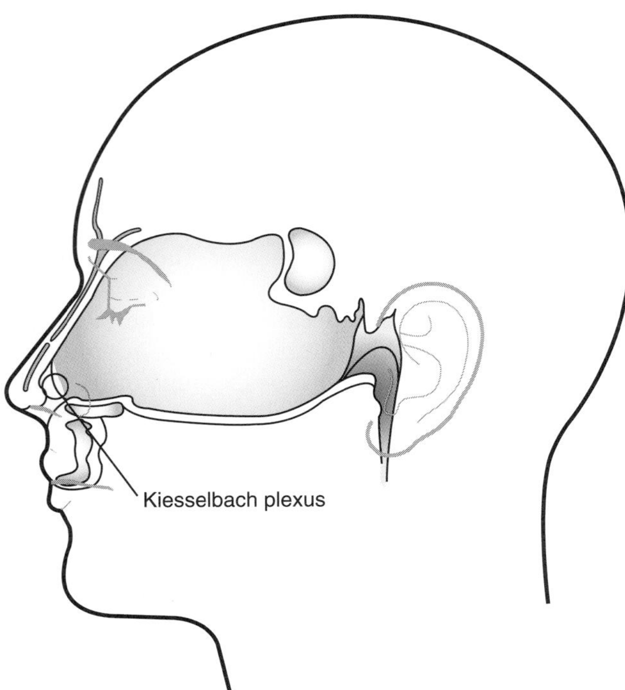

Figure 23.7 ■ Nasal septum at Kiesselbach's plexus. (Illustration by Traci Feldman)

Nursing Actions

- Apply continuous pressure on the anterior nares by thumb and finger for 10 minutes (Tunnessen, 1999).
- If direct pressure does not work, apply an upward pressure to the labial artery by placing a cotton compress beneath the upper lip and putting upward pressure on it while keeping pressure on the anterior nare.
- Have the student sit up with head learning forward to avoid swallowing blood (Gluckman et al., 2002).
- Teach parents about the importance of humidification and saline sprays to prevent drying of nasal tissue in Kiesselbach's plexus.
- Teach parents and student about use of KY jelly to the area inside of the nose to decrease friability of nasal vessels and promote healing (Hay et al., 2003).
- Work with school administration and custodial staff regarding environmental problems such as air humidification of the classrooms. Interventions could be part of the individual health plan that the school nurse develops for a particular student (see Chapter 9).
- Teach students about the problems with nose-picking behavior. Encourage parents to keep the student's fingernails short.
- Work with physical education teachers about the importance of wearing protective face gear during contact sports (see Chapter 24).
- If bleeding fails to stop with direct pressure on anterior nares followed by the addition of upward pressure on the labial artery, contact the parent. The student may need to be transported to an emergency setting, depending on the severity of the bleeding.
- If protocol permits and bleeding fails to stop, Neo-Synephrine or Afrin nasal sprays can be put on a gauze and put in the anterior nares to shrink the blood vessels. Then, with gauze in the nares, squeeze nose for 10 minutes (Gluckman et al., 2002).
- Inform the parents that the child may vomit a little blood or have a dark stool because of blood swallowed (Schmidtt, 2002).

Nasal Trauma

The nose is the third most common broken bone in the body (Byrne, Tawfilis, & Kim, 2003) and it is the most frequently injured organ in the body (Toback, 2003). Injuries need to be evaluated to avoid cosmetic damage. Blunt trauma from falls, altercations, and auto accidents are the cause of 85% of nasal fractures (Rubinstein & Strong, 2000). Nasal trauma must be considered part of the assessment for a concussion. Injury to the nose may result in nasal septal hematomas as well as fractures (Toback, 2003).

Key History Points

- Ask about the mechanism of injury in any trauma, including nasal trauma.
- Ask teachers or staff who may know the student well to indicate if there is any difference in the appearance of the nose.
- Ask if there was any bleeding previously, which has now stopped.
- Query about any loss of consciousness or the presence of headache.
- Inquire about associated complaints, such as vomiting, clear nasal discharge, vision changes, or any difficulty breathing.

Physical Assessment

- If there is no bleeding, do a vision screening and compare to the last vision screen.
  - Evaluate the orbital bones by doing extraocular movements.
  - Check for pupil reactivity to light.
- Observe for deviation of the nasal septum.
- Look for septal hematoma, which would present as bulging of the nasal septum into the nasal cavity.
  - Accumulation of blood in the septal cartilage and overlying mucoperichondrium can deprive the cartilage of blood supply.
  - Observe the fluid coming from the nares. If there is a persistent clear fluid leak of cerebrospinal fluid (CSF), there may be a skull fracture through the cribriform plate.
- Look in the oral cavity for any injury from the trauma.
- There may be fractures of midface region so the eyes and mouth must also be included in this assessment.

Nursing Actions

- Have the student sit upright without hyperextending his or her head to avoid swallowing blood.
- Avoid applying pressure when applying a cool compress to reduce swelling.
- Educate parents about head injury precautions.

Foreign Body in the Eyes, Ears, and Nose

It is not uncommon for children and adolescents to put small toy parts, beads, food, seeds, nuts, paper, cotton, foam, stones, beads, or wads of tissue in their nose and ears. Similarly, other objects can get in the eyes, ears, and nose, either by accident or on purpose. These might include environmental dust, dirt, sand, insects, or toys. Students can present with a foreign body or a foreign body sensation in the eye, ears, and nose. Allergy can also present with a foreign body sensation. It is important to determine if there is any history of trauma for eye complaints.

A student who has nasal foreign body may visit the health office with other complaints or may be sent to the nurse for evaluation relating to a foul odor around the face and nose, or have a visible purulent discharge. School-age students may be embarrassed to admit that they put an object in their nose or ear. Therefore, the foreign body may be in the nose or ear for a few days before an odor or discharge is detected. While it is usually a unilateral nasal discharge, students can put objects up both nares. (Be advised that objects can also be inserted into the urethra, vagina, and rectum. If these are reported, it is suggested that the parents be notified and take their child to their primary care provider.)

Key History Points

- It may be difficult to obtain a history from a student who would insert a foreign object. Phrase questions in an indirect way, “Sometimes students put things in their nose or ears; have you ever thought about that?”
- What is the history before the foreign body sensation?
- Was the student playing in an area where he or she might have gotten sand or dirt in the eye, ear, or nose, such as a playground?
- Did the student put something in the ear or nose or poke the eye? What was the nature of the inserted object? (If sharp, is there bleeding?)

- Is there pain?
- Are there any vision or hearing changes the student can describe?
- Has the student had this problem before? What helped the student?
- Is there a discharge or an odor? When did the odor or discharge begin?
- Flies and bugs can get caught in the ear and the student may complain of a noise or fluttering sound.

Physical Assessment

Eye

- Remove contact lenses if in place.
- Examine the eye as suggested above looking for a foreign body.
- Look for any redness or localized area of irritation.
- Gently invert the upper lid to see if you can see any foreign object. (Do not assume that if a foreign object cannot be visualized it does not exist.)

Nose

- Follow the procedure for looking in the nose (outlined in section on nasal congestion). Despite not visualizing a foreign body, something may still be present.

Ear

- Follow the procedure for physical assessment of the nose (outlined in the section on earache).

Nursing Actions

- Shield the eye if there is any history of eye trauma with foreign body sensation. Have the student rest with the unshielded eye shut to decrease movements.
- If you can see an eyelash or a piece of sand, carefully flush with warm water.
  - With warm water, gently flush out an obvious eyelash or nonpenetrating foreign body such as sand or dirt, running the water from the inner to the outer part of the eye.
  - If it is in the corner of the eye, use a moistened cotton swab to try to remove.
  - If it is in the lower lid, pull the lower lid out by depressing the skin above the cheekbone; touch the particle with a moistened cotton swab. If that doesn't work, try pouring water onto the speck while holding the lid out (Schmidtt, 2002).
- If the particle cannot be seen, it is probably under the upper lid. Have student open and close the eye multiple times while the eye is submerged in a pan or sink of water, or use an eye cup. If this fails, pull the upper lid out and draw it over the lower lid; this maneuver, and tears, will sometimes dislodge the particle (Schmidtt, 2002).
- If you cannot see anything, but the student is still complaining of a foreign body sensation, or if vision does not return, the student needs to be referred to an eye care specialist.
- If the student is cooperative and the foreign body is anterior in the nose, have him or her gently blow out the nose after taking a breath through the mouth while in a sitting position. Do not remove the nasal foreign body unless it is right at the anterior nare ready to come out.
- Advocate for the student. Foreign objects in the nose can present with an extremely foul odor. Classmates may make fun of the student because of the smell. Allow him or her to wait in the office until the parent arrives.
- If there is a bug in the ear, take student into a dark room and shine a bright light into the ear; the insect may come out on its own.
  - If there are no ear tubes and if policy allows, fill the ear canal with mineral oil (baby oil) or soapy water; after 10 minutes, turn onto the affected ear and wiggle the upper lobe by pulling back (Schmidtt, 2002).
  - Do not use tweezers, cotton swabs, or fingers, as these often push the implement in further.

MOUTH AND THROAT PROBLEMS

Tooth Pain

Many conditions can cause mouth and tooth pain. The origin of toothache complaints can include caries, infections, debris between the teeth, and trauma. Medical conditions are rarely the result of dental problems. However, the teeth and gums are sensitive and can cause significant pain for a student. Most dental complaints can be resolved only by an evaluation and treatment program by a dental professional. A healthy, pain-free mouth is important for good overall health (Jones et al., 2000). However, statistically fewer than one out of every five children who are enrolled in Medicaid use the preventative dental services available in any one year (Mofidi, Rozier, & King, 2002); finding competent dental health professionals is also a problem for those with chronic conditions. Treatment and preventive dental care for students is affected by economics, past experiences, phobias, and cultural beliefs.

Key History Points

- Does the student visit a dentist regularly?
- What is the student's brushing habit, including flossing?
- Does the student use mouthwash?
- What are the student's previous dental care experiences, including phobias?
- Is there any ongoing dental work/orthodontia in progress?
- Is there recent trauma to the face and/or teeth?
- Does the student have insurance or access to a dental clinic program?
- Does the student complain of sensitivity to cold?
- Is there pain when biting down?
- Is pain dull, sharp, throbbing, or radiating into the ear?
- Has the student had a tongue or lip piercing?

Physical Assessment

- Assess vital signs, especially temperature, to rule out dental abscess.
- Asses if student can open mouth wide enough for visual assessment.
- Examine the gum line for any swelling, pus, or redness.
- Is there evidence of halitosis?
- Look at the teeth for any plaque or caries. Is there evidence of a crack in enamel or a broken tooth?
- Is there a loose tooth?
- Examine the jaw and neck lymph nodes for any enlargement.
- Is there food lodged between the teeth?

Nursing Actions

- Apply cold compresses to jaw for 20 minutes. Use warm water or saline rinses to clean inside of mouth and teeth.
- Teach student brushing and flossing skill if absence of severe pain permits this action.
- Know community resources for dental care for emergency needs. Is there a dental school or clinic that assists school-age students? Have knowledge of dentists in the area who may be willing to work with families on payment plans.
- Provide floss or help student use it.
- If appropriate, administer analgesic for pain.

Oral Lesions

Children and adolescents can have oral lesions due to trauma, infections, poor dental care, and the use of smokeless tobacco. Oral lesions can be painful and cause distress for the student, thereby interfering with learning. Most are referred to as canker sores or benign mouth ulcers. Some oral lesions are recurrent, such as aphthous ulcers/stomatitis (Leung & Kao, 2003) or ulcers related to chronic illnesses such as inflammatory bowel disease or lupus erythematosus (Olive-Hemker, 1999). Aphthous ulcers are painful, shallow, pseudomembranous depressions with an erythematous halo. They can vary in size and number and are more common in the oral mucosa (Zitelli & Davis, 2002).

Oral candidiasis can occur in children who are immunocompromised or young children who have been on courses of antibiotics (Zitelli & Davis, 2002). These white lesions will be on an erythematous base and will bleed when gently scraped. They are uncommon in well school-age students. Ulcers on the outer lips are often referred to as fever blisters and are usually due to herpesvirus.

Key History Points

- How long has the student had the lesions? Are they painful?
- Does the student know what they are from?
- Has the student been chewing any smokeless tobacco or other drugs?
- Has the student eaten acidic foods?
- Has the student been dehydrated?
- Has the student bitten his or her cheek recently?
- Has the student had mouth or tongue piercings recently?
- Does the student have any joint pain, diarrhea, red eyes, or other associated complaints?
- Is there a family member with these lesions?
- How long has the student had the same toothbrush?

- What are the student's brushing habits? (*The lesions may be caused by strenuous brushing.*)
- Ask the adolescent about oral sex. It is important to ensure confidentiality and make sure that this is asked in privacy. The nurse must be in touch with her own feelings about adolescent sexuality and not act shocked or surprised.
- Is the student complaining of recurrent abdominal pain?

Physical Assessment

- Carefully examine the oral mucus membranes in the mouth, looking at the sides, top, back, and under the tongue.
- Describe the size, depth, color, and location of the ulcer(s) as well as the pain level.
- Assess hands and feet for blisters and peeling to rule out hand–foot disease caused by coxsackie virus.

Nursing Actions

- Discuss bland diet and liquids that will not burn the lesions.
- Advise parents to change the student's toothbrush after the lesions have resolved.
- Infection control measures such as proper hand washing and using a separate or disposable bathroom cup for each family member should be taught to students and parents.
- Although these lesions may not require students leaving school, some form of communication with the parent about the lesions is advised, perhaps by an information sheet.
- If allowed by policy, use 1 tsp of liquid antacid as a mouthwash after meals to decrease the pain (Schmidtt, 2002).

Throat Pain

Sore throat or pain on swallowing is a common complaint in the pediatric population. Tonsils and adenoids are lymphoid tissues that are found in the nasopharynx and oropharynx (Gross & Harrison, 2000). Students who have throat pain can present with tender cervical nodes, halitosis, fever, or pain on swallowing (Gross & Harrison, 2000).

Most sore throats are caused by viruses with 15% to 30% of infections due to Group A streptococcus (Schroeder, 2003). A history of a close contact with Group A streptococcus and a high prevalence rate in the community can be a significant history point. An acute onset of sore throat with fever, associated with headache, nausea, vomiting, and abdominal pain also increases the likelihood of Group A streptococcus (Schroeder, 2003). Viral sore throats are more likely to be associated with upper respiratory symptoms along with cough, conjunctivitis, and diarrhea (Schroeder, 2003). The throat can also become sore related to overuse of the voice, persistent cough, mouth breathing, dust, and dry weather (Lafferty & Baird, 2001).

Key History Points

- How did the pain begin? Is it the same intensity? Has it increased?
- How long has the throat pain been present?
- Is the pain usually present before leaving for school and does it get better as the day progresses?
- Can the student point with one finger to the pain region?
- Did the student choke on something or swallow something that got stuck in his or her throat?
- Is the pain sharp or dull? Where does the student rate the pain on a pain scale?
- Is the student allergic; does he or she have a postnasal drip?
- Is the sore throat associated with fever, headache, or abdominal pain?
- Does the student have upper respiratory tract symptoms/or distress?
- Is the student sexually active and having oral sex?
- More serious causes of throat pain are indicated if the following questions are positive.
    - Is the student's head tilted because of massive enlargement of the cervical nodes?
    - Can the student swallow? Inability to swallow may indicate a more serious cause for the sore throat.
    - Is the student drooling or is there a change in voice quality/muffled voice? Changes in vocal quality, an inability to swallow, drooling, and an ill appearing child may indicate a retropharyngeal abscess (epiglottitis). *If this is the case, DO NOT ATTEMPT TO VISUALIZE THE THROAT; CALL 9-1-1 AND ACCOMPANY CHILD TO AN EMERGENCY ROOM.*
    - Is there a history of recent travel to a country where diphtheria is present?
- Is there anything that provokes the pain—smoking, inhalant abuse, drug abuse?

- Is there exposure to dry air or smoke in the household?
- Is there a possibility of a foreign body in the posterior pharynx?

Physical Assessment

- *If the student is drooling or cannot swallow,* ***do not*** *use the tongue blade to view the tonsils, since hyperextension of the neck can cause the swollen epiglottis to rise and block the airway.*
- Assess vital signs; rule out respiratory distress.
- Examine the color of the skin around the mouth for circumoral pallor and for any nail bed cyanosis.
- Look at the oral mucosa for any white patches/lesions.
- Examine the buccal mucosa and oral membrane for any ulcerative lesions.
- Examine the teeth for any caries or inflammation of the gum.
- Examine the palate for any oral lesions, petechiae, or papular pattern.
- Examine the posterior pharynx.
  - Reassure the student that you are not going to use a tongue blade.
  - Tell the student you are going to play the "ha-ha" game. Ask the student to open his or her mouth and say, "ha, ha" loudly. If this does not work, ask the student to open his or her mouth and pant like a puppy.
  - Two other approaches that may assist in this examination are asking the student to make his or her tongue touch the chin or say "ah ah" in short sounds rather than long ones.
- Examine the tonsils; the size of the tonsils is measured as:

  +1 visible

  +2 halfway between the tonsillar pillars and the uvula

  +3 touching the uvula

  +4 touching each other (Colyar, 2003)
- Look for erythema or swollen tonsils with or without exudate. Heavy, gray malodorous exudates can be from Epstein Barr virus (Gross & Harrison, 2000).
- Note if one tonsil is much larger than the other.
- Look for ulcerative or vesicular lesions that suggest viral illnesses
- Note any enlargement or hyperplasia of the lymphoid follicles on the posterior pharynx that makes the posterior pharynx look pebbled.
- Is there a postnasal drip? What is the color and quantity?
- Examine the neck for any adenopathy.
- How is the student positioned? Does the student insist on sitting up and refuse to lie down, or stay fixed in a position of comfort?

Nursing Actions

- Depending on protocol, give antipyretic if fever is present or provide lozenges or analgesic for pain.
- Encourage adequate fluid intake to keep mucus thin.
- Observe the student until you are confident that there is no respiratory distress.
- Allow the student to rest while awaiting guardian or parent.
- Teach student gargling with warm salt water to relieve throat irritations; or remove secretions, and promote healing (1/4 tsp. salt in 8 oz. water) (Lafferty & Baird, 2001).
- Provide student with lemon and honey in warm tea.
- Eliminate irritants from the environment (hairspray, perfumes, fumes, smoke).
- Encourage the student to discard his or her toothbrush and use a new one when symptoms resolve.

NECK PROBLEMS

Torticollis

Torticollis or head tilt can be divided into congenital or acquired. It is a physical sign that can be from a cold draft or infection of the lymph nodes to a serious problem of tumors in the CNS (Kautz & Skaggs, 1998). Torticollis may be the result of trauma and can be a serious manifestation of vertebral subluxation or dislocations (Berlin, 2000; Tunnessen, 1999). Torticollis can be confused with nuchal rigidity or stiff neck.

Key History Points

- Ask about any trauma in the past week.
- Does the student have any genetic conditions that may predispose to subluxation such as

Down syndrome, dwarfism syndromes, or bone dysplasias?

- Has the student had a viral infection over the past week?
- Is this a congenital problem?
- Has the student been prescribed neuroleptic medications (antipsychotics such as phenothiazines, haloperidol) that can cause acute, painful dystonic reactions?
- Does the student have strabismus, nystagmus, or a disorder of ocular motility that causes the student to tilt his or her head to avoid double vision?
- Does the student have any changes in gait, bladder function, increased clumsiness, or neck pain indicating a CNS problem?
- Does the student have a sore throat?
- Does the student have neck pain with the torticollis?
- Is there early morning headache or any episodes of vomiting or nausea prior to the onset of torticollis?
- Does the student have a history of rheumatoid arthritis or any other systemic disease involving joints?

Physical Assessment

- Assess vital signs; is a fever present?
- If there is a history of trauma, allow the student to be in a position of comfort and activate EMS.
- If this is not the result of acute trauma, evaluate the eyes, throat, and neck, and do a quick overview of the student as well.
  - Do not force a student to move the neck in a direction that he or she does not want to turn.
  - Evaluate the neck range of motion by manual examination.
  - Evaluate the student's vision for any changes and compare with previous screenings; evaluate for extraocular movements; do a cover test to evaluate for strabismus.
  - Examine the throat.
  - Evaluate for lymphadenopathy in the head and neck region.
  - Evaluate for neck pain by gentle palpation on the cervical spine.
  - Is there any difficulty in gait or bladder control?
  - Is there any pain or swelling in any joint?
  - Look for tremor or weakness of the extremity.

Nursing Actions

- If this is not the result of acute trauma and if protocol allows, warmth (wet or dry) may be applied to neck muscle.
- Neck torticollis or pain may respond to gentle massage on the sternocleidomastoid muscle.
- Allow the student to rest in a position of comfort.
- If permitted, provide analgesics.

Neck Pain

Neck pain can overlap with torticollis but can present as an isolated complaint. The student with neck pain following a trauma is an emergency and are not discussed in this section. When the student presents with neck pain, the nurse needs to determine whether the child is systemically ill, has a trauma with neurological symptoms, is asymptomatic neurologically, or is in a high-risk category for atlanto-axillary dislocation (Braganza & Adam, 2003). Common neck injuries are sustained during contact sports resulting from brachial plexus trauma. Sports injuries may not be reported if the child feels pressure to continue to play (Patel, Greydanus, & Pratt, 2001). This chapter discusses the child with neck pain without a history of trauma.

Key History Points

- How long has the pain existed?
- Did the pain occur just on waking this morning?
- Is there any recent trauma?
- Was the student in a car accident (*whiplash*)?
- How long is the student engaged in computer time or playing video games?
- Ask about a previous history of neck pain.
- Ask about arm weakness.
- Are there other symptoms, such as chest pain, drowsiness, dyspnea, headache, nausea, vomiting, or tinnitus (ringing in the ears)?
- Is there pain while chewing or with jaw movement?
- Is student taking medications for pain or fever? (Analgesics taken at home can mask symptoms once the student arrives at school.)

- Is the student being followed by an orthopedist or chiropractor for neck pain or scoliosis?
- For athletes, ask about "stingers" or "jolts" or "burners" (burning waves of pain).

Physical Assessment

- Assess vital signs and level of consciousness.
- Evaluate hand and arm strength/weakness bilaterally.
- Assess for swollen glands.
- Evaluate the skin for any sign of injury, even if the student does not report it.
- Evaluate the student for point tenderness over the cervical spine.
- Evaluate the student for range of motion of the neck.
- Assess for scoliosis (see Chapter 20). Is there difference in the height of one shoulder due to difference in the sternocleidomastoid muscle?

Nursing Actions

- If protocol allows, apply moist heat to the neck.
- If protocol allows, administer analgesics.
- Do not force range of motion of neck.
- Use a folded towel under the neck to support it while lying down.

RESPIRATORY PROBLEMS

Cough

Cough is a symptom that results from a reflex phenomenon in the cough receptors in the airways of the lung, pharynx, paranasal sinuses, and external auditory canal and controlled by the cough center in the medulla. The result is a short breath followed by a release under pressure with a forceful expiratory phase. Cough involves the forceful expulsion of air from the respiratory tree (Wubbel & Faro, 2003). However, the cough may be absent even in the presence of a foreign body in the airway since there is not a uniform stimulus threshold in the respiratory tree. "A coughing spasm is $>$ 5 minutes of continuous coughing" (Schmidtt, 2002). Coughs can be productive (where mucus is expectorated or swallowed) or dry and nonproductive. Children with productive coughs rarely spit out mucus and usually swallow mucus.

Cough can result from irritation from the environment, an infectious process, allergic problems, foreign bodies, genetic diseases, congenital or acquired disorders, or cardiac disease as well as extrinsic and intrinsic mechanical factors (Wubbel & Faro, 2003). A psychogenic cough is a loud, explosive, seal-like cough that occurs during the day (Goodman & Brady, 2000).

Key History Points

- Does the student have fever?
- How long has the student had the cough?
- How does the student describe the cough?
- Is the cough productive? What are the color, consistency, and odor of the mucus produced by the cough? Is the mucus swallowed?
- Did the cough begin suddenly/overnight?
- When does the cough occur?
- What makes the cough better or worse? What triggers the cough?
- Does a body position alleviate or exacerbate the cough?
- Does the student feel pain when coughing? Is there severe chest pain? (*pneumothorax*)
- Is the cough related to eating a large meal? Does the student complain of heartburn?
- Is the cough associated with a specific time of day or activity?
- Have there been any changes in appetite, energy, or weight?
- Is there a change in tolerance with exercise, such as climbing stairs?
- Does the student have a sore throat?
- Does the student have a cold with a rhinorrhea?
- Is there is a known history of asthma?
- Does the student have any other symptoms?
- Has there been exposure to fumes, chemicals, or cleaning equipment?
- Has the student initiated smoking, is actively smoking, or is exposed to second hand smoke?
- Is the student using any inhalant drug or chemical?
- Are there adults in the house with history of a cough or present cough?
- In younger students, is the cough related to any choking?

- Are immunizations up to date, especially pertussis? When was the last TB test and what were the results?

Physical Assessment

- Is student flushed, pale, anxious, agitated, fearful, nervous, and lethargic?
- Is skin cool, cold, clammy, or dry?
- Assess temperature and respiratory rate. Respiratory rate is one of the most sensitive indicators of acute respiratory distress. Watch chest configuration when the student is coughing. Note quality of cough (dry, congested, productive or not), paroxysmal (*multiple coughs in rapid succession without a breath between them; may indicate pertussis*).
- Evaluate the overall appearance of the student—does the student have allergic shiners or signs of allergies such as mouth breathing, allergic crease across the nose, or a bumpy or cobblestone appearance to the back of the throat?
- Evaluate the nose and throat for any signs of dryness, crusting, swelling, congestion, or boggy mucosa. Is the throat sore?
- Palpate the neck for masses or lymphadenopathy.
- Look at the nails for any signs of clubbing or color changes around the lips during and after coughing.
- Inspection
  - How does the student appear?
  - Are there signs of respiratory distress—flaring, retractions of the ribs, or retraction of the supraclavicular notch?
  - Is the student using accessory muscles?

  (Signs and symptoms of respiratory distress are outlined in Box 23.1.)
- Palpation and percussion of the chest are difficult to perform within school settings but dullness, flatness, and tympany can be heard.
- Auscultate the chest.
  - Listen to the chest: front, back, and sides.
  - Are the breath sounds equal bilaterally?
  - Can you hear good air entry?
  - Note any adventitious sounds—crackles (rales and rhonchi), friction rubs, wheezing; describe exactly what you hear.

  (Table 23.3 describes various breath sounds and possible associated problems.)

Box 23.1 ■ ■ ■

SIGNS AND SYMPTOMS OF RESPIRATORY DISTRESS

Nasal flaring

Increased heart rate and respiratory rate in absence of fever or drug/medication use

Expiratory grunting

Retractions:

Only isolated intercostals retractions: Mild respiratory distress

Subcostal, suprasternal and supraclavicular retractions: Moderate distress

Use of accessory muscles and rib retractions: Severe distress

Lack of synchronous chest and abdominal movement with inspiration (paradoxical breathing)

If student has inspiratory stridor, the obstruction is in the upper airway or upper pharynx, larynx, or subglottic area.

If student has expiratory stridor, the obstruction is in the trachea or upper bronchus.

If the student has a muffled voice and respiratory distress, the child may have a supralaryngeal obstruction, supraglottitis (epiglottitis), or retropharyngeal abscess.

Child is unable to talk.

Child is sitting forward.

Changes in color to cyanosis as well as confusion are late signs.

- If allowed by policy, obtain the oxygen level via a pulse oximeter.
- If the student is using peak flow to monitor asthma, assess the peak flow.

Nursing Actions

- Assess vital signs, especially respiratory rate, and color
- Administer p.r.n. medications prescribed for this situation. Notify parents of administration of the medication.

Table 23.3 ■
BREATH SOUNDS AND POSSIBLE PROBLEMS

ADVENTITIOUS SOUND	WHAT YOU HEAR	LOCATION OF THE PROBLEM
Heterophonous wheezing	High pitched musical sounds of different pitches	Indicates problem with the small airways (asthma, cystic fibrosis)
Homophonous wheezing	Single pitched honking expiratory wheezes	Indicates problems with trachea and upper airway (tracheomalacia, foreign body, obstruction of upper airway)
Coarse crackles	Intermittent low pitched, high intensity with long duration	Indicates secretions in large airways
Fine crackles	Intermittent, high pitched, low intensity sounds with short duration	Indicates problems with bronchioles (pneumonia, bronchitis)
Pleural friction rubs	Harsh, intermittent, grating sound varying with respiration	Indicates pleural effusion or pleuritis
Cardiac friction rub	Harsh, continuous, grating sound varying with respiration	Indicates cardiac effusion

Source: Adapted from Wubbel, C., & Faro, A. (2003). Chronic cough in children. *Pediatric Case Reviews*, *3*(2), 95–104; Colyar, M. (2003). Well-student assessment for primary care providers. Philadelphia: F. A. Davis.

- If a beta agonist is prescribed under protocol for this student, administer medication as directed and record time/response.
- Do not permit the student to be alone—monitor until the parent or guardian arrives if there is mild wheezing.
- Assist the student to maintain a position of comfort. The student may want to sit and lean forward over a table or with the head extended slightly back in a "sniffing" position.
- Provide warm liquids to help soothe the throat or cough drops if student is old enough and protocol allows. Do not give anything by mouth if danger of choking exists.
- Provide the student with emotional support during an acute episode.
- If the student is well and comfortable, he or she can return to class with a note for the parents.
- Initiate environmental controls to decrease irritants.
- If cough is a chronic complaint over 3 weeks, it may indicate a chronic lung condition like asthma (Wubbel and Faro, 2003). Encourage the guardian or parent to seek the advice of the primary care provider, noting time and date of referral.

Chest Pain

Chest pain occurs in students of all ages. The most common age at occurrence is 12 years (Selbst, 1997). The younger the student with chest pain, the more likely there is an organic cause for pain. Adolescents and children may have cardiac, gastrointestinal, pulmonary, psychogenic, musculoskeletal, or idiopathic causes of chest pain (Berman & Brayden, 2003). There is no racial or sexual predilection (Kocis, 1999). Chest pain can be from referred or local sources; the pain may come from the structures within the thorax or it can be referred from visceral organs.

Chest pain has significance for the student and the family, as it tends to be associated with cardiac disease and death. However, chest pain during exercise is a red flag for organic disease. Fever with chest pain requires a workup for organic etiology such as myocarditis or pneumonia and needs a prompt referral (Berman & Brayden, 2003).

Key History Points

- Adolescents may worry that their heart is causing the chest pain. Depending on past familial experiences, the adolescent with chest pain may fear death. Inquire about the student's fears.
- Ask what the student thinks precipitates the pain.
- Ask about the length, severity, frequency, and location of the pain.
- Are there associated complaints?
- Does the chest pain disrupt the student's normal activities?
- When did the chest pain begin?
- Did the student tell his or her parents? Did the student seek any medical attention?
- Is there a history of blunt trauma?
- Is there a history of carrying heavy books?
- Is there a history of participation in contact sports?
- Is there a history of doing excessive exercise or starting an exercise program that includes lifting weights?
- Can the student reproduce the pain with a position, activity, or touch? Does the student only complain of pain when he takes a deep breath?
- Does the pain present at a particular time of day or class activity?
- Ask specifics about the pain
  - Rate the pain—use pain scales for age.
  - Does the pain improve when the student sits up and sits forward?
  - Is the pain dull and increased when taking a deep breath?
- Is there new breast development or breast tenderness?
- Does the student complain of funny feelings or paresthesias in his or her arms?
- Is there a history of a family member with recent chest pain related to cardiac disease? (*Cardiac or psychogenic origin*)
- Is there increased stress in the student's life? (*Psychogenic pain*) (Berman & Brayden, 2003).
- Is there a past or present history of huffing or smoking?
- Is there cough and fever, dyspnea or night cough with interrupted sleep?
- Does the student complain of burning midsternally, worsened by reclining or eating spicy food? Does the student get relief with antacids or an H2 blocker? Is there a history of using an antacid medication over the counter? (*Gastroesophageal reflux*)
- Ask female adolescents about birth control pills and smoking-associated acute onset of sudden severe chest pain (*pulmonary emboli*) (Neinstein, 2002).
- Is there a history of an eating disorder associated with purging? Is there a history of tetracycline use (*esophagitis*) (Neinstein, 2002)?
- Ask about drug usage with cocaine, crack, or any other sympathomimetic agent (*cardiac or pulmonary source*).
- Does the student have sickle cell disease? Acute chest syndrome can be life threatening (Tanyi, 2003).
- Does the student have chest pain with signs of a rash following a dermatome on one side of the chest (Bodemer, 2003) (*herpes zoster or shingles*)?
- Is there a history of choking on an object? Does the student have a history of an acute onset of vomiting and inability to hold down food (*foreign body in esophagus*)?

Physical Assessment

- Assess vital signs.
- Note any sweating or pallor.
- Examine the ribs and thorax.
  - Inspect for soft tissue hematoma. Are there any visible signs of trauma?
  - Palpate the costochondral border to evaluate for costochondritis, which causes tenderness with palpation of the costochondral junction.
  - Palpate for point tenderness over the ribs that may indicate a fracture.
  - If the mechanism of injury is significant, refer to the ED. There may a bruise to the great vessels or heart.

- Pull the lower rib cage anterior to elicit pain associated with slipping rib syndrome. This occurs due to irritation of the eighth, ninth, and tenth ribs (Berman & Brayden, 2003).
- Assess the lungs.
  - Count respiratory rate for a full minute looking at regularity and the use of accessory muscles.
  - Listen for decreased breath sounds or adventitious sounds such as wheezing, or listen for prolonged expiratory phase.
- Breast buds may be noted on physical assessment.
- Assess cardiovascular system.
  - Evaluate pulses for strength.
  - Listen to the heart in both sitting and sitting forward positions as well as left lateral position to increase the sound of the heart sounds (Brumond & Strong, 2002).
  - Evaluate cardiac rate and rhythm. Note any irregularity of the heartbeat not associated with respirations.
  - Listen for any friction rubs, murmurs, or distant heart sounds. If the friction rub is continuous, it may be pericarditis (Marinella, 1998).
- Assess skin for petechiae of nearby muscles related to increased strenuous use.

Nursing Actions

- Visually observe the student at all times.
- Administer oxygen if indicated according to policy/protocol or the health plan for that student.
- Advise the parents of the student's complaint of chest pain while seeking parental input. If pain has resolved, offer directions about keeping a diary of the episodes to bring to the healthcare provider.
- If pain continues, advise seeking immediate medical attention.
- If the source is musculoskeletal, have the student avoid activities that reproduce the pain.
- Reassure the student if an assessment is normal.
- If chest pain occurs with exercise, provide the student with written clearance before he or she resumes participation in gym or other exercise.
- For an anxious student, teach relaxation techniques or yoga classes to alleviate the chest pain.
- Administer analgesic such as Tylenol, if allowed by protocol or parental consent.
- Full documentation on a progress note is important for future comparisons.
- Administer oxygen if indicated according to policy/protocol or health plan for that student.

GASTROINTESTINAL PROBLEMS

Abdominal Pain

Abdominal pain can be divided into acute and chronic. This section discusses the student with recurrent abdominal pain (RAP). The chapter on acute emergent problems (see Chapter 22) will discuss acute abdominal pain. However, it should always be kept in mind that the student with chronic abdominal pain may have an acute episode. Therefore, it is imperative that the student presenting with abdominal pain multiple times be evaluated each time and the complaint taken seriously and documented for comparison purposes.

Apley (1975), in his classic work, found that one out of every nine students has abdominal pain that lasts for 3 months at least three times growing up. RAP is reported to occur in 10% to 15% of all students between 4 and 16 years of age (Thiessen, 2002). The peak age is between 10 and 12 years. Rhee, Miles, Halpern, and Holditch-Davis (2005) found that stomachache was the fourth most prevalent symptom (18%) reported by middle and high school students. Recent thinking about RAP is that the pain results from an alteration in the transmission of messages from the enteric nervous system to the central nervous system causing visceral hypersensitivity (Stickler, 2002). The visceral hypersensitivity is expressed depending on the sociocultural, emotional, and mental state of the student (Theissen, 2002; Zeiter & Hyams, 2001). Some students express emotional stress and anxiety with RAP or recurrent headaches (Theissen, 2002; Zeiter & Hyams, 2001).

A student younger than 4 years of age who has recurrent abdominal pain is more worrisome than an older student who does not have the red flags of organic recurrent abdominal pain.

Key History Points

- Be an empathetic listener, especially if this student is a frequent visitor to the health office.
- Ask when and how much did the student last eat. (The student may simply be hungry.)

- Ask about the intake of spicy foods or foods high in lactose or sorbitol.
- What are the student's eating habits related to fast food or restaurant fare?

- Evaluate the symptoms.
  - What provokes the symptoms?
  - What makes the symptoms better or worse?
  - Where does the pain start and go to?
    - A red flag is that the further the pain is away from the umbilicus, the more likely it is to be organic.
  - Ask the student to point to where it hurts with one finger.
  - Ask about the relationship of the pain to activity, meals, and time of day. (*Pain after eating suggests dyspepsia or gastroesophageal reflux.*)
  - How severe is the pain? (*Use a pain scale appropriate for the student's age.*)
- How long has the student had pain? What happened the last time the student had this pain? Is this pain different from other abdominal pain the student has had? How?
  - Red flags include weight loss associated with the abdominal pain or a change in appetite associated with the new onset of abdominal pain.
- When did the student last have a bowel movement? Students of all ages experience difficulty using school bathrooms because of privacy issues and/or lack of toilet paper.
  - A red flag is if the student has diarrhea or wakes up at night to have a stool.
- Ask about sleep pattern.
  - A red flag is if the pain wakens the student from sleep.
- What is the absentee record of the student?
  - What else is going on with the student in school?
  - What is the student's school performance?
  - How is the student getting along with classmates?
  - Listen carefully for concerns the student offers about school facilities and teaching environments.
  - If there are excessive visits to the school health office, consider what is happening at home and after school. Are there recent changes in the student's life, such as a divorce or a new baby?
- If female, does the student have menses?
- What medications does the student take?
  - Side effects of many medications may be abdominal pain.
- If the student seems sad or withdrawn, ask about the possibility of physical or sexual abuse.
  - Ask the student: Does anyone touch you or hurt you? Does anyone do things that make you upset?
- Is the guardian or parent on vacation or business trip? Does the child feel homesick?

Physical Assessment

- Assess vital signs.
- Determine weight and height.
- Complete a nutritional assessment.
- Are there any extraintestinal manifestations of a medical problem?
  - Look for red eyes and ulcers in the mouth
- Listen to the chest for adventitious sounds, such as wheezing or rales.
- See if the student has normal range of motion of the extremities, especially at the hip.
  - Does the student have joint pain?
- Inspection
  - Note position.
    - Does student appear comfortable and move with ease?
    - Is the student rolled into a fetal position with flexion of the hips in an attempt to avoid movement or does the student "guard" movement of the abdomen with the arms?
    - Is the student having episodes of restlessness, which is associated with intestinal cramps or gas pains?
  - Does abdomen appear distended?
- Auscultate.
  - Ask the student's permission to listen to the abdomen.
  - Listen to the abdomen for bowel sounds in all four quadrants before doing any palpation.
  - The absence of bowel sounds does not rule out appendicitis (Pisarra, 1999).
- Palpate.
  - Always stress privacy and confidentiality.
  - Palpate away from area of pain. Have the child flex at the knees to decrease tension from abdominal muscles. (One relaxation mechanism when palpating the abdomen is to tell the student you can tell him what he ate yesterday.) Determine if pain is localized or diffuse.

  - Does the student allow palpation despite the statement of pain?
  - Healthy students will have pain if palpated deeply in the left lower quadrant in the area of the descending colon, especially if there is a large amount of stool there.
  - Ask the student to jump up and down or have him hop down from the table since students with appendicitis may have pain when doing this. (You may explain why you request this.) Also check for rebound tenderness.

Nursing Actions

- If pain is acute, have the student lie down in a comfortable position.
- Closely monitor for any changes or for what things improve the pain.
- Help the student identify stressors that cause abdominal pain.
  - Help the student use imagery to deal with stress.
  - Refer to the school counselor if simple techniques do not work (with parental permission and guidance).
  - Try relaxation exercises in stressful situations.
- Notify parent of situation and pain existence/change.
- Notify the child protective services and the school social worker (if there is one), if hunger pains are a chronic problem and the nurse is concerned about lack of food.
- Notify child protective services and the school social worker (if there is one), if there is any concern about physical or sexual abuse.

Constipation

Constipation is defined as the passage of pellet-like stools or defecation less than two times a week lasting for two weeks (Arce, Ermochilla, & Costa, 2002; DiPalma & Gremse, 2003). It also is defined as being unable to pass a bowel movement after straining and pushing for >10 minutes (Schmidtt, 2002). Students can present to the school heath office with complaints of abdominal pain or discomfort or feelings of distention or fullness. Students with constipation can have pain, rectal bleeding, and soiling due to overflow incontinence, caused by liquid stool leaking around a large piece of impacted stool. The younger the student, the more difficult it is in the school setting to obtain a history of bowel habits.

Constipation frequently occurs due to a diet that is low in roughage and fiber, lack of time for defecation, or lack of activity due to increased computer time or TV watching (Roma, Adamidis, Nikolar, Constantopoulos, & Messaritakis, 1999). There are medical conditions and treatments that can present with constipation. If there is no identifiable reason for the constipation, the school nurse may want to consider providing student and family education to increase exercise, as well as fiber, fruit, vegetable, and fluid intake (Nurko, 2001). It is important to reassure and support the student, while allowing privacy and time for defecation so that the issue can be resolved with time.

Key History Points

- What medications is the student taking, including alternative medications and vitamins, especially iron?
  - High caffeine intake can be associated with constipation in some students.
- What are the color, size, frequency, ease, and consistency of the movements? Is there a history of bleeding with the passage of a hard stool? Is there fresh blood on the stool or is the blood only on the toilet paper after wiping?
- Is there pain associated with defecation?
- Is there any vomiting?
- Does the student have recurrent urinary tract infections?
- Are there any stressful events in the student's life or is the student overscheduled? Are there psychological factors resulting from restricted use/lack of privacy with toileting, which can result in constipation?
- Is there a myth/belief that the student must have a bowel movement every day?
- Is there any description of laxative abuse/enemas being advocated by caretakers?
- What is the dietary pattern?
  - Have there been social changes in the home?
  - Where are meals eaten?
  - Does the student drink excess amounts of milk?
  - Which fluids are consumed each day, and in what volume?
- Is there a weight gain with fatigue, eye puffiness or dry, doughy, rough skin with orange color (Young, 2001)? (*May indicate a thyroid problem.*)

- Is there any history of unsteady or clumsy gait? Is there a recent change in urination with dribbling of urine? (*May indicate a neuromuscular problem.*)

Physical Assessment

- Does the student look ill?
- Assess vital signs.
- Assess the abdomen as outlined above. Is it distended?
- Palpate the left lower quadrant; does it reveal sausage-shaped stools?
- Note any gait abnormalities.

Nursing Actions

- Educate the family and the student regarding which foods are constipating, such as rice and bananas.
- Educate about the importance of high-fiber foods (bran, graham crackers, oatmeal, brown rice, popcorn), and appropriate fluid intake for age. Carbohydrates, especially sorbitol, can increase water content and frequency of defecation (Nurko, 2001).
- Promote consumption of fruits and vegetables. Promote apple, pear, cherry, grape, and prune juices; citrus juices are not helpful for constipation. Decrease intake of milk products (Schmidtt, 2002).
- A low-carbohydrate diet can contribute to constipation because of lack of dietary fiber.
- Encourage the student to increase his or her activity level.
- To ease rectal pain, encourage the student to take a warm bath at home.
- Families may want instant results but frequently this is a chronic problem that needs adequate fluids, fiber, and a regular pattern of defecation.
- Evaluate the student's school and play schedule looking for private time to allow for defecation, both in school and at home.
- Work with school administration to make sure bathrooms are safe and clean, with an ample supply of toilet paper and soap. Bathrooms need to be monitored for privacy and security.
- Educate the family and student about the dangers of chronic laxative use and enemas.
- Educate staff about many students' sensitivity to this subject. Asking invasive questions can have adverse effects.

Diarrhea

Diarrhea is an increase in frequency, volume, or liquidity of stool (Berman, 2003). Diarrhea can be acute or chronic. Acute diarrhea can be from gastrointestinal infections and infections outside the gastrointestinal tract (Berman, 2003). Chronic diarrhea is the persistence of loose stools for more than 2 weeks. Acute episodes of diarrhea can be related to food intake, juice intake, infections, medications, allergic diseases, and endocrine disorders as well as chronic or acute diseases including tumors.

Key History Points

- Does the student feel acutely sick?
- Are there any other gastric problems such as recurrent abdominal pain, abdominal distention, or epigastric pain?
- How long has the student had diarrhea?
- Does any other family member have diarrhea?
- Is the student using any over-the-counter medications for diarrhea?
- Has the student traveled recently? If yes, has the student noted any worms in the stools?
- What regular prescribed medications does the student use?
- Does the student have any abdominal pain or cramping? If so, can the student point to one area that is painful?
- Are there are any other symptoms of illness?
- Is the diarrhea related to food, juice, chewing gum, or candy with high fructose or sorbitol content? Is the diarrhea related to intolerance of certain foods, such as milk, high fruit intake, and beans?
- Is there a recent history of weight loss? What are the growth parameters and have they changed?
- Is there any systemic disease?
- Have the student describe his or her bowel movement.
- Is there blood, mucus, or pus in the stool or is there anal pain (*to rule out GI infection and Crohn's disease*) (Olive-Hemker, 1999)?
- Is there any redness of the student's eyes, blurred vision, or joint pain indicating Crohn's disease (Baron, 2002)?
- Is there incontinence of stool (*Shigella*)?

- Has the student had any recent camping trips (*giardiasis*)?
- Has the student voided? Does the student have saliva? Is the student thirsty? (*signs of dehydration*)

Physical Assessment

- Assess vital signs.
- Is there an evidence of systemic illness?
- Evaluate state of hydration. Observe tongue color/dryness and offensive breath odor.
- Examine the throat for any signs of ulcers that indicate a viral illness.
- Inspect for any abdominal distention or asymmetry.
- Listen for bowel sounds in all four quadrants.
- Palpate the abdomen for any pain or areas of tenderness, evaluating from areas of no tenderness to areas of tenderness.

Nursing Actions

- Recognize the student's need for privacy.
- Provide resting area for student while awaiting the parent or guardian.
- Provide easy access and privacy to use lavatory. Provide the student with toilet tissue and demonstrate hand-washing techniques.
- Discourage use of over the counter antidiarrhea medications unless discussed with the primary care provider.
- Provide fluid intake to prevent dehydration; fruit drinks or soft drinks will make the problem worse as a result of the high osmotic load (Schmidtt, 2002). Give pretzels or salty crackers to replace sodium; promote starchy foods.
- Teach parents about foods and fluids that can affect diarrhea. If the child is not vomiting, early feeding can help repair the mucosal intestine following injury and is recommended in simple diarrhea.

Nausea and Vomiting

Nausea and vomiting can be acute or chronic and be the presenting symptoms of many disorders. This symptom complex can be from medications, anatomical problems, a foreign body, obstruction, neurological problems, infectious diseases, endocrine disorders, respiratory problems, allergies, and other causes including pregnancy and eating disorders. It can be the first indication of asthma, a sign of migraine, or the result of swallowing increased mucus related to post nasal drip. Chronic recurrent vomiting clearly needs evaluation by the primary care provider.

Key History Points

- Ask when the vomiting started.
- How many episodes of vomiting and how much emesis? What is in it (food, blood, bile)?
- How often has the student voided today and is the amount more or less than usual?
- Is there any pain and is the pain intermittent or continuous?
- Is the pain relieved by the vomiting?
- Does the student have any other symptoms?
- What medications or drugs is the student taking presently?
- Ask about weight loss or self-induced vomiting.
- Is the student sexually active and is there a chance a female student might be pregnant?
- Is the emesis forceful and bilious or green? Review the student's surgical history.
- Has the student been medicated for fever prior to coming to school?
- Does the student have a developmental delay with known pica behavior? (*Consider foreign body in the esophagus.*)
- Does the vomiting occur in the morning and is it associated with headache? (*May indicate a brain tumor.*)
- Does the student have a cough associated with vomiting? Does the student swallow large amounts of mucus?
- Is there associated dizziness with and continuing after the vomiting?

Physical Assessment

- Assess vital signs.
- Assess for any signs of dehydration—increased pulse rate, dry, flushing of skin, stringy saliva, sunken orbits, delayed capillary refill, quiet behavior with lack of interest in surroundings (Berman, 2003).
- Inspect the skin for any changes in color—observe for any jaundice by looking at sclera, mucous membranes, and tympanic membrane; check chest for rash.
- Palpate for abdominal masses indicative of GI obstruction.

- Assess for neck pain or stiffness.
- Evaluate the student for large parotid glands, thinning hair, sallow color, dental erosions, palatal scratches, or callous on knuckles (Russell's sign). (*May indicate an eating disorder*) (AAP, 2003d).
- Evaluate the student's chest for any adventitious sounds or respiratory distress.
- Listen for bowel sounds and any localized area of tenderness, especially in the right lower quadrant. (*May indicate appendicitis.*)
- Assess orientation/level of consciousness to rule out encephalitis or drug overdose.

Nursing Actions

- Let the student rest in a well ventilated quiet room.
- Provide easy access to pail or toilet in case of vomiting.
- If student has vomited, allow student to rinse out mouth (swish and spit).
- Do not allow the student to drink fluid if you have concerns about appendicitis or an acute abdomen.
- With active vomiting, make NPO; then start with rehydration ice pops if available (CDC, 2003). If not available, water or ice chips can be started as "water is directly absorbed across the stomach wall" (Schmidtt, 2002); progress to small amounts of Gatorade (1 tsp. every 5 minutes).
- Until the problem is resolved, instruct the student to avoid dairy products, caffeine, carbonated drinks, and spicy, greasy foods.
- For nausea, have the student "take slow, deep breaths (about 5 seconds each in, hold, out)" (Lafferty & Baird, 2001, p. 368).

GENITOURINARY/GYNECOLOGICAL PROBLEMS

Genital Discharge/Itch

The most common gynecological complaint in children and adolescents is vaginal discharge or itch (Tunnessen, 1999). A school-age student who presents with this complaint may need a professional, confidential, and sensitive school nurse for emotional support, guidance and a noninvasive reflection of what is being said. Maintaining eye contact with the student is a valuable tool. This complaint may be the result of an overgrowth of bacteria from obesity, poor hygiene, tight clothing, or nonabsorbent underwear. *Candida* infections may result from antibiotic use or diabetes in prepubescent students. Occasionally, students can get a Group A streptococcal infection in the perianal and genital region from an untreated strep throat. A vaginal foreign body or a retained tampon may also lead to bacterial overgrowth and result in itch, discharge, and foul odor. Young students may have pinworms that present as a genital itch. Pinworms can also present as vaginal or rectal itching, which will be worse at night.

Pubertal females may become concerned when they note a discharge on their underwear. This vaginal discharge is clear or white and generally is odorless and relatively normal. Genital itch from sand, nylon, pantyhose, or tight fitting underwear, bubble baths, soaps, or detergent leading to both vaginal irritation and urinary tract infections is common in young students. Older students may be sexually active and have a sexually transmitted infection with presentation of vaginal discharge (Burstein & Murray, 2003) (see Chapter 42). Young students who have been sexually abused may not know how to explain their complaint of vaginal itching and discharge. Emotional support is needed to guide the student offering this complaint.

Key History Points

- Is there burning or itching? When did the itch or discharge start? Did the student note it started after taking any medication?
- Ask about the recent medication history.
- Ask about the onset of menarche.
- Has the student been to the beach or sitting in a sand box?
- Has the student been in a wet bathing suit for a time or a swim team member?
- In what recreational activities does the student participate, such as wearing tight dance clothing?
- What is the overall hygiene of the student?
- Does the student use bubble bath, sit in a bathtub, or use any vaginal preparations such as douches? (*These may cause local irritation of genital tissues.*)
- Ask about sexual activity.
- Has the student had a recent sore throat?
- Ask the student about her playtime and eating habits, looking for the possibility of ingestion of the pinworm egg.
- Has another household member been treated for pinworms?

- Has the student been using any treatment for the problem?
- Is there pain on urination?

Physical Assessment

- Physical assessment of the genital region is not usually performed in the school setting.
- Evaluate for any signs of fever, or underlying systemic disease via history.

Nursing Actions

- Teach the importance of proper hygiene and discourage use of bubble bath, oils, sprays, and powders for students of all ages; teach females to wipe the vaginal region from front to back after urination and defecation.
- If the student is sexually active, suggest the use of condoms.
- Educate adolescents about the broad causes of vaginal infections.
- Instruct the student to avoid tight fitting clothing, sitting in wet bathing suits, or sitting in sand piles or boxes.
- Suggest females wear cotton-lined underpants and remove them before sleeping.
- Teach adolescents to abstain from sexual activities with partners who may have infections. Use of condoms is suggested, along with appropriate hygienic measures after sexual activities.
- Educate females about the avoidance of feminine hygiene sprays, douches, powders, and deodorant tampons; remove tampons after a few hours and replace with a new one.
- Encourage adequate fluid intake.
- Applying cool moist compresses to the labia may be soothing to areas of irritation.
- Support the student/adolescent in a nonjudgmental manner
- Approach the parent or guardian with sensitivity and understanding. The parent or guardian must understand that complaint is physical and assure parent of confidentiality. Refer to the primary care provider.

Dysmenorrhea

Dysmenorrhea is a cramping pain in the lower abdomen that is associated with menstruation (Coco, 1999) and is experienced by 50% of girls (Schmidtt, 2002). Although the exact mechanism is not understood, the uterine prostaglandins are responsible for the symptoms (Neinstein, 2002). Pain may be intermittent, sharp, and extend from the suprapubic area to the back of the legs as well as to the lower back (Coco). Nausea, vomiting, fatigue, and headache may also be presenting complaints. The student develops this problem within the first 3 years of menarche (Coco, 1999). Adolescent females with dysmenorrhea may experience increased absenteeism, which can affect their school performance.

Key History Points

- Obtain a complete menstrual history including:
  - Onset of menstruation
  - Onset of pain with menses
  - Interval and length of menses
  - How dysmenorrhea interferes with daily schedule
  - Is student menstruating now? If not, when is it due?
  - Is there heavy menstrual bleeding?
- Ask about sexual history, including if the student has been treated for sexually transmitted disease or may be pregnant.
- Ask about bowel habits to evaluate if pain may be related to problems of the GI tract.
- Ask about nausea or any associated vomiting or diarrhea with the dysmenorrhea.
- Is pain of the same character as the last time student had menses?
- Does the student take medication for relief of menstrual cramps? What is used?
  - When is medication taken? Does the doctor prescribe this?
  - Does the mother suffer from menstrual cramps?
  - Are any alternative medicines used?
  - Is pain more intense when voiding?

Physical Assessment

- When the student walked into the health office, was she able to walk unaided or was she doubled over clutching her abdomen?
- Assess vital signs.
- Listen for normal bowel sounds and gently palpate the abdomen for GI causes, such as appendicitis.
- Evaluate need for hydration if vomiting is present.

Nursing Actions

- Allay the student's difficulty and embarrassment sometimes associated with discussing menstruation.
- Educate about normal menstruation; provide emotional support and reassurance.
- Educate the student that the problem is physiological and can be treated by the primary care provider.
- Educate the adolescent about simple measures for relief including use of warmth and resting in a comfortable position.
- As an advocate for the student, the nurse should help provide the parent or guardian with education and resources.
- Teach student that regular exercise can decrease the severity of symptoms to varying degrees.
- If allowed by policy, administer ibuprophen 400 to 600 mg q.i.d. (Do not administer if the student might be pregnant.) The use of an over-the-counter nonsteroidal anti-inflammatory agent does limit prostaglandin synthesis and can be helpful with dysmenorrhea, whereas acetaminophen does not affect prostaglandin synthesis.
- It is important for the school nurse to be aware that oral contraceptives are often effective as treatment; alternative therapies such as magnesium and vitamin B_1 may also have some effect (Proctor and Murphy, 2001).
- Provide herbal teas that may release uterine cramping. It is recommended that the student not drink alcoholic beverages, as these release vasopressin and can worsen cramping (Lafferty & Baird, 2001).
- The use of imagery and relaxation techniques was found to be helpful in treating chronic pain by a National Institutes of Health Panel (1996).
- Allow the adolescent to assume a comfortable position. Use local heat on a low setting for 20 minutes, if allowed by protocol. Elevate hips with pillows, putting feet up on the wall to decrease the pressure of the bleeding against the cervical wall (Lafferty & Baird, 2001).

Excessive Menstrual Bleeding

The menstrual cycle normally comes every 28 days +/- 7 days and lasts between 2 and 7 days (Rimsza, 2002). Excessive bleeding is most common in the first 2 years after menarche (Neinstein, 2002; Rimsza, 2002). The blood loss during the entire cycle should be approximately 30 ml with a high range of 80 ml. During the initiation of menstruation, the cycle may be anovulatory and there is disruption of the normal menstrual buildup of the endometrium. This lack of maturity of the hypothalamic–pituitary axis is the most common reason for excessive bleeding but systemic chronic illness, endocrine disorders, gynecological abnormalities, and poor nutrition can be factors (Haven & Sullivan, 2002). It is estimated that 17% of total body fat is need to initiate menses and that 22% is needed to maintain it (Rimsza, 2002). Excessive bleeding can present with short frequent cycles of heavy bleeding or long periods of bleeding.

Key History Points

- Ask about the onset of menses, changes in the length of cycles, number of pads per day, type of pads used, level of saturation, any new changes in bleeding, use of double pads, and accidental breakthroughs.
  - The longer the time between the onset of menses and the onset of excessive bleeding, the less likely it is related to anovulatory cycles.
- Inquire about the use of tampons as well as any possibility that the student may have forgotten to remove the tampon.
- Review all medications being used including contraceptives, acetaminophen, ibuprofen, aspirin, antidepressants, tranquilizers, vitamin E, anticoagulants, and ergogenic products.
- Is the student sexually active?
- Ask about the possibility of pregnancy to rule out a miscarriage.
- Does the student bruise or bleed easily?
- Is there any milk production from the breast?
- Is there any weight loss or gain?
- Is the menstrual cycle of a regular length with a normal interval but with increased bleeding? This is more related to a blood dyscrasia or abnormality of the uterus (Neinstein, 2002).
- Is bleeding prolonged or are menstrual periods more frequent (*associated with anovulatory cycles*).
- Does the adolescent exercise excessively as part of an eating disorder?
- Are menstrual cramps associated with the excessive bleeding?

Physical Assessment

- Assess vital signs, with attention to changes in pulse rate and blood pressure sitting and standing.
- Compare the present height and weight with previously recorded height and weight.
- Calculate the Body Mass Index (BMI).
- Assess the neck for any obvious goiter.
- Assess the back of the neck for hyperpigmentation around the neck or acanthosis nigricans that may indicate insulin resistance (Freeman, 2002).
- Look for signs of eating disorder—emaciated appearance, slow heart rate or bradycardia, dull or thinning hair, sunken cheeks, dry or sallow skin, mouth sores, scratches at the palate or on the fingers (Russell's sign), damaged nail beds, or erosion of the tooth enamel (AAP, 2003d).

Nursing Actions

- Discuss normal menstruation. Have education pamphlets available regarding menstruation.
- Serve as resource for all adolescents; understand the need for sensitivity and confidentiality.
- Teach the student that use of hot tubs during menses may increase blood flow (Schnare, 2002).
- Stress follow-up and routine care with the student. Know community resources for practices that will accommodate all students.

Urinary Frequency

Healthy students without any symptoms may have urinary frequency due to acute or chronic emotional stress (Green, 1998). The student with extraordinary daytime urinary frequency syndrome or pollakiuria may go to the bathroom as frequently as every 5 minutes during the day but sleep through the night (Green, 1998). Students who are cold or excited may also have urinary frequency (Green, 1998). Teachers usually discuss with the school nurse their concern about students who visit the lavatory frequently. However, since diabetes, neurological problems, urological abnormalities, and infections can present with frequency, the nurse has an important role in educating school personnel about problems of urinary frequency so that support for students can be provided. Students with urinary tract infections can present with frequency and burning while urinating. One study estimated that 8.4% of girls and 1.7% of boys have suffered at least one episode by the age of seven (Williams, Lee, & Craig, 2003).

Key History Points

- Review the medical records for any history of spinal bifida occulta or medical problems.
- Has student had recent illness or fever?
- Allow time to establish a relationship to encourage student to talk with you about new stresses including any possible sexual assault.
- Has the student used any prescription medications or over-the-counter drugs recently?
- Ask about burning on urination, especially at the end of voiding.
- Ask whether the student is waking up at night to void.
- Inquire whether the student has noted any blood in the urine.
- Is the student thirsty? How much does he or she drink?
- Has the student lost weight?
- Is there an underlying change in feelings of sadness or mania?
- Has student had sexual intercourse?
- Does the student complain of any symptoms of sexually transmitted diseases?
- Ask all female adolescents about the possibility of pregnancy since this may present with urinary frequency.
- Review the family medical history as appropriate.

Physical Assessment

- Assess the vital signs for any signs of infection.
- Assess for weight changes.
- Does the student look ill?
- Evaluate for signs of diabetes such as acanthosis nigricans (darkening at the back of neck) and obesity.
- Can student point with one finger to area of pain—note the suprapubic region and elicit tenderness in the costovertebral region. (*May indicate pyelonephritis.*)

Nursing Actions

- Discuss with the adolescent female the nature of urinary frequency.

- Teach the family the importance of follow-up with a primary care provider.
- Make sure the student has adequate access to the bathroom until the problem is resolved.
- Educate the teachers and staff about promotion of health and evaluation of common complaints including urinary frequency and about diabetes and the relationship to obesity.
- Notify child protective services about any suspicion of sexual assault.

NEUROLOGICAL PROBLEMS

Headache

Headache is a common symptom in pediatrics. Ninety percent of headaches are benign, usually caused by muscle contraction and/or vascular factors (Lafferty & Baird, 2001). Those due to muscle tension feel like a vise around the head; these may worsen during the day. Headaches can be divided into isolated acute, recurrent acute, chronic nonprogressive, or chronic progressive. Approximately 75% of students will have a headache by the time they are 15 (Forsyth & Farrell, 1999), and headaches are the most prevalent symptom experienced by adolescents (Rhee at al., 2005). Burton et al. (1997) identified the frequency of presenting etiologies to the emergency department as viral illness, sinusitis, migraine, posttraumatic headache, pharyngitis, tension headaches, and psychosocial causes. Migraine headaches account for 1 million school days lost each year (Mao-Draayer & Bingham, 2003). Headaches can be associated with fatigue, hunger, eating certain foods and additives, allergens, light, fever, head injury, sinus problems, and stress (Lafferty & Baird, 2001).

Over-the-counter medications to treat headaches can actually result in a rebound headache, and thus a vicious cycle. The International Headache Society suggests that if analgesics are used more than 9 days each month for headache, the person should be assessed by a physician. Migraine headaches are thought to result from spasm and vasodilation of extracerebral cranial arteries (Lafferty & Baird, 2001). They may be accompanied by nausea and vomiting, photosensitivity, and vision changes.

Key History Points

- Always ask about the quality (dull, aching, acute, throbbing, pressure), radiation, severity, location (unilateral, bilateral, anterior, posterior, facial), exacerbating or alleviating factors, duration and timing, and associated neurological and other symptoms.
- Try to determine if the headache is acute, acute recurrent, or chronic. Is it progressive or not progressive?
- What aggravates the head pain? Does bright light or noise make the headache worse?
- Elicit the names and dosages of over the counter and prescribed medications used, including vitamins, oral acne treatments, or street drugs.
- Ask specifically about the use of oral contraceptives; many adolescents do not associate or consider them as medications.
- What lessens the headache pain?
- What time of day do the headaches occur?
- When and what was the last meal?
- Ask if there is any history of certain foods, such as chocolate, alcohol, and tyramine-cheeses, triggering a headache.
- Are there factors such as stress or anxiety that precipitate the headache?
- Is there a relationship to the menstrual cycle, lack of sleep, excitement, or exercise?
- Is there any reported or observable head trauma?
- Are there recent visual changes?
- Is headache associated with dental work or the need for dental work?
- What is the family's attitude about the headaches?
- Has treatment been initiated for past headaches?
- Have there been recent changes in school performance and attendance?
- Is there a family history of headaches?
- Has there been a recent change in body weight?
- Has the student ever been diagnosed with migraines?
- Does the student have nausea, vomiting, or abdominal pain?
- Are there any visual or auditory auras noted before or after the headache occurs?
- Are there any changes in the family structure?
- Are there any other associated problems since the headaches began?
- Ask open-ended questions about "feelings" to determine relationship to sadness or

anhedonia (the inability to have pleasure from normally pleasurable experiences).

- Red flags in headaches include:
  - Headaches that disrupts sleep. (*May indicate an organic process such as brain tumor.*)
  - Headaches associated with change in academic performances. (*May indicate a brain tumor.*)
  - Headaches that are not helped by analgesics (*may indicate complex migraines, brain tumors, infectious processes*).
  - Early morning headache associated with vomiting. (*May indicate a brain tumor*).
  - Headache associated with stiff neck. (*May indicate meningitis.*)
  - Headaches associated with impaired consciousness. (*May indicate head trauma or brain tumor.*)
  - The student reports, "This headache is the worse headache I ever had." (*May indicate stroke, migraine.*)

Physical Assessment

- Assess vital signs, especially blood pressure changes, fever, and level of consciousness.
- Does the student look ill?
- Assess the eyes, ears, nose. and throat.
  - Evaluate the teeth for any severe caries.
  - Assess for blurred or double vision.
  - Look in the nose for any purulent discharge with foul odor.
  - Look for red eardrum with loss of landmarks.
  - Reevaluate vision screening, if applicable.
- Neck: Are there any signs of nuchal rigidity or spasms of cervical neck muscles?
- Evaluate for any changes in the student's mental status.
- Is there any confusion or problems with speech?
- Are there changes in the student's gait and general motor skills?
- Assess chest and extremities for purpura or other rashes.

Nursing Actions

- Have the student rest in a dark quiet room for a short period unless the student appears acutely ill with a change in mentation.
- Activate the EMS system if headache is associated with significant head trauma and change of level of consciousness.
- Encourage the student to discuss feelings using open-ended questions.
- Offer a snack if the student indicates he or she is hungry or has not eaten.
- Offer the student fluids, especially if the student has not had adequate fluid during the day.
- Educate the parents and student about the need to maintain a diary about headaches to help the primary healthcare provider in the diagnosis.
- Massage the neck and temples.
- Apply cold washcloths over the eyes for 20 minutes.
- If permitted, administer analgesics.

Dizziness

Dizziness is classified into four categories: vertigo, presyncope, disequilibrium, and lightheadedness. Vertigo is a feeling that one is moving either in circles or linearly. The student may have pallor, nausea, vomiting, or perspiration with the vertigo. Students may complain of dizziness by saying they feel like they are on a merry-go-round or that their head is spinning. Students may also complain of feeling off balance (MacGregor, 2002). Vertigo can indicate inner ear disease or another neurological problem. Students may complain of dizziness in order to describe lightheadedness from hyperventilation or from lack of fluid or food (Green, 1998). Many terms can be used by students and adolescents to describe these feelings with each complaint implying a need for a different nursing action.

Key History Points

- Obtain a description of the episode and of any previous attacks. It is helpful to get a description from witnesses.
- What preceded the episode?
- What was the student doing when the episode happened?
- Was the student sitting or standing when the episode occurred?
- Are there any recent illnesses or stressful occurrences in the student's life?
- What medications is the student taking? (*Aspirin or excessive alcohol use can increase symptomatology.*)
- Has the student experienced a change in hearing? Does the student complain of ringing or fullness in the ears?

- Has there been any loss of consciousness or signs of seizure activity?
- Does the student complain of a headache associated with the vertigo?
- Is there a history of trauma to the temporal bone region? Note the locations of point of origin.
- Is the student huffing/sniffing? (*Dizziness can result from toxic fumes, inhalation of gasoline, or solvent sniffing.*)
- Has there been exposure to sun and exercising without fluid replacement? Is there evidence of sweating/diaphoresis?
- Is there possible exposure to carbon monoxide? Do other family members or school peers have chronic headaches?
- Does the student tire easily? Is this a new onset of syncope that may indicate cardiac problems (Ackerman, 1998; Benditt, Lurie, & Fabian, 1997)?

Physical Assessment

- Assess vital signs: Note the rate and rhythm of respirations and pulse. Is the heart rate out of proportion with the temperature? Take blood pressure lying down, sitting, and standing.
- Evaluate the student's affect.
- Note level of anxiousness and/or if there is hyperventilation.
- Observe the student's gait. How does he walk or place his feet?
- Look at extraocular movements of the eye, that is, for nystagmus (rhythmic, rapid eyeball movements).
- Perform a Romberg test. The student should stand with one foot in front of the other with the arms extended, crossed in front, or at the sides. The student does this with the eyes open first and then shut for 30 seconds. Note if the student demonstrates a loss of positional sense.
- Perform a current hearing screening and compare with most recent screening. Document results. A loss of hearing may indicate a labyrinthitis.

Nursing Actions

- Action will depend on the cause:
  - If the student lacks fluid or food, provide adequate fluid replacement.
  - If the student has a fever from environmental problems, cool down and provide fluid.
  - If the student has an inner ear disorder, allow the student to rest in a position of comfort while awaiting arrival of a parent or guardian.
  - If substance abuse is suspected, follow school procedure/policy while offering support and education for referral, safety, and security.
  - If there is a concern about carbon monoxide exposure in the classroom, immediately notify the administration. Provide fresh air to the involved class or relocate them to another area of the school.

Syncope (Fainting)

Syncope is a reversible, acute, transient loss of consciousness and muscle tone (McLeod, 2003). In early adolescents, syncope is reported to be as high as 25%, with peak ages being 15 to 19 years (Rollinson, 2005). Cardiac arrhythmias, vasovagal stimulation, seizures, migraines, breath-holding spells, hypoglycemia, hysteria, and orthostatic and situational events can cause syncope (Lewis & Dhala, 1999). A syncopal episode causes significant anxiety for the family, playmates/peers, and school personnel.

The most common reason for syncope is neurally mediated (Rollinson, 2005); it includes vasovagal and neurocardiogenic syncope (Narchi, 2000). Vasovagal syncope is caused by an autonomic dysfunction of increased vagal tone causing a decrease in heart rate with peripheral vasodilatation (Willis, 2000). This vasodepressor response causes a decrease in cerebral perfusion pressure due to hypotension resulting in a syncopal episode.

Cardiac syncope is associated with little or no prodrome and occurs suddenly even when the student is lying down. However, students with syncope during exercise, with complaints of palpitations, or with chest pain during exercise need emergent medical evaluation (Allen, Golinko, & Williams, 1994). Cardiac syncope may be associated with exercise. There may be a history of palpitations. Students younger than 6 years of age with syncope are more worrisome unless there is an explaining situational problem, such as fear, anxiety, pain, hunger, crowding, fatigue, injection, or the sight of blood.

Syncope can occur when adolescents or preadolescents have been in a warm place, have not eaten, have had limited fluid intake, or stand up too quickly. Situational syncope is common with this age group, especially when seeing blood, fearing immunizations, and so forth. If the student was stretching the arm upward with the spine extended when a syncopal episode occurred, there may be a spine injury as well. A syncopal episode can actually be temporal lobe epilepsy or cough-induced because of poor asthma control.

Key History Points

- Assess the airway first to ensure patency. If the student is still unconscious after 2 minutes, call EMS.
- Does the student have a history of anaphylaxis?
- What happened before the event? What activity was being performed? Was the student exercising at the time?
- What environmental conditions existed when the syncopal event occurred (odors, site, and temperature)?
- What was the position of the patient (sitting, standing, changing positions, running)?
- What is the student's recollection of how he felt or what he saw or heard (aura) before the syncopal episode?
- After the event, the history should include any deficits noted and the time length for recovery and sequelae.
- Witnesses to the event should tell you the length of the episode and the student's appearance. Ask specifically about any cyanosis. Was there incontinence? Were there any unusual eye or limb movements or sounds made by the student during the episode?
- Ask the student about any associated symptoms such as dizziness, palpitation, chest pain, tunneling of vision, headache, belching, yawning, weakness, cold hands, sweating, or nausea prior to the event.
- When was the last time the student ate?
- Does the student engage in breath-holding?
- Inquire about medication or any illicit drug use, including:
  - What was the last medicine or drug taken and at what time?
  - What weight reduction medications, herbal remedies, or over–the-counter (OTC) medications are used? Does student combine prescribed or OTC drugs?
  - Does the student engage in any huffing?
- Is there a history of sudden death in the family?
- Does the medical history include diabetes, cardiac surgery, or Kawasaki's disease?
- What is the social history?
  - Have there been any new stressors in the student's life?
  - Is there a secondary gain that might result from a syncopal episode?

Physical Assessment

- Assess cardiac and neurological systems.
- Assess vital signs.
  - Compare blood pressure in each arm sitting, standing, and supine.
  - Heart rate should be assessed sitting, standing, and supine.
    - Positive orthostatic changes are changes of 20 mm of mercury or more when moving from supine to standing position.
- If the student has diabetes or suspected diabetes and has orders for blood glucose, check blood glucose levels.
- Evaluate the head and neck for any signs of trauma, bruising, or pain on palpation.
- Evaluate cerebral function by asking age-appropriate questions.
- Evaluate for any signs of postictal state.
- Evaluate muscle strength and motor skills by asking student to walk and hop.
- Evaluate lung sounds. (*Cough syncope can be associated with poor control of asthma.*)
- Assess hydration status.
- Evaluate psychological status. Hyperventilation can cause syncope. The student may report feeling anxious, depressed, unable to sleep, or having sensations of unreality.

Nursing Actions

- After a vasovagal episode, allow the student to lie down with the feet elevated (without a pillow under the head) for at least 10 to 20 minutes to increase blood flow to the brain. Continue to offer support and reassurance.
- Allow the student to rest if acutely ill.
- Do not cover the student if he or she was warm before episode.
- Give fluids if the student has not been drinking or eating. Recovery can be prompt with carbohydrate intake, such as fruit juice.
- Educate the student about the importance of fluids and salt in simple syncope (Rollinson, 2005).
- Apply a cold washcloth to the student's forehead.

- Keep the environment free of stimuli.
- Discuss stressors for the particular student and the particular age.

Weakness

Weakness can be a vague symptom that heralds underlying problems in the endocrine, hematological, musculoskeletal, and neurological systems, or that signals the presence of infectious diseases or exposure to toxic substances. Weakness should be differentiated from ataxia. Weakness involves the inability to resist normal strength whereas ataxia is difficulty coordinating movements in a smooth, accurate fashion but with normal strength (Jacobson, 1998). Weakness is a common chronic symptom (Mowad, 1997).

Key History Points

- Ask about the amount and quality of sleep and fluid and food intake.
- Ask about any weight loss or changes in food intake.
- Ask about constipation.
- Is there difficulty in climbing stairs or riding a bike—Is the student able to keep up with his peers when he does this? (*May indicate myopathy or anemia.*)
- Ask the teacher about changes in the student's academic performance.
- Distinguish between acute or chronic weakness. Are the symptoms new or has the student felt weak for prolonged periods?
- Is the weakness symmetrical?
- Does the child have difficulty writing?
- Are there other associated problems that the student can describe aside from weakness?
- Is there any difficulty with swallowing?
- Is there a history of anemia or bruising?
- Is there any new onset of rash on extensor surfaces or on the fingers (*may indicate dermatomyositis*)?

Physical Assessment

- Assess vital signs—note heart rate abnormalities.
- Note any weakness getting up from the floor. The student should not get from sitting to standing using legs or table for support (*Gower's sign indicating myopathy*).
- Note bilateral hand strength.
- Can the student jump up and down?
- Have the student write his or her name or draw.
- Have the student sit and hold the legs out. The student should be able to keep the legs extended for 60 seconds without difficulty.
- Is there generalized laxity of the joint that may present as weakness?
- Do the extremity muscles appear equal or different in size?
- Does the child have unexplained bruising? Are there other signs of anemia, such as paleness? (*May indicate hematological problems, such as leukemia.*)

Nursing Actions

- Encourage the student to eat meals on a regular basis.
- Allow the child to rest and evaluate improvement.

MINOR TRAUMA

Scrapes, Cuts, and Splinters

Many students have minor cuts that do not require any medical intervention other than local first aid. These scrapes are minor and are not deep enough for suturing. Therefore the subcutaneous fat will not be visible in these wounds. These wounds need thorough irrigation with saline or water (Bansal, Wiebe, Perkins, & Abramo, 2002;. Valente, Forti, Freundlich, Zandieh, & Crain, 2003). Abrasions with tattooing of dirt and gravel imbedded into the skin and subcutaneous tissue that cannot be removed with irrigation may need to be cleaned after local injection of lidocaine and therefore will need medical care (Trott, 2002). Organic foreign bodies in the skin, for example, wood or thorns, "usually become infected if they are not removed. Nonorganic slivers (e.g., metal or glass) generally do not" (Schmidtt, 2002).

Key History Points

- Does the student have any medical history that would interfere with wound healing, such as bleeding disorders, diabetes, or immunosuppression?
- What is the mechanism of injury?
  - Get a description of the wounding agent (metal, glass, wood, plants, playground asphalt, dirt, pencil graphite, etc.)
  - Ask about potential contaminants.

- When did the injury happen? How long has the wound been bleeding?
- Was anythinrg put on the wound?
- Is the student on any medication that interferes with normal healing?
- Does the student have a medical condition that may interfere with normal healing, such as diabetes?
- Did the child hit his head?
- When was the last diphtheria and tetanus (dT) immunization?
- Are there any associated symptoms such as pain, paresthesia or funny feelings, or weakness?

Physical Assessment

- Do a brief secondary survey looking for an underlying injury such as other cuts, underlying fracture, or areas of tenderness (see Chapter 22). Make sure to evaluate for point tenderness on the head.
- Look for any problems with motor strength distal to the laceration.
- Inspect the area that is injured.
  - Look at the type and size of scrape or abrasion.
  - Evaluate the depth.
  - Look for foreign bodies, such as splinters.
  - Evaluate the ease in which the bleeding is controlled.

Nursing Actions

For scrapes and cuts:

- Clean the wound using spiral technique described in Box 23.2. Clean the wound away from the area of injury going from inside to outside. Never bring dirt toward the wound.
- Thoroughly irrigate the wound with a physiological solution such as normal saline. However, if you do not have normal saline, a recent study found no difference in healing between water or normal saline in the rate of infection (Fernandez, Griffiths, & Ussia, 2003).
- Do not use agents that are cytotoxic to human fibroblasts, lymphocytes, and inhibit collagen tissue, such as povidone iodine 10%, acetic acid, hydrogen peroxide, and Zephiran (Trott, 2002).
  - The stronger the cleanser, the more toxic it is to cells.
- Using nonionic surfactants such as Shur-Clens or Pharm-Clens which have the cleaning properties of soap avoids tissue toxicity. However, they have no antibacterial activity.
- Apply topicals if allowed by school protocol. Silvadene (silver sulfadiazine RX) and other topical antibiotics have been shown to reduce the bacterial counts of wounds. Topicals do not sterilize the wound, but rather control bacterial growth. However, topicals promote wound reepithelialization (Trott, 2002).
- Let the parent know that the student has a scrape but there is no need to come in.

For splinters:

- Remove splinters before they become hidden by swollen tissue or embedded in issue. These will need to be seen by the primary care provider.
- Superficial splinters may be washed off; some can be removed by using very sticky tape. If using tweezers, sterilize them, wash area

Box 23.2 ■■■

SPIRAL TECHNIQUE FOR WOUND CLEANING

Irrigation is the foundation of good wound cleaning.

Begin at the center and move away to the periphery without crossing back over the wound.

Do not cross over the wound as you work away from it.

Clean the area around the wound until all the debris and dried blood is removed.

Do not scrub the wound since this damages the dermis and other wound tissue.

Do not use soap, hydrogen peroxide, povidone iodine scrub, zephiran, Hibiclens, or pHisoHex on the wound.

In a dirty wound, 1% povidone iodine can be used with minimal toxicity to tissue but irrigation is key.

Information from:
Bansal, B., Wiebe, R., Perkins, S., & Abramo, T. (2002). Tap water for irrigations of lacerations. *The American Journal of Emergency Medicine, 20* (5), 469–472.
Trott, A. (2002). *Wounds and lacerations: Emergency care and closure.* St. Louis: C. V. Mosby.
Valente, J. H. Forti, R., Freundlich, L., Znadieh, S., & Crain, E. (2003). Wound irrigation—Saline vs. tap water? *Annals of Emergency Medicine, 41*, 609–614.

with soap and water (unless the foreign body is wood, since it will swell with water).

- Using a good light source, expose the foreign body, grasp with tweezers and pull out at the same angle it went in (Schmidtt, 2002).
- Wash with soap and water; apply antibiotic ointment if appropriate.

Puncture Wounds

Puncture wounds can be superficial or deep. Puncture wounds are reported to have a high infection rate after animal bites, possibly because of the deposition of bacteria deep in the skin (Medeiros & Saconato, 2003). Wounds that involve the chest, abdomen, neck, and eye are considered serious penetrating trauma (Baldwin & Colbourne, 1999).

Key History Points

- What is the mechanism of injury?
- Where is the wound located?
- What kind of object penetrated the skin and is the object intact?
- Was it through foam rubber inner soles of foot wear? Infection rate is higher if a nail went through tennis shoes.
- When did the student last receive a tetanus shot?

Physical Assessment

- Evaluate the depth of the wound.
- Assess the wound and wound area.
- Assess circulation and motor function distal to the wound.
- Look for any retained foreign body.
- If the puncture occurred hours or days ago, assess for signs of infection: erythema, swelling, and persistent pain.

Nursing Actions

- Clean and irrigate the wound. (Refer to Box 23.2.)
- If the student has stepped on a nail, the student should be referred to the primary care provider. Let the parent know that the student has a puncture wound.
- The usage of antibiotics to prevent infection after such puncture wounds remains controversial, with no clear study pointing to their effectiveness (Harrison, 2002).

CONCLUSION

This chapter has reviewed the common problems that can present to the school nurse office. However, some children will present with unusual complaints that will challenge the nurse. An organized approach to history and physical assessment, well documented to the primary care provider, allows the nurse the opportunity to have a positive impact on the health of the child.

Acknowledgment

The authors would like to thank Tracy Feldman for her contributions of the drawings in this chapter.

Resources

Web site related to the eyes
http://www.ophthalmologyresource.com/

Web sites related to the ears
http://www.vh.org/pediatric/provider/otolaryngology/otitismedia/index.html
http://www.entlink.net (go to education, click on COOL for tutorials)

Information about otitis media and treatment
http://www.rcsullivan.com/www/ears.htm
http://www.kyent.com/eardrum_and_middle_ear. htm

Web site related to the nose
http://www.entusa.com/nose_photos.htm

Web site with content on the oral cavity and the throat
http://www.entusa.com/oral_photos.htm

Web sites related to lung sounds
http://www.rale.ca/
http://www.medstudents.com.br/pneumo/lungsounds/lungsou.htm
http://www.vh.org/adult/provider/internalmedicine/LungSounds/LungSounds.html

References

American Academy of Ophthalmology (AAO). (2002). *Pediatric eye evaluations*. Retrieved April 12, 2003 from http://www.aap.org http://www.aao.org/aao/education/library/loader.cfm?url=/ commonspot/security/getfile.cfm&PageID=16439

American Academy of Pediatrics (AAP). (1996). *The management of acute diarrhea in young children*. Retrieved September 12, 2003 from http://www.aap.org/policy/gastro.htm

American Academy of Pediatrics (AAP). (2003a). Eye examination and vision screening in infants, children, and young adults. *Pediatrics, 111*(4), 902–907.

American Academy of Pediatrics (AAP). (2003b). *Red Book: 2003 Report of the Committee on Infectious Diseases*. Elk Grove Village, IL: American Academy of Pediatrics.

American Academy of Pediatrics (AAP). (2003d). *Identifying and treating eating disorders*. Retrieved September 12, 2003 at http://www.aap.org/policy/020003.html#table3

American College of Asthma, Allergies, and Immunology (ACAAI). (2003). *Summertime: Peak season for seasonal allergies*. Retrieved September 10, 2003 from http://www.pcipr.com/newsroom_archive/ACAAI/screen2001/ACAAI_EdBackgr nd.html

Ackerman, M. (1998). The long QT syndrome. *Pediatrics in Review, 19*(7), 3232–3238.

Allen, H., Golinko, R., & Williams, R. (1994). Heart murmurs in children: When is a workup needed? *Contemporary Pediatrics, 11*(11), 29–52.

Allen, P., & Vessey, J. (2004). School and the child with a chronic condition. In P. Allen & J. Vessey (Eds.), *Primary care of the child with a chronic condition*. St. Louis: C. V. Mosby.

Apley, J. (1975). *The child with abdominal pain* (2nd ed). Oxford: Blackwell.

Arce, D., Ermochilla, C. & Costa, H. (2002). Evaluation of constipation. *American Family Physician, 65*(11), 2283–2290.

Baldwin, G., & Colbourne, M. (1999). Puncture wounds. *Pediatrics in Review, 20*(1), 21–19.

Bansal, B., Wiebe, R., Perkins, S., & Abramo, T. (2002). Tap water for irrigations of lacerations, *The American Journal of Emergency Medicine, 20*(5), 469–472.

Baron, M. (2002). Crohn disease in children. *American Journal of Nursing, 102*(10), 26–31.

Behrman, R., & Kliegman, R. (2002). *Nelson essentials of pediatrics*. Philadelphia: W. B. Saunders.

Benditt, D., Lurie, K., & Fabian, W. (1997). Clinical Approach to diagnosis of syncope: An overview. *Cardiology Clinics, 15*, 165–176.

Berlin H. (2000). The differential diagnosis and management of torticollis in children. *Physical Medicine & Rehabilitation: State of the Art Reviews, 14*(2), 197–206.

Berman, J. (2003). Heading off the dangers of acute gastroenteritis. *Contemporary Pediatrics, 20*(6), 57–66.

Berman, S., & Brayden, R. (2003). Chest pain. In S. Berman (Ed.), *Pediatric decision making* (pp. 286–289) Philadelphia: C. V. Mosby.

Bodemer, C. (2003). Varicella-Zoster Infections. In L. Schachner & R. Hansen (Eds.), *Pediatric dermatology* (pp. 1080–1086). Philadelphia: C. V. Mosby.

Braganza, S., & Adam, H. (2003). Atlantoaxial dislocation. *Pediatrics in Review, 24*(3), 106–107.

Brumund, M., & Strong, W. (2002). Murmurs, fainting, chest pain: Time for a cardiology referral? *Contemporary Pediatrics, 3*, 155–164.

Byrne, P., Tawfilis, A., & Kim, D. (2003). *Facial trauma, nasal trauma*. Retrieved April 12, 2003 from http://www.emedicine.com/plastic/topic482.htm

Burstein, G., & Murray, P. (2003). Diagnosis and management of sexually transmitted diseases among adolescents. *Pediatrics in Review, 24*(4), 119–127.

Burton, L, Quinn, B., Pratt-Cheney, J., & Pourani, M. (1997). Headache etiology in a pediatric emergency department. *Pediatric Emergency Care, 13*, 1–4.

Centers for Disease Control and Prevention (CDC). (2002, October 25). *Guidelines for hand hygiene in Healthcare Settings*. Retrieved September 12, 2003 from http://www.cdc.gov/mmwr/PDF/rr/rr5116.pdf

Centers for Disease Control and Prevention (CDC). (2003, November 21). *Managing Acute Gastroenteritis Among Children*. Retrieved October 24, 2004 from http://www.cdc.gov/mmwr/pdf/rr/rr5216.pdf

Childs, C., Harrison, R., & Hodkinson, C. (1999). Tympanic membrane temperature as a measurement of core temperature. *Archives of Disease in Children, 80*, 262–266.

Coco, A. (1999). Primary dysmenorrhea. *American Family Physician*. Retrieved July 23, 2003 from http://www.aafp.org/afp990800ap/489.html

Colyar, M. (2003). *Well-student assessment for primary care providers*. Philadelphia: F. A. Davis.

Cuculino, G., & DiMarco, C. (2002). Common ophthalmologic emergencies: A systematic approach to evaluation and management. *Emergency Medicine Reports, 23*(13), 164–178.

DiPalma, J., & Gremse, D. (2003). Chronic constipation in children: Rational management. *Consultant for Pediatricians*, 2(4), 151–156.

Elden, L. & Potsic, W. (2002). Screening and prevention of hearing loss in children. *Current Opinion in Pediatrics, 14*, 723–730.

Fernandez, R., Griffiths, R., & Ussia, C. (2003). Water for wound cleansing. [Systematic Review] Cochrane Wounds Group. *Cochrane Database of Systematic Reviews*. 1.

Forsyth, R., & Farrell, K. (1999). Headache in childhood. *Pediatrics in Review, 20*(2), 39–45.

Freeman, S. (2002). Polycystic ovary syndrome: Diagnosis and management. *Women's Health Care, 1*(4), 15–20.

Gluckman, W., Barricella, R., & Quraishi, H. (2002). *Epistaxis*. Retrieved August 30, 2003 from http://www.emedicine.com/ped/topic1618.htm

Goodman, M., & Brady, M. (2000). Respiratory disorders. In C. Burns, M. Brady, A. Dunn, & N. Starr (Eds.), *Pediatric primary care: A handbook for nurse practitioners* (pp. 858–891). Philadelphia: W. B. Saunders.

Green, M. (1998). *Pediatric diagnosis*. Philadelphia: W. B. Sanders.

Gross, C., & Harrison, S. (2000). Tonsils and adenoids. *Pediatrics in Review, 21*(3), 75–78.

Harrison, M. (2002). Antibiotics after puncture wounds to the foot. *Emergency Medicine Journal, 19*(1), 49–53.

Haven, C. S., & Sullivan, N. D. (Eds.) (2002). *Manual of outpatient gynecology*. Baltimore: Lippincott Williams & Wilkins.

Hay, W., Hayward, A., Levin, M. & Sondheimer, J. (2003). *Current pediatrics: Diagnosis & treatment*. New York: Lange Medical Books/McGraw-Hill.

Hertle, R., & Bacal, D. (1997). Traumatic hyphema: Evaluation and management. *Contemporary Pediatrics*. Retrieved April 2, 2003 from http://www.contemporarypediatrics.com

Hoffman, R. (1997). *Evaluating and treating eye injuries. Contemporary Pediatrics*. Retrieved April 2, 2003 from http://www.contemporarypediatrics.com

Irvin, S. M. (1999). Comparison of oral thermometers versus the tympanic thermometer. *Clinical Nurse Specialist, 13(2)*, 85–89.

Jackson Allen, P., & Vessey, J. (2004). *Primary care of the child with a chronic condition*. St. Louis: C. V. Mosby.

Jacobson, R. (1998). Approach to the child with weakness or clumsiness. *Pediatric Clinics of North America, 45*(1), 145–168.

Jones, C. M., Tinanoff, N., Edelstein, B. L., Schneider, D. A., De-Berry-Sumner, B., Kanda, M. B., Brocato, R. J., Blum-Kemelor, D., & Mitchell, P. (2000). Creating partnerships for improving oral health of low-income children. *Journal of Public Health Dentistry, 60*(3), 193–195.

Kautz, S. M., & Skaggs D. L. (1998). Getting an angle on spinal deformities. *Contemporary Pediatrics, 15*(9), 111–112, 114, 117–118.

Kocis, K. C. (1999). Chest pain in pediatrics. *Pediatric Clinics of North America, 46*, 189–197.

Lafferty, S., & Baird, M. (2001). *Tele-Nurse: Telephone triage protocols*. Clifton Park, NY: Thomson Delmar Learning.

Lai, S., & Tom, L. (2001). Allergic rhinitis in children. *Current Opinion in Otolaryngology and Head and Neck Surgery, 9*, 359–364.

Leicke-Rude, M. K., & Bloom, L. (1998). A comparison of temperature taking methods in neonates. *Neonatal Network, 17*(5), 21–36.

Leung, A., & Kao, P. (2003). Oral lesions in children, *Consultant for Pediatricians, 2*(2), 81–82.

Lewis, D., & Dhala, A. (1999). Syncope in the pediatric patient: The cardiologist's perspective. *Pediatric Clinics of North America, 46*(2), 205–219.

Lorin, M. I. (2000). Fever in critically ill patients. *Seminars in Pediatric Infectious Diseases, 11*(1), 13–18.

MacGregor, D. (2002). Vertigo. *Pediatrics in Review, 23*(1), 11–16.

Mao-Draayer, Y., & Bingham, P. (2003). Two teenagers with headaches. *Pediatric Case Review, 3*(3), 117–126.

Marinella, M. (1998). *Electrocardiographic manifestations and differential diagnosis of acute pericarditis. American Family Physician*. Retrieved September 10, 2003 from http://www.aafp.org/afp/980215ap/marinell.html

Matz, P. (2002). Acute otitis media. *Pediatric Case Reviews, 2*(4), 209–217.

McLeod, K. A. (2003). Syncope in childhood. *Archives of Diseases in Studenthood, 88*, 350–353.

Medeiros, I., & Saconato, H. (2003). Antibiotic prophylaxis for mammalian bites. [Systematic Review]. *Cochrane Wounds Group Cochrane Database of Systematic Reviews*. 1.

Mofidi, M., Rozier, G., & King, R. (2002). Problems with access to dental care for Medicaid-insured children: What caregivers think. *American Journal of Public Health, 92*(1), 53–58.

Mowad, E. (1997). Chronic weakness. In J. C. Gartener & B. Zitelli (Eds.), *Common and chronic symptoms in pediatrics* (pp. 143–160). St. Louis: C. V. Mosby.

Narchi, H. (2000). The student who passes out. *Pediatrics in Review, 21*, 384–388.

Neinstein, L. (2002). *Adolescent health care: A practical guide*. Philadelphia: Lippincott Williams & Wilkins.

National Institutes of Health (NIH) Panel. (1996). Integration of behavioral and relaxation approaches into the treatment of chronic pain and insomnia. NIH Technology Assessment Panel on integration of behavioral and relaxation approaches into the treatment of chronic pain and insomnia. *Journal of the American MedicalAssociation, 276*(4), 313–318.

Niskar, A. S., Kieszak, S. M., Holmes, A. E., Esteban, E., Rubin, C., & Brody, D. J. (2001). Estimated prevalence of noise-induced hearing threshold shifts among children 6 to 19 years of age: The Third National Health and Nutrition Examination Survey, 1988–1994, United States. *Pediatrics, 108*(1), 40–43.

Nurko, S. (2001). CME: Managing constipation: Evidence put to practice. *Contemporary Pediatrics, 12*, 56–65.

Olive-Hemker, M. (1999). More than a gut reaction: Extraintestinal complications of IBD. *Contemporary Pediatrics, 10*, 45–53.

Osterhoudt, K. (2002). Experiencing ectasy: Is it all the rave? *Pediatric Case Reviews, 2*(2), 126–129.

Patel, D., Greydanus, D., & Pratt, H. (2001). Youth sports: More than sprains and strains. *Contemporary Pediatrics, 18*, 45–54.

Pisarra, V. (1999). Recognizing the various presentations of appendicitis. *The Nurse Practitioner, 24*(8), 42–53.

Proctor, M., & Murphy, P. (2001). Herbal and dietary therapies for primary and secondary dysmenorrhoea. [Systematic Review] Cochrane Menstrual Disorders and Subfertility Group. *Cochrane Database of Systematic Reviews*. 1.

Rhee, D. J., & Pyfer, M. D. (Eds). (1999). *The Wills eye manual* (3rd ed.) Philadelphia: Lippincott Raven.

Rhee, H., Miles, M., Halpern, C., & Holditch-Davis, D. (2005). Prevalence of recurrent physical symptoms in U.S. adolescents. *Pediatric Nursing, 31*(4), 314–319, 350.

Rimsza, M. (2002). Dysfunctional uterine bleeding. *Pediatrics in Review, 23*, 227–233.

Rollinson, N. (2005). Understanding and managing neurally mediated syncope in the adolescent. *Journal of School Nursing, 21*(4), 200–207.

Roma, E., Adamidis, D., Nikolara, R., Constantopoulos, A., & Messaritakis, J. (1999). Diet and chronic constipation in children: The role of fiber. *Journal of Pediatric Gastroenterology and Nutrition, 28*, 169–174.

Rubinstein, E., & Strong, E. B. (2000) Management of nasal fracture. *Archives of Family Medicine, 9*, 738–742.

Rudolph, A., Kamei, R., & Overby, K. (Eds). (2002). *Rudolph's fundamentals of pediatrics*. New York: McGraw-Hill.

Schmidtt, B. (2002). *Pediatric telephone protocols*. Evanston, IL: American Academy of Pediatrics.

Schnare, S. (2002). Abnormal and dysfunctional uterine bleeding. *Women's Health Care, 1*(5), 25–31.

Schroeder, B. (2003, February 13). *Practice guidelines: Diagnosis and management of Group A streptococcus infections*. Retrieved September 6, 2003 from http://www.aafp.org/afp/20030215/practice.html

Selbst, S. (1997). Chest pain in children. *Pediatrics in Review, 18*(5), 169–173.

Simons, J., & Kaw, P. (2001). Vision screening performed by the pediatrician. *Pediatric Annals, 30*, 446–452.

Sokol, J., & Hyde, M. (2002). Hearing screening. *Pediatrics in Review*, 23, 155–161.

Stickler, G. (2002). Recurrent abdominal pain. *Pediatric Case Reviews, 2*(2), 95–99.

Stockard-Pope, J. (2001). Auditory development and hearing evaluation in children. *Advances in Pediatrics, 48*, 273–299.

Taketomo, C., Hodding, J. H., & Kraus, D. (2004). *Pediatric dosage handbook* (11th ed.). Hudson, OH: Lexi-comp.

Tanyi, R. (2003). Sickle cell disease: Health promotion and maintenance and the role of primary care nurse practitioners. *Journal of the American Academy of Nurse Practitioners, 15*(9), 389–397.

Teoh, D., & Reynold, S. (2003). Diagnosis and management of pediatric conjunctivitis. *Pediatric Emergency Care, 19*(1), 48–55.

Thiessen, P. (2002). Recurrent abdominal pain. *Pediatrics in Review, 23*(2), 39–45.

Toback, S. (2003). Nasal septal hematoma in an 11-month-old infant: A case report and review of the literature. *Pediatric Emergency Care, 19*(4), 265–267.

Trott, A. (2002). *Wounds and lacerations: Emergency care and closure*. St. Louis: C. V. Mosby.

Tunnessen, W. (1999). *Signs and symptoms in pediatrics* (3rd ed.). Philadelphia: Lippincott Williams & Wilkins.

U.S. Food and Drug Administration (FDA). (2003). *2003 Safety alerts for drugs, biologics, medical devices, and dietary supplements*. Retrieved August 17, 2003 from http://www.fda.gov/medwatch/SAFETY/2003/safety03.htm pama

Valente, J. H. Forti, R., Freundlich, L., Znadieh, S., &Crain, E. (2003). Wound irrigation: Saline vs. tap water? *Annals of Emergency Medicine, 41*, 609–614.

Watts, R., Robertson, J., & Thomas, G. (2003). Nursing management of fever in children: A systematic review. *International Journal of Nursing Practice, 9*(1), S1–S8.

Williams, G. J., Lee, A., & Craig, J. C. (2003). Long-term antibiotics for preventing recurrent urinary tract infection in children. [Systematic Review]. Cochrane Renal Group. *Cochrane Database of Systematic Reviews*. 1.

Willis, J. (2000). Syncope. *Pediatrics in Review, 21*, 201–204.

Wilshaw, R., Beckstrand, R., Waid, D., & Schaalje, G. B. (1999). A comparison of the use of tympanic, axillary, and rectal thermometers in infants. *Journal of Pediatric Nursing, 14*(2), 88–93.

Wong, D., Hockenberry-Eaton, M., Wilson, D., Winkelstein, M., & Schwartz, P. (2001). *Wong's essentials of pediatric nursing*. St. Louis: C. V. Mosby.

Wright, K. (2003). *Pediatric ophthalmology for primary care*. Evanston, IL: American Academy of Pediatrics.

Wubbel, C., & Faro, A. (2003). Chronic cough in children. *Pediatric Case Reviews, 3*(2), 95–104.

Young, M. (2001). *Dermatologic signs of systemic disease. Patient Care*. Retrieved September 15, 2002 from http://www.patientcareonline.com

Zeiter, D., & Hyams, J. (2001). Clinical aspects of recurrent abdominal pain. *Pediatric Annals, 30*(1), 17–21.

Zitelli, B. & Davis, H. (2002). *Atlas of pediatric physical diagnosis*. Philadelphia: C. V. Mosby.

Chapter 24

Athlete Health Promotion

JANICE DENEHY

Chapter Outline

INTRODUCTION

Approximately 30 million children and adolescents participate in organized sports each year (CDC, 2002); millions more engage in sporting activities with friends. Students may participate in recreational, club, or competitive athletic activities from the time they enter preschool through their high school years. There are numerous opportunities for both girls and boys to engage in a wide variety of sports. With this participation, there are many benefits, but there are also health risks to consider. As advocates for student health, school nurses play an important role in advising and educating students, parents, staff, coaches, administrators, and the community regarding developmentally appropriate activities and environments that promote health and fitness of young athletes.

A Consensus Statement from the National Athletic Trainers' Association, Appropriate Medical Care for Secondary School-Age Athletes suggests that the Athletic Health Care Team should include trainers, team physicians, school nurses, physical therapists, emergency medical services, dentists, and other healthcare professionals (NASN, 2002). Appropriate care of the student athlete goes beyond basic emergency care that may be needed during participation, but also includes the prevention and rehabilitation of athletic injuries.

There is no shortage of literature on sports and health-related concerns for athletes of all ages and levels, from the very young child to the elder athlete, from recreational activities to organized sport, as well as from amateur players to the professional athlete. There are hundreds of articles in the health-related literature that speak to sports from golf, skiing, bicycling, diving, bowling, table tennis, badminton, bungee jumping, rodeo, and baton twirling to the more common sports seen in school athletic programs, such as football, baseball, track, volleyball, and basketball. This chapter focuses on the more common concerns that can apply to students participating in recreational activities as well as the needs of the student athlete participating in school-sanctioned programs.

Because school nurses are in the position to address parental questions about athletic participation on issues related to appropriateness for age and developmental level, the benefits and risks of participation, as well as how the time invested in sport may affect their child's family life and academic achievement, it is essential that school nurses have up-to-date information on which to base anticipatory guidance, policy development, and care of the student athlete. School nurses also need to be well informed about the potential risks involved in participation so they can provide appropriate education to students, parents, coaches, administrators, and the community in order to prevent injuries and promote athlete health. They also may monitor students who have been injured during practice or competition and make recommendations for treatment, rehabilitation, and safe return to play.

The purpose of this chapter is to present an overview of the benefits and risks of participation in sports, to discuss the major developmental, physiological, psychological, and environmental perspectives related to athlete health, and to outline the role of the school nurse in promoting the health of student athletes.

Box 24.1 ■ ■ ■

BILL OF RIGHTS FOR YOUNG ATHLETES

Right to participate in sports

Right to participate at a level commensurate with each child's maturity and ability

Right to have qualified adult leadership

Right to play as a child and not as an adult

Right of children to share in the leadership and decision-making of their sport participation

Right to participate in safe and healthy environments

Right to proper preparation for participation in sports

Right to an equal opportunity for success

Right to be treated with dignity

Right to have fun in sports

(Martens & Seefelt, 1979)

THE BENEFITS AND RISKS OF PARTICIPATION

The American Academy of Pediatrics (AAP) states: "Participation in organized sports can have physical and social benefits for children" (AAP, 2001a). Today, with the concern about the lack of exercise among children and the epidemic of obesity, participation in sports is one avenue to generate interest in physical activity and life-long involvement in activities that would promote health. Parents may enroll their young school-age children in recreational sport programs to increase their physical activity and to develop skills in a particular sport. Participation in a sport should be fun for young children, reinforcing physical activity early in life. As children get older, participation in sports helps the student develop and refine skills, learn to cooperate as a team member, and develop collegiality and school spirit. The Bill of Rights for Young Athletes (Box 24.1) lists the rights of students to participate at a level appropriate to their age and ability in a safe and healthy environment (Martens & Seefelt, 1979).

Although benefits are gained with involvement in sports, there are also potential risks to the student athlete. The American Academy of Pediatrics (AAP, 2001a) cautions parents and healthcare professionals about involvement when the demands of the sport exceed the child's cognitive and physical development. The AAP also cautions that parental involvement and pressure can be discouraging to the young child.

While the American Academy of Pediatrics recommends that children and adolescents participate in a variety of different activities to develop a wide range of skills and interests, many young athletes are specializing in one sport at an early age (AAP, 2000b). These student athletes may practice year around at a high intensity level to achieve "elite" status. A number of high-profile sports, such as gymnastics, swimming, figure skating, and tennis, include many talented young athletes performing at the amateur, professional, and Olympic levels. Young athletes and their parents, in their quest for a college scholarship or professional career, spend an inordinate amount of time practicing a single sport at all hours of the day, limiting their time for family, school, and peer-related activities, and increasing the risk of overuse trauma.

In younger children, the risk of serious injury is low. As students begin to engage in competitive sports, the number of injuries rises, especially during practice and competition. While the number of injuries is highest during practice sessions because of the greater number of athletes participating, injuries suffered during competition tend to be more serious. It is estimated that 20% of young people involved in a sport are injured each year. The majority of these injuries are bruises; inflammation of bones, joints, or muscles; muscle strains; ligament sprains; or minor bone fractures (National Safe Kids Campaign, 1996). For most, these injuries are not serious, and full recovery is expected. For others, an injury may mean a long recovery period, missed practices and competition, or an end to the athletic season.. The older and bigger the athlete and the more contact that is involved in the sport, the greater the risk of injury. Baseball has the greatest risk of serious injury, including injury to the eye or chest from direct contact with the ball. Basketball, soccer, wrestling, and gymnastics also have high rates of injury. Fortunately, most sports injuries are preventable (Bennett, 2001).

The school nurse needs to educate all involved in student sports that the physical and psychological benefits need to be balanced with the needs of the growing student. Student athletes and parents need to be aware of the potential problems with intense physical training and competition. Primary healthcare providers should monitor the physical and psychological health of these athletes and intervene to prevent long-term effects of overuse and stress associated with performing at a high level (AAP, 2000b).

DEVELOPMENTAL PERSPECTIVES

Elementary School Children

Parents are encouraging their children at younger and younger ages to become involved in organized sports, including T-ball, soccer, dance, softball, and gymnastics. This encouragement stems from the belief that by enrolling their children in a specific program, they will develop the physical skills and experience needed to become proficient in that sport as well as the social sense of commitment and belonging. There may be the feeling that this is an expectation for children today. However, many children have been enrolled in programs without considering their cognitive readiness or developmental level.

Children generally express a desire to participate, anticipating fun and the opportunity to play with their friends. They enjoy being part of a team and the action involved. However, many younger children do not have the cognitive maturity to understand the rules or strategy involved in many sports. Their coping skills may not be developed to the point where they can deal with stress, disappointment, or success or failure. Elementary school children should focus on the fun, participation, and trying out a variety of sports. The emphasis should be on learning basic skills and teamwork—not on winning.

School nurses can help students and parents find a good fit for the individual child by considering the growth and development of the child and the opportunities available in the community. Young children should have the opportunity to engage in free play and explore multiple areas. The school nurse can share this information in conjunction with physical education teachers via newsletters home to parents.

Middle School Children

As students mature in their physical ability, they are able to refine their skills and handle the stress of team play and competition. Middle school students are ready for new challenges, both individually and as members of a team. These student athletes may emulate a particular professional sports figure they admire. This may promote the formation of goals for future performance and participation in a particular activity. This is also a time when competition rather than participation becomes the focus, often resulting in students dropping out of athletic activities because they feel that participating is no longer fun. Parents, coaches, and other significant adults can have a major impact on encouraging or dissuading young people in their athletic participation. Fear of "performing" and feeling they are not good enough can inhibit a student's participation in sports, as can the destructive power of teasing.

Middle school students are still concrete thinkers and "live in the moment." They understand about rules of the game and begin to understand about strategy. Physically, they are beginning puberty, with significant growth in their bones and muscles as well as changing body proportions. Flexibility may decrease, making them more prone to overuse injury.

School nurses are in a position to give anticipatory guidance to parents and children about the psychological effects on those who are not physically gifted or may not have the competitive drive or discipline needed to succeed in a particular sport. Of particular concern is that many middle school students, especially girls, drop out of sports, which may influence their attitude about physical activity and interfere with the establishment of healthy practices that should carry into adulthood (Petlichkoff, 1992). At a time when health professionals are concerned about the lack of opportunities for physical activity by today's youth, school nurses can be resources for other options that give students age 11 to 14 an opportunity to be physically active. This may include lifetime physical activities, such as running, biking, fitness activities, skating, dancing, walking, martial arts, skateboarding, and skiing.

High School Students

School-sponsored high school athletics offers an opportunity for students to further develop their physical and leadership skills and compete with school teams from neighboring communities. School spirit and loyalty provide an opportunity to promote teamwork and to widen the horizons of the student athlete. Participation in organized high school sports gives students the opportunity to refine specific sport-related skills and gain recognition among their peers. However, the drive to win may overshadow proper training and reporting injuries. It may also result in feelings of frustration and failure by those who may find themselves on the bench or cut from the team. At this level, there may be limited places, for participants in team sports; therefore, only the most talented secure a place on the team. The emphasis clearly moves from participation to competition and winning. The number of students participating in sports declines as the less talented athletes may not make the teams, while others may drop out because of the time required or intensity of practice sessions, the stress related to competition, or because they are not comfortable with the pressure to win or the persons running the program.

However, there are still physical activities in which all students participate. Physical education class is a requirement for almost all students at some point during high school. Work-out rooms and swimming pools are very popular in some schools and provide an ideal site for students to see faculty and staff also engaging in healthy behaviors. School dances are an excellent venue for encouraging activity. Students may be encouraged to bike to school or walk around the track during lunchtime or after school.

THE PREPARTICIPATION PHYSICAL EXAMINATION

Prior to participation in any sport, a preparticipation physical examination (PPE) is recommended for younger student athletes and required for those engaging in competitive sports. This screening exam is designed to determine general health status, maturity, readiness for participation, and performance capacity (Mills & Muscari, 1998). Although the preparticipation examination may identify some individuals who may require treatment, the intent is to ensure that students are medically cleared for the activity in which they wish to participate. Therefore, 4 to 6 weeks prior to the first practice is an ideal time for the exam. Physical fitness may be tested, and limitations for participation identified and treated prior to participation (American College of Sports Medicine [ACSM], 1994). The American Academy of Pediatrics (2001a) recommends that physicians and other health professionals use this exam as an opportunity to assess developmental readiness and medical suitability of students to participate in organized sports, as well as "matching the child's physical, social, and cognitive maturity with appropriate sports activities."

While the PPE should not be a substitute for routine health care, for many students it is their only contact with healthcare providers. Therefore, it is an ideal time for screening, evaluation, and health teaching (Myers & Sickles, 1998). Questions about allergies, the use of nutritional supplements, menstrual history, and any existing chronic conditions will guide the healthcare provider and the school nurse in providing relevant information to the student in order to maintain nutritional and physical safety or make adjustments in athletic activities. This information might also identify areas where the athletic staff needs inservice education in order to prevent problems or modify the athletic experience.

The PPE is a good time to talk to parents about the benefits and potential risks involved in sports participation, such as the change in nutritional needs, the need for protective equipment and sunscreen, and the need to balance the sport with the student's educational and recreational goals. Strategies to promote health and prevent sports injuries should be discussed with both the student athlete and the parents. The school nurse can partner with nurse practitioner programs to have detailed PPE of students accomplished at no cost on site. In many school districts, it is the responsibility of school nurses to review the PPE and to ensure that recommended measures are initiated.

PHYSIOLOGICAL ISSUES

Nutrition for Student Athletes

An important component of athlete health promotion is emphasis on good nutrition and appropriate caloric intake needed for the increased activity level during practice and competition. This is particularly important during adolescence, a time of rapid growth second only to the rapid growth experienced during infancy. Not only does good nutrition support normal growth and activity, but the nutritional practices developed in childhood and adolescence often persist into adulthood. Therefore, healthy nutritional practices are essential to set the stage for healthy nutritional choices throughout life. This is particularly challenging at a time when fast-paced family life and the full schedules of student athletes may make snacks and fast foods particularly attractive. In addition, adolescents are not known for their healthy diets, preferring high-fat, high-calorie, and high-sodium foods readily available and acceptable to this age group.

Another barrier faced by student athletes in getting adequate nutrition is their daily schedule. Many students come to school early in the day, eat during an early lunch period, and practice until dinnertime. Early school start times may prevent many students from eating a nutritionally adequate breakfast, an important meal to fuel the body for the day's activities. Students who rely on school buses for transportation to school, especially in rural areas, may need to rise an hour earlier to catch the bus, making breakfast time rushed or skipped altogether. Lunchtimes often occur from 10:30 to 1:30 and range from 20 to 45 minutes. While the schedule may depend on school start time, often it is random or based on class schedule.

The main concern is that an early lunch and after school practice or competition for student athletes results in a long time interval between lunch and the family dinner hour. Under these circumstances, the student athlete will require caloric and fluid intake prior to and during practice, particularly if practice is intense or the weather is hot. Too often, however, the most available foods to be found after school are located in vending machines that dispense snack foods that are high in calories, but low in nutritional value. Although there is a trend to limit non-nutritious foods in vending machines and substitute them with healthy alternatives, these options are expensive if used as a regular source of nutrition and fluid supplementation.

Other athletes may practice early in the morning before school, thus making it difficult for them to eat breakfast prior to the practice or going to classes directly after practice without adequate intake to cover the calories burned during practice or to prepare for the activities of the day. Taking healthy food with them to eat prior to the start of classes is a good practice to encourage. This may include fresh fruit, cereal bars, sandwiches, milk, fruit juices, or other foods high in protein and carbohydrates needed to provide energy.

It is generally accepted "that physical activity, athletic performance, and recovery from exercise are enhanced by optimal nutrition" (ACSM, 2000, p. 2130). While student athletes may need more calories because of increased energy expenditure due to exercise, they do not require a special diet. They may require extra carbohydrates for energy and protein for cell repair and endurance. A normal healthy diet and a variety of foods representing all food groups in the food pyramid are critical for maintenance of normal weight and mineral stores, just as for any other student. Fat should not be restricted, as it provides energy and essential nutrients. There is no evidence that a diet high in carbohydrates, protein, or fats has a positive effect on performance (ACSM, 2000).

To promote health and performance, it is important to consider not only the selection of nutrients and fluids, but also the timing of one's intake. During periods of high activity, such as practice or competition, energy and nutrition needs must be met to restore energy stores, maintain body weight, and repair muscle tissue. Adequate intake of carbohydrates and proteins, as well as an adequate fat intake, are necessary to assist in weight maintenance and the absorption of fat-soluble vitamins.

Prior to practice, a meal or snack should provide carbohydrates necessary for energy, fluids to maintain hydration, and a moderate amount of protein. The preparticipation meal needs to be easily digested and low in fat and fiber to reduce gastric distress. During practice and competition, adequate energy (calories) needs to be consumed to maintain body weight and maximize performance. Inadequate energy reserves during exercise may result in loss of muscle mass, menstrual dysfunction, fatigue, injury, or illness. Carbohydrate consumption during exercise is essential to maintain blood glucose levels and to restore glycogen stores. After heavy exertion (training, practice, or competition), adequate carbohydrates need to be consumed to replace glycogen stores and to promote rapid recovery, and proteins are needed to repair and build muscles. Therefore, a meal with a variety of nutrients is recommended post exercise. All of this information needs to be taught to student athletes (and coaches, if necessary) to assist them if maximizing their performance both in the sport and in the classroom.

Hydration

In addition to good nutrition, adequate hydration is essential to athlete health, especially when the temperature and/or humidity are high (Vepraskas,

2002). Remember, even though it may be cool outdoors, when practice and competition take place indoors, the temperature in these venues may be higher for active students. Student athletes need to replace fluids regularly during workouts, practice, or competition. Water breaks should be incorporated into practice sessions and monitored by coaches, with the knowledge that adequate hydration not only promotes the health of athletes, but also enhances their performance and endurance.

Dehydration decreases athletic performance and increases the risk of fatigue, injury, and illness (ACSM, 2000). Athletes need to consume sufficient fluids to replace fluid losses. Again, timing of consumption is critical. Fluid intake before, during, and after practice or competition is essential. Two hours prior to exercise, athletes should consume 14 to 22 oz. of fluids. During practice or competition, 6 to 12 oz. should be consumed every 15 to 20 minutes, and after exercise, athletes should drink sufficient fluids to replace sweat and weight loss (ACSM, 2000). Adequate hydration after exercise promotes recovery. Hydration requirements may vary for individual athletes based on gender, size of the individual, nature of the sport, intensity of the exercise, and environmental conditions.

Although water is often the preferred liquid to maintain hydration, athletes who participate in vigorous exercise or compete in extreme weather conditions will benefit from sports drink with carbohydrates with a concentration of 4% to 8%. Higher concentrations may reduce gastric emptying and bioavailability (ACSM, 2000). Many sports drinks contain only sugars, sucrose, fructose, and corn syrup that provide energy but do not replace electrolytes lost in sweat. These drinks are *not* the best choice for extended activity, but "the sweetness of energy drinks may be more appealing to children than water (and)... may be helpful in getting the child to consume more fluids" (MayoClinic.com, n.d.). Although hyponatremia may occur after vigorous exercise, there appears to be no advantage to replacing electrolytes after intense exercise lasting less than an hour, especially if salt was in the preparticipation meal. For longer exercise sessions, including sodium seems to enhance the drive to drink, increasing the amount of fluids consumed during exercise (ACSM, 2000).

Many intense sports are played under conditions that could potentially result in heat cramps, heat exhaustion, and heat stroke. Football, cross country running, and soccer are played in late summer and fall, while track, soccer, and softball are played in the spring and summer. In many geographical locations, any season may present the potential for heat-related illness in athletes who do

Table 24.1 ■

HEAT-RELATED ILLNESS: SYMPTOMS AND TREATMENT

HEAT DISORDER	SYMPTOMS	TREATMENT
Heat cramps	Painful cramping usually in the legs or abdomen; heavy perspiration; nausea	Move to a cool, shady area; firm, gentle massage to cramp; drink at least 4 oz. of fluid every 15 minutes
Heat exhaustion	Dizziness, headache; normal temperature possible; weakness and fatigue; heavy perspiration; nausea; cold, pale, clammy skin	Move to a cool, shady area; loosen clothing; fan student; drink at least 4 oz. of fluid every 15 min; apply cool, wet cloths to neck, forehead, and underarms
Heat stroke	Hot, red and dry skin; absence of sweating; rapid, strong pulse; nausea/vomiting; confusion, incoherent speech; possible seizures; possible loss of consciousness; body temperature ranges from 102° to 106°	Call 911, medical emergency; move to a cool or air-conditioned area; fan student; loosen clothing; cool with cool bath or sponging; take temperature, if able; lie supine with feet elevated; if vomiting, turn on the side; do not give fluids if unconscious, confused or seizing.

Source: Vepraskas (2002, p. 239).

Temperature	Relative Humidity (%)									
(F)	90.0	80.0	70.0	60.0	50.0	40.0	30.0	20.0	10.0	
75	79.7	76.7	75.8	74.8	73.9	72.9	72.0	71.1	70.1	Green Zone Below 80
80	88.2	85.9	84.2	82.8	81.6	80.4	79.0	77.4	76.1	
85	101.4	97.0	93.3	90.3	87.7	85.5	83.5	81.6	79.6	
90	119.3	112.0	105.8	100.5	96.1	92.3	89.2	86.5	84.2	
95	141.8	131.1	121.7	113.6	106.7	100.9	96.1	92.2	89.2	Yellow Zone 80 to 100
100	168.7	154.0	140.9	129.5	119.6	111.2	104.2	98.7	94.4	
105	200.0	180.7	163.4	148.1	134.7	123.2	113.6	105.8	100.0	Red Zone Above 100
110	235.6	211.2	189.1	169.4	151.9	136.8	124.1	113.7	105.8	

Green Zone : Outdoor conditions ideal.
Yellow Zone: Heat exhaustion possible with prolonged exposure & activity
Red Zone: Heat cramps & exhaustion likely with prolonged exposure. Heatstroke possible. Limit or cancel outdoor rehearsals.

Figure 24.1 ■ Heat index chart. (From Vepraskas, 2002, p. 240.)

not take precautions to maintain adequate hydration. The National Weather Service has developed guidelines to assist coaches and athletes in making decisions about the safety and wisdom of practicing or competing in extreme weather conditions (FIGURE 24.1). Vepraskas (2002) recommends that school nurses educate student athletes, parents, band directors, and coaches about the potential health dangers of dehydration. She developed a chart outlining the symptoms and treatment of heat-related illness (TABLE 24.1). In addition to concern about athletic participation in heat, there are also concerns about participation in dry, cold weather and at high altitudes.

Weight Management

Of special concern are student athletes participating in those sports in which weight is an issue—either when weight gain is desired, as in football, or when weight is restricted, as in rowing, wrestling, cheerleading, diving, ski jumping, or gymnastics. Wrestling can fall into either category. Major concern has been expressed about the health of students when weight requirements are a prerequisite to competition. In sports in which maintaining or attaining a certain weight determine eligibility to compete, athletes may resort to extreme methods to achieve the desired weight goal without regard to the effects such methods may have on their health as well as their performance. Ideally, this weight change should be accomplished slowly, and during the off-season or the beginning of the season prior to the start of competition in consultation with a registered dietitian or healthcare provider.

For athletes who participate in sports that may encourage fast weight gain, a well balanced diet from all food groups is essential. It is important to make sure quality foods are ingested. Diets high in protein may encourage muscle growth, but also may be high in cholesterol. High intake of refined carbohydrates may be detrimental to dental health and provide minimal nutrients.

There is a great emphasis by many sports coaches on body weight of athletes. It is often these coaches who mandate that students lose weight to attain specific weight limits without regard to the student's percentage of body fat. There has been considerable discussion about the appropriateness of weight restrictions, especially for high school wrestlers, at a time when adolescent growth is normal and expected, and adequate nutrition is essential to support the physical and sexual development characteristic of this developmental period.

Practices resulting in rapid weight loss have been common among wrestlers for decades, despite documentation of the potential harmful effects of such practices and the development of guidelines to regulate unhealthy practices (ACSM, 1996). The American College of Sports Medicine has developed recommendations of body fat percentages as measured by body composition testing; it recommends that male wrestlers 16 years of age and younger with a body fat percentage less than 7% and those older than 16 with a body fat percentage of less than 5% not be allowed to compete without medical clearance, noting that a body fat percentage of over 5% is necessary for normal physiological functioning. The average body fat for high school males is 15%, while the average percentage for wrestlers is 8% to 11% during the off-season and 6% to 7% during the season (ACSM, 1996).

When student athletes restrict energy (caloric) intake, "fat and lean muscle mass will be used by the body for fuel" (ACSM, 2000, p. 2132), resulting in loss of strength and endurance. Athletes who participate in sports where maintaining or attaining an unusually low weight for body size is desired need extra care in selecting a well-balanced diet. Students who severely restrict dietary intake may require a multivitamin and mineral supplement to ensure adequate intake of micronutrients (ACSM, 2000). The diets of many adolescents, particularly females, may be deficient in calcium, iron, and zinc (ACSM, 2000). Monitoring the diets of athletes for adequate nutrient intake is essential, particularly those restricting their diets or participating in vigorous endurance training and competition.

To "make weight," as many as 25% to 67% of high school wrestlers restrict caloric and fluid intake. In addition, some resort to the use of diuretics, laxatives, saunas, rubber suits, and excessive exercise to promote quick weight loss (ASCM, 1996). Some wrestlers will attempt to rehydrate after they weigh in prior to competition. However, it takes 24 to 48 hours to reestablish fluid homeostasis, 72 hours to replace glycogen stores, and even longer to replace muscle mass (ACSM, 1996). The use of diuretics and laxatives may cause the body to retain more fluid during rehydration, causing greater weight gain (IAHSAA, 1998). Finally, there is concern about the effects of repeated "weight cutting" practices on normal growth and development, academic performance, and immune function (ACSM, 1996).

Most state high school athletic associations have guidelines for wrestlers and coaches about safe practices in "making weight" prior to competition. The Iowa High School Athletic Association (IAHSAA) (1998), for example, posts guidelines for safe weight loss and lists dangerous practices that would exclude athletes from participation. These specific guidelines emphasize that not only are some practices designed to restrict weight gain or to lose weight prior to a weigh-in unsafe, but they are actually detrimental to performance and against the rules. This association stresses wellness for athletes, including information about substance abuse, strength training, overuse injuries, asthma and athletics, and mouth guards, as well information for parents, being a good sport, character development, and the reality of college athletics.

Healthier guidelines recommend that athletes restrict weight loss to two pounds a week through decreased caloric intake and increased exercise. This will result in weight loss primarily through fat. Rapid weight loss over the period of a few days through other methods will result in weight loss due to fluid, energy reserves, and lean muscle loss, resulting in a decrease in performance strength and endurance and lack of concentration (IAHSAA, 1998).

School nurses should play a key role in monitoring the weights and resulting health status of athletes to ensure safe practices and to educate both athletes and coaches regarding the above information. They should also be an integral player in developing or ensuring that existing policies that affect the weight status of players are followed. They must explore resources in their state in order to provide education that is consistent with and complementary to state recommendations for athletic participation.

Chronic dietary restriction may result in malnutrition and disordered eating, such as variations of anorexia nervosa and bulimia. This is especially a concern during adolescence when physical and sexual maturation may be affected and calcium stores are being laid down in bone. Eating behaviors learned in adolescence can have a life-long impact on weight management practices in adulthood as well as on one's perception of body image and self-esteem.

Female Athlete Triad

The long-term health effects of intense training on the female athlete have recently come under scrutiny (AAP, 2000a; Sherman & Thompson, 2004; Smith, 1996). In the last 30 years, there has been tremendous growth in the number of females participating in organized athletics both at the high school and college levels. While this has promoted female competition at a high level, it has also increased the possibility of serious health risks associated with intensive training and competition (Sherman & Thompson, 2004). Females who participate in sports where there is emphasis on appearance, a lean physique, or weight categories for participation, such as dance cheerleading, swimming, rowing, or cross country running, are at greater risk for experiencing a cluster of symptoms now known as the Female Athlete Triad.

The three characteristic components are: (1) disordered eating, (2) amenorrhea, and (3) osteoporosis (ACSM, 1997). Disordered eating may take many forms, from occasional restriction of food intake to anorexia nervosa or bulimia nervosa. While the incidence of disordered eating is 5% to 10% in the general population, it is 16% to 72% among female athletes, depending on the sport (Sherman & Thompson, 2004). Amenorrhea is usually due to deficient estrogen that can then lead to a decrease in bone mass. Osteoporosis is exacerbated by inadequate nutrition and lack of estrogen and may contribute to stress fractures in female athletes (ACSM, 1997). The triad of symptoms may also create cardiac problems in the future.

Athletes may perceive that weight loss will make them more attractive and enhance their performance, when, in fact, the opposite may be true. Poor nutrition may result in decreased endurance, strength, speed, and ability to concentrate, and consequently, increases the risk for injury (APA, 2000a). Not only does physical performance suffer, but there is also psychological morbidity. The internal and external pressures to maintain an unrealistic body weight underlie the development of body image and disordered eating (ACSM, 1997). The presence of disordered eating among female athletes is often denied and not recognized by parents and coaches.

School nurses need to identify female athletes at risk and educate student athletes, parents, trainers, coaches, administrators, other healthcare professionals, and the public about the female athlete triad and the magnitude and seriousness of the health risks involved. All trainers and coaches should receive education about the importance of training that is physically and psychologically sound and not putting emphasis on weight or appearance. Female athletes should be monitored regularly by their physicians to evaluate nutrition status, normal growth and development, as well as menstrual history, especially when even one sign of the female athlete triad is present. School nurses should be prepared to recommend community resources for nutritional counseling, as well as medical and psychological evaluations. In addition to the negative effects on performance and health of female athletes, the long-term effects of disordered eating and osteoporosis are a serious concern for women's health during their reproductive and elder years.

Nutritional Supplements and Performance-Enhancing Drugs

An important issue that has surfaced more recently is the use of nutritional supplements and performance-enhancing drugs by student and professional athletes. The fact that research over the last 20 years has supported the positive effect of good nutrition on athletic performance and recovery has increased interest in enhancing performance through dietary supplements. Athletes who consume a diet consisting of a variety of foods should have adequate energy to participate in sports and should not require nutritional supplementation. However, athletes who restrict intake to meet weight requirements, those who lose weight rapidly, and vegetarians or others who eliminate specific food groups from their diet may require supplementation (ACSM, 2000). Before supplementation is implemented, the need must be documented and the effectiveness, safety, and legality of the supplements considered. This should be in collaboration with experts in nutrition and sports medicine who are knowledgeable about current treatments and issues.

Many dietary supplements are available on the market today. Advertisements on the Internet and television have increased public awareness and availability of these products. Too often manufacturers of dietary supplements make unsubstantiated claims about their product's effectiveness in enhancing athletic performance and provide little information about product safety. Because many of these substances are classified as nutritional supplements, they are not regulated by the Food and Drug Administration. They may be dangerous in the hands of students or coaches whose goal is added strength and peak performance rather than the long-term health of athletes. There is no evidence these supplements enhance performance, and there have been no studies on the long-term effects of these supplements, particularly literature to support the safety of their use in growing adolescents.

Energy or sports food bars are attractive because of their convenience, especially to student athletes because they are portable, and do not require refrigeration. Many of these bars do provide a good source of energy (about 200 to 250 calories), but tend to be high in fat. Other bars supplement with a variety of micronutrients (vitamins and minerals) without substantiated benefit. These sports bars are expensive alternatives to less expensive food items that provide the same nutrients.

Protein supplements are also popular among student athletes. While protein supplements may be of value to athletes whose diets provide inadequate protein, the highly active athlete who is getting sufficient intake to maintain weight will not benefit from extra supplementation. Most students who consume a varied healthy diet have an adequate protein intake. Some protein supplements advertise the benefits of a specific amino acid. However, "the body has a pool of amino acids that it can use to build muscle...concern is that if you eat large quantities of one amino acid, it may interfere with the absorption of others" (MayoClinic.com, 2002). The body can only use about 1 gram of protein per pound of body weight. Amounts greater than this are flushed through the kidneys. Water is essential for protein synthesis; therefore, adequate hydration is critical. If a student has diabetes or altered kidney function, protein supplementation is potentially dangerous.

Another widely used supplement is creatine. Many players and coaches desiring increased strength or endurance are drawn to the promises of this product. While manufacturers, vendors, and coaches argue this is a naturally occurring substance in the body, the doses recommended are not natural and are potentially harmful (IAHSAA, 2000, 2001). Although an initial weight gain may occur when taking creatine, this weight gain is often due to water retention rather than increased muscle mass. Creatine use has been "shown to provide small improvements in short-burst 'power' activities, such as maximal bench press and cycling sprint speed" (MayoClinic.com, 2002). However, there is little evidence it enhances strength or endurance. Until there is more evidence about the safety and efficacy of nutritional supplements, especially in adolescents, many state high-school athletic associations have taken the position that coaches are not to endorse, recommend, or dispense nutritional supplements to student athletes.

Of greater concern is the use of anabolic steroids and ephedra. The American Academy of Pediatrics (1997) condemns the use of either of these performance enhancers, and provides information to healthcare professionals about their dangers and uses. Anabolic steroids, now banned by many professional sports, are taken to enhance muscle and strength and decrease recovery time after a hard workout (MayoClinic.com, 2002). The more common adverse physiological effects of long-term use of steroids include baldness, breast enlargement, and shrunken testicles in males and increased body hair, deepened voice, and decreased breast size in females (National Institute on Drug Abuse, 2000). However, increases in blood cholesterol, acne, and psychiatric disorders, including aggression, have been reported. An additional hazard for teens is that "steroids can halt their normal pattern of growth and development and put them at risk of future health problems" (MayoClinic.com, 2002).

Ephedra has received considerable attention because of recent deaths of high profile professional athletes and the move to ban this product. Sold over the counter and marketed to increase energy and promote weight loss, Ephedra "speeds metabolism and increases the rate at which a person burns calories. It also drives up blood pressure and heart rate" (Health and Health Care in the Schools, 2003). In January 2004, the Food and Drug Administration moved to ban the sale of ephedra in the United States.

School nurses need to be informed about the wide range of supplements available and their claims. They then will be in a position to educate coaches, students, and parents about these products.

Alcohol Use

Alcohol is a common drug that may be used by student athletes (see Chapter 40). Alcohol is the most widely used and abused drug in America. Billions of dollars are spent annually to promote alcohol products and their use, many of which are sports-event related. Media messages relate alcohol consumption to success in athletics, sociability, sex appeal, and happiness. Even though consuming alcohol is illegal until adulthood, a large percentage of teens report drinking alcohol. Studies report student athletes drink at least as much as nonathletes, although many drink much more (IAHSAA, 1999).

Many athletes consume alcohol because of peer pressure or the need to assert their independence, despite the risk of disciplinary action for violating school or team policies that would limit or prohibit their participation in athletics. There is some evidence that alcohol may increase self-confidence, but research shows that alcohol has a negative effect on psychomotor skills. A moderate amount of alcohol has repeatedly been shown to slow reaction time, reduce hand–eye coordination, impair mental processing, and affect balance and coordination (ACSM, 1982). Student athletes need to understand the effects of alcohol not only on their athletic performance, but also the potential effects on the entire team. They need to explore how to celebrate victories without alcohol and how to avoid situations where alcohol may be served. These messages need to be reinforced by parents, teachers, coaches, and others in the community.

Transmission of Bloodborne Infections

While participation in sports in which contact occurs puts students at risk for transmission of bloodborne pathogens, the American Academy of Pediatrics (1999) has determined that the risk is small. It is possible, however, that some students may have bloodborne infections, such as hepatitis B, hepatitis C, or human immunodeficiency virus (HIV). Although some students may be aware they are infected, it is likely that many others who are infected are not aware (Kukka, 2004). Boxing, a sport not recommended by the American Academy of Pediatrics, and wrestling present the greatest risk for transmission of pathogens via injured skin, blood, and other body fluids.

The American Academy of Pediatrics published a Policy Statement on bloodborne pathogens in the athletic setting that states, "Because of the very low probability of transmission of their infection to other athletes, athletes infected with HIV, HBV, or HCV should be allowed to participate in all sports" (AAP, 1999). The testing of student athletes for these infections is not indicated. Confidentiality about a student athlete's bloodborne infection is essential to protect student and family privacy and to avoid unnecessary fears among others and possible discrimination or exclusion. Information about a student's infection status should not appear on preparticipation physical examination forms in order to prevent violation of the student's confidentiality.

To prevent the possibility of the spread of bloodborne pathogens, coaches and trainers should be trained in first aid, emergency procedures, and how to implement standard precautions to prevent the spread of bloodborne infections in the athletic setting. Latex or vinyl gloves should be worn when cleaning mats or equipment or when dealing with injured students to prevent contact with blood or other body fluids. Equipment and playing surfaces contaminated with blood should be cleaned and disinfected with an appropriate germicide (1 part bleach to 10 parts water) and allowed to air dry (AAP, 1999). Athletes should cover existing cuts or wounds with a dressing prior to practice or participation. Those injured during participation should be removed from play and not return until the wound has been cleansed, the bleeding has stopped, and the wound covered. If the player's uniform or equipment has been contaminated with blood, it should be replaced or cleaned before the player returns to competition. Those handling equipment and laundry, such as student trainers and janitors, should be trained in proper handling of washable and disposable equipment. It is the school nurse's responsibility to train the trainers and coaches so that they can stress (and reinforce) this information with students and other staff.

Coaches and trainers should educate student athletes and their parents about the potential risks and prevention strategies used to protect student athletes from bloodborne infections. School nurses and coaches should stress the importance of HBV immunization for players, coaches, trainers, equipment handlers, janitors, and others at risk for exposure to athletes' blood (AAP, 1999). Student athletes should be discouraged from sharing personal items, such as razors, nail clippers, and toothbrushes, that may be contaminated with blood. They also need to be educated about the risk of transmitting HIV and other bloodborne infections through sexual activity and needle sharing, including anabolic steroid injections (AAP, 1999).

Skin Infections

Skin infections are a common occurrence in athletes. Since 2000 there have been reports of methicillin-resistant *Staphylococcus aureus* (MSRA) infections among athletes participating in a wide variety of sports, such as football, wrestling, and volleyball. Occurrences of MSRA infections used to be restricted to patients in hospitals and long-term care settings. The treatment and recuperation from MRSA can be long and debilitating; some infected athletes have required debridement, hospitalization for intravenous therapy, and even skin grafts.

School nurses and athletic coaches need to educate students and parents about the importance of reporting any skin infections to ensure early and adequate treatment as well as protecting against further spread. They need to be alert to the signs of infection, swelling, purulent drainage, pain, or fever. Students with draining wounds should keep them covered with a dressing. These dressings may need to be changed frequently, depending on the amount of drainage. Good hand washing technique and proper disposal of soiled dressings needs to be emphasized. Clothing, towels, and linens that come in contact with the wound should be isolated from other laundry, washed in hot water and dried on the highest setting. Linens and towels need to be changed frequently. Students with draining wounds should be restricted from participation in contact sports until the wound is no longer draining or the primary care provider clears the student for participation.

Skin-to-skin contact with other athletes, inherent in some sports, increases the risk of transmission. In addition, abrasions, floor burns, and shaving provide an opportunity for microorganisms to enter the skin. Even students participating in sports that have less physical contact may suffer abrasions or chafing from protective clothing or sweating. Sharing towels, clothing, and equipment is another way infection can be spread from a symptomatic student or an asymptomatic carrier. "The use of shared equipment or other personal items that are not cleaned or laundered between users could be a vehicle for *S. aureus* transmission" (CDC, 2003).

The school nurse is the school's infection control expert and, as such, needs to play a proactive role. Since MRSA does not respond to penicillin or other methicillin-related antibiotics, treatment often involves the use of more expensive agents for a longer period of time. "This underscores the need for aggressive control and prevention measures for all antibiotic resistant organisms" (Texas Department of Public Health [TDPH], 2003). Primary prevention begins with frequent and thorough hand washing. All students and teachers need to understand that the use of warm water, soap, and a clean cloth or paper towel provides the best defense against the spread of germs. School facilities and athletic locker rooms need to be adequately equipped to prevent and control the spread of infections. Hand washing needs to be instituted after coughing or sneezing, after using the bathroom, and when leaving the athletic facility. If soap is not available, the use of an alcohol hand sanitizer is recommended. Athletes should shower after practice or competition and use a clean towel to dry. Towels should not be shared, even on the field, nor should there be sharing of other athletic equipment, clothes, balms, or ointments.

Student athletes should wear clean clothes or uniforms for practice and competition. If students are responsible for their own equipment and uniforms, they should be transported home in a plastic bag, washed in hot water with regular detergent, and dried on a high setting; if they go home in a duffel bag, the bag should also be washed, if possible. Sports equipment and areas need to be disinfected regularly, using a solution of 1 part bleach to 10 parts water. This should be done at least weekly, if not more often (TDPH, 2003).

Ringworm is another common skin infection among athletes. Ringworm is the lay term for any fungal skin infection (see Chapter 25). "Ringworm of the scalp is called tinea capitis; of the body, tinea corporis; of the groin, tinea cruris; of the hand, tinea manus; ...and of the feet, tinea pedis or athlete's foot" (Venes, 2001, p. 1896). The root word *tinea* comes from the Latin term for intestinal worm, or ringworm, as the lesions exhibit characteristic worm-like borders (McLeod, 2004). Infected students need to be treated with over-the-counter antifungal preparations that should be applied twice daily. For those infections that do not respond, a prescription medication may be required. It is important to note that the lesions may take 6 weeks to completely clear. Because ringworm is rarely contagious to other students in the school setting, it is not necessary to exclude the student from school. However, wrestlers should not wrestle until the lesions have been treated for 24 hours. After that time, the lesions should be completely covered during practice and competition (McLeod, 2004).

School nurses, coaches, and athletic trainers need to monitor student athletes for skin infections and educate them about prevention of skin infections. Students with infected skin lesions should be encouraged to see their primary care provider to have the wound cultured and appropriate antibiotic therapy instituted as indicated. School nurses then need to monitor the lesions' status to determine when the student can return to active participation.

SPORTS INJURIES

In 2001, there were approximately 1.8 million nonfatal sports- and recreation-related injuries among 5- to 19-year-olds that required treatment in an emergency room (CDC, 2002). The injury rate was highest for 11- to 14-year-old boys. For children younger than 10, most injuries involved playgrounds, bicycles, scooters, and trampolines. For males 10 to 19 years of age, "football-, basketball-, and bicycle-related injuries were most common. For females aged 10 to 19 years of age, basketball-related injuries ranked highest" (CDC, 2002, p. 737).

Preparation for Participation

Adequate physical preparation is a key strategy for the prevention of sports injuries. Sports participation demands flexibility, coordination, strength, and endurance. Each sport has its own requirements; for example, cross country athletes need to develop cardiovascular fitness and muscular endurance, while cheerleading demands flexibility and upper body strength for the difficult and complex stunts performed. The endurance, flexibility, skills, and strength needed for sport cannot be developed the week before the season begins; it must be developed over time with a properly structured program. Many student athletes engage in preseason workouts, summer camps, and training to prepare for athletic participation. All athletes need to stretch, warm up, and cool down after practice and competition to improve flexibility. Investing time in warm up and cool down exercises will reduce injuries and enhance performance.

Strength Training for Student Athletes

Strength training has become an integral part of physical fitness programs and athletic training. Training for strength and endurance is often sport specific and an important part of sports injury prevention. Recommendations for strength and endurance training are based on age, gender, body composition, and physical maturity. Questions have been raised about the appropriateness of strength training for children and adolescents, especially prepubescent athletes. More repetitions with less resistance (weight) should be the norm until sexual maturity (Tanner Stage 5) (Bennett, 2001).

Strength training may involve the use of resistance machines, free weights, elastic tubing, or body weight (APA, 2001b). While many athletes participate in strength training to increase strength, prevent injuries, rehabilitate from injuries, and improve physical appearance, there is little evidence that strength training actually enhances athletic performance or reduces sports-related injuries. "Young people who desire to improve sports performance will generally benefit more from practicing and perfecting skills of the sport than from resistance training" (AAP, 2001b).

Strength training has the potential to increase bone mineral density, improve motor skills, and prepare students for the rigors of athletic participation and competition (Faigenbaum, 2000). Strength training programs should begin slowly, with emphasis on developing proper technique before adding increased weight and repetitions. There is a risk of muscle strain injuries, most commonly to the lumbar spine, from strength training. Most injuries, however, can be prevented by using proper technique, having adequate supervision, and avoiding maximal lifts or excessive repetitions (AAP, 2001b).

For those who desire long-term health benefits, a strength-training program should be augmented with an aerobic exercise program. For those whose goals are to increase muscle mass and strength, education about the effects of nutritional supplements and anabolic steroids is appropriate to encourage athletes to avoid their use.

Musculoskeletal Injuries

About 40% to 50% of sports injuries in children and adolescents are the result of overuse (Shell & Miller, 1996). Overuse injuries can be prevented through proper training and use of equipment. When they occur, treatment usually involves some combination of rest, immobilization, cryotherapy (ice), and occasionally the use of nonsteroidal anti-inflammatory agents to control inflammation. Referral to the student's primary care provider can determine the extent of the injury and ensure appropriate treatment and follow-up.

Traumatic injuries can occur at any time during practice or competition and commonly involve the ankle or knee. "Unrecognized and inappropriately managed foot and ankle injuries can lead to significant long-term functional disability" (Title & Katchis, 2002, p. 587). Although the student athlete may be anxious for a quick return to practice and competition, it must be emphasized that injuries require significant time to recover. A well-planned rehabilitation program that maintains fitness during recovery ensures optimal healing with quick return to participation while prolonging the career of the young athlete.

The growth plate is weaker than surrounding ligaments during adolescence, making the growth plate more susceptible to fracture. "Immediate swelling and inability to bear weight suggest fracture" (Ganley, Flynn, Pill & Hanlon, 2000, p. 311). If the student is not able to bear weight, has a limp, or exhibits significant pain or tenderness, he or she should be referred to the primary care provider for further assessment.

The most significant risk factor for an ankle sprain is a previous sprain. Methods commonly used to prevent future sprains include taping the ankle, using orthotics, wearing high top shoes or an ankle brace, or a combination of these methods (Thacker et al., 1999). While it appears that none of these methods have an effect on athletic performance, athletes who have sprained an ankle should undergo supervised rehabilitation before returning to competition. Ankle taping is frequently used post ankle injury to immobilize or restrict movement of the joint, as well as to prevent swelling and to provide a splint. It should be performed only by someone trained in proper application techniques. Taping is also used to prevent injury as well as to prevent reinjury and protect the injury as it heals (Birrer & Poole, 1994). Thacker and colleagues (1999) recommend that both student athletes and coaches take responsibility for the prevention of ankle injuries. This involves education, supervision, reporting of suspected injuries, early identification of injuries, and proper rehabilitation before returning to practice after an injury.

Shin splints are another common musculoskeletal overuse injury seen in student athletes. Researchers have studied the use of shock absorbing insoles, foam heel pads, alternative footwear, heel cord stretching, and graduated running programs in preventing or treating this disorder. While there is no research support for the use of any of these strategies, the use of shock-absorbing insoles seems to have the most promise in preventing shin splints (Thacker, Gilchrist, Stroup, & Kimsey, 2002).

Knee injuries are of great concern to athletes, parents, and coaches because of the long recovery period and the potential for season- or career-ending injuries. In addition, many athletes continue to experience knee problems into adulthood.

Anterior cruciate ligament (ACL) tears are common in student athletes but can occur in anyone; they can be a serious life-changing injury for an athlete (Ireland, 2002). ACL tears often occur when a student athlete lands unbalanced, on one foot, or out of control. Cutting movements or changing direction, which are commonplace in basketball, football, soccer, or volleyball may precipitate such injuries. The player reports hearing a "pop" before falling to the ground unable to continue play (Jonides, Walsh, & Rudy, 1993). Immediate immobilization, compression with ice, and elevation are the first aid responses. Current surgical procedures can repair the trauma, but rehabilitation is a long process.

ACL injuries are four to eight times higher in female athletes than male athletes. Neuromuscular performance varies during the menstrual cycle. A research study described the relationship between the menstrual cycle and ACL injuries in female athletes. Wojtys, Huston, Lindenfeld, Hewett, and Greenfield (1998) found that noncontact ACL injuries were higher than expected during the ovulatory phase of the cycle, and fewer injuries occurred during the follicular phase. It appears that hormones may play a part in ACL injuries in female athletes.

Today many children grow up with limited physical activity or training, which may have an effect on their physical coordination and skills. Coaches need to make sure student athletes receive the proper conditioning and sport-specific skills needed, such as safe landings and foot movement skills for basketball and other sports, to ensure safe participation.

Overuse injuries can result in tendonitis and stress fractures. Athletes who participate in volleyball are likely to have injuries related to blocking or spiking—skills that relate to vertical jump and landing. The most common overuse injuries are "patellar and shoulder tendonitis, suprascapular neuropathy, and low-back injury" (Briner & Benjamin, 1999, p. 53). "Certain aspects of the growing athlete may predispose the child and adolescent to repetitive stress injuries such as traction apophysitis (Osgood-Schlatter disease, Sever disease, medical epicondylitis [Little League elbow]), injuries to developing joint surfaces (osteochondritis dissecans), and/or injuries to the immature spine (spondylolysis, spondylolisthesis, vertebral apophysitis)" (AAP, 2000b). The weak musculature of the immature athlete contributes to these overuse disorders. Treatment involves medical management, as well as rehabilitation. Coaches, trainers, and health professionals need to become educated about these disorders and prevention measures that can be implemented to protect student athletes from developing overuse injuries.

When student athletes, regardless of level, are injured, they need to give the affected area time to rest and heal. Prevention and early identification of sports injuries can minimize disability and time lost from practice and competition. "Children and adolescents should never be encouraged to 'work through' such injuries (tendonitis, apophysitis, stress fractures, 'shin splints')" (AAP, 2000b). The suggested injury-related policy of the AAP includes the following:

- Encourage student to report pain and assure young athletes that their position on a team is rarely in jeopardy because of an injury.
- Prohibit students in pain from continued participation in any activity that might exacerbate the injury. If pain relievers are required to continue playing, the activity should not be permitted.
- Develop alternative activities that help maintain fitness or develop skills without involving an injured limb or body system for students who temporarily cannot participate because of an injury.
- Require parent notification about injuries. Do not rely on a student's self-report. This is particularly important for head, chest, and abdominal injuries.
- Record all injuries, including data on time of day, nature of sport, site of injury, nature of collision or other description, level of supervision, age and sex of the injured student, and the geographic location within the school or off-campus activity.
- Routinely monitor the following:
  - Student's level of conditioning and nutritional practices, particularly hydration;
  - Status of previous injuries, particularly those that might not have completely healed;
  - Student's psychological and motivational status;
  - Number of available, experienced adult supervisors with CPR and first aid training;
  - Availability, status, and use of personal protective equipment; and
  - Status of district equipment and field facilities.
- Establish an effective communication system with emergency paramedic help. (AAP, 2004, p. 183)

Nurses can assist the families and students to understand the RICE principle to treat soft tissue injury. This includes:

- *R*est of the injured area for 48 hours
- *I*ce placed on the injured area for 20 minutes at a time, 4 to 8 times per day
- *C*ompression with elastic bandages, splints, or special appliances
- *E*levation of the injured part

Rehabilitation and Return to Play

Another concern of school nurses is determining when it is safe for the athlete to return to practice or competition. It is difficult for students and coaches to follow recommendations to cut down practice or miss competition during a short season. Students would rather compete with pain than miss the BIG game or meet (and it seems that all games and meets are big!) than consider the long-term effect on their health or ability to perform. School nurses need to work with student athletes, parents, and coaches to protect the health of their student athletes and prevent reinjury to the musculoskeletal system by ensuring that athletes do not return to practice or competition too soon after an injury.

Dental Injuries

Students participating in contact sports, such as football, soccer, and ice and field hockey, and sports that include apparatuses or other equipment, such as gymnastics or baseball, are at risk for dental injury. More than 500,000 to 750,000 sports-related dental injuries occur each year (Krasner, 2000). If a tooth is knocked out during practice or competition, students, coaches, and school nurses need to know what actions need to be taken to save the tooth. When a tooth is knocked out or avulsed, the periodontal ligament (PDL) that holds the tooth in place is stretched and breaks. While part of the ligament remains in the tooth socket, part of it is attached to the avulsed tooth. The key to successful replantation is preserving the cells of the periodontal ligament on the avulsed tooth during transport to the dental office.

Acting quickly is essential because every minute that passes with the tooth out of the mouth, results in more of these cells dying. The ideal treatment would be to replant the avulsed tooth in its socket immediately after the injury, as this is the ideal medium to protect the cells of the PDL. This is rarely done, however, because the individuals present do not know what to do or are afraid to do this for fear of blood, infection, or hurting the child. In addition, the child may be bleeding, in pain, uncooperative, or even hysterical (American Association of Endodontists, n.d.).

If the avulsed tooth is to be transported extraorally to the dental office, it must be handled very carefully to minimize the damage to the PDL cells. First, the tooth should be picked up by the crown—not the root. Next, it should be placed in an appropriate transport medium in a specimen jar or cup. The tooth should *not* be rinsed with water or cleaned off with a tissue or other object because this will damage the PDL cells. It should *not* be wrapped in a tissue or gauze for transport. The tooth needs to be kept moist and transported quickly with the child so that it can be reimplanted. One hour's time is the optimal window for successful reimplantation. This information should be communicated to coaches and trainers.

The ideal solution for transport is Hank's Balanced Salt Solution (HBSS), a tissue culture medium that is available from biological research supply companies. HBSS contains all the metabolites necessary to maintain normal cell metabolism of the PDL. Small containers of HBSS are included in some dental first aid kits or can be purchased over-the-counter from many pharmacies. Ideally, small containers of HBSS should be readily available at playgrounds and athletic events where dental injuries are likely to occur. Parents may want to include a small container of HBSS in their family first aid kit. If HBSS is not available, the next best transport solution is milk, followed by normal saline, saliva, or water (AAE, n.d.). If there are other serious facial injuries, such as lacerations or possible fractures, the child may be transported to the emergency room.

Many dental injuries are preventable when appropriate equipment, such as mouth guards, helmets and facemasks, is used regularly and correctly (Ranalli, 2000). Coaches and parents must insist that student athletes have and use protective gear in both practice and competition. Mouth guards need to be fitted to the individual athlete. Many local dentists fit student athletes with mouth guards as a community service, although very affordable customizable mouth guards are available at most sporting goods stores. Other protective equipment should fit the athlete and be in good repair. Coaching staff need to monitor equipment to ensure its fit is secure and that it will protect the athlete from oral injury.

Eye Injuries

Ocular injuries can be particularly devastating because vision is a person's primary way of interacting with the environment. Thirteen percent of all eye injuries are due to sports and recreational activities; nearly two thirds of these injuries are related to blunt trauma, as in baseball and basketball, and impalement, as in fishing. "Eighteen percent of eyes with sport-related injuries remain legally blind even after treatment" (Witherspoon, Kuhn, Morris, & Mann, 1999, p. 333). The consistent use of proper fitting facial and ocular protection is the key to prevention of these devastating injuries.

Head Injuries

The sports injuries that have the most serious potential consequences are head and spinal cord injury. While cervical spinal cord injuries can be devastating, they are relatively uncommon; proper and prompt treatment is similar for that of head injuries (McAlindon, 2002). The most common head injury is concussion, which is most frequently associated with football, ice hockey, soccer, martial arts, and boxing; however, it can occur in a wide variety of sports (Powell, 2001). Concussions can be mild to severe and are caused by jarring or shaking of the head, resulting in an alteration in mental status that is not necessarily associated with a loss of consciousness. However, confusion and retrograde amnesia are common. Mild traumatic brain injury or concussion can also be the result of collisions and falls (Kushner, 2001), as well as resulting from blunt trauma to the head with sticks and balls.

The evaluation and management of concussion as well as when it is safe to return to play is a controversial topic among sports medicine professionals (Oliaro, Anderson, & Hooker, 2001). There are three widely used grading systems for concussion and return-to-play guidelines: (1) Cantu Guidelines (revised 2001); (2) Colorado Medical Society Guidelines (1991); and (3) American Academy of Neurologists (AAN) Guidelines (1997) (Cantu, 2004a).

Table 24.2 ■
CONCUSSION SCALES

	CANTU	COLORADO	AAN
Grade 1			
LOC	None	None	None
PTA	< 30 minutes	None	None
Neurological signs and symptoms	< 30 minutes	Transient confusion	Transient confusion
Return to play after first concussion	After 1 week symptom free	After 20 minutes symptom free	After 15 minutes symptom free
Return to play after subsequent concussions	End season	End season	End season
Grade 2			
LOC	< 1 minute	None	None
PTA	> 30 minutes; < 24 hours	Confusion with PTA	
Neurological signs and symptoms	> 30 minutes; < 24 hours		> 15 minutes
Return to play after first concussion	After 1 week symptom free	After 1 week symptom free	After 1 week symptom free
Grade 3			
LOC	> 1 minute	Any LOC	Any LOC
PTA	> 24 hours		
Neurologic signs and symptoms	> 7 days		
Return to play after first concussion	One month symptom free	One month, with 2 weeks being symptom free	1–2 weeks symptom free

Source: Cantu (2004g).
LOC, loss of consciousness; PTA, posttraumatic amnesia.

Although there are some differences among these scales (TABLE 24.2), they are similar in many ways. The Cantu scale is the most widely used scale and is more conservative than the others regarding mild concussion, recommending that the athlete not be allowed to play in the same game and return to play only after a symptom-free week. The Colorado Guidelines, although endorsed by the NCAA, are viewed as impractical because of the long time recommended for return to play after a concussion involving any loss of consciousness (LOC) (Table 24.2). (The AAN Guidelines are similar to the Colorado Guidelines but are less conservative about when to return to play. The AAN Guidelines require a formal sideline evaluation to differentiate between a Grade 1 and Grade 2 concussion, an important factor in determining readiness to return to play (Cantu, 2004a).

Factors used in grading concussion include loss of consciousness (LOC), posttraumatic amnesia (PTA), and other neurological signs and symptoms. According to the Cantu Concussion Grading Guidelines, a Grade 1 or mild concussion involves no LOC or PTA or postconcussion signs or symptoms lasting no longer than 30 minutes (see Table 24.2). A Grade 2 or moderate concussion involves LOC lasting less than 1 minute and PTA and postconcussion signs or symptoms lasting longer than 30 minutes but less than 24 hours. A Grade 3 or severe concussion includes LOC that lasts longer than 1 minute and PTA that lasts more than 24 hours or postconcussion signs or symptoms lasting longer than 7 days (Cantu, 2004b).

It is important to note that concussions can occur without loss of consciousness (Grade 1). Determining the amount of time for LOC is essential because it differentiates between a moderate (Grade 2) and severe (Grade 3) concussion, which in turn determines when an athlete is allowed to return to play. One challenge in determining LOC is when a player also experiences posttraumatic amnesia, he/she is unable to reliably report LOC; therefore, this will need to be determined by a reliable eyewitness or a videotape if available (Cantu, 2004c). Prolonged LOC represents a neurological emergency and requires prompt medical attention and evaluation (Kelly, 2001).

Posttraumatic amnesia, probably more accurately called posttraumatic confusional state, is the most reliable indicator of severity of brain injury and in predicting outcomes. The mildest form of PTA is retrograde, the partial or total loss of ability to recall events immediately before the injury. The second type, anterograde amnesia, is reduced ability to form new memories after the trauma "which may result in decreased attention and inaccurate perception" (Cantu, n.d.). This anterograde memory is the last function to be restored after LOC. Determining the presence of PTA on the field is important to ascertain the injured player's orientation to time, immediate memory, and concentration. Checking for both retrograde and anterograde amnesia can be done on the sidelines by using simple word or number recall tests, included on standardized assessment tools for concussion (Cantu, 2004d, 2004e).

Box 24.2 ■ ■ ■

SIGNS AND SYMPTOMS OF POST-CONCUSSION SYNDROME

- Headache
- Nausea/vomiting
- Dizzy, tinnitus (ringing in ears), vacant stare
- Drowsy, excessive sleep, or sleep disturbances
- Memory problems; loss of orientation
- Altered balance or coordination
- Poor concentration, easily distracted
- Personality change or inappropriate emotions
- "Feel different"
  - Nervous, irritable
  - Feel "in a fog", "slowed down"
  - Depressed, sad
  - Hypersensitive to light and noise

(Cantu, 2004f)

It is important to systematically assess the neurological status of a student athlete to determine if there has been a concussion. The Standardized Assessment of Concussion is a brief screening tool that can be performed on the sidelines in about 5 minutes. It includes measures of orientation, memory, neurological status, exertion maneuvers, and delayed recall. This screening tool is helpful in identifying mild concussions even in cases where there is no LOC or obvious signs of a concussion (Cantu, 2004e). Post-concussion signs and symptoms checklists are available to determine neurological status after a concussion. These can be used immediately after the posttraumatic event and in monitoring neurological status during the follow-up period (Cantu, 2004f). (See Box 24.2.)

Deciding when a student is ready to safely return to play post concussion is difficult. There are a number of return-to-play guidelines available to give guidance in making this decision. The three concussion grading systems mentioned previously also have return-to-play guidelines that relate to the grade of the concussion as well as the number of concussions the athlete has suffered in the past. There is some variability among these guidelines that has led to confusion and controversy about when return-to-play is advisable. For example, after a Grade 1 (mild) concussion, Cantu recommends return to play after one symptom-free week; the Colorado Guidelines state the player may return if symptom free for 20 minutes, and the AAN Guidelines allow return to play after 15 symptom-free minutes (Cantu, 2004g). It is important that coaches and trainers be familiar with these guidelines when talking to athletes and parents about return to play. However, the final decision should be made in consultation with the team physician or the athlete's physician.

The reason the return-to-play decision is so important is to prevent Second-Impact Syndrome (SIS), a second head injury that occurs before the symptoms associated with the first injury have subsided (Cobb & Battin, 2004). It is important to note that the symptoms of head injury, such as headache, mental changes, thought and memory processes, as well as visual, motor, and sensory changes, often take hours, days, or weeks to clear (Cantu, 2004h). However, there is wide agreement that athletes should not return to play until all symptoms have resolved. A second head injury does not have to be severe to produce serious neurological effects. The athlete may appear stunned momentarily, but is typically able to resume play or walk off the field. Some athletes will continue to play in a dazed state, similar to those who experience a Grade 1 concussion without LOC. However, "within seconds to minutes of the second impact, the athlete – conscious but stunned – suddenly collapses to the ground, semi-conscious with rapidly dilating (widening) pupils and loss of eye movement, and stops breathing" (Cantu, 2004h). The return-to-play guidelines are cautious when recommending return to play after a second or third concussion, often recommending ending the season after a second Grade 2 or Grade 3 concussion, and encouraging the athlete to consider withdrawal from contact sports after a third Grade 3 concussion (Cantu, 2004g).

Recently, there has been discussion about the effect of purposeful heading in soccer and its effect on cognitive functioning. A review of the literature on the topic revealed that soccer players as well as other athletes have selective cognitive deficits, but the reasons for these deficits are many. "Concussions are a common head injury in soccer (mostly from head-head and head-ground impact) and a factor in cognitive deficits and are probably the mechanism of the reported dysfunction" (Kirkendall & Garrett, 2001, p. 328).

Data about catastrophic head injuries from high school and collegiate sports are compiled and maintained by the National Center for Catastrophic Sports Injury Research. From this extensive database, injury trends can be monitored and recommendations made about policies and injury prevention procedures. "A football-related fatality has occurred every year from 1945 through 1999, except for 1990" (Mueller, 2001, p. 312). Head injuries accounted for 69% of the deaths, 16.3% related to cervical spinal cord injuries, and other injuries accounted for 14.7% of the deaths. The greatest percentage of deaths occurred at the high school level. From 1984 to 1999, there were 69 football head injuries that resulted in permanent disability. Although football head injuries have received the most attention, permanent disabilities and deaths have been reported in other sports, including baseball, track, and cheerleading. This reinforces the role of protective headgear and the need to ban illegal maneuvers involving the head and neck.

PSYCHOLOGICAL PERSPECTIVES

There are many psychological benefits of participating in sports. Student athletes gain satisfaction from the acquisition of new skills, they develop a sense of belonging with a group of individuals who share similar interests, and they learn to contribute as a member of a team. The goal of athletic participation is to provide a supportive, positive learning environment. However, there are psychological as well as physiological injuries. Although there are statistics gathered to determine physical injury rates, similar data are not reported for psychological repercussions from these injuries. The psychological impact may produce long-term effects on self-esteem and attitudes about sports and fitness participation for years to come. Because of their holistic perspective, school nurses need to consider psychological as well as physical injuries. They should explore the reasons why the student enjoys or avoids a sport in order to better counsel them.

Many students, especially during their elementary years, participate because they enjoy the social aspect of the activity. As the focus moves from participation to competition that demands a higher level of performance, the stress of trying to meet these demands increases, thus decreasing the enjoyment of the activity. There is also the stress of meeting the expectations of parents and coaches and of disappointing their classmates. Consequently many students drop out of athletic participation. Participation in sports that demands individual performance is much more stressful than team sports, such as soccer or volleyball, where there is less pressure on the individual and more emphasis on the team working together to achieve its goals. It is important that student athletes participate in a sport that is compatible with their personal goals and provides a positive experience with opportunities to grow in skills, as well as to participate as a member of a team. In other words, there needs to be a good fit between the student and the athletic endeavor.

The Psychological Impact of Injury

When an athlete becomes injured, there is often great concern about the physiological injury and recovery, and its effect on future participation. However, there is evidence that there are emotional effects on the injured athlete that need to be recognized and treated as appropriate. While many of the research studies do not focus exclusively on student athletes, the findings have implications for those who work with injured athletes of all ages. Pearson and Jones (1992) found that many injured athletes were frustrated, depressed, and bored. Subjects also had a more negative mood profile, exhibiting tension, hostility, tiredness, and confusion. Another study (Johnston & Carroll, 1998) reported that frustration and depression were common during rehabilitation. In early rehabilitation, this was attributed to disruption to normal functioning; during middle rehabilitation it was attributed to a negative appraisal of progress in rehabilitation; and during the final phase of rehabilitation, these reactions were linked to impatience and readiness to return to sport participation.

Striegel, Hedgpeth, and Sowa (1996) examined the relationship between the severity of the injury and the length of rehabilitation to the psychological effects on the athlete. During the first few weeks of recovery, athletes focus on "resiliency and coping with the stress associated with injury" (p. 330). Support should focus on stress management and the development of coping strategies. For more serious injuries requiring longer rehabilitation, the focus should be on motivation and compliance with the rehabilitation regime. Treatment includes goal setting and support. For those with severe injuries that end an athlete's participation in a particular sport, treatment should focus on grief counseling and the transition to a new identity and lifestyle. Students need to identify other positive strengths that can be nurtured during rehabilitation to maintain a positive mindset.

Depression is a common response to athletic injury. This depression can be significant and last throughout the recovery period (Smith & Milliner, 1994). Adolescents with depression are at risk for suicide, a leading cause of death among those 15 to 24 years of age. A study of five injured student athletes who attempted suicide identified five common themes: (1) the injured athlete had experienced considerable success prior to the injury; (2) the student experienced a serious injury that required surgery; (3) the nature of the injury required a long rehabilitation period with restrictions from participating in their sport during this time; (4) upon return to the sport, the skill level of the athlete was not at preinjury level; and (5) teammates had replaced them or taken their position on the team during their rehabilitation (Smith & Milliner, 1994). It is important to recognize depression in injured athletes and determine if the athlete is at risk for suicide. Keep injured athletes involved with the team activities; they can go to games, be in the locker room, and provide team support (see Chapter 34).

ENVIRONMENTAL PERSPECTIVES

Safety and Equipment

School nurses are concerned about student safety, beginning with playground safety in the preschool years. Nurses are aware of the importance of safe equipment, proper surfaces, and adequate supervision on their school playground (Hudson, Thompson, & Mack, 1999). Records of playground injuries should be maintained to note trends so that recommendations for playground changes for the health and safety of children can be made (Peterson, 2002). Many of these same principles apply to the prevention of sports injuries.

First, safe equipment is essential for any sport, whether it be gymnastics, football, or track. To ensure the safety of equipment, regular inspection and ensuring proper use are fundamental. The consistent use of protective equipment, such as shin guards for soccer, face masks for soft ball, and mouth guards for football, is essential to prevent injuries. School nurses must emphasize to students, parents, and coaches the importance of safe equipment and use of protective gear to promote safety and student performance. Although many student athletes have been issued protective equipment, they often do not use it properly or regularly (Ward, 2004).

Proper surfaces are also essential for injury prevention. This includes not only gym floors, but also football, baseball, and soccer fields, cross country running areas, as well as cushioned landing areas for track and gymnastic events. These surfaces needed to be maintained and monitored regularly to ensure student safety (ACSM, 1994). The school district should identify a person to be responsible for inspecting and maintaining equipment and playing areas; however, the school nurse must be an advocate for change if she identifies a potential safety hazard (Peterson, 2002).

Supervision

Supervision by qualified adults is instrumental in ensuring safety in organized sports. Coaches, managers, and trainers must be knowledgeable not only about the sport, but of growth and development, the potential physical and psychological risks involved, recognition of common injuries, first aid, and injury prevention (AAP, 2001a). Many sports organizations offer education for coaches, have standards for competencies, and offer certification for those who meet educational requirements and competencies.

School nurses can provide education to coaches and athletic staff on growth and development, injury prevention, first aid, and CPR classes. Today, many schools are purchasing automatic electronic defibrillators (AED) that are available in gymnasiums and at sporting event venues. Coaches, trainers, and athletic staff need to be trained to use AEDs in case of a cardiac emergency. The portability of the AED allows it to be taken to away games and practices.

The school nurse has a significant role in the development of emergency plans. The development of an emergency plan for responding to a variety of medical emergencies, especially those involving the musculoskeletal, neurological, or cardiovascular systems, needs to be developed by the school athletic health team. The plan should include triage, first aid, and immobilization procedures, necessary equipment, and appropriate contact information. Language used in the plan must be comprehensible to non-medical personnel who are likely to be present. Training should be provided regularly so that all involved in sports are familiar with the plan; the school nurse may have a role in this training. It is recommended that a healthcare professional be available during competition to assist in case of a medical emergency.

ROLE OF THE SCHOOL NURSE IN ATHLETE HEALTH PROMOTION

The school nurse has an important role in promoting the health of student athletes. However, because student participation in recreational and school-sponsored athletic programs usually occurs after school hours, school nurses are not likely to be directly involved with students or coaches during athletic practice or competition. Therefore, their role focuses more on education, advocacy, monitoring, and sports injury prevention.

Because of their specialized knowledge of growth and development, health, and mechanisms of injury, school nurses are a vital part of the athletic healthcare team. A Consensus Statement from the National Athletic Trainers' Association, *Appropriate medical care for* secondary *school-age athletes* (NASN, 2002), states that appropriate care of the student athlete goes beyond basic emergency care that may be needed during participation, but also includes the ongoing care of student athletes as well as the prevention and rehabilitation of athletic injuries. School nurses are able to monitor the health of student athletes beyond the practice field in the school setting. By contributing their unique knowledge to the athletic healthcare team, there is a focus on athlete health promotion.

School nurses should monitor injury trends among athletes in school-sponsored sports to determine the safety of equipment, the playing surface, and the adequacy of appropriate supervision during practice sessions as well as competition. They should have copies of all accident reports involving students. Documentation of sport-related injuries provides the data necessary to make recommendations about equipment, supervision, and policies. As student health advocates, school nurses have an obligation to be aware of potential risks to the health of student athletes and follow up on recommendations that would prevent injuries and promote the health of student athletes.

The American Academy of Pediatrics (2001a) states that qualified coaches should be the key factor in ensuring a safe experience for student athletes. Many coaches are quite knowledgeable about the sport they coach, but are not as familiar with the physiological and psychological risks. It is not within the scope of practice for most coaches to manage injury or rehabilitation, or make educated objective decisions about an injured athlete's physiological readiness to return to play. Short competitive seasons often do not allow injured athletes sufficient time for the rest and healing needed before returning to practice and competition, thus increasing the pressure on the athlete to return to play. This puts them at a greater risk for reinjury or disability.

School nurses have a role in monitoring the status of injured athletes to ensure they do not return to participation prematurely. School nurses can also monitor injury trends that may indicate the need for closer supervision, enforcement of wearing protective equipment, safer playing surfaces, and attention to risk factors in implementing preventive strategies by coaches, trainers, and other athletic staff. A strong relationship between the school nurse and coaches will promote cooperation in planning for the health of student athletes.

The nursing intervention, Sports-Injury Prevention: Youth, from the *Nursing interventions*

(text continues on page 586)

Box 24.3 ■ ■ ■

SPORTS-INJURY PREVENTION: YOUTH

Definition: Reduce the risk of sport-related injury in young athletes.
Activities:

- Encourage general fitness as prerequisite to participation in sports.
- Encourage modification of game rules according to age and ability of participants.
- Inform parents of the differences between recreational and organized competitive sports.
- Assist athlete in finding a sport that is a good fit with interests and abilities that will promote the development of life-long fitness behaviors.
- Assist parents and athletes to set realistic goals for participation.
- Provide resources for parents, athletes, and coaches concerning the psychosocial aspects of sports involvement.
- Encourage appropriate matching of competitors by age, weight, and stage of physical maturation.
- Monitor adherence to recommended training guidelines and correct biomechanics.
- Monitor compliance with safety rules.
- Monitor field of play for safe playing conditions.
- Monitor proper use and condition of safety equipment.
- Encourage appropriate supervision for training, recreation, and competitive events.
- Monitor sports physicals to ensure they are complete before participation.
- Encourage use of warm-up and cool-down activities to prevent injuries.
- Use certified athletic trainers for competitive sports at the junior and senior high school levels.
- Ensure medical coverage at competitive sporting events, as appropriate.
- Develop an emergency plan in case of serious injury.
- Coordinate preseason seminars for athletes, families, and coaches, to increase awareness of injury prevention.
- Collaborate with other professionals in planning programs related to injury prevention.
- Inform parents and athletes of steps they can take to prevent injuries.
- Inform parents and athletes of signs and symptoms of overuse injuries, dehydration, heat exhaustion, use of performance-enhancing drugs, eating disorders, menstrual dysfunction, and stress.
- Collect data on injury type, rate, treatment, and referrals.
- Monitor the long-term health of athletes.
- Monitor return of injured athletes to participation to prevent reinjury.
- Provide emotional support for athletes experiencing injury.
- Arrange for coaches to get annual CPR and first aid training.
- Communicate with coaches the importance of emphasizing "fun" in sports.
- Ensure that coaches are well informed of normal childhood development and the physical, emotional, and social needs of children.
- Communicate information about special healthcare concerns of individual athletes, as appropriate.
- Develop oversight groups to ensure education of school and volunteer coaches.
- Inform parents of qualifications and behavior expected of coaches.
- Encourage parents to become involved in their children's sports programs.
- Monitor athletes for sport-related stress and provide referrals for athletes with emotional/psychosocial concerns.
- Teach relaxation techniques and coping strategies to athletes, coaches, and parents.
- Advocate for the health of young athletes.

(Dochterman & McCloskey, 2004, pp. 667–668)

classification (Dochterman & Bulechek, 2004) provides a concise list of activities the school nurse can implement to reduce the risk of sports-related injuries (Box 24.3). These activities give school nurses guidance in planning specific strategies to promote healthy practices and environments for student athletes in the school setting.

CONCLUSION

The school nurse is in a unique position to promote the health of student athletes through education, advocacy, and monitoring. A good understanding of growth and development is the basis for care delivered to students in the school. This information needs to be shared with those who work with student athletes to ensure a positive growth experience that may affect their attitude about sports and physical activities that will last a lifetime. School nurses also need to be aware of sports injury trends nationwide and in their school district in order to develop education programs aimed at sports injury prevention. Specific knowledge of the physical demands of various sports aids the school nurse's educational efforts.

School athletics is often associated with the high profile sports, such as football, basketball, and baseball. However, many students participating in less visible or popular sports also have health risks relative to the nature of the sport, the age of the participant, or the conditions where practice and competition occur. Today schools are providing opportunities for males and females to participate in a multitude of sports, such as soccer, cross country running, crew, wrestling, volleyball, lacrosse, golf, and field and ice hockey. In addition, other groups, such as cheerleaders (Hutchinson, 1997), dance teams, and marching band (Vepraskas, 2002), consider themselves student athletes because of the unique demands and risks of injury of their sport. School nurses need to have knowledge of the risks unique to each sport and appropriate sports injury prevention strategies so they can educate students, athletes, and coaches.

Good health practices as well as sensible training and competition are essential to the physical and psychological health of student athletes. Who is better positioned than school nurses in providing health education for students, families, coaches, and the community about athlete health? School nurses are also tireless advocates for the health of children. Being informed about strategies to promote the health of student athletes of all ages who participate in a variety of sports is essential. Being involved in a sport provides a valuable opportunity for students to develop physical, social, and leadership skills. It also gives them an opportunity to have fun, work together as a part of team, as well as develop a lifetime interest in physical activity so necessary for health. These physical endeavors are not without the potential for injury. By becoming involved with student athletes and athletic programs, school nurses can ensure that these opportunities are achieved.

References

American Association of Endodontists (AAE). (n.d.). *Treating the avulsed permanent tooth*. Retrieved September 22, 2003 from http://www.aae.org/ws94ecfe.html

American Academy of Pediatrics (AAP). (1997). *Adolescents and anabolic steroids: A subject review*. Retrieved August 24, 2002 from http://www.aap.org/policy/970601.html

American Academy of Pediatrics (AAP), Committee on Sports and Fitness. (1999). Policy Statement: Human immunodeficiency virus and other blood-borne viral pathogens in the athletic setting (RE9821). *Pediatrics, 104*(6), 1400–1403. Retrieved January 18, 2004 from http://www.aap.org/policy/re9821.html

American Academy of Pediatrics (AAP). (2000a). *Medical concerns in the female athlete*. Retrieved August 24, 2002, from http://www.aap.org/policy/re0003.html

American Academy of Pediatrics (AAP). (2000b). *Policy Statement: Intensive training and sports specialization in young athletes. Pediatrics, 106*(1), 154–157. Retrieved September 24, 2002 from http://www.app.org/policy/RE9906.html

American Academy of Pediatrics (AAP). (2001a). *Organized sports for children and preadolescents, Policy Statement*. Retrieved September 24, 2002 from http://www.aap.org/policy/re0052.html

American Academy of Pediatrics (AAP). (2001b). *Policy Statement: Strength training by children and adolescents. Pediatrics, 107*(6), 1470–1472. Retrieved September 24, 2002 from http://www.aap.org/policy/re00048.html

American Academy of Pediatrics (AAP). (2004). *School health policy and practice*. Elk Grove Village, IL: Author

American College of Sports Medicine (ACSM). (1982). *Position Statement: The use of alcohol in sports*. Retrieved October 13, 2003 from http://www.acsm-msse.org

American College of Sports Medicine (ACSM). (1994). The prevention of sport injuries of children and adolescents. *Journal of the American Academy of Physician Assistants, 7*(6), 437–442.

American College of Sports Medicine (ACSM). (1996). *Position Stand: Weight loss in wrestlers*. Retrieved October 13, 2003 from http://www.acsm-msse.org

American College of Sports Medicine (ACSM). (1997). *The female athlete triad. Position stand. Medicine and Science in Sports and Exercise, 29*(5), i–ix. Retrieved October 13, 2003 from http://www.acsm-msse.org

American College of Sports Medicine (ACSM). (December 1, 2000). *Joint Position Statement with the American Dietetic Association and Dietitians of Canada: Nutrition and athletic performance. Medicine & Science in Sports & Exercise*, 2130–2145. Available at http://www.acsm-msse.org

Bennett, C. (2001). Athlete health promotion. In M. Craft-Rosenberg & J. Denehy (Eds.), *Nursing interventions for infants, children, and families* (pp. 573–592). Thousand Oaks, CA: Sage Publications.

Birrer, R. B., & Poole, B. (1994). Taping of sports injuries: Review of a basic skill. *Journal of Musculoskeletal Medicine, 11*(6), 56–58, 61–63, 66–68.

Briner, W. W., & Benjamin, H. J. (1999). Volleyball injuries: Managing acute and overuse disorders. *Physician & Sportsmedicine, 27*(3), 48–49, 53–54, 57–60.

Cantu, R. C. (2004a). *Concussion grading systems and return-to-play guidelines: A comparison.* Retrieved January 20, 2004 from http://www.momsteam.com/ alpha/features/health_safety/concussion_grading. shtml#cantu

Cantu, R. C. (2004b). *Comparison of 1986 and 2001 Cantu concussion grading guidelines*. Retrieved January 20, 2004 from http://www.momsteam.com/alpha/features/health_safety/drcantu_revised_guidelines.shtml

Cantu, R. C. (2004c). *Determining loss of consciousness in athletes*. Retrieved January 20, 2004 from http://www.momsteam.com/alpha/features/health_safety/determining_loss.shtml

Cantu, R. C. (2004d). *Post-traumatic amnesia*. Retrieved January 20, 2004 from http://www.momsteam.com/ alpha/features/health_safety/post_traumatic_amnesia.shtml

Cantu, R. C. (2004e). *Standardized assessment of concussion*. Retrieved January 20, 2004 from http://www.momsteam.com/alpha/features/health_safety/standard_assessment.shtml

Cantu, R. C. (2004f). *Post-concussions signs & symptoms A checklist*. Retrieved January 20, 2004 from http://www.momsteam.com/alpha/features/health_safety/post_concussion_signs.shtml

Cantu, R. C. (2004g). *Concussion grading systems and return-to-play guidelines: A comparison*. Retrieved January 20, 2004 from http://www.momsteam.com/alpha/features/health_safety/concussion_grading4.shtml#returntoplay

Cantu, R. C. (2004h). *Second-impact syndrome: What is it?*. Retrieved January 20, 2004 from http://www.momsteam.com/alpha/features/health_safety/second_impact_syndrome.shtml

Centers for Disease Control and Prevention (CDC). (2002). Nonfatal sports- and recreation-related injuries treated in emergency departments—United States, July 2000–June 2001. *Morbidity and Mortality Weekly Report, 51*(33), 736–740.

Centers for Disease Control and Prevention (CDC). (2003). Methicillin-resistant *Staphylococcus aureus* infections among competitive sports participants—Colorado, Indiana, Pennsylvania, and Los Angeles County, 2000–2003. *Morbidity and Mortality Weekly Report, 52*(33), 793–795. Retrieved September 23, 2003 from http://www.cdc.gov/mmwr/preview/mmwrhtml/mm5233a4.htm

Cobb, S., & Battin, B. (2004). Second-impact syndrome. *Journal of School Nursing, 20*(5), 262–267.

Dochterman, J., & Bulechek, G. M. (2004). *Nursing interventions classification (NIC)* (4th ed.). St. Louis: C. V. Mosby.

Faigenbaum, A. D. (2000). Strength training for children and adolescents. *Clinics in Sports Medicine, 19*(4), 593–619.

Ganley, T. J., Flynn, J. M., Pill, S. H., & Hanlon, P. A. (2000). Ankle injury in the young athlete: Fracture or sprain? *Journal of Musculoskeletal Medicine, 17*(6), 311–313, 317–319, 323–325.

Haywood, H., & Boyce, W. (1996). Knee overuse injuries in the skeletally immature athlete. *Physiotherapy Canada, 48*(3), 190–196, 202.

Health and Health Care in the School. (March, 2003). *Dietary supplement under scrutiny. 4(1)*. Retrieved March 3, 2003 from http://www.healthinschools.org/ejournal/2003/mar03_4.htm

Hudson, S., Thompson, D., & Mack, M. G. (1999). The prevention of playground injuries, *Journal of School Nursing, 15*(3), 30–33.

Hutchinson, M. R. (1997). Cheerleading injuries: Patterns, prevention, case reports. *The Physician and Sportsmedicine, 25*(9), 83–93.

Iowa High School Athletic Association (IAHSAA). (1998). *Safe weight loss*. Retrieved October 8, 2002 from http://www.iahsaa.org/wu98–1.htm

Iowa High School Athletic Association (IAHSAA). (1999). *Alcohol and athletes*. Retrieved October 13, 2003 from http://www.iahsaa.org/wu99–6.htm

Iowa High School Athletic Association (IAHSAA). (2000). *Creatin supplementation*. Retrieved October 8, 2002 from http://www.iahsaa.org/wu20–4.htm

Iowa High School Athletic Association (IAHSAA). (2001). *Nutritional supplements: Separating fact from fiction*. Retrieved October 8, 2002, from http://www.iahsaa.org/wu01–6.htm

Ireland, M. L. (2002). The female ACL: Why is it more prone to injury? *Orthopedic Clinics of North America, 33*(40), 637–651.

Johnston, L. H., & Carroll, D. (1998). The context of emotional responses to athletic injury: A qualitative analysis. *Journal of Sport Rehabilitation, 7*(3), 206–220.

Jonides, l., Walsh, S., & Rudy, C. (1993). Knee pain in school-aged girls. *Journal of Pediatric Health Care, 7*(4), 185–196.

Kelly, J. P. (2001). Loss of consciousness: Pathophysiology and implications in grading and safe return to play. *Journal of Athletic Training, 36*(3), 249–252.

Kirkendall, D. T., & Garrett, W. E. (2001). Heading in soccer: Integral skill or grounds for cognitive dysfunction? *Journal of Athletic Training, 36*(3), 328–333.

Krasner, P. (2000). Management of sport-related tooth displacements and avulsions. *Dental Clinics of North America, 44*(1), 111–135.

Kukka, C. (2004). Bloodborne infections: Should they be disclosed? Is differential treatment necessary? *Journal of School Nursing, 20*(6), 324–330.

Kushner, D. S. (2001). Concussion in sports: Minimizing the risk for complications. *American Family Physician, 64*(6), 1007–1014.

Martens, R., & Seefelt, F. (1979). *Guidelines for children's sports*. Reston, VA: American Alliance for Health, Physical Education, Recreation and Dance.

MayoClinic.com. (n.d.). *Helping young athletes eat to play well: Questions and answers*. Retrieved February 24, 2003 from http://www.mayoclinic.com/invoke.cfm?objectid=2FB18747-D235-4B35-BE5E284F705C72B8

MayoClinic.com. (June 1, 2002). *Banned substances enhance athletic performance, but at a price*. Retrieved February 24,2003 from http://www.mayoclinic.com/invoke.cfm?objectid=36414434-DF76-46A4-BA2854D093590AF4

McAlindon, R. J. (2002). On field evaluation and management of head and neck injured athletes. *Clinics in Sports Medicine, 21*(1), 1–14.

McLeod, R. P. (2004). Lumps, bumps, and things that go itch in your office! *Journal of School Nursing, 20*(2), 359–360.

Mills, D., & Muscari, M. E. (1998). Preventing sports injuries, *American Journal of Nursing, 98*(7), 58, 60.

Mueller, F. O. (2001). Catastrophic head injuries in high school and collegiate sports. *Journal of Athletic Training, 36*(3), 312–315.

Myers, A., & Sickles, T. (1998). Preparticipation sports examination. *Primary Care: Clinics in Office Practice, 25*(1), 225–236.

National Association of School Nurses (NASN). (2002). *Appropriate medical care for secondary school-age athletes consensus statement*. Retrieved March 1, 2003 from http://www.nasn.org/positions/positions.htm

National Institute on Drug Abuse. (April, 2000). Anabolic steroids. *Community Drug Alert Bulletin*. Bethesda, MD: US Department of Health and Human Services/National Institutes of Health.

National Safe Kids Campaign. (1996). *Fact sheet promoting sports safety. A Program of children's National Medical Center*. Washington, DC: Author

Oliaro, S., Anderson, S., & Hooker, D. (2001). Management of cerebral concussion in sports. *Journal of Athletic Training, 36*(3), 257–262.

Pearson, L., & Jones, G. (1992). Emotional effects of sports injuries; Implications for physiotherapists. *Physiotherapy, 78*(10), 762–770.

Peterson, B.(2002). School injury trends. *Journal of School Nursing, 18*(4), 219–225.

Petlichkoff, L. M. (1992). Youth sport participation and withdrawal: Is it simply a matter of FUN? *Pediatric Exercise Science, 4*, 105–110.

Powell, J. W. (2001). Cerebral concussion: Causes, effects, and risks in sports. *Journal of Athletic Training, 36*(3), 307–311.

Ranalli, D. N. (2000). Prevention of sport-related traumatic dental injuries. *Dental Clinics of North America, 44*(1), 35–51.

Shell, D., & Miller, K. (1996). Managing overuse injuries in young athletes. *Family Practice Recertification, 18*(3), 51–54, 59–60, 62.

Sherman, R. T., & Thompson, R. A. (2004). The female athlete triad. *Journal of School Nursing, 20*(4), 197–202.

Smith, A. (1996). The female athlete triad: Causes, diagnosis, and treatment. *The Physician and Sportsmedicine, 24*(7), 67–69, 70, 75–76, 86.

Smith, A. M., & Milliner, E. K. (1994). Injured athletes and the risk of suicide. *Journal of Athletic Training, 29*(4), 337–341.

Striegel, D. A., Hedgpeth, E. G., & Sowa, C. J. (1996). Differential psychological treatment of injured athletes based on length of rehabilitation. *Journal of Sport Rehabilitation, 5*(4), 330–335.

Texas Department of Public Health (TDPH). (2003). *Antibiotic resistance*. Retrieved September 23, 2003 from http://www.tdh.state.tx.us/ideas/ antibiotic_resistance/mrsa/school_athletic_departments.asp

Thacker, S. B., Gilchrist, J., Stroup, D. F., & Kimsey, C. D. (2002). The prevention of shin splints in sports: A systematic review of the literature. *Medicine & Science in Sports & Exercise, 34*(1), 32–40.

Thacker, S. B., Stroup, D. F., Branche, C. M., Gilchrist, J., Goodman, R. A., & Weitman, E. A. (1999). The prevention of ankle sprains in sports: A systematic review of the literature. *American Journal of Sports Medicine, 27*(6), 753–760.

Title, C. I., & Katchis, S. D. (2002). Traumatic foot and ankle injuries in the athlete. *Orthopedic Clinics of North America, 33*(3), 587–598.

Venes, D. (Ed). (2001). *Taber's cyclopedic medical dictionary* (19th ed.). Philadelphia: F.A. Davis.

Vepraskas, C. (2002). Beat the heat: Managing heat and hydration in marching band. *Journal of School Nursing, 18*(4), 237–243.

Ward, C. (2004). Teens' knowledge of risk factors for sports injuries. *Journal of School Nursing, 20*(4), 216–220.

Witherspoon, C. D., Kuhn, F., Morris, R., & Mann, L. (1999). Epidemiology of general and sports eye injuries. *Ophthalmology Clinics of North America, 12*(3), 333–343.

Wojtys, E. M., Huston, L., Lindenfeld, T. N., Hewett, T. E., & Greenfield, M. L. V. (1998). Association between the menstrual cycle and anterior cruciate ligament injuries in female athletes. *American Journal of Sports Medicine, 26*(5), 614–619.

Chapter 25

Skin Disorders

LEATHA ROSS ▪ MARGARET CLARK GRAHAM

Chapter Outline

INTRODUCTION

Skin lesions, including rashes, lumps, and bumps, can cause alarm among teachers, healthcare providers, and parents. The school nurse is in an ideal position to provide an accurate assessment of these problems and, when necessary, suggest treatment or recommend a referral. Some of the most common skin problems seen in the school setting are discussed in this chapter, including pruritus, urticaria, eczema, impetigo, molluscum, tinea or various fungal infections, candidiasis, pediculosis, scabies, Fifth disease, poison ivy and poison oak, acne, sun exposure, body art, and self-mutilation. A discussion of the assessment and management of these conditions, including patient education, is included. Chapter 26 covers a full description of the assessment and management of pediculosis.

THE BASICS

Health History

The school nurse is often the first person who receives a report or concern from a teacher or parent, or the students themselves, regarding a skin problem. Despite the myriad of conditions affecting the skin, a very organized approach to the evaluation of a rash or skin problem simplifies the process of developing a list of differential diagnoses. The term "differential diagnosis" is a list of potential causes of a presenting problem. The health history and physical assessment of the skin will provide the information needed to develop the differential diagnosis.

The most important tool in assessing any body system is an accurate and thorough health history. The health history associated with skin alterations will help the school nurse identify the problem in about 90% of the presenting conditions. The nurse should assess any presenting skin problem by asking about the onset, or when the problem started. This question will help determine both the onset and the duration of the skin problem. In determining the duration, it will be important to identify if it "comes and goes" or if the lesion or rash has been present since the onset. The nurse should ask where the lesion is located; if more than one is present, the nurse should determine their distribution. Questions to help determine the location and distribution include: Is there only one lesion? Are there several lesions in one area of the body? Are the skin lesions in some type of distribution, such as linear, circular, or is there a general distribution over the entire body? In determining the onset, duration, and location, the nurse needs to determine if new lesions are developing. Did the lesion begin in one spot or as one lesion and has it spread to other areas?

Next, the school nurse will need to determine "characteristics" of the skin lesion. Questions related to characteristics include: Does the lesion itch, burn, or hurt? Has there been any bleeding or weeping of the lesion? Alleviating and aggravating factors need to be identified; what makes the skin lesion worse and what makes it better? It is important to find out what treatments have been used on the skin lesion. Remember, many times people will use home remedies on skin lesions, so be sure to assess for any type of treatment including conventional and unconventional therapies. A thorough history of over-the-counter and prescription medications that the student may be using for other conditions should be included in the history related to skin lesions. It is also essential to assess whether other symptoms are present that might indicate a systemic problem.

An exposure history is important to identify contact with poisonous plants or any animals that have had contact with these plants. Even gardening and visiting parks put people at risk. Being in areas where new insecticides or cleaning agents are used, as well as science classes or tanning booths, may provide a clue. Identifying what medications the student is taking as well as the activities in which the student has engaged while on the medication might also prove important.

The school nurse will also need to assess for a past history of skin problems. Identifying whether anyone else at home might have the same symptoms is also important; a skin problem could be contagious and other family members may be experiencing the same condition. Questions related to the family health history will help develop a differential diagnosis of the presenting problem.

Physical Exam

A basic knowledge of primary and secondary lesions is also necessary in developing the differential diagnosis. Primary lesions are the basic beginning lesions of most skin problems. The presence of a primary lesion provides initial assessment data and allows the formulation of a differential diagnosis (Habif, Quitadamo, Campbell, & Zug, 2001). One should be able to distinguish between a macule, papule, patch, plaque, nodule, wheal, tumor, hives, vesicle, cyst, pustule, or bulla (TABLE 25.1).

Table 25.1 ■
PRIMARY SKIN LESIONS

PRIMARY LESION	DESCRIPTION
Macule	Rounded, flat, <1 cm. Examples: freckle or petechiae
Papule	Palpable, solid, elevated, rounded, <1 cm. Examples: wart or mole
Patch	Same description as a macule but >1 cm. Examples: Mongolian or café au lait spots
Plaque	Combined papules that form an elevated surface; wider than 1 cm. Examples: psoriasis, lichen planus
Nodule	Hard or soft, solid, elevated area measuring >1 cm. Examples: neurofibroma, hard cyst or keloid
Wheal	Transient, firm edematous papule or plaque. Example: mosquito bite or hives

(continued)

PRIMARY LESION	DESCRIPTION
Tumor	Firm or soft lesion, deep in dermis, greater than a few centimeters. Examples: lipoma, hemangioma
Hives (urticaria)	Coalesced wheals; formation of extensive reaction, very itchy
Vesicle	Rounded collection of fluid, elevated cavity, up to 1 cm. Examples: herpes simplex, varicella (chickenpox), contact dermatitis
Cyst	Encapsulated, subcutaneous, fluid-filled cavity. Example: sebaceous cyst
Pustule	Circumscribed, elevated cavity; containing pus. Example: carbuncle
Bulla	Rounded collection of free fluid, >1 cm in diameter. Example: friction blister, contact dermatitis

Source: Adapted from Jarvis (2004).

Secondary lesions are lesions that arise from primary lesions. For example, in acne, a primary lesion may begin as a papule but then it may become pus filled which would make it a secondary lesion. Table 25.2 gives examples of commonly seen secondary lesions.

Following the determination of the type of lesion, the school nurse should assess the color of the lesion; red or pink (erythema) rashes can be differentiated from honey-colored crusts. The margins and centers of the lesions should also be noted. Are there different colors between the edges of the lesion compared to its center? Does it resemble a bulls-eye? The location on the body should be noted as well as the distribution of the lesions; lesions are described as scattered or clustered, linear, confluent (run

Table 25.2 ■
SECONDARY LESIONS

SECONDARY LESION	DESCRIPTION
Scales	Compact, dry flakes of skin, silvery or white in color. Example: psoriasis, seborrhea
Crust	Thickened, dried exudate left when a vesicle or pustule bursts or dries up. Example: impetigo
Ulcer	Deep depression extending into dermis, irregular shape
Scar	A permanent fibrotic change that occurs after a skin lesion is replaced with collagen
Keloid	A hypertrophic scar; excess scar tissue, looks smooth, rubbery; higher incidence among blacks (may look like a cyst at first glance)
Fissure	Linear crack, break in skin. Example: athlete's foot.

Source: Adapted from Jarvis (2004).

together) or discrete. Identify if the location is directly related to contact with creams, jewelry, or clothing or if the lesion is heavier in areas of higher body heat.

Full body rashes are often due to viral illness. The school nurse should be aware that 6 to 12 days after receiving the measles vaccine, a child may break out in a fine pink maculopapular rash; the rash is harmless and the student is not contagious (Schmitt, 2002). Large areas of macular rash might also be due to a reaction to medication; if this is the case, the school nurse should assess for respiratory problems and notify the parent so that the prescribing provider is called before the next dose is to be given.

Assess for pain or pruritus associated with the skin lesion (see below). Some rashes may have no discomfort; others may produce intense itching at the site of the lesion. Some skin lesions, such as those that are infected or are in the genital region and have contact with urine, may cause pain.

When examining the skin, the school nurse should pick a few lesions that look like primary lesions. Describe them as clearly as possible using correct terminology. After examining a few lesions, look for the lesions on other parts of the body. After a thorough assessment of the skin, the school nurse should palpate the lesion for consistency (McLeod, 2003); sometimes the use of a glove is warranted.

Other signs of illness should be noted; signs of allergy and anaphylaxis will direct care in one direction, whereas fever, lethargy, and general discomfort would result in interventions focused in another direction. **Please note: if the rash is really purpura (large reddish-purple areas) or petechiae (tiny red dots indicative of decreased platelets) not related to injury or friction, the student needs to be assessed immediately by a physician to rule out meningococcemia and bleeding disorders, respectively** (Schmitt, 2002). Emergency services need to be called for those having an anaphylactic reaction (see Chapter 28 on allergies). For a non-emergency situation, ask about contact with plants or walks in the woods (i.e., poison ivy), chemicals (solvents or insecticides), fiberglass, or animals. Animals can have contact with poison ivy and bring it into the home; simply petting the animal can transfer the irritant to the individual.

Children with the following symptoms need to be seen by a primary care provider within a few hours of the identification of the skin problem: painful rashes (possibly due to a spider bite), if fever is present, if severe itching is present, or if there are signs of an infection at the site of the lesion.

Pruritus

Pruritus, or itch, is a very common, unpleasant sensation associated with many skin lesions; it is often followed by a scratching or rubbing response that can lead to a disruption of the skin's integrity causing infection and scarring. Causes of pruritus include a direct irritation by the offending substance or the histamine released. Most commonly, dry skin is the cause of pruritus, in which case no skin lesion may be present.

It is necessary to assess for the cause of the pruritus. Chemicals, physical causes, or cold, dry weather can cause irritation and itching of the skin. Ask about soaps or body creams used, and the type of fabric in contact with the skin. Some students have an increased sensitivity to natural fibers such as wool and mohair. These may result in an allergic or atopic dermatitis (see Chapter 28 on allergy). Excessive bathing, especially with hot water and harsh soap, can also cause dry skin (Hooper &

Box 25.1 ■■■

INTERVENTIONS FOR PRURITUS

- Limit baths to no more than once a day, and preferably lasting less than 10 minutes. Use tepid water rather than hot water.
- Keep the use of soap to a minimum. Use a mild perfume-free soap, such as Dove.
- Apply moisturizer to wet skin.
- Parents may use calamine lotion or a baking soda solution (1 tsp. baking soda in 4 oz. of water).
- If a steroid cream has been recommended by the healthcare provider (usually a 1% hydrocortisone over the counter product), it can be applied every 2 hours initially and then four times a day (Schmitt, 2002).
- An environment low in humidity can cause dry skin; therefore, a humidifier in the home may be helpful.
- For histamine-related pruritis, antihistamines may be recommended by the primary care provider. Some are sedating (diphenhydramine HCl [Benadryl], Brompheniramine maleate [Dimetapp], chlorpheniramine [Chlor-Trimeton], and hydroxyzine HCl [Atarax]) and others are not (cetirizine HCl [Zyrtec], loratadine [Claritin], and fexofenadine HCl [Allegra].

Goldman, 1999). Dry skin (xerosis) may present as slightly scaly with variable erythema and superficial fissuring, most commonly on the extremities. In many cases, dry skin may be either the cause or a contributing factor to pruritus.

If the cause can be identified, the obvious solution is to avoid the cause. A mild soap can be used to remove the irritant from the skin, but then soap should be avoided until the situation resolves; warm water can be used to cleanse an area. Cool compresses can be applied for 20 minutes every 3 to 4 hours or the pruritic part can be soaked in cool water for 20 minutes. The goal is to decrease the discomfort and prevent scratching.

Suggestions can be made to students and their parents for home care related to generalized skin problems. These are included in Box 25.1. If these approaches do not alleviate the problem, the student should be referred for further evaluation and treatment.

The following is a brief discussion of common skin lesions seen in the school setting. Information related to the presenting history and physical exam and management will be included.

ALLERGIC CONDITIONS

Urticaria

Urticaria is also known as hives. Approximately 25% of the American population will have at least one episode of hives; some patients will have chronic urticaria lasting for years. Urticaria usually involves the dermis and subcutaneous tissue (angioedema). The release of mediators such as histamine from mast cells will cause vasodilation with extravasation of fluid and edema into the interstitial region. The etiology of urticaria may be unknown but causative factors may include exposure to sun, cold (occurs within minutes of rewarming the affected site), or pressure, or an allergic reaction to medication, an inhalant, or food. Common food allergens include milk, eggs, wheat, shellfish, and nuts (see Chapter 28 on allergy). If allergy is the cause, the reaction occurs from within minutes to hours after contact. Students who are infected with parasites also may present with urticaria (Fitzpatrick, Johnson, Wolff, & Suurmond, 2001; Goldsmith, Lazarus, & Tharp, 1997).

Assessment

The student with urticaria usually presents with intense itching. Edema of the lips, eyes, hands, and feet may be present. The nurse should initially assess for respiratory involvement by asking about shortness of breath or any difficulty breathing. The physical findings may include hives that are transient red raised plaques with sharp borders varying in size from 1 to 8 cm. They can occur anywhere on the body. Angioedema is manifested by skin-colored soft tissue enlargement, such as the eyelids, lips, tongue, ears, genitals, palms, and soles. Wheezing may be present (Fitzpatrick et al., 2001). Aquagenic (a reaction to immersion) and cholinergic (in response to an increase in one's core temperature for any number of reasons) urticaria present as flesh-colored small papules (Habif, Rothe, & Grant-Kels, 1997).

Management

Students who present with signs of anaphylaxis, including hypotension, wheezing, tachycardia, coughing, severe anxiety, or cyanosis need immediate referral to emergency services. Administer epinephrine if the situation warrants. Students who present with hives and no indication of respiratory distress may be managed with over-the-counter or prescriptive antihistamines, although cold compresses may also be helpful. Most cases are self- limiting and disappear without treatment (Goldsmith et al., 1997).

Obviously, the first intervention is to remove the underlying cause. The school nurse should encourage the student who has chronic recurring urticaria (lasting longer than 6 weeks) to identify any associated patterns that may help identify the precipitating factor and to see his or her healthcare provider. However, many times it may not be possible to determine the etiology.

Eczema

Eczema is a general term used to describe a condition of redness, scaling, vesicles, and crusting (Hoekelman, Adam, Nelson, Weitzman, & Wilson, 2001). It may present as allergic contact dermatitis, irritant dermatitis, nummular eczema, atopic dermatitis, and seborrheic dermatitis (Nicol & Bradley, 1999). Atopic dermatitis is a common, chronic, relapsing, pruritic type of eczema and usually occurs in individuals who themselves have allergies or a family history of such. Stress can cause eczema to flare, especially among good students who put added stress on themselves to do well in school. For more in-depth information regarding allergic conditions, see Chapter 28.

Assessment

A thorough history of the presenting complaint and treatments used is imperative in eczema. This includes a review of the student's allergies. The student may complain of itching, which is one of the major criteria for a diagnosis of eczema.

Examination of the involved skin areas with eczema will reveal erythema, edema, vesicles, and weeping. Tiny, clear, fluid-filled vesicles are seen on the skin surface. The development of bullae can occur (Habif et al., 2001). The most common sites are areas that are warmer and wetter, such as the antecubital and popliteal spaces, thighs, neck, and hands. Younger children often have eczema on their cheeks and scalp.

If this is a chronic condition, the skin pattern changes over time and a thickened skin with deeper skin lines may develop with some hypo- or hyper-pigmentation (Hoekelman et al., 2001). During adolescence and with chronic episodes, lichenification (thickened skin) and increased markings as a result of chronic rubbing and scratching may be seen (Hoekelman et al., 2001).

Management

The goal of treatment is to break the inflammatory and itch–scratch cycle. Daily skin care that hydrates and lubricates is of primary importance. Families can be educated to avoid wool or other itch-provoking fabrics and to use a humidifier in the home. In the school setting, cool wet compresses can be applied. Other treatment regimens include the application of topical steroid creams, topical immunomodulators, oral antihistamines, and the management of secondary infections that may develop. The student should be referred for further evaluation and treatments.

Sixty percent of cases of eczema are resolved by adulthood but other allergic conditions may appear in its place, such as asthma (Goldsmith et al., 1997). Students with atopic eczema and chronic forms of dermatitis are at "risk for a particular severe form of primary herpes simplex infection and thus should avoid contact with people with active herpetic infections" (Zitelli & Davis, 2002).

INFECTIOUS CONDITIONS

Impetigo

Impetigo is a common, contagious, superficial skin disorder caused by bacterial infection. The infection is caused by Group A beta-hemolytic streptococcus, *Staphylococcus aureus*, or a combination of both bacteria limited to the skin (Fitzpatrick et al., 2001; Habif et al., 2001). Exposed parts of the body such as the face, extremities, hands, and neck are the most commonly involved sites. It can be spread by biting and stinging insects such as mosquitoes and flies (Hooper & Goldman, 1999). The infection often starts in an area of trauma or skin lesion, including bug bites. Students in close physical contact with others can also spread the infection. The incidence is increased in individuals with poor hygiene.

Assessment

The student who presents with impetigo usually states that the problem began as a single lesion that may be described as a macule, papule, or plaque. Staphylococcus-induced impetigo frequently has blisters. The primary lesion may become a secondary lesion with a crust or scaling. Lesions can be either bullous or nonbullous. These thin-walled vesicles on an erythematous base expand laterally with the formation of satellite lesions (Hooper & Goldman, 1999). The lesions rupture easily and "the dried serum forms a characteristic golden brown or honey-colored crust" (Hooper & Goldman, p. 74).

On inspection of the skin the nurse may find localized or widespread bullous type lesions with crusting. Regional adenopathy and pruritis may or may not be present. It should be noted that infections with other organisms, such as tinea capitis, can present an identical picture to impetigo (Zitelli & Davis, 2002). If impetigo is suspected, treat the lesions as contagious.

Management

Local, limited infections of impetigo may be effectively treated with an over-the-counter antibiotic preparation such as Bactroban (cream or ointment). Students with widespread infections or recurrent infections should be referred for systemic antibiotic treatment. It is important to explain the contagious nature of impetigo to the parents or guardians. Good hand washing practices and isolation of the student's towels, washcloths, and linens should be emphasized.

In addition to antibiotics, treatment usually consists of soaking the lesions in warm water 10 to 15 minutes three or four times a day in order to remove the crusts and hasten the healing. Then they should wash with gentle antibacterial soap, such as Dial. "The prognosis is more severe in adults than in children" (Hooper & Goldman, 1999, p. 73).

Molluscum Contagiosum

Molluscum contagiosum is a common skin disorder caused by a poxvirus infestation that affects the top layer of the skin. Similar to warts, the virus enters the skin through small breaks of hair follicles. The infection is usually localized and self-limiting. However, it can spread through self-inoculation and is also transmitted to others by skin-to-skin contact. Wrestlers in school programs are particularly susceptible. The incubation period is 2 to 7 weeks (Hooper & Goldman, 1999).

Assessment

The history associated with molluscum may be a complaint of lesions that have been present for a few months. These lesions may be found alone or in clusters on exposed skin surfaces, especially the face in children and near the genitals in sexually active teens. It can also be seen on the face, trunk and limbs; the palms and soles are not involved. The initial skin findings of molluscum begin as a small shiny papule, 1 to 2 mm in diameter. The lesions may appear white to flesh-colored, dome-shaped, firm, and have a tiny dimple or umbilicated area in the center. Over weeks, these papules may increase to 5 mm in diameter. They become softer, pink in color with a more obvious dimpling in the center. Secondary impetigo-type excoriations may occur (Habif et al., 2001).

The student may complain of tenderness and itching, associated with mild inflammation. The school nurse must keep in mind that a differential diagnosis to consider is warts or herpes lesions. For confirmation, a referral for a biopsy may be considered.

Molluscum may be sexually transmitted in young adults. Lesions occurring on skin normally covered by clothing should raise suspicion of sexual abuse. Individuals with atopic dermatitis appear to be prone to numerous lesions that are difficult to clear until the atopic dermatitis is under control (Habif et al., 2001).

Management

The school nurse should teach those with the infection to avoid skin-to-skin contact to minimize transmission of the virus. Students should keep the areas of infection covered with clothing, if possible. The lesions resolve spontaneously in healthy individuals; therefore, treatment is usually not necessary. However, many of the treatment options lead to significant scarring, so treatment considerations should be individualized. The treatments are aimed at destroying the lesion and virus by freezing it with liquid nitrogen or surgically removing it (Goldsmith et al., 1997). Reassurance to wait and watch the normal course of the disease is appropriate.

Cutaneous Fungal Infections

Fungal infections of the skin are caused by various dermatophytes that infect the nonviable keratinized cutaneous tissues including the skin, nails, and hair. The term tinea is specific to the part of the body infected with a fungus, such as tinea capitis (hair), tinea corporis or ringworm (trunk, legs, and arms excluding the feet hands and groin), tinea cruris or jock itch (groin, pubic area, and thighs), tinea facialis (face), and tinea manuum (hands) (Fitzpatrick et al., 2001). Technically, all could be considered ringworm, although that designation is usually limited to tinea corporis (Hooper & Goldman, 1999).

Tinea capitis

Tinea capitis occurs in school-age children with a decreasing incidence after puberty. It is transmitted by personal contact and occasionally by pets, although the infecting spores can remain viable for long periods of time and can be cultured from combs, brushes, blankets, hats, theater seats, and telephones (Hooper & Goldman, 1999). For unknown reasons, infection is endemic among black students and is five times more common in boys (Hooper & Goldman, 1999; Zitelli & Davis, 2002).

Assessment

The student usually presents complaining of scaling of the scalp or patchy hair loss. In other cases, the fungal organism invades the hair shaft and the student may present with hair breakage with a “salt and pepper” appearing scalp. In more severe cases, the assessment may reveal erythema, edema, and pustular lesions. The areas of weeping and gold colored crusting can resemble and be confused with impetigo (Zitelli & Davis, 2002).

Management

Management requires oral medication for treatment. Topical preparations may be used to prevent transmission. The school nurse should refer students with tinea capitis for evaluation and management. Parent and student education regarding the transmission and prevention of the infection is important. Shampooing with selenium sulfide 1% (Selsun Blue) can reduce the risk of shedding spores. All household contacts should be encouraged to shampoo with selenium sulfide. Scrupulous cleaning of all possibly contaminated objects helps prevent reinfection. Usually following successful treatment, normal hair growth will occur. However, in more severe cases of tinea capitis, hair regrowth may not occur, causing permanent alopecia.

Tinea Cruris

Tinea cruris, commonly referred to as jock itch, is an infection of the crural folds of the groin area. The infection is not contagious; therefore, spread from person to person is rare.

Assessment

The student will usually complain of itching in the groin area, especially when he or she has been sweating after vigorous exercise or during warm days. The history may also include tinea pedis or prior tinea cruris infection. Often the infection is found on the groin (Habif et al., 2001). Plaques form as well-defined scaling and sometimes a vesicular border advances out of the crural fold onto the thigh and may involve the scrotum. The skin becomes less scaly and red papules may develop. Inflammation occurs with continued wearing of occlusive clothing. Over time, if untreated, the infection may migrate to the buttock and gluteal areas.

Management

Over-the-counter antifungal powders, creams, or lotions may be used for treatment. The student should be advised to avoid tight-fitting clothing and to wear loose-fitting underwear, such as boxers instead of briefs. Teach students to change their underwear frequently, especially after tasks that leave them hot and sweaty. Following a workout, the student should be taught to bathe or shower right away and to apply an antifungal preparation. The use of a drying powder, such as miconazole nitrate, may be of benefit. The student should be taught to avoid storing damp clothing in a locker or gym bag. Washing workout clothing after each wearing will help to avoid reinfection. For resistant infections, the school nurse should refer the student for evaluation and further treatment.

Tinea Pedis

Tinea pedis, commonly called athlete's foot, is more frequently seen following puberty. The most common form of tinea pedis is interdigital. Other forms may be the moccasin type (which is common in atopic individuals), vesicular, ulcerative, and dermatophytid (Fitzpatrick et al., 2001).

Assessment

The student may present with itching and/or pain between the toes or on other areas of the foot. In interdigital tinea pedis, the student may have fissures between the toes with underlying erythematous skin that may weep. In moccasin type tinea pedis, there is a well-demarcated erythema with white scaling on the soles and lateral edges of the foot, giving it a moccasin-like appearance. Other forms of tinea pedis may present as vesicles, bulla, and ulcers.

Management

All students, especially those with tinea pedis, should be instructed to wear shoes while showering in public facilities to try to decrease the spread of the fungus. Students may use over-the-counter antifungal cream, powder, or spray. The moccasin type tinea is more resistant to treatment and students with this type of infection may need a referral (Fitzpatrick et al., 2001).

Tinea Corporis and Tinea Facialis

Tinea corporis or ringworm is a dermatophyte infection of the trunk and limbs, excluding hands and feet, face, and groin. Tinea corporis may be transferred from other parts of the body affected with tinea, from household contacts or from animals. Tinea facialis, a fungal infection on the face, is frequently misdiagnosed. It is common in children (Fitzpatrick et al., 2001).

Assessment

The student presenting with tinea corporis may have one lesion or more than one. The size of the lesion varies. Physical findings usually include annular (ring-shaped) scaling erythematous plaques with sharply marginated, indurated, hyperkeratotic borders; the center of the ring may also be clear, and the ring may consist of pustules or vesicles (Hooper & Goldman, 1999). The initial lesion may be either a macule or a plaque and varies in size from less than a centimeter to greater than 8 cm. The student presenting with tinea facialis may be asymptomatic or they may complain of pruritis (Fitzpatrick et al., 2001). The student should be assessed for dermatophyte infections involving other body areas.

Management

Prescriptive or topical antifungal medications may be used for treatment. Medication is applied to the lesion and the surrounding skin, since this fungus spreads outward; "subclinical infection with the dermatophyte may extend up to 8 cm from the clinically active border" (Hooper & Goldman, 1999, p. 118). Therapy is continued for a few weeks after the clinical symptoms have resolved.

Tinea Manus

Tinea manus, a fungal infection of the hand, may be associated with tinea pedis or tinea cruris (Fitzpatrick et al., 2001).

Assessment

The student with tinea manus may present with itching and thickened dry scaling of one hand. The infection may be bilateral but frequently is found on the dominant hand. Scaling is usually found in the palmar creases of the hand.

Management

Tinea manus may be managed with antifungal creams or powders. The student needs to be assessed for tinea involving other body locations and all affected areas need to be treated.

Candidiasis

Candidiasis is usually caused by *Candida albicans*, a yeast-like fungus that is normally found in the gastrointestinal tract and vagina, and on the skin. The yeast infects the outer layers of the epidermis of the mucous membrane and skin (Habif et al., 2001). Yeast tends to grow in moist, warm areas and is usually found on mucous membranes and in folds of skin and other areas of the skin that provide this environment. Candidiasis may be seen in obese children who have excessive body creases that create the dark moist environment necessary for the growth of the fungus. Oral antibiotic therapy can predispose individuals to genital candidiasis.

Assessment

The student may complain of itching, burning, and irritation. The appearance of candidiasis is dependent on the location. If there is an infection of the mouth, the lesions are white plaques with an underlying bright red surface. These lesions may extend to the esophagus so an assessment of problems related to swallowing is important. Skin lesions can appear as red, moist, and occasionally peeling with areas of maceration (i.e., axillary, perianal, gluteal, and inframammary folds and any other areas of skin-to-skin contact, especially in those who are obese) (Habif et al., 2001). Secondary lesions caused by fungus may appear pustular.

Management

Several topical treatment options are available for treatment of candidiasis. Treatments may be in the form of powders, creams, or ointments. For oral fungus or thrush, or vaginal candidiasis, oral treatments in the form of oral suspensions, tablets, and troches may be used. Usual superficial infections are treated with topical therapy. The school nurse should refer for management of this condition.

Students can be encouraged to use a blow dryer after bathing to ensure drying of the skin, especially in skin folds. Cool water or Burrow's solution soaks are often soothing. Students should be encouraged to wear loose-fitting cotton clothing and to have the humidity lowered in their home environment. Since obesity and hyperglycemia can predispose one to candida infection, these risk factors should be addressed (Hooper & Goldman, 1999).

Pediculosis (Lice)

Pediculosis is an infestation of a blood-obligate parasite. There are three species of lice that infest humans (head, body, and genital region). Head lice infestation is endemic among millions of school-aged children and is more prevalent than all other communicable diseases combined (Estrada & Morris, 2000). Pediculosis is an annoyance to the students, parents, healthcare providers, and school personnel. A comprehensive discussion of pediculosis is in Chapter 26.

Scabies

Scabies is caused by a contagious mite infestation that causes intense itching. Scabies is usually contracted by close body contact with an infected individual. While it is rare, infection can occur by the use of contaminated towels, bed linen, and clothing. The mite burrows into the skin and deposits its eggs there. The eggs hatch and over the next 30 days or so, the mites mature and travel on the skin. Therefore, the incubation period is 1 to 2 months (Hooper & Goldman, 1999).

Assessment

The history associated with scabies is intense itching that is worse at night and a rash that affects the hands, wrists, genital area, waist, buttocks, and areas around the knees and elbows. The pruritis is related to a reaction to the mite or to the feces of the mite. The student who has scabies will not have complaints of facial itching, as scabies does not affect the face. Many times, more than one person in the household will have symptoms. Skin lesions associated with scabies may include macules, papules, and linear erythematous lesions that represent the areas where the mite has burrowed. A burrow is linear, curved, or S-shaped and is the classic lesion of scabies. Common sites of infection include the finger-webs, popliteal fossa, wrists, axillae, lower abdomen, and buttock. Eczematous type lesions are most commonly seen and at times these lesions mimic impetigo with honey-colored crust (Habif et al., 2001).

Management

Application of a scabicide such as Elimite is curative. Elimite is a prescription drug so the student may need to be referred to obtain the prescription. When treating the skin with Elimite, the skin below the neck should be covered with the lotion. Elimite should be left on the skin for 8 to 12 hours. Elimite is removed by washing. One re-treatment in 1 to 2 weeks may be necessary.

Household contacts should be educated on the nature of the infection. Because scabies is contagious, all family members should be treated even if they are asymptomatic. All clothing and linens should be washed and dried in the hot cycle. Articles that may not be washed in hot water such as blankets, coats, and stuffed animals can be placed in a dark plastic bag, sealed and put aside for 3 weeks. If the mite does not have human contact, it will die in 10 to 18 days.

Erythema Infectiosum (Fifth's Disease)

The skin disorder erythema infectiosum is an infection caused by parvovirus B19 that primarily affects preschool and young school-age students. The peak incidence of this infection is usually late winter and early spring. It is slightly contagious and can appear randomly or in epidemics. Asymptomatic infections are common. Infections during pregnancy may cause miscarriages (Hooper & Goldman, 1999).

Assessment

The history associated with Fifth's disease includes headache, nausea, and muscle aches. The school nurse usually sees a rash that begins on the face with a large, bright red patchy rash over the cheeks resembling "slapped cheeks." These patches are warm but nontender and have rounded borders that are usually macular (Zitelli & Davis, 2002). This "slapped cheek" appearance fades in 4 days. Two days following the rash, the student develops a lacy reddened rash that begins on the extremities and extends to the face and buttock. This rash fades in 6 to 14 days without any scaling or pigmentation.

Management

The school nurse can reassure the student and parents that the rash will fade and no treatment is required. Pregnant students should be referred to their healthcare provider for assessment of fetal hydrops. The school nurse is advised to check with the local health department for recommendations. Most health departments do not recommend exclusion from school for students with Fifth's disease.

POISON IVY AND POISON OAK

Poison ivy, oak, and sumac are caused by a reaction to the sap-like material (urushiol) from the Rhus genus of plants. Trauma to the leaves of these plants releases material that is often dragged across the skin or transferred by another vehicle, usually a pet. The urushiols bind rapidly to the skin on contact. Approximately 25% to 60% of the population is sensitive to these plants. The body's reaction to the plants is a delayed, cell-mediated hypersensitivity; therefore the incubation period after the first exposure is 5 to 21 days, although reexposure can result in a reaction within 12 to 48 hours, depending on the dosage and past exposure (Hooper & Goldman, 1999). Burning vines can release the particles into the air and this can affect sensitized individuals (Tunnessen, 1994).

Assessment

The usual presentation is linear papulovesicular lesions, but it can also be nonlinear. The itching is intense. The vesicles drain serous fluid and the skin surface becomes moist and crusted; the fluid from the vesicles does not spread the lesions.

Management

Because of the delayed reaction, "scrubbing areas that are known to have come in contact with the plants can prevent the development of lesions if it is done early enough" (Tunnessen, 1994, p. 915). While the lesions are not contagious to others, the student's clothing and anything else that has had contact with the plant resin, such as animal fur, can continue to transfer the sap. Once the lesions appear, treatment usually consists of cool soaks, calamine lotion to assist in drying the lesions, and antihistamines to decrease the itching. More intense reactions may require steroids.

ACNE VULGARIS

Acne is the most prevalent skin disorders among school-age students (Rudy, 2003). This condition frequently causes significant embarrassment and anxiety in affected individuals. Acne commonly starts in the early teen years when the oil glands in the body start making more sebum (oil). Acne can occur with varying degrees of severity (Feldman, Careccia, Barham, & Hancox, 2004). Some students will present with noninflammatory blackheads (open comedones) and whiteheads (closed comedones), while other times there may be inflammatory papules, pustules, nodules, or cysts (Rudy, 2003).

Impacted sebum and cellular debris leads to sebaceous gland swelling (Figure 25.1) This prevents the normal shedding of follicular keratinocytes that then obstruct the follicle. Accumulated debris encourages colonization of bacteria, which precipitates an immune response, leading to further inflammation (Feldman et al., 2004).

Assessment

If a student presents with acne, a thorough history is indicated. Sometimes the condition may be triggered or worsened by sweating, wearing helmets, menses, or stress. Some emollients, cosmetics, and medications may also worsen the problem (Feldman et al., 2004). On physical exam, evaluate the areas of the face, neck, chest, upper arms, and back. The skin findings consists of papules smaller than 5 mm in diameter, pustules with visible purulent material, nodules or cystic areas, and sometimes scarring. Some of the areas may be reddened and painful if touched.

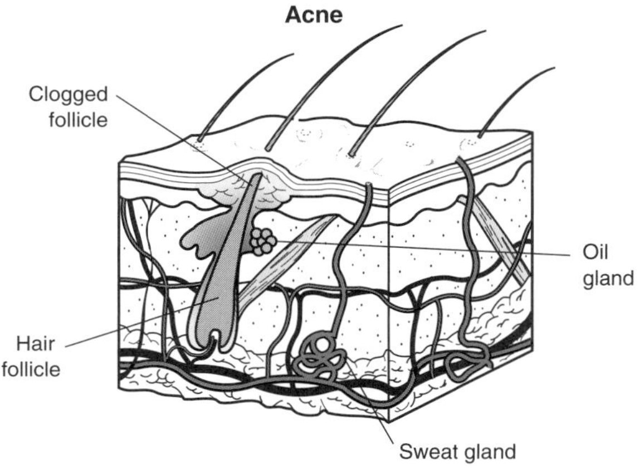

Figure 25.1 ■ Acne.

Management

Acne treatment depends on the severity and location of the lesions. The goal of therapy is to control acne lesions and to prevent scarring. Many topical medications are available for those suffering from this disorder. If the person has facial acne, the face should be washed twice a day. Benzoyl peroxide is an inexpensive keratolytic agent effective against acne and is available over-the-counter. There are other topical applications that are keratolytic that include an antibiotic such as Benzamycin, BenzaClin, or Cleocin T solution which have been found to be effective against acne, but these preparations require a prescription (Feldman et al., 2004). As an initial step, the school nurse can safely recommend these over-the-counter products.

Acne sufferers should be encouraged not to pick or squeeze eruptions, which can lead to skin damage. Students with persistent acne should be referred to their primary care provider for the prescriptive medications. If the student has severe recalcitrant nodular acne that is unresponsive to other therapy, he or she may be referred to a dermatologist for treatment with a retinoid such as Accutane. This is reserved only after the basic oral antibiotics have not been successful. Female students who are treated with a retinoid are usually required to have two negative pregnancy tests and be using two effective forms of contraception 1 month prior to the initiation of the drug and for 1 month after the cessation of the retinoid. Because of the extreme teratogenic properties of retinoids, these precautions are a requirement even if the student denies engaging in sexual activity.

SUN EXPOSURE ISSUES

The incidence of skin cancer has been rapidly increasing worldwide for the last two to three decades. UV light exposure plays a role in the development of skin cancers. Many skin cancers are preventable, especially if prevention measures start at an early age. Nearly 80% of a person's lifetime sun exposure occurs before age 21 (Laughlin-Richard, 2000).

Early diagnosis is an important component in decreasing morbidity and mortality from skin cancer. However, prevention will have the greatest impact (Laughlin-Richard, 2000). Starting prevention habits at a young age will help ensure less resistance to change in later years. Nurses and educators should focus on promoting avoidance of this hazard. "Protective measures should include sun avoidance from 10 am to 3 pm when the sun's rays are strongest, wearing protective clothing, use of sunscreens, and avoiding tanning beds" (Laughlin-Richard, 2000, p. 24).

School nurses are in a prime position to provide education and guidance regarding sun exposure risk to the greatest number of children and adolescents. They can assist communities to conduct periodic skin cancer screening clinics and can be instrumental in the development of school-based sun protection policies (Laughlin-Richard, 2000). Many preschools and elementary schools now have parents provide sunscreen with a signed consent so that teachers apply it to students prior to outside activities. For assistance and information on skin cancer prevention and educational initiatives, the reader is referred to the Centers for Disease Control and Prevention website (http://www.cdc.gov/ cancer. html).

BODY PIERCING, TATTOOING, AND BRANDING

Body alteration, whether by piercing, tattooing, cutting, or branding, is covered in Chapter 40. Included in that chapter is information on where it is done, how it is done, why it is done, and the complications that can occur. However, in this section, the care of the body alteration will be covered, both the normal after-care and the care of complications.

Piercing

After a piercing, it is essential that appropriate care be provided to prevent infection and other sequelae. Ice may be applied to decrease swelling. Emphasis should be placed on hand washing to keep unclean hands away from the piercing site. Clothing, bedding, and hair should also be kept clean, depending on the area of the piercing. The site should be washed with antibacterial soap and water twice a day and rotated at that time. Alcohol and hydrogen peroxide should not be used on piercings, as they interfere with healing. Oral piercings can be cleaned after eating by rinsing with antiseptic mouthwash that does not include alcohol (Armstrong & Kelly, 2001). Students should be encouraged to wear the jewelry until the piercing is healed. This may range from 4 weeks to 8 months, depending on the piercing site; a pierced navel may take up to 1 year to heal because of the increased irritation by the waistband and the warmth of the area increasing the risk for infection (Armstrong & Kelly, 2001).

Piercings done incorrectly have the potential to cause bleeding. The amount of bleeding associated with piercing is site dependent, with the tongue presenting the greatest threat to life. Bleeding may require pressure and an ice pack.

Infection is the most common complication related to piercing. Any break in the skin may result in either a local or systemic infection. The most common organisms associated with body piercing include *Staphylococcus aureus*, Group A streptococcus, and *Pseudomonas* (Stirn, 2003). While slight redness is normal the first few days after piercing, redness, edema, pain, heat, and yellow or green discharge may indicate an infection. If an infection is suspected, *do not remove the jewelry,* as this may prevent drainage and increase the risk of developing an abscess at the site. Systemic infections occurring following piercing may include fever, night chills, weakness, myalgia, arthralgia, lethargy, or malaise (Goldrick, 2003).

An allergic reaction to the metal of the piercing is possible, especially to nickel. Localized allergic signs and symptoms will be present, including edema and pruritis. If an allergic reaction is suspected, remove the jewelry immediately in order to stop the allergic response.

Tattooing

Tattooing causes superficial bleeding. After the tattoo is applied, a dressing is used until the bleeding stops. The dressing is removed after a few hours. From that point, the area should be treated like a burn. The area needs to be kept clean by using antibacterial soap and water twice daily and applying a thin coat of antibiotic ointment or Vaseline for a few days. The purpose of keeping the tattoo moist is to prevent a scab from forming in order to preserve the art work. If drainage continues for more than a few days or if it has the characteristics of infection, the primary care provider should be notified by the parent. As healing proceeds, the lesion may itch as scabbing occurs; the nurse should advise the student to avoid scratching as this has the potential to interfere with the art. The healing takes approximately 3 to 4 weeks (Armstrong & Kelly, 2001).

A new tattoo is at risk for infection; students should avoid swimming, hot tubs, or saunas and steam rooms until it is healed. In addition, sunlight fades the ink; therefore, students need to be constantly reminded to wear sunblock on the lesion.

Tattoo pigments are not FDA approved for intermdermal use; therefore there is no standardization of the inks used in applying tattoos. Hypersensitivity reactions have been reported with the use of tattoo ink used for permanent tattoos and henna used for temporary tattoos. If the student is having an allergic reaction to particular colors, the only way to stop the reaction is to have the tattoo artist "re-tattoo" over the affected site (which is very painful) to allow the offending color to ooze out of the skin.

Branding

Branding results in a second- or third-degree burn. A "strike" consists of touching the skin with a steel design. Healing following branding may take up to one year. Skin that has been branded will change color, going from the original erythematous skin from the newly acquired burn to the desired brown or grey color (Armstrong & Kelly, 2001).

The site must be cleaned twice daily and a non-adhesive bandage should be applied. Some burns will require an antibacterial ointment for prophylaxis. The student must understand there is a risk of keloid scars with branding.

SELF-MUTILATION

Self-mutilation is frequently referred to as "cutting" by adolescents. Self- mutilation is repeated superficial cutting with a sharp object; it includes burning, carving, or scratching of the skin. Self-mutilation may be in areas readily seen by the school nurse, including extremities, or the sites may be hidden by clothing. The scars are the presenting symptom and range from one to hundreds of scars. The scars are usually superficial and may present in a pattern or symbol. Students who participate in self-mutilation may be more likely to wear clothes that cover their arms and legs and avoid participation in events that would require exposing their skin (Derouin & Bravender, 2004). Management of cutting involves nonjudgmental active listening to the student who is a self-mutilator and prevention of infection. Referral for counseling may be appropriate (Derouin & Bravender, 2004).

CONCLUSION

The school nurse is often the first person the student seeks when there is a problem. Parents and teachers will also come to the school nurse for guidance to address skin disorders. Acquiring a history using nonjudgmental therapeutic communication and performing a physical exam of the involved areas will help the school nurse determine the etiology and appropriate management of the presenting skin problem.

References

Armstrong, M. L., & Kelly, L. (2001). Tattooing, body piercing, and branding are on the rise: Perspectives for school nurses. *Journal of School Nursing, 17*,(1), 12–24.

Derouin, A., & Bravender, T. (2004). Living on the edge : The current phenomenon of self multilation in adolescents. *The American Journal of Maternal / Child Nursing, 29*(1), 12–18.

Estrada. J., & Morris, R. (2000). Pediculosis in a school population. *The Journal of School Nursing, 16*(3), 32–38.

Feldman, S., Careccia, R. E., Barham, K. L., & Hancox, J. (2004). Diagnosis and treatment of acne. *American Family Physician, 69*(9), 2123–2130.

Fitzpatrick, T. B., Johnson, R. A., Wolff, K., & Suurmond, D. (2001). *Color atlas and synopsis of clinical dermatology* (4th ed.). New York: McGraw-Hill.

Goldsmith, L., Lazarus, G., & Tharp, M. (1997). *Adult and pediatric dermatology. A color guide to diagnosis and treatment.* Philadelphia: F. A. Davis.

Goldrick, A. B. (2003). Endocarditis associated with body piercing. *American Journal of Nursing, 103*(1), 26–27.

Habif, T., Quitadamo, M., Campbell, J., & Zug, K. (2001). *Skin disease: Diagnosis and treatment*. St. Louis: C. V. Mosby.

Habif, T., Rothe, M., & Grant-Kels, J. (1997). *Diagnostic algorithms in dermatology: disease and treatment pathways for the primary care physician*. Westwood Squibb.

Hoekelman, R. A, Adam, H. M, Nelson, N. M, Weitzman, M. L., & Wilson, M. H. (2001). *Primary pediatric care* (4th ed.). St. Louis: C. V. Mosby.

Hooper, B., & Goldman, M. (1999). *Primary dermatologic care*. St. Louis: C. V. Mosby.

Jarvis, C. (2004). *Physical examination and health assessment* (4th ed.). Philadelphia: W. B. Saunders.

Laughlin-Richard, N. (2000). Sun exposure and skin cancer prevention in students and adolescents. *Journal of School Nursing, 16*(2), 20–26.

McDonald, L. L., & Smith, M. L. (1998). Diagnostic dilemmas in pediatric/adolescent dermatology: Scaly scalp. *Journal of Pediatric Health Care, 12*, 80–84.

McLeod, R. P. (2003). Lumps, bumps, and things that go itch in your office! *The Journal of School Nursing, 19*(6), 359–360.

Nicol, N. H., & Bradley, B. J. (1999). *Nursing assessment of school age youth: Dermatologic*. Scarborough, MA: National Association of School Nurses.

Rudy, S. (2003). Overview of the evaluation and management of acne vulgaris. *Pediatric Nursing, 29*(4), 287–293.

Schmitt, B. (2002). *Pediatric telephone protocols*. Evanston, IL: American Academy of Pediatrics.

Stirn, A. (2003). Body piercing: Medical consequences and psychological motivations. *The Lancet, 361*, 1205–1215.Tunnessen, W. (1994). Pediatric dermatology. In F. Oski, C. DeAngelis, R. Feigin, J. McMillan, & J. Warshaw (Eds.), *Principles and practice of pediatrics* (pp. 898–948). Philadelphia: Lippincott.

Zitelli, B. J., & Davis, H. W. (2002). *Atlas of pediatric physical diagnosis* (4th ed.). St. Louis: C. V. Mosby.

Chapter 26

Pediculosis Infestation

LAURA JANNONE ▪ BARBARA KRIVDA

Chapter Outline

INTRODUCTION

Lice are a great concern to school nurses. Every school nurse knows how parents react to a phone call or a note sent home about infestation; the nurse is also the best resource for accurate information about lice. Although the school nurse assumes the leadership role, managing lice infestation in the school population is a responsibility that needs to be shared among school administrators, teachers, school physicians, local physicians, public health departments, other community groups, and families (Vessey, 2000).

Infestation with lice is termed pediculosis. Three different species of lice infest the human body: head lice, body lice, and pubic lice (Vessey, 2000). These insects are ectoparasites, insects that feed on the human host but live outside the body. Infestations of ectoparasites are common in children, primarily by head lice (Potts, 2001).

HEAD LICE

The most common lice in the United States are head lice (*Pediculus humanus capitis*). Each year approximately six to twelve million Americans, most of these between ages 3 and 12, are infested with head lice (Williams, Reichert, MacKenzie, Hightower, & Blake, 2001), although there seems to be no basis for this number. There is also no agreement as to what constitutes an infestation.

It is important to remember that *Pediculus humanus capitis*, unlike other species of lice, is *not* associated with disease transmission or with one's hygiene. However, the words "head lice" cause a high level of anxiety among parents of school-age children (Frankowski, Weiner, the Committee on School Health, and the Committee on Infectious Diseases, 2002).

Head lice are small parasitic insects that reside mainly on the scalp and neck hairs of a human host, but feed off of the host's capillary blood through the scalp from every few hours to once a day (Burgess, Pollack, & Taplin, 2003; Frankowski et al., 2002); therefore, they must live close to the scalp. Having head lice is an annoying but relatively harmless condition.

Head Louse Life Cycle

The life cycle of adult head lice is from 23 to 30 days (Burgess et al., 2003). The female louse lays approximately 10 eggs or nits per day or as many as 400 eggs in its lifespan. When the eggs are released, a cement-like substance is also released, allowing the egg to stick to the hair shaft within 6 mm of the scalp (Burgess et al., 2003). The eggs hatch in 10 to 14 days; at this point they are called nymphs and are about the size of a period (Burgess et al., 2003). On about the third day of life, the nymphs leave the eggshell casings and continue to grow until day 9 to 12, when they mature to the adult stage (Frankowski et al., 2002). At this point, the females are 2.4 to 3.3 mm in size and the male is 2.1 to 2.6 mm, about the size of a sesame seed (Burgess et al., 2003). The adults mate and the cycle is repeated (FIGURE 26.1). The color of the louse may vary from tan through

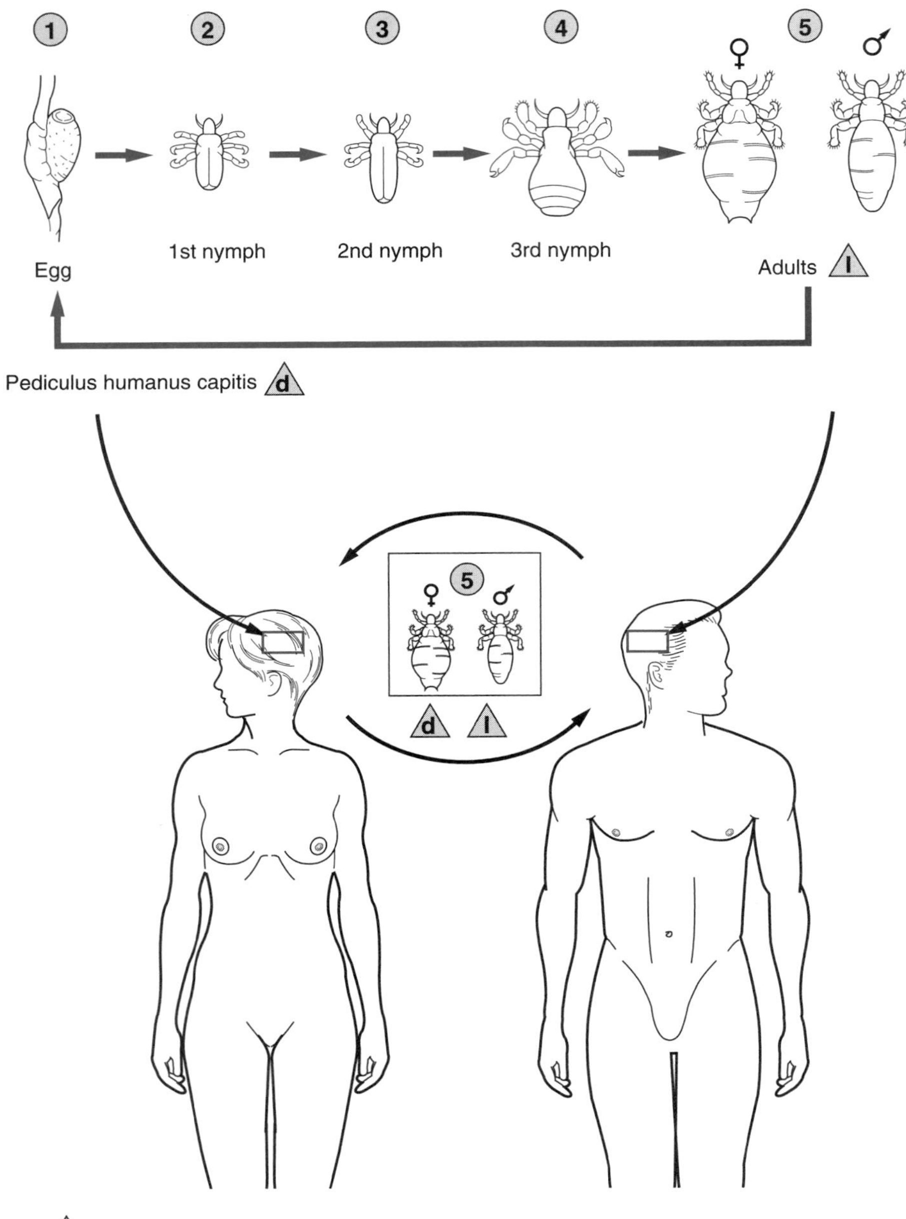

Figure 26.1 ■ Head lice life cycle. (From CDC, 2002, p. 1.)

gray. With its six legs, the louse can grasp the human hair shaft and scurry between hairs on the scalp (Frankowski et al., 2002).

Nits are the eggshell casings of the lice eggs and are about 1 mm long; they are shaped like a teardrop. It is difficult to tell if the nits contain developing embryos or if they are empty casings; only the former may produce a live louse and need to be treated. Williams et al. (2001) examined the likelihood of becoming infested with lice as a result of having nits. They found that just 18% (9 out of 50) of children presenting with nits converted to lice within 14 days. While the number of nits was not significant, the distance of the nits to the scalp was considered a risk factor, especially for those very close to the scalp.

Viable nits may be pigmented and camouflaged to match the host's hair color (Frankowski et al., 2002), whereas empty nit casings are white and easier to see except, perhaps, on a person with white or light blond hair. The nits are laid close to the scalp, as body heat is needed to incubate the eggs. Egg production occurs at a temperature that is warmer than room air but in some parts of the world, scalp temperatures may be the same or even cooler than ambient air temperature; therefore, most eggs are laid on the hair shaft within 1/2 inch of the scalp (Frankowski et al., 2002).

When the louse feeds, it injects a small amount of saliva, which can cause a pruritic reaction. Sensitivity to the saliva can take 4 to 6 weeks to develop (Frankowski et al., 2002). An adult louse can survive up to 30 days on a host's scalp. If the louse falls off the host, it will die within 2 days (Centers for Disease Control and Prevention [CDC], 2001).

Transmission

"It is probably impossible to totally prevent head lice infestations" (Frankowski et al., 2002, p. 639). The primary mode of transmission is direct physical contact, especially head-to-head. Lice have no wings, and therefore cannot fly or jump between individuals; they can only crawl (Burgess et al., 2003). Static electricity and the charges that result, especially those caused with low temperatures and low humidity and the use of a plastic comb, can cause a louse to appear to move great distances. "Presumably, a person would also need to pick up at least one male and one female–or a pregnant female- to launch a perpetuating population" (Frankowski et al., p. 4).

Transmission via personal belongings of the infected host, or fomites, is less likely but is possible (Frankowski et al., 2003). The danger in not wearing shared protective headgear for contact sports has a significantly higher risk of significant sequelae than is the risk of getting lice. Therefore, there is no excuse for not using these protective items. Also, "pets do not spread head lice" (Frankowski et al., p. 4).

Head Lice: Who's at Risk?

While everyone is susceptible to infestations, some groups are at greater risk than others:

- Children between 3 and 10 years of age and their families are infested most often (CDC, 2001). Females have more head lice than males, in a 2:1 ratio. One possible reason is that girls tend to share more hair implements than boys, such as combs, brushes, and hats (CDC, n.d.).
- Whites have a greater likelihood of having head lice than African Americans, by almost 99%. This lower prevalence among African Americans in the United States is probably attributable to the North American species of lice that cannot grip the oval-shaped hair shaft characteristic of African Americans (Meinking, 1999).

Avoiding the Spread of Head Lice

To prevent or lessen the risk of contracting head lice, instruct students, teachers, and families as follows:

- Avoid head to head contact, whether in the classroom when students are working on projects together or in sports, such as wrestling.
- Do not share clothing, hats, or towels.
- Do not share combs, brushes, or hair accessories, including those made available during picture-taking sessions.
- Do not lie on beds, couches, pillows, carpets, or stuffed animals of someone who is infected.
- Use caution when multiple persons use headphones, helmets, patrol hats, or hats worn as props for plays.
- In schools or other places where children gather, separate belongings into lockers, cubbies, or separated hooks. Do not put clothing into piles (CDC, 2002; Hootman, 2004).

Identification

"The gold standard for diagnosis of head lice is finding a live louse on the head" (Frankowski et al., 2002, p. 638). Finding a live louse can be difficult as the louse crawls rapidly. Nits attached to the hair shaft are easier to see than a moving louse (FIGURE 26.2). Nits within 1/2 inch of the scalp are most likely to be viable. The live nits are most often seen at the

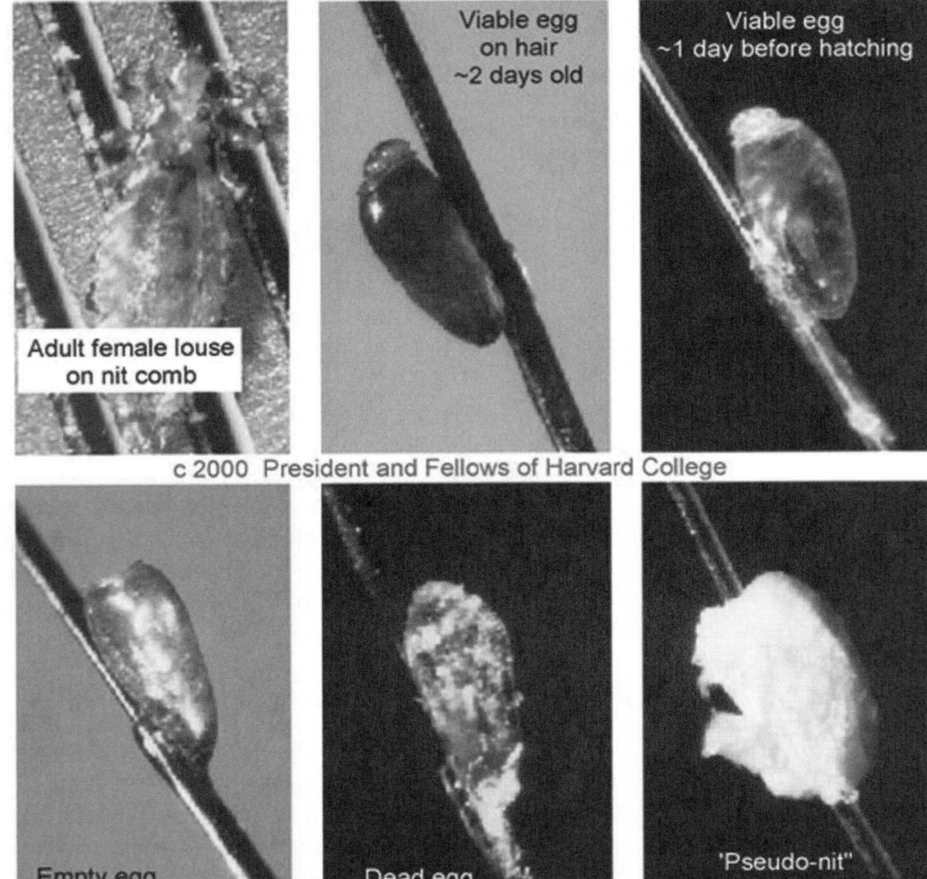

Figure 26.2 ■ Images to assist in the identification of head lice and their eggs. (http://www.hsph.harvard.edu/headlice.html; Pollack et al., 2000.)

posterior hairline and behind the ears. Dandruff, hair casts, hair spray droplets, scabs, dirt, and aphids have all been misidentified as nits (Pollack, Kiszewski, & Spielman, 2000).

The person infested with head lice may feel a tickling sensation of something moving in the hair. Itching of the scalp begins as a result of the sensitivity reaction from the louse bites. Sores caused by scratching may be present on the head (CDC, 2002). Secondary bacterial infections, such as pyoderma and impetigo, can occur related to scratching, but systemic infections are rare. Posterior cervical and suboccipital lymphadenopathy may be present (Potts, 2001).

The School Nurse's Role

The American Academy of Pediatrics does not recommend screening for head lice. Screenings result in unnecessary absenteeism with little effect on the incidence of head lice (Frankowski et al., 2002). However, during the time of a widespread outbreak in a school, screening in classrooms affected may be necessary.

A student may be sent to the nurse when an observant teacher notices the student scratching his or her head. When a student with a possible case of head lice comes to the school nurse, the role of the school nurse is to:

- Identify if pediculosis exists.
- Document the problem.
- Contact, educate, and support the family (Figure 26.3).
- Facilitate the student's return to school, or if your school does not have a "no-nit" policy, to ensure the student remains in school.
- Maintain confidentiality (Estrada & Morris, 2000).

Parent Bulletin
Head Lice

____
Date

A case of head lice (pediculosis) has been reported in your child's school. Lice are a common occurrence in schools. Head lice do not transmit disease.

When a child gets lice, it does not suggest that the child is not clean. It only indicates that the child has been near someone with lice.

All families are being informed so that parents examine their children's scalp and hair carefully each day for head lice.

Lice may cause itching and scratching of the scalp.

Head lice are insects the size and color of a sesame seed. They do not fly or jump but scamper on the scalp. Lice are spread by head-to-head contact or shared items.

Lice eggs (nits) are tear drop shaped and white or hair color. They are tightly attached to the hair shaft, usually behind the ears and at the back of the neck. Nits cannot be "flicked off."

If a head louse is found on your child, treatment is required before the child is permitted to return to school. All treatments need careful attention to directions to decrease any risk of side effects and to ensure elimination of the infestation. Use only treatments recommended for head lice as products intended for animals or for other purposes will not be effective. Please contact your school nurse or healthcare provider for recommendations on treatment. The school nurse can also provide more information about head lice and school district policies.

________________School Nurse

Figure 26.3 ■ Example notification for parents in a school with an exclusion policy.

The school nurse first needs to consider the student's privacy, as head lice can cause embarrassment and misunderstanding (Frankowski et al., 2002). The nurse or screener needs to be educated as to how to recognize head lice in order to avoid misidentification of dandruff or other debris as nits or lice (Pollack et al., 2000); nits adhere to the hair and will not fall off with shaking, while dandruff will fall off with movement. In a private setting with good lighting, the nurse or screener uses applicators or other thin disposable instruments to separate hair into small sections with special attention to the area behind the ears and at the nape of the neck. The applicators or instruments are disposed of after each head inspection.

The nurse observes for live lice, nits, rash, head scratching, and enlarged lymph nodes (Hootman, 2004). If a living nymph or adult head louse is found in the hair, the child is considered actively infested (Keoki, Reichert, Blake, MacKenzie, & Hightower, 2001). The nurse needs to observe any nits for location and color of egg casing. Viable nits are usually located within a half inch of the scalp because of their need for a warm ambient temperature. A found louse or nit can be placed on a 3×5 card and secured with clear tape for documentation. After the screening, discuss the findings with the student and inform the student's parents (Hootman, 2004).

Once a live louse or nit is discovered, the school nurse must follow the school district's policy on head lice. School district policies vary widely in response to pediculosis. National organizations give disparate recommendations on the subject of head lice. The American Academy of Pediatrics (AAP) recommends the "child with active head lice should remain in class but be discouraged from close direct head contact with others" and the parent contacted and educated as to how to deal with the lice (Frankowski et al., 2002, p. 641). However, the AAP does note that head lice may be more readily transmitted at child care centers because of the close head-to-head contact (Frankowski et al., 2002) and these sites may need stricter measures.

Some school districts have "no nit" policies that require a student who has even one nit to be dismissed from school until the problem is resolved. No Nit policies are recommended by the National Pediculosis Association. A No Nit policy states that children must be free of lice and nits to attend school (National Pediculosis Association, n.d.). Under a No Nit policy, a child identified with nits is excluded until all nits are removed. The results of the study by Williams et al. (2001) as well as the American Academy of Pediatrics discourage No Nit policies. Their reason for this position is that children have had unnecessary prolonged absences due to nit free school policies (Frankowski et al., 2002). Scott, Gilmer, and Johannessen (2004) suggest that a nit rating scale be used and that if lice are identified, the family be notified at the end of the school day, so that the student can be treated that evening and would not miss any class time. As long as the student's nit score continues to decrease each day, he or she should be allowed to stay in school.

Hootman (2004) recommends that only those students who need treatment be dismissed. This requires the school nurse to differentiate between nits that are empty casings and those that contain eggs. She recommends that those with lice should be excluded and that students should be rechecked immediately on return to school. "Removal of nits is not mandatory unless directed by school policy" (Hootman, 2004, p. III-HEADL-1).

After identification of an individual with active head lice infestation, all persons in close contact with that individual within the previous week need to be inspected. This includes the individual's family, friends, and classmates. When it is known that students in one school have possibly exposed students in neighboring schools, the school nurses for those schools should be notified. The principal should be notified if three students in one classroom or 3% of the student population is infested within two consecutive weeks (Hootman, 2004). Mass screening for the school can then be scheduled.

The school nurse in the leadership role needs to be involved in the development or revision of the school district's pediculosis policy. School board policies should be in place before an outbreak. The head lice policy needs to be evidence based, not based on unfounded fears, anecdotal information, or misinformation. The policy should address screening procedures, notification procedures, requirements for return to school, and any special procedures for a widespread outbreak.

By providing education using accurate available information, the school nurse can address the concerns of the school community. Teachers report that they need more information about head lice and that they would prefer to receive information from the school nurse in the form of videos and brochures (Kirchofer, 2001). Head lice education is recommended for students, families, and staff on a regular basis. The school nurse can speak at faculty meetings and parent organization meetings. The school nurse is the primary source of information on treatment of head lice. In her role as educator, the school nurse needs to stay up-to-date on the recommended treatments.

Treatment

Any persons found to be infested with live lice or viable nits need to be treated (Vessey, 2000). There are three schools of thought for head lice treatment: common pediculicides (TABLE 26.1), alternative natural products, and systematic nit removal (Vessey, 2000).

Pediculicides

Permethrin 1% (Nix by Pfizer) is the current recommended treatment for head lice (Frankowski et al., 2002). Permethrin is a synthetic pyrethroid. It comes as a cream rinse and is applied to towel-dried hair after shampooing. The cream rinse is left on the hair for 10 minutes and then rinsed off. All topical pediculicides should be rinsed off with cool water rather than hot to limit absorption from vasodilation. The product should be rinsed into the sink, rather than during a shower, to limit exposure. Permethrin leaves a residue on the hair that kills nymphs emerging from unhatched eggs; therefore, it needs to be used only once. This product reports low toxicity and does not cause an allergic reaction in individuals with plant allergies. Resistance to permethrin has been reported (Frankowski et al., 2002).

Pyrethrin (Rid by Bayer, A-200 by Hogill Pharmaceutical, R&C by GlaxoSmithKline, Pronto by Del Laboratories and Clear Lice Systems by Care Technologies) is manufactured from natural extracts of chrysanthemums. This product is neurotoxic to lice and has low toxicity for humans. However, the label warns of possible allergic reaction in persons sensitive to ragweed. Most products are shampoos applied to dry hair and left on for 10 minutes and then rinsed out. Twenty to thirty percent of eggs remain viable after treatment. Repeat application is recommended in 7 to 10 days in order to kill the newly hatched nymphs. Resistance has been reported (Frankowski et al., 2002). If that second treatment is delayed, a new crop of lice will have been born.

Failure of over-the-counter products has been attributed to two causes: improper use or insecticide resistance (Burgess, 2003). Improper use includes inappropriate use due to misidentification of lice or nits, not using enough product to cover the scalp and hair or not repeating the treatment in 7 to 10 days (for pyrethrin only). It is important to remember that no pediculicide kills 100% of viable nits. For continued infestation (observed live lice and not just the presence of nits) after treatment, referral to the family's healthcare provider is recommended to ensure accurate diagnosis and determine whether there is a need for further treatment.

Malathion (Ovide by Taro Pharmaceuticals) has been recently reintroduced in the United States. This organophosphate is available only by prescription. The lotion is applied to the hair, left to air dry

Table 26.1 ■
COMMON PEDICULICIDES

PEDICULI-CIDE	BRAND NAME	OVICIDAL ACTIVITY	APPLI-CATION	ADVANTAGES	DISADVANTAGES
Permethrin	Nix	High	Crème rinse	Low toxicity Residual ovicidal activity Nonprescription	Possible resistance Allergic reaction risk
Pyrethrin	Rid Clear R&C Pronto	Low	Shampoo	Low toxicity Nonprescription	Possible resistance No residual ovicidal activity Allergic reaction risk
Lindane	Kwell	Low	Shampoo	None	CNS toxicity Known resistance No residual ovicidal activity Do not use with pregnant or nursing mothers.
Malathion	Ovide	High	Apply to dry hair; leave on 12 hours	Kills lice and eggs. Residual effect for 1 week	Prescription only Smells bad. Flammable

for 8 to 12 hours, and then washed off. It should be reapplied only if live lice are seen in 7 to 10 days. Malathion is highly ovicidal. The product has a high alcohol content and is highly flammable. If accidentally ingested, there is a risk of severe respiratory depression. This product is recommended for use only in instances of lice resistance to other products. Caution is recommended (Frankowski et al., 2002).

Skin reactions may occur with topical application. Itching or a mild burning sensation caused by inflammation of the skin may last for several days after all lice have been killed. It is important to differentiate this reaction to the topical product from the itching due to head lice so as not to recommend overtreatment.

Lindane (by Morton Grove Pharmaceuticals) is an organochloride insecticide like DDT. This product is available only by prescription and because of the availability of safer products, is no longer indicated for the first line treatment of pediculosis in the United States (Lindane, 2005). It can be toxic to humans if used incorrectly, leading to seizures or death (Burgess et al., 2003). Worldwide resistance has been reported. For these reasons, lindane should be used only if a physician decides it is really needed.

Natural Alternatives

Products marketed by health food stores as natural products do not need to meet FDA standards for safety and effectiveness. Lice Freee claims to be the number one nontoxic head lice solution. This product's active ingredient is mineral sodium chloride (Tec Labs, n.d.). Pronto lice killing shampoo by Del Pharmaceuticals contains natural extracts and oils. Hair Clean 1-2-3 by Quantum Health contains anise, ylang ylang, coconut oils, and isopropyl alcohol. One researcher found this product to be as effective as Nix (Frankowski et al., 2002).

Occlusive agents used to treat head lice include mayonnaise, petroleum jelly, pomades, and food oils.

These products are massaged into the scalp and the hair is coated. A shower cap is worn overnight. Diligent shampooing is required to remove the products. In theory, these substances may obstruct the respiration of the louse, but need to be kept on for hours in order to even theoretically be effective. No research on effectiveness or safety has been reported.

Families should not use kerosene, insect repellents, flea control sprays or shampoos, or other items not labeled for human use (Hensel, 2000). These pose great hazards and have no proven efficacy.

Nit Removal

Manual nit removal or systematic combing to remove nits can be effective in eliminating head lice (Pollack et al., 2000). This is a time consuming and difficult task, which requires a nit picker with good eyesight and a cooperative child. Once per day with a head lice comb or gloved fingers, the hair needs to be separated and nits within 1/2 to 1 inch of the scalp removed. It is very important to clean the head lice comb frequently during the process (Vessey, 2000). A number of school nurses indicate that bare fingers and washing after work better for nit removal than latex gloves. It is believed that the gloves prevent the fingers from sliding along the hairs, thus causing pain.

Battery-powered head lice combs have not shown an advantage over traditional fine tooth lice combs (Frankowski et al., 2002). There are commercial products, which claim to loosen the glue that attaches nits to the hair shaft, thus making the process of nit picking easier. Clear Lice Egg Remover Gel by Care Technologies is a vinegar-based product. No clinical benefit has been shown. This product has been tested with over-the-counter pediculicides; its use is not recommended as it may interfere with the residual activity of the lice-killing product. Acetone, bleach, vodka, and WD-40 have all proved to be ineffective in loosening nits from the hair shaft and present an unacceptable risk to the individual (Frankowski et al., 2002).

Environmental Control

Transmission of head lice by environmental surfaces is less likely than transmission by head-to-head contact. However, it is prudent to clean items that have been in contact in the previous two days with the head of the person with the infestation. Personal items can be washed, soaked, or dried at a temperature greater than 130°F. Nonwashable items such as stuffed animals can be sealed in plastic bags for 10 to 14 days or dry-cleaned. Carpeting, overstuffed furniture, pillows, and car seats that have been in contact with the head of the person with head lice should be vacuumed. Students' coats can be isolated by putting them in plastic bags and hanging them on the backs of chairs (Hootman, 2004).

Pediculicide sprays should not be used because exposure cannot be controlled. Also, sprays are hazardous to children with asthma and to pets. They are expensive and have little or no effect on the lice. Head lice cannot be transmitted to pets, and animals do not need to be included in the cleaning measures. Whole house fumigation or the services of pest control companies are unnecessary (Frankowski et al., 2002).

Outbreaks

True epidemic outbreaks of head lice are rare (Vessey, 2000). However, if an outbreak occurs the result may be "outraged parents, concerned school administrators and puzzled children" (Hall, 2003, p. 13).

The school nurse, in her leadership role, is vital to the school's response to the problem. During the time of the outbreak, the nurse can recommend that dress-up clothing, especially hats, be put away in plastic bags. The students' hats should be stuffed into their coat sleeves. Sports helmets and earphones may need to be individually labeled and not shared. Close contact sports such as wrestling may require head inspections during the outbreak. Carpeting, especially in rooms with younger students, requires daily, thorough vacuuming. Teaching staff, families, and students need to be provided, with evidence-based information about head lice. The county board of health, neighboring school districts, and the school physician can provide assistance. When the school reacts in a calm manner, parents can focus on treatment and not become overly upset (Frankowski et al., 2002).

Family Support

The school nurse needs to consider that families affected by pediculosis are impacted physically, emotionally, financially, and socially (Hensel, 2000). Families have varying access to information and may encounter barriers to successful treatment. The school nurse can provide the needed support for effective treatment outcomes. "Without trust, families are often not ready to accept and apply health information" (Hootman, 2002, p. 85).

BODY LICE

Infestation with body lice (*Pediculus humanus corporis*) is common worldwide. However, in the United States, body lice infestations are rare (CDC, 2003).

The body louse affects primarily those living in squalid conditions and who do not wash or change their clothes regularly (Potts, 2001).

Body lice live on the skin, and in the clothing and bedding of infested humans (CDC, 2003). The mature lice lay eggs in their host's clothing seams. The body louse emerges, usually at night, to feed on the host's blood. Poor hygiene contributes to the transmission of body lice through infested clothing and linens. To prevent outbreaks or eliminate body lice infestation, simple hygiene and laundering of clothes and bed linens is usually sufficient (Potts, 2001).

Body lice are acquired mainly through direct contact with an infested person or his or her clothing, or their bed linens. Unlike head lice, body lice can transmit diseases. Typhus and other louse-borne diseases have become epidemic at times of war, during disasters, or within prisons or refugee camps (CDC, 2003).

Body lice have a life cycle similar to that of head lice. The nits are generally easy to see in the seams of clothing and around the armpits and waistline. The nits are usually yellow to white (CDC, 2003). The louse is similar in appearance to head lice, only larger (Potts, 2001).

Body lice infestation causes itching and a rash. The louse bite causes a hypersensitivity reaction in the host. Bite sites may be visible on the body, particularly on the trunk, axilla, and groin. Hands and feet are usually not affected (Potts, 2001). Areas of lice bites may develop secondary infections (CDC, 2003). School nurses should refer these students to a healthcare provider if secondary infections are present. Body lice can be treated when the infested person washes and changes clothes and launders all clothing and linens. Laundering requires use of the hot wash cycle and dryer cycle. Permethrin or pyrethrin lice shampoo may be applied to the body, as directed by the healthcare provider.

PUBIC LICE

Pubic lice (*Pthirus pubis*) or crabs are parasites that infect the genital region of humans. Infection is common worldwide (CDC, 2003). Pubic lice have short crab-like bodies, which are very different from head lice or body lice. The pubic louse has a life cycle similar to that of the head and body louse. The nits are attached to the hair shaft usually in the genital region and are hard to see (CDC, 2003).

Crabs are most frequently found in the genital area on pubic hair of the infested person, but may also be found elsewhere on the body. Infestation of young children is usually on the eyebrows and eye lashes. Sexual contact is the usual mode of transmission. "Infection in a young child or teenager may indicate sexual activity or abuse." If sexual abuse is suspected, the school nurse should call protective services. If the student is an emancipated adult, appropriate referral to a heath care provider should be made (CDC, 2003, p. 1). Pubic lice transmission through an infested person's bed linens, towels, or clothing is unlikely. The toilet seat is not a probable place for transmission of pubic lice because of the cool temperature and the crab's lack of feet to walk on or hold onto smooth surfaces (CDC, 2003).

Pubic lice are treated with pediculicidal shampoo. It is recommended that nits be removed and bedding as well as underwear and clothing worn within the previous three days should be laundered on the hot cycle or dry cleaned. Sexual partners need to be informed. Any sexual partner needs to be treated and sexual contact needs to be avoided until the infestation has been cured (CDC, 2003).

CONCLUSION

The school nurse is in the position to be a student advocate and a healthcare expert. "The school nurse's goals are to contain infestation, provide appropriate health information for treatment and prevention, prevent overexposure to potentially hazardous chemicals and minimize school absence" (National Association of School Nurses [NASN], 2004). NASN's position statement on pediculosis states, the management of pediculosis should not disrupt the education process. Children found with live head lice should be referred to parents for treatment. Data do not support school exclusion for nits. Because no disease process is associated with head lice, schools are not advised to exclude students when nits remain after appropriate lice treatment, although further monitoring for signs of reinfestations is appropriate. The school nurse, as student advocate and nursing expert, should be included in school district-community planning, implementation, and evaluation of vector control programs for the school setting. The school nurse retains an important role in educating all constituencies about pediculosis and dispelling myths and stigmas regarding lice infestation" (NASN, 2004).

Resources

Educational Materials

Web sites: These Web sites provide information for professionals and the public on head lice, body lice, and pubic lice.

Centers for Disease Control and Prevention
http://www.cdc.gov/ncidod/dpd/parasites/headlice/default.htm

Harvard School of Public Health
http://www.hsph.harvard.edu/headlice.html
This Web site provides comprehensive information about head lice, plus a recommendation for practice.

National Association of School Nurses
http://www.nasn.org/positions/2004pediculosis.htm
NASN position statement on no-nit policies

Videos

"Removing Head Lice Safely"—Watch On-Line—University of Nebraska, Lincoln. FREE on-line video for parents or professionals in English, Spanish and Arabic.
http://www.lancaster.unl.edu/enviro/HeadLice/Video.htm—19

"Head Lice: An Itchy Problem"
Coastal Video Commercial video to present to staff and/or families. 1.800.725.3418
http://www.coastal.com/coastalACB/showdetl.cfm?&DID=7&Product_ID=7215

Pharmaceutical Companies Providing Educational Materials

(Note: these generally advocate the use of their brand of pediculicide.)
Tec Laboratories
1 800 ITCHING
http://www.licefreee.com

Bayer
Web site covers Rid and head lice
Links to information on body lice and pubic lice
http://www.ridlice.com
coupon on site

Woodridge Labs, Inc.
16217 Kittridge St.
Van Nuys, CA 91406
http://www.safetek4lice.com
(888) 766–7331

Organizations

National Pediculosis Association (NPA)
P.O. Box 610189
Newton, MA 02161
http://www.headlice.org

Treatment Aids

LiceMeister™ Comb available through the National Pediculosis Association
This comb meets the standards for nit removal.

Lice Guard Robi-Comb
ARR Health Technologies, Inc. Available through pharmacies
800 739 9883
http://www.liceguard.com

References

Burgess, I. (2003). Commentary: How to advise a patient when over the counter products have failed. *British Medical Journal, 326*, 1257.

Burgess, I., Pollack, R., & Taplin, D. (2003). *Cutting through controversy: Special report on the treatment of head lice*. Morristown, NJ: Premier Healthcare Resource.

Centers for Disease Control and Prevention (CDC). (2001, July). *Fact sheet: Head lice infestation*. Retrieved September 14, 2003 from http://www.cdc.gov/ncidod/dpd/parasites/headlice/factsht_head_lice

Centers for Disease Control and Prevention (CDC). (2002, September 12). *Parasites and health: Head lice*. Retrieved October 4, 2003 from Division of Parasitic Diseases Web site: http://dpd.cdc.gov/dpdx/HTML/G-L/Headlice/body_HeadLice_page1.htm

Centers for Disease Control and Prevention. (CDC). (n.d.). *Fact Sheet: Body lice*. Retrieved October 4, 2003 from Division of Parasitic Diseases Web site: http://www.cdc.gov/ncidod/dpd/parasites/lice/ factsht_body_lice.htm

Centers for Disease Control and Prevention. (CDC). (n.d.). *Fact sheet: Pubic lice or "crabs."* Retrieved October 4, 2003 from Division of Parasitic Diseases Web site: http://www.cdc.gov/ncidod/dpd/parasites/lice/factsht_pubic_lice.htm

Estrada, J. S., & Morris, R. I. (2000). Pediculosis in a school population. *The Journal of School Nursing, 16*(3), 32.

Frankowski, B. L., Weiner, L. B., the Committee on School Health, & the Committee on Infectious Diseases (2002). Head lice: Clinical report. *Pediatrics, 110*, 638–643.

Hall, D. (2003). The school nurse and oh, no—head lice. *NASN Newsletter, 18*(5), 13–14.

Hensel, P. (2000). The Challenge of choosing a pediculicide. *Public Health Nursing, 17*, 300–304.

Hootman, J. (2002). Quality improvement projects related to pediculosis management. *The Journal of School Nursing, 18*, 80–86.

Hootman, J. (2004). *Quality nursing interventions in the school setting: Procedures / models / guidelines*. Scarborough, ME: National Association of School Nurses.

Keoki, W. L., Reichert, A., Blake, P. A., MacKenzie, W. R., & Hightower, A. W. (2001). Lice, nits and school policy. *Pediatrics, 107*, 1011.

Kirchofer, G. M. (2001). Primary grade teachers' knowledge and perceptions of head lice. *Journal of School Health, 2001*, 448–452.

Lindane (topical). (2005). Retrieved September 2005 from http://www.drugs.com/MMX/Lindane.html

Meinking, T. A. (1999). Infestations. *Current Problems in Dermatology, 11*, 73–120.

National Association of School Nurses. (NASN). (2004). *Pediculosis in the school community*. Retrieved September 7, 2005 from http://www.nasn.org/positions/ 2004pediculosis.htm

National Pediculosis Association. (n.d.). *The no nit policy: A healthy standard for children and their families*. Retrieved October 11, 2003 from http://www.headlice.org/downloads/nonitpolicy/htm

Pollack, R. J., Kiszewski, A. E., & Spielman, A. (2000). Overdiagnosis and consequent mismanagement of head louse infestations in North America. *Pediatric Infectious Disease Journal, 19*, 689–693.

Potts, J. (2001). Eradication of ectoparasites in children. *Postgraduate Medicine, 110*(1), 57.

Scott, P., Gilmer, M., & Johannessen, W. (2004). The Nit Rating Scale. *Journal of School Health, 74*(3), 108–110.

Tec Labs. (n.d.). *Lice freee! Homeopathic pediculicide*. Retrieved October 12, 2003 from http://www.licefreee.com

Vessey, J. (2000). *Current Concepts in Pediculosis Management*. Scarborough, ME: NASN.

Williams, L.K., Reichert, A., MacKenzie, W., Hightower, A., & Blake, P. (2001). Lice, nits, and school policy. *Pediatrics, 107*(5), 1011–1015.

PART VI

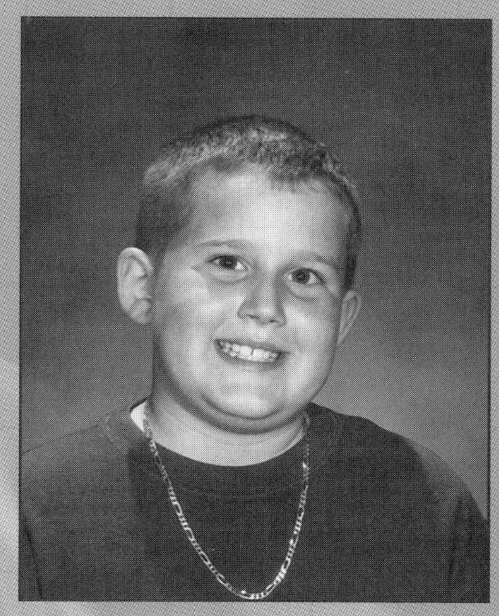

Chronic Conditions of School Children

Chapter 27

Children with Chronic Conditions

JANICE SELEKMAN ▪ MICHAEL GAMEL-McCORMICK

Chapter Outline

INTRODUCTION

Children with chronic conditions make up a significant proportion of today's school children. Depending on the definition used, prevalence rates of chronic conditions in children younger than the age of 18 in the United States range from 2% to 32% (Centers for Disease Control and Prevention [CDC], National Center for Health Statistics, 2003; Ireys, 2001). Some of the children with chronic conditions are considered disabled because of their condition, but not all. Some have a diagnosis of a chronic condition, but are minimally affected by it. A major study demonstrated that while only 18% of children between the ages of 3 and 18 have a disability, at least 24% and perhaps up to 32% have chronic conditions, but they are not officially labeled as having disabilities (Kuhlthau, Ferris, Beal, Brotmaker, & Perrin, 2002).

The school nurse needs to be aware of both the subset of those with disabilities who receive services under the Individuals with Disabilities Education Act (IDEA) and Section 504 of the Rehabilitation Act (see Chapter 14) as well as the larger population of children with chronic conditions. For some of these students, taking intermittent medications or treatments is sufficient to function in the school setting. However, when a crisis occurs, such as a seizure or an acute allergic reaction, the student needs the interventions of the school nurse. All of these students need an Individualized Health Plan (IHP). It is the school nurse who must anticipate complications, provide interventions, treat exacerbations, provide anticipatory guidance, and evaluate care.

As mortality rates associated with chronic conditions continue to decrease and life expectancy increases, there is a corresponding increase in morbidity. This will increase the healthcare and service needs of these students and their families. The prevalence of chronic conditions increases with age; therefore older children and adolescents have a greater chance of having a chronic condition than younger children (Mudrick, 2002). Boys younger than age 18 have a higher incidence than females; Caucasians have a higher incidence than black American children. Poor children not only have a higher incidence rate, but the severity of their disabilities is also greater (Newacheck, Hung, & Wright, 2002; Perrin, 2002).

It is very difficult to determine the prevalence because of the variation in definitions of what constitutes a chronic condition. The primary conditions include (1) respiratory conditions, for example, asthma (Chapter 29) and cystic fibrosis (Chapter 32); (2) impairments of speech, vision, and hearing; (3) alterations in intelligence (Chapter 35) and learning (Chapter 30); (4) mental and nervous system disorders (Chapters 34 and 37); and (5) motor and mobility disorders (Chapter 31) (Mudrick, 2002).

During the past few decades, there has been a significant decrease in the incidence of the chronic conditions of polio and rheumatic fever. Most cardiac conditions and anomalies are treated as acute rather than chronic conditions. However, there has been a significant increase in the incidence of asthma (Chapter 29), allergies (Chapter 28), type 2 diabetes (Chapter 33), attention deficit hyperactivity disorder (ADHD) (Chapter 30), and autism (Chapter 34) in children. As the healthcare profession saves more and more babies with extreme prematurity and as new viruses and environmental toxins emerge, it appears there will always be children with chronic conditions. The purpose of this chapter is to define the multiple terms associated with chronic conditions and to describe the breadth of conditions included in this category and how they impact on the educational setting and on school health.

CLARIFICATION OF TERMS

Chronic conditions include both physical and mental health disorders. Problems due to chronic conditions account for 24% of all school absences, 19% of all physician contacts, and 33% of all hospital days. Half of these children have a mild form of their disorder (CDC, National Center for Health Statistics, 2003). **Chronic conditions** are defined as: "any physical or mental conditions that require long-term (>6 months) monitoring and/or management to control symptoms and to shape the course of the disease" (Corbin, 2001, p. 1). The term refers to any condition that meets the following criteria: (1) relative permanence; (2) lasts at least 6 months (although some say 1 year); (3) requires special training of the client or those who provide the client's care; (4) is caused by a nonreversible pathological alteration, (5) is usually not curable by short-term treatment, and (6) is often characterized by remissions and exacerbations.

A great deal of confusion exists regarding the terms used in discussing this population of children. Many people use the words **chronic condition** and **chronic illness** interchangeably. An illness implies being sick and needing to recover. While some chronic conditions are in fact chronic illnesses, such as cancer, from which recovery is desired, the vast majority are conditions that will be permanent for the life of the individual. They may be genetic/chromosomal or the result of birth defects or injury. Examples include a student with Down syndrome, a student born without an extremity or without vision, or a student with cerebral palsy or ADHD. Although these students may also acquire or become infected with the common illnesses of childhood, their chronic conditions are *not* illnesses. Therefore, they are not ill because of their condition and should not be treated as such, except perhaps during periods of exacerbation. For this reason, the term *chronic condition* is used throughout this chapter and includes chronic illnesses.

Disability is another term that promotes confusion. Disability is defined in at least two different ways, based on whether or not the student qualifies for special education services under the Individuals with Disabilities Education Act (IDEA). IDEA (Chapter 14) defines disability by the condition. It states that a child with a disability "means a child with mental retardation, hearing impairments (including deafness), speech or language impairments, visual impairments (including blindness), serious emotional disturbance, orthopedic impairments, autism, traumatic brain injury, other health impairments or specific learning disabilities; and who, by reason thereof, needs special education and related services" (IDEA, 1997). A myriad of conditions that may significantly affect a child's ability to be alert and able to learn are included in the "other health impairment" category, such as Attention Deficit Hyperactivity Disorder and selected metabolic disorders.

The Americans with Disabilities Act (ADA) of 1990 has a broader interpretation of the term disability and defines it as the inability to perform some key life functions that are normally expected of individuals at that age. An "individual with a disability is a person who has a physical or mental impairment that substantially limits a "major life activity" *or* has a record of such impairment, *or* is regarded as having such an impairment" (ADA, 1990). The specific conditions identified in this law include contagious and noncontagious diseases; orthopedic, visual, speech and hearing impairments; cerebral palsy; epilepsy; muscular dystrophy; multiple sclerosis; cancer; heart disease; diabetes; mental retardation; emotional illness; specific learning disabilities; human immunodeficiency virus (HIV) disease; tuberculosis; drug addiction; and alcoholism. Major life activities include the ability to care for oneself, perform manual tasks, walk, see, hear, speak, breathe, learn, or work.

The implications are that the definition used will determine who is identified as meeting the criteria and there is a risk of under-identification (Westbrook, Silver, & Stein, 1998). While these two definitions identify a disability in only approximately 18% of the entire pediatric population using federal guidelines, there are many others with chronic conditions.

Disabilities can be physical, cognitive, psychological, or social. They are on a continuum from mild to severe and rarely stay static. Exacerbations and remissions as well as the changing nature of conditions with age will result in students moving back and forth along the continuum as they grow toward adulthood. Regardless of the degree of severity, the school nurse will interact with most of these students.

Any disability that impacts on the development of children is called a **developmental disability**. Federal legislation considers a developmental disability "a substantial chronic disability likely to continue indefinitely that results from a physical and/or mental impairment manifested in a person before 22 years of age. The developmentally disabled person has substantial limitations in at least three of the following life activities: self-care, mobility, learning, capacity for self-direction, capacity for independent living, receptive and expressive language, and economic self-sufficiency" (Developmental Disabilities Assistance and Bill of Rights Act Amendments, 1996).

The 1997 amendments to IDEA give states and local educational agencies the discretion to identify children younger than the age of 9 years as developmentally delayed, rather than "disabled" (IDEA, 1997). This includes delays in the areas of physical, cognitive, communication, social or emotional, or adaptive development. It is estimated that 17% of US children under 18 have a developmental disability (Administration on Developmental Disabilities, 2004). Therefore, many students with chronic conditions are not yet considered to have a disability, especially if their condition is mild and they are younger than age 9. Under these definitions, sickle cell disease might not be considered a disability, but it most certainly is a chronic condition. Conditions are disabilities only if they interfere with a life act. Therefore, chronicity is not synonymous with disability.

One term that should be avoided is the word **handicap**. A handicap is a limitation imposed on the individual by environmental demands and is related to the individual's ability to adapt or adjust to those demands. Individuals never are born with or have a corresponding handicap with a condition unless one is imposed on them by society. Treating them differently, calling them names or giving them derogatory labels, preventing their access to accommodations, and placing physical and psychological barriers in their way all result in the development of handicaps. School nurses can play a major role in decreasing barriers and therefore eliminating the concept of handicap.

Other terms commonly used in reference to children with chronic conditions include **compromised children** and special needs children. Children with chronic conditions are *not* compromised. A compromise is a settlement in which each party gives up something he or she wants; the individuals make concessions or settle for something. No person wants to be considered a compromise. While parents may *feel* compromised by their lot in life, the children are *not* compromised as human beings.

While it sounds "nice" to refer to children with chronic conditions as special, all children want to be considered special. The concept of children with special healthcare needs may take on a different tone depending on how it is used. Is it an entitlement or an excuse? According to the American Academy of Pediatrics, children with special healthcare needs are "those who have or are at increased risk for a chronic physical, developmental, behavioral, or emotional condition and who also require health and related services or a type or amount beyond that required by children generally" (McPherson et al., 1998, p. 138). This definition focuses on the need for services and the concept of "risk." Biological risks include premature birth, metabolic deficiencies, chromosomal abnormalities, HIV, trauma, or use of technical support. Environmental risks may include social and economic factors, abuse or neglect, and second-hand smoke or other pollutants. The concept of "children with special healthcare needs" is used as a descriptor for those who qualify for state Title V programs.

Regardless of the terminology used, those with disabilities generally prefer to use **person-first language** (American Speech-Language-Hearing Association [ASHA], 1992). This means that school health personnel should always refer to the student as someone with a chronic condition rather than as the condition itself. Nurses and other healthcare providers sometimes have a bad habit of referring to children and adolescents as "diabetics," "asthmatics," and "cystics" rather than as individuals who also happen to have one of these conditions; an individual is not the disorder. There is a greater risk of treating individuals as "sick" if they are identified as having or being a disease; rather, they should be viewed as being in the state that is normal for these individuals.

ETIOLOGY

Chronic conditions can originate in every organ system in the body. They may have been passed genetically from the parents; have occurred in utero due to poor prenatal care, poor maternal nutrition, or maternal use of drugs, alcohol, or tobacco during the pregnancy; have occurred during the perinatal period; be the result of immunological processes or trauma, such as child abuse or anoxia; have been caused by environmental factors, such as poor child nutrition or lead poisoning; or they may be idiopathic, for which the cause is not known.

EXAMPLES OF CHRONIC CONDITIONS AFFECTING CHILDREN AND ADOLESCENTS

Any body system can be affected by chronic conditions. Some are present at birth and treated before the child starts school. Others continue to have implications as the child ages. The more common conditions are covered in separate chapters later in this text (asthma, allergies, ADHD and learning disabilities, cerebral palsy, cystic fibrosis, diabetes, epilepsy, and mental retardation, and obesity). Many conditions impact on multiple body systems, resulting in the need for comprehensive interventions so that students can take full advantage of the learning environment.

Genetic Conditions

An increasing number of conditions are being attributed to a genetic etiology. As the Human Genome Project continues to relate the identified rungs of the DNA ladder with disorders, more will be known about the cause and perhaps ways to prevent these conditions. Genetic conditions can refer to conditions caused by a deviation in just one "rung" of the DNA ladder (as in sickle cell disease), a deviation or omission of one or more genes (representing hundreds of rungs within a chromosome, as in inborn errors of metabolism, for example, phenylketonuria or maple sugar urine disease), or an alteration in the number of chromosomes.

Four of the 23 chromosome pairs are implicated in chromosomal disorders. These are chromosome 13 (trisomy 13), chromosome 18 (trisomy 18), chromosome 21 (trisomy 21/Down syndrome), and the sex-linked chromosomes. (A trisomy means that the individual received three chromosomes instead of two on a pair because one parent's pair failed to separate [nondisjunction] during meiosis. Therefore, the offspring has 47 chromosomes in every cell instead of 46.)

Children with trisomy 13 and 18 are often severely disabled and often need total care. They are severely delayed cognitively and physically and often die before the school-age years. These conditions are rare. Trisomy 21, on the other hand, is very common, being present in approximately one in every thousand births (Roizen, 2002) (see Chapter 35).

Chromosomal conditions affecting the sex-linked chromosomes are Turner syndrome and Klinefelter syndrome. All of those with Klinefelter syndrome are males with three chromosomes rather than two on the sex-linked pair. The XXY is due to nondisjunction from either the mother (XX) or father (XY) during meiosis, resulting in 47 chromosomes. In Turner syndrome, all those affected are female and the condition is due to a deletion of a chromosome (monosomy) on the sex-linked pair, resulting in only 45 chromosomes, again due to nondisjunction. In the past, it was thought that individuals with these conditions had an associated mild mental retardation. However, it is now known that most of these individuals usually have normal intelligence, but do have significant learning disabilities (Robinson, Bender, & Linden, 2001; Sybert, 2001).

Genetic conditions may be due to one or more genes passed at conception to the child. These include type 1 diabetes (Chapter 33), cystic fibrosis (Chapter 32), sickle cell disease, phenylketonuria (PKU), achondroplasia, fragile X syndrome (Chapter 35), Duchenne muscular dystrophy, hemophilia A, and thalassemia. Asthma (Chapter 29) and type 2 diabetes are thought to be due to a combination of genetic and environmental factors. ADHD and learning disabilities (Chapter 30) also have a genetic component in more than half of those affected. The school nurse needs to keep updated on basic genetics in order to provide accurate information and to clarify misinformation of students and staff. Explaining genetic causes is an effective way to reinforce that these conditions can never be "caught" by anyone else and that they are no one's "fault."

Sensory Deficits

Sensory deficits usually include difficulty with hearing, vision, and speech. They can be congenital or acquired, unilateral or bilateral. Students identified with these conditions often use assistive technology in the classroom. These are devices that help the student accommodate for senses they do not have.

Hearing Loss

Hearing is mature at birth and therefore screening can be done in the first week of life. Identifying hearing loss is now a routine part of newborn screening in many hospital nurseries across the country. Consequently, more and more children will enter the school system already identified as having a hearing loss. Hearing affects the initial development of speech and is certainly a major component of communication. Therefore, having a decrease or absence in the ability to hear will affect the child's safety and the ability to speak, and will delay the ability to communicate and interact socially. Hearing loss also has an impact on one's performance on IQ tests, although it does not affect one's potential or ability to learn (ASHA, 2002; National Information Center for Children and Youth with Disabilities [NICHY], 2003).

The deaf community wants to be referred to as "deaf" or "hard of hearing." They do not want to be labeled "hearing impaired" because the word "impaired" denotes that something is wrong with them. However, IDEA does refer to hearing impairment. IDEA differentiates hearing impairment from deafness by defining the former as an impairment that adversely affects a child's educational performance, whereas deafness prevents a person from receiving most forms of sound (NICHY, 2003).

Approximately one million children have some degree of hearing loss. This represents approximately 1.3% of all students in school (Herer, Knightly, & Steinberg, 2002). Almost 72,000 students in the United States receive special education services in the schools because of a hearing impairment (NICHY, 2003). However, one study estimated that 15% of children 6 to 19 years of age have a unilateral or bilateral hearing loss (ASHA, 2002).

Hearing loss can be due to problems in the middle ear (conductive hearing loss), in the inner ear (cochlea or eighth cranial nerve) (sensorineural hearing loss), or both. Conductive hearing loss interferes with sound moving from the outer ear to the inner ear. It usually affects the *loudness* of sound, also referred to as the amplitude or intensity of sound. This is measured in *decibels* (dB). Thus, this type of hearing loss is most responsive to amplification measures. Hearing loss due to problems in the inner ear results in problems related to sound discrimination. This involves the *pitch or frequency* of sound and is measured by sound cycles per second or *hertz* (Hz). Vowel sounds usually have a low frequency (Hz) but a higher intensity (dB) than consonants, which are usually of higher frequency and a lower intensity (Herer et al., 2002). A low or deep sound would have a frequency of 250 Hz; a sound with a 4,000-Hz frequency would be high pitched, such as a whistle.

An audiogram measures both the pitch and the loudness. The softest level at which a person can hear the various frequencies being tested is called the threshold; this is what is recorded on the audiogram. Hearing loss is evaluated as a reduction in loudness and/or pitch. It can range from mild to profound. Usually, charts of the degree of hearing loss are only identified by the decibel level (TABLE 27.1). For a child, a reading of 0 to 15 db is normal (Northern & Downs, 1991). A person with a hearing loss of more than 90 decibels is considered to be deaf, whereas someone with a hearing loss of less than that is labeled "hard of hearing" (NICHY, 2003). Normal conversational speech is approximately 40 to 70 decibels. The labels indicate the impact of a loss of hearing in the educational setting, and, for the younger child, on the development of speech.

Hearing loss has numerous causes. Perinatal cytomegalovirus (CMV) or rubella; prematurity; chronic middle ear effusions and otitis media; the sequelae of meningitis, mumps, or ototoxic drugs; and high noise levels have all been implicated. Alteration in the location or shape of the ears may impact on one's ability to hear. A number of craniofacial conditions have also been identified as a structural cause of hearing loss. These conditions include cleft palate and Treacher Collins syndrome.

"At least half of hearing loss in children is caused by genetic factors" (Herer et al., 2002, p. 201), as more than 70 genetically caused syndromes are associated with deafness. However, in at least one third of the cases, there is no identifiable cause (Fox, 1997).

Table 27.1 ■
HEARING LOSS MEASUREMENTS (IN DECIBELS) FOR CHILDREN

0–15	Normal	
16–25	Slight hearing loss	May miss unvoiced consonant sounds.
26–40	Mild hearing loss	Hears only some speech sounds.
41–65	Moderate hearing loss	Misses most speech sounds at conversational level.
66–95	Severe hearing loss	Hears no speech sounds of normal conversation.
>95	Profound hearing loss	Hears no sounds.

There is also a genetic form of hearing loss that occurs during late adolescence and early adulthood. The school nurse may have an integral role in identifying these young adults during school screenings (Chapter 20) or other times when faculty note changes in a student's behavior or decreasing attention in the classroom. While hearing loss is often permanent, decreased hearing due to an accumulation of cerumen or a foreign body can be resolved as soon as the obstruction is removed.

Assessments of students who are suspected of having a hearing loss include observing that they may focus on the speaker's lips and may not respond to questions if the speaker's lips cannot be seen. Speech development, especially in the young child, may be a key finding in identifying hearing loss. Students who need high volumes on appliances or those who cup their ears with their hands may need to be evaluated. Even students with a unilateral hearing loss need a full evaluation.

There are different modes of amplification depending on the degree and cause of the hearing loss. The goal is to provide the student with access to as much speech as possible while still maintaining comfort. The most common is the use of hearing aids. These devices are battery-operated and work by picking up sound via a microphone and amplifier and changing it to electrical energy. "The receiver changes the electric signal back to acoustic energy so the sound can be heard" (Gregory, 1998, p. 23). However, they amplify all sound, including background/environmental noise and therefore work best in a quieter environment.

Amplification of the decibel level can be controlled by a volume control dial. The school nurse, teachers, and speech-language specialist need to periodically check that the hearing aid is being worn, that it is turned to the appropriate volume, and that the batteries are working. Batteries last for approximately 100 to 150 hours of wear. Extra batteries can be kept in the school nurse's office; care should be taken to store them in a childproof container and to dispose of them safely because of their hazardous acid content and size.

Hearing aids come in different shapes and sizes. Some are worn behind the ear (BTE) and are connected to a plastic ear mold that fits inside the outer ear. "Poorly fitting BTE ear molds may cause feedback, a whistle sound caused by the fit of the hearing aid or by buildup of earwax or fluid" (National Institute on Deafness, 2002, p. 4). A second type is in the ear (ITE). This harder plastic holds all of the components within the outer ear. These are not as common in children because of the need to continuously change them as the child's ear grows. This is also true of the types of aids that fit completely into the ear canal. When a child does not respond to the other options, a body hearing aid is used. The earpieces are attached by wires to a box that is strapped to the child. This type is becoming less common as other options become available. For the child who has persistent ear drainage, a bone conduction hearing aid can be used. This one-inch vibrator is attached to a headband, which holds it in place over the mastoid bone. The sound is sent by a signal via bone conduction to the cochlea.

Three different types of circuitry are available for hearing aids: analog/adjustable, analog/programmable, and digital/programmable. The analog/adjustable is the least expensive; in this form, the audiologist determines the volume and specifications needed and these are built into the device. The analog/programmable device comes with a remote control that allows the student to change to predetermined computer-generated programs, based on environmental needs. The digital hearing aid is the most expensive (thousands of dollars) and comes with a microphone, receiver, battery, and computer chip. It can be adjusted for the individual's best sound quality (National Institute on Deafness, 2002).

Care of hearing aids involves avoiding heat and moisture. Earmolds are prone to break down and clog with ear wax. If needed, the earmold can be removed and cleaned in warm soapy water; "use a pipe cleaner or air blower to remove wax or moisture from tubing. Dry completely before reattaching it to aid. Never use alcohol or cleaners as they can cause cracking and drying" (Gregory, 1998, p. 23). If a whistling noise is heard, it may indicate that the hearing aid is no longer working or is not fitting correctly. Earmolds should fit comfortably and securely. However, as the child grows, the earpiece may not fit and may irritate the child. The fit should be checked at least annually.

Some students with hearing aids also use a personal frequency-modulated transmission device, referred to as FM systems. The transmitter unit is clipped to the shirt of the speaker, usually the teacher or parent, and the student wears the receiver unit. This allows the speaker to move about the room and the student does not have to rely on reading the teacher's lips. It also assists the student to separate out the speaker's voice from background noise.

Cochlear implants are now being surgically embedded under the skin behind the ear in children with profound hearing loss. Wires are surgically inserted into the inner ear to transmit electrical impulses that the brain interprets as sound. They provide a substitute for the hair cells of the cochlea. A headpiece is worn behind the ear that can easily be removed; it is attached to the speech processor, which is worn either behind the ear or on a belt. While it does not restore normal hearing, it does allow the student to "hear" environmental sounds and to begin to interpret them.

In 2002, the Centers for Disease Control and Prevention ruled that people with cochlear implants were at increased risk for developing bacterial meningitis, especially those younger than 7 years of age during the first year post transplant (CDC, 2002), although it can occur at any age and at any point following transplant. The school nurse should remain alert to this possibility. In addition, the computer chip in the implant can be erased when in the presence of a strong magnet. Therefore, students with these implants need to exercise caution related to magnets in the environment. Static electricity, such as that caused by wearing a sweater in a building with low humidity or going down a plastic slide, can also interfere with the functioning of the implant.

The earlier the hearing loss occurred, the more it will impact on the development of language. Consequently, the earlier intervention is started, the better the student will do in learning to communicate. There are two different communication approaches for children with significant hearing loss: sign language and oral speech. Sign language incorporates signs made with the hands with facial expressions and body postures. American Sign Language (ASL) is not a universal language, so it may not be applicable for children from other countries who are deaf. ASL has its own rules for grammar, punctuation, and sentence order. It will be important for the school nurse to know a few signs such as pain, stomachache, "where," and "how long" and to have pictures to check for understanding.

Some individuals believe that since this is a hearing world, it is best to learn to communicate the way hearing people do. Those raised according to this philosophy do not use sign language. They depend on lip reading and speech skills to communicate. Cued speech is an offshoot of the oral–auditory approach and breaks language down phonetically. It uses eight configurations and four positions of the hand around the face to supplement visible manifestations of natural speech.

Students with mild hearing loss may not need any accommodations other than sitting in the front of the room. However, other measures that can be instituted include making sure that the teacher or other speaker faces them when talking so that the student can read lips. Students with more involved hearing loss may rely on lip reading. Speakers need to make sure that their back is not to windows, as the glare of the sunlight may make it more difficult for the student to see the speaker's face. It is recommended that those with coclear implants be seated in the middle of the room. In that way, they can hear not only the teacher, but also the comments of their classmates.

Additional interventions to assist students with a hearing loss include the following: speak clearly and distinctly, but do not exaggerate the pronunciation of words; do not shout; interact in a well-lit environment; wait for the child's attention before speaking; decrease additional noise in the room; allow only one person to speak at a time; keep sentences short; use multisensory approaches (especially demonstration) to develop speech and to teach content; and promote peer interactions (Kohler, Schweikert-Stary, & Lubkin, 1998).

The teacher and the school nurse must be aware of the ambient noise that exists in their rooms from outside traffic, heating and cooling systems, and the activity within the room. Also remember that a hearing loss will be exaggerated when the student has a cold or ear infection.

Establish a buddy system for emergencies to ensure that students with hearing deficits are alerted in case of an emergency and know where to go and what to do. A telecommunication device for the deaf (TDD) also needs to be available within the school, especially if a parent is hard of hearing as well. When a school does not have a TDD, a deaf relay service is available that provides telephone communication between one hearing person and one who has a TDD. Fax machines may also be used as a source of communication.

One national program that promotes noise reduction to prevent hearing loss is WISE EARS. This program is sponsored by the National Institute of Health and includes classroom activities and materials for schools, the public, and parents to increase awareness about noise-induced hearing loss and to promote interventions to decrease the risk (National Institute on Deafness, 2003).

Vision Loss

As with hearing, degrees of visual acuity range across a spectrum. The term "functional vision" refers to the sight a person has, and is capable of using, rather than focusing on the deficit and therefore goals can be to optimize the sight available to the student (Davis, 2003). The term "totally blind" is used for those who have no sight at all as well as for those who can decipher light, form, and movement but cannot see large print. The term "legally blind" or "functionally blind" is used to describe central visual acuity of 20/200 or less in the better eye, *after* correction. The term "low vision" is used for individuals who have visual acuity of worse than 20/70 in the better eye *after* correction (Miller, Menacker, & Batshaw, 2002). They are often referred to as partially sighted. (An acuity of 20 over 200 means that a person standing 20 feet away from an object will see that object as if it is 200 feet away.) While the above groups are considered to have visual impairments, the school nurse is more often on the lookout for students who may be visually impaired *before* correction but who can be helped with the aid of glasses. About 1 in 3,000 children are blind and 1 in 20 require visual correction with glasses (Miller et al., 2002). Of those who are blind, 46% were born blind and another 38% lost their vision before their first birthday. However, when students lose or forget their glasses, they are just as visually impaired as their peers with more serious vision losses.

Vision does not reach adult maturity until age 8; therefore it is essential to initiate treatments for eye conditions prior to this time to allow for correction to occur (Miller et al., 2002). Failure to treat conditions such as amblyopia (lazy eye) during the preschool years can result in significant vision loss in the affected eye, despite later optical correction. It is often the responsibility of the school nurse to screen children for suspected vision deficits and to refer for follow-up.

Vision loss may be due to congenital defects, such as a cataract, retinoblastoma and other brain tumors, or it may be the result of maternal infections and medications or prematurity. "Retinoblastoma is the most common ocular tumor of childhood" (Fox, 1997, p. 386). Vision loss can also be the result of trauma. In addition, visual deficits are found in one-half to two-thirds of individuals with developmental disabilities (Miller et al., 2002).

A child who is blind from birth has no visual memories; the child cannot see perspective or reflection and does not have the visual sensory cues to explore his or her environment. When these children do attempt to move about, they are at increased risk of being injured by contact with furniture and other obstructions. Children who are legally blind should already have been identified before entering the school system. However, those with visual deficits may not always be identified early. Assessments are appropriate for students who are slow to acquire certain behavior patterns; they may have a head tilt, engage in frequent eye-rubbing, blinking, squinting, or cover or close one eye while reading; and they may put their face very close to their book or work. Assess for a film developing over the eye or deviating eyes when trying to focus. (See Chapter 20 on screening for vision.)

Eyeglasses are the intervention of choice for those with refractive errors. They should be made of "polycarbonate plastic rather than glass. Although plastic lenses scratch more easily, they are impact resistant, lighter, and last longer. For smaller children, frames with cable temples and spring hinges tend to fit best" (Miller et al., 2002, p. 179). Students should be professionally reevaluated at least annually to see if any changes are needed in the prescription for their glasses.

Interventions to enhance vision include seating the student closest to the blackboard and using large type if he or she has partial vision, or sitting at a table with the teletype machine in order to take notes and participate in assignments. Using magnifiers or high-intensity lamps may be of benefit to some students. Books on tape and voice recognition software can also be helpful. Bright lines on the floor throughout all of the corridors and handrails will assist some students with their independent mobility. Some may use a tapping stick, which is now being replaced by devices with lasers to detect objects.

For students with no sight, explain strange sounds as well as what is being seen; announce yourself when approaching and especially before you touch the child; give explicit explanations before, during, and after an activity; and provide as much hands-on learning or instruction as possible. Use the student's name often during conversations so that the child knows he or she is included. The school nurse and the teacher need to ensure that a buddy system is in place to be certain that students with vision difficulties are guided to a safe place in case of an emergency.

Teachers need to focus on the purpose of the lesson and to consider alternative ways for the student to accomplish the learning objective, as well as associated tasks including school-based daily living tasks, such as mealtimes and changing clothes for physical education class. Classrooms, as well as hallways, need to be configured to ensure safety as the student moves about. The teacher can encourage good listening skills among the other students to support the student who is blind.

Be aware that a child may feel eyestrain and develop headaches as the eyes get tired. Therefore, allow the student time to rest their eyes throughout the day. Some optical aids may include computer programs that read text. Some children are taught Braille, which is a code using raised dots that are read from left to right. Having small children handle various objects and textures prepares them for the sensation of "reading" the letters. Children with visual impairment need to be taught computer typing skills early.

Students with significant vision loss are eligible for services under IDEA so that an Individualized Education Program is developed for them (Chapter 9). They also need an Individualized Health Plan as well as an Emergency Plan (Chapter 9).

Communication Deficit

Many conditions can result in the inability of the student to verbalize words. A language disorder can result from problems with any of the components of language: memory, learning, message reception and processing, and expressive skills (Hardman, Drew, & Egan, 2002). Receptive language disorders involve getting the words to the brain and making sense of those words. Conditions such as a hearing loss, in which an individual cannot perceive the sounds of the words, and mental retardation, in which the words may have no meaning, are two examples.

Expressive language disorders involve difficulty in producing speech. The cause of the problem may be that the larynx (voice box) is not functioning properly. Since air must flow from the lungs across the larynx, a student with a tracheostomy will not be able to speak without an adaptor on the tracheostomy. The trach tube may be necessary because of congenital tracheal malasia, in which the trachea is soft and cannot stay open to maintain an airway; or because a child is on a portable ventilator; or because of damage from lye ingestion. Inability to speak may also be due to respiratory problems. A student on a ventilator or who has extreme shortness of breath may not have enough airflow to produce speech.

Other expressive language deficits are due to problems of the muscles of the face and airway. A student with spastic cerebral palsy may have difficulty with the motor activity of forming words and sentences (see Chapter 31). Muscles of the face, lips, and tongue that have altered sensation may make it difficult to form words. A defect in the structure of the mouth, such as a cleft palate, will interfere with articulation of words. Some children with Down syndrome (Chapter 35) have a small oral cavity, although it may appear that they have a large tongue, which they protrude in order to maintain an adequate airway. This makes the process of speech difficult.

A number of psychiatric conditions appear to lock children into a nonverbal or an altered-verbal world. These may include autism (Chapter 34) and some forms of mental retardation (Chapter 35).

Aphasia may be a combination of both receptive and expressive language difficulty. An injury or stroke may result in a lesion that prevents the understanding of and expression of language.

Communication disorders are common. Nineteen percent of all children and adolescents who receive services for a disability have a communication problem. "Speech disorders are identified in about 12% to 15% of children in kindergarten through grade 4" (Hardman et al., 2002, p. 343). One should never assume that someone who cannot speak has difficulty hearing or understanding. There is no need to raise one's voice or to speak slower when speaking to this student. Assuming he or she has some cognitive ability to respond, a number of communication devices are available. These include picture boards and voice synthesizers that speak what the person types. (One example is Speaking Dynamically Pro by Mayer-Johnson.) The school nurse must know which communication style the student uses.

THE STUDENT WHO IS TECHNOLOGY DEPENDENT OR RECEIVES TECHNOLOGY ASSISTANCE

Children with chronic conditions frequently use technological devices to attain or maintain health and quality of life, and, in some cases, to maintain life. Many students depend on technology and yet are not considered to be technology dependent, for example, students with glasses, hearing aids, or insulin pumps. The types of equipment usually referred to when speaking of dependence on technology are ventilators/oxygen/tracheostomy tubes, feeding tubes, and mobility devices. The Assistive Technology Act of 1998 defines these devices as "any item, piece of equipment, or product system, whether acquired commercially, modified, or customized, that is used to increase, maintain, or improve functional capabilities of individuals with disabilities" (1998, Section 3a(3)). They are also used to "minimize deterioration in functioning, to maintain a level of functioning in any major life activity" (Assistive Technology Act, 1998, Section 3a(9)(A)(ii)). Consequently, all forms of technology that assist students in participating in and receiving an education are included.

Bryant and Bryant (2003) provide the following list of questions that can help to determine the need for a specific technology to compensate for any chronic needs in addition to those that assist in oxygenation, nutrition, and elimination:

- What tasks are needed in the school setting? (These can be as major as hearing/seeing, communicating, and getting from one classroom to another to more mundane needs such as being able to hold a pencil, needing larger keys on a calculator, or needing a different classroom chair.) Keep in mind that the special technological needs go beyond the classroom; they include transportation to and from school, cafeteria needs, as well as adaptations for physical education, art, and music classes.
- What abilities does the student have?
- What abilities does the student need in order to complete the task or meet the expectation?
- What adaptations are needed to bridge the difference between the previous two questions in the school setting?
- What adaptations are available to the school/student? Does the adaptation require special training by the student? By the teacher? By the school nurse?
- What supplies need to be kept in the school for this equipment (batteries, tubing, cleaning agents)?
- Will the family provide the needed supplies or cleaning agents?
- What kind of maintenance is needed for this equipment?
- Will the adaptation have an impact on the environment, such as space needed, noise made, and electricity needed?
- How will the school evaluate the effectiveness of this technology? (Modified from Bryant & Bryant, 2003, pp. 31–33.)

It is the responsibility of the school nurse to be educated in the use of specific technological devices used by the students. One resource is the Advanced Practice Nurse (APN) in the specialty clinic the student attends. The APN is well aware of the need for a continuum of care and can be an excellent resource in providing hands-on training as well as literature regarding the technology, its uses, and how to troubleshoot when problems arise. Some devices are used continuously, while others are used on a routine basis or intermittently as needed; some are simple and some are complex. It is estimated that one in every thousand children requires technological assistance for health-related reasons (Levy & O'Rourke, 2002). Another resource for the school nurse is the Rehabilitation Engineering and Assistive Technology Society of North America. Their Web site is in the resource section of this chapter and their role is to provide guidance regarding assistive technology.

Mobility Devices

A wide range of technological devices are used to enhance mobility. These include prostheses, crutches, braces, walkers/gait trainers, and wheelchairs. The school nurse's role with regard to these devices is to ensure that they (1) are used correctly and safely (especially for students who continuously lean on their crutches pressing the top of the crutch into the axillary area or the child in a wheelchair doing "wheelies"); (2) are in good working order (e.g., ensuring that the rubber on the bottom of crutches and walkers is in good condition); (3) they are not causing skin breakdown, especially related to the student growing, sweating, or not wearing the appropriate underclothing to protect the device; and, further, (4) if batteries are used to charge the device, they are charged. It is important to know how long the charge lasts and what should be done if there is no charge.

There are different sizes and types of wheelchairs. They may be manual or motorized. Junior wheelchairs are available for smaller children and there are sports wheelchairs for teens who wish to engage in sports such as basketball and tennis. There are also racing wheelchairs. It is essential that brake locks be checked and used when the chair has stopped. A wheelchair that is too small will cause rubbing and skin irritation; the student should be able to reach the wheels of the wheelchair or the electronic controls in order to be self sufficient at some point. While the initial fitting for a wheelchair is done by either an occupational therapist or a physical therapist, it is often the nurse who has the opportunity to identify that a change in wheelchair size is needed. Either the parent or the school nurse can contact the wheelchair vendor to adjust the wheelchair for a proper fit.

Increasing in popularity are motorized carts, especially for older children and teens. Safety is always an issue with these devices, especially related to stairs and the potential of running into classmates.

Seating and Positioning Devices

To maintain safety and efficacy, it may be necessary to use cushions to attain enough height to sit at a desk or in a chair. "The desk height should be about two inches above the level of the elbows when the elbows are bent and the child is sitting upright in the chair" (Ball, 2002, p. 18). Raised seats may also be used to transfer the student from a wheelchair to a chair. Straps may be necessary to secure a student to the chair, especially in the case of paralysis of the chest and abdominal areas. Some students who have poor head and neck control need a high-backed chair or one with cushions to maintain their head in proper alignment.

Positioning devices may be as minor as a splint for the hand and wrist, a brace or cushion for the spine, either for scoliosis or to maintain an erect position, or cushions between the legs in order to maintain alignment and prevent future problems. Other students may need devices such as standers to help them maintain an upright position.

Feeding Devices

Feeding devices are usually used because of the child's inability to ingest food, resulting from conditions that interfere with the coordination between speaking and swallowing, such as structural problems of the esophagus or spasticity. They may also be used for those students who have oral intake that is insufficient to promote growth. A gastrostomy tube (referred to as a G-tube or a peg tube) is the most common device and enters percutaneously directly into the stomach via a tube through the abdominal wall, but a jejunostomy tube (J-tube) may also be present and used for feeding. These devices are anchored to the abdominal wall or a balloon filled with saline may be used to keep it in the stomach. A written protocol may be needed in order for the school nurse to reinsert the tube if it should come out and reinflate the balloon.

Some students may have a nasogastric or nasojejunal tube in place, which is inserted through the nose into the stomach and taped to the face. Replacing these devices is within the nurse's scope of practice in all states and the school nurse can receive education and practice sessions regarding the care of these devices as well as how to reinsert them if they come out. Feeding protocols will vary based on the type of device and whether the feeding is continuous or intermittent, including whether or not feeding pumps are used, the timing of the feedings, and the amount of water needed to flush the tubing. Feeding tubes are also used for the administration of medications, which need to be in liquid form or crushed in order to be administered through the tube.

Some students with spasticity or neuromuscular deficits will need special eating utensils. Occupational therapists associated with the school can assist in devising or obtaining the needed equipment, such as silverware with wide grips or straps to stay on the hands, dishes with lips that assist in scooping food against it in order to get the food on a spoon, special cups, or mats that keep the plate from slipping.

Elimination Devices

Ostomies (colostomy, ileostomy) may be permanent, such as those needed for short bowel syndrome, or temporary so that the bowel can have a rest in conditions such as ulcerative colitis and Crohn disease. In a vesicostomy, the bladder exits onto the abdominal wall, and in a ureterostomy, the ureters exit onto the abdominal wall. Either way, the care is similar with the use of a collecting device. Care of the stoma and routine emptying of the bags is essential to maintaining optimal skin health. In many cases, the student can be taught to care for his or her own elimination needs, but may need the privacy of the health office bathroom because of the equipment needed and the extra space needed to facilitate this process.

Urinary and/or bowel incontinence may require the use of diapers. This can be very difficult for students who are older, especially if there is a significant odor problem. Attention should be paid to ensure that frequent diaper changes occur to keep the odor to a minimum. The Advanced Practice Nurse in the specialty clinic/office can provide the student with a list of foods that make the odor worse and those that lessen it, and this information may need to be incorporated into the student's IHP.

Catheterization for the purpose of emptying the bladder is a common skill for school nurses. Sometimes the catheterization is through the stoma on the abdominal wall, but usually it is through the urethra. Young children are taught to complete this task on their own, with the nurse available for problems. Typically, a clean technique is used, rather than the sterile process used in hospitals. Students may rinse out their catheters after each use and leave them in the health office until they are needed again. Some students may actually have a four-inch metal catheter that they keep in something resembling an eyeglass case that allows them to use regular bathroom facilities and void directly into the toilet.

For students who may be receiving dialysis because of the loss of all kidney function, catheters are used in the exchange of fluids. Whether the child is receiving hemodialysis (in which the shunts may be in the forearm) or peritoneal dialysis (in which the shunts are in the abdomen), it is the nurse's responsibility to ensure that the shunts are protected from trauma and to anticipate emergency measures should they be dislodged.

Cardiopulmonary Devices

Cardiopulmonary devices include ventilators, oxygen supplementation by nasal cannula, positive airway pressure devices, tracheostomy tubes, surveillance devices such as a cardiopulmonary monitor, and pulse oxygenation and peak flow monitoring, and treatments to enhance pulmonary function, such as the various appliances that can now assist with percussion and postural drainage (see Chapter 32). Some of the devices have alarms that indicate highs and lows; since these may go off in the classroom, the teacher must be educated as to what should be done. Checking to make sure that the student is breathing comfortably is always the first step.

The school nurse's responsibilities may include recording readings of the pulse oximeter, peak flow meters, and vital sign data on a schedule agreed on in the development of the IEP and IHP as well as times when the student is having difficulties. Often, alarms will indicate a problem. The school nurse should check the placement of probes and tubing both at the machinery end and where they are attached to the student, the setting of the alarms and the amount of oxygen being delivered. The pulse oximeter easily clips onto a finger, toe, or ear; "because this device reflects how well oxygen is being delivered to vital organs, it is an important monitor; unfortunately, it is quite susceptible to false alarms resulting from probe displacement, movement of the extremity, or electrical interference" (Levy & O'Rourke, 2002, p. 634).

For a student with a tracheostomy tube, it is essential that the school nurse has an extra tracheostomy tube with all necessary equipment for a trach change and a change of the trach ties. The school nurse will need special training by personnel in the child's healthcare setting regarding the technique for a trach change. They should also provide an opportunity to practice this skill in a controlled environment. Suction equipment must be available in the school. A number of creative suctioning apparatuses can be easily adapted to the school setting.

All school nurses must maintain current CPR certification, including the use of external defibrillation devices. These devices are becoming more common in schools throughout the country and school nurses are the prime individuals to educate the rest of the staff on their use.

The presence of a trach tube may interfere with the development of language and may interfere with communication. If a student cannot speak with their trach, they will need to utilize the communication equipment mentioned earlier. Behavior problems have been noted in some children with a trach tube who are frustrated in their attempts to communicate and may respond with aggressive and acting-out behavior (Levy & O'Rourke, 2002).

Intravenous Lines

Peripherally inserted central venous catheter (PICC) lines and implanted vascular access devices for antibiotics, fluids, or hyperalimentation/total parenteral nutrition (TPN), Broviac lines for chemotherapy, and shunts for dialysis are the most common intravenous lines seen in the school setting. Although administering medications in these lines is usually not the responsibility of the school nurse, protecting the tubing from trauma is. A hemostat should be available in the health office should one of these lines become detached. The IHP should be developed with the family and healthcare provider in order to know what emergency measures should be taken should a problem with the tubing occur.

Other Devices

There are other technological and assist devices that are not usually considered when speaking of assistive technology. Adaptations to computers are needed for some students. These may include the size or shape of the keyboard, the size of the keys (whether they will be pushed by fingers, toes, or a stick in the mouth or attached to a head piece), the speed of the machine when a key is pressed (preventing the letter from being repeated until the pressure has been released), the size and shape of the mouse, whether or not moisture on the keyboard will interfere with the working of the computer, and if a voice recognition system or touch screen is needed. In addition to the computer, using a tape recorder and having notes transcribed, having a reader, using magnification aids, or making large-print materials available are other technological adaptations that may be used.

Some students are embarrassed by their dependence on technology and try to conceal it so that they will not appear "different" to their peers. They may also try to conceal it from teachers and the school nurse. This can be a problem, especially if the school nurse and teacher do not know that tubing exists that must be protected and that certain activities may not be appropriate for the student. This is particularly a concern in the high schools. An example is a 10th grade boy who had a central line for a hematological problem. It was only by accident that the school nurse found out. He informed her that when he didn't feel good, he would sit in the back of the darkened auditorium because he did not want people to know.

The presence of technology in the maintenance of students with chronic conditions adds additional strain on the family. Not only must they be attentive to the needs of the child regarding their condition, but there is also a significant financial strain. Because it is helpful, and in some cases essential, to have a set of equipment in the school building, there is the added expense of buying and maintaining this equipment. School nurses must be kept updated by parents and the primary care provider regarding changes in the child's prescribed technological interventions. The need to emphasize this to the parents should be taken into account when developing the IHP.

Because of their dependence on technology, children with chronic conditions are referred to as "medically fragile" by some. However, identifying them as "fragile" may underestimate their ability to participate in educational and social opportunities and their potential contribution to society. Therefore, it is preferred that this term not be used.

THE STUDENT WITH MYELODYSPLASIA/SPINA BIFIDA

The terms *myelomeningocele, spina bifida, myelodysplasia*, and *neural tube defect* are often used interchangeably, but they refer to different parts of the same process. Neural tube defect is the broadest of the terms. It refers to malformations in the development of the skull and spinal cord caused by failure of the neural tube to close during early embryonic development. Those defects that affect the brain include *encephalocele* (in which brain tissue herniates and protrudes outside the body into a sac, usually in the occipital region) and *anencephaly* (in which the cranium is not closed and brain tissue above the brainstem is not present).

Myelodysplasia is the general term for neural tube defects of the spinal cord. This condition occurs during embryonic development when a part of the spinal cord fails to fuse. The mildest and most common form, *spina bifida occulta*, is characterized by failure of fusion of the posterior vertebral arches, usually in the 5th lumbar or 1st sacral vertebrae. No herniation of the spinal cord or meninges is present, although the child may have a dimpling or tuft of hair along the spinal cord in the affected area. A second type of myelodysplasia is a *meningocele.* In this defect, a fluid-filled sac (filled with cerebrospinal fluid and meninges) protrudes at the point of the spinal cord where the fusion failed. No spinal nerves are present in this sac, and removal of the sac shortly after birth usually is not followed by any symptoms other than a scar along the spine, although hydrocephalus is a possibility (Farley & Dunleavy, 2000).

When the myelodysplasia involves a sac that includes the meninges, cerebrospinal fluid, *and* spinal nerves, it is referred to a *myelomeningocele or meningomyelocele*. It is this condition that many refer to as spina bifida. The surgery to reduce or remove the myelomeningocele is performed within days of birth; however, there is no way to return the spinal nerves to their correct position. Therefore, the signs and symptoms vary depending on where the lesion occurred, the size of the lesion, and the amount of spinal nerves within the sac. The higher up the lesion is, the more nerve-related deficits are present. Myelomeningocele occurs in approximately 60 out of every 100,000 births (Liptak, 2002).

Signs and symptoms vary from complete flaccid paralysis caused by a high lesion down through the lower extremities, including respiratory compromise and absence of bowel and bladder control, to normal mobility and bowel and bladder function from a sacral lesion. It is important for the school nurse to evaluate the degree of impact on mobility and bowel and bladder continence.

Hydrocephalus usually accompanies spina bifida. In 85% of cases, a shunt needs to be implanted into the lateral ventricle of the brain to drain the fluid, usually into the abdominal cavity where it is absorbed (Farley & Dunleavy, 2000). This form of hydrocephalus is not caused by an increase in the amount of spinal fluid formed; rather, it is due to decreased absorption space from scarring from the repair and the decrease of spinal nerves innervating the lower part of the body. It may also be due to Chiari II malformation (Green, 2003), in which the brainstem and part of the cerebellum are downwardly displaced toward the neck.

The implications for the school nurse include awareness of the symptoms that may be present if the shunt stops functioning. These include headache, lethargy, irritability, and vomiting, which are the symptoms of increased intracranial pressure. The parents should be notified immediately, as standard treatments for headache or abdominal discomfort will not be effective. There is the small possibility that the neurological impact of the hydrocephalus and the internalized shunt, including infections that may develop, can result in a seizure disorder as well as limited intellectual functioning.

If the lower extremities are affected, the student may need to use leg braces or a wheelchair. If paralysis is present, attention must be paid to safety concerns regarding heat, cold, and compression. Mobility devices, such as those mentioned earlier, and seating devices may be necessary. If bowel and/or bladder dysfunction (referred to as neurogenic bowel and bladder in which the nerves fail to innervate those structures) is present, there will be incomplete emptying of the bladder and possible incontinence of the bowel. In this case, catheterization and a bowel program may be necessary.

Possibly because of a significant amount of early exposure to latex during early procedures, 18% to 40% of students with myelodysplasia develop sensitivity to latex (Farley & Dunleavy, 2000). This has significant implications for the school nurse and the school regarding equipment in the health office and in the rest of the school.

Additional health-related concerns for the student with spina bifida include the possibility of spinal curvatures as a result of the spinal herniation and the initial surgical correction and short stature. These young people are also at an increased risk for obesity, perhaps because of their decreased activity (Liptak, 2002); the school can implement an altered physical education program for these students to enhance strength and also increase energy expenditure. It is essential that a comprehensive IHP be developed.

THE STUDENT WITH ORTHOPEDIC/ MUSCULOSKELETAL PROBLEMS

In addition to the motor deficits common with myelodysplasia noted in the preceding section and the problems in motor activity related to cerebral palsy (Chapter 31), other types of musculoskeletal problems are commonly seen in the pediatric population. *Scoliosis* occurs in approximately 4% of adolescents (Hill & Sullivan, 1999). There are different types of spinal curvature, depending on the direction of the curve. Scoliosis is a lateral curvature, whereas kyphosis is convex protrusion of the spine (rounded out) and lordosis is a concave curvature of the spine (curved in—otherwise referred to as swayback). The curvature, which ranges from mild to severe, is measured in degrees of angulation. The principles of scoliosis screening are described in Chapter 20. In some cases, the degree of curvature is so severe that it may result in respiratory compromise on the affected side, as the lung is compressed by the ribs.

The treatment for scoliosis, initially, is bracing, with the goal being to stop the progression of the spinal curving. The most common brace is a molded plastic shell worn around the chest and attached with Velcro straps. The brace is worn *over* a tee shirt; however, the school nurse should be aware that skin irritation is possible and the skin should be assessed to ensure proper fit, especially as growth continues. For many, the brace is worn non-stop during the school day and removed only for showering. Others are allowed to attend school without the brace but need to put it on as soon as they return home.

In some cases, spinal fusion surgery is needed to stop the progression. This usually involves bone grafting and insertion of a rod along the spine. The school nurse should be aware that once the student returns to school, he or she often has a significant increase in height, which should be noted on the student's school record. He or she also will have some types of activity restrictions, especially contact sports and those that require extreme bending and twisting. Regardless of whether surgery is done, it is essential to obtain recommendations from the student's healthcare provider regarding modifications in activity and physical education.

A progressive and ultimately fatal condition is *muscular dystrophy* (MD). Multiple forms of MD exist, all of which are genetically transmitted. The most common form, Duchenne MD, is seen only in males and is caused by a deficit in the production of a muscle fiber. Children with this form of MD appear normal during their infancy. It is during the early years that muscle weakness is observed, especially as the child moves from a sitting to standing position. By early adolescence, the youth may not be able to ambulate and may require a wheelchair. By mid to late adolescence, the teen may have muscle weakness so severe that it interferes with self-care activities and even breathing. Ultimately, death is due to respiratory failure. Schools have had to deal with "no code" requests by family members for young men with MD who chose to attend classes until the day they died. NASN (2004) has issued a position statement that recommends how to proceed when parents request a "no code" for their child. (See Chapter 47 for further discussion of this issue.)

There are implications for the school nurse related to the progressive nature of this condition. As

Table 27.2 ■
SELECTED MUSCULOSKELETAL CONDITIONS

CONDITION	DESCRIPTION
Achondroplasia	Dwarfism with short extremities compared to the trunk size with tibial bowing; spinal stenosis with spinal cord compression
Arthrogryposis	Multiple joint contractures, often present from birth, requiring multiple surgeries, OT and PT
Juvenile rheumatoid arthritis	Autoimmune inflammation of the synovium; three forms (pauciarticular—few joints involved; polyarticular—many joints involved; systemic); affects connective tissue; associated with inflammation of the uvea of the eye that could lead to blindness (annual ophthalmologic exams are needed)
Osteogenesis imperfecta	Deficient collagen results in brittle bones, frequent fractures of any bone with normal daily activity; blue sclera; poor dentition

the student's musculature weakens, adaptive equipment may be needed to lift the student, for assisting the student in academic activities, and in providing for eating and elimination needs. Coordination with other members of the health team will help facilitate this plan. Additional orthopedic/musculoskeletal conditions are listed in TABLE 27.2. Many of them have a genetic cause.

THE STUDENT WITH HEMATOLOGICAL PROBLEMS

A multitude of chronic conditions affecting children are caused by problems of the hematological system. These include conditions affecting the platelets and clotting factors, such as idiopathic thrombocytopenic purpura and hemophilia; those affecting the red blood cells, such as sickle cell disease and anemia; and those affecting the white blood cells, as in HIV disease and leukemia. While the school nurse may not have daily contact with these students, he or she must be vigilant for side effects of treatments and potential threats to the student's status as well as have plans in place in case of an acute episode. Other students with hematological problems may need frequent rest periods during the day, adaptations to how much they can eat or when they eat, and specific treatments during the day.

Hemophilia

Hemophilia is a genetically caused condition that affects the development of clotting factors. The type of hemophilia is determined by the type of clotting factor affected. Regardless of the type, the result is an alteration in the clotting cascade. Parents are often taught to administer the clotting factor or DDAVP (desmopressin acetate), a synthetic vasopressin, to the child at home; an implanted venous access device may be in place. However, the school nurse must conduct a comprehensive assessment and initiate immediate measures to decrease bleeding should an insult occur. Assessments that are commonly made include a detailed description of what parts of the body were injured, even if no symptoms are apparent, and noting excessive bruising or splinting of body parts.

Attention needs to be paid to minor cuts and trauma, especially head trauma because of the danger of intracranial bleeding. Even minor injuries, such as nose bleeds and those caused by teeth loss, should be attended to with more vigilance than usual. Medications are available to maintain a clot and therefore decrease the bleed. For extremities, elevate affected areas, apply an elastic bandage and a lightweight ice pack, and apply firm pressure for 10 to 15 minutes to the bleeding. While no signs may determine that there is bleeding into a joint, the student will complain of pain that may require the administration of acetaminophen (Karp, 2000).

The specific interventions should be part of the student's IHP, including whether clotting factor needs to be administered. Any head trauma requires a medical evaluation. All interventions should require notification of the parent. A regular exercise program is important for these students. However, contact sports are strongly discouraged; swimming without diving and golf are acceptable activities. Wearing medical identification bracelets is strongly encouraged.

Sickle Cell Disease (SCD)

Sickle cell disease (SCD) is also genetically transmitted. It is the most common genetic disease in the United States, with an incidence of 1 in 500 African-American births. It occurs because of an alteration in one rung of the DNA ladder that makes hemoglobin. Consequently the hemoglobin formed is significantly less effective than normal adult hemoglobin. Hemoglobin is in red blood cells (RBCs) and it is in the RBCs via hemoglobin that oxygen received from the alveoli is carried throughout the body. Normal RBCs can live 120 days; sickled RBCs can survive only 10 to 20 days (Carroll, 2000).

Normal, RBCs have a round, pliable shape so that they can move into smaller vessels. In SCD, certain events change the shape of RBCs into that of a crescent moon, which prevents them from moving through the vessels. They back up on each other, which results in an obstruction, referred to as a vasoocclusive crisis. This obstruction results in pain. The conditions that can cause sickling are primarily dehydration, acidosis, and deoxygenation. Dehydration can occur during illness or overheating. Consequently, the first interventions are often administration of oxygen and fluids in an attempt to reverse the sickling process. Then pain management is addressed. These measures should be determined ahead of time when the IHP is being developed.

Because school-age children and adolescents probably have functional asplenia due to obstruction and destruction of the spleen after years of SCD, they are at high risk for bacterial infections and should be encouraged to receive the pneumococcal vaccine. Anemia is commonly present, resulting in a persistently low hemoglobin level. This may become evident in the student who appears to have no energy for activity or even for schoolwork.

Additional problems that may arise in children and adolescents as a result of SCD include the potential for leg ulcers, priapism (a painful prolonged erection not associated with sexual arousal), delayed puberty, biliary colic caused by gallstones, retinopathy, and stroke. "The chances of a child with SS [Sickle Cell Disease] having a first stroke by age 20 years is estimated at 11%" (Carroll, 2000, p. 816). Acute chest syndrome is another major complication of SCD, especially in younger children. The only symptoms may be fever, cough, and tachypnea (Carroll, 2000); school nurses should be more attentive to these symptoms in young children with SCD.

Anemia

Anemia is a symptom of another problem; it can be due to any hematological condition or may be due to a poor iron-enriched diet. Students who are anemic, regardless of cause, will be pale, may appear to have shortness of breath, will be tired and unable to participate vigorously, and may perhaps experience more difficulty learning. Any suspicion of anemia should be shared with the parents with a recommendation to seek an assessment from their healthcare provider.

HIV Disease

HIV disease is caused by a virus that attacks the helper T cell of the white blood cells (WBC). WBCs are the cells that regulate and produce antibodies that attack foreign invaders. There are helper and suppressor T cells. Normally there are two helper T ($CD4^+$) cells to keep the immune system vigilant to every one suppressor T cell ($CD8^+$) that turns the system off. Since HIV attacks the CD4 cells, and makes them decrease or stop their function, the level of CD4 T cells is an indication of the student's ability to mount an attack against any foreign invader. Therefore the student may be susceptible to infection.

HIV is transmitted by blood and body secretions. It is not transmitted by casual contact, nor is it airborne. Because the school nurse will probably not know which students or staff in the school are HIV positive, it is essential to practice standard precautions (Chapter 21) when caring for *all* students and *all* blood and body secretions. "No case of person-to-person transmission of HIV infection has ever been documented in child care centers or schools" (Spiegel & Bonwit, 2002, p. 135).

It should be noted that even though the student who is HIV positive may have received all immunizations, the student remains at risk for all childhood contagious diseases, since the immune system may not be able to mount an effective attack against an invading organism. Therefore, families must be notified immediately if any infections are identified in the school environment. Healthcare providers may want to administer passive antibodies (hyperimmune globulin) to protect those who are HIV positive against the offending agent within 72 hours of contact.

Leukemia

Leukemia is the primary type of cancer affecting children. Leukemia is the abnormal proliferation of white blood cells (WBCs). The WBCs are produced too rapidly to mature; thus, these immature cells (blast cells) are released into the circulation and are ineffective in their role. Blast cells cannot fight infection and multiply continuously without respect to the body's needs. Normally, the population of blast cells is less than 5% in the bone marrow and they are never in the peripheral blood. In leukemia, their levels may be as high as 95% of the bone marrow and they are seen in the peripheral blood. Therefore, children and adolescents often speak of their blast cell count as a measure of how they are progressing in their treatment.

The bone marrow often hypertrophies as a result of this mass production of leukemic cells; this can lead to pathologic fractures, which can occur spontaneously. A student with leukemia who comes to the school nurse complaining of bone pain without trauma should receive a complete assessment in case a fracture might be present. Children who are being treated for leukemia are also susceptible to developing anemia and bleeding disorders, as the RBCs and platelets are also affected by the deficient function of the bone marrow.

There are different types of leukemia; some are more common for different ages and they have varying prognoses. Acute lymphocytic leukemia (ALL) is the most common type and usually is seen in preschool and school-age children. In this age group, it also has the best prognosis. Ninety percent to 95% of children with ALL achieve a first remission, in which all symptoms abate and there is no more hematological evidence of the cancer. Almost 80% live at least 5 years (Westlake & Bertolone, 2002). The child between ages 3 and 7 with ALL and an initial WBC count of less than 10,000/mm^3 at the time of diagnosis has the best prognosis. Acute myelogenous leukemia (AML) is more common in adolescents. Of those teens with AML, 50% to 70% reach a first remission and 15% live at least 5 years.

Box 27.1 ■ ■ ■

COMMON FORMS OF CANCER SEEN IN CHILDREN AND ADOLESCENTS

(from most common to least common)

- Leukemia
  - Acute lymphoblastic leukemia
  - Acute myelogenous leukemia
- Brain and central nervous system
  - Infratentorial (medulloblastoma, ependymoma)
  - Brainstem glioma
  - Supratentorial (astrocytomas, craniopharyngioma, gliomas)
- Lymphoma
  - Non-Hodgkin's (lymphoblastic lymphoma, Burkitt's lymphoma)
  - Hodgkin's lymphoma
- Neuroblastoma
- Soft tissue sarcomas (rhabdomyosarcoma)
- Nephroblastoma/Wilms' tumor
- Bone tumors (osteosarcoma, Ewing's sarcoma)
- Retinoblastoma

(Ruccione, 2002)

THE STUDENT WITH CANCER

Other types of cancers affect children and adolescents. In fact, pediatric cancer is the second most common cause of death in the school-age population. While the incidence of cancer in children has only slightly increased during the past quarter century, there has been a significant increase in the five-year survival rate, which is now greater than 80% (Moore, 2002). Box 27.1 lists the most common pediatric cancers. Any tumor in a child is considered to be malignant until it is histologically identified, even if it is encapsulated. Childhood tumors grow faster than adult tumors because body tissues are normally in a state of rapid growth and high metabolic rate during childhood and adolescence. The incidence of pediatric cancers increases with age.

Students with cancer are treated with the same interventions as for adults: chemotherapy, radiation, surgery (if appropriate), bone marrow or stem cell transplantation, and immunotherapy. Occasionally, biotherapy is used in the form of biologic response modifiers; these are naturally occurring or synthesized substances that can enhance, regulate, or restore functions of the immune system. Students still in active treatment may be in school. They may have infusion ports that must be protected from trauma. They may be immune suppressed and require vigilance on the part of the school nurse in informing the family of potential infectious outbreaks, especially varicella, so that the child will stay home during those periods. Also, it may be necessary for the student to wear a mask while in school. It may be necessary to provide education to the entire class, which may also be required if the student has developed alopecia as a side effect of the chemotherapy. There are many reports in the lay literature of classrooms where all the boys in the class shaved off their hair to give support to their classmate or where a class organized a hair drive to collect long hair that could be made into a wig for their classmate.

Months or years after the initial treatment, there is a significant risk for what is referred to as "late effects." These include "the development of second malignancies, impaired growth, diminished cognitive functioning, and organ damage" (Dragone, 2000, p. 283).

THE STUDENT WITH EARLY ONSET OR CONGENITAL CONDITIONS

With advances in medicine, more and more children will be entering the educational setting who will have survived serious congenital anomalies as well as prematurity. Cardiac anomalies used to be considered a chronic condition in children. With surgical advances, repair of many of these conditions is completed during the early years of life. In many cases, no treatment or medication is needed. It is important that the school nurse inquire about any limitations on activity and sports as the student moves through the educational setting. Their cardiac repair may have resulted in some mixing of arterial and venous blood, resulting in a slightly cyanotic color. It is important for the school nurse to know what the student's baseline color and heart rate are.

Cleft lip and palate are commonly repaired during infancy and toddlerhood. However, the residual impact on speech may result in the continued need for speech therapy. The potential scarring and facial disfiguration and the speech deficits may have an impact on the student's body image.

The presence of necrotizing enterocolitis due to a premature birth may have resulted in the removal of much of the gastrointestinal track. The resulting short bowel syndrome may have created the need for permanent ostomies and the need for total parenteral nutrition by a central line. Other potential gastrointestinal problems may be due to repaired congenital anomalies of esophageal atresia, tracheoesophageal fistula, or imperforate anus. The resulting impact on the student's dietary needs and toileting needs should be part of the student's IHP.

Other problems associated with prematurity include intracranial bleeds and respiratory distress syndrome (RDS). Intracranial bleeds may have resulted in learning disabilities (Chapter 30). RDS, resulting from insufficient surfactant production and difficulty keeping the alveoli open, is treated, in part, by placing the infant on a ventilator. One of the dangers of ventilation is a lack of elasticity of lung tissue and difficulty in oxygen perfusion. This is known as bronchopulmonary dysplasia. Even when infants or toddlers are weaned from the ventilator, they may continue to have increased respiratory problems throughout childhood.

COMORBIDITY/MULTIPLE DISABILITIES

Since the 1990s, it has been recognized that many children and adolescents appear to have more than one chronic condition. In fact, 21% of children have two chronic conditions and 9% have 3 or more chronic conditions (Hayes, 2001; U.S. Department of Education [U.S. DOE], 2000). As children with chronic conditions survive into adulthood, the potential for having more than one chronic condition increases. It is especially common to see comorbidity with the psychiatric conditions and in students who have had severe neurological insults. IDEA defines "multiple disabilities" as "concomitant impairments (such as mental retardation-blindness-orthopedic impairment, etc.), the combination of which causes such severe educational needs that they cannot be accommodated in special education programs solely for one of the impairments. The term does not include deaf-blindness" [34 C.F.R. 300.7C (7) (1999)].

The nursing implication with regard to comorbidity is that students rarely present to a healthcare provider with only one condition; therefore the school nurse may experience difficulty differentiating symptoms and knowing to which condition the symptoms should be attributed. In addition, the student may be receiving medications for both conditions and therefore there is an increased chance of drug reactions when the student is being treated for yet a third, perhaps acute, condition.

In some cases, one condition may significantly affect the student's response to the second condition. Examples include students with myelomeningocele that resulted in significant scoliosis. These students may have more compromise with respiratory infections and may have more difficulty recovering from these. Other examples are students with epilepsy who develop a febrile illness which may place them at greater risk of having febrile seizures; students with cystic fibrosis who develop a cold or become pregnant; students with diabetes who develop gastroenteritis, which has an impact on their food intake and insulin needs; and students who are developmentally delayed and have difficulty describing their symptoms regarding abdominal pain to the nurse.

Perhaps the most severe example is the student who has sustained a traumatic or acquired brain injury, whether due to an accident, a period of anoxia, or to bleeding into the brain following a premature birth. This type of trauma may result in cognitive deficits of memory, concentration, problem- solving, and learning; seizures, headaches, and vision problems; and/or severe deficits in the activities of daily living—eating, communicating, eliminating wastes, walking and using their hands.

REHABILITATION

Rehabilitation is a common component of the lives of children and adolescents with chronic conditions, yet it is never defined. In adult healthcare, it usually represents a process of helping individuals regain or accommodate functions that have been lost. It is almost exclusively focused on mobility, dexterity, and cognitive functioning. This is a very narrow view, especially when the needs of children and adolescents are considered. Selekman (1991) identified the following concepts that should be included in any theory of pediatric rehabilitation.

Habilitation

The term rehabilitation in the pediatric setting is a misnomer. Children are either born with a disability or chronic condition or develop it as a result of trauma or an immune insult. As they engage in the activities to attain and maintain function, they are aiming toward developmental skills that they have not previously achieved. Their expected performance will be at a level expected for their new age and not the one prior to their trauma or the initiation of therapy. Therefore, children are often experiencing *habilitation*.

Etiology

The causes of childhood chronic conditions are very different than those experienced by adults. Most adult conditions requiring rehabilitation are due to stroke, heart disease, and trauma, as well as debilitating acquired conditions, such as diabetes, smoking-related pulmonary problems and arthritis. In contrast, those conditions affecting children are usually due to genetic or congenital conditions, prematurity, or trauma.

Growth and Development

There is a significant impact of growth and development on the chronic condition and there is an impact of the chronic condition on growth and development. The rapid growth that occurs in childhood and adolescence impacts on nutritional needs and sleep needs. These areas are also important for those with chronic conditions, perhaps more so. Some conditions, such as cerebral palsy, utilize excess energy, thus decreasing the nutrients available to support growth at the expected rates. Some interfere with the growth process, such as chronic renal failure and myelomeningocele. Growth impacts on insulin needs; the onset of puberty; as well as the fit of prostheses, braces, and wheelchairs.

Students who are hospitalized frequently or homebound may also experience a delay in their development. Children attached to ventilators have decreased opportunity to explore their environment, to play hide-and-seek, to catch lightning bugs, and interact with others their age. Adolescents with chronic conditions are often treated like younger children and are not afforded adult responsibilities and independence. They are not provided with sex education and genetic counseling specific to their needs.

Coping

Coping is usually an activity for the parents. Since children are usually born with their condition, or develop it early in life, the condition is a part of them. Their degree of acceptance will be strongly influenced by how their parents and those in the schools treat them and whether or not they have been treated as "handicapped." Coping is different in the pediatric years, because it is usually "revisited" by parents at *every* developmental stage. It is common to hear them say, "If only my child didn't have this condition, they would be able to do _____."

Influence of Family

The family is essential as a source of support and an adjunct to treatment. Often, the bulk of the care as well as the financial responsibility falls on the family and impacts on what the family can do as a unit. Normal family activities are often out of the question or take considerable planning and assistance. Qualified babysitters may not be available to allow parents some time for themselves or quality time with the siblings. Parents may have to quit jobs in order to provide care, or if they do work, they rely on the school to provide care during the hours they work. Many of these families are ideal candidates for respite care and home health nursing services. School nurses should be aware of the criteria to access state Social Security Disability Insurance (SSDI), Medicaid waivers, and/or Early Periodic Screening, Diagnostic, and Treatment (EPSDT) programs.

Acute versus Chronic Care

There is a debate in adult rehabilitation whether rehabilitation is an acute process needed to attain skills or whether it is a chronic process. The premature infant who is now the preschool child on a ventilator has probably needed multiple habilitation services and will probably need more during the transition into a regular school setting. The chest physiotherapy done two to four times a day for a student with cystic fibrosis, the speech therapy needed by students with hearing impairments, and the exercises needed by the adolescent with rheumatoid arthritis in order to decrease stiffness and prevent contractures are all components of the same process to assist these individuals to attain, maintain, and regain health.

Educational Needs

School not only offers the advancement of knowledge and skills, but it is also a testing ground for children. This is the setting where they learn rules and values, perhaps different from those in the home. They learn to interact with others and respect the differences in others. It is a place for them to be treated like all other children in the class, usually with the same expectations. The law empowers them to attend class and be included in school activities with the accommodations needed for them to be successful (see below).

The Psychology of Habilitation

Adults often ask when rehabilitation will be over. For many children and adolescents, habilitation continues indefinitely. Those who provide the habilitation services have to be careful not to imply that the child is not "normal" and therefore requires additional services. For many, the presence of these activities is normal, much like putting glasses on before one starts the day. However, it is important for children and adolescents to often hear that you like them "just the way they are." Care must be taken to prevent making a chronic condition into a handicap.

Chronic Pain

Some chronic conditions are accompanied by pain, such as arthritis, or painful treatments, such as finger sticks. There is very little literature that explores the impact of chronic pain in children and how it might affect their future.

Children with Chronic Conditions Are Children First

Perhaps the most important concept is that children need to be children. The child is not his or her condition. These are not disabled children, but rather children who happen to also have a chronic condition.

SPECIAL EDUCATION

Some children with chronic conditions (approximately 7%) (U.S. DOE, 2004) receive special education through their local school districts. To understand the impact of the special education system on this group, it is important to understand the principles of special education, the number of children served and their types of disabilities, services and supports available for children and their families, and the typical outcomes for students with disabilities.

Principles of Special Education Services

Special education in the United States is authorized based on the federal Public Law 94-142, known as the Education for All Handicapped Children Act (EHA) of 1975, now known as IDEA (the Individuals with Disabilities Education Act). IDEA originally was created with the intent to ensure that all children of school age be provided with a free, appropriate public education. Until 1975, children were routinely denied access to schools based on their physical condition, their mental condition, or their medical and health needs (Turnbull & Turnbull, 1990). It was not unusual to find a child with moderate to severe cerebral palsy or Down syndrome staying at home because the principal of a neighborhood school stated that the school could not serve the child (Hardman, Drew, & Egan, 2002). With the passage of EHA and the reauthorization of the law as IDEA, those instances have changed and the United States became, and remains, the only country in the world that provides free public education to virtually 100% of its children. As of 2002, more than 5.6 million children with disabilities were served in public schools and more than one million of those children have severe physical, sensory, or cognitive disorders (U.S. DOE, 2004).

Based on the goal to provide education to all children, IDEA consists of six provisions or principles. These principles are listed in Box 27.2 and discussed below.

Zero Reject

The zero reject principle addresses the primary goal of IDEA: to educate all children no matter what their disability. This provision of IDEA states that no matter what the type or level of disability, schools are responsible for providing educational services to the child. This includes *all* children, including those

Box 27.2 ■ ■ ■

SIX PRINCIPLES OF SPECIAL EDUCATION SERVICES

1. Zero reject
2. Nondiscriminatory evaluation
3. Free and appropriate public education (FAPE)
4. Least restrictive environment (LRE)
5. Parent and student participation
6. Procedural due process

with the most severe disabilities and children with significant health and medical needs. The zero reject principle acknowledges the belief that all children can gain skills and learn and that society has a responsibility to provide those services to all children (Turnbull, 1998).

In recent years, this has meant that children and adolescents with complicated and chronic health conditions have been present in schools on a routine basis. This includes children with ventilators, central lines, gastrostomy tubes, and tracheotomies, who 20 years ago may not have been discharged from the hospital. They, along with children with chronic respiratory disorders, children who are HIV positive, and children with severe cognitive impairments and severe social-emotional disorders, are now routinely found in any large school district and in many small or rural school districts. While the needs of these students are often challenging to school districts, their presence in schools is an acknowledgment that both society and government have taken a stand to educate every child in the country and recognize that every child can benefit from a well-planned and implemented curriculum.

Nondiscriminatory Evaluation

This principle is tied closely to the zero reject principle. It is designed to ensure that all children who are referred to determine their eligibility to receive special education services will receive an evaluation that is bias-free (IDEA, 1997). This means that the evaluation process should determine whether or not a child is eligible for special education services and then identify the types and amount of services needed to ensure that the child learns to the best of his or her ability. To ensure that a bias-free evaluation of the student's skills is conducted, a multidisciplinary team of professionals and family members collects information about the child. In cases where there are chronic conditions, a nurse or other health professional should be included on this assessment team. The assessment procedures used by the team should be free of bias, particularly when it comes to socioeconomic status, ethnicity, and language of the child and family. Assessments of children should be conducted in the native language of the child and should use instruments that have been standardized in that language (Turnbull, 1998).

Free Appropriate Public Education (FAPE)

The third principle of IDEA is that all children must be provided with a free and appropriate public education. As implemented today, this principle states that all children with disabilities who are 3 to 21 years of age must be provided with an appropriate education plan and that plan must be provided free of charge to the family, as would any public school service to any other child. While many children with mild disabilities do not require education services during their preschool (age 3 to 5) years or during their young adult years (age 18 to 21), those students with moderate to severe disabilities often do require services and supports that begin prior to entry into kindergarten and extend beyond the typical time of high school graduation. An optional component of IDEA allows states to provide services to children with disabilities ages birth to 36 months. All states and territories of the United States currently provide these services (Turnbull, 1998).

A critical aspect of FAPE is the development of an appropriate education plan for the student. For most students (3 to 21 year olds), the vehicle for this plan is the individualized education program (IEP) and for young children (birth to 3 years of age) the vehicle is the individualized family services plan (IFSP) (see Chapter 9).

Least Restrictive Environment (LRE)

The least restrictive environment (LRE) provision of IDEA has proven to be the most controversial since the original passage of the law (Mayberry, 2002). LRE means that a student with a disability must be provided education in the setting that is most like the setting in which his or her peers without disabilities receive education services *and* that will best provide for his or her educational development. During the late 1970s and the 1980s, this principle was manifested in the movement entitled *mainstreaming*, meaning that students with disabilities were placed with students without disabilities; they were placed in the mainstream of their schools (Turnbull, 1998). The goal of the mainstreaming movement to ensure that students with disabilities received their special education services in settings with students who did not have disabilities was rarely achieved. The reality was that children with disabilities were often placed in educational settings with children without disabilities but they did not receive the services or supports necessary for them to integrate into those settings. Consequently, they did not achieve well and there were often conflicts between the needs of students with disabilities and the needs of students without disabilities (Leyser & Lessen, 1985). Based on the backlash that occurred in the late 1980s, the LRE provision of IDEA was not strongly enforced (Turnbull, 1998).

In the early 1990s, partly in response to the segregation into separate schools and programs of students with chronic medical conditions, groups of parents, advocates, students, and legislators began to call for the reimplementation of the LRE provision of IDEA (Arnold & Dodge, 1994; Schultz, 1994). This movement became known as the *inclusion* movement. Its proponents stated that all students should be included in the typical educational setting and that the support services necessary for the students should be provided in those typical settings. The strongest proponents of this movement stated that all students, no matter what their disability or service need, should be educated in typical settings. This movement recognized that all students, particularly those with chronic conditions, often have aspects of their development that are typical. The student with severe cerebral palsy may have typical or even advanced cognitive skills. The student in need of a ventilator may have the same social and cognitive needs and abilities as a student without a ventilator.

The proponents of inclusion also pointed to the detrimental effects of segregating students, especially students with disabilities. Much of the research of the past 20 years examining the effects of inclusive schooling with students with sensory, physical, and cognitive disabilities has found that the students' social, communication, and cognitive outcomes are typically better than the outcomes for their peers who received education in segregated, self-contained special education settings (McMillian, 1996; Morse & Santos, 1995; Odom & Beckman, 2002).

Based on the inclusion movement and the research of the late 1980s and 1990s, IDEA 1997 strengthened the LRE provision of the law. Since 1997, school districts have been expected to provide therapeutic, health, assistive technology, and other services for students with chronic conditions in their typical school settings (Davis & Hopwood, 2002; Sandler, 1999; Wood, 1998). The expectation has had a significant impact on where students with disabilities receive their education. In 1986, only 26% of students with disabilities received their education services in general education classrooms. In 2000, almost 48% of students with disabilities received their education service in general education classrooms and another 30% received their services in a general education school through a resource room (U.S. DOE, 2004). In 2000, fewer than 2% of students were in a specialized school compared to more than 9% 15 years earlier (U.S. DOE, 2004).

Proponents of the inclusion movement have argued that students benefit in numerous ways. They are, first and foremost, afforded access to the standard curriculum that all other students receive and therefore can advance their academic skills. Historically, students receiving special education services have not been able to participate in the standard curriculum and consequently numerous students who have had the ability to learn to read, write, and compute have been denied that education (Turnbull, Turnbull, Shank, Smith, & Leal, 2002).

In addition to access to the general education curriculum, students with disabilities also benefit from the social peer contact that occurs in inclusive settings. While some studies indicate that students with disabilities, particularly those with behavioral or attentional disabilities, are targets for teasing and bullying, the preponderance of empiric evidence indicates that students with disabilities in inclusive settings benefit socially (Turnbull et al., 2002).

Critics of the LRE provision of IDEA and of the inclusion movement have serious concerns about the services provided to students with disabilities, particularly for students with chronic health and medical needs. Moving students with moderate to significant service needs from specialized schools to neighborhood schools can reduce the services provided to the student. These reductions in services can come in the areas of reduced nursing services, therapeutic services, and assistive technology services. Critics also indicate that moving students with complex medical and health needs to neighborhood schools inefficiently disperses limited medical and health services and limits the contact with students needed by specialized service providers. Finally, critics state that decentralized services in neighborhood schools makes it difficult to develop team relationships with the teachers, aides, and other educators providing services to these students (Sandler, 1999).

Missing Services

A common concern of families as well as professionals regarding students with disabilities is the availability of services to address students' needs. Both in specialized and inclusive settings, the concern expressed is whether or not children will have the health, therapeutic, and medical support necessary so that they can take advantage of the educational process in the setting they are attending. This is true for mild chronic conditions as well as for more significant ones.

For example, in the late 1990s, a number of school districts throughout the country refused to provide services for insulin injections for children with diabetes. Without this support, a child could not attend the school and his or her life could be threatened. However, with support, the child can easily participate in almost all school activities and certainly benefit from the educational programming being provided. It is a relatively easy process to provide nursing support so that a child can receive his or her insulin injections and therefore be a part of the educational settings (Lightfoot, Mukherjee, & Sloper, 2001; Reiter, 2000).

A more complex situation might include a student who has a tracheotomy. Because of the need for constant monitoring and frequent suctioning, a school or district may argue that it is not possible to serve a child with a tracheotomy in its educational settings. However, the child may be developing completely normally in the cognitive and receptive communication domains and may best be served in the setting of a general education classroom. If the support services are not available for this student, he or she may need to move to a more restrictive setting for children with chronic conditions.

In some cases, school nurses have been called upon to train teachers, volunteers, and other professionals to provide health services in their classrooms. Services might include gastrostomy feeding, gavage feeding, and tracheostomy suctioning. This may be the only way that students can be placed in the educational setting that best fits their academic and social needs. However, before this teaching occurs, it is essential that the school nurse check the state's nurse practice act to ensure that these skills can be delegated to unlicensed assistive personnel.

Parent and Student Participation

A primary principle of services to students with disabilities has been the involvement of families and the student in the education process. From the passage of the first law in 1975, parents have had an active part in the evaluation of their child, the development of their education plan, and the implementation of that plan. With the passage of IDEA 1997, families, educators, therapists, and healthcare workers have recognized that the student, too, must take an active role in the development of his or her education program. Beginning as early as 8 or 9 years of age, students are asked to participate in their education planning meetings and asked what services and supports they need to ensure that their educational development proceeds as far as possible. As with all healthcare provision, the active participation of the client improves outcomes. In the case of special education services of students with chronic conditions, this is also true (Turnbull, 1998).

Procedural Due Process

The final principle of IDEA and special education is procedural due process. When passed in 1975, the U.S. Congress expressed the concern that the set of services and principles stated above would be difficult to implement and that families and students needed a process to ensure that their rights were being protected. Written into the law was a provision to ensure that families and students have a process to petition independent groups if they feel that school personnel or school districts are violating their rights.

This procedural due process portion of the law has proven to be valuable to students with chronic medical conditions. For example, it was used in the late 1980s and early 1990s to ensure that students who were HIV positive were afforded education services in the least restrictive environment. A number of schools in the late 1980s barred students who were HIV positive from attending school. Federal courts found, based on the IDEA principles, that schools could not bar students from attending because of their health status (Harvey, 1994).

The procedural due process provision of the law has also been the vehicle through which families have secured more inclusive education services for their children who need medical supports and healthcare services. Clean intermittent catheterizations, respiratory therapies, gastrostomy feedings, and tracheotomy suctioning were unheard of in the 1980s in general school settings. In the early 2000s, it is not unusual to see these procedures taking place in an elementary or secondary school with the support of school nurses or other healthcare professionals. Access to these medical and health supports was secured through families who claimed that their children were being denied educational services based solely on their medical and healthcare needs. The school nurse can empower parents to use this provision to obtain the services they need for their child.

Who Are the Children Receiving Special Education Services?

Under IDEA, children from birth to 21 years of age who have a qualifying disability are eligible for special education services. While children from birth to

36 months are provided those services through various agencies in the different states (e.g., Department of Public Welfare in Pennsylvania; Department of Education in South Dakota; and Department of Social and Health Services in Washington), for children 3 to 21 years of age with a disability, services are provided by the state Departments of Education, local school districts, and state Departments of Public Health (U.S. DOE, 2004).

In 2003, more than 5.7 million students in schools throughout the country received special education services (U.S. DOE, 2004). Just under 50% of these, or more than 2.88 million, were eligible for special education services because of their specific learning disabilities. In addition to the students with learning disabilities, there were numerous students with chronic conditions. More than 73,000 students had chronic orthopedic impairments (i.e., physical disabilities), approximately 100,000 had sensory impairments, more than one million had speech and language impairments, and more than 612,000 had mental retardation (see TABLE 27.3).

Of the more than 5.7 million students ages 3 to 21 years receiving special education, more than 500,000 are between the ages of 3 and 5. Another 2.5 million are between the ages of 6 and 11 and 2.3 million are between the ages of 12 and 17. Almost 250,000 students are between the ages of 18 and 21.

Table 27.3 ■

CATEGORIES OF STUDENTS ELIGIBLE FOR SPECIAL EDUCATION SERVICES IN SCHOOL YEAR 2002–2003

	IDEA, PART B SERVICES TO STUDENTS	
DISABILITY	NUMBER	PERCENTAGE
Specific Learning Disabilities	2,887,217	49.99
Speech and Language Impairments	1,093,808	19.01
Mental Retardation	612,978	10.61
Emotional Disturbance	473,662	8.20
Other Health Impairments	291,850	5.05
Multiple Disabilities	122,559	2.12
Autism	78,749	1.36
Orthopedic Impairments	73,057	1.26
Hearing Impairments	70,767	1.23
Developmental Delay	28,935	0.50
Visual Impairments	25,975	0.45
Traumatic Brain Injury	14,844	0.26
Deaf-blindness	1,320	0.02
Total	5,775,722	100.00

Source: U.S. Department of Education. (2004). *24th Annual Report to Congress on the Implementation of the Individuals with Disabilities Education Act*. Author: Washington, DC.

The needs of students with chronic conditions vary significantly by age group. Many preschool children and their families are still in the diagnostic process and are trying to identify the syndrome, condition, or disability affecting the child's health and educational development. For these children, coordinating medical and health information to identify services and support is critical. For young adults ages 18 to 21, transition services to community, employment, housing, and social/recreational activities are important.

Students with disabilities in 13 different categories are eligible for special education services (see Table 27.3); however, the characteristics of the children within each of these categories vary significantly. Two students in the same category may not need the same specialized healthcare services. The variation in the types and intensity of medical and health services for students receiving special education emphasizes the importance of individualized education programs and determination of the services to support the student's educational development.

Box 27.3 ■■■

SPECIAL EDUCATION SERVICES POSSIBLE TO INCLUDE IN A STUDENT'S INDIVIDUALIZED EDUCATION PROGRAM

SERVICE
Specialized instruction
Speech and language instruction
Occupational therapy
Physical therapy
Psychological testing and counseling services
Diagnostic and evaluation services
Social work services
Assistive technology devices and services
Family counseling and education services
Transportation services
Health services necessary for the child to participate in educational activities
Coordination of services

Who Is Missing from this Group?

While students eligible to receive special education services are clearly defined by IDEA and the definition is further refined by each state education agency, there are numerous students with chronic health concerns who are missing from this group. Students with asthma, allergies, cystic fibrosis, hemophilia, muscular dystrophy, sickle cell disease, and other chronic health concerns are not eligible for special education services or the due process protections of IDEA. The number of children excluded from services by IDEA but with chronic health conditions is difficult to determine. Some estimates are as high as five million students, essentially doubling the number of students with chronic health and developmental concerns who are in schools.

One area of confusion involves students with attention deficit hyperactivity disorder (ADHD). Some of these students are eligible for services and supports under IDEA, if their ADHD has a significant enough impact on their cognitive processing and their academic achievement. Under these conditions, students may be eligible for special education services. In other cases, students with ADHD are found not eligible for special education services and may go without the support, accessibility, technology, or curriculum adaptations they might need to succeed. In at least two court cases, students with ADHD were denied their medication by the schools based on the fact that they had not qualified for special education services (Forness & Kayale, 2001).

Services and Supports for Students Receiving Special Education

The services and supports available for students receiving special education services vary. The most important factor in determining services is that the service must advance the student's ability to learn new educational skills and knowledge (IDEA, 1997). This distinction is made in order to ensure that services are linked to the educational development of the child and that health and medical services continue to be provided by the healthcare community. Despite this distinction, it is critical to bridge the health services provided by the healthcare community and the health needs of students with disabilities in schools. It is this intersection at which the school nurse often finds herself.

There are 12 specific services that are provided to students under IDEA and the special education umbrella (Box 27.3). These services are designed to ensure that students are able to participate in educational activities that will advance their skills and knowledge. Services that do not provide students with access to educational services are not the responsibility of schools.

THE MULTIDISCIPLINARY (M-D) TEAM

In many schools where there are students with chronic conditions, a multidisciplinary team plans, implements and evaluates the services and supports for those students (IDEA, 1997). M-D teams are often comprised of general educators, special educators, nurses, physical therapists, school psychologists, speech–language pathologists, occupational therapists, and other professionals necessary to address the students' needs. Other professionals might include orientation and mobility specialists, nutritionists, assistive technology specialists, and audiologists.

The school nurse often has a special place on the M-D team as the lead team member when medical and health issues need to be addressed (Knight, 1996). This necessitates at least five key roles, which are listed in Box 27.4 and described below.

First, the nurse must collect information about the student's chronic condition through contacts with the student's family and healthcare professionals. This is a critical role that will allow the team to make the best possible decisions for the student.

A second role of the school nurse on the M-D team is as translator or interpreter. While many of the professionals on the M-D team will have an extensive background in human development, educational interventions, and psychological interventions, it is the school nurse who will be most familiar with the medical and health information. It is his or her responsibility to be able to translate the information collected from community health and medical providers so that the rest of the team has an understanding of that information *and* its impact on the educational, social, and recreational goals of a student.

A third major role is to document sequelae of the conditions presented in the school. Whether the health event is minor or major, the school nurse must capture that information and ensure that it is communicated back to the M-D team. If, for instance, a student with asthma begins to increase the rate at which she needs to use her inhaler, the school nurse should be documenting the rate of inhaler use and communicating that to the team. Medical and health conditions often manifest in classrooms as behavioral and academic concerns. Without information from the school nurse, teachers, therapists, and psychologists may misinterpret the actions of students.

The fourth major role is as communicator back to the student's family and healthcare providers. Important medical and health events that take place in the school should be communicated by the nurse to the student's healthcare providers and to the student's family.

Finally, the school nurse ensures quality medical and healthcare services to the students in the school setting and continuing evaluation of those services as they impact the special education process. Without the ongoing monitoring and evaluation of healthcare services, the special education interventions and related services may be compromised or ineffective.

Box 27.4 ■ ■ ■

MULTIDISCIPLINARY EDUCATION TEAM: THE SCHOOL NURSE'S KEY ROLES

1. Collect information.
2. Translate or interpret health information for the M-D team members.
3. Document sequelae.
4. Communicate with students' families and healthcare providers.
5. Ensure quality medical and healthcare services are provided to students.

TRANSITIONING

When most healthcare professionals speak of transition services, they speak of adolescents making the change from secondary education to employment, continued education, and/or independent living. By law, transitioning refers to a coordinated set of activities. It is mandated by IDEA that the process of transitioning MUST begin at age 14 with career exploration activities, meeting with the school counselor, participating in vocational assessment activities, and finding out other resources regarding careers. An Individualized Transition Plan must be incorporated into the IEP by the time the student is 16 and include the services needed and the interagency responsibilities or linkages before the student leaves secondary education. Vocational Rehabilitation, a nation-wide federal–state program, is an excellent resource for assisting eligible people with disabilities to define a suitable employment goal and to explore available training and support options.

The Department of Health and Human Services developed a consensus statement regarding healthcare transitions for adolescents from pediatric healthcare services to adult services using the same parameters as those mandated in IDEA (Blum, 2002). "Healthy People 2010 established the goal that all young people with special healthcare needs will receive the services needed to make necessary transitions to all aspects of adult life, including healthcare, work, and independent living" (Blum, 2002, p. 1305). They acknowledge that transition is a multifaceted active process, that it precedes at different rates for different individuals, and that it is more complex for those with more severe disabilities.

The factors identified as being associated with more successful transitioning include the following: "(1) the family, young adult, and provider have a future orientation; (2) transition is started early; (3) family members and healthcare providers foster personal and medical independence; (4) planning occurs for the future; (5) the young adult verbalizes the desire to function in the adult medical world; (6) reimbursement for services is not interrupted; (7) pediatric providers continue to provide care into adulthood, but change the location of service delivery to adult clinics or practice; and (8) individuals continue to receive services from the same health care system" (Reiss & Gibson, 2002, p. 1312).

The concept of transitioning, however, needs to be defined in a broader sense. The real meaning of the word transitioning implies passing from one state, stage, or place to another. It therefore occurs at every stage of development and in every change in one's educational setting, including entry and exit to the educational system (Ralabate, 2002). This includes the transition from early intervention services and using the Individualized Family Service Plan as a starting point for the Individualized Educational Program.

It is just as important for the kindergarten teacher to know what communication patterns and adaptive equipment a child used in preschool as it is to plan for a child's future at age 18. Knowing a child's needs for adaptations and exactly what works will save the new school time and money for assessments and trying different equipment and will assist the student by not missing class time and educational experiences. Making sure that prerequisite tests or evaluations have been completed and the results included will facilitate the transition process.

Advanced planning is required. One approach is for the family, school teachers and school nurses to develop a transition portfolio for the child as they prepare to transition from one level or school to another (Demchak & Greenfield, 2003). A portfolio is described as a folder that documents strategies that work for a particular student. It includes personal and medical information about the student, as well as educational programming suggestions, ideas for adaptations and supports, including communication strategies and behavioral support plans, and notes on what has worked and what has not. It goes without saying that parental approval (and the student's assent) is needed before this information is shared.

The portfolio may contain information on medications the student receives and the best way to give those medications; communication modalities; special health-related equipment needed; alteration in hearing, vision or mobility; special feeding or elimination needs; coping skills and what helps the student adapt; and educational needs. In can also include those approaches/interventions that the school should avoid. It also is a medium to identify the student's strengths.

PROGNOSIS

Most children and adolescents do not outgrow their chronic condition as they age; however, the symptoms and sequelae may change. In 1980, 80% of children with chronic conditions lived to age 20; by 1997, 95% lived to age 20 (Bittles et al., 2002; Hutton, Cooke & Pharoah, 1994; Strauss & Shavell, 1998). For example, the average age of a person with cystic fibrosis is 31 years, compared to 7 years in 1973; while 33% of those with myelomeningocele reached the age of 20 in the 1970s, now more than 80% reach that age (Reise & Gibson, 2002). Therefore, it can be seen that children with chronic conditions grow up to be adults with chronic conditions.

While 90% of students without disabilities receive a high school diploma, only 61% of those with disabilities receive a diploma (U.S. DOE, 2000). These figures impact on the individual's ability to become gainfully employed. It is also more difficult for these young adults to access needed services once they reach their 22nd birthday.

ISSUES

Stigma/Labels

Some parents are hesitant for a student to be diagnosed with a chronic condition, especially one involving their child's mental health status, fearing that the label of the condition will affect their child's academic and social opportunities. Once a diagnosis is made, parents, and even students themselves, do not want to identify themselves as disabled, and therefore forgo the services that would be available to them under IDEA. The strongest message that can be given to these families is "No label—no service." In other words, no accommodations can be mandated for students if they have not received a diagnosis of a condition that warrants those accommodations. Failure to obtain needed services will put the student's academic performance in jeopardy; therefore the risk/benefit ratio leans strongly toward the benefit side if school personnel take action.

The problem of labels is made worse when descriptors are attached to the students with particular conditions. Referring to individuals as "retarded" or "mentally ill" will affect how staff and peers interact with the individuals and will affect the students' images of themselves.

Being "Different"

Discomfort or embarrassment regarding the technology or aspects of conditions can occur for both the student with the disability and the rest of the class. Classmates are often curious as to what it is like to live with that device or to not have a particular life skill. It is important for the school nurse and the classroom teacher to work together to provide books and have discussions with the class regarding the specific disability and the technology used. Role-play is especially effective; getting around in a wheelchair, being blindfolded, and not using one extremity allows peers to understand the need for and function of various pieces of equipment. One of the reasons students do not want others to know is because it implies that they are different during a period of their lives when fitting into the group is essential.

Need for Primary Care

Children with chronic conditions are usually followed by specialists for their particular condition. Because healthcare visits are so common, the parents often forget to ensure that the primary care needs of the child are met. The school nurse can help by keeping updated on these students for their growth and development needs, as well as their immunizations.

Late Effects/Sequelae

It is important to recognize that some young people who are treated for a chronic condition may demonstrate late effects of the treatments or of the disease many years later. Examples are the emergence of leukemia in those with Down syndrome, the development of osteopenia in those who are wheelchair dependent, and the appearance of diabetes late in adolescence in the individual with cystic fibrosis.

Financial Constraints

One of the problems facing schools and the healthcare industry is the lack of financial resources available for children with chronic conditions, especially those whose conditions require costly appliances/treatments or the need for attendants in the schools. It has been estimated that 5% of children use 80% of the resources. When these children's needs are met, there is very little left to distribute to the other 95% of the children and their schools. A major study found that approximately 13% of those with special healthcare needs were responsible for 45% of the pediatric healthcare expenditures (CDC, National Center for Health Statistics, 2003). For those students eligible for Medicaid reimbursement, the school district can recoup some of the costs of the services provided by the school nurse. Therefore documentation of services provided as well as progress made is essential (Chapter 44).

NASN RESPONDS

Because of the great prevalence of children with chronic conditions in the school environment, the National Association of School Nurses, along with multiple other pediatric health-related groups, developed an action plan for schools, students, and families (Students with Chronic Illnesses, 2003). This plan identifies some of the family's responsibilities, such as communicating with the school about their child's health condition and what is needed to make accommodations for the child in the school setting, participating in the development of the IEP, providing the medication or supplies needed by their child, and providing a way for the parent to be contacted by the school at all times. The school and school district are expected to have comprehensive guidelines and protocols in place for students with chronic conditions, especially for those with the most common conditions, to identify, plan, and implement accommodations for these students, to provide nondiscriminatory opportunities to students with chronic conditions, to communicate with families, and ensure proper record keeping. Students are expected to participate in their care and to notify an adult about any concerns.

CONCLUSION

According to the Assistive Technology Act of 1998, "disability is a natural part of the human experience and in no way diminishes the right of individuals to a) live independently; b) enjoy self-determination and make choices; c) benefit from an education; d) pursue meaningful careers; and e) enjoy full inclusion and integration in the economic, political, social, cultural, and educational mainstream of society in the United States" (Title IV, Section 2a1). The school nurse is the constant in the student's school experience over the years. It is the nurse who can see the whole picture of what is happening with a student over time in his or her assessments, planning, and interventions. The nurse is their advocate, the coordinator of care, and the one person who both can meet their health-related needs and build their self-esteem at the same time.

Resources

ABLEDATA (Assistive Technology and Rehabilitation Equipment Information Clearing House)
8455 Colesville, Rd., Suite 935
Silver Spring, MD 20910
800-227.0216 (voice/TTY)
http://www.abledata.com

Alexander Graham Bell Association for the Deaf and Hard of Hearing
3417 Volta Place NW
Washington, DC 20007
202-337-5220
http://www.agbell.org

American Foundation for the Blind
15 W. 16th Street
New York, NY 10011
800-232-5463

American Society for Deaf Children
P.O. Box 3355
Gettysburg, PA 17325
717-334-7922
http://www.deafchildren.org

American Speech-Language-Hearing Association
10801 Rockville Pike
Rockville MD 20852
301-897-5700
http://www.asha.org

Exceptional Parent Resource Guide
555 Kinderkamack Road
Oradell, NJ 07649
877-372-7368
http://www.eparent.com

National Association of the Deaf
American Society for Deaf Children
814 Thayer Avenue
Silver Spring, MD 20919-4500
301-587-1788
TTY: 301-587-1789
http://www.nad.org

Children with Disabilities
Online Guide to Resources for Parents and Children
U.S. Department of Justice
http://www.childrenwithdisabilities.ncjrs.org

National Center for Youth with Disabilities
Adolescent Health Program
University of Minnesota
Box 721-UMHC
Harvard Street at East River Road
Minneapolis, MN 55455
800-333-6293

National Council on Disability
1331 F St. NW, Suite 1050
Washington, DC 20004
202-272-2004 (voice)
202-272-2074 (TTY)
http://www.ncd.gov

National Eye Institute
Building 31, Room 6A32
31 Center Drive, MSC 2510
Bethesda, MD 20892
301-496-5248
http://www.nei.nih.gov

National Information Center for Children and Youth with Disabilities (NICHCY)
P. O. Box 1492
Washington, DC 20013
800-695-0285 (voice/TTY)
http://www.aed.org/nichcy

National Institute of Neurological Disorders and Stroke
P. O. Box 5801
Bethesda, MD 20824
800-352-9424
http://www.ninds.nih.gov

National Organization for Rare Disorders
100 Route 37, P.O. Box 8923
New Fairfield, CT 06812
800-999-6673 (voice)
203-746-6927 (TTY)
http://www.nord_rdb.com/~orphan

Rehabilitation Engineering and Assistive Technology Society of North America
1700 North Moore Street
Suite 1540
Arlington, VA 22209
703-524-6686
http://www.resna.org

References

Administration on Developmental Disabilities. (2004). Retrieved October 26, 2004 from http://www.acf.hhs.gov/programs/add/

American Speech-Language-Hearing Association (ASHA). (1992). *Resource on person-first language*. Retrieved June 16, 2003 from http:// professional.asha.org/resources/journals/person_first.cfm

American Speech-Language-Hearing Association (ASHA). (2002). *Communication facts: Incidence and prevalence of communication disorders and hearing loss in children – 2002 edition*. Retrieved May 10, 2003 from http://professional.asha.org/resources/factsheets/children.cfn

Americans with Disabilities Act. (1990). PL 101-336, 42 U.S.C. §§12101 et seq.

Arnold, J., & Dodge, H. (1994). Room for all. *American School Board Journal, 181*(10), 22–26.

Assistive Technology Act of 1998. (1998). S.2432, 105th Congress. Retrieved May 21, 2003 from http://www.section508.gov/docs/AT1998.html

Ball, M. (2002). *Developmental coordination disorder*. London: Jessica Kingsley.

Bittles, A., Petterson, B., Sullivan, S., Hussain, R., Glasson, E., & Montgomery, P. (2002). The influence of intellectual disability on life expectancy. *The Journals of Gerontology. Series A, Biological Sciences and Medical Sciences, 57* (7), 470–472.

Blum, R. (2002). Improving transition for adolescents with special health care needs from pediatric to adult-centered health care. *Pediatrics, 110*(6 Suppl.), 1301–1306.

Bryant, D., & Bryant, B. (2003). *Assistive technology for people with disability*. Boston: Pearson Education.

Carroll, B. (2000). Sickle cell disease. In P. Jackson & J. Vessey (Eds.), *Primary care of the child with a chronic condition* (pp. 808–836). St. Louis: C. V. Mosby.

Centers for Disease Control and Prevention (CDC). National Center for Health Statistics. (2002). *Cochlear implants and meningitis*. Retrieved July 26, 2004 from http://www.cdc.govncbdd/ehdi/cochlear/CochlearImplantQ&As.pdf

Centers for Disease Control and Prevention (CDC), National Center for Health Statistics. (2003). *National survey of children with special health care needs*. Maternal and Child Health Bureau. Retrieved September 7, 2005 from http://www.cdc.gov/nchs/about/major/slaits/cshcn.htm

Corbin, J. (2001). Introduction and overview: Chronic illness and nursing. In R. Hyman & J. Corbin (Eds.), *Chronic illness: Research and theory for nursing practice* (pp. 1–15). New York: Springer.

Curry, H. (2004). Bleeding disorder basics. *Pediatric Nursing, 30*(5), 402–405, 428–429.

Davis, P. (2003). *Including children with visual impairment in mainstream schools: A practical guide*. London: David Fulton.

Davis, P., & Hopwood, V. (2002). Including children with a visual impairment in the mainstream primary school classroom. *Journal of Research in Special Educational Needs, 2*(3), 1–11.

Demchak, M., & Greenfield, R. (2003). *Transition portfolios for students with disabilities*. Thousand Oaks, California: Corwin Press.

Developmental Disabilities Assistance and Bill of Rights Act Amendments of 1996, P.L. 104-183, 42 USC 6000, et seq.

Dragone, M. (2000). Cancer. In P. Jackson and J. Vessey (Eds.), *Primary care of the child with a chronic condition* (pp. 266–304). St. Louis: C. V. Mosby.

Farley, J., & Dunleavy, M. (2000). Myelodysplasia. In P. Jackson & J. Vessey (Eds.), *Primary care of the child with a chronic condition* (pp. 658–675). St. Louis: C. V. Mosby.

Forness, S., & Kayale, K. (2001). ADHD and a return to the medical model of special education. *Education and Treatment of Children, 24*(3), 224–247.

Fox, J. (1997). *Primary health care of children*. St. Louis: C. V. Mosby

Green, A. (2003). Update on Chiari malformation: Clinical manifestations, diagnosis, and treatments. *Pediatric Nursing, 29*(4), 331–335.

Gregory, E. (1998). *The ear and hearing: A guide for school nurses*. Scarborough, ME: National Association of School Nurses.

Hardman, M., Drew, C., & Egan, M. (2002). *Human exceptionality: Society, school and family*. Boston: Allyn & Bacon.

Harrison, B., Faircloth, J., & Yaryan, L. (1995). The impact of legislation and litigation on the role of the school nurse. *Nursing Outlook, 43*(2), 57–61.

Harvey, J. (1994). Confidentiality and public policy regarding children with HIV infection. *Journal of School Health, 64*(1), 18–19.

Hayes, V. (2001). Families' and children's chronic conditions: Knowledge development and methodological considerations. In R. Hyman & J. Corbin (Eds.), *Chronic illness: Research and theory for nursing practice* (pp. 106–143). New York: Springer.

Herer, G., Knightly, C., & Steinberg, A. (2002). Hearing: Sounds and silences. In M. Batshaw (Eds.), Children with disabilities (pp. 193–227). Baltimore: Paul H. Brookes.

Hill, N., & Sullivan, L. (1999). *Management guidelines for pediatric nurse practitioners*. Philadelphia: F.A. Davis.

Hutton, J., Cooke, T., & Pharoah, P. (1994). Life expectancy in children with cerebral palsy. *British Medical Journal, 309*, 431–435.

Individuals with Disabilities Education Act Amendments of 1997. (1997). PL 105-17, 20 U.S.C. §§1400 et seq.

Ireys, H. (2001). Epidemiology of childhood chronic illness: Issues in definitions, service use, and costs. In H. Koot & J. Wallander (Eds.), *Quality of life in child and adolescent illness: Concepts, methods and findings* (pp. 123–150). London: Brunner-Routledge.

Karp, S. (2000). Bleeding disorders. In P. Jackson & J. Vessey (Eds.), *Primary care of the child with a chronic condition* (pp. 212–241). St. Louis: C. V. Mosby.

Kenefick, J. (2002). Vision. In L. Porter (Ed.), *Educating young children with special needs* (pp. 81–95). Crows Nest, Australia: Allen & Unwin.

Knight, S. (1996). Defining a model for team leader development. *Nurse Education Today, 16*(5), 309–315.

Kohler, K., Schweikert-Stary, M., & Lubkin, I. (1998). Altered mobility. In I. Lubkin (Ed.), *Chronic illness: Impact and intervention* (pp. 122–148). Boston: Jones and Bartlett. Kuhlthau, K., Ferris, T., Beal, A., Gortmaker, S., & Perrin, J. (2002). Who cares for medicaid-enrolled children with chronic conditions? *Pediatrics, 108*(4), 906–912.

Levy, S., & O'Rourke, M. (2002). Technological assistance: Innovations for independence. In M. Batshaw (Ed.), *Children with disabilities* (pp. 629–645). Baltimore: Paul H. Brookes.

Leyser, Y., & Lessen, E. (1985). The efficacy of two training approaches on attitudes of prospective teachers toward mainstreaming. *Exceptional Child, 32*(3), 175–183.

Lightfoot, J., Mukherjee, S., & Sloper, P. (2001). Supporting pupils with special health needs in mainstream schools: Policy and practice. *Children & Society, 15*(2), 57–69.

Liptak, G. (2002). Neural tube defects. In M. Batshaw. *Children with disabilities* (pp. 467–492). Baltimore: Paul H. Brookes.

Mayberry, S. (2002). *Teaching students with special needs in the 21st century classroom*. Lanham, MD: Scarecrow Press.

McMillian, D. (1996). Full inclusion: An empirical perspective. *Behavioral Disorders, 21*(2), 145–159.

McPherson, M., Arango, P., Fox, H., Lauver, C., McManus, M., Newacheck, P., Perrin, J., Shonkoff, J., & Strickland,

B. (1998). A new definition of children with special health care needs. *Pediatrics, 102*(1), 137–140.

Miller, M., Menacker, S., & Batshaw, M. (2002). Vision: Our window to the world. In M. Batshaw (Ed.), *Children with disabilities* (pp. 165–192). Baltimore: Paul H. Brookes.

Moore, I. (2002). Cancer in children. In R. Hyman & J. Corbin (Eds.), *Chronic illness: Research and theory for nursing practice* (pp. 80–103). New York: Springer.

Morse, T., & Santos, K. (1995). Full inclusion: Dream or reality? *Journal for a Just and Caring Education, 1*(4), 449–457.

Mudrick, N. (2002). The prevalence of disability among children: Paradigms and estimates. *Physical Medicine and Rehabilitation Clinics of North America, 13*(4), 775–792.

National Association of School Nurses (NASN). (2004). *Position statement: Do Not Resuscitate*. Retrieved September 7, 2005 from http://www.nasn.org

National Information Center for Children and Youth with Disabilities (NICHY). (2003). *Deafness and hearing loss*. Retrieved May 10, 2003 from http://www.nichy.org/pubs/factshe/fs3txt.htm

National Institute on Deafness and Other Communication Disorders. (2002). *Hearing aids. Retrieved May 11, 2003 from http://www.nidcd.nih.gov/health/hearing/hearingaid.asp*

National Institute on Deafness and Other Communication Disorders. (2003). *WISE EARS!* Retrieved June 13, 2003 from http://www.nidcd.nih.gov/health/wise

Newacheck, P., Hung, Y., & Wright, K. (2002). Racial and ethnic disparities in access to care for children with special health care needs. *Ambulatory Pediatrics, 2*(4), 247–254.

Northern, J., & Downs, M. (1991). *Hearing in children*. Baltimore: Williams & Wilkins.

Odom, S., & Beckman, P. (2002). *Widening the circle: Including children with disabilities in preschool programs*. New York: Teachers College Press.

Perrin, J. (2002). Health services research for children with disabilities. *The Milbank Quarterly, 80*(2), 303–324.

Ralabate, P. (2002). *Meeting the challenge: Special education tools that work for all kids*. Washington, DC: National Education Association.

Reiss, J., & Gibson, R. (2002). Health care transition: Destinations unknown. *Pediatrics, 110*(6 Suppl.), 1307–1314.

Reiter, S. (2000). Society and disability: A model of support in special education and rehabilitation. *Focus on Exceptional Children, 32*(8), 1–14.

Robinson, A., Bender, B., & Linden, M. (2001). Klinefelter syndrome. In S. Cassidy & J. Allanson (Eds.), *Management of genetic syndromes* (pp. 195–206). New York: Wiley-Liss.

Roizen, N. (2002). Down syndrome. In M. Batshaw (Ed.), *Children with disabilities* (pp. 307–320). Baltimore: Paul H. Brookes.

Ruccione, K. (2002). Biologic basis of cancer in children and adolescents. In C. Baggott, K. Kelly, D. Fochtman, & G. Foley (Eds.), *Nursing care of children and adolescents with cancer* (pp. 24–63). Philadelphia: W. B. Saunders.

Sandler, A. (1999). Short-changed in the name of socialization? Acquisition of functional skills by students with severe disabilities. *Mental Retardation, 37*(2), 148–150.

Schultz, J. (1994). Inclusion: The debate continues. *Instructor, 104*(4), 55–56.

Selekman, J. (1991). Pediatric rehabilitation: From concepts to practice. *Pediatric Nursing, 17*(1), 11–14.

Spiegel, H., & Bonwit, A. (2002). HIV infection in children. In M. Batshaw (Eds.), *Children with disabilities* (pp. 123–139). Baltimore: Paul H. Brookes.

Strauss, D., & Shavelle, R. (1998). Life expectancy of adults with cerebral palsy. *Developmental Medical Child Neurology, 40*, 369–375.

Students with chronic illnesses: Guidance for families, schools, and students. (2003). *Journal of School Health, 73*(4), 131–132.

Sybert, V. (2001). Turner syndrome. In S. Cassidy & J. Allanson (Eds.), *Management of genetic syndromes* (pp. 459–484). New York: Wiley-Liss.

Turnbull, A., & Turnbull, H. (1990). *Families, professionals, and exceptionality: A special partnership* (2nd ed.). Columbus, OH: Merrill.

Turnbull, H. (1998). *Free appropriate public education: The law and children with disabilities*. Denver, CO: Love Publishing.

Turnbull, H., Turnbull, A., Shank, M., Smith, S., & Leal, D. (2002). *Exceptional lives: Special education in today's schools*. Upper Saddle River, NJ: Pearson Education.

U.S. Department of Education (U.S. DOE), Office of Special Education Programs. (2000). *20th Annual Report ot Congress on the Implementation of the Individuals with Disabilities Education Act*. Author: Washington, DC.

U.S. Department of Education (U.S. DOE), Office of Special Education Programs. (2002). *24th Annual Report to Congress on the Implementation of the Individuals with Disabilities Education Act*. Author: Washington, DC.

U.S. Department of Education (U.S. DOE), Office of Special Education Programs. (2004). *24th Annual Report to Congress on the Implementation of the Individuals with Disabilities Education Act*. Author: Washington, DC.

Westbrook L., Silver, E., & Stein, R. (1998). Implications for estimates of disability in children: A comparison of definitional components. *Pediatrics, 101*(6), 1025–1030.

Westlake, S., & Bertolone, K. (2002). Acute lymphoblastic leukemia. In C. Baggott, K. Kelly, D. Fochtman, & G. Foley (Eds.), *Nursing care of children and adolescents with cancer* (pp. 466–490). Philadelphia: W. B. Saunders.

Wood, M. (1998). Whose job is it anyway? Educational roles in inclusion. *Exceptional Children, 64*(2), 181–195.

Chapter 28

Allergy

JANICE SELEKMAN ▪ CAROL GRAY

Chapter Outline

INTRODUCTION

Allergy is the most common chronic condition of childhood. At least 20% of the pediatric population in the United States, and perhaps up to 40%, has some type of allergy, although the exact number affected is unknown (Wills-Karp & Hershey, 2003). Allergy "refers to an acquired potential to develop immunologically mediated adverse reactions to normally innocuous substances" (American Academy of Allergy, Asthma, & Immunology [AAAAI], 2000a, p. i). To understand how allergy affects students (and staff), knowledge of some immune system basics is essential.

THE IMMUNE SYSTEM AS IT RELATES TO ALLERGY

Functions of the Immune System

The primary role of the immune system is to identify "self" cells and those that are "nonself" (Shearer & Fleisher, 2003). Almost all cells of the body carry a code on their outer shell that identifies them as belonging to either that individual or to an "invader." The "invaders" often take the form of pathogens, but could also be foreign bodies or transplanted organs. Once the body identifies something as "nonself," the role of the immune system is to inactivate the foreign element and eliminate it, hopefully without damage to its own tissues. The destruction and elimination involve multiple cells of the immune system.

The three basic functions of the immune system are (1) *defense* against nonself antigens, (2) *homeostasis* to clean up (phagocytosis) and eliminate dead or injured cells, and (3) *surveillance*—for cells that are nonself, including those that mutate (Table 28.1). The difficulty arises when one of these three systems is either overactive or underactive. If the *surveillance* function is *underactive*, it does not identify cells that have mutated and does not alert the other cells to act, and *cancer* will develop and spread. If the *homeostasis* function is *overactive*, it not only cleans debris of the "war" against the invaders and normal body cells that have aged and died, but also begins to attack good healthy cells; this results in *autoimmune disease*. If the *defense* component is *underactive*, it cannot stimulate the cells to fight invaders, and *immunodeficiency* results, with the possibility of opportunistic infections. Finally, and most important to this chapter, if the *defense* component is *overactive*, it not only fights "nonself" invaders, but also begins to attack items to which the body does not normally react, and this is the basis for *allergy*.

The Immune Cells (White Blood Cells/Leukocytes)

There are three main types of white blood cells: granulocytes (neutrophils, eosinophils, and basophils), monocytes, and lymphocytes (T and B). Neutrophils go by many names. Officially, they are polymorphonuclear leukocytes, or polys; they are in the category of granulocytes and also are called segs (mature neutrophils) and bands (immature neutrophils). Neutrophils are the first cells that arrive at the site of trauma or invasion. They are the most numerous of the white blood cells (approximately 60%) but they are short lived. They attack bacteria and fungi and function by phagocytosis. Once they leave the blood vessel, they stay in the general area of the trauma or invasion (Eales, 2003). Their presence at the site results in some of the symptoms of inflammation. While not usually associated with allergy, they are always present following initiation of the allergic response and are the cause of many of the secondary symptoms of inflammation that are observed, especially edema.

Eosinophils are another type of granulocyte. While they can also engage in phagocytosis, their primary focus is to release toxic granules to destroy parasites. Eosinophils release multiple products that stimulate inflammation, especially in response to mast cell degranulation, and therefore have an increased presence during an allergic attack that involves a histamine reaction. This is referred to as eosinophilic infiltration. They make up only 4% of the white blood cells (Eales, 2003).

Basophils are the third category of granulocytes. Basophils (in the blood) and mast cells (in the tissues) have very similar functions; they are intimately involved in the allergic reaction and their role is described in the next section. Mast cells are found throughout the body, but are more prevalent under the epithelial surface of the skin, in the mucosal linings of the nose and upper airways, and in the conjunctival lining of the eyes and along the

Table 28.1 ■ FUNCTIONS OF THE IMMUNE SYSTEM

FUNCTION	EXAMPLE	ALTERATIONS: HYPO-	ALTERATIONS: HYPER-
Defense	Protection against nonself antigens	Increased susceptibility to repeat infections	Allergy
Homeostasis	Removal of worn out or damaged "self" components	—	Autoimmune disease
Surveillance	Perception and destruction of cell mutants	Malignancy	—

Source: Selekman (1990).

gastrointestinal tract. They lie near blood and lymphatic vessels. All of these sites are prime entry sites for antigens/allergens.

Monocytes are another type of white blood cell that engage in generalized phagocytosis. However, they arrive much later than the neutrophils and stay much longer. Consequently, they are more numerous in chronic inflammatory conditions. Monocytes also have the important role of taking the specific markers (referred to as antigenic markers) of the "nonself" product to the lymphocytes so that antibodies can be made. They also can release a vast array of chemical mediators (called bioactive substances or cytokines) that attract other immune cells to the site of the trauma or invasion. A macrophage is a monocyte that has left the circulation and entered the tissues; it does not circulate back to the blood (Eales, 2003). Macrophages are known by many different names, including Kupffer cells in the liver and histiocytes in connective tissue.

Granulocytes and monocytes respond the same way regardless of the type of organism that has invaded or the type of trauma that has occurred (Eales, 2003). Their response is nonspecific and leads to the same general signs of inflammation. Lymphocytes, however, respond specifically to the individual markers of the offending antigen.

There are two types of lymphocytes: T and B. B lymphocytes are responsible for making antibodies. When the B cell receives the antigenic marker from the monocyte, it travels to the closest lymph node, which then turns into a factory to make antibodies specific to that marker. (That is why lymph nodes are enlarged near the site of infection; it also explains why antibodies against one organism will not protect an individual against a different organism.)

Antibodies fall into five immunoglobulin classes: IgM, IgG, IgA, IgD, and IgE. (These immune components are found in the globulin or plasma protein part of the blood plasma.) Their functions are listed in TABLE 28.2. The one with the most relevance to this chapter is IgE, for it is this class that stimulates the most common allergic reactions. What is special about immunoglobulins is that they have memory. Years, and even decades after their first contact with the antigenic marker, they can remember to make the antibodies against it when stimulated.

While B lymphocytes are responsible for making antibodies, it is the T lymphocytes that control the manufacturing process via products (lymphokines) contained within their cell wall (Eales, 2003). All hematological cells are made in the bone marrow; those that then pass through the thymus are called T cells. CD4 cells (previously called helper

Table 28.2 ■
IMMUNOGLOBULINS

IMMUNOGLOBULIN TYPE	PERCENTAGE OF IG	NORMAL SERUM CONCENTRATION	OTHER
IgM	10	60–170 mg/dl	Largest Ig; makes first antibodies to antigen; activates complement; contains antibodies for ABO groups
IgG	70–75	700–1,500 mg/dl	Smallest Ig; only one to cross placenta to provide immunity to fetus; activates complement; primary antibodies
IgA	15–20	150–400 mg/dl	In all body secretions, especially respiratory and GI tract; prevents virus from entering through mucous membrane; matures during school-age years.
IgD	>1.0	3 mg/dl	Unclear role
IgE	.002–.004	.01–.03 mg%	Primarily seen in allergy; binds to mast cells and causes release of histamine; attacks parasites

T cells) are the "on" switch that tell the B cells to make more antibodies; CD8 cells (previously called suppressor and cytotoxic cells) are the "off" switch and indicate that the production can stop. Normally, there are twice as many CD4 cells as there are CD8 cells. (The virus that causes acquired immunodeficiency syndrome [AIDS] attacks the CD4 cells, resulting in more CD8 cells than CD4 cells and a system that is suppressed, or turned off.)

The different T cells release various substances (lymphokines) that have different roles in regulating the immune process. T cell subsets called Th1 and Th2 have a role in allergy. Individuals with more Th1 do not appear to develop allergic symptoms, whereas the presence of more Th2 "sets into motion a complex series of events leading to IgE production, the development, recruitment, and activation of effector cells such as mast cells, basophils, eosinophils and effector T cells and a variety of downstream effector cascades" (Wills-Karp & Hershey, 2003, p. 1442).

All of the cells identified in this section are included in a white blood count and differential. This information will assist the healthcare provider to identify the cells involved in the immune insult and give beginning clues about what is going on in a patient.

Tolerance

Tolerance has multiple meanings. It refers to the body's acceptance (immunologically) of itself. The body does not usually mount an immune response to its own body parts. However, most humans are also nonresponsive (immunologically) to common environmental components, such as pollen, wool, animal dander, and foodstuffs. This nonreactivity to nonself products is also referred to as tolerance (Eales, 2003). The development of tolerance or resistance to a substance, especially after increased exposure, is the goal of immunotherapy (allergy shots). One hypothesis is that allergy shots "induce T cells capable of turning off IgE responses to allergens that likely represent a switch from Th2 to Th1 allergen-specific T cells" (Shearer & Fleisher, 2003, p. 11). In the medical field, tolerance also refers to a situation in which someone had responded to a particular drug or dose of a drug in the past and now does not, for example, a bacterium developed a tolerance for penicillin.

CLASSIFICATION OF ALLERGIC REACTIONS

Allergy is an overreaction of the defense role of the immune system resulting in a hypersensitivity to nonself components of the environment on reexposure (Shearer & Fleisher, 2003). Nonself molecules that result in an allergic reaction are referred to as *allergens*. Allergies are described in multiple ways, including the type of white blood cell involved, the timing of the allergic reaction, the organ system involved, and the route or source of the allergen.

Allergic Reactions by Immunological Reaction

A classification system for allergic reactions was initially developed by Gell and Coombs in the 1950s (Eales, 2003) and has since been modified. Type I hypersensitivity, also known as IgE-mediated immediate reaction, is the type typically associated with allergy. It involves IgE and is the type seen in allergic rhinitis (hay fever), atopic dermatitis, bronchial asthma, food allergy, and anaphylaxis.

In an IgE allergic reaction, the allergen enters the body either by contact, ingestion, inhalation, or injection. The macrophages take the allergenic markers from the wall of the allergen and present them to the B cell and a helper T cell. The B cell then makes the IgE antibodies. All immunoglobulins are in the shape of the letter "Y." The tail of the "Y" for IgE is perfectly suited to fit into receptor sites on basophils or mast cells. All of this happens the first time the individual is exposed to the antigen, yet the symptoms of an allergic reaction are not commonly seen until the second exposure. The arms of the "Y" are shaped to fit the specific allergenic markers. When the IgE antibodies that are connected to the basophils or mast cells have contact with the allergenic markers on their subsequent reentry into the body, a reaction occurs that results in the release of products from basophils and mast cells. These include histamine, heparin, and other substances that result in the symptoms seen in an allergic reaction and its inflammatory sequelae (Eales, 2003; Wills-Karp & Hershey, 2003). The role of histamine is to dilate and increase the permeability of the blood vessels so that immune cells can exit the vessel and enter the area of tissue damage with resulting edema, erythema of the skin, and respiratory symptoms. This reaction can occur in the GI tract as well; as a result, the individual may then experience cramps, bloating, diarrhea and vomiting (AAAAI, 2000a).

In addition to increasing vessel permeability, histamine also causes constriction of bronchiolar and vascular smooth muscle (resulting in wheezing), as well as increased nasal and bronchial secretions (AAAAI, 2000a). When the substances are released in excess, anaphylaxis occurs. In anaphylaxis, the individual will experience the above respiratory distress as well as other signs of generalized vascular permeability. The bronchoconstriction may result in dyspnea and cyanosis with the possibility of complete airway occlusion. Individuals may complain of "itching all over" and feeling hot and flushed, and experience hypotension with vascular collapse. As the blood pressure falls, the pulse rate will increase and the individual may lose consciousness as they go into anaphylactic shock. "Up to 20% of students who will have an anaphylactic reaction have their first one in school" (AAAAI, 2002, p. 8).

The typical symptoms commonly seen in a type I reaction are due to the histamine. Histamine is irritating and causes sneezing and an "itchy" sensation in the ears and in the back of the throat. Those afflicted try all types of vocalizations, coughing, and pulling on the ears to decrease this sensation. As the permeability increases because of the histamine, fluid and substances are released from the vessels into the tissue, resulting in edema and erythema of tissues. (See a more complete description of the signs and symptoms in the sections on allergic rhinitis.) Structural changes occur in response to repeated exposure to allergens of already inflamed tissue. Examples include thickening of smooth muscle, fibrosis of tissue, and mucous cell hyperplasia (Wills-Karp & Hershey, 2003).

Other typical responses to a type I reaction include urticaria and angioedema which occur as a result of the vascular permeability. Urticaria is more commonly known as hives. It is an "intensely itchy rash that consists of raised, irregularly shaped wheals. The wheals have a blanched center, surrounded by a big red flare" (Scruggs & Johnson, 2004, p. 78). A flare is a red halo of dilated vessels around the wheal. Angioedema, on the other hand, is defined as "an area of circumscribed swelling of any part of the body. It may be caused by the same mechanisms that cause hives except that the immunologic events occur deeper in the cutis or in the submucosal tissue of the respiratory or gastrointestinal tract" (Scruggs & Johnson, p. 78). Because the edema of angioedema occurs at a deeper level, "the skin may appear normal, and the patient usually complains of pain or burning rather than itching. Angioedema most often involves the face, tongue, extremities, or genitalia whereas urticaria can occur virtually anywhere on the body" (AAAAI, 2000a, p. xiii).

Type II hypersensitivity, also known as a cytotoxic reaction, involves IgG and IgM antibody production against cell-surface receptors or receptor sites; they activate complement that results in cell lysis. (Complement is a component of the immune system that is initiated after there is contact between antigen and antibody. Specific proteins connect to the tail of the antibody and then connect to each other and then with the antigen, ultimately causing the antigen to be destroyed.) The autoimmune conditions that result from this cytotoxicity include hemolytic anemia, thrombocytopenic purpura, Graves' disease (antibodies are made against the thyroid), and myasthenia gravis (antibodies are made against acetylcholine receptors) (Wills-Karp & Hershey, 2003).

Type III hypersensitivity is known as immune complex–mediated reaction because IgG and IgM antibodies attack body tissues such as heart valves (rheumatic fever), the glomerulus of the kidney (acute glomerulonephritis and nephrotic syndrome), or connective tissue (systemic lupus erythematosus or rheumatoid arthritis) and stimulate the action of complement, which results in tissue damage. Another example is type 1 diabetes mellitus, in which beta cells of the pancreas are attacked. Since hypersensitivity types II and III are generally considered autoimmune conditions, they are not covered further in this chapter.

Type IV hypersensitivity, also known as delayed hypersensitivity, is due to sensitized T cell activity and the lymphokines they release and is not due to immunoglobulins. Examples include contact dermatitis (as with poison ivy) or the reaction to tuberculosis or the purified protein derivative (PPD) (Eales, 2003). Graft-versus-host disease is also an example of delayed response.

Timing of the Allergic Reaction

In addition to the four types of allergic reaction described in the preceding section, allergies are described as immediate or delayed. A type I hypersensitivity reaction begins "within seconds of exposure to the antigen. The early phase of the response (occurring up to 30 minutes post-allergen challenge) is manifest by local edema, smooth muscle contraction, vasodilation and increased permeability of post-capillary venules" (Eales, 2003, p. 161). These symptoms are due to the IgE-mast cell contact with the allergen and the release of histamine and the other substances. A secondary inflammatory response, or later phase response, occurs 4 to 12 hours later and can last for up to 2 days as a result of the influx of other white blood cells and the inflammation that results (Wills-Karp & Hershey, 2003). However, type I is still referred to as "immediate."

Type IV hypersensitivity is referred to as delayed type hypersensitivity. Because T cells respond later than sensitized IgE, reactions may not be seen for 24 hours or longer (Eales, 2003).

Organ Systems Involved

The three main organ systems involved in type I and type IV allergic responses are respiratory, gastrointestinal, and dermatologic. Examples of each are given at the end of this chapter.

Sources of Allergen

Allergens refer to any substance that initiates the allergic response; they can include **inhalants** (pollen, dust [mites], mold spores, animal dander [including rodents], cockroach droppings, and latex particles), **injectable substances** (insect and bee stings and some medications), **ingestants** (foods and some medications), and **contactants** (plants, chemicals/cosmetics, topical drugs, metals, latex, and animal dander). Animal dander can be spread by direct contact with an animal or exposure to the dander of an animal, such as on someone else's clothes. It can also be spread by the airborne route. The severity of the reaction is directly proportional to the dose of the allergen. When people are allergic to animals, the allergen may not be the fur, but rather a protein within the pet's saliva and dander (the sloughed epithelial skin cells). When cats groom themselves, they deposit saliva onto their fur and skin. The dander is shed onto carpets or clothing or becomes airborne when the animal rubs against furniture or brushes against someone. Dander is also a food supply for dust mites.

Pollens are fine powdery grains of plant sperm that vary widely based on the locale and the season. In some parts of the country, "allergy season" can be predicted based on when trees, grasses, and weeds pollinate. Airborne concentration of pollens depends on the weather. Levels tend to be highest at midday during warm, slightly windy conditions (Sicherer & Eggleston, 2000) and when grass is being mowed.

Molds can be either from indoor or outdoor sources. Indoor sources include damp areas, such as basements and shower areas; outdoor sources may include wooded areas, compost, and mulch. Some mold spores are more prevalent with rain and high humidity while others present a higher risk of exposure in dry windy weather (AAAAI, 2000a). Dust mites can be found in carpeting, stuffed toys, mattresses, pillows, and upholstered furniture. Routine dusting and vacuuming "have little effect on reducing dust mites" (AAAAI, p. 17). Other rarer causes of allergic reactions may include rapid changes in the ambient temperature and the sun.

Allergic reactions to medications account for 5% to 10% of all adverse drug reactions (Ditto, 2002). Dermatologic reactions represent the most common form of allergic drug reactions. Anaphylaxis is the classic clinical picture of an IgE-mediated drug reaction, which requires the presence of IgE antibodies specific to the drug allergen. However, all types of allergic reactions are seen in response to various medications.

The Seasonal Nature of Allergy

In most cases, individuals who have allergies are aware of when during the year their symptoms are worse. The symptoms may last 1 to 2 months at a time. It is important for school nurses to understand the particular pattern of pollination of their geographical region. Tree pollens are more common during January to June, depending on the region of the United States, grass pollens are present from March to October, depending on the region, and ragweed is seen from July to November, although it persists until the first frost (FIGURE 28.1). The weather station that serves the school district will be able to indicate which days have high pollen counts.

Dust allergies occur year round, referred to as perennial, but are more prevalent during the fall and winter when heating systems are turned on, windows are closed, and students are spending more time indoors.

ETIOLOGY

There is a genetic predisposition to allergies. If both parents have allergies, their offspring have a 66% to 75% chance of developing an allergy; if only one parent has allergies, there is a 50% chance that their offspring will develop allergies (AAAAI, 2000a; Eales, 2003). The term "atopy" "refers to the genetic tendency to develop the "classical" allergic diseases, namely, allergic rhinitis, asthma, and atopic dermatitis" (AAAAI, 2000a, p. vi). In addition to the genetic cause, the timing of the introduction of foods can result in food allergies. The gut is immature for the first few months of life and if certain proteins are given too early, they may be absorbed through a permeable bowel leading to the initiation of the allergic response. Also, because IgA does not reach its adult level of protection of mucous membranes until the school-age years, children are at a greater risk of developing respiratory allergies, especially following high levels of allergen exposure in the environment.

Other suspected risk factors include early use of antibiotics, early introduction of foods in infancy, and even the excessive cleanliness of the environment. Exhaust smoke and passive smoke exposure are not causes of allergy, but they can "enhance allergic sensitization" (AAAAI, 2000a, p. 18).

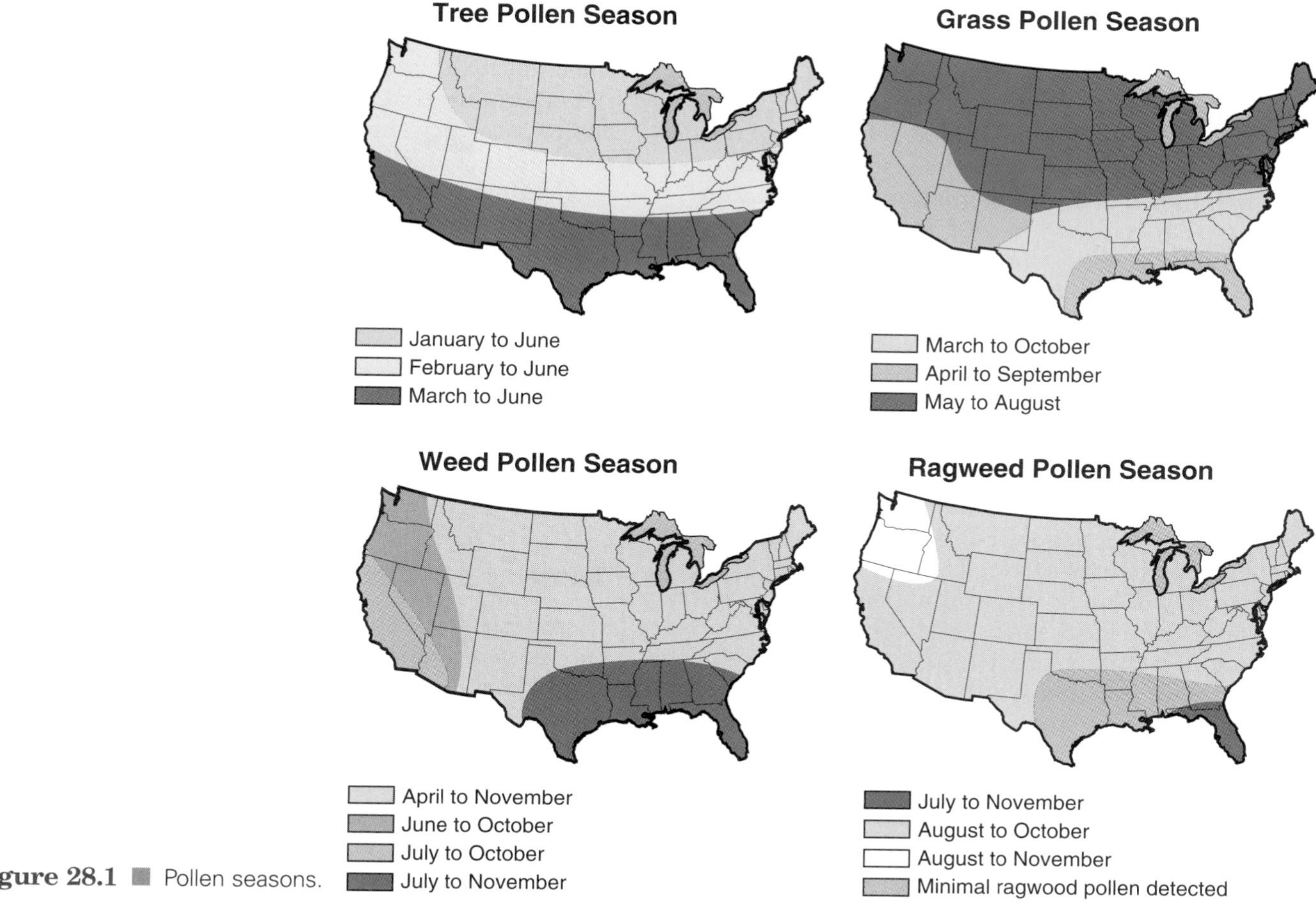

Figure 28.1 ■ Pollen seasons.

INCIDENCE

Allergy affects from 20% to 40% of children in the United States each year, most of which occurs as allergic rhinitis and asthma (AAAAI, 2000a). Atopic dermatitis affects between 10% and 15% of the pediatric population; half of these occur in the first year of life and another 30% occur before the age of 5 years (AAAAI). Of interest, half of the infants and young children with atopic dermatitis will later develop asthma. In addition, 35% of those with atopic dermatitis also have a food allergy (AAAAI). Approximately 2 million children and adolescents have food allergies (Munoz-Furlong, 2003).

The mean age at onset of seasonal allergic rhinitis is 10.6 years of age, whereas it is 9.1 years for perennial rhinitis (Berger, 2002). While some types of allergy decrease during the early years, such as eczema, and may even disappear during childhood, respiratory allergies increase with age and reach a peak between ages 12 and 15 (Berger, 2002).

DIAGNOSIS OF ALLERGIES

Diagnostic testing for allergic disease differentiates the allergic disorder from other diseases, uncovers previously unsuspected allergens, and guides treatment. The two testing modalities are in vivo via skin testing and in vitro blood studies. "The most common allergy tests in the United States are prick/puncture tests, which detect IgE antibodies" (AAAAI, 2000a, p. ix). The results should correlate with the patient's history and can generally be performed on patients of any age.

Skin testing usually involves skin pricks or punctures using a very small needle that passes through an allergen extract and scratches or punctures the skin. These tests are usually performed on the forearms or back. At times, a second step to skin testing is needed; this intradermal method injects allergen extract intradermally, creating a small bleb, similar to giving a PPD. Intradermal tests are usually performed on the upper outer arms. Positive tests react as a wheal with erythema and itch like a mosquito bite, usually within 20 minutes (Ownby, 2000).

The most common aeroallergens that can be tested using skin testing include trees, grasses, weeds, and molds. The individual selections of these aeroallergens are specific to the area of the country in which they are more commonly found. Skin testing can also be done to test for allergies to dust mites, cockroaches, stinging insects, and animals, such as cats, dogs, horses, hamsters, guinea pigs, and mice. Skin testing for food allergies focuses on a large variety of vegetables, seafood, fruits, eggs, milk, wheat, soybean, nuts, and meats. Skin testing is also done to identify allergies to specific medications, such as penicillin, which is the most common allergic drug reaction (AAAAI, 2000b).

Young children may have a numbing topical cream (i.e., EMLA) applied prior to skin testing to decrease the pain associated with the needle pricks. Itching may occur at the sites of positive skin tests. Low-dose hydrocortisone cream may be ordered after skin testing to reduce the local itching; oral antihistamines will also reduce the local itching and resolve the wheal and erythema from the positive reactions more quickly.

If a student has had skin testing for allergies in the morning and returns to school, the school nurse may notice areas on the arms and back with markings in pen where positive reactions occurred. Should the student complain of itching at the site, the school nurse might apply cool compresses or ice until the parents can be contacted to identify if steroid creams were ordered. An antihistamine will reduce the local reactions and itching, if available for p.r.n. use. A nonsedating antihistamine is usually chosen to prevent drowsiness in school.

In vitro testing involves allergen-specific immunoassays to detect IgE antibodies in the serum of patients who respond clinically to those allergens. The interpretation requires correlating the patient's history with environmental exposures and the results of in vivo testing. In vitro testing requires a venous blood sample and is more expensive and time consuming than skin testing, but may be preferable for patients who have dermagraphism, ichthyosis, or generalized edema, take tricyclic antidepressants, are at undue risk if their medications (i.e., antihistamines and beta blockers) are discontinued, or have a clinical history suggesting a higher risk of anaphylaxis with skin testing to a specific allergen (Ownby, 2000).

Two in vitro tests are ImmunoCAP (clinical assay Pharmacia) and RAST (radioimmunoassay); they measure IgE against specific allergens. These tests are reported as class scores 0 to 6. Class 0 represents undetectable IgE in the patient's blood. The higher the class score, the higher the quantity of IgE to the specific antigen (Ownby, 2000). The choice of selection for in vitro testing is available by calling the laboratory that will be performing the tests. The choices are very similar to those on the skin testing list identified earlier. The panel of specific allergens used differs based on the area of the country in which the test is given; therefore, a student tested in Vermont who then moves to Virginia may not have been tested for the allergen specific to Virginia. While the school nurse will not be in a position to interpret the test results, she may be asked by parents or the student to explain how the testing works and what the results might mean.

UPPER RESPIRATORY ALLERGIES

Anatomy and Physiology

Disorders of the nose and nasal function are among the most common causes of medical disability, with an estimated 17% of the population suffering with allergic rhinitis and 10% with vasomotor (nonallergic) rhinitis during the course of each year (Kaliner, 2001).

The normal functions of the nose are to purify the inhaled air by trapping and eliminating particles by mucociliary action. Mucus lines the nose and contains proteins, such as lysozymes, that kill bacteria, and IgA antibodies, which kill both viruses and bacteria. The normal color of mucus is clear or light yellow, but it may become a darker yellow with a cold. With a bacterial infection, the color reflects the presence of many neutrophils as well as bacteria and may become green or dark gray. Normal mucus is odorless, but if bacteria are present, may have a rank smell (Kaliner, 2001). The nose also humidifies and warms the inhaled air, provides the sense of smell, and contributes to the sense of taste (FIGURE 28.2).

The paranasal sinuses are four paired cavities in the skull superior, medial, and inferior to the orbits. The maxillary sinuses are below the eyes in the cheeks, the ethmoid sinuses are between the eyes, the frontal sinuses are above the eyes, and the sphenoid sinuses are posteromedial to the eyes. Each sinus contains between 10 ml and 60 ml of air. The roof of the maxillary sinus is the floor of the eye while the floor of the maxillary sinus is the roof of the mouth.

The maxillary and ethmoid sinuses are present at birth, but the frontal sinuses develop during the first year of life, and the sphenoid sinus develops during the first several years of life. Sinuses are well developed by age 7 to 8 and reach their adult size and shape at puberty (Eccles, 2003).

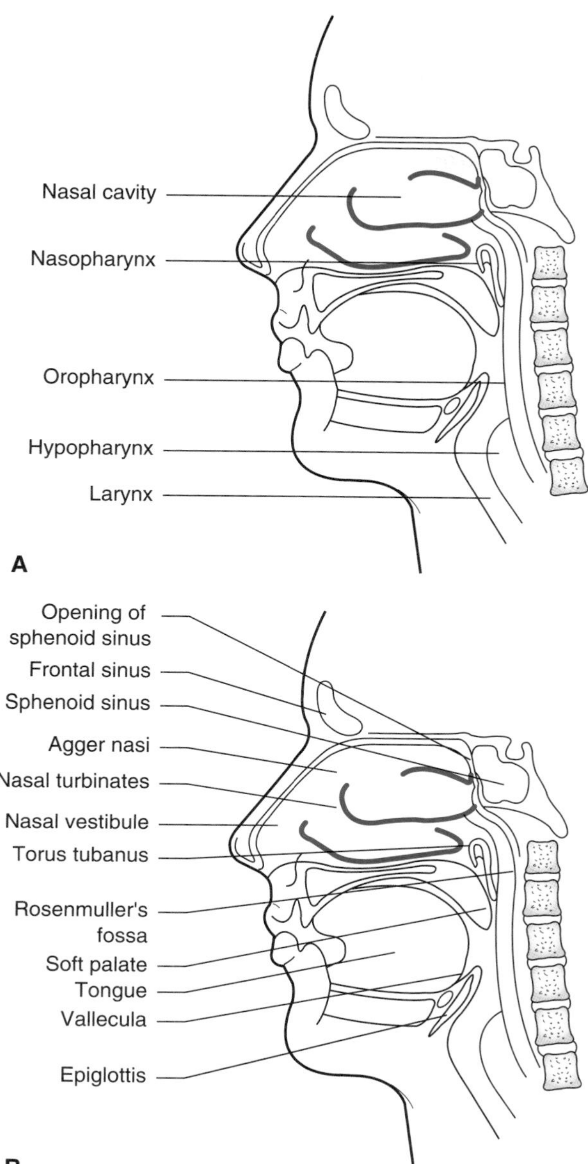

Figure 28.2 ■ Schematic of the upper airway with designation of anatomical structures.

The physiological function of the sinuses are not clear. The sinuses communicate with the nose through small openings known as ostia, located in narrow, convoluted channels. The sinuses are ventilated with each breath, they lighten the weight of the skull and provide resonance to the voice, as well as produce some of the mucus that constantly clears the nose of trapped particulate materials, preventing it from being inhaled into the lungs. Mucus is cleared against the force of gravity by the action of cilia (Chandra, Conley, & Kern, 2002), which constantly move mucus along the walls of the sinus to and through the ostia and then toward the back of the nose. Approximately two quarts of mucus are made every day by the nose and sinuses, most of which is swallowed (Kaliner, 2002) (FIGURE 28.3).

Drainage from the maxillary sinus is facilitated when a person is in a recumbent position; this explains why some individuals experience postnasal drip and coughing when they lie down. The posterior ethmoid air cells and the sphenoid sinuses drain further back in the nose, and the drainage from these sinuses goes down the throat. Thus, the posterior sinuses are more likely to produce postnasal drip, while the more anterior sinuses may cause rhinorrhea (Kaliner, 2001).

Allergic Rhinitis

Perhaps the most common chronic condition that afflicts children and adolescents is allergic rhinitis (inaccurately called hay fever, as hay is not the problem and there is no fever). It is possible that one or two in every five students has this type of allergy (Blaiss, 2002; Wills-Karp & Hershey, 2003). Allergic rhinitis affects more than 6 million children, who are absent from approximately 2 million school days each year (Berger, 2002). The average allergic patient is symptomatic for 5 months of the year.

Rhinitis is a universally experienced symptom of an upper respiratory infection, the "common cold," chronic rhinosinusitis with complications, or allergy. When allergy is the cause, early phase response triggers are allergens, such as pollens, dander, mites, molds, and cockroaches (Kaliner, 2002); however, allergic nasal symptoms can also be triggered by

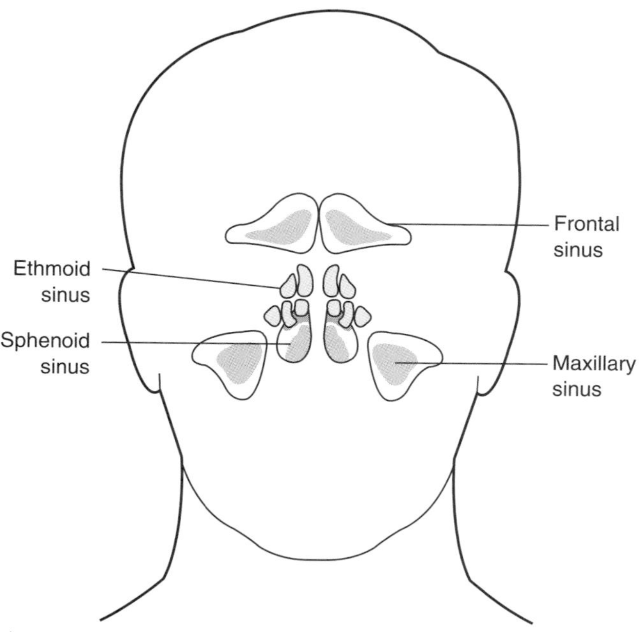

Figure 28.3 ■ Sinuses.

irritants such as tobacco smoke, air pollutants, perfumes, ammonia, changes in temperature relative to humidity or barometric pressure, exercise, emotions (particularly depression), foods (such as spicy hot food, beer, and wine), and spraying of pesticides in the school, especially if they have an odor. The major sources of the airborne allergens are wind-pollinated trees, grasses, and weeds.

Allergic rhinitis usually develops by the time a student exits elementary school and peaks during mid- to late adolescence. "Because immunoglobulin E (IgE) levels are highest during puberty, symptoms are often the most severe during that time" (Economides & Kaliner, 2002, p. 35).

Signs and Symptoms of Allergic Rhinitis

As noted earlier, numerous immunological processes are active in the eyes, ears, nose, throat, and respiratory system. All of these mucous membranes have an abundance of mast cells and are prime sites for a type I allergic reaction. Histamine is irritating when it is released into the tissues. The irritation causes repeated sneezing and persistent "itching" in the back of the throat, the ears, and eyes. Watery eyes and clear watery rhinorrhea, postnasal drip, and a gelatinous conjunctival discharge are common symptoms for the student with an *allergic rhinitis*.

As histamine is released, the vessels at the sites dilate and their permeability increases. This results in congestion in the nose; the nasal turbinates are pale blue and boggy, which is a classic sign of allergic rhinitis (Wolf, 2000). In an attempt to relieve the itching and congestion, the student will often rub his or her nose, pushing it up with the heel of a hand. This is often referred to as the "allergic salute." Persistence of this behavior will result in a transverse crease above the tip and below the bridge of the nose (see FIGURE 28.4).

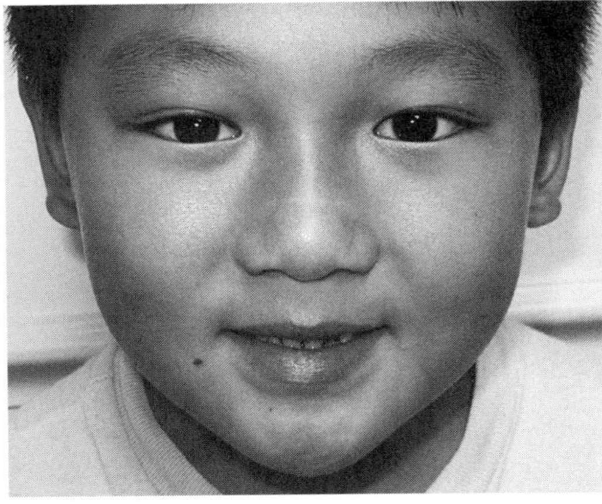

Figure 28.4 ■ Nasal crease caused by continual upward rubbing of the nose to relieve itching.

The congestion leads to mouth breathing, which results in altered smell and taste and a dry mouth, which, if persistent, can increase the chances of getting a respiratory infection. Mouth breathing can also lead to facial abnormalities, such as retrognathic maxilla and mandible, increased facial length, high arched palate, and dental malocclusions (Berger, 2002). (It is helpful to resolve the nasal congestion prior to removing any orthodontia in order to maintain correct teeth alignment.) If severe, nasal obstruction can cause sleep apnea with resultant daytime somnolence and decreased attentiveness.

Another indication of congestion is "allergic shiners" (see Figure 28.4), which is "a darkening of the infraorbital skin resulting from venous dilation and indicative of chronic nasal congestion" (AAAAI, 2000b, p. 9). Headaches, sinus pressure, and snoring are other symptoms noted. Adolescents report feeling embarrassed by their symptoms and may demonstrate increased irritability, impatience, and anger (Economides & Kaliner, 2002).

Conjunctivitis may be manifested along with the other symptoms of respiratory allergies, or it may be the only indication. The predominant symptom of allergic conjunctivitis is itching, which is intensified by rubbing the eye. Usually, allergic conjunctivitis is bilateral, but it may be unilateral when manual contamination occurs, such as with foods or animal dander. The conjunctiva may be injected, edematous, and, if severe, swollen shut. Ocular signs are minimal despite the significant symptoms. Symptoms are less severe if allergic conjunctivitis has become chronic (Lieberman & Blaiss, 2002).

Rhinosinusitis (inflammation of the paranasal sinuses) may be seen concurrent with or as a result of allergic rhinitis. Rhinosinusitis, rather than sinusitis, is the more appropriate term, because sinus inflammation is often preceded by rhinitis (Chandra et al., 2002). The symptoms include increased mucus production, blocked nasal passages, and poor drainage of the mucus normally produced by the sinuses and middle ear. Viruses and bacteria flourish in the trapped mucus, resulting in sinusitis and ear infections. However, 98% of sinus infections are viral and do not need to be treated with antibiotics.

Symptoms of acute rhinosinusitis are persistent "cold" symptoms, without fever; symptoms usually last beyond 7 to 10 days. Students usually present with cough and nasal discharge, whereas adults have discolored nasal discharge, facial pain, headache, and cough. Long-standing inflammation is accompanied by chronic nasal congestion, thick post-nasal drip, sore throat, facial fullness, and sometimes hearing problems (Corren & Rachelefsky, 2000). TABLE 28.3 compares allergic rhinitis with allergic rhinosinusitis.

Table 28.3 ■
COMPARISON OF SYMPTOMS OF ALLERGIC RHINITIS AND RHINOSINUSITIS

	CONGESTION	SNEEZING	ITCHING	COUGH	FEVER	POST-NASAL DRIP	CLEAR MUCUS	PURULENT MUCOUS	HEADACHE
Allergic rhinitis	****	***	***	*	—	* or **	****	—	*
Rhino sinusitis	****	*	—	***	**	****	—	****	***

Number of asterisks indicates the degree of symptomatology.

When a student comes to the health office frequently with undiagnosed allergic symptoms, it is the responsibility of the school nurse to identify a pattern of the symptoms; it may be that symptoms occur in a particular classroom (such as one with rugs or pets), when the student is engaged in a particular activity (such as lunch or outdoor physical education), during a particular season, or when the student is with particular people (who may have pets or use perfumes). Identification of a family history of atopic disease helps support the diagnosis.

Differential Diagnosis

The "common cold" is often difficult to distinguish from allergic rhinitis and rhinosinusitis. The cold is a viral infection of the upper respiratory tract, which causes inflammation of the mucosa of the nose down to the bronchi. The symptoms usually last 7 to 10 days. Symptoms include sneezing, coughing, nasal obstruction or congestion, rhinorrhea, malaise, low-grade to no fever, and watery or inflamed conjunctiva. On nasal exam, it is noted that the nasal mucosa is erythematous and inflamed rather than pale to bluish as with allergic rhinitis (Uphold & Graham, 1998).

It is always possible for a foreign body to be present in a child's nose. A key differentiating symptom would be unilateral nasal discharge which could be purulent and malodorous versus bilateral symptoms with rhinosinusitis (Uphold & Graham, 1998).

Environmental Interventions

Management of allergic rhinitis includes environmental control and avoidance, use of medication, and, if needed, immunotherapy. Environmental control needs to address the common allergens, unless specific allergens have been identified that are amenable to environmental control. Allergists provide families with these suggestions, but many can be implemented in the school environment (TABLE 28.4).

Airborne concentration of pollens depends on the weather. Levels tend to be highest at midday during warm, slightly windy conditions (Sicherer & Eggleston, 2000). Avoiding peak pollen exposure times of the day helps limit the exposure. Students with allergies who spend a great deal of time outside during times of high pollen counts should be encouraged to wash their hair before going to bed in order to reduce contact with the pollen that has landed on their hair.

Molds can be found both indoors and outdoors. The only control one has for mold exposure is with the indoor molds. Outdoor exposure, however, is highest in wooded areas, hay, and when cutting grass as this "kicks up" the mold growing under the cut grass from previous cuttings. Wearing a mask over the nose and mouth would be helpful when outdoors, or in a barn. Mold likes to hide indoors, usually in warm, dark, and damp places, so one has to "seek and find." Basements and crawl spaces are ideal places for mold growth. Dehumidifiers need to be used in these areas. Black growth on shower curtains or around windowsills in bathrooms is evidence of mold growth. Household plants can also be a common substrate for mold growth. Live Christmas trees should be avoided, as mold lives on the live bark of trees and in the water in the tree holder.

Dust mites are microscopic skin-eating creatures. They feed off the skin scales that humans shed daily. Dust mites like dark, warm, and moist places. To avoid inhaling the dust mites, it would be prudent to remove carpeting; this is the most effective way to eliminate the dust mite exposure from this source. If this cannot occur, treat the carpets with mite-killing agents and then vacuum the car-

Table 28.4 ■

ALLERGEN AVOIDANCE AND CONTROL MEASURES FOR THE HOME AND SCHOOL

Dust Mites

Remove carpeting from floors.
Damp dust often when the student is not in the immediate area.
No curtains or blinds; window shades are preferable.
No stuffed chairs (unless they can be wiped down)
Decrease clutter; remove non-washable dust collectors from classrooms, i.e., stuffed animals; use plastic, metal, and wood toys that can be wiped down.
Replace feather pillows and comforters or encase in allergy proof duvet; encase mattress and pillow in allergy proof covers; no wool blankets (cotton or synthetic only).
Wash bed sheets weekly on the hot cycle ~130 degrees.
Keep indoor humidity less than 50%.

Pollens and Outdoor Molds

Avoid being outdoors when grass is being cut and close classroom windows.
Stay indoors with the windows closed.
Use air conditioning with regular changing of filters to reduce indoor exposure to outdoor pollen.
Reduce outdoor exposure during times of high pollen counts in season.
Shower after outdoor activity to remove pollen from self.
Do not hang clothes on a clothes line.
Wipe the fur of outdoor animals before they come indoors to remove the pollen.
Avoid outdoor gym class when the pollen or mold count is high.

Indoor Mold

Clean visible mold growth in bathrooms, showers, locker rooms, concrete, or cement block walls (especially in basements) and damp wood surfaces with bleach-based agents.
Keep showers and locker room cleaned daily and well ventilated with the appropriate-sized ventilation exhaust system.
Repair indoor leaks and seepage (besides mold, cockroaches like humid moist areas).
Reduce humidity in the school building below 50% to avoid excess humidity.
In some areas with high relative humidity, the use of dehumidifiers may be necessary.
Remove carpets in the classroom if able as these are a good source of mold.
Classroom walls should have washable paint.

Animals

Remove pets from home if able or keep outdoors.
Keep furry pets out of classroom (turtles and fish are OK).
Assure that rooms are swept daily and garbage is removed to prevent food from attracting cockroaches.
Use a HEPA filter (Studies on the effects of air cleaners on clinical symptoms have been inconclusive) (Zoratti, 2000).
Keep cat allergen low by bathing cats twice a week.

Irritants that may *not* be beneficial to students

Live flowers in the classroom
Sprays, paints, cleaners, insecticides used while students are in the area
Smoking allowed in the school environment or at entry ways
Perfumes or other strong smells

casses and excrement. Also, vacuum the carpet once a week utilizing a HEPA (high-efficiency particulate arrester) filter, which is very efficient in removing both dust and animal dander. A study by Almqvist and colleagues (1999) demonstrated that the level of cat allergen is high in a classroom where many students are cat owners; cat dander is present on the clothing of students who are cat owners. This could result in significant exposure and contamination of the clothing of students who do not own cats.

Medical Management—Pharmacotherapy

The goals of pharmacotherapy in allergic diseases are to relieve symptoms, prevent progression of the disease, prevent morbidity and mortality, and minimize the potential for adverse effects of the medication. Since cure of the disease is probably not achievable, the goal in the use of medication is to minimize the impact of the disease on the student's life. The most common medications given for allergy include antihistamines, decongestants, intranasal steroids, leukotriene receptor agonists, and nonsteroidal nasal sprays. These may be administered systemically or locally.

Antihistamines

The mainstay for treatment in allergic reactions is the antihistamine. These are histamine receptor agonists and compete for the histamine receptor sites. Histamine causes vasodilation of the vascular system, an increase in heart rate and contractility, and contraction of the smooth muscle of the lungs (Bernstein, 2002). Antihistamines provide relief of itchy nose and eyes, rhinorrhea, sneezing, urticarial reactions, and pruritis. They are not very helpful for nasal congestion and edema.

Antihistamines are H1 and H2 blockers. H1 receptors are involved in allergy by mediating the increased vascular permeability; they block histamine-induced hypotension and bronchoconstriction. In addition to their antiallergic properties, H1 blockers are used for varying degrees of sedation, as antiemetics, for motion sickness, and as antitussives. H2 blockers inhibit food-induced, gastrin-induced, and acetylcholine-induced gastric secretion of acid induced by histamine (Bernstein, 2002). H2 blockers are used in the management of peptic ulcer or reflux disease (i.e., cimetidine, ranitidine, nizatidine); they are also used in the management of immediate hypersensitivity reactions to block cardiac and vascular H2 responses to histamine and to prevent anaphylactic shock (Simons, 2002).

Antihistamines are prescribed for allergic rhinitis, allergic conjunctivitis, urticaria, allergic food reaction, insect anaphylaxis, latex allergy, and angioedema. Common examples of antihistamines are in TABLE 28.5. Their main action is to reduce

(text continues on page 661)

Table 28.5 ■
FORMULATIONS AND DOSAGES OF REPRESENTATIVE H_1 ANTIHISTAMINES

GENERIC (BRAND) NAME	FORMULATION	RECOMMENDED DOSE
First-Generation H_1 Antihistamines		
Chlorpheniramine (Chlor-Trimeton)	Tablets 4 mg, 8mg,* 12mg* Syrup 2.5 mg/5 ml Parenteral solution 10 mg/ml	Adult: 8–12 mg bid* Pediatric†: 0.35 mg/kg/24 hr
Diphenhydramine (Benadryl)	Capsules 25 or 50 mg Elixir 12.5 mg/5 ml Syrup 6.25 mg/5 ml Parenteral solution 50 mg/ml	Adult: 25–50 mg tid Pediatric: 5 mg/kg/24 hr
Doxepin (Zonalon)	Capsules 10–75 mg	Adult: 25–50 mg tid or od (hs)
Hydroxyzine (Atarax)	Capsules 10 mg, 25 mg, 50 mg Syrup 10 mg/5 ml	Adult: 25–50 mg tid or od (hs) Pediatric: 2 mg/kg/24 hr

(continued)

Table 28.5 ■ *(Continued)*

GENERIC (BRAND) NAME	FORMULATION	RECOMMENDED DOSE
Second-Generation Oral H_1 Antihistamines		
Acrivastine (Semprex)	Tablets 8 mg	Adult: 8 mg tid
Cetirzine (Reactine, Zyrtee)	Tablets 10 mg Syrup 5 mg/5ml	Adult: 5–10 mg od Pediatric (6–11 yr): 5–10 mg od; 6 mo-5 yr: 5 mg od
Desloratadine (Aerius, Clarinex)	Tablets 5 mg	Adult and pediatric ≥ 12 yr: 5 mg od
Ebastine (Ebastel)‡	Tablets 10 mg	Adult: 10–20 mg od Pediatric (6–12 yr): 5 mg od Pediatirc (2–5 yr): 2.5 mg od
Fexofenadine (Allegra, Telfast)	Tablets 60 mg, 120 mg, 180 mg	Adult and pediatric ≥ 12 yr: 60 mg bid or 120 or 180 mg od
Levocetirizine (Xyzal, Xusal)‡	Tablets 5 mg	Adult and pediatric ≥ 6 yr: 5 mg od
Loratadine (Claritin)	Tablets 10 mg Rapidly disntegrating tablets (Reditabs) 10 mg Syrup 5 mg/5 ml	Adult: 10 mg od Pediatric: (6–10 yr): 10 mg od Pediatric (2–9 yr): 5 mg od
Mizolastine (Mizollen)‡	Tablets 10 mg	Adult: 10 mg od
Topical H_1 Antihistamines		
Azelastine (Astelin)	Nasal solution 0.1% (0.137 μg/spray)†	Adult and pediatric ≥ 12 yr: 2 sprays/nostril bid
Ketotifen (Zaditor)	0.025% Ophthalmic solution†	Adult and pediatric ≥ age 3 yr: 1 drop in each eye bid
Levocabastine (Livostin)	Intranasal microsuspension 50 μg/spray Ophthalmic suspension 0.05% (0.5 mg/ml)	Adult nasal: 2 sprays per nostril bid-qid Ophthalmic: 1 drop in each eye bid-qid
Olopatadine (Patanol)	0.1% Ophthalmic solution	Adult and pediatric ≥ 3 yr: 1 drop in each eye bid (6–8 hr apart)

od, Once daily; *bid,* twice daily; *tid,* three times daily: *qid,* four times daily; *hs,* at bedtime; *mo,* months.
* Timed-release.
† For individuals weighing ≤ 40 kg.
‡ Not approved in the United States at time of publication.
§ Azelastine and ketotifen are also available as oral formulations in some countries: azelastine tablets 2 mg (dose 2–4 mg b.i.d.); ketotifen tablets 1 mg or 2 mg (dose, adult and pediatric ≥ 3 yr: 1 mg bid or 2 mg od).
Source: Simons (2002, p. 849). Reprinted with permission.

itching and sneezing, rhinorrhea, and hives. Side effects of antihistamines include CNS depression and sedation (more so in first-generation antihistamines) (Bernstein, 2002). Other clinical problems associated with antihistamines include dryness of the mouth, blurred vision, urinary retention, and constipation. School nurses should know that paradoxical excitation can occur in children taking antihistamines.

"Second generation antihistamines have been well documented to cause less impairment of cognitive and psychomotor skills, such as learning, reaction times, driving, memory, tracking, perception, recognition, and processing" (Bernstein, 2002, p. 74). School nurses should advise high school students who drive to avoid first-generation antihistamines. Children undergoing evaluations for school learning issues should be assessed as to whether they are using first-generation antihistamines. The Joint Task Force on Practice Parameters for the diagnosis and management of rhinitis recommended that "second-generation, non-sedating antihistamines should be first-line treatment of perennial and seasonal allergic rhinitis to avoid potential CNS side effects" (Bernstein, 2002, p. 74). If side effects or tolerance occurs, switching to another antihistamine may be beneficial. Nonsedating antihistamines allow for continued daily activities and are preferred.

Topical H1 antihistamine ophthalmics relieve itchy eyes that accompany allergic conjunctivitis. Antihistamines are sometimes combined with vasoconstrictors, for example, Vasocon C and Naphcon A. Vasoconstrictors make the eye look better than it really is. Avoid contamination of the medication bottles. Astelin Nasal Spray (azelastine) is the only antihistamine with decongestant and anti-inflammatory properties. There are also mast cell stabilizers without antihistamine action, such as cromolyn sodium (Intal/Nasalcrom) and nedocromil (Tilade).

Students who are pregnant or who are breast feeding should make sure their primary care provider is aware of their condition. Certain antihistamines may be safe for use during pregnancy, for example, Loratadine (Claritin) and cetirizine (Zyrtec), which have shown no evidence of producing birth defects in animals. Tripelennamine (Pyribenzamine), chlorpheniramine (Chlor-Trimeton), and diphenhydramine (Benadryl) cause no greater risk of birth defects than in the normal population, but place the pregnant student at risk due to sedation. All antihistamines are excreted in the breast milk. Mothers who are taking first-generation antihistamines and breast-feed may have infants who experience drowsiness and irritability (Bernstein, 2002).

Nasal Topical Inhaled Corticosteroids

Inhaled and intranasal corticosteroids are extremely effective in their anti-inflammatory role in the allergic airway (Lipworth & Jackson, 2000); they reduce mucosal inflammation by reducing fluid movement from the vascular space into tissues by decreasing inflammatory cell recruitment. They also minimize nasal irritant receptor sensitivity and reduce inflammatory cell activation (Ledford, 2000). They may decrease the mast cell histamine pool, possibly via inhibition of the intracellular synthesis of histamine. These actions decrease vascular permeability, decrease recruitment of secondary inflammatory cells, and decrease mucus production.

The nasal corticosteroids are most effective if instituted 5 to 7 days prior to the onset of the allergy season. Table 28.6 lists nasal topical inhaled corticosteroids. Side effects include drying of the nasal passages, epistaxis, and septal perforation. To reduce complaints of dry nasal passages, use saline nose drops or KY Jelly on a Q-tip and gently roll it inside the nostril openings twice a day. This also helps reduce epistaxis. To reduce or prevent epistaxis and septal perforation, direct the spray away from the septum and completely insert the snout of the nasal spray into the nostrils. Using the right hand to spray the left nostril and the left hand to spray the right nostril helps facilitate the correct direction of the spray.

Concerns about the safety of long-term inhaled corticosteroid use have been allayed by multiple studies that have demonstrated minimal absorption of the steroid into the systemic circulation. Studies have also supported that the inhaled steroids have no effect on the physical growth of children (Lipworth & Jackson, 2000). If the allergic reaction is severe enough, oral corticosteroids may be needed.

Nonsteroidal Nasal Sprays

Cromolyn sodium is a mast cell stabilizer; it binds to the mast cell receptors and prevents the release of histamine. It blocks both immediate and delayed allergic reactions. Therefore, it is best when it is given *before* the allergen binds to the mast cell. In this way, it manages the previously identified symptoms of allergic rhinitis; it is more effective as a preventative rather than as a treatment for occurring symptoms (Kemp, 2000). It also needs to be used four times a day compared to once daily dosing with the above-mentioned nasal sprays. Another nonsteroidal spray is Ipratropium (Atrovent) Nasal Spray; it is an anticholinergic and relieves rhinorrhea. Appropriate for any school environment is the use of saline nasal washes. The saline can be pre-

Table 28.6 ■
TOPICAL CORTICOSTEROIDS USED TO TREAT ALLERGIC RHINITIS

DRUG	DELIVERY	AGE	DOSE
Beclomethasone			
Beconase (Glaxo Wellcome, Research Triangle Park, NC)	42 μg fluorocarbon aerosol	6–12 years 12 years	1 spray/nostril tid 1 spray/nostril bid-qd
Beconose AQ (Glaxo Wellcome, Research Triangle Park, NC)	42 μg liquid spray	6 years	1 or 2 sprays/nostril bid
Vancenase (Schering, Kenilworth, NJ)	42 μg fluorocarbon aerosol	6–12 years	1 spray/nostril tid
	Pockethaler	12 years	1 spray/nostril bid–qd or 2 sprays/nostril bid
Vancenase AQ (Schering, Kenilworth, NJ)	84 μg liquid spray	6 years	2 sprays/nostril qd
Budesonide			
Rhinocort (Astra, Westborough, MA)	32 μg fluorocarbon aerosol	6 years	2 sprays/nostril bid or 4 sprays/nostril qd
Flunisolide			
Nasarel (Dura Pharmaceuticals, San Diego, CA)	25 μg aqueous aerosol	6 years	1 spray/nostril tid or 2 sprays/nostril bid
Fluticasone propionate			
Flonase (Glaxo Wellcome, Research Triangle Park, NC)	50 μg aqueous spray	12 years	2 sprays/nostril qd or 1 spray/nostril bid; maintenance: 1 spray/nostril qd
Triamcinolone acetonide			
Nasacort (Aventis Pharmaceuticals, Parsippany, NJ)	55 μg fluorocarbon aerosol	>6 years	2 sprays/nostril qd-bid or 1 spray/nostril qid; maintenance: 1 spray/nostril qd
Nasacort AQ (Aventis Pharmaceuticals, Parsippany, NJ)	55 μg aqueous spray	>12 years	2 sprays/nostril qd; 1 spray/nostril qd
Mometasone furoate monohydrate			
Nasonex (Schering, Kenilworth, NJ)	50 μg aqueous spray	12 years 3–11 years	2 sprays/nostril qd; 1 spray/nostril qd

bid, twice daily; qd, daily; tid, three times daily
Source: Kaliner (2002, p. 85). Reprinted with permission.

pared by the school nurse using the directions in Box 28.1.

Oral and Topical Decongestants

Decongestants stimulate alpha-adrenergic receptors resulting in blood vessel constriction and reduced blood flow to the nasal mucosa. Therefore, decongestants reduce nasal congestion that is interfering with nasal airflow. Side effects may include insomnia, irritability, dry mouth, impairment of bladder emptying, and jitteriness. Lowering the dosage helps control these symptoms most of the time. Of note, topical application to the nose or eye can cause rebound congestion if used for a prolonged period. This is often referred to as being "addicted to the nasal spray" and is usually treated with oral

Box 28.1 ■■■

NASAL-SINUS CARE USING SALINE

IMPORTANCE

Patients with chronic rhinitis have swelling and inflammation of the nasal membranes and increased mucus production. This inflammation causes blocked nasal passages and poor drainage of the mucus normally produced by the sinuses and middle ear. Viruses and bacteria flourish in the trapped mucus, resulting in sinusitis and ear infections. The drainage of excess mucus from the nose and sinuses can trigger chest symptoms in asthmatic patients as well. To help prevent these events from occurring, it is extremely important to keep the nose free of excess mucus. The goal of nasal-sinus irrigation is to keep the nasal passages open, wash out excess mucus, allergens, and germs, and promote the natural healing process of the nasal membranes.

SALINE

Saline (salt water solution) is used for nasal-sinus irrigations. Sterile saline may be purchased in liter bottles from a pharmacy or it can be made at home or at school. To make saline, add 1/2 teaspoon of table salt to 8 oz. of warm water and stir until the mixture is dissolved. If desired, a pinch of baking soda can be added to buffer the saline.

IRRIGATION METHOD FOR OLDER CHILDREN AND ADOLESCENTS

Method 1 (the simplest method): Pour some saline solution into the palm of your hand and "snuff" up each nostril, one at a time. Then spit the fluid out of your mouth and blow your nose *lightly* afterward. This is best done with the head down, bent far over the sink.

Method 2 (a more effective method): Purchase a large all-rubber syringe (the blue baby syringe at the drugstore). Fill the syringe completely. Insert the syringe tip just inside one nostril and pinch the nostril around the tip to keep the solution from running out of the nose. Gently squeeze the bulb and release several times to swish the solution around in the nose. Then squeeze the bulb hard enough to make the saline solution go up and over the palate in the roof of the mouth. Allow the fluid to run out of the mouth. Repeat for the other nostril. While doing this, sniff air through the open nostril to assist the movement of the liquid. Directing the stream toward the eye is the most effective way to flush the large sinuses under the eyes.

IRRIGATION METHOD FOR YOUNGER CHILDREN

Use a dropper and put 10 to 20 drops of saline in each nostril. If necessary, use a bulb syringe to suction the mucus out of each nostril. For older children (those who can blow their nose with coaching), use a clean, empty squeeze bottle, such as a nasal spray bottle. Fill the bottle with saline and gently squeeze the solution into each nostril, one at a time. Have the child blow his nose after each squeeze.

Clean equipment using hot tap water after each use. Draw hot water into the bulb syringe, swish and empty completely. Always stand bulb tip-down after rinsing (e.g., in a clean glass) to allow the syringe to drain completely. At least once daily, fill bulb with a fresh solution of mild detergent and hot water, swish, and empty completely. Rinse well with tap water; then draw a 70% solution of isopropyl alcohol into the syringe (seven parts rubbing alcohol and three parts tap water). Swish and then empty completely. Stand bulb tip-down to drain.

steroids and topical nasal corticosteroids (Settipane & Settipane, 2002). Because there may be a relationship between decongestants and elevated blood pressure, it is recommended that the decongestant be stopped if an increase in blood pressure is noted.

Examples include pseudophedrine hydrochloride, Neo-synephrine, phenylpropanolamine hydrochloride, phenylephrine hydrochloride, and Afrin Nasal Spray. Pseudophedrine is found in many over-the-counter products. These should not be used in pregnancy because of the potential to reduce blood flow to the uterus owing to its vasoconstrictive properties (Greenberger, 2002). Astelin, an antihistamine, has decongestant properties without the side effects of other decongestants.

Leukotriene Receptor Antagonists

Since cysteinyl leukotrienes induce nasal congestion in allergic rhinitis, leukotriene receptor antagonists may block the effects of leukotrienes on congestion; thus, this is another approach to congestion in addition to using decongestants. However, the drug does not significantly improve the three other characteristic symptoms of allergic rhinitis (sneezing, rhinorrhea, and nasal itching). An example is montelukast (Singulair). Side effects include headache and stomach pains, which are relieved by discontinuing the medication. While these drugs are primarily used in the management of asthma, be careful not to label all students on a leukotriene antagonist as children with asthma.

Other Agents

In addition to the medications noted previously, it is also possible for a student to be on a tricyclic antidepressant for his or her allergic symptoms. Tricyclic antidepressants were originally developed as an antihistamine. Doxepin has a high H1 receptor affinity and can be used for management of chronic urticaria (Bernstein, 2002).

Medical Management—Immunotherapy

Allergen immunotherapy, also referred to as "allergy shots" or "hyposensitization," is a series of allergen-vaccine injections over a defined period, which results in decreased sensitivity or tolerance to inhaled or injected allergens; this change in response can be measured both clinically and immunologically (Fox & Lockey, 2000). This therapy is used for the management of allergic rhinitis, stinging insect hypersensitivity (discussed later in this chapter), and allergic asthma (Chapter 29). It works by inducing an IgG response against the allergen so that the IgG will attach to it before the fixed IgE can, thus preventing or decreasing the release of histamine. It also down-regulates Th2 lymphocytes and moderates the allergic reaction by a variety of mechanisms.

Immunotherapy is only about 80% effective, but should be considered for individuals who fail to respond to environmental control or to pharmacotherapy. Those who have difficulty or are inconvenienced in using the medications or need them year round would be good candidates for immunotherapy (Fox & Lockey, 2000). It is most effective against the allergens that result in allergic rhinitis and for reactions to insect stings. Immunotherapy is not effective for intrinsic causes of asthma, atopic dermatitis, and food allergies or urticaria.

The most frequent side effect is local reaction at the site of injection, but the size of the local reaction does not predict the likelihood of a systemic reaction. Most systemic reactions occur within 20 minutes after an injection. Therefore students need to be monitored during this time. While most school nurses do not administer immunotherapy, some do. However, sometimes students return to classes without waiting in the physician's office and therefore react at school. Risk factors for systemic reactions include symptomatic asthma, highly sensitive patients, starting a new vaccine vial, dosing errors, injections during the pollen season, and use of beta-blockers.

If giving immunotherapy, one must have emergency medication readily available; this includes injectable epinephrine and diphenhydramine. The school nurse must know the appropriate dosage for the student. For local reactions, relief can be obtained with ice application and oral antihistamines (Grammer, 2002). Serum should be kept upright in the refrigerator to prevent leakage and contamination. The vial should be rotated gently in the hands rather than shaken and a TB syringe used. The aim of the dosing regimen is to increase the dose according to a set schedule in order to prime the body to "tolerate" the allergen. Therefore, students must have regular contact with their allergist in order to have the serum and dosage changed. Records need to be kept of the dose given, the date, the site used, and any reaction that occurred.

Treatment for Anaphylaxis

Anaphylaxis is an emergency and usually involves more than one body system. Symptoms may start as itchy skin or hives and progress to swelling of the lips and tongue and signs of respiratory distress. Anxiousness may be noted and the dyspnea may result in a loss of consciousness. Death can occur within minutes, so immediate treatment is necessary. Fatalities "are associated with the absence or delayed use of epinephrine" (National Association of Student Nurses [NASN], 2001).

Epinephrine (adrenaline) is the single most important agent for treating anaphylactic reactions. It counters the effects of histamine by constricting blood vessels and relaxing smooth muscles of the respiratory tract.

Schools frequently receive standing orders to keep this drug on hand in case of emergency. It comes in a prefilled auto-injector syringe in two doses and is given right through the clothing. EpiPen contains 0.3 mg; EpiPen Jr. contains .15 mg. (The adult dose is 0.2 ml to 0.5 ml of a 1:1,000 dilution intramuscularly or subcutaneously; for children, the dose is 0.01 mg/kg body weight up to a maximum of 0.03 mg/kg, or 0.03 ml/kg of 1:1,000 by syringe [Simons, 2002]). *The effects of an epinephrine dose disappear in 20 minutes; therefore doses may be repeated every 15 minutes for up to three doses.* Intramuscular administration is preferred over subcutaneous injection and should be given in the lateral thigh for best absorption.

When storing epinephrine, keep at room temperature. Do not expose it to direct sunlight or a very hot environment. The solution should be clear and colorless; make sure to check the expiration date.

The side effects of epinephrine may include increased heart rate and nausea. Children on betablockers, usually for migraine management or hypertension, are at higher risk of anaphylaxis because of the danger of epinephrine resistance. This may be countered with glucagon (available in a prefilled syringe kit). Of note, delayed, biphasic, or prolonged anaphylaxis occurs in more than 20% of cases. Therefore, extended observation in the emergency room is required in all cases (AAAAI, 2000a). Late reoccurrence of anaphylaxis can be prevented by prednisolone administered within 1 hour of the reaction. Directions on how to use the EpiPen are provided in Figure 28.7.

Other medications that may be used during a significant reaction may include antihistamines and steroids.

Rhinosinusitis

Because the etiology of the symptoms is inflammation and mucus production, whether viral or bacterial, the best treatment strategy is to utilize saline nasal lavages three times a day, and decongestants (oral or nasal topical) for 3 to 4 days only. If purulent colored mucus is persistent beyond 7 to 10 days, an antibiotic should be considered.

Allergic Conjunctivitis

The allergic diseases of the eye include contact dermatoconjunctivitis, acute allergic conjunctivitis, and vernal conjunctivitis. When the causative agent has contact with the conjunctiva and the eyelid, a dermatoconjunctivitis occurs (Bielory, 2000). Vesiculation may occur early, but by the time a student seeks care, the presenting appearance is thickened and chronically inflamed reddened lids. If the conjunctiva is involved, there is tearing and erythema. Pruritis is the cardinal symptom and a burning sensation may also be present. Rubbing the eye intensifies the itch.

Treating allergic conjunctivitis is the same as with allergic rhinitis as it includes avoidance, medications for symptomatic relief, and immunotherapy. Six classes of topical agents are available for medication management of allergic eye diseases. They are vasoconstrictors, "classic" antihistamines, "classic" mast cell stabilizers, new agents with multiple "antiallergic" activities, nonsteroidal anti-inflammatory agents, and corticosteroids (Bielory, 2000).

FOOD ALLERGY

Before a discussion of food allergy can begin, it is essential to differentiate a food allergy from food intolerance. Food intolerance is NOT an allergy and does not initiate an IgE or other immune response. Food intolerance is an adverse reaction to a specific food or an ingredient due to an inability of the body to handle that substance. Decreased intestinal enzymes to denatured food proteins, altered acid levels or gastric flora, or the status of the mucosal barriers may all make it difficult to digest and metabolize specific foodstuffs. These may result in the same gastrointestinal discomfort as seen with allergy, but no immune process is occurring. Examples include lactase deficiency and reactions to caffeine or monosodium glutamate.

Food allergies occur in 6% to 8% of children. The most common foodstuffs that result in an allergic reaction are the proteins in cow's milk, eggs, peanuts, soybeans, wheat, fish, and tree nuts (such as pecans, cashews, and walnuts) (Astwood, Bannon, Dobert, & Fuchs, 2003). Milk, eggs, and peanuts account for 80% of pediatric allergies to food. While food allergies to milk, eggs, soy, and wheat tend to resolve in most children by the time they are in school, allergies to peanuts, fish, and tree nuts may persist for life (Astwood et al., 2003). Cross-reactivity can occur in foods that have similar antigenic markers, such as different crustaceans or mollusks, or fish or different nuts. In the "pollen-fruit cross-reactivity syndrome," pitted fruits cross-react with birch pollen or melons and bananas cross-react with ragweed (Bock & Sampson, 2003). Therefore, a child who has an allergy to one product but has never eaten a particular food may have an allergic reaction to it on first contact (see FIGURE 28.5).

The most common type of food allergy is a type I IgE-mediated reaction (Astwood et al., 2003). It can result in gastrointestinal symptoms of nausea, vomiting, diarrhea, or abdominal cramps as the allergic reaction and the resulting inflammation occur in the gastrointestinal tract or an intense local reaction can occur on the lips on contact with food. This may start with itching of the lips and tongue, followed by edema. It is possible to develop a dermatitis on physical contact with the food allergen but not have gastrointestinal symptoms following ingestion of the food. However, it is also possible to have the food allergy to ingested foods present as a skin allergy (with urticaria, angioedema, or atopic dermatitis) or as allergic rhinitis and asthma. As with any IgE reaction, food allergy can also result in anaphylaxis and death (Bock & Sampson, 2003) and is the leading cause of anaphylactic reactions outside of the hospital (Sampson, 2003).

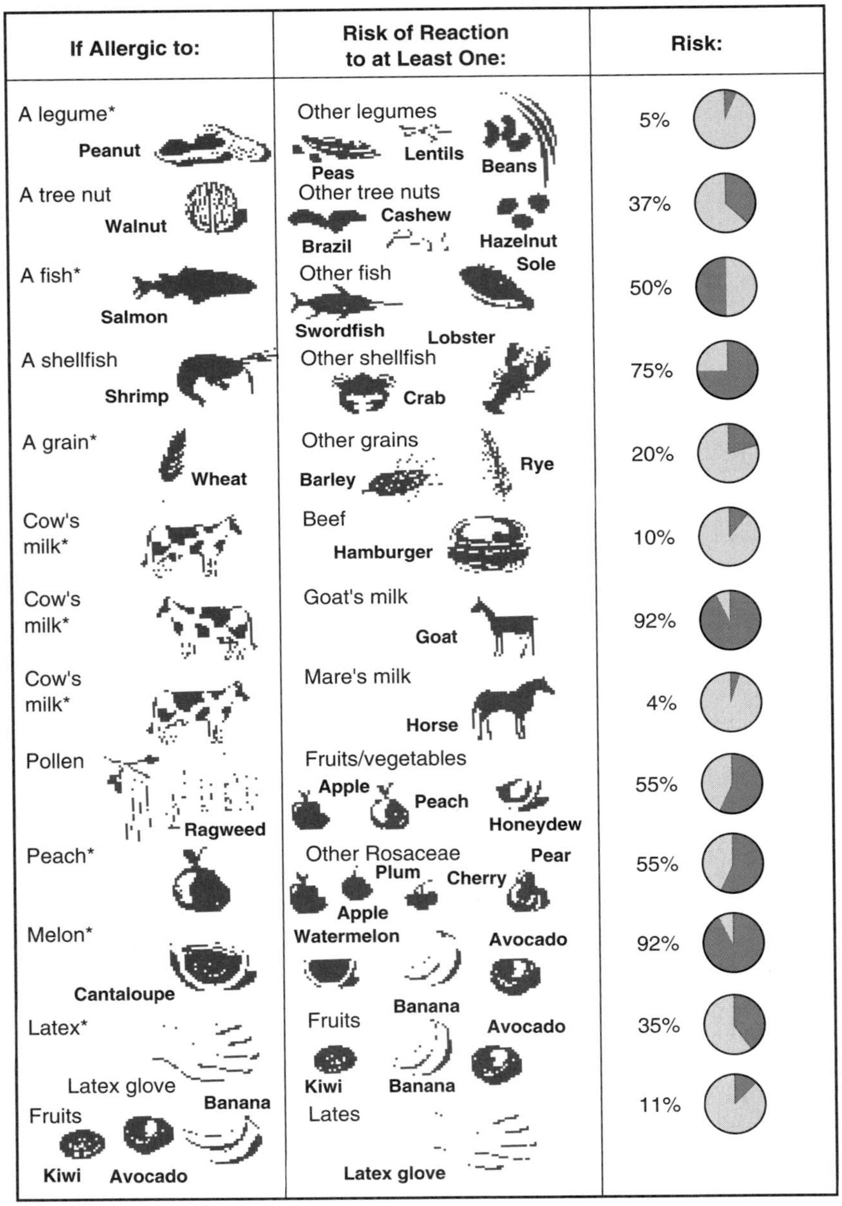

If Allergic to:	Risk of Reaction to at Least One:	Risk:
A legume* Peanut	Other legumes Lentils Peas Beans	5%
A tree nut Walnut	Other tree nuts Cashew Brazil Hazelnut	37%
A fish* Salmon	Other fish Sole Swordfish	50%
A shellfish Shrimp	Other shellfish Lobster Crab	75%
A grain* Wheat	Other grains Barley Rye	20%
Cow's milk*	Beef Hamburger	10%
Cow's milk*	Goat's milk Goat	92%
Cow's milk*	Mare's milk Horse	4%
Pollen Ragweed	Fruits/vegetables Apple Peach Honeydew	55%
Peach*	Other Rosaceae Pear Plum Cherry Apple	55%
Melon* Cantaloupe	Watermelon Avocado Banana	92%
Latex* Latex glove	Fruits Avocado Kiwi Banana	35%
Fruits Banana Kiwi Avocado	Lates Latex glove	11%

Figure 28.5 ■ Approximate rate of clinical reactivity to at least one other related food.

While some symptoms will be seen immediately on contact with the food, other symptoms may not be seen for hours postingestion (Wills-Karp & Hershey, 2003). It is important for the school nurse to know the usual pattern for a student, including how the symptoms usually present and in what time frame. There are even reports of anaphylaxis occurring as a result of the fumes released by cooking certain foods, such as fish or peanuts.

Diagnosis

In addition to the foods that can be tested by in vitro or skin testing, an elimination diet may be used as a method to observe reactions to certain food groups. This process usually takes 1 to 2 weeks and involves removing selected foods and then adding a food every 3 to 4 days to observe for a reaction. The school nurse may be asked to participate in this process by observing for symptoms and notifying the parent should any be observed.

Interventions

The only effective management of food allergies is avoidance of the food. Both the parents and those who work in food preparation must read labels carefully. The school nurse should check on the preparation of food to make sure that utensils and table surfaces are properly cleaned so that the allergen is not transferred unknowingly. It is also essential to prevent food trading by children, an event that occurs frequently during the day. Policies should be in place in the school regarding "no trading" of food as well as what foods can be brought into the school for celebrations.

The school nurse needs to educate faculty and staff so that all are vigilant. Celebrations should involve nonfood items, such as books, stickers, or trinkets. Those who monitor art and science projects need to be aware of the products used. Most reactions in schools from peanuts or tree nuts have been caused by food used in class projects (Munoz-Furlong, 2003). In addition, children with specific food allergies who receive free meals at school must receive allergen-free foods at no additional cost to the families. Communication among all participants, including parents, is essential.

NASN endorses the School Guidelines for Managing Students with Food Allergies (FIGURE 28.6) as well as the development of a Food Action Allergy Plan (FIGURE 28.7). Resources for the school nurse related to food allergies are the FAAN School Food Allergy program, which is a multimedia program for school staff, and "Be A PAL: Protect A Life From Food Allergies" program (Munoz-Furlong, 2003).

ATOPIC DERMATITIS

Allergic reactions that involve the skin can be grouped into contact dermatitis and atopic dermatitis, the latter of which is often synonymous with eczema. Atopic dermatitis is defined as "a chronic or recurrent atopic inflammatory skin disease that usually begins in the first few years of life" (AAAAI, 2000a, p. xi). This form of allergy is seen in approximately 10% of all children and is often the first indication of an allergic predisposition, with 80% of those afflicted having symptoms before the age of 5 (AAAAI, 2000a). For most young children, atopic dermatitis begins to subside and allergic rhinitis or asthma may develop in its place (Nicol, 2003). There is a significant correlation between food hypersensitivity and atopic dermatitis, especially in young children (Wills-Karp & Hershey, 2003).

Atopic dermatitis can be caused by either a type I or a type IV hypersensitivity reaction. It can be caused by inhaled allergens, food allergens, or contactants. In some cases, it can occur following rapid changes in the ambient temperature and, more rarely, after exposure to the sun during certain seasons.

IgE-mediated atopic dermatitis usually begins "as erythematous papular eruptions that evolve over time into scaly, lichenified dermatitis" (Hanifen, 2003). For contact dermatitis, the rash occurs in the area of contact. Regardless of the cause, inflammation and pruritus are present. Metals containing nickel are associated with a higher rate of contact dermatitis, especially inexpensive rings and necklaces. It may become evident after new body piercings.

In some instances, the etiology of the offending agent is readily apparent as it is used for the first time or just changed, such as make-up (eyebrow pencil or brush-on products, eye shadow, eye liner, mascara, artificial lashes, and lash extenders). Ask about new brushes and pads for make-up application. The reaction may cause the eye to look as though it has conjunctivitis. Face soaps and creams can also produce the same results. The substances in these agents that cause these reactions are usually the coloring agents, lanolin, paraben, sorbitol, paraffin, petrolatum, and other vehicles and perfumes. Cosmetic formulations are frequently altered and therefore a cosmetic that did not cause a problem before can at any time become a sensitizing agent (Bielory, 2000).

The intermittent scratching can occur at any time during the day, but it is usually worse in the evening and can disrupt sleep. The danger in the scratching is the potential to develop secondary bacterial, fungal, and viral infections in areas of skin excoriation.

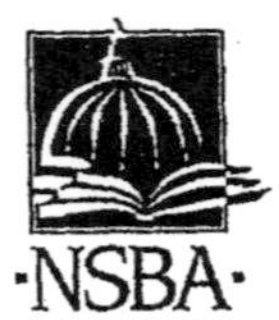

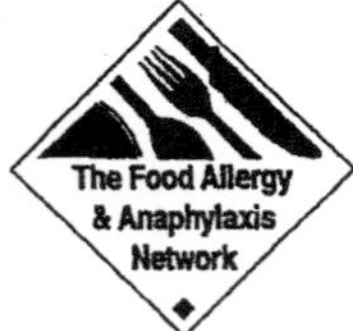

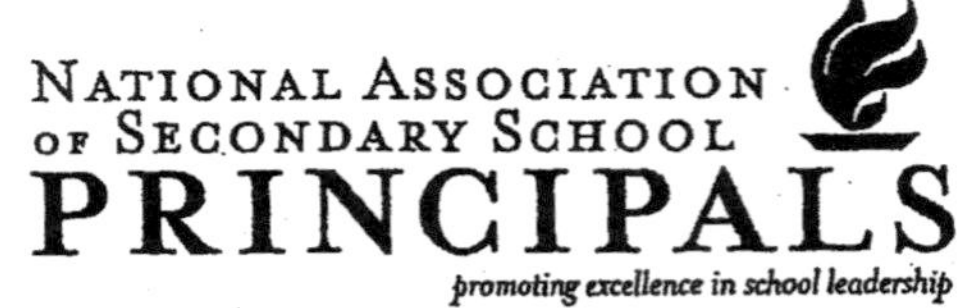

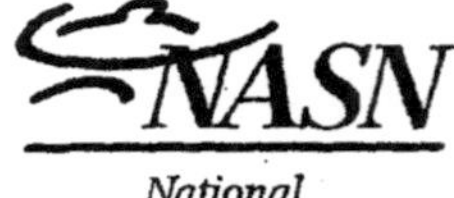

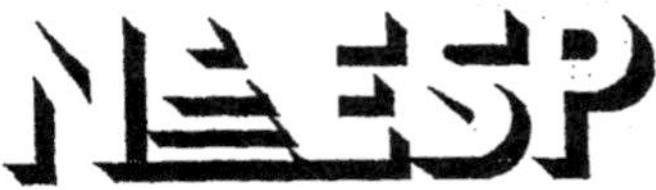

SCHOOL GUIDELINES FOR MANAGING STUDENTS WITH FOOD ALLERGIES

Food allergies can be life-threatening. The risk of accidental exposure to foods can be reduced in the school setting if schools work with students, parents, and physicians to minimize risks and provide a safe educational environment for food-allergic students.

Family's Responsibility

- Notify the school of the child's allergies.
- Work with the school team to develop a plan that accommodates the child's needs throughout the school including in the classroom, in the cafeteria, in after-care programs, during school-sponsored activities, and on the school bus, as well as a Food Allergy Action Plan.
- Provide written medical documentation, instructions, and medications as directed by a physician, using the Food Allergy Action Plan as a guide. Include a photo of the child on written form.
- Replace medications after use or upon expiration.
- Educate the child in the self-management of their food allergy including:
  - ☐ safe and unsafe foods
  - ☐ strategies for avoiding exposure to unsafe foods
  - ☐ symptoms of allergic reactions
  - ☐ how and when to tell an adult they may be having an allergy-related problem
  - ☐ how to read food labels (age appropriate)
- Review policies/procedures with the school staff, the child's physician, and the child (if age appropriate) after a reaction has occurred.

School's Responsibility

- Be knowledgeable about and follow applicable federal laws including ADA, IDEA, Section 504, and FERPA and any state laws or district policies that apply.
- Review the health records submitted by parents and physicians.
- Include food-allergic students in school activities. Students should not be excluded from school activities solely based on their food allergy.
- Identify a core team of, but not limited to, school nurse, teacher, principal, school food service and nutrition manager/director, and counselor (if available) to work with parents and the student (age appropriate) to establish a prevention plan. Changes to the prevention plan to promote food allergy management should be made with core team participation.
- Protect students from offending allergens.
- Assure that all staff who interact with the student on a regular basis understands food allergy, can recognize symptoms, knows what to do in an emergency, and works with other school staff to eliminate the use of food allergens in the allergic student's meals, educational tools, arts and crafts projects, or incentives.
- Practice the Food Allergy Action Plans before an allergic reaction occurs to assure the efficiency/effectiveness of the plans.
- Coordinate with the school nurse to be sure medications are appropriately stored, and be sure that an emergency kit is available that contains a physician's standing order for epinephrine. Keep the medications easily accessible in a secure location central to designated school personnel.
- Designate school personnel who are properly trained to administer medications in accordance with the State Nursing and Good Samaritan Laws governing the administration of emergency medications.
- Be prepared to handle a reaction and ensure that there is a staff member available who is properly trained to administer medications during the school day regardless of time or location.
- Review policies/prevention plan with the core team members, parents/guardians, student (age appropriate), and physician after a reaction has occurred.
- Work with the district transportation administrator to assure that school bus driver training includes symptom awareness and what to do if a reaction occurs.
- Recommend that all buses have communication devices in case of an emergency.
- Enforce a "no eating" policy on school buses with exceptions made only to accommodate special needs under federal or similar laws, or school district policy. Discuss appropriate management of food allergy with family.
- Discuss field trips with the family of the food-allergic child to decide appropriate strategies for managing the food allergy.
- Follow federal/state/district laws and regulations regarding sharing medical information about the student.
- Take threats or harassment against an allergic child seriously.

Student's Responsibility

- Should not trade food with others.
- Should not eat anything with unknown ingredients or known to contain any allergen.
- Should be proactive in the care and management of their food allergies and reactions based on their developmental level.
- Should notify an adult immediately if they eat something they believe may contain the food to which they are allergic.

More detailed suggestions for implementing these objectives and creating a specific plan for each individual student in order to address his or her particular needs are available in The Food Allergy & Anaphylaxis Network's (FAAN) *School Food Allergy Program.* The *School Food Allergy Program* has been endorsed and/or supported by the Anaphylaxis Committee of the American Academy of Allergy Asthma and Immunology, the National Association of School Nurses, and the Executive Committee of the Section on Allergy and Immunology of the American Academy of Pediatrics. FAAN can be reached at: 800/929–4040.

The following organizations participated in the development of this document:

American School Food Service Association
National Association of Elementary School Principals
National Association of School Nurses
National School Boards Association
The Food Allergy & Anaphylaxis Network

Figure 28.6 ■ School guidelines for managing students with food allergies.

Food Allergy Action Plan

ALLERGY TO: ______________________

Place Child's Picture here

Student's Name: ______________ D.O.B: ______________ Teacher: ______________

Asthmatic Yes* ☐ No ☐ *High risk for severe reaction

◆ SIGNS OF AN ALLERGIC REACTION ◆

Systems:	Symptoms:
• MOUTH	itching & swelling of the lips, tongue, or mouth
• THROAT*	itching and/or a sense of tightness in the throat, hoarseness, and hacking cough
• SKIN	hives, itchy rash, and/or swelling about the face or extremities
• GUT	nausea, abdominal cramps, vomiting, and/or diarrhea
• LUNG*	shortness of breath, repetitive coughing, and/or wheezing
• HEART*	"thready" pulse, "passing-out"

The severity of symptoms can quickly change. *All above symptoms can potentially progress to a life-threatening situation.

◆ ACTION FOR MINOR REACTION ◆

1. If **only symptom(s)** are: ______________, give ______________
medication/dose/route

____

Then call: Include home/work/ & cell phone #s

2. Mother______ Work phone:______ Home phone:______, Father______ Work phone:______ Home phone:______, or emergency contacts.
3. Dr.______________ at______________

If condition does not improve within 10 minutes, follow steps for Major Reaction below.

◆ ACTION FOR MAJOR REACTION ◆

1. **If ingestion is suspected and/or symptom(s) are:** ______________,
give ______________ IMMEDIATELY!
medication/dose/route

Then call:

2. Rescue Squad (ask for advanced life support) Transport to what ER?
3. Mother______________, Father______________, or emergency contacts.
4. Dr.______________ at______________

DO NOT HESITATE TO CALL RESCUE SQUAD!

Parent's Signature______________ Date______ Doctor's Signature______________ Date______

EMERGENCY CONTACTS	TRAINED STAFF MEMBERS
1. ______________	1. ______________ Room______
Relation:______ Phone:______	2. ______________ Room______
2. ______________	3. ______________ Room______
Relation:______ Phone:______	
3. ______________	
Relation:______ Phone:______	

EPIPEN® AND EPIPEN® JR. DIRECTIONS

1. **Pull off gray safety cap**

2. **Place black tip on outer thigh (always apply to thigh)**

3. **Using a quick motion, press hard into thigh until Auto-Injector mechanism functions. Hold in place and count to 10. The EpiPen® unit should then be removed and discarded. Massage the injection area for 10 seconds.**

For children with multiple food allergies, use one form for each food.

Figure 28.7 ■ Food allergy action plan.

Interventions

Once the offending allergen has been identified, the goals include eliminating the exacerbating factors, hydrating the skin, controlling pruritus, decreasing inflammation and infection, and ensuring that ointments are being applied correctly (Nicol, 2003). The treatment of choice is removal of the offending agent if it can be identified. Recommend that any newly used product be discontinued or changed. If a medication has just been started, the parents and physician should be informed of the symptoms.

Reactions to contact lenses and to the chemicals used to treat them can also occur. Usually it is the preservatives, such as thimerosal, or the bacteriostatic agents, such as chlorhexidine, in these solutions that cause the cell-mediated contact dermatitis. EDTA, which is a chelating agent for the lens can produce the same reaction. If the eyes are red and irritated, recommend stopping the use of contact lenses until the symptoms clear. If unable to quickly and easily remedy the situation, then the student should be referred to an appropriate physician, possibly including an allergist or dermatologist.

While bathing routines are done at home, skin creams may be prescribed to be applied during the school day. Skin solutions come in ointments, creams, lotions, and gels. (*Lotions consist of suspensions of a powder in water; creams are semisolid emulsions of oil in water; ointments consist of water droplets suspended in the continuous phase of oil or petrolatum; and gel is a transparent and colorless semisolid emulsion that liquefies on contact with the skin [Arndt & Bowers, 2002].*) Symptomatic relief can be obtained using topical corticosteroid creams and ointments. The percentage of medication in these substances differs; therefore it is important to know the potency of the product. The school nurse should ensure that he or she has directions on where to apply the products, how much to apply, how often it can be applied, and when it should not be used.

When a student is seen for increased pruritus caused by excessive dry skin or eczema, the nurse can lubricate the skin as directed by the healthcare provider's office. Used appropriately, moisturizers can restore water to the skin for a short period of time or can help the skin retain moisture when applied after bathing. The most effective lubricants are petrolatum, mineral and baby oil, Albolene, or Eucerin (Arndt & Bowers, 2002). Oral antihistamines are useful in reducing itching (Fitzpatrick, Johnson, Wolff, & Saurmond, 2001). Another goal of therapy is to alleviate anxiety, as emotional support is beneficial in the relief of pruritis (Arndt & Bowers, 2002).

The steroids used are of mid to high potency and used for a short duration; they include mometasone furoate (Elocon), fluticasone propionate (Cultivate), or triamcinolone (Aristocort). Topical immunomodulators (topical calcineurin inhibitors) are an alternative to topical steroids. These nonsteroidal topical creams include pimecrolimus (Elidel) and tacrolimus (Protopic).

Eczema

It is often difficult to differentiate between atopic dermatitis and eczema. Eczema has often been called the "itch that rashes" (see Chapter 25). It is a chronic condition with remissions and exacerbations, the latter often brought about by contact with an allergen, stress, dry air, temperature changes, sweating, or bathing too frequently. Sebaceous gland activity and fat content are decreased, which causes increased sweat retention and itchy skin. This leads to the scratching that starts the cyclical pattern. The results are weeping vesicles, leading to crusting, lichenification, and infections. It is especially prevalent on sweaty areas of the body: cheeks, scalp, flexor surfaces, and postauricular areas. The rash is not infectious.

Latex Allergy

The prevalence of latex allergy is increased in healthcare workers and individuals who have had multiple surgical procedures early in life (Wills-Karp & Hershey, 2003). Latex can result in an allergic reaction either by direct contact with products that contain it or it can be airborne; therefore it can affect either the skin or the respiratory tract. Anaphylaxis has been known to occur. Those with allergies to certain fruits, for example, banana, avocado, kiwi, and chestnut, may have a crossover allergic reaction to latex because of similar antigens (Wills-Karp & Hershey, 2003). Latex can be a component of everything from adhesive tape and pencil erasers to the rubber on your stethoscope or rubber gloves. It can be in condoms, the elastic in clothes, rubber bands, and balloons. *Alternatives to these products must be sought.* Nonlatex gloves, bandages, and adhesive tape should be available. A valuable Web site is the American Latex Allergy Association in the resource section of this chapter.

INSECT STINGS (BEES, WASPS, HORNETS, FIRE ANTS)

Children may be allergic to one or all stinging insects. Allergic reactions to insect stings are common. The acute reactions are due to IgE antibodies reacting with insect venom. The incidence of anaphylaxis in the general population ranges from 0.3% to 3%, or about 40 deaths per year (Reisman, 2000). These insects are from the order of Hymenoptera of the class Insecta and divided into three families. The vespids include the yellow jacket, hornet, and wasp; the aphids include the honeybee and bumblebee; and the fire ants. Identification of the responsible stinging insect in a severe reaction is important for directions on avoidance and for venom immunotherapy. Of note, biting insects such as the mosquito rarely causes serious allergic reactions.

Different stinging insects are more common in different parts of the country. For example, the African honeybee is now present in Texas, Arizona, and California. The wasp is more common in Texas and honeybees are more common in farm areas where they are used for plant fertilization (Reisman, 2000). The fire ant is found primarily near the Gulf Coast and is spreading slowly northwest.

Insect stings can result in local or systemic reactions, the latter of which can progress quickly to anaphylaxis. "Any swelling that is contiguous to the sting site, no matter how large, in absence of systemic symptoms, is considered a local reaction" (AAAAI, 2002, p. 14). Therefore, no matter how large the swollen extremity gets, it is still considered a local reaction. Be prepared for a sting on the hand to cause the entire forearm to swell. The swelling may be limited by cold compresses or ice on the sting site, or using a baking soda and water paste to reduce the reactions. If the stinger and venom sac are still attached to the skin, carefully remove it by scraping with a fingernail. Analgesics may be given for the local pain and antihistamines may be prescribed, as may topical steroid creams. These symptoms may last for 7 to 10 days.

If a systemic reaction is suspected, administration of epinephrine may be needed. Symptoms of anaphylaxis after an insect sting usually start within 10 to 30 minutes, the most common of which are hives, flushing, and angioedema. Respiratory distress with upper airway swelling, circulatory collapse, and shock may follow. Other symptoms may include nausea, abdominal cramps, diarrhea, and a feeling of "impending doom" (Reisman, 2000).

Management and treatment of stinging insect anaphylaxis include prevention, immunotherapy, medic alert identification, and epinephrine, if needed. The success rate for venom immunotherapy is better than 98% (Reisman, 2002). Antihistamines, such as diphenhydramine, are recommended for hives and edema. When an older child is participating in an outdoor event or on a field trip, a fanny pack containing preloaded epinephrine is recommended. An adult should be designated and educated about the student's plan of care before the event occurs.

To decrease the chance of insect stings, the following measures should be followed:

1. Wear long-sleeve shirts, long pants, and shoes when outside; avoid loose clothes (they trap insects), black and bright colors, or flowery prints (wear light colors: white, green, tan, khaki).
2. Don't drink sweet liquids outdoors, and wash hands and face after drinking these. Keep beverages capped, especially soda cans.
3. Keep garbage covered outside; if picnicking, do not sit near garbage cans.
4. Avoid flowering bushes.
5. Avoid perfumes, hair spray, hair tonic, suntan lotion, and cosmetics.
6. Keep hair short.

ALLERGY TO MEDICATION

Allergic reactions account for 6% to 10% of all adverse drug reactions (Ditto, 2002). Dermatologic reactions represent the most common form of allergic drug reaction (Anderson, 2000). Anaphylaxis is the classic clinical picture of an IgE-mediated drug reaction that requires the presence of IgE antibodies specific for the drug allergen. The drug allergen binds to IgE antibodies that are bound to the surface of mast cells or basophils.

The clinical manifestations of delayed dermatologic reactions include macropapular, morbilliform, or erythematous rashes, exfoliative dermatitis, photosensitivity reactions, and eczema (Ditto, 2000). Usually these reactions are caused by penicillin and sulfonamides. Contact dermatitis is common with neomycin.

Common Drug Reactions

Penicillin reactions are the most common allergic drug reactions. The reaction presentation may include urticaria, pruritis, and morbilliform rash, and rarely presents as angioedema, laryngeal edema, wheezing, anaphylaxis, and hypotension. In vitro, cross-reactivity between penicillin and cephalosporins is well established but clinical relevance is not clear. Skin tests are effective in the diagnosis of a penicillin reaction and desensitization is effective if the drug is needed (Wills-Karp & Hershey, 2003).

Insulin reactions generally occur at the injection site and do not require treatment. These frequently occur when reinstituting therapy following a gap in treatment. The reaction may involve the insulin itself or formulation additives such as protamine (Anderson, 2000).

Reactions to vaccines have been attributed to proteins cross-reactive with eggs, hydrolyzed gelatin, sorbitol, and neomycin, all of which may be found in some vaccines. True anaphylactic reactions are rare. Current measles–mumps–rubella (MMR) vaccines are derived from cultures that contain insignificant amounts of proteins cross-reactive with eggs. The recommendation of the American Academy of Pediatrics Committee on Infectious Disease suggests that children with egg allergy may routinely be given MMR without prior skin testing (Centers for Disease Control and Prevention [CDC], 1998). If there is concern, skin testing should be considered. Influenza vaccine should be avoided for patients with severe systemic sensitivity to eggs (AAAAI, 2000b).

IMPACT OF ALLERGIES ON CHILDREN AND ADOLESCENTS

The two most prevalent sequelae of allergic reactions include physical discomfort from the reaction and the side effects of medications. Children with allergic rhinitis consistently report lower quality of life than do their nonallergic peers. Their symptoms lead to embarrassment, frustration, decreased cognitive function, slower psychomotor speed, and decreased verbal learning and memory during the allergy season (Kaliner, 2002). Medications used to manage symptoms of allergy may cause side effects that make the student appear sleepy or uninterested in class work. Other side effects of allergy medicine may cause the child to be more active and seen as disruptive. Without medication for allergy, the student may appear overactive; to scratch what itches, the student is constantly moving. If the student continues to scratch, there is the potential for bleeding and infection.

"Allergic rhinitis accounts for over 2 million days of school missed yearly in the United States (Berger, 2002). This means that on a typical school day, 10,000 children are absent because of allergic rhinitis (Blaiss, 2002, p. 1). In 1996, in the United States, the overall cost of allergic rhinitis was $5.3 billion dollars. This includes 10 million office visits related to allergic symptoms and medications. It would follow that the children need caretakers when home ill, which then leads to loss of work productivity.

Some characteristics seen in children with allergies include shyness, anxiety, anger, depression, and possibly low self-esteem (Nicol, 2003). Those with atopic dermatitis may have a poor body image. Interruption in sleep can occur as a result of the allergic symptoms or from the side effects of medications, resulting in chronic fatigue, or increased irritability, daytime somnolence, or behavior problems. Whether due to the symptoms of allergy or the first-generation antihistamines, the lack of sleep may interfere with cognitive function and learning (AAAAI, 2000b; Berger, 2002). "Patients with allergic rhinitis are more likely than matched controls to have snoring, disturbed sleep, sleep apnea, and daytime sleepiness" (Wolfe, 2002, p. 802).

Recent data have supported that snoring is associated with daytime sleepiness (Wolfe, 2002). It is also associated with poor school performance, sleep problems such as parasomnias, and upper respiratory infections. Radioallergosorbent testing (RAST) is positive in 40% of children who snore and in 57% of children with sleep apnea (Wolfe, 2002).

SCHOOL NURSE ACTION PLAN

The school nurse must develop an emergency plan for students who have allergies, especially related to anaphylaxis. Knowing what symptoms are typical of an allergic reaction in a particular student is helpful, as are the symptoms that might indicate the student is in trouble.

Trouble swallowing, feeling like something is caught in their throat, or a hoarse voice may be the first indication of swelling of the respiratory tract. It is important to administer medication as soon as possible. Once epinephrine is administered, call 911 so that the student can be transported for follow-up care. Check with the local ambulance service to ensure that epinephrine is available when they are called, especially if the school is not permitted to keep this medication available (FIGURE 28.8).

CONCLUSION

Allergies are increasing in prevalence among school-age children with increasing implications for school nurses. Allergic symptoms must be differentiated from other upper respiratory, dermatological, and gastrointestinal symptoms. Most important is the nurse's role in environmental management to control or decrease the incidence of allergens. Because the allergic reaction may result in anaphylaxis, the school nurse must be prepared to identify and provide appropriate emergency measures.

EMERGENCY ACTION PLAN

Name:	
School:	**Birth Date:**
Parent/guardian:	**Grade:**
	Phone: (H) **(W)**
HealthCare Provider:	**Phone:**
Known Allergies:	
Health Problem:	

In a Health Emergency the student appears:

Please do the following:

______________ **Parent** ______________ **School Nurse** ______________ **Date**

Copy to: ☐ **Principal** ☐ **Secretary** ☐ **Parent** ☐ **Playground Aid** ☐ **Cafeteria Aid** ☐ **Teacher,**
Other ______________

Copy location: ☐ **Health File** ☐ **Substitute teacher**

Figure 28.8 ■ Emergency action plan.

Resources

American Academy of Allergy, Asthma, and Immunology
http://www.aaaai.org

American Academy of Dermatology
http://www.aad.org

American Academy of Pediatrics
http://www.aap.org

American College of Allergy, Asthma, and Immunology
http://www.acaai.org

American Latex Allergy Association
http://www.latexallergyresources.org

Asthma & Allergy Foundation of America
http://www.aafa.org

Food Allergy and Anaphylaxis Network
http://www.foodallergy.org

Food Allergy Initiative.
http://www.foodallergyinitiative.org

Food Contents, U.S. Department of Agriculture
http://www.nalusda.gov/fnic/index.html

School Asthma and Allergy
http://www.schoolasthmaallergy.com

References

Almqvist, C., Larsson, P., Egmar, A., Hedren, M., Malmberg, P., & Wickman, M. (1999). School as a risk environment for children allergic to cats and a site of transfer of cat allergen to homes. *Allergy Clinical Immunology, 103*, 1012–1017.

American Academy of Allergy, Asthma, & Immunology (AAAAI). (2000a). *The allergy report: Overview of allergic diseases* (Vol. I). Milwaukee, WI: Author.

American Academy of Allergy, Asthma, & Immunology (AAAAI). (2000b). *The allergy report: Diseases of the atopic diathesis* (Vol. II). Milwaukee, WI: Author.

American Academy of Allergy, Asthma, & Immunology (AAAAI). (2002). *School nurse allergy and asthma tool kit*. Milwaukee, WI: Author.

Anderson, J. (2000). Allergic and allergic-like reactions to drugs and other therapeutic agents. In P. Lieberman & J. Anderson (Eds.), *Allergic diseases: Diagnosis and treatment* (pp. 303–322). Totowa, NJ: Humana Press.

Arndt, K., & Bowers, K. (2002). *Manual of dermatologic therapeutics*. Philadelphia: Lippincott Williams & Wilkins.

Astwood, J., Bannon, G., Dobert, R., & Fuchs, R. (2003). Food biotechnology and genetic engineering. In D. Metcalfe, H. Sampson, & R. Simon (Eds.), *Food allergy: Adverse reactions to foods and food additives* (pp. 51–70). Malden, MA: Blackwell.

Berger, W. (2002). Pediatric rhinitis. In W. Kaliner (Ed.), *Current reviews of rhinitis* (pp. 83–91). Philadelphia: Current Medicine, Inc.

Bernstein, J. A. (2002). Antihistamines. In L. Grammer & P. Greenberger (Eds.), *Patterson's allergic diseases* (pp. 65–79). Philadelphia: Lippincott Williams & Wilkins.

Bielory, L. (2000). Diagnosis and treatment of ocular allergy. In P. Lieberman & J. Anderson (Eds.), *Allergic diseases: Diagnosis and treatment* (pp. 195–212). Totowa, NJ: Humana Press.

Blaiss, M. (2002). Costs of allergic rhinitis. In M. Kaliner (Ed.), *Current review of rhinitis* (pp. 1–6). Philadelphia: Current Medicine, Inc.

Bock, S., & Sampson, H. (2003). Immediate reactions to foods in infants and children. In D. Metcalfe, H. Sampson, & R. Simon (Eds.), *Food allergy: Adverse reactions to foods and food additives* (pp. 121–135). Malden, MA: Blackwell.

Centers for Disease Control and Prevention (CDC). (1998). Retrieved 2004 from http://www.cdc.gov/travel/diseases/measles.htm

Chandra, R., Conley, D., & Kern, R. (2002). Chronic sinusitis: Role of rhinoscopy and surgery. In L. Grammer & P. Greenberger (Eds.), *Patterson's allergic diseases* (pp. 773–784). Philadelphia: Lippincott Williams & Wilkins.

Corren, J., & Rachelefsky, G. (2000). Sinusitis and otitis media. In P. Lieberman & J. Anderson (Eds.), *Allergic diseases: Diagnosis and treatment* (pp. 183–193). Totowa, NJ: Humana Press.

Ditto, A. (2002). Drug allergy. In L.Grammer & P. Greenberger (Eds.), *Patterson's allergic diseases* (pp. 295–385). Philadelphia: Lippincott Williams & Wilkins.

Eales, L. (2003). *Immunology for life scientists*. West Sussex, England: John Wiley & Sons.

Eccles, R. (2003). Anatomy and physiology of the nose and control of nasal airflow. In N. Adkinson, J. Yunginger, W. Busse, B. Bochner, S. Holgate, & F. Simons (Eds.), *Middleton's allergy: Principles & practice* (pp. 775–787). St. Louis: C. V. Mosby.

Economides, A., & Kaliner, M. (2002). Allergic rhinitis. In M. Kaliner (Ed.), *Current review of rhinitis* (pp. 35–51). Phildelphia: Current Medicine, Inc.

Fitzpatrick, T., Johnson, R., Wolff, K., & Saurmond, D. (2001). *Color atlas and synopsis of clinical dermatology*. New York: McGraw-Hill.

Fox, R., & Lockey, R. (2000). Allergen immunotherapy. In P. Lieberman & J. Anderson (Eds.), *Allergic diseases* (pp. 421–436). Totowa, NJ: Humana Press.

Grammer, L. (2002). Principles of immunologic management of allergic diseases due to extrinsic antigens. In L. Grammer & P. Greenberger (Eds.), *Patterson's allergic diseases* (pp. 183–194). Philadelphia: Lippincott Williams & Wilkins.

Greenberger, P. (2002). Allergic disorders and pregnancy. In L. Grammer & P. Greenberger (Eds.), *Patterson's allergic diseases* (pp. 581–593). Philadelphia: Lippincott Williams & Wilkins.

Hanifin, J. (August, 2003). An overview of atopic dermatitis. *Dermatology Nursing*, (Suppl.), 6–9.

Kaliner, M. (2001). Allergic rhino-sinusitis. In *AAAAI. Allergy & immunology 2001: Six lectures in the treatment of allergy, asthma, & immunology* (pp. 37–89). Milwaukee, WI: American Academy of Allergy, Asthma & Immunology

Kaliner, M. A. (2002). *Current review of rhinitis*. Philadelphia: Current Medicine, Inc.

Kelly, H., & Raissy, H. (2003). Principles of pharmacotherapeutics. In N. Adkinson, B. Bochner, J. Yunginger, S. Holgate, W. Busse, & F. Simons (Eds.), *Middleton's allergy: Principles & practice* (pp. 789–802). St. Louis: C. V. Mosby.

Kemp, S. (2000). Cromolyn and neocrom. In P. Lieberman & J. Anderson (Eds.), *Allergic diseases: Diagnosis and treatment* (pp. 367–375). Totowa, NJ: Humana Press.

Ledford, D. (2000). Rhinitis. In P. Lieberman & J. Anderson (Eds.), *Allergic diseases: Diagnosis and treatment* (pp. 159–182). Totowa, NJ: Humana Press.

Lieberman, P., & Blaiss, M (2002). Allergic diseases of the eye and ear. In L. Grammer & P. Greenberger (Eds.), *Patterson's allergic diseases* (pp. 195–223). Philadelphia: Lippincott Williams & Wilkins

Lipworth, B., & Jackson, C. (2000). Safety of inhaled and intranasal corticosteroids. *Drug Safety*, 23(1), 11–33.

Munoz-Furlong, A. (2003). Daily coping strategies for patients and their families. *Pediatrics, 111*(6), 1654–1661.

National Association of School Nurses (NASN). (2001). *The role of school nurses in allergy/anaphylaxis management: Position statement*. Retrieved from http://www.nasn.org/positions/allergy.htm

Nelson, H., & Rachelelefsky, G. (2000). Anaphylactic and anaphylactoid reaction. In *The allergy report 2000* (pp. 115–130). Milwaukee: The Academy of Allergy, Asthma & Immunology, Inc.

Nicol, N. (August, 2003). Evolution in the treatment of atopic dermatitis: New approaches to managing a chronic skin disease. *Dermatology Nursing*, (Suppl.), 4–5.

Ownby, D. (2000). Diagnostic tests in allergy. In P. Lieberman & J. Anderson (Eds.), *Allergic diseases: Diagnosis and treatment* (pp. 29–39). Totowa, NJ: Humana Press.

Reisman, R. (2000). Insect sting allergy. In P. Leiberman & J. Anderson (Eds.), *Allergic diseases: Diagnosis and treatment* (pp. 73–83). Totowa, NJ: Humana Press.

Sampson, H. (2003). Anaphylaxis and emergency treatment. *Pediatrics, 111*(6), 1601–1608.

Scruggs, K., & Johnson, M. (2004). *Pediatric treatment guidelines: American Academy of Pediatrics*. Laguna Hills, CA: Current Clinical Strategies Publishing.

Settipane, R., & Settipane, G. (2002). Nonallergic rhinitis. In M. Kaliner (Ed.), *Current reviews of rhinitis* (pp. 53–66). Philadelphia: Current Medicine, Inc.

Shearer, W., & Fleisher, T. (2003). The immune system. In N. F. Adkinson, B. Bochner, J. Yunginger, S. Holgate, W. Busse, & F. E. Simons (Eds.), *Middleton's allergy: Principles & practice* (pp. 1–14). St. Louis: C. V. Mosby.

Sicherer, S., & Eggleston, P. (2000). Environmental allergens. In P. Lieberman & J. Anderson (Eds.), *Allergic diseases: Diagnosis and treatment* (pp. 41–51). Totowa, NJ: Humana Press.

Simons, F. (2002). *Histamine and H1-antihistamines in allergic disease*. New York: Marcel Dekker.

Uphold, C., & Graham, M. (1998). *Clinical guidelines in family practice*. Gainesville: Barmarrae Books.

Wills-Karp, M., & Hershey, G. (2003). Immunological mechanisms of allergic disorders. In W. Paul (Ed.), *Fundamental immunology* (pp. 1439–1479). Philadelphia: Lippincott Williams & Wilkins.

Wolf, B. (2000). Approach to the allergic patient. In P. Lieberman & J. Anderson (Eds.), *Allergic diseases: Diagnosis and treatment* (pp. 17–27). Totowa, NJ: Humana Press.

Wolfe, L. (2002). Sleep disorders in the allergic patient. In L. Grammer & P. Greenberger (Eds.), *Patterson's allergic diseases* (pp. 797–806). Philadelphia: Lippincott Williams & Wilkins.

Zoratti, E. (2000). Environmental control of respiratory irritants and allergens. In P. Lieberman & J. Anderson (Eds.), *Allergic diseases: Diagnosis and treatment* (pp. 405–420). Totowa, NJ: Humana Press.

Chapter 29

Asthma

MICHELLE FICCA ■ CAROL MURPHY MOORE

Chapter Outline

INTRODUCTION AND PREVALENCE

Asthma is one of the most common chronic condition in childhood; it affects nearly nine million children or approximately 12% of children under the age of 18 (Centers for Disease Control and Prevention [CDC], 2004a). Therefore, in a typical school classroom, approximately two or three students are likely to have asthma. Asthma affects slightly more males than females. More than four million children and adolescents (6% of that population) had an asthma attack in 2002.

Non-Hispanic black children have an incidence more than twice that of Hispanic students. Those living in poverty have a higher rate of asthma (16%) compared to those who are not poor (11%). Children living in families headed by a single mother have an asthma prevalence rate higher than that of two-parent families (17% versus 11%). Of interest, only 10% of children living with single fathers have asthma. Finally, "children in fair or poor health were almost seven times as likely to have had an asthma attack in the past 12 months as children in excellent or very good health (29% versus 4%)" (CDC, 2004a, p. 11).

The incidence of asthma increases with age, with 16% to 18.9% of high school students indicating that they have been diagnosed with asthma (CDC, 2005). Therefore, asthma can develop at any age. Asthma can result in significant morbidity during childhood and adolescence. It accounts for 14 million lost school days per year (CDC, 2004b), or about 25% of all school absenteeism (Reilly, 2000). It is not unusual for a student with asthma to miss 10 or more school days per year. Asthma is the third leading cause of hospitalization among children younger than 15 years of age; 214,000 in this age group were hospitalized with the complications of asthma in 2002. In addition, symptoms of asthma accounted for 728,000 Emergency Room visits in 2002 (CDC, 2004b).

Mortality resulting from asthma attacks continues to threaten young people. In 1999, there were 144 deaths from asthma in the 5- to 14-year-old age group, which is an annual rate of 3.6 per million children (CDC, 2002a).

These statistics highlight the fact that asthma prevalence and the complications associated with asthma continue to affect school-age youth and adolescents. To address these concerns, Healthy People 2010 (U.S. Department of Health and Human Services, 2000) identifies eight objectives related to the reduction of the mortality and morbidity associated with asthma (TABLE 29.1).

The American Lung Association (2003) reported that while school nurses were very experienced in dealing with asthma in the schools, asthma was poorly understood by students, parents, and school staff; this results in significant problems in the schools and increases the responsibilities of the school nurse. Quality asthma management requires seamless collaboration by the school, home, and healthcare providers. As a student spends 7 to 9 hours a day in school, optimal management must involve the school nurse.

PATHOPHYSIOLOGY OF ASTHMA

Asthma is a chronic inflammatory disorder of the airways. The primary manifestations of asthma are bronchospasm leading to bronchoconstriction, increased bronchial mucus, and inflammation of bronchial tissue leading to edema. These cause recurrent episodes of "wheezing, breathlessness,

Table 29.1 ■

HEALTHY PEOPLE 2010 OBJECTIVES RELATED TO ASTHMA

24–1 Reduce asthma deaths in children 5 to 14 years from 3.2 per million to 1 per million and adolescents from 5.9 per million to 3 per million.

24–2 Reduce hospitalization for asthma in children 0–5 years of age from 60.9 per 10,000 to 25 per 10,000, and 5 years to adulthood from 13.8 per 10,000 to 8 per 10,000.

24–3 Reduce hospital Emergency Room visits for asthma for children younger than 5 years of age from 150 per 10,000, and for those 5 years of age through adulthood, from 71.1 per 10,000 to 50/10,000.

24–4 Reduce activity limitations among those who have asthma from 19% to 10%.

24–5 Reduce the number of school days missed due to asthma.

24–6 Increase the proportion of those with asthma who receive formal patient education, including information about community and self-help resources as an essential part of the management of the condition, from 10% to 30%.

24–7 Increase the proportion of those with asthma who receive appropriate asthma care
- a. Receives written asthma management plans.
- b. Receives instructions on how to use prescribed inhalers properly.
- c. Receives education in order to recognize early signs and symptoms of asthma episodes and how to respond appropriately, including instruction on peak flow monitoring for those who use daily therapy.
- d. Receives medication regimen that prevents the need for more than one canister of short-acting inhaled beta agonist each month for relief of symptoms.
- e. Receives medical follow-up care for long-term management of asthma after any hospitalization related to asthma.
- f. Receives assistance with assessment; assesses and reduces exposure to environmental risk factors in their home and school environment.

24–8 Develop a state-wide tracking system related to asthma deaths, as well as tracking the impact of this condition, the way it presents, and its impact on the student.

(U.S. Department of Health and Human Services, 2000).

chest tightness, and cough … that is associated with widespread but variable airflow obstruction that is often reversible either spontaneously or with treatment" (National Asthma Education and Prevention Program Expert Panel Report, 2002).

Regardless of cause, the bronchi appear to be hyperreactive to stimuli, resulting in increased immunoglobulin E (IgE) production; increased mast cell degranulation (IgE connects to mast cells); and increased release of inflammatory mediators, such as histamine, prostaglandins, and leukotrienes (Brashers, 2002). (See Chapter 28.) The hyperactivity of the lung tissue results in some referring to asthma as reactive airway disease. Because of the bronchial irritation, white blood cells (neutrophils, eosinophils, and lymphocytes) are stimulated and infiltrate the bronchial tissue, resulting in inflammation. The irritation causes mucus to be produced in increased amounts, which impedes the functioning of the cilia (Brashers, 2002). Meanwhile, histamine causes the smooth muscles in the bronchi to constrict. All of these processes lead to airway obstruction and air trapping. A full description of this pathophysiological process is provided in Chapter 28 under the description of a type I allergic response.

SYMPTOMATOLOGY

The multiple immune processes result in early and late stages of asthma. It is this latter stage that is most often ignored by healthcare providers. The early stage occurs within 10 to 20 minutes of exposure to an inhaled allergen (Porth, 2005) or whatever may cause the bronchospasm; the bronchoconstriction that results is due to the release of histamine from the mast cells (see Chapter 28). There is dyspnea and increased respiratory effort. The student may complain that he or she is having trouble breathing or that his or her chest feels "tight." The nurse may observe retractions caused by use of accessory muscles, open mouth breathing, and a position of comfort that involves sitting upright. Auscultation may reveal decreased breath sounds and wheezing, especially expiratory wheezing. This is caused by air that gets in with the help of accessory respiratory muscles, but then has difficulty exiting; because the air is forced through a narrow airway, the wheeze may be heard. If air is trapped in the alveoli by the swollen airways, there will be decreased breath sounds in that area.

The late stage can occur 4 to 12 hours after the initial attack "due to persistent eosinophil and lymphocyte activation…and it can be even more severe than the initial attack" (Brashers, 2002, p. 1123). The inflammation results in "increased airway responsiveness that prolongs the asthma attack and sets into motion a vicious cycle of exacerbations" (Porth, 2005, p. 696). This late stage can last for days as the inflammatory process continues, causing increased respiratory compromise. This inflammatory response occurs in all patients, regardless of the severity of the disease state. Persistent untreated inflammation can result in long-term, irreversible damage to the airway, referred to as airway remodeling. Examples include mucus gland hyperplasia, smooth muscle hypertrophy, and loss of elastic fibers (American Academy of Allergy, Asthma and Immunology [AAAAI], 2000).

Up to 80% of children with asthma develop their first symptoms before the age of 5 (AAAAI, 2000). Symptoms manifest in different ways depending on the child's age. Common asthma symptoms include:

- Wheezing (more often, expiratory wheezing), accompanied by a prolonged expiratory phase. Note: wheezing may not be present.
- Coughing (nighttime or early morning). Starts with a nonproductive cough; only as the bronchoconstriction resolves does the cough produce thick stringy mucus that can cause even more respiratory distress.
- Shortness of breath, tachypnea, and tachycardia
- Chest tightness
- Retractions (suprasternal, substernal, intercostal, subcostal), including nasal flaring
- If remodeling has occurred, barrel chest may be present (hyperinflation of the thorax).

Associated symptoms may include fatigue and difficulty eating. Students may slow down or stop playing or become irritated easily. They may avoid certain activities and indicate that they don't have the stamina for them any more. Tachypnea may make it difficult to eat. It is important for the school nurse to recognize that the signs and symptoms of asthma can vary widely from student to student. In addition, coughing may be the only symptom present.

ETIOLOGY

The primary causes of asthma are genetics and environment. There is an increased risk for the allergic response if there is a family history of allergy; however, the process is thought to involve multiple genes. "Genetic factors account for up to one half of an individual's susceptibility to asthma"

(Guilbert & Drawiec, 2003, p. 527). One theory gaining popularity involves the helper T cells (Th). There are two types of helper T cells: Th1 and Th2. Th1 stimulates B cells to produce immunoglobulin G (IgG) and IgM in response to microbes (see Chapter 28). However, Th2 increases the body's response to allergy and parasites and stimulates the production of IgE. In addition, Th2 stimulates production of cytokines that increases those cells that cause and exacerbate an allergic response. Genetics may predispose individuals to a hyperreactive response of the bronchial tissue, regulation of Th1 and Th2, and an increased production of IgE (Brashers, 2002).

Environmental causes of asthma include allergens and viruses, as well as anything that irritates or affects the respiratory tract. Exposure to high allergen counts can precipitate the development of IgE. Viral infections, especially early exposure to respiratory syncytial virus (RSV), puts one at risk for developing asthma (Gern & Lemanske, 2003). However, the time of exposure to these viruses is essential. One etiological hypothesis that combines genetics and environment is the "hygiene hypothesis." This theory postulates that exposure to pathogens during the first year of life increases the chance of developing Th1 and suppresses Th2. Absence of this exposure supports the development of Th2 and predisposes to asthma. Therefore early, repeated viral infections, especially those that do not lead to lower respiratory infections, lead to a decreased risk of asthma (except for exposure to RSV) (Guilbert & Krawiec, 2003).

Multiple products can irritate or exacerbate the respiratory tract, stimulating it to go into spasm and begin the process of an asthma attack (Porth, 2005). These are referred to as "triggers" and include respiratory tract infections, cigarette smoke, air pollution, cold air, exercise, emotional upset, and possibly hormonal changes prior to the menstrual cycle. In some cases, asthma occurs during a type I allergic response to a common allergen (AAAAI, 2000). Triggers can change over time.

Exercise-induced asthma (EIA), or exercise-induced bronchospasm, is thought to be caused by changes in airway temperature, and loss of heat and water from the airway. An increased respiratory rate, resulting from exercise, "of air that is cooler and dryer than that of the respiratory tree precipitates the bronchospasm" (Baker, Friedman, & Schmitt, 2002, p. 129). This reaction can occur during physical activity or immediately following vigorous activity. The bronchospasm peaks within 10 minutes of stopping the activity and resolves within the next 30 minutes (Baker et al., 2002). EIA occurs in 70% to 90% of those with persistent asthma; however, it also occurs in 10% of the general population (Sheth, 2003).

DIAGNOSIS

Diagnosis is typically made based on the presence of symptoms and confirmed by spirometry. The school nurse should suspect asthma when the student displays the symptoms described earlier. The school nurse should be sure to obtain a careful and complete history regarding symptom patterns. The school nurse's referral to the student's healthcare provider (or information given to the parent to take to the healthcare provider) should include objective data collected by the nurse and subjective history obtained from the student, parents, and teachers. The objective data include respiratory rate; lung auscultation; color; chest movement; assessment of the ear, eye, nose, and throat; history of upper respiratory infections; exercise tolerance; and history of visiting the health office. Subjective data include the reported history of allergies, triggers, and responses to interventions. The school nurse can use the referral process to initiate the diagnostic process and to foster collaboration between the school and the healthcare provider.

The gold standard for the diagnosis of asthma is spirometry (Kelly, 2003). Spirometry utilizes a machine that measures lung function, recorded as the FEV1 (forced expiratory volume in 1 second). It provides an accurate analysis of any airway obstruction and the body's response to bronchodilators; it is given before and 15 minutes after the person receives a short-acting inhaled bronchodilator. Based on the FEV1 reading, the asthma can be classified as mild, moderate, or severe; less than 80% of predicted FEV1 is indicative of difficulty (Kelly, 2003).

Peak flow measurements are not recommended as a diagnostic measure, as they are not a sensitive measure to airflow obstruction; their results are more variable and less reliable than those of the FEV1 (Kelly, 2003). As a primary measure of large airway function, peak flow measures can be used for monitoring, but not for diagnosis (AAAAI, 2000). Peak flow measurements are usually lowest in the early morning hours and highest in the late afternoon. The most effective way to utilize peak flow measures is to measure it on awakening before using a bronchodilator and again testing after the bronchodilator is used in the late afternoon. "A greater than 20% difference between the morning and evening measurements suggests inadequately controlled asthma" (AAAAI, 2000, p. 41). However, routine monitoring of asthma by using peak flow measurements is "of limited value for predicting adverse outcomes from asthma" (Kelly, 2003, p. 599).

In addition to measurements of lung function, it is necessary to identify the triggers for the asthma. Many students will need to be tested for allergies

(Chapter 28). If these are negative and the symptoms continue, it is possible that another type of condition is present that needs additional work-up.

CLASSIFICATION

The classification system for asthma is based on severity and frequency of symptoms during the day and at night, as well as lung function (as measured by spirometry or peak flow) and response to short acting beta-2 agonists (AAAAI, 2000). The four categories of asthma severity are mild intermittent, mild persistent, moderate persistent, and severe persistent (TABLE 29.2).

The classification system measures severity before treatment. Only one criterion in a category qualifies an individual for that category. "An individual should be assigned to the most severe grade in which any feature occurs" (AAAAI, 2000, p. 44).

Table 29.2 ■

ASTHMA CLASSIFICATION SYSTEM

Classification	*Clinical Features BEFORE Treatment*			
ASTHMA SEVERITY	SYMPTOM SEVERITY	NIGHTTIME SYMPTOMS	LUNG FUNCTION IN PATIENTS WHO CAN USE A SPIROMETER OR PEAK FLOW METER	SHORT-ACTING BETA$_2$-AGONIST USE
Severe persistent	• Continual symptoms • Limited physical activity • Frequent exacerbations interfere with normal activities	Frequent	• FEV_1 or PEF ≤ 60% predicted • PEF variability > 30%	qid use daily does NOT completely relieve symptoms
Moderate persistent	• Daily symptoms • Exacerbations ≥ 2 times/week; may last days; may affect activities	> 1 time/week	• FEV_1 or PEF > 60% to < 80% predicted • PEF variability > 30%	Daily
Mild persistent	• Symptoms > 2 times/week but < 1 time/day • Exacerbations may affect activities	> 2 time/month	• FEV_1 or PEF > 80% predicted • PEF variability 20% to 30%	> 2 times/ week but < 1 time/day
Mild intermittent	• Symptoms ≤ 2 times/week • Asymptomatic and normal PEF between exacerbations • Exacerbations brief (from a few hours to a few days); intensity may vary	≤ 2 times/month	• FEV_1 or PEF ≥ 80% predicted • PEF variability < 20%	≤ 2 times/ week

Source: American Academy of Allergy, Asthma, and Immunology (2000, p. 44)

Children classified at a particular category may have episodes that involve mild, moderate or severe exacerbations (Burns, Brady, Dunn, & Starr, 2000). Furthermore, it is important to note that the child's asthma classification may change over time.

MANAGEMENT

Asthma management involves environmental measures and pharmacotherapy. Education is also a component of the total picture. The goals of asthma management are to have the student lead as normal a life as possible and to respond to symptoms early to prevent morbidity. The school nurse is an essential partner in the coordinated care for these students.

Asthma Action Plan

One of the first actions following diagnosis is to develop an Asthma Action Plan. This is usually completed by the healthcare provider in conjunction with the family. It is individualized for the student with the goal of preventing or helping to manage asthma episodes. It also provides the beginning component of education for the family. The environmental measures include recommendations of how to alter the home or activities, especially if allergy or exercise is the cause of the asthma. The pharmacologic component includes not only the daily medication to keep the asthma under control, but also the actions to take in an emergency. This includes directions as to when the student should be brought to the emergency room. TABLE 29.3 lists the components of a typical asthma action plan. These plans should be made in triplicate so that a copy can be given to the school nurse. It is essential that there be consistency in the measures taken between the home and school. Asthma action plans should be revised at least annually with the healthcare provider and more often if the plan is not effective in controlling asthma episodes.

Table 29.3 ■
ASTHMA ACTION PLAN

Asthma Action Plan for ____________________
Date ____________________
Healthcare Provider's Name ____________________
Healthcare Provider's Phone Number ____________________

Allergies ____

Asthma triggers: what makes asthma worse?
Recommended modifications of the environment
____
____
____
____
____

Asthma symptoms: Early indicators of an impending asthma attack
____
____

Green Zone: Indicators that the child is doing well
No cough, wheeze, chest tightness, or shortness of breath during the day or night
Can do usual activities.

If a peak flow meter is used, more than ____________________ (80% or more of my best peak flow)
My best peak flow is: ____________________

(continued)

Take these medications each day (include an anti-inflammatory)

Medicine	How much to take	When to take it

Yellow Zone: Asthma is getting worse.

Cough, wheeze, chest tightness, or shortness of breath, or
Waking at night due to asthma, or
Can do some, but not all, usual activities

If a peak flow meter is used: ____________________ to ______________________
(50% to 80% of my best peak flow)

FIRST: Keep taking the Green Zone medications, and ADD the following quick-relief medicine:

_____________________________ (short-acting beta2-agonist)
(Circle one of the following and cross out the other two)
Take 2 puffs every 20 minutes for up to 1 hour
Take 4 puffs every 20 minutes for up to 1 hour
Use a nebulizer, once

SECOND: If symptoms (and peak flow) return to the Green Zone after 1 hour.

(circle one)
Take the quick-relief medicine every 4 hours for 1–2 days

Double the dose of your inhaled steroid for ________(7–10) days

OR

If symptoms (and peak flow, if used) do NOT return to Green Zone after 1 hour of above treatment (healthcare provider must determine what medications are to be taken, in what dosage, and for what period of time).

Take _______(2 or 4) puffs of _____________(short-acting beta-2 agonist)
Add __________________(oral steroid) mg/day for ___________(3–10) days
Call your healthcare provider before ________hours after taking the oral steroid.

Red Zone: Medical Alert

Very short of breath, or
Quick-relief medicines have not helped, or
Cannot do usual activities, or
Symptoms are same or get worse after 24 hours in Yellow Zone, or
Peak flow is less than ___________(50% of my best peak flow).

Take this medicine__________________(short-acting beta2-agonist) _______(number of puffs [2 or 4] or use of nebulizer)
And/or (circle one)
___________________(oral steroid) _____mg

Then, call your healthcare provider NOW.

Go to the hospital or call an ambulance if you are still in the red zone after 15 minutes AND you have not reached your healthcare provider

DANGER SIGNS:

Trouble walking and talking due to shortness or breath
Lips or fingernails are blue

GET TO A HOSPITAL NOW.

Individualized Health Plan

From the Asthma Action Plan, the school nurse should develop an Individualized Health Plan (IHP) for the student (see Chapter 9). This plan should be developed in collaboration with the parents, the student, if appropriate, and the healthcare provider. Within that plan, there should also be information related to daily management and emergency care, as per the guidelines provided in the Asthma Action Plan. The IHP should include the following information:

- Triggers
- Peak flow monitoring schedule and personal best number, if recommended
- Daily medication plan
- Any special instructions
- Limits to activity

The emergency portion of the IHP should provide:

- Emergency contact names and phone numbers
- Specific symptoms to look for when the student is in trouble
- A peak flow reading that signals trouble for the student
- Steps to take during an asthma episode
- Emergency asthma medications, both the dose and the number of times to be taken

Assessment of the student's technique in the use of inhalers is crucial. Other information for inclusion in an IHP includes:

- Location of medications
- Student's ability to self-medicate
- Assessment of effectiveness of treatment
- Name and contact information of healthcare provider
- Student's knowledge level about asthma

See Chapter 9 for an example of an Individualized Health Plan and an Emergency Action Plan related to asthma. Box 29.1 is an example of a Student Asthma Action Card.

Environmental Measures

One approach to reduce episodes of asthma is to reduce exposure to offending allergens or irritants. It is the school nurse's responsibility to assess environmental conditions of the school. For asthma management, this assessment includes specific allergens and irritants that are known or suspected triggers to the student with asthma. A trigger is anything that causes airway irritation or inflammation and leads to the development of asthma symptoms. Some triggers found in the school may include:

- Air pollutants (cigarette smoke)
- Animal dander from dogs, cats or other furred animals
- Chalk dust
- Cleaning agents
- Cockroaches
- Dust (dust mites)
- Feathered animals
- Mold
- Pesticides
- Strong odors (dry erase markers, magic markers, perfumes, glue or chemicals)
- Sudden temperature changes

Once the triggers are identified, the goal is to remove or reduce them. Removing the potential triggers from the school environment requires a collaborative effort with school nurses, teachers, administration, and custodial staff. It also involves compliance by the school body and their families. The AAAI (2003) has identified actions the school nurse can take to reduce environmental triggers. These are:

- Discourage keeping furred or feathered pets in classrooms.
- Discourage use of carpet and upholstered furniture in classrooms to decrease dust.
- Recommend that indoor humidity be reduced to less than 50%.
- Recommend that outdoor activities be limited when pollen counts are high.
- Recommend that the environment be kept clean and dust free.
- Recommend avoidance of smoke from wood burning stoves or camp fires.
- Recommend against using strong smelling cleansers and heavy perfumes.
- Recommend that grass is cut and pesticides sprayed when children are not in school.
- Recommend that heating and ventilation systems are cleaned regularly.
- Recommend to teachers that the child wear a scarf around his or her face during cold weather.
- Recommend to teachers that classroom windows should be kept closed when pollen counts are high.

(text continues on page 687)

Box 29.1 ■ ■ ■

STUDENT ASTHMA ACTION CARD

Name: ______________________ Grade: ________ Age: ______

Homeroom Teacher: ______________________ Room: ____________

Parent/Guardian Name: ______________________ Ph:(h): ____________

Address: ______________________ Ph:(w): ____________

Parent/Guardian Name: ______________________ Ph:(h): ____________

Address: ______________________ Ph:(w): ____________

Emergency Phone Contact #1 ____

Name Relationship Phone

Emergency Phone Contact #2 ____

Name Relationship Phone

Physician Treating Student for Asthma: ______________________ Ph: ____________

Other Physician: ______________________ Ph: ____________

EMERGENCY PLAN

Emergency action is necessary when the student has symptoms such as, ____________, ____________, ____________, ____________ or has a peak flow reading of ______________________.

- **Steps to take during an asthma episode:**
  1. Check peak flow.
  2. Give medications as listed below. Student should respond to treatment in 15–20 minutes.
  3. Contact parent/guardian if ____
  ____
  4. Re-check peak flow.
  5. Seek emergency medical care if the student has any of the following:
     - ✓ Coughs constantly
     - ✓ No improvement 15–20 minutes after initial treatment with medication and a relative cannot be reached.
     - ✓ Peak flow of ____________
     - ✓ Hard time breathing with:
       - Chest and neck pulled in with breathing
       - Stooped body posture
       - Struggling or gasping
     - ✓ Trouble walking or talking
     - ✓ Stops playing and can't start activity again
     - ✓ Lips or fingernails are grey or blue

IF THIS HAPPENS, GET EMERGENCY HELP NOW!

- **Emergency Asthma Medications**

	Name	Amount	When to Use
1.			
2.			
3.			
4.			

See reverse for more instructions

(Continued on the following page)

Box 29.1 ■■■

STUDENT ASTHMA ACTION CARD *(Continued)*

Daily Asthma Management Plan

- **Identify the things which start an asthma episode (Check each that applies to the student.)**

☐ Exercise
☐ Respiratory infections
☐ Change in temperature
☐ Animals
☐ Food ______________
☐ Strong odors or fumes
☐ Chalk dust/dust
☐ Carpets in the room
☐ Pollens
☐ Molds
☐ Other ______________

Comments ______________

- **Control of School Environment**

(List any environmental control measures, pre-medications, and/or dietary restrictions that the student needs to prevent an asthma episode.) ______________

- **Peak Flow Monitoring**

Personal Best Peak Flow number: ______________
Monitoring Times: ________ ________ ________ ________

- **Daily Medication Plan**

	Name	Amount	When to Use
1.			
2.			
3.			
4.			

Comments / Special Instructions

____

For Inhaled Medications

☐ I have instructed ______________ in the proper way to use his/her medications. It is my professional opinion that ______________ should be allowed to carry and use that medication by him/herself.

☐ It is my professional opinion that ________ should not carry his/her inhaled medication by him/herself.

______________ Physician Signature ______________ Date

______________ Parent/Guardian Signature ______________ Date

Asthma & Allergy Foundation of America • 1233 20th Street, N.W., Suite 402, Washington, DC 20036 • www.aafa.org • 1-800-7-ASTHMA

The school nurse has a significant role in assessment of indoor air quality, if necessary, and advocating for change. The Environmental Protection Agency (EPA) provides resources for schools in the assessment of indoor air quality and other potential asthmatic triggers. Much of the information can be downloaded from the EPA Web site, http://www.epa.gov/schools. The accommodations needed by the student should be identified and an accommodation plan developed. An example of an asthma accommodation plan for a student with asthma is in Chapter 9.

While non-allergy–related factors can trigger an asthma attack, it is essential for the school nurse and the school staff to be aware of the possibility. Therefore stress or strong emotions may stimulate hyperventilation and the initiation of an attack; stress-reducing measures (breathing exercises or distraction) may be appropriate to lessen the chance of an attack. Intense laughing or crying may also be the trigger for an attack. Again, awareness will promote earlier assessment and use of rescue treatments, if needed.

If students are more sensitive to cold, teachers may need to rethink outdoor recess, or modify the environment to protect the affected student. The student with upper respiratory infections may need increased vigilance on the part of the school nurse and teachers. This is another reason to educate students about the importance of hand washing and the prevention of illness. Students with asthma should be strongly encouraged to receive annual flu vaccine.

For students with **exercise-induced asthma**, multiple factors must be taken into consideration. Students who follow their asthma action plan and keep their asthma under good control can usually participate in all sports, even the most vigorous ones, including running around during recess. Allowing students with asthma to have convenient access to their medications is the key to participation in physical activity/sports/exercise. The other important component is to ensure that the student is compliant with his or her maintenance therapy; sport participation may be an incentive for these students. Sports that are more intense and sustained may provoke an asthma episode, but having access to medications and good asthma control should allow for full participation.

All sports coaches and trainers, as well as physical education teachers must be aware of what actions need to occur before the student participates in the activity, the symptoms that might indicate an attack, and the immediate actions that must be taken (see Box 29.2). Some students may benefit from using their inhalers 5 to 10 minutes before physical activity/sports/exercise, in addition to a warm-up period before more vigorous exercise. Each student is different and the key to good control is to have an up-to-date Asthma Action Plan for each student. Once permission from the parent/guardian is obtained, the student's action plan should be shared with the coach and physical education teacher.

Physical activity can be beneficial to the student with asthma. "With appropriate warm-up, pacing, hydration, and preventive pharmacologic therapy, almost all children with asthma will be able to participate in active school activities on a regular basis" (Kieckhefer & Ratcliff, 2004, p. 192). There are times when physical activities may need to be adjusted for any student with asthma, especially during their allergy season to outdoor allergens. These include:

- On a severe allergy day
- On an extremely windy day
- On an extremely cold day
- During and/or after an upper respiratory infection

Box 29.2 ■■■

QUICK REFERENCE SHEET FOR COACHES

- Have a copy of the student's Emergency Action Plan.
- Know where the rescue medications are kept.
- Allow the student to use his or her inhaled medication when needed.
  - Do not expect or require the student to "tough it out".
- Know the acute symptoms that require prompt action:
  - Coughing or wheezing
  - Difficulty breathing
  - Student reporting chest tightness
- Know when to **get Emergency Help**
  - If the student fails to improve
  - If the student is hunched over, with shoulders lifted and straining to breathe
  - If the student has difficulty completing a sentence without pausing for breath
  - If the student's lips or fingernails turn blue

(American College of Sports Medicine, 2000).

The school nurse must assume the role of advocate and change agent to ensure that the student gets the care he or she requires, including appropriate anti-inflammatory pharmacotherapy. Once diagnosed, the school nurse plays the role of detective in attempting to identify triggers. Perhaps most challenging is getting school administrators to initiate changes that will benefit the student. This requires teamwork, as the student will qualify for accommodations and the development of a 504 plan (see Chapter 14).

Pharmacological Measures

Pharmacological treatment focuses on inflammation control in order to regulate airflow obstruction and the associated symptoms. The control of inflammation can improve asthma control and normalize lung function (NAEPP, 2002). The goals of therapy are:

- No or minimal symptoms during the day and night
- No or minimal asthma exacerbations
- Minimal use of short-acting beta-2-agonists
- PEF (peak flow) > 80% of personal best
- Minimal adverse effects from medications
- Normal activities (including no school days missed)

The approach to pharmacological therapy follows the guidelines of the National Asthma Education and Prevention Program (USDHHS, 2003) and is based on the classification of asthma; it is a stepwise approach. Use of this approach is recommended in order to gain and maintain control of symptoms. The goal of the stepwise approach is to manage the student at a step in which control of symptoms is maintained. If symptoms are not managed at a particular step, pharmacological management at the next step would be instituted. Once the symptoms are controlled, management would be returned to the lowest step possible. While use of the step-wise approach is useful, management strategies should be reviewed as often as every 1 to 6 months. TABLE 29.4 presents the stepwise approach to asthma management.

Multiple categories of medications are used in treating asthma (see TABLE 29.5): quick relievers (also called rescue medications), nonsteroidal anti-inflammatory agents, inhaled corticosteroids, long-acting beta2-agonists, systemic corticosteroids, leukotriene modifiers, and methylxanthines. Because the underlying inflammation is so significant in the process, long term controllers are essential, with quick-acting rescue medication being used for acute symptoms caused by the bronchoconstriction (USDHHS, 2003). The long-term control medications are taken on a daily basis in order to achieve and maintain control of persistent asthma. It is important for the student to recognize that these medications need to be taken on a regular basis and should not be used to attain control of acute symptoms of asthma.

Quick-relief medications are taken to give rapid relief of acute symptoms of an asthma exacerbation by dilating the bronchial tree. These include short-acting beta-2 agonists, oral corticosteroids, and anti-cholinergics. The overuse of quick-relief medications may indicate poorly controlled asthma and requires reevaluation of the treatment plan. Furthermore, overuse is a risk factor associated with mortality from asthma. The school nurse should assess for excessive use of short-acting beta-2-agonists or lack of response when these medications are used for acute symptom management.

Inhaled corticosteroids are the preferred medications for long-term therapy for children over 5 years of age and adolescents who have persistent asthma. The use of inhaled corticosteroids improves asthma control when compared to use of short-acting beta2 agonists (USDHHS, 2003). The use of long-acting inhaled beta-2 agonists in combination with inhaled corticosteroids is the preferred therapy for moderate and severe persistent asthma.

Controversy exists over the use of steroids and their potential for growth velocity reduction. Overall, the data suggest that while the use of inhaled corticosteroids may have the potential of decreasing growth, "the effects are small, nonprogressive and may be reversible" (NAEPP, 2002). With this in mind, the school nurse should monitor the growth of students taking corticosteroids, every 3 to 4 months (AAAAI, 2000).

Leukotriene modifiers are alternative therapies for the treatment of persistent asthma. They may be used to treat mild persistent asthma or in combination with inhaled corticosteroids to treat moderate persistent asthma.

Medications to treat asthma are typically given by inhalation and the oral route. The inhaled route is preferred because higher concentrations of the medication can be delivered to the small airways (AAAAI, 2000). Furthermore, the systemic side effects of the medication are minimized. For the school-age student, inhaled medications using metered-dose inhalers (MDI), dry-powder inhalers (DPI), and nebulizers are the preferred routes of

(text continues on page 698)

Table 29.4 ■

STEPWISE APPROACH FOR MANAGING ASTHMA IN ADULTS AND CHILDREN OLDER THAN 5 YEARS OF AGE: TREATMENT

Classify Severity: Clinical Features Before Treatment or Adequate Control			***Medications Required to Maintain Long-Term Control***
	SYMPTOMS/DAY / **SYMPTOMS/NIGHT**	**PEF OR FEV_1** / **PEF VARIABILITY**	**DAILY MEDICATIONS**
Step 4 Severe Persistent	Continual / Frequent	≤ 60% / > 30%	• Preferred treatment: – High-dose inhaled corticosteroids AND – Long-acting inhaled $beta_2$-agonists AND, if needed, – Corticosteroid tablets or syrup long term (2 mg/kg/day, generally do not exceed 60 mg per day). (Make repeat attempts to reduce systemic corticosteroids and maintain control with high-dose inhaled corticosteroids.)
Step 3 Moderate Persistent	Daily / > 1 night/week	> 60% – < 80% / > 30%	• Preferred treatment: – Low-to-medium dose inhaled corticosteroids and long-acting inhaled $beta_2$-agonists. • Alternative treatment (listed alphabetically): – Increase inhaled corticosteroids within medium-dose range OR – Low-to-medium dose inhaled corticosteroids and either leukotriene modifier or theophylline. If needed (particularly in patients with recurring severe exacerbations): • Preferred treatment: – Increase inhaled corticosteroids within medium-dose range and add long-acting inhaled $beta_2$-agonists. • Alternative treatment (listed alphabetically): – Increase inhaled corticosteroids within medium-dose range and add either leukotriene modifier or theophylline.

(continued)

Table 29.4 ■ *(Continued)*

	SYMPTOMS/DAY SYMPTOMS/NIGHT	PEF OR FEV_1 PEF VARIABILITY	DAILY MEDICATIONS
Step 2 Mild Persistent	> 2/week but < 1 × /day > 2 nights/month	≥ 80% 20–30%	• Preferred treatment: – Low-dose inhaled corticosteroids. • Alternative treatment (listed alphabetically): cromolyn, leukotriene modifier, nedocromil, OR sustained release theophylline to serum concentration of 5–15 mcg/mL.
Step 1 Mild Intermittent	≤ 2 days/week ≤ 2 nights/month	≥ 80% < 20%	• No daily medication needed. • Severe exacerbations may occur, separated by long periods of normal lung function and no symptoms. A course of systemic corticosteroids is recommended.
Quick Relief All Patients	• Short-acting bronchodilator: 2–4 puffs short-acting inhaled $beta_2$-agonists as needed for symptoms. • Intensity of treatment will depend on severity of exacerbation; up to 3 treatments at 20-minute intervals or a single nebulizer treatment as needed. Course of systemic corticosteroids may be needed. • Use of short-acting $beta_2$-agonists >2 times a week in intermittent asthma (daily, or increasing use in persistent asthma) may indicate the need to initiate (increase) long-term control therapy.		

⇩ Step down
Review treatment every 1 to 6 months; a gradual stepwise reduction in treatment may be possible.

⇧ Step up
If control is not maintained, consider step up. First, review patient medication technique, adherence, and environmental control.

Goals of Therapy: Asthma Control

- Minimal or no chronic symptoms day or night
- Minimal or no exacerbations
- No limitations on activities; no school/work missed
- Maintain (near) normal pulmonary function
- Minimal use of short-acting inhaled $beta_2$-agonist (< 1x per day, < 1 canister/month)
- Minimal or no adverse effects from medications

Note

- The stepwise approach is meant to assist, not replace, the clinical decisionmaking required to meet individual patient needs.
- Classify severity: assign patient to most severe step in which any feature occurs (PEF is % of personal best; FEV_1 is % predicted).
- Gain control as quickly as possible (consider a short course of systemic corticosteroids); then step down to the least medication necessary to maintain control.
- Provide education on self-management and controlling environmental factors that make asthma worse (e.g., allergens and irritants).
- Refer to an asthma specialist if there are difficulties controlling asthma or if step 4 care is required. Referral may be considered if step 3 care is required.

Source: U.S. Department of Health and Human Services (2003).

Table 29.5a ■

USUAL DOSAGES FOR QUICK—RELIEF ASTHMA MEDICATIONS

MEDICATION	DOSAGE FORM	ADULT DOSE	CHILD DOSE*	COMMENTS
Short-Acting Inhaled Beta$_2$-Agonists				
	MDI			
Albuterol (Proventil, Ventolin) Albuterol HFA Pirbuterol (Maxair)	90 mcg/puff, 200 puffs 90 mcg/puff, 200 puffs 200 mcg/puff, 400 puffs	• 2 puffs 5 minutes prior to exercise • 2 puffs tid-qid prn	• 1–2 puffs 5 minutes prior to exercise • 2 puffs tid-qid prn	• An increasing use or lack of expected effect indicates diminished control of asthma. • Not generally recommended for long-term treatment. Regular use on a daily basis indicates the need for additional long-term-control therapy. • Differences in potency exist but all products are essentially comparable on a per puff basis. • May double usual dose for mild exacerbations. • Nonselective agents (i.e., epinephrine, isoproterenol, metaproterenol) are not recommended due to their potential for excessive cardiac stimulation, especially in high doses.
	DPI			
Albuterol Rotahaler	200 mcg/ capsule	1–2 capsules q 4–6 hours as needed and prior to exercise	1 capsule q 4–6 hours as needed and prior to exercise	
	Nebulizer solution			
Albuterol	5 mg/ml (0.5%) 2.5 mg/ml 1.25 mg/3 ml 0.63 mg/3 ml	1.25–5 mg in 3 cc of saline q 4–8 hours	0.05 mg/kg (min 1.25 mg, max 2.5 mg) in 3 cc of saline q 4–6 hours	May mix with cromolyn or ipratropium nebulizer solutions. May double dose for severe exacerbations.

(continued)

Table 29.5a ■ *(Continued)*

MEDICATION	DOSAGE FORM	ADULT DOSE	CHILD DOSE*	COMMENTS
	Nebulizer solution			
Bitolterol (Tornalate)	2 mg/ml (0.2%)	0.5–3.5 mg (0.25–1 cc) in 2–3 cc of saline q 4–8 hours	Not established	May not mix with other nebulizer solutions.
	Nebulizer solution			
Levalbuterol (Xopenex)	0.31 mg/3 ml 0.63 mg/3 ml 1.25 mg/3 ml	0.63 mg–2.5 mg q 4–8 hours	0.025 mg/kg (min. 0.63 mg, max. 1.25 mg) q 4–8 hours	0.63 mg of levalbuterol is equivalent in efficacy and side effects to 1.25 mg of racemic albuterol. The product is a sterile-filled preservative-free unit dose vial.
Anticholinergics				
	MDI			
Ipratropium Bromide (Atrovent)	18 mcg/puff, 200 puffs	2–3 puffs q 6 hours	1–2 puffs q 6 hours	Evidence is lacking for anticholinergics producing added benefit to beta$_2$-agonists in long-term-control asthma therapy.
	Nebulizer solution 0.25 mg/ml (0.025%)	0.25 mg q 6 hours	0.25–0.5 mg q 6 hours	
	MDI			
Ipratropium with albuterol (Combivent)	18 mcg/puff of ipratropium bromide and 90 mcg/puff of albuterol. 200 puffs/ canister	2–3 puffs q 6 hours	1–2 puffs q 8 hours	

(continued)

MEDICATION	DOSAGE FORM	ADULT DOSE	CHILD DOSE*	COMMENTS
	Nebulizer solution			
	0.5 mg/3 ml ipratropium bromide and 2.5 mg/3 ml albuterol	3 ml q 4–6 hours	1.5–3 ml q 8 hours	Contains EDTA to prevent discoloration of the solution. This additive does not induce bronchospasm.
Systemic Corticosteroids				
	(Applies to the first three corticosteroids)			
Methylprednisolone (Medrol)	2, 4, 6, 8, 16, 32 mg tablets	• Short course "burst": 40–60 mg/day as single or 2 divided doses for 3–10 days	• Short course "burst" 1–2 mg/kg/day, maximum 60 mg/day, for 3–10 days	• Short courses or "bursts" are effective for establishing control when initiating therapy or during a period of gradual deterioration. • The burst should be continued until patient achieves 80% PEF personal best or symptoms resolve. This usually requires 3–10 days but may require longer. There is no evidence that tapering the dose following improvement prevents relapse.
Prednisolone (Prelone, Pediapred)	5 mg tablets, 5 mg/5 cc, 15 mg/5 cc			
Prednisone	1, 2.5, 5, 10, 20, 50 mg tablets; 5 mg/cc, 5 mg/5 cc			
	Repository Injection			
(Methylprednisolone acetate)	40 mg/ml 80 mg/ml	240 mg IM once	7.5 mg/kg IM once	May be used in place of a short burst of oral steroids in patients who are vomiting or if adherence is a problem.

*Children ≤ 12 years of age.
Source: U.S. Department of Health and Human Services (2003, pp. 120–121).

Table 29.5b ■ ESTIMATED COMPARATIVE DAILY DOSAGES FOR INHALED CORTICOSTEROIDS

	Low Daily Dose		*Medium Daily Dose*		*High Daily Dose*	
DRUG	**ADULT**	**CHILD***	**ADULT**	**CHILD***	**ADULT**	**CHILD***
Beclomethasone CFC (Vanceril Beclovent Beconase) 42 or 84 mcg/puff	168–504 mcg	84–336 mcg	504–840 mcg	336–672 mcg	> 840 mcg	> 672 mcg
Beclomethasone HFA (Qvar) 40 or 80 mcg/puff	80–240 mcg	80–160 mcg	240–480 mcg	160–320 mcg	> 480 mcg	> 320 mcg
Budesonide DPI (Pulmicort) 200 mcg/ inhalation	200–600 mcg	200–400 mcg	600–1,200 mcg	400–800 mcg	> 1,200 mcg	> 800 mcg
Inhalation suspension for nebulization (child dose)		0.5 mg		1.0 mg		2.0 mg
Flunisolide (Aerobid) 250 mcg/puff	500–1,000 mcg	500–750 mcg	1,000–2,000 mcg	1,000–1,250 mcg	> 2,000 mcg	> 1,250 mcg
Fluticasone MDI (Flovent, Advair): 44, 110, or 220 mcg/puff	88–264 mcg	88–176 mcg	264–660 mcg	176–440 mcg	> 660 mcg	> 440 mcg
DPI: 50, 100, or 250 mcg/inhalation	100–300 mcg	100–200 mcg	300–600 mcg	200–400 mcg	> 600 mcg	> 400 mcg
Triamcinolone acetonide (Azmacort) 100 mcg/puff	400–1,000 mcg	400–800 mcg	1,000–2,000 mcg	800–1,200 mcg	> 2,000 mcg	> 1,200 mcg

*Children ≤ 12 years of age

Notes

- The most important determinant of appropriate dosing is the clinician's judgment of the patient's response to therapy. The clinician must monitor the patient's response on several clinical parameters and adjust the dose accordingly. The stepwise approach to therapy emphasizes that once control of asthma is achieved, the dose of medication should be carefully titrated to the minimum dose required to maintain control, thus reducing the potential for adverse effect.
- Comparative dosages in the EPR-2 were based on a limited number of published comparative clinical trials and extrapolation of differences in topical potency and lung delivery. This updated comparative dosage chart is based on review of recently published clnical trials involving more than 5,000 patients and published reviews. The key differences from the EPR-2 include a higher dosage of budesonide and recommendations for two newly available medications: beclomethasone HFA and budesonide suspension for nebulization. The rationale for these changes is summarized as follows:
  - The high dose is the dose that appears likely to be the threshold beyond which significant hypothalamic-pituitary-adrenal (HPA) axis suppression is produced, and, by extrapolation, the risk is increased for other clinically significant systemic effects if used for prolonged periods of time.
  - The low and medium dose reflects findings from dose-ranging studies in which incremental efficacy within the low-to-medium dose ranges was established without increased systemic effect as measured by overnight cortisol excretion. The studies demonstrated a relatively flat dose-response curve for efficacy at the medium-dose range; that is, increasing the dose to high-dose range did not significantly increase efficacy but did increase systemic effect.
  - The dose for budesonide dry powder inhaler (DPI) is based on recently available comparative data with other medications, rather than the comparison to budesonide metered-dose inhaler (MDI) that was used in the EPR-2. These new data, including a meta-analysis of seven studies, show that budesonide DPI is comparable to approximately one-half the microgram dose of fluticasone.
  - The dose for beclomethasone HFA is one-half the dose for beclomethasone CFC, based on studies demonstrating that the different pharmaceutical propeties of the medications result in enhanced lung delivery for the HFA (a less forceful spray from the HFA propellant and a reengineered nozzle that allows a smaller particle size).
  - The dose for budesonide nebulizer suspension is based on efficacy and safety studies, but no comparative studies with other inhaled corticosteroids are available. It is noted that the efficacy studies did not demonstrate a clear or consistent dose-response, although the high dose of 2.0 mg was effective in a placebo-controlled study in 40 infants with severe asthma. In a small open-label long-term safety study, the ACTH stimulated cortisols appeared lower in the 13 infants receiving the high dose of 2.0 mg budesonide compared to infants receiving lower doses, but this was not statistically significant due, perhaps, to the small study size.
- Some doses may be outside package labeling, especially in the high-dose range.
- MDI dosages are expressed as the actuater dose (the amount of the drug leaving the actuater and delivered to the patient), which is the labeling required in the United States. This is different from the dosage expressed as the valve dose (the amount of drug leaving the valve not all of which is available to the patient), which is used in many European countries and in some scientific literature. DPI doses are expressed as the amount of drug in the inhaler following activation.

Source: U.S. Department of Health and Human Services (2003, p. 119).

Table 29.5c ■

USUAL DOSAGES FOR LONG-TERM-CONTROL MEDICATIONS

MEDICATION	DOSAGE FORM	ADULT DOSE	CHILD DOSE*	COMMENTS
Inhaled Corticosteroids ***(See Estimated Comparative Daily Dosages for inhaled Corticosteroids)***				
Systemic Corticosteroids				
				(Applies to all three corticosteroids)
Methylprednisolone	2, 4, 8, 16, 32 mg tablets	7.5–60 mg daily in a single dose in a.m. or qod as needed for control	0.25–2 mg/kg daily in single dose in a.m. or qod as needed for control	• For long-term treatment of severe persistent asthma, administer single dose in a.m. either daily or on alternate days (alternate-day therapy may produce less adrenal suppression). If daily doses are required, one study suggests improved efficiency and no increase in adrenal suppression when administered at 3 p.m.
Prednisolone	5 mg tablets, 5 mg/5 cc, 15 mg/5 cc	Short-course "burst": to achieve control 40–60 mg per day as single or 2 divided doses for 3–10 days	Short-course "burst": 1–2 mg/kg/day, maximum 60 mg/day for 3–10 days	• Short courses or "bursts" are effective for establishing control when initiating therapy or during a period of gradual deterioration.
Prednisone	1, 2.5, 5, 10, 20, 50 mg tablets; 5 mg/cc, 5 mg/5 cc			• The burst should be continued until patient achieves 80% PEF personal best or symptoms resolve. This usually requires 3–10 days but may require longer. There is no evidence that tapering the dose following improvement prevents relapse.
Long-Acting Inhaled Beta$_2$-Agonists				
Salmeterol (Serevent)	MDI 21 mcg/puff DPI 50 mcg/blister	2 puffs q 12 hours 1 blister q 12 hours	1–2 puffs q 12 hours 1 blister q 12 hours	• Should not be used for symptom relief or exacerbations. Use with corticosteroids. • May use one dose nightly for symptoms.
Formoterol (Foradil)	DPI 12 mcg/ single-use capsule	1 capsule q 12 hours	1 capsule q 12 hours	• Efficacy and safety have not been studied in children <5 years of age.

(continued)

MEDICATION	DOSAGE FORM	ADULT DOSE	CHILD DOSE*	COMMENTS
				• Each capsule is for single use only; additional doses should not be administered for at least 12 hours. • Capsules should be used only with the Aerolizor™ inhaler and should not be taken orally.
Combined Medication				
Fluticasone/ Salmeterol	DPI 100 mcg. 250 mcg, or 500 mcg/50 mcg	1 inhalation bid; dose depends on severity of asthma	1 inhalation bid; dose depends on severity of asthma	• Not FDA approved in children <12 years of age. 100/50 for patient not controlled on low-to-medium dose inhaled corticosteroids. 250/50 for patients not controlled on medium-to-high dose inhaled corticosteroids.
Cromolyn and Nedocromil				
Cromolyn Sodium (Intal)	MDI 1 mg/ puff Nebulizer 20 mg/ampule	2–4 puffs tid-qid 1 ampule tid-qid	1–2 puffs tid-qid 1 ampule tid-qid	• One dose prior to exercise or allergen exposure provides effective prophylaxis for 1–2 hours.
Nedocromil Sodium (Tilade)	MDI 1.75 mg/puff	2–4 puffs bid-qid	1–2 puffs bid-qid	• See cromolyn above.
Leukotriene Modifiers				
Montelukast (Singulair)	4 mg or 5 mg chewable tablet 10 mg tablet	10 mg qhs	• 4 mg qhs (2–5 years of age) 5 mg qhs (6–14 years of age) 10 mg qhs (> 14 years of age)	• Montelukast exhibits a flat dose-response curve. Doses >10 mg will not produce a greater response in adults.
Zafirlukast (Accolate)	10 or 20 mg tablet	40 mg daily (20 mg tablet bid)	• 20 mg daily (7–11 years of age) (10 mg tablet bid)	• For zafirlukast, administration with meals decreases bioavailability: take at least 1 hour before or 2 hours after meals.
Zileuton (Zyflo)	300 or 600 mg tablet	2,400 mg daily (give tablets qid)		• For zileuton, monitor hepatic enzymes (ALT).

(continued)

Table 29.5c ■ (Continued)

MEDICATION	DOSAGE FORM	ADULT DOSE	CHILD DOSE*	COMMENTS
Methylxanthines				
Theophylline (Slo-Bid) (Theo-Dur)	Liquids, sustained-release tablets, and capsules	Starting dose 10 mg/kg/day up to 300 mg max; usual max 800 mg/day	Starting dose 10 mg/kg/day; usual max: • <1 year of age: 0.2 (age in weeks) + 5 = mg/kg/day • ≥1 year of age: 16 mg/kg/day	• Adjust dosage to achieve serum concentration of 5–15 mcg/mL at steady state (at least 48 hours on same dosage). • Due to wide interpatient variability in theophylline metabolic clearance, routine serum theophylline level monitoring is important.

*Children ≤12 years of age
Source: U.S. Department of Health and Human Services (2003, pp. 117–118).

administration. Many older than 5 years of age can use the MDI and DPI; however, because of the difficulty children have in coordinating the release of the medication from the MDI with breathing, the use of a spacer or holding chamber is recommended (AAAAI, 2000). In addition to making it easier to use the MDI, spacers decrease the oropharyngeal deposit of medication and possible side effects of the medication. Box 29.3 includes guidelines for the use of these delivery systems.

To assist the school nurse in assuring appropriate pharmacological management of asthma, the school should have a policy for the administration of medications. School health professionals, in conjunction with medical advisory committees, school boards, school superintendents and legal personnel, should be involved in the development of such guidelines. The National Association of School Nurses (2004) issued a position statement recommending that every school district assess its need for the school nurse to have a standing order for rescue medication, especially epinephrine. Further, NASN's 2002 issue brief indicated that "Children have the right to easily accessible quick relief inhalers, including the right to carry these inhalers and self-administer medications when developmentally able." (See Chapter 47.)

Peak Flow Monitoring

Peak flow monitoring, which primarily measures large airway functioning, helps determine how well a student's asthma is controlled. Peak flow monitoring measures pulmonary airflow; thus when airflow is obstructed, peak flow monitoring measures the extent of the obstruction. Each student should know his or her personal best peak flow and this baseline reading should be recorded in the student's asthma action plan. During an acute asthma attack, a peak flow reading can be compared to the personal best or baseline reading to provide some idea as to the severity of airway obstruction. To establish a student's personal best peak flow, the student needs to take his or her peak flow twice a day for 2 weeks (or every morning on awakening before using a short-acting bronchodilator), use the same peak flow meter, and measure at the same time each day (AAAAI, 2000). Ideal times for establishing a personal best record are mornings and early afternoon. The nurse should ensure the student's asthma is under good control while establishing this baseline information.

A peak flow monitoring program can help monitor the effectiveness of preventive medications,

(text continues on page 700)

Box 29.3 ▪▪▪

DIRECTIONS FOR USING METERED DOSE INHALER (MDI), DRY POWDER INHALERS (DPI), NEBULIZER, AND SPACERS

METERED DOSE INHALER

1. Remove the cap and shake the inhaler. (Contents crystallize and need to be shaken vigorously a few times so that each dose contains the right mixture of the medication.)
2. Hold the inhaler upright.
3. Tilt your head back slightly and breathe out all the way.
4. Use one of these methods:
   a. Open mouth with inhaler 1 to 2 inches away.
   b. Use a spacer or holding chamber (attached to the inhaler).
   c. Put inhaler in mouth and seal lips around the mouthpiece.
5. As you start breathing in slowly through your mouth, press down on the inhaler one time to release the medication.
   a. Breathe in slowly for 3 to 5 seconds, then hold your breath for 10 seconds (count slowly to 10) to allow the medicine to get to the lungs.
   b. For a spacer or holding chamber, press down on inhaler one time; within 5 seconds begin to breath in slowly as deeply as you can.
6. Wait ONE MINUTE before repeating the process for the next puff if the medicine is a quick-relief beta 2 agonist. This will allow the second dose to get even lower in the lung than the first dose.
7. Cleaning the inhaler: If there is powder in or around the hole, remove the metal canister from the L-shaped plastic mouthpiece. Rinse in warm water and let dry overnight. In the morning, put the canister back inside and put the cap on.
8. Check amount in canister: The number of puffs is listed on the canister. Figure out how many puffs you take each day and divide that number into the number of puffs in the canister. This tells you how many days the canister should last. Write the date on a new canister.

HOW TO USE A SPACER

(This device is especially helpful with younger children. It holds the medicine in the chamber so it can be inhaled in one or two slow deep breaths):

1. Shake canister well.
2. Attach the inhaler to the spacer or holding chamber.
3. Press the button on the inhaler so that one puff of medicine is pushed into the holding chamber.
4. Breath out.
5. Place the mouthpiece of the space in the mouth and inhale slowly.
6. Hold your breath for a few seconds and then exhale.
7. Repeat steps 5 and 6.
8. *To clean*: Remove back piece (but do not tamper with valve during cleaning). Soak both parts for 15 minutes in lukewarm water with liquid detergent. Agitate gently. Rinse in clean water. Shake out excess water (Do not rub dry). Air dry in vertical position.

DRY POWDER INHALER AEROLIZER

1. Remove one capsule from a blister card immediately before using.
2. Remove inhaler cover and twist mouthpiece open exposing the chamber. Place capsule in chamber and twist closed.
3. Hold aerolizer vertically with the open end up. Depress side buttons once, both at same time and listen for click. Release buttons.
4. Move aerolizer into horizontal position with buttons on the sides.
5. Exhale away from mouthpiece.
6. Tilt head back, place mouthpiece in mouth, close lips tightly and breathe in quickly and steadily.
7. Hold breath as long as possible…and then exhale.
8. Open inhaler to check if any powder remains in chamber; if it does, repeat steps 4 to 8 but do not push the buttons again.
9. Do NOT wash this device and do not swallow capsules.

(Continued on the following page)

Box 29.3 ■■■

DIRECTIONS FOR USING METERED DOSE INHALER (MDI), DRY POWDER INHALERS (DPI), NEBULIZER, AND SPACERS *(Continued)*

DPI DISKUS

1. Note number of doses that appears on the dose counter.
2. Keep inhaler in a horizontal position at all times; do not shake.
3. Place thumb in thumb rest and pull cover fully open until click is heard and mouthpiece is exposed.
4. Move lever back until click is heard.
5. Exhale away from mouthpiece.
6. Tilt head back, place mouthpiece in mouth, close lips tightly and breathe in quickly and steadily.
7. Hold breath as long as possible...and then exhale.

DPI TURBUHALER

1. Look for red dot in dose window. If it occurs, there are 20 or fewer doses remaining. When red dot is fully exposed at bottom of dose window, the device is empty.
2. Twist cover counterclockwise off inhaler while holding brown base.
3. Hold inhaler vertically; holding the base, grip and twist inhaler to right and then left until a click is heard.
4. Move Turbuhaler into horizontal position.
5. Exhale away from mouthpiece.
6. Tilt head back, put mouthpiece in mouth, close lips tightly, and breathe in quickly and steadily.
7. Remove from mouth and hold breath as long as possible...and then exhale.
8. Rinse mouth and spit after use.

NEBULIZER (USED FOR YOUNG CHILDREN WITH THE ASSISTANCE OF THE SCHOOL NURSE)

1. Measure correct dose of medication and place in the cup of the machine.
2. Fasten the mouthpiece to the T-shaped part and then fasten this unit to the cup.
3. Put mouthpiece in mouth. Seal lips tightly around it.
4. Turn on air compressor machine.
5. Take slow deep breaths in through the mouth.
6. Hold each breath 1 to 2 seconds before breathing out.
7. Continue until the medicine is gone from the cup (about 10 minutes).
8. Clean: remove mouthpiece and T-shaped part from cup and rinse in warm running water. Do not wash or rinse tubing. Shake off excess water and air dry on a clean paper towel.

determine how the student is responding to asthma treatments, identify an early warning sign of an asthma exacerbation for children older than 5 years of age, and provide evidence in seeking emergency treatment (AAAAI, 2003). Directions for use of peak flow meters are provided in Box 29.4.

A peak flow zone system is usually used to monitor control and determine pharmacological and, if needed, emergency action. A difference of greater than 20% from baseline data indicates poor control. Any time a student's peak flow level falls below 50% of the personal best reading, immediate action must be taken. This includes administration of the prescribed medication and calling 911 if the peak flow remains in the Red Zone level after taking the medication (AAAAI, 2003).

EDUCATION

The role of the school nurse includes education of students, parents, and faculty and staff. Teachers need to understand the disease process, the signs and symptoms of the disease, triggers for the individual student, and management of an asthma attack in order to be able to identify when a student is having difficulty (see Box 29.5). Coaches also need to have the same information as teachers and know

(text continues on page 702)

Box 29.4 ■ ■ ■

HOW TO USE A PEAK FLOW METER

Follow these steps:

1. Put the sliding marker or arrow at the bottom of the numbered scale.
2. Stand up straight.
3. Take a deep breath (as deep as you can). Put the mouthpiece of the Peak Flow Meter into your mouth and close your lips tightly around the mouthpiece. (Be sure to keep your tongue away from the mouthpiece.)
4. In one breath, blow out as hard and as fast as possible until you have emptied almost all of the air from your lungs.
5. Write down the number where the marker is.
6. Repeat steps 1 to 5 two more times and write down the numbers you get
7. Record the highest reading (NOT the average of the 3). This highest number is what is recorded in the daily log.
8. The number can then be compared to your personal best:
   a. Green Zone if it is 80% to 100% of your personal best
   b. Yellow Zone if it is 50% to 79% of your personal best
   c. Red Zone if it is below 50% of your personal best.
9. Check your Asthma Action Plan as to the action you should take based on your results.

Box 29.5 ■ ■ ■

LESSON PLAN FOR TEACHERS

OBJECTIVES	CONTENT	INSTRUCTIONAL STRATEGIES	EVALUATION
1. Teachers will describe what asthma is and what triggers an asthma attack.	Asthma is characterized by: • Airway inflammation • Airway hyperresponsiveness • Airway obstruction	Pictures of the respiratory system Handouts with lists of symptoms Have teachers breathe through a straw after running in place for 2 minutes	Teachers will complete a post-test with 100% accuracy
	Signs and symptoms of an asthma attack: • Wheezing • Tightness/pain in the chest • Coughing throughout the day • Difficult breathing and shortness of breath • Little energy	Case study of a child with asthma at recess on a cold, windy day	

(Continued on the following page)

Box 29.5 ■■■

LESSON PLAN FOR TEACHERS *(Continued)*

OBJECTIVES	CONTENT	INSTRUCTIONAL STRATEGIES	EVALUATION
	Triggers: • Mold, pollen, dander, feathers, dust • Respiratory infections, colds • Vigorous exercise • Exposure to cold • Fumes, strong odors • Excitement, stress	Examples of triggers in the school that may be in the school or classroom	
2. Teachers will list what needs to be done when a child is symptomatic.	Response to the signs and symptoms of an asthma attack: • Know where the child's rescue medication is kept • Allow the child to use the medication • If sent to the nurse's office, send another student along • If the nurse is not available and the medication is not working (wheeze, cough, or shortness of breath worsens), activate the emergency response system • Serious symptoms: trouble breathing, walking or talking, chest is sucked in with each breath, lips and fingernails are blue	Brainstorming about what would work in school, at recess, and on field trips	Teachers will complete a post-test with 100% accuracy.

who on the team has a diagnosis of asthma and what they should do if the student complains of symptoms. Arrangements should be made to allow the student immediate access to rescue medications for all sporting events, including practices. Both teachers and coaches need to be made aware that asthma is a serious disease that can result in death if not properly managed. In addition, classmates need to understand when to tell an adult that a student needs help and to reinforce that asthma is not contagious.

Parents may be overwhelmed with a child's diagnosis of asthma and may lack knowledge about the disease process, the manifestations of the disease, and the proper use of medications. Meeting with the parents at the time the Asthma Action Plan is developed in order to develop the Individualized Health Plan and then at least annually, are perfect times to assess the parents' knowledge level. Including the student in these meetings provides the school nurse with the opportunity to also assess the student's knowledge level and technique for medication administration.

Various resources are available for teaching students about asthma. The American Lung Association has updated the *Open Airways for Schools* program and it is available in English and Spanish. The program is geared to parents and children and provides six interactive, 40-minute sessions that are led by the school nurse or trained volunteers. The American Lung Association also provides *AsthmaBusters*, an on-line club (AsthmaBusters.org) for children ages 7 to 14 who have asthma. The STARBRIGHT Foundation also offers educational materials for students, including a CD-ROM game: *Quest for the Code*.

EMERGENCY MANAGEMENT

When a student presents with symptoms that indicate respiratory distress or complaints of chest tightness, the school nurse should respond immediately. Assess the respiratory status for degree of distress (coughing, wheezing, shortness of breath, tachypnea, retractions, decreased breath sounds, circumoral cyanosis, tachycardia, agitation, exercise intolerance, orthopnea, inability to talk (number of breaths needed to complete sentence), increased use of short-acting bronchodilators, and decreased PEF into the yellow or red zones).

During an acute exacerbation, the school nurse should consult the student's asthma action plan and administer a quick relief medication, usually a short-acting beta-2 agonist, such as albuterol. Prior to administering the medication, the student's peak flow reading should be taken, although this may not be possible if the student is in respiratory distress. Position the student in an upright position that will allow for ease of breathing. The child should also be encouraged to take slow, deep breaths. If the distress remains severe and the student does not respond to the medication within 20 to 30 minutes, or as directed by the Asthma Action Plan, emergency care should be sought. Note: asthma and allergy may be present simultaneously; an anaphylactic reaction may appear as an asthma attack and an Epi-Pen may be needed (see Chapter 28).

CONCLUSION

Asthma management is an ideal example of how the Coordinated School Health Model (Chapter 3) can be effective. It involves not only health services in school and through the healthcare provider, but also includes managing the environment to be asthma-friendly, providing health education to students and staff, involving the community and family, promoting physical activity with safety measures insured, advocating for the rights of students by making appropriate accommodations, and assuring that students have emotional support as they cope with a chronic condition (CDC, 2002b).

The student with asthma can have a positive experience in school with limited interruptions from a chronic health problem if there is collaboration and cooperation of students, parents, school nurses, teachers and administrators. The school nurse is in the unique position to coordinate this effort and ensure its success.

Resources

Allergy and Asthma Network/Mothers of Asthmatics, Inc.—resources related to asthma especially geared to children and parents
http://www.aanma.org

American Academy of Allergy, Asthma, and Immunology—source for current information and tools for education
http://www.aaaai.org

American Academy of Pediatrics—source for information on asthma and children
http://www.aap.org

American Camping Association—information about camps for children with special healthcare needs
http://www.acacamps.org

American Lung Association—source for *Open airways for schools, an education program for students with asthma* and The School Nurse Tool Kit
http://www.lungusa.org/school

Asthma and Allergy Foundation of America—source for educational materials for the school
http://www.aafa.org

Centers for Disease Control—statistical data and information related to asthma
http://www.cdc.gov/asthma

Environmental Protection Agency—a source for information related to assessment and management of indoor air quality
http://www.epa.gov/schools

National Association of School Nurses—source for educational materials related to asthma
http://www.nasn.org

National Asthma Education and Prevention Program-Expert Panel Report—updated guidelines for asthma
http://www.nhlbi.nih.gov/guidelines/asthma

National Heart, Lung and Blood Institute—a source for the most current information related to asthma
http://www.nhlbi.nih.gov

SchoolAsthmaAllergy.com for those caring for school-age children with asthma and allergy
http://www.schoolasthmaallergy.com

STARBRIGHT Foundation—nonprofit organization that provides information to children, parents, professionals about chronic illnesses
http://www.starbright.org

References

American Academy of Allergy, Asthma and Immunology (AAAAI). (2000). *The Allergy Report: Diseases of the atopic diathesis* (Vol. 2). Milwaukee, WI: AAAAI.

American Academy of Allergy, Asthma and Immunology (AAAAI). (2003). *School nurse tool kit*. Retrieved on

August 15, 2003 from http://www.aaaai.org/members/allied- health/tool-kit

American College of Sports Medicine (2000). *Exercise-induced asthma*. Retrieved November 19, 2003, from http://www.acsm.org/health+fitness/pdf/currentcomments/EIA.pdf

American Lung Association (2003). *Report on the results of the Asthma Awareness Survey*. Retrieved on October 6, 2003 from http://www.lungusa.org/press/asthma/asthma-091003.html

Baker, V., Friedman, J., & Schmitt, R. (2002). Asthma management: Part I: An overview of the problem and current trends. *Journal of School Nursing, 18*(3), 128–137.

Brashers, V. (2002). Alterations of Pulmonary Function. In K. McCance & S. Huether (Eds.), *Pathophysiology: The biologic basis for disease in adults and children* (pp. 1105–1144). St. Louis: C. V. Mosby.

Burns, C. E., Brady, M. A., Dunn, A. M., & Starr, N. B. (2000). *Pediatric primary care. A handbook for nurse practitioners.* Philadelphia: W. B. Saunders.

Centers for Disease Control and Prevention (CDC). (2002a). Surveillance for Asthma— United States, 1980–1999. *Morbidity and Mortality Weekly Report, 51*(SS-1), 1–13.

Centers for Disease Control and Prevention (CDC). (2002b). *Strategies for addressing asthma within a coordinated school health program*. Atlanta: CDC.

Gern, J., & Lemanske, R. (2003). Infectious triggers of pediatric asthma. *The Pediatric Clinics of North America, 50*(3), 555–576.

Centers for Disease Control and Prevention (CDC). (2004a). *Summary health statistics for U.S. children: National Health Interview Survey, 2002*. Series 10, Number 221. Hyattsville MD: U.S. Department of Health and Human Services. Retrieved September 10, 2005 from http://www.cdc.gov/nchs/data/series/sr_10/sr10_221.pdf

Centers for Disease Control and Prevention. (2004b). *Addressing asthma in schools*. U.S. Department of Health and Human Services. Retrieved December 2004 from http://www.cdc.gov/HealthyYouth/Asthma

Centers for Disease Control and Prevention. (2005). Self-reported asthma among high school students—United States, 2003. *Morbidity and Mortality Weekly Report, 54*(31), 765–767.

Guilbert, T., & Krawiec, M. (2003). Natural history of asthma. *The Pediatric Clinics of North America, 50*(3), 523–538.

Kelly, H. (2003). The assessment of childhood asthma. *The Pediatric Clinics of North America, 50*(3), 593–608.

Kieckhefer, G., & Ratcliffe, M. (2004). Asthma. In P. Jackson Allen & J. Vessey (Eds.), *Primary care of the child with a chronic condition* (pp. 174–197). St. Louis: C. V. Mosby.

National Association of School Nurses (NASN). (2002). *Issue brief. Asthma management in the school setting*. Retrieved September 10, 2005 from http://www.nasn.org

National Association of School Nurses (NASN). (2004). *Position statement: Rescue medications in school*. Retrieved September 10, 2005 from http://www.nasn.org/positions/2004rescuemeds.htm

National Asthma Education and Prevention Program Expert Panel Report. (2002). Guidelines for the diagnosis and management of asthma: Update on selected topics. *Journal of Allergy and Clinical Immunology, 110*(5), S141–220.

Porth. C. (2005). *Pathophysiology: Concepts of altered health states*. Philadelphia: Lippincott Williams & Wilkins.

Reilly, D. (2000). *Managing asthma triggers training manual*. Scarborough, ME: National Association of School Nurses.

Sheth, K. (2003). Activity-induced asthma. *Pediatric Clinics of North America, 50*(3), 697–716.

U.S. Department of Health and Human Services (USDHHS), Office of Disease Prevention and Health Promotion (2000). *Healthy People 2010*. Washington, DC: USDHHS.

U.S. Department of Health and Human Services (USDHHS). (2003). *Expert panel report: Guidelines for the diagnosis and management of asthma*. Update on selected topics 2002. NIH publication No. 02–5074.

Chapter 30

Attention Deficit Hyperactivity Disorder and Learning Disabilities

JANICE SELEKMAN

Chapter Outline

INTRODUCTION

The condition that is now known as attention deficit hyperactivity disorder (ADHD) has been known by many names over the past 100 years. A German physician wrote a poem in 1854 called "Fidgety Phil" in which hyperactivity is described ("…he turns and churns, he wiggles and jiggles…"); the identified problem was behavior and the implied treatment was discipline (Wender, 2000). In 1902, Still described a correlation between learning and attentional problems (Stubbe, 2000). The problem behaviors described were aggression, defiance, resistance to discipline, and overactivity.

In the 1920s, the condition was called postencephalitic behavior disorder when a correlation was made that children who had recovered from encephalitis often developed behavior problems that impacted on attention and learning. Names then changed to minimal brain damage, minimal brain dysfunction, and hyperkinetic reaction to childhood. During the 1930s, the first report on the efficacy of amphetamine in treating these children was published, and in 1956, methylphenidate was developed (Wilens & Spencer, 2000). In 1980, the name was changed to attention deficit disorder (ADD) with and without hyperactivity and in 1987 to its current name of ADHD. Many families continue to use the term ADD rather than ADHD, but ADHD is the accepted terminology.

The term *learning disabilities* (LDs) was first defined in 1963. According to the *Diagnostic and Statistical Manual of Mental Disorders*, fourth edition (DSM-IV), LD is categorized as a "learning disorder"; ADHD is in a category called "Attention-Deficit and Disruptive Behavior Disorders" (American Psychiatric Association [APA], 2000). There is great heterogeneity in both conditions, so that the signs and symptoms vary among different individuals and neither is considered a single entity. Up through the 1980s, these two conditions were often merged together in the literature and the terms were used interchangeably. This accounts for much of the confusion about how they differ. Only in the late 1980s was a clear distinction made between the two conditions. "A Learning Disability affects the student's ability to process and use information, thus interfering with his or her ability to learn. ADHD results in behaviors that make it difficult for the student to sit, attend, or reflect, thus interfering with the student's availability to learn" (Silver, 1999, p. 10). This is a crucial distinction when it comes to the law and the student's rights related to education.

DEFINITION AND DIAGNOSTIC CRITERIA FOR ADHD

According to the DSM-IV, ADHD is defined as "a persistent pattern of inattention and/or hyperactivity–impulsivity that is more frequent and severe than is typically observed in individuals at a comparable level of development.... These manifestations occur in all facets of a child's life and frequently worsen in situations requiring sustained attention" (APA, 2000, p. 85). There are four subtypes: predominantly inattentive, predominantly hyperactive– impulsive, a combined subtype, and a category called ADHD Not Otherwise Specified.

Nine characteristics are listed by the DSM-IV for both the inattention and hyperactivity-impulsivity categories (Box 30.1). To be diagnosed with ADHD, an individual must have at least six of the nine characteristics in a category. If an individual has at least six in each category, he or she is considered to have the combined type of ADHD. Symptoms must be present for at least 6 months to a degree that is maladaptive and inconsistent with the child's developmental level. Some impairment must be seen before the age of 7 and some impairment must be seen in two or more settings. This means that the child who is described as fine at home but having symptoms of ADHD at school (or vice versa) may not have the condition.

Box 30.1 ■ ■ ■

DIAGNOSTIC CRITERIA FOR ATTENTION DEFICIT HYPERACTIVITY DISORDER

I. Either A or B
   A. Six (or more) of the following symptoms of **INATTENTION** have persisted for at least 6 months to a degree that is maladaptive and inconsistent with developmental level:
      1. Often fails to give close attention to details or makes careless mistakes in schoolwork, work, or other activities.
      2. Often has difficulty sustaining attention in tasks or play activities.
      3. Often does not seem to listen when spoken to directly.
      4. Often does not follow through on instructions and fails to finish schoolwork, chores, or duties in the workplace (not due to oppositional behavior or failure to understand instructions).
      5. Often has difficulty organizing tasks and activities.
      6. Often avoids, dislikes, or is reluctant to engage in tasks that require sustained mental effort (e.g., schoolwork or homework).
      7. Often loses things necessary for tasks or activities (e.g., toys, school assignments, pencils, books, or tools).
      8. Is often easily distracted by extraneous stimuli.
      9. Is often forgetful in daily activities.
   B. Six (or more) of the following symptoms of **Hyperactivity–Impulsivity** have persisted for at least 6 months to a degree that is maladaptive and inconsistent with developmental level.

      Hyperactivity:
      1. Often fidgets with hands or feet or squirms in seat.
      2. Often leaves seat in classroom or in other situations in which remaining seated is expected.
      3. Often runs about or climbs excessively in situations in which it is inappropriate (in adolescents or adults, may be limited to subjective feelings of restlessness).

4. Often has difficulty playing or engaging in leisure activities quietly.
5. Is often "on the go" or often acts "as if driven by a motor."
6. Often talks excessively.

Impulsivity:

7. Often blurts out answers before questions have been completed.
8. Often has difficulty awaiting turn.
9. Often interrupts or intrudes on others (e.g., butts into conversations or games).

II. Some hyperactive–impulsive or inattentive symptoms that caused impairment present before age 7 years.

III. Some impairment from the symptoms present in two or more settings (e.g., at school or work and at home).

IV. Clear evidence of clinically significant impairment in social, academic, or occupational functioning

V. Symptoms do not occur exclusively during the course of a pervasive developmental disorder, schizophrenia, or other psychotic disorder and are not better accounted for by another mental (e.g., mood disorder, anxiety disorder, dissociative disorder, or a personality disorder).

(American Psychiatric Association, 2000, pp. 92–93)

Those who manifest some of the symptoms but do not meet all of the criteria are often considered under the category "ADHD Not Otherwise Specified." This category is more common for those diagnosed as older adolescents or adults who cannot document symptoms before the age of 7 and who may have variations of the symptoms, such as daydreaming and hypoactivity (APA, 2000). Symptoms of ADHD cannot be due to other psychiatric conditions and are in no way related to a child's intelligence quotient (IQ). ADHD is a nonprogressive condition. The manifestations occur in all facets of a child's life and frequently worsen in situations requiring sustained attention, such as a school setting.

There is a major belief that the core deficit of ADHD is both a lack of inhibition of behavior and impaired "executive functioning"; the latter includes the ability to organize and analyze information that is presented, prioritize the information, make a plan based on the information, and complete the task in a timely manner (Barkley, 2000). Most believe that ADHD is a neurodevelopmental rather than a psychiatric condition (Accardo & Blondis, 2000a). It may be found that ADHD is actually more than one condition.

The diagnosis of ADHD is purely clinical and is one of exclusion. There is no definitive test, although research is in progress to attempt to develop a neurological scan that can assist in the diagnosis. "To date, no individually administered test or group of tests has demonstrated an acceptable degree of ecological validity to be helpful in the diagnostic process" (DuPaul & Stoner, 2003, p. 29). A developmental history is essential in the diagnostic process to help identify alternative and additional conditions. The diagnosis for a majority of students with ADHD is based on difficulties experienced in a structured school setting, with the average age at diagnosis being 9.8 for the inattentive form and 8.5 for the combined (Carlson & Mann, 2000). The school nurse should play a significant role in the diagnostic process. She can be an independent observer of the student's behavior on more than one occasion in both structured and unstructured activities and can also assist in ruling out other causes for the behavioral characteristics. While the school nurse has a significant knowledge base related to normal growth and development and would be a wonderful asset in behavioral assessments of students, it is recognized that many school nurses do not have the time to engage in this diagnostic activity.

The diagnostic process starts with a complete physical including a developmental history, a history of medications used, and information about the home environment and living arrangements. A number of rating scales (TABLE 30.1) are used to assist in the diagnosis, most of which have both a teacher and parent variation and compare the student to his or her same-age peers as well as measuring symptom frequency. As long as the rating scales identify the 18 criteria from the DSM-IV and are used consistently, they can be used to evaluate the student on an intermittent basis to determine symptomatology and efficacy of treatment modalities. Inattention cannot be measured directly; therefore the evaluator infers it. However, it is estimated that in the population of those with ADHD, the inattentive form makes up 35% to 50% of the cases (Buitelaar, 2002).

Many of the behaviors on the checklists are commonly seen in all students intermittently. The ability to pay attention, have impulse control, and control activity all mature with age. Therefore, it is not just "the presence of these behaviors, but their intensity, their time courses, and their negative impact on other areas of behavior and functioning

Table 30.1 ■

SELECTED BEHAVIOR RATING SCALES FOR SCREENING FOR ADHD AND THE EFFICACY OF TREATMENT

BEHAVIOR RATING SCALE	AGES FOR WHICH VALIDITY IS ESTABLISHED	REASON TO USE
Achenbach's Child Behavior Check List	4–18	To assess for concurrent psychosocial problems
Attention Deficit/Hyperactivity Disorder Rating Scale IV	5–18	To diagnose and monitor
Conners Rating Scales	3–17	To diagnose and monitor
Attention Deficit Disorder–Hyperactivity Comprehensive Teacher Rating Scale (ACTeRs)	5–13	To monitor progress
Attention Deficit Disorder Evaluation Scale (ADDES)	5–18	To monitor
Behavior Assessment System for Children (BASC-PRS)	4–18	To assess for emotional and behavioral disorders

Most have parent and teacher rating scale versions; some also have self assessments.
Source: Selekman and Moore (2004).

that compel a diagnosis of Attention Deficit Hyperactivity Disorder" (Accardo & Blondis, 2000a, p. 11). Input from both parents and teachers is essential to the diagnostic process (American Academy of Pediatrics [AAP], 2004). Report cards and other information provided by the school counselor, reports of vision and hearing screening by the school nurse, as well as any history of abuse are necessary information for the evaluator.

Possible differential diagnoses include seizure disorders, especially absence seizures; sensory disorders, such as vision and auditory deficits; thyroid abnormalities; learning disabilities; mental retardation; brain tumor; lead poisoning; family disruption, such as in abuse, neglect, and parental separation; and multiple other psychiatric conditions. The intermittent inattentiveness or increased motor activity of a student with hypoglycemia, significant allergies, pruritis, the side effects of allergy medication, or who has skipped breakfast may also produce the symptoms seen in ADHD. The school nurse should also pay particular attention to those students with a high accident rate, high impulsivity in unsafe situations, a history of insufficient sleep, and persistent discipline problems.

Issue: The teacher indicates to the school nurse that she thinks a student has ADHD. She repeatedly sends the student to the principal's office or to the nurse for "not listening" in the classroom and disrupting the class. The principal wants the parents to medicate the child. What are the issues?

1. Teachers are *not* qualified to diagnose ADHD. However, their input is important and they may be asked to participate in the diagnostic process by being asked to fill out behavior rating scales on the student periodically.
2. Teachers and principals *may not* require the use of medication by a student as a condition of returning to the classroom. They do not

have the medical knowledge or authority to determine medical treatments.

3. School nurses also do not usually have the diagnostic background to diagnose ADHD. Their role is to refer the family to an appropriate source. Some school districts do not want the school nurse to make a referral for ADHD to the school psychologist. Therefore, a line that can be used by the school nurse with the parents is as follows: "The next time you see your child's doctor, you may want to mention that your child is exhibiting the following symptoms at school. These include… If the child is also demonstrating these signs at home, you may want to mention that as well."
4. The student needs to be evaluated by medical personnel qualified to diagnose ADHD, such as a child psychologist or a developmental pediatrician.
5. For the Federal law regulations, see Chapter 14.

DEFINITION AND DIAGNOSTIC CRITERIA FOR LEARNING DISABILITIES

LDs are defined in different ways, as both the definition and the criteria for LDs are controversial. The term was first used in 1963 and a definition was developed by the National Joint Committee on Learning Disabilities in 1997. It states that LDs refer to "a heterogeneous group of disorders manifested by significant difficulties in the acquisition and use of listening, speaking, reading, writing, reasoning, or mathematical skills."

Federal legislation defines a learning disability as a "disorder in one or more of the basic psychological processes involved in understanding or in using language, spoken or written, which…may manifest itself in an imperfect ability to listen, read, write, spell or do mathematical calculations" (Individuals with Disabilities Education Act Amendments [IDEA], 1997, p. 13). It includes dyslexia, learning problems resulting from brain injury, aphasia, and perceptual disabilities. It does not include learning problems that result from vision and hearing deficits, mental retardation, motor handicaps, or other psychiatric or emotional disturbances. Thus, an individual must have at least a normal IQ to be diagnosed with an LD. The learning problems can also not be due to the educational environment, the individual's culture, or economic disadvantage (IDEA, 1997). It should be noted that learning problems are not necessarily learning disabilities.

A third definition of LDs comes from the DSM-IV. It states that LD is a disorder "characterized by academic functioning that is substantially below that expected given the person's chronological age, measured intelligence, and age-appropriate education" (APA, 2000, p. 49). The DSM-IV presents LD only as a deficit in academic functioning. The four types identified are the following: (1) reading disorders (which include dyslexia), (2) mathematics disorders, (3) disorders of written expression, and (4) learning disorders not otherwise specified. This last category is for any individuals with learning problems who do not fit into the first three.

While the schools use these categories, school nurses know that learning as well as social interactions continue throughout the day, whether or not the student is in school. Therefore, another way to consider LDs is to view them according to the functions of the central nervous system in its sensory/receptive, integrative, motor/expressive, and diffuse roles (Selekman, 2002b).

Sensory–Receptive Deficits

These sensory processing disabilities involve difficulty in processing and/or interpreting information received by one of the senses. These include visual perceptual deficits, auditory perceptual deficits, and tactile perceptual deficits. *Visual perceptual deficits* do not result from difficulty with vision, but rather with the brain's ability to interpret what is seen. This may manifest itself as (1) dyslexia, where letters or words are reversed; (2) difficulty copying or matching; (3) difficulty differentiating a figure from the background; (4) difficulty judging distance and speed; (5) difficulty reading social signals, such as facial expressions; (6) the inability to track a sentence across the line, resulting in reading part of one line and part of the next; and (7) difficulty with visual memory and symbols, such as remembering which keys on the piano go with which notes on the page or learning foreign languages when the letters are not written using the English alphabet (Selekman, 2002b). It is certainly the responsibility of the school nurse to check the student's visual acuity to rule out the need for eyeglasses.

Auditory perceptual deficit is also not a hearing deficit, although it is a responsibility of the school nurse to check students' hearing acuity and refer to appropriate practitioners if a problem appears to exist. It is a problem with how the brain interprets what it hears. Signs of this deficit may be difficulty

(1) differentiating the sounds of words or notes (b and d may sound the same); (2) reciting from memory; (3) differentiating a sound from the noise of the background; (4) interpreting the tone of voice of the speaker; and (5) following oral directions, especially those that involve multiple steps (Selekman, 2002b).

Students with *tactile perceptual* deficits may have difficulty with interpreting the cues that indicate the need to void or defecate or the sensations related to the initiation of one's monthly menses. A student with this deficit who also has asthma may be unaware of the initial sensations of dyspnea in order to take early measures to stop an attack. As with the student with ADHD, they may also be hypersensitive to certain fabrics against their skin or the tags on their clothes (Silver, 1999).

Integrative Deficits

Once the stimuli get to the brain, they must be processed and stored so that they can be retrieved if needed. Individuals with this type of deficit have difficulty with such cognitive functions as (1) sequencing, (2) problem solving and analyzing information in order to develop a plan, (3) organizing and prioritizing, (4) abstract thought, and (5) concepts of science and math (Smith, 2002), including dyscalculia and the concepts of parts and whole, distance, time, and cause/effect. Students with this type of deficit may have a poor sense of direction and get lost easily. They are limited in the general knowledge they process from the environment. They also have difficulty understanding jokes or interpreting sarcasm and teasing; these may certainly interfere with social relationships.

Motor/Expressive Deficits

Deficits in hand–eye coordination may be evident in dysgraphia, or difficulty writing, especially within a certain space. Students may have "sloppy" handwriting; they may have difficulty lining up rows of numbers; and may not do well in activities that require hand–eye motor skills, such as hitting a ball. They also may be identified as being "clumsy" as they attempt motor activities. A student with diffuse learning disabilities has characteristics from more than one category.

There is no single test that is best to diagnose LDs. Contrary to the list of symptoms for ADHD, there is no list of characteristic behaviors that assist in diagnosing a learning disability. LDs can be diagnosed by psychometric and psychological testing on multiple parameters, most often the Wechsler Intelligence Scale for Children (WISC) and the Wechsler Individual Achievement Tests (WIAT). These measure general intelligence or cognitive functioning and also have verbal and performance (motor) scales, each of which has multiple subtests.

One of the keys in diagnosis is to find inconsistencies in performance among and between the components of the scales and subtests of the WISC (Fletcher, Shaywitz, & Shaywitz, 1999). Typically, the condition is diagnosed by demonstrating a "*significant* discrepancy between a measure of intelligence (i.e., IQ score) and the student's academic ability as measured by a standard achievement test" (Pliszka, Carlson, & Swanson, 1999, p. 189). It is actually the definition of the word "significant" that causes variation from state to state and from one school district to another regarding whether or not a student is diagnosed as having an LD. "The most widely accepted criterion for determination of LD calls for a difference of at least 22 points or 1.5 standard deviations between intelligence test scores and achievement test scores" (Mather & Goldstein, 2001, p. 39). However, different states have different cutoff points. Therefore, it is possible for two students to have the same scores on testing, but only one to be diagnosed as LD. It should be remembered that intellectually gifted children might also have an LD. Although often not identified because they have not failed in school, they still may demonstrate a significant difference in scores between IQ and performance and deserve the same services as for other children with LDs. Often, they are denied the services they need, resulting in behavior problems (Montgomery, 2003).

LDs can be diagnosed at any point in the life span. There is no minimum or maximum age by which someone must be identified as having an LD. Some LDs may not become apparent until course material becomes more complex and more abstract. Because individuals with LD have at least a normal IQ, they can learn; they just learn differently (Selekman, 2002b).

INCIDENCE

ADHD has been identified as the most common neurobehavioral disorder of childhood, yet learning disabilities are more common. In the 1990s, it was estimated that 3% to 5% had ADHD and 5% to 10% of children and adolescents had a learning disability. The literature now indicates that the prevalence rates range from 5% to 17.8% for ADHD, with most now indicating that the prevalence is between 5% and 10% of children between 5 and 18 years of age (Buitelaar, 2002). While the hyperactive–impulsive type is the least common form of ADHD, it is diagnosed more in younger children (McBurnett, Pfiffner, & Ottolini, 2000).

Some indicate that the prevalence of LDs may be 10% to 20% (MacMillan, Gresham, & Bocian, 1998; Turkington & Harris, 2002). A study by the Centers for Disease Control (CDC) found that 7% of children 6 to 11 years of age were diagnosed with ADHD and 8% were diagnosed with an LD (Pastor & Reuben, 2002). Turkington and Harris (2002) indicate that 120,000 children are diagnosed each year with an LD, and thousands more are not diagnosed or identified. Those with ADHD account for 4% of physician visits by children and up to 50% of child mental health clinic populations (Stubbe, 2000). Therefore, it is estimated that there are two students with LD and/ or ADHD in every classroom.

Children with LDs make up the largest category for special education programs under IDEA (Hallahan & Keogh, 2001). The U.S. Department of Education estimates that 2.8 million students in the United States are currently receiving special education services for learning disabilities (National Center for Learning Disabilities, 2002). Since many children with ADHD are not receiving special education services, it is estimated that approximately 4.5 to 9 million children and adolescents in the United States have either LD or ADHD (U.S. Department of Health and Human Services, 2002). Fifty-four percent of students receiving special education services through the public schools are identified as having LDs (Pastor & Reuben, 2002). The prevalence of ADHD appears to decrease somewhat with age after the elementary grades (NIH Consensus Statement, 1998).

The male/female ratio for ADHD is approximately 3:1, with a larger percentage of males having the hyperactive–impulsive form and a larger percentage of females having the inattentive form (Solanto, 2001). The incidence of LD ranges from being similar in males and females (Pastor & Reuben, 2002) to being twice as common in males (Sousa, 2001). Those with the inattentive form of ADHD (primarily females) have fewer conduct problems but are more likely to exhibit depression and anxiety.

Both LDs and ADHD are seen in all cultural groups. While the percentage of students with LDs does not vary significantly by race or ethnicity, ADHD is more commonly diagnosed in Caucasian children than in other groups (Pastor & Reuben, 2002).

ETIOLOGY

While there are many proposed causes of ADHD, the two primary areas of study are neurological function and genetics. The neurological causes are divided into the neurobiological and the neuroanatomical. The neurobiological hypothesis focuses on the dysregulation of neurotransmitters; these include the catecholamines dopamine, epinephrine, norepinephrine, and possibly serotonin (Anastopoulos & Shelton, 2001). Because most of the medications with proven efficacy for ADHD stimulate receptors to increase dopamine release and inhibit reuptake of neurotransmitters, deficits in this system seem to be supported as one of the primary causes of ADHD (Barkley, 2000). It is thought that a deficit in the amount of available catecholamines interferes with one's ability to hold onto a task, such as attention (Solanto, 2001).

The prefrontal cortex is the neuroanatomical site that is rich in dopamine receptors and is responsible for inhibiting behavior and regulating attention. It is referred to as the executive control center and is the site that assists in planning, problem solving, higher order thinking, and emotional restraint (Sousa, 2001). In some studies, the frontal lobes have been found to be smaller and have decreased blood flow in children with ADHD compared to controls (Castellanos 2001; Spencer, Biederman, & Wilens, 2002). Stimulant medications appear to increase the blood flow to this area, thus allowing normal brain function (Anastopoulos & Shelton, 2001).

ADHD is thought to be transmitted genetically from parent to child in at least 50% of all cases, possibly by an autosomal dominant transmission with reduced penetrance (Solanto, 2001). While the condition is probably polygenic, there appears to be up to an 82% concordance rate for monozygotic twins and 37.9% concordance rate for dizygotic twins (Anastopoulos & Shelton, 2001; Solanto, 2001). "Siblings of children with ADHD are between five and seven times more likely to develop the syndrome than children from unaffected families…and the children of a parent who has ADHD have up to a 50 percent chance of experiencing some difficulties" (Barkley, 1998). The primary genes suspected are the dopamine transporter gene (*DAT1*) and dopamine receptor gene (*DRD4*) (Spencer et al., 2002). While these genes encode for the receptors and transporters of the neurotransmitters, other genes are also being evaluated.

LDs are believed to be intrinsic to the individual and due to some type of dysfunction of the central nervous system, although no pathology has yet been identified. Since symptoms result from control centers throughout the brain, no one site is viewed as the prime cause. Neurotransmitters are not implicated in the cause of learning disabilities.

A myriad of conditions can result in learning disabilities. These include CNS insults resulting from prematurity, hypoxic/anoxic episodes, and the late effects from cranial irradiation. Other "causes" of ADHD and LDs include the sequelae of traumatic brain injury and brain infections; lead poisoning; thyroid dysfunction; complications during pregnancy; and alcohol, nicotine, or narcotic use by the mother during pregnancy (Anastopoulos & Shelton, 2001, Barkley, 2000). In addition, the incidence of ADHD or LDs in children who are adopted is five times higher than would be expected (Silver, 1999).

LDs are also thought to be genetic in a significant number of cases, although the specific genes have not yet been identified. A gene associated with dyslexia has been located on chromosome 15; the gene associated with Tourette syndrome is thought to be located on chromosome 18 (Thapar, 2003; Whitman, 2000a). It should be noted that while many LDs are genetic, the parent's LD may not present the same way or in the same category as the child's (Sousa, 2001).

While there is no empiric support that certain dietary chemicals, such as sugar, refined carbohydrates, aspartame, salicylates, preservatives, and food additives and colors, cause inattention and behavior problems, some children may demonstrate a high degree of sensitivity to these products. Withdrawal of the suspected cause should resolve the symptoms (Weyandt, 2001). Parenting styles and teaching modalities do not cause ADHD or LDs, although they may exacerbate or lessen symptomatology (Wender, 2000). Other myths implicate video games, fluorescent lights, and stress as causes, none of which is true.

COMORBIDITIES WITH ADHD

Both LD and ADHD have been found to occur with other psychiatric conditions concomitantly. It is estimated that from 12% to 50% of children with ADHD also have another psychiatric condition (Hechtman, 2000b; Pliszka, 2000). This fact has complicated both the diagnosis of ADHD and the development of a treatment plan. The most common conditions seen with ADHD include LDs, oppositional defiant disorder (ODD), and conduct disorder (CD). Other comorbid conditions seen with ADHD include mood disorders and depression, anxiety disorders, obsessive–compulsive disorder, Tourette syndrome, pervasive developmental disorders, and mental retardation (Brown, 2000; DuPaul & Stoner, 2003; Pliszka, Carlson, & Swanson, 1999).

Approximately 25% of students with ADHD also have an LD (Pliszka, 2000). However, Willcutt et al. (2003) indicate that ADHD and reading disabilities co-occur in 25% to 40% of children with one of the conditions, and Fletcher, Aram, Shaywitz, and Shaywitz (2000) indicate that there is an overlap of from 33% to 50% between LD and ADHD. As many as 50% of students with ADHD may appear to have LDs as their distractibility results in a lower percentage of work completed and poor test-taking skills and therefore impairment in their ability to demonstrate what they know (Trapani, 2000).

Approximately 20% of students with CD also have ADHD and between 10% and 42% of students with ADHD have CD (Scahill & Schwab-Stone, 2000; Ward & Guyer, 2000). Between 19% and 44% of students with ADHD also have ODD (Scahill & Schwab-Stone, 2000). It is this combination of either ADHD and CD or ADHD and ODD that significantly increases the risk of later delinquency, substance abuse, and antisocial behaviors (Hechtman, 2000b; Wilens, Spencer, & Biederman, 2000). The prevalence of both CD and ODD in girls with ADHD is half of what is reported in boys with ADHD (Biederman et al., 2002).

Tic disorders usually peak during the school-age years and then the incidence decreases during adolescence. Although fewer than 7% of individuals with ADHD have tics, 25% to 85% of those with Tourette syndrome have ADHD (Comings, 2000; Ward & Guyer, 2000).

TREATMENT—ADHD AND LD

ADHD is a chronic condition that requires long-term treatment (Spencer et al., 2002); LDs are lifelong and require individuals to learn how to compensate for their disability. According to a major study exploring the most effective treatment options for children and adolescents with ADHD, it was determined that the best treatment approach to ADHD must be multimodal, consisting of medication, behavior modification, and environmental modification (Jensen, Arnold, Richters, et al., 1999; MTA Cooperative Group, 2004). The results of this landmark longitudinal study suggest that pharmacological management and behavioral interventions are more effective than intensive behavioral treatment alone. However, nonpharmacological interventions should always be tried first.

Effective treatment must address the behavioral, educational, and healthcare needs of the student, who thus benefits from a team effort. The family must have a significant role in developing a treatment regimen. Also participating on the treatment team should be teachers, administrators, the school psychologist, the psychiatrist or treating healthcare provider, social workers, if needed, and of course, the school nurse. The American Academy of Pediatrics (AAP) released evidence-based treatment guidelines in 2001. The key components are that (1) there be a collaborative approach with the clinician, parents, child and school personnel; (2) stimulant medication and/or behavioral therapy may be used as appropriate to achieve the desired outcomes; and (3) lack of improvement in symptom management needs to be thoroughly evaluated in terms of adherence and potential comorbidities.

Unfortunately, for many students with LDs, interventions are not identified until after a student fails a subject in school; in some school districts, services are not initiated until after the student has failed in two subjects. This puts the student at even more of a disadvantage than one who is identified early and has interventions in place to prevent failures and ensure success. Medication is *not* part of the treatment plan for the student who only has an LD. Many of the nonpharmacological interventions for LD are similar to those for ADHD, although these will depend on the extent and the type of the disability. Therefore, nonpharmacological interventions for both LD and ADHD will be covered together. Regardless of the type of intervention initiated, the goals of treatment include academic success, improved quality of life, higher self-esteem, enhanced emotional well-being, better social functioning, and positive peer relationships.

Behavioral Nonpharmacological Interventions: ADHD and LD

Behavioral interventions (Box 30.2) include measures that can be initiated in the home and/or in the school; the measures should be clearly identified and implemented consistently in all settings by parents, caregivers, and teachers. This requires open lines of communication among all parties. The plan must be individualized to the student's special needs.

Box 30.2 ■ ■ ■

NONPHARMACOLOGICAL INTERVENTIONS

- CLASSROOM INTERVENTIONS
  - Reduce environmental stimuli.
    - Color of walls should match floors.
    - Windows should be opaque.
    - Decrease materials on walls and hanging from ceilings.
  - Clear desks except for the current assignment and pencil.
    - Use work cubicles if possible.
  - Request smaller class size, if possible.
  - Place student in class near teacher; near appropriate on-task peer; away from doors, windows and high traffic areas; in front of classroom.
  - Maintain a structured classroom.
  - Post specific daily schedule; call attention to any schedule changes; give advance warning of transitions to start planning for what is needed next.
  - Teach the more demanding content when medication is at its peak.
  - Post classroom rules in prominent place; make sure students understand them.
    - No laughing when someone makes a mistake.
    - Come prepared.
    - Be courteous.
    - Cooperate.
  - Explain rationales for everything (rules, correct answers, protocols).
- ASSISTIVE TECHNOLOGY
  - Combine multimodal methods of learning content (see, write, trace, say, do).
  - Use interactive computer programs, especially as a reward for positive behaviors.
  - Allow computer/typewriter instead of handwriting; electronic spellers/calculators/word processing/voice recognition.
  - Encourage the development of keyboard typing skills.
  - Allow tape recorders.
  - Encourage books on tape or by video.
  - Use graph paper for math in order to line up columns.
  - Allow student to use headphones or ear plugs to block out room noise.
- TEACHING INTERVENTIONS
  - Maintain consistency.
  - Set specific goals; have clear expectations; list all steps necessary to complete assignment.
  - Post assignments in a clear manner; have a peer check that the assignment is written down correctly.
  - Pace the student; do not let the student get overloaded.
  - Give student frequent opportunities to get up and move around.

(Continued on the following page)

Box 30.2 ■■■

NONPHARMACOLOGICAL INTERVENTIONS *(Continued)*

- Help student organize with a list of materials needed for a given class or assignment; color code materials; use calendars and check-off lists.
- Break assignments up into manageable pieces.
- Outline material.
- Highlight important material; emphasize key words.
- Consider allowing sign language or computer language classes rather than foreign language.
- Create "what if" questions to encourage problem solving.
- For testing:
    - Allow alternative methods of demonstrating knowledge.
    - Allow taking tests in an alternative site.
    - Provide extra time for tests so that content and not reading speed is measured.
    - Permit breaks during tests or lessons; allow student to walk around the room when needed.
    - Decrease competition; no timed tests; give enough time so that students can figure out the answer.
- Use rewards and consequences consistently (pick rewards and consequences that are meaningful to the student).
- Provide an extra set of textbooks for the home.
- Provide more hands-on/experiential learning.
- Allow children with dysgraphia to print rather than use cursive writing.
- Teach self-monitoring behaviors; encourage use of a timer to complete tasks.
- Use token reinforcers, with opportunities to achieve these several times each day.
- Give simple decisions to make during the day with rationales.
- Ignore minor misbehaviors.

- COMMUNICATION
    - Maintain frequent teacher–student/teacher–parent communication.
    - Develop daily/weekly journal for assignments and report of progress.
    - Notify parents immediately if assignments are missing.
    - Develop nonverbal discrete clues or cue cards to assist student to refocus (e.g., hand on shoulder).
    - Have a signal for student to give teacher when he or she knows the answer.
    - Find out what he or she already knows.
    - Provide immediate and frequent feedback.
    - Get the student's attention with eye contact before giving instructions; repeat instructions if needed and check for understanding
    - State the behavior desired.
    - Give one instruction/request at a time.
    - Provide visual cues when giving directions.

- PSYCHOSOCIAL
    - Identify strengths and support these and build on them.
    - Give positive recognition often.
    - Build the student's self-esteem and self-confidence at every opportunity.
    - Encourage peer coaching and the use of peer role models; have a study-buddy.
    - Provide opportunities for success.
    - Separate the behavior from the person.
    - Encourage small group supervised activities with peers.
    - Help them identify what they need in order to accommodate to their disability.
    - Help them advocate for their needs.
    - Let them know that they have rights.
    - Make sure that they understand about their disability and understand that it is not their fault.
    - Help the student differentiate between feelings and actions.
    - Seat student near front of bus near window, so to decrease contact with students getting on and off bus.
    - Supervise play.
    - Encourage noncompetitive sports.
    - Acknowledge the student's feelings.
    - Help to develop a sense of humor about his or deficits.

Behavior management interventions for the student with ADHD must be age appropriate, but are generally based on the principles of positive reinforcement, withdrawal of privileges (cost–response intervention), and token economies (see Chapter 38). "Tangible reinforcers are more effective at improving…behavior and academic performance than are teacher attention or other social reinforcers"

(Anastopoulos & Shelton, 2001, p. 174). Lack of compliance to directions from teachers, parents, or other authority figures and not completing tasks are examples of problems for which these interventions may be useful. The same behavioral rating scales used in the diagnostic process can be helpful in periodically evaluating the efficacy of treatment modalities. The school nurse can play an integral role in this evaluation.

It is essential that the student, his or her parents, and school personnel decide on the target outcomes, for these will guide the intervention plan and set priorities. It is equally important for the teacher to set up classroom rules and insist that all students follow them. These should include that all students (1) come to class prepared, (2) be courteous, (3) cooperate, and (4) not be allowed to laugh or make a negative comment when someone makes a mistake (Selekman, 2002a).

The more predictable the school environment is, the more likely it is that the student with LD or ADHD will be successful. Daily routines should be as consistent as possible, allowing extra time for the student to overcome his or her frequently limited organizational skills. For the younger child, picture charts or written reminder lists can be helpful. Students with LDs and ADHD benefit from small structured classes. While this is not always available, other measures can assist in making the environment more conducive to student achievement.

To decrease the stimuli of too many directions, activities can be broken down into their component parts so that a task does not appear to be overwhelming. Teachers and school staff can provide a short list of directions or use checklists or check-off sheets to assist in their organization or understanding of what is expected. Calendars are helpful with the assignments listed for the given date and an indication of where the current date is. The day's schedule can also be placed on the blackboard in the classroom, so that students know what will happen when during the day. These may assist students to be more aware of their behavior and may prevent the student from becoming overloaded.

Structured social and extracurricular activities also may be beneficial to students with ADHD. They allow a student to develop new strengths and thus enhance his or her self-esteem, to interact in a modality that has boundaries, and to have adult supervision to avoid teasing and promote acceptance of differences. In this regard, the concept of peer coaching has been very effective in school settings. Students with ADHD are assigned a peer who can provide guidance to them in ensuring that they are taking the books they need to the next class, ensuring that they stay on task, and allowing the student with ADHD to see a positive role model in their interactions with others (Barkley, 2000; Weyandt, 2001).

Specific learning disabilities require specific interventions. The goal for students with LDs is to learn to compensate for their disability. For the student with a visual perceptual deficit, such as dyslexia, it may be helpful to have material presented on an audiotape or using hands-on demonstration. Checklists may need to use pictures rather than words. Adolescents who want to participate in driver education may need additional assistance in judging distance or may need to delay getting their licenses until they have learned to compensate for this deficit. For the student with an auditory perceptual deficit, directions need to be written or in picture form. Hands-on learning is also effective.

Students with integrative deficits will benefit from multisensory approaches to learning. The student who is overwhelmed by stimuli or who has difficulty identifying important material from the text may need to have sections of the text highlighted to identify key points or use lists or calendars. Feedback should be elicited often to check comprehension. Testing often needs to be modified for students with ADHD or LDs. They need extra time to process the question and need to develop creative ways to demonstrate their knowledge. The student with motor deficits should be encouraged to use the computer to present his or her work rather than to rely on handwriting. Computer skills should be encouraged.

For most students with ADHD and many with LDs, accommodations may be sufficient to allow them to be successful in the academic setting. Accommodations are any modifications to the individualized educational program or 504 Plan (see Chapter 14).

Pharmacological Interventions: ADHD

Psychostimulants are the first line drug of choice for those with ADHD. There has been a significant increase in the number of students taking stimulants for treatment of ADHD over the past two decades. Studies indicate that from 1.3% to 10% of school-age children are taking this category of medication (Barkley, Fisher, Smallish, & Fletcher, 2003), with regional variations. Between 74% and 97% of school-age children with ADHD who are on stimulants respond favorably to the medications (Barkley et al., 2003). "Psychostimulant medications are the most commonly prescribed psychotropic treatment for children in the United States" (Wilens & Spencer, 2000, p. 573). The effects of these drugs on children have been studied extensively and found to be safe and effective in more than 200 controlled studies with school-age children.

Stimulants are thought to work as endogenous catecholamines by binding to the dopamine transporter protein and blocking the reuptake of dopamine and other neurotransmitters by the presynaptic nerve endings, resulting in the release of monoamines into the extraneuronal space (Wilens & Spencer, 2000). Because of this action, the student is better able to pay attention and focus; stimulants assist students to block out extraneous stimuli, thus making them more receptive to learning. In addition to being effective for the core symptoms of ADHD, stimulant medications may help with oppositional behavior and aggression (Pelham, Gnagy, Burrows-Maclean, et al., 2001). Contrary to myths, stimulant medications do not "control" the behavior of students, nor do they improve their intelligence (Accardo & Blondis, 2000b). They simply make the student more "available" for learning to take place and often result in increased school-based productivity. Stimulants are not a cure for ADHD; their use is frequently compared to the use of insulin for a diabetic individual or the use of glasses for the child who has visual difficulties.

The dosage of stimulant medications (Table 30.2) is not usually related to body weight, as it is for most other medications, except for Atomoxetine. The goal is to maximize the desired effect while at the same time minimizing the side effects of these medications (Accardo & Blondis, 2000b). However, as children age and their body metabolism changes, their medications or the dosages may need to be changed. The recommended premise for dosage is to start with a low dose and to slowly titrate it upward at intervals of approximately one week until the desired effects are achieved or until side effects appear that are unacceptable to the student and his or her family.

Table 30.2 ■
PSYCHOSTIMULANTS USED FOR ADHD

DRUG	DOSAGE	RANGE	DURATION (H)	NOTES
Methylphenidate				
Ritalin/Methylin	5, 10, 20 mg	5–60 mg/day Divided doses	3–4	Onset 20–30 min; peak 1–2 h
Focalin	2.5, 5, 10 mg	2.5–30 mg/day	3–4	
Ritalin LA	20, 30, 40 mg		6–8	Do not chew or crush.
Methylin ER	10, 20 mg		3–8	
Concerta	18, 36, 54 mg		9–12	Slow constant release; do not chew
Metadate-CD	20-mg capsules	20–60 mg/day	8–12	6 mg released immediately; 14 mg over next 12 hours
Metadate-ER	10, 20 mg	10–60 mg/day	up to 8 hours	Half released immediately; One fourth 4 hours later

(continued)

DRUG	DOSAGE	RANGE	DURATION (H)	NOTES
Dextroamphetamine				
Dexedrine/Dextrostat	5-, 10-mg tablet; 5-, 10-, 15-mg capsules	10–40 mg/day	4–6 6–8	Do not chew or crush.
Mixed salts of dextro- and levo-amphetamine				
Adderall	5, 7.5, 10, 12.5, 15, 20, 30 mg	10–40 mg/day	6–8	
Adderall XR	5-, 10-, 15-, 20-, 25-, 30-mg capsules	10–60 mg/day	10–12	Half released immediately; half over time
Amphetamine				
Desoxyn	2.5, 5 mg	2.5–25 mg/day	8–10 hours	
Nonstimulant				
Strattera	5, 10, 18, 25, 40, 60 mg	1.2–1.4 mg/kg or 100 mg, whichever is less	Half-life is 5 hours; peaks 1–2 hours	

NOTE: Pemoline (Cylert) is no longer given to new patients because of the significant incidence of liver toxicity. However, patients for whom pemoline continues to be effective are being maintained on that drug with careful follow-up of liver function tests (Accardo & Blondis, 2000b).
Sources: American Academy of Pediatrics (2001); Naparstek (2002); Solanto, Arnsten, Castellanos (2001).

It is usually suggested that dose changes or medication changes occur on Saturday, so that parents can observe the effects on their child for the first two days; school personnel can then evaluate the student on Thursday, so that the prescribing healthcare provider can be contacted on Friday to again change the dose by Saturday (Anastopoulos & Shelton, 2001). The effectiveness of stimulants is measured by behavioral changes (e.g., decreased motor activity and increased attention span and concentration). Teacher input is essential in evaluating the effectiveness of this treatment. The school nurse can collect data from the teachers in order to identify patterns of drug efficacy. Behavioral changes can often be identified within 30 to 90 minutes of ingestion.

If a student does not respond as desired to one stimulant or has serious side effects, other stimulants should be tried before moving to a second-line agent (Accardo & Blondis, 2000b). It has been demonstrated that some students respond to one stimulant and not others (American Academy of Child and Adolescent Psychiatry [AACAP], 1997).

The most commonly used stimulant medications include methylphenidate (MPH) products (Ritalin, Methylin, Concerta, Metadate, and Focalin) and amphetamines and their derivatives (Adderall, Adderall-XR, Dexedrine, and Dextrostat). Contraindications to the use of stimulant medications include symptomatic cardiovascular disease, moderate to severe hypertension, marked anxiety or agitation, hyperthyroidism, glaucoma, a history of psychosis, or a history of drug abuse. Because a rare side effect of stimulant medications is the development or worsening of tics, there is debate as to whether individuals with tic disorders should receive stimulants (Popper, 2000).

Short-acting medications usually require several daily doses; thus students need to come to the school nurse's office for a mid-day dose. Longer acting sustained release preparations often require only a morning dose, although some individuals will need a short-acting dose once they return home to be able to attend to the activities required of them through the evening. During the past two decades, school nurses have spent a good part of their day administering stimulant medications to those with ADHD. It is hoped that as more students switch to long-acting preparations, this activity will decrease. One concern is that students will forget to take (or be given) their medications before they get to school; this concern should be addressed in communication with the parents and several doses can be kept at school, with the accompanying MD order to give as needed when the student forgets and the parent requests it. This can also be written into the IEP or 504 plan.

For some students, medication effects don't last as long as is typical for that medication. Thus, a stimulant that usually lasts 4 hours may stop working after 3 hours, causing an increase in negative behaviors or a rebound effect. In some students, the dose may last 5-6 hours (Accardo & Blondis, 2000b). However, if a student is only taking a short acting stimulant in the morning and has physical symptoms in the afternoon, these are probably not the direct result of the stimulant. If, however, signs and symptoms occur during the peak of the medication, it is important to relay this information to the student's healthcare provider.

Long acting preparations should never be crushed into powder in order to facilitate administration. Adderall XR is the only long acting stimulant in capsule form that can be opened and sprinkled to aid in administration for children who are unable to swallow tablets whole; however, the granules cannot be chewed.

A newer medication for ADHD is Atomoxetine (generic) or Strattera. This selective noradrenergic enhancer has a different mechanism of action but an effect similar to MPH; it is a "potent inhibitor of the presynaptic norepinephrine transporter, with minimal affinity for other noradrenergic receptors or for other neurotransmitter transporters or receptors" (Biederman et al., 2002, e75). However, its exact mechanism of action is unknown. It is not a stimulant drug and it is not a controlled substance (Eli Lily, 2002). Its main side effects are abdominal pain, vomiting, drowsiness or insomnia, anorexia and weight loss, and headache. It is also more expensive than the other stimulants. However, in 2005, the Food and Drug Administration issued a Public Health Advisory to alert physicians of increased reports of suicidal thoughts in children and adolescents on Strattera (U.S. Food and Drug Administration, 2005).

The most common adverse effects of stimulant medications are appetite suppression and sleep disturbances. Parents who administer medication too late in the afternoon or evening may have children unable to sleep. Consequently, students may come to school sleep deprived, making it difficult to tell if their symptoms are due to the ADHD or a lack of sleep. Rebound behavioral problems may be seen in some students as the medication is wearing off, resulting in an exacerbation of symptoms of the condition, possibly accompanied by irritability, anger, or frustration. Rebound is not as much of a problem with the long-acting preparations.

Other side effects include irritability, stomachache, nausea, headache, dizziness, tachycardia, weight loss, nervous mannerisms or nervousness with tremors, tics, excessive crying, and rarely, growth problems (Barkley et al., 2003; Spencer et al., 2002). All of these have implications for the school nurse when the student comes to her office with one of these complaints. If nausea or stomachache is a problem, it may be helpful for students to take their medication on a full stomach, requiring that they come for their stimulants after lunch rather than before. Taking medications after meals is also an effective approach if the medication causes anorexia (Spencer et al., 2002). Headaches are usually mild and do not require acetaminophen for their resolution. Allowing the student to lie down for a short period should help (Accardo & Blondis, 2000b). Emotional lability or a "spacey" behavior may indicate an overdose.

Because the stimulant medication causes anorexia, it is essential to ensure that the student is getting not only enough calories to support growth because of the hyperactivity, but also getting quality calories. These students may also be easily distracted from the meal and leave the table before they are finished eating, especially in the school cafeteria. The school nurse can keep a careful record of the student's height and weight throughout the year at approximately 6-month intervals. While stimulant medication may initially slow growth, there are no significant differences in height by the time the child reaches adolescence (Greenhill, 2001).

There is discussion as to whether students should take a "drug holiday," or a break from their medication regimen to be able to evaluate the status of baseline behavior. This should certainly never be recommended at the beginning or end of the school year when first impressions, classroom rules, and evaluation testing are occurring. School vacations and weekends are the best times for these, if they are taken. However, if there are expectations of class work or activities that require sustained attention or if family interactions or peer socialization is negatively affected, taking a drug holiday may place the student at a disadvantage.

There has been a great deal of press regarding concerns that children were being "drugged" with these stimulants. This has not been demonstrated to be the case. While the stimulants do not make a student smarter or control behavior, they do give the student a chance to make a choice. A consensus development conference held by the National Institutes of Health (1998) concluded that stimulants were effective as treatment for ADHD but that long-term studies were needed.

Research also does not support parental fears that taking stimulants as treatment for ADHD will lead to alcohol or drug addiction. The stimulants are not addictive when taken by students diagnosed with ADHD in the doses prescribed. Students with ADHD do not get high from the stimulants they take (Wender, 2000). Studies have shown that treatment of ADHD with stimulants significantly decreases the risk for subsequent substance use disorders (Barkley et al., 2003; Wilens, Faraone, Biederman, & Gunawardene, 2003). The only exception to this finding is the individual who also has conduct disorder (CD). The combination of CD and ADHD does put the student at a higher risk for later drug abuse.

For the small percentage of students who do not respond to stimulants or for those with comorbid psychiatric conditions, nonstimulant second-line medications are frequently prescribed (Table 30.3). These include tricyclic antidepressants (TCAs) [with imipramine being the drug of choice in this category], alpha-adrenergic agonists (such as clonidine and guanfacine), and selective serotonin reuptake inhibitors (SSRIs). Clonidine is not abusable and comes in a patch that lasts for 5 to 7 days (Wender, 2000). It is sometimes given later in the day for students on stimulants because of its sedative effect to assist in falling asleep.

The research data are limited regarding the safety and efficacy of these nonstimulant medications for children with ADHD (Guevara, Lozano, Wickizer, Mell, & Gephart, 2002). However, these drugs have more serious side effects than the stimulant drugs and it may take a few weeks for these drugs to achieve the desired effect (Wender, 2000).

Students being treated with psychotropic medications should be followed closely by their healthcare provider. This is especially true for those taking second-line medications because of the cardiotoxicity that is possible. TCAs can prolong the conduction of electrical activity of the heart (Wender, 2000). Second-line medications should not be withdrawn suddenly as withdrawal symptoms will appear; 2 to 3 weeks should be allowed for this process (AACAP, 1997).

"Although in clinical practice ADHD patients commonly receive more than one psychotropic, little

Table 30.3 ■

NONSTIMULANT MEDICATION PRESCRIBED FOR CHILDREN WITH ADHD

Antidepressants	Imipramine (Tofranil) Desipramine (Norpramin) Nortriptyline (Pamelor) Bupropion (Wellbutrin) Serotonin-based antidepressants (Prozac, Zoloft, Paxil, Effexor, and Celexa)
Antihypertensives	Clonidine (Catapres) Guanfacine (Tenex)

Sources: American Academy of Pediatrics (2001); Naparstek (2002).

Issue: The adolescent does not come to the nurse's office to get his lunchtime dose of stimulant medication.

1. With the emphasis on "drug-free schools" and "Say no to drugs," students may feel self-conscious or guilty about being dependent on medication.
2. The student doesn't want to be different from peers.
3. The student "forgets."

Approaches:

1. The student and family may not know about the extended/long-acting medications. The school nurse could say, "The next time you see your physician, you may want to ask about some of the long-acting preparations; this might eliminate this middle-of-the-day dose." For students who do not have regular check-ups with their healthcare provider, this may be a way to stimulate a visit.
2. Comparing stimulant medications to insulin or introducing students with ADHD to those with diabetes may assist them in seeing the similarities in their need for medication in order to stay healthy and alert in the classroom.
3. For students who forget to come to the nurse's office, peer mentors can be used to remind students of the need to get their medication before or after they have had their lunch.

is known about combined pharmacotherapy in ADHD" (Spencer et al., 2002, p. 249). Most of the medications prescribed for ADHD have not been tested in children younger than the age of 6. Regardless of the category of medication prescribed, communication between the healthcare provider and the school nurse enhances the success of any program of care.

Alternative Therapies

Dietary modifications have often been suggested as one means to regulate a child's behavior. Dietary supplements and herbal preparations are not regulated for safety, efficacy, or standardized contents (Wender, 2000) and are not recommended for children. The Feingold diet has now lost favor when its results could not be replicated in repeated studies; this diet eliminates sorbitol, caffeine, and refined sugars (Barkley, 2000). While some children are more sensitive to chemicals than others, this diet cannot hurt the child, but rarely produces positive results. Megavitamin therapy has also not been demonstrated to be beneficial to children with ADHD; it may actually be harmful and make the behaviors exhibited with ADHD appear worse (Barkley, 2000).

Other controversial therapies have been proposed for both ADHD and LDs, although most were specifically developed for those with learning disabilities. These include patterning, cognitive therapy, EEG biofeedback/neurofeedback (attention training), sensory integration training, and visual training or tinted lenses or prisms on glasses. According to Wender, "there is no evidence whatsoever that coordination training will help the ADHD child's learning difficulties. The same statement applies to specific treatment programs of eye exercises" (2000, p. 132). Biofeedback is based on programs that change the electrical activity of the brain, yet no deficit in the EEG has been identified for ADHD. This lengthy, time-consuming, costly program does not have scientific evidence supporting its efficacy (Barkley, 2000), but studies are currently in progress. None of these programs are recommended by the American Academy of Pediatrics (AAP, 2004).

PSYCHOSOCIAL IMPLICATIONS OF HAVING ADHD OR AN LD

The more years a student experiences academic failures and rejection, the more psychological sequelae will result. A delayed diagnosis or improper or inadequate intervention strategies can result in poor self-esteem, anxiety, depression, psychosomatic complaints, school absenteeism or resignation (Greenhill, 1998). Teachers and other school personnel may inappropriately negatively label students; this may further aggravate the psychological sequelae.

Once a diagnosis is made, parents often are concerned about having the label of ADHD or LD attached to their child's record. The school nurse can help to allay these concerns by stressing that without the diagnosed label, the student would not be able to receive the services he or she needs to compensate for and deal with the deficits of the conditions. The labels that hurt are those that mark the student as "dumb", "lazy", or "unmotivated"; the school nurse can work with the school psychologist and the teachers to assure that these terms are not used by either the staff or the student's classmates.

Social problems may result from motor or language deficits or as a result of students' low frustration tolerance, impulsivity, and difficulty perceiving nonverbal social cues (Weyandt, 2001). These same behaviors may affect relationships within the family as well. Therefore, social interactions are more negative and more stressful. The students experience more peer rejection because they are viewed as exhibiting undesirable behaviors. The school nurse needs to be aware of the teasing and social rejection experienced by the student with a disability.

Having a child with ADHD can be extremely difficult for the parents. Frequently they feel (or are told by others) that they are at fault for their child's behavior; they believe that they are not good parents. They may feel they have tried everything. Children with ADHD may not respond to conventional discipline strategies, as the symptoms of ADHD may make it difficult, if not impossible, for the student to respond to cues, learn from past disciplinary actions, or generalize one set of rules to a different setting (Selekman & Moore, 2004). Parents rely on the school to assist them in working with their child, but frequently the school dismisses their concerns or blames the parents. Perhaps the most telling of these frustrations is the line from one parent who said, "Every time I send my child out into the world, the world sends him back."

There are ways to view the student's hyperactive or inattentive behaviors in a more positive way that can be shared with the student and the parents. Comments such as "responds well when highly motivated," "a concrete thinker," "imaginative," "creative," "energetic," "showing signs of effort in spite of difficulties" will go a long way in turning a negative situation into something more positive. Psychological support may be needed by the student with ADHD or LD related to the stress of having a disability. Students need to understand that even though they failed a course or an examination, they are not failures.

The school nurse can assist the family by recommending community resources available for students with ADHD and their families. Parents need continued education regarding ADHD and interventions that may be appropriate for their child. In addition, there are books and other resources for children, adolescents, parents, and teachers to assist in understanding about the condition as well as planning interventions. There are also parent support groups through ChADD (Children and Adults with Attention Deficit Disorder). The primary roles of the school nurse for the family are being a support person and an advocate to ensure that the school meets the students' needs.

Be aware of the needs of siblings. Some may be embarrassed by their sibling's disability; others may be protective of them. Some siblings are angry at what is perceived as extra time and attention given to the child with special needs or a leniency in homework assignments and chores. They need special explanations; they also need to be assured that they do not have the same problem (assuming that that is the case). Other family members also need attention. Grandparents often do not understand about the disorders and once they hear it is genetic, may tend to blame the other spouse. Remembering that both ADHD and LDs are biological problems and not character defects will help to keep the problems in their proper perspective.

SAFETY IMPLICATIONS

Students with LDs and ADHD have a higher risk of accidents than those without these conditions, especially in the evening when the effect of medications had worn off (Cox, Merkel, Penberthy, Kovatchev, & Hankin, 2004). They have a decreased ability to tolerate delays or to think before acting; they often act without considering potential outcomes. Their impulsive behavior may therefore alter their judgment, placing them at a higher risk for engaging in unsafe activities. This is also true for adolescents as they begin learning to drive. Altered judgments of speed, space, and distance, plus distractibility place them at an increased risk for motor vehicle accidents (Barkley, 2000). It may be recommended that adolescents who have difficulty in these areas delay driving for a few years. The high accident rate and the resulting effect on insurance may be a stimulus to encourage some reluctant teens to continue taking their medication.

Medication safety is an essential component for the school nurse. Because many of the stimulants are easily abused by those without the diagnosis of ADHD, and because students with ADHD may be asked to sell their medications on the way to school prior to them getting to the school nurse's office, it is essential that a pill count occur both from the parent sending in the pills and the school nurse administering them. The school nurse must be aware of district policies regarding handling and storing controlled substances; if a policy is not in place, the school nurse should participate in its development. They need to be kept in a locked site within the office. There are reports of Ritalin being stolen directly from the nurse's office. On the street, Ritalin is referred to as "Vitamin R," "Rids," "Skittles," or "Smarties." The tablets can be crushed and inhaled. The long acting preparations do not allow for the same response and therefore are not attractive to those seeking a "high." Some non-ADHD students use stimulants in order to stay up all night to complete assignments or prepare for exams.

SCHOOL IMPLICATIONS

The educational plan for any student with either ADHD or LD needs to be individualized. The school nurse or someone from the staff needs to coordinate services regarding the student's IEP or 504 Accommodation Plan. While students with LDs are covered under IDEA guaranteeing them the development of an Individualized Education Program, those with ADHD are covered under Section 504 of the Rehabilitation Act, thus guaranteeing them reasonable accommodations and the development of an accommodation plan. Students who are severely affected with ADHD may also qualify under IDEA as "other health impaired" (U.S. Department of Education, 1999) (see Chapter 14).

In addition to the IEP, the school nurse should develop an Individualized Health Plan for these students. This can be a valuable tool for the nurse, counselor, and classroom teacher, and can, at times, lead to nursing services being added to the IEP that can assist in Medicaid Reimbursement for a school district.

Working with students with ADHD can be labor intensive for the teacher as well as the family. "Children with ADHD are more frequently off-task, are less able to sustain compliance, and do not complete chores" (Whitman, 2000b, p. 445). Students with ADHD and LDs may be educated in regular classrooms, use the resource room, attend special education classes, be tutored, or use a combination thereof. The goal is to include them in normal classroom functioning as much as possible. These students do better in small structured classrooms. They also benefit from classrooms that have a minimum of visual and auditory stimulation.

If a student is suspected of having an LD or ADHD, the school nurse can refer him or her to the school psychologist for an evaluation. She can advocate for the student to ensure that he or she gets the accommodations needed in order to be successful in the school environment.

Students with persistent poor performance need to be assured that they are not stupid and they need to be taught how to be advocates for themselves and to ask for a repeat of directions or clarification of content. As part of the educational plan, students' strengths must be identified as well as their special needs. It is essential to teach them how to compensate for and deal with their particular disability. They need to understand what accommodations work best for them and to share this information with each teacher they have. The special education teacher can serve as a resource person to the classroom teachers. The school nurse can be an advocate for these students to provide information to the faculty on LDs and ADHD. A number of books are available to provide educators with teaching approaches that best meet the needs of students with ADHD or LDs. School personnel can try to "catch" the student doing appropriate behaviors and to recognize and reinforce those behaviors (Whitman, 2000b).

Discipline is a component of the educational process. As for all students, the discipline used should fit the seriousness of the misbehavior. Students with ADHD and some learning disabilities do not learn well from past experiences and may not be able to control their behavior. They require clarification as to why what was done was wrong and why they are being punished. Frequent feedback related to improvement and what they are doing right is important. The students needs to hear that it was the "behavior" that was bad or wrong, not the "student" being bad; the student needs to know that adults care about him or her. The mainstay of discipline is that it must be consistent and part of the daily routine. Limit setting is effective for students with ADHD. Although behavior modification helps to improve targeted behaviors and skills, it does not reduce inattention, hyperactivity or impulsivity (AACAP, 1997). Rewards for good behavior are effective, especially if given immediately after the behavior is identified or the short-term task completed.

Certain interventions have been demonstrated to be more effective in the academic arena (see Box 30.2). These include maintaining a routine, handling situations consistently every time they occur, communicating directly with the student, modeling, providing positive reinforcement, and allowing for decision making. Peer tutoring, where two students work together can be effective for both learning and modeling of appropriate behaviors. The use of thematic units to relate content being taught by multiple subjects may help to present similar content from multiple perspectives.

Extra care must be taken when teaching about menstruation and high-risk behaviors. Girls may need a calendar to predict and mark the dates for monthly menstruation. Role-playing may help in learning resistance behaviors. Because of impulsivity and poor problem-solving skills on the part of some of these students, education needs to be individualized to the needs of the student and repeated often. When "accidents" happen, students need to know which staff member to approach for assistance.

For students who have difficulty with organization, a second set of books can be obtained as part of their accommodation plan so that one set stays at home and one set stays in school. This may also be true for medical equipment for other special needs they may have. The school nurse needs to follow up closely to ensure that information gets home to the parents and that medication and equipment gets to the school. It may also be important for the school nurse to know which students are taking long-acting stimulants, so that even though he or she is not administering them in the school, she can be aware when the student has not taken their dose, is having side effects during the peak of the drug's activity, and noticing the efficacy of its action.

Some students are super-sensitive to certain fabrics against their skin or the tags in the back of shirts. These can cause the student to focus only on these sensations rather than on what is going on in the classroom; if the nurse is astute to this possibility, a note home to the parents may resolve this stimulus.

Students with specific learning disabilities who come to the school nurse's office need to have the same teaching modalities used there as in the classroom. Directions may need to be given one at a time. Skills being taught in the nurse's office may need to be broken down into smaller parts. Praise needs to be given at every opportunity.

The student's motivation to overcome or compensate for their disability plays a significant role in their potential for success. To keep motivation high, the student must experience success in the classroom and feel special and appreciated.

OTHER IMPLICATIONS FOR THE SCHOOL NURSE

1. A diagnosis of ADHD has no implications for the student's immunization requirements.
2. If a learning disability is suspected, it is essential that careful hearing and vision screenings be completed on a routine basis.

3. If a student demonstrates receptive or expressive language disorders, speech and language assessments should be initiated.
4. Enuresis and encopresis may occur in students with ADHD and LDs. They may be unaware of the cues their body puts out or they may be too distracted to include toileting into their schedule. Therefore, the teacher needs to incorporate toileting into the day's activities.
5. The stimulants are Schedule II controlled substances with a high abuse potential for individuals without ADHD in the school. Therefore, these drugs need to be counted daily and kept double locked.
6. Students taking stimulants, tricyclics, clonidine, or guanfacine may have mild alterations in their blood pressure. It would be wise to have baseline blood pressure readings on these students, and to perform blood pressure checks every few months for those taking medications other than the stimulants.
7. Students taking TCAs and clonidine may have mild increases in their pulse rate within the first month of taking these medications (Greenhill, 2001).
8. Some of the symptoms of ADHD may be similar to multiple illnesses, such as irritability and inability to attend to a task. The question to ask is whether the student is ill or whether the medications or other interventions are just not working.
9. Side effects of stimulant medications may mask symptoms of illness, such as stomachache, headache, insomnia, anorexia, and weight loss.
10. The lack of appetite, insomnia, and difficulty resting the body may interfere with the healing process as well as taking in the fluids and nutrients needed in recovering from an illness.
11. Psychological conditions in the student's life due to other life events (e.g., divorce, illness, death in the family, poverty, malnutrition, rejection by friends) may result in difficulty attending to tasks but should not be confused with a worsening of the disability.
12. Beware of labeling the student and parents as "noncompliant" without first finding out if the lack of follow-through was due to the characteristics of LD or ADHD for both the child and the parents.

PROGNOSIS

Many individuals with ADHD and LDs grow up to become successful adults in spite of their disability. While learning disabilities stay with an individual for life (National Joint Committee on Learning Disabilities [NJCLD], 1997), one of the goals of childhood is to learn to compensate for these deficits. There are wonderful reports of individuals with LDs who "made it" in society (Table 30.4).

Table 30.4 ■

FAMOUS INDIVIDUALS WHO MAY NOT HAVE BEEN OFFICIALLY DIAGNOSED BUT WHO ARE SUSPECTED OF HAVING ADHD OR AN LD

Artists/musicians/actors	August Rodin, Leonardo DaVinci, Mozart, Cher, Tom Cruise, Ty Pennington
Military/national leaders	Woodrow Wilson, Nelson Rockefeller, Gen. George Patton, Winston Churchill
Inventors/scientists	Albert Einstein, Henry Ford, Thomas Edison
Athletes	Bruce Jenner, "Magic" Johnson, Babe Ruth
Authors	Hans Christian Anderson, William Butler Yeats
Other corporate leaders	Walt Disney, Charles Schwab

Source: Guyer (2000).

Schools may want to use these individuals' stories as examples of success stories.

Approximately 20% of children do appear to outgrow ADHD. However, up to 80% of children with ADHD still manifest symptoms as adolescents and 50% to 65% still meet all or part of the criteria into adulthood (Barkley, 2000). While many will become successful adults, 18% to 53% "will be academic underachievers, performing significantly below their level of intelligence" (Anastopoulos & Shelton, 2001, p. 49). They become undereducated and underemployed. The presence of CD is associated with a poorer prognosis and a significant risk for developing addictions (Spencer et al., 2002). Adults report increased interpersonal problems resulting in having fewer friends and increased job terminations (especially in jobs requiring problem-solving, prioritizing, task completion, and self control). They also have significantly less formal schooling (Anastopoulos & Shelton, 2001; Mannuzza & Klein, 2000). The symptoms of ADHD appear to change as the child becomes an adult. Some of the hyperactivity may demonstrate itself as restlessness.

CONCLUSION

The near future offers great hope in the diagnosis and management of children and adults with ADHD. New scanning techniques will provide clearer diagnostic abilities; new nonstimulant medications are being developed that may prove to be equally effective without the negative societal messages of taking stimulant medications; and better clarification will be developed to differentiate the various forms of ADHD and their comorbidities.

LDs and ADHD affect all components of a child's life, including his or her family. They affect the student's self esteem and feelings of achievement and success. They are valid conditions with a range of symptoms from mild to severe and from a single entity to one that is combined with numerous other psychiatric conditions (Selekman, 2002a). The school nurse plays an integral part in their care and can help set the stage for their future.

Resources

Books for Children, Parents, and Teachers

ADDitude Magazine. Box 421, 2476 Bolsover, Houston, TX 77005-2518
800-856-2032 additude@additudemag.com

Adelezzi, J., & Goss, D. (2001). *Parenting children with learning disabilities*. Westport, CT: Bergin and Garvey.

Barkley, R. (2000). *Taking charge of ADHD: The complete authoritative guide for parents*. New York: Guildford Press.

Cooper, P., & Ideus, K. (1996). *Attention deficit/ hyperactivity disorder: A practical guide for teachers*. London: David Fulton.

Fisher, G., & Cummings, R. (2002). *The survival guide for kids with LD*. Minneapolis, MN: Free Spirit Publications.

Fowler, M. (1999). *Maybe you know my kid: A parents guide to identifying, understanding, and helping your child with attention deficit hyperactivity disorder.* New York: Birch Lane Press.

Galvin, M. (2001). *Otto learns about his medicine: A story about medication for children with ADHD*. Washington, DC: Magination Press.

Gantos, J. (2000). *Joey Pigza loses control*. New York: Farrar, Straus, & Girout.

Greenbaum, J., & Markel, G. (2001). *Helping adolescents with ADHD and learning disabilities*. Paramus, NJ: The Center for Applied Research in Education.

Greene, R. (1998). *The explosive child*. New York: Harper Collins.

Levine, M. (2002). *A mind at a time*. New York: Simon & Schuster.

Mangrum, C., & Strichart, S. (2000). *Peterson's colleges with programs for students with learning disabilities or ADDs*. Princeton, NJ: Peterson's Guides.

McEwan, E. (1998). *The principal's guide to attention deficit hyperactivity disorder*. Thousand Oaks, CA: Corwin Press.

Nadeau, K., & Dixon, E. (1997). *Learning to slow down and pay attention: A book for kids about ADD* (2nd ed.). Washington, DC: Magination Press.

Osman, B. (1997). *Learning disabilities and ADHD: A family guide to living and learning together.* New York: John Wiley & Sons.

Quinn, P., & Stern, J. (1991). *Putting on the brakes: Young people's guide to understanding attention deficit hyperactivity disorder*. New York: Magination Press.

Silverstin, A., Silverstein, V., & Nunn, L. (2001). *Attention deficit disorder*. New York: Franklin Watts.

Smith, M. (1997). *Pay attention, Slosh!* Morton Grove, IL: Albert Whitman & Co.

Strip, C. (2000). *Helping gifted children soar: A practical guide for parents and teachers*. Scottsdale, AZ: Gifted Psychology Press.

The ChADD information and resource guide to Attention Deficit/Hyperactivity. (2001). Landover, MD: Children and Adults with Attention-Deficit/Hyperactivity Disorder.

Resource Groups

National Attention Deficit Disorder Association (ADDA)
P.O. Box 543
Pottstown, PA 19461
(484) 945-2101
http://www.add.org

ADD Warehouse
300 Northwest 70th Avenue, Suite 102
Plantation, FL 33317
(800) 233-9273
www.addwarehouse.com

Children and Adults with Attention Deficit Disorder (CHADD)
8181 Professional Place, Suite 150
Landover, MD 20785

(800) 233-4050
http://www.chadd.org

Learning Disabilities Association of America
4156 Library Road
Pittsburgh, PA 15234-1349
(412) 341-1515
http://www.ldanatl.org

National Center for Learning Disabilities (NCLD)
381 Park Ave. S., Suite 1401
New York, NY 10016
(888) 575-7373
http://www.ncld.org

National Information Center for Children and Youth with Disabilities (NICHCY)
PO Box 1492
Washington, DC 20013-1492
(800) 695-0285
http://www.nichcy.org

National Institute of Mental Health
NIMH Public Inquiries
6001 Executive Boulevard, Rm. 8184, MSC 9663
Bethesda MD 20892-9663
(301) 443-4513
http://www.nimh.nih.gov/publicat/adhdmenu.cfm

References

Accardo, P., & Blondis, T. (2000a). The Strauss syndrome, minimal brain dysfunction, and the hyperactive child: A historical introduction to attention deficit hyperactivity disorder. In P. Accardo, T. Blondis, B. Whitman, & M. Stein (Eds.), *Attention deficits in children and adults: Diagnosis, treatment and management* (pp. 1–11). New York: Marcel Dekker.

Accardo, P., & Blondis, T. (2000b). Pediatric management of ADHD medication. In P. Accardo, T. Blondis, B. Whitman, & M. Stein (Eds.), *Attention deficits in children and adults: Diagnosis, treatment and management* (pp. 513–533). New York: Marcel Dekker.

American Academy of Child and Adolescent Psychiatry (AACAP). (1997). Practice parameters for the assessment and treatment of children, adolescents, and adults with attention-deficit/hyperactivity disorder. *American Academy of Child and Adolescent Psychiatry, 36*(10), 85S–112S.

American Academy of Pediatrics (AAP). (2000). Clinical practice guideline: Diagnosis and evaluation of the child with attention-deficit/hyperactivity disorder. *Pediatrics, 105*(5), 1158–1170.

American Academy of Pediatrics (AAP). (2001). Clinical practice guideline: Treatment of the school-aged child with attention-deficit/hyperactivity disorder. *Pediatrics, 108*(4), 1033–1044.

American Academy of Pediatrics (AAP). (2004). *ADHD: A complete and authoritative guide*. Elk Grove Village, IL: American Academy of Pediatrics.

American Psychiatric Association (APA). (2000). *Diagnostic and statistical manual of mental disorders: Text revision. Edition IV*. Washington, DC: Author.

Anastopoulos, A., & Shelton, T. (2001). *Assessing attention-deficit/hyperactivity disorder*. New York: Kluwer Academic/Plenum.

Barkley, R. (September, 1998). Attention-deficit hyperactivity disorder. *Scientific American*. Retrieved from http://www.sciam.com/1998/0998issuebarkley.html

Barkley, R. (2000). *Taking charge of ADHD*. New York: The Guilford Press.

Barkley, R., Fischer, M., Smallish, L., & Fletcher, K. (2003). Does the treatment of attention-deficit/hyperactivity disorder with stimulants contribute to drug use/abuse? A 13-year prospective study. *Pediatrics, 111*(1), 97–109.

Biederman, J., Heiligenstein, J., Faries, D., Galil, N., Dittmann, R., Emslie, G., Kratochvil, C., Laws, H., & Schuh, K. (2002). Efficacy of atomoxetine versus placebo in school-age girls with attention-deficit/hyperactivity disorder. *Pediatrics, 110*(6), e75.

Brown, T. (2000). *Attention-deficit disorders and comorbidities in children, adolescents, and adults*. Washington, DC: American Psychiatric Press.

Buitelaar, J. (2002). Epidemiological aspects: What have we learned over the last decade? In S. Sandberg (Ed.), *Hyperactivity and attention disorders of childhood* (pp. 30–63). Cambridge, UK: Cambridge University Press.

Carlson, C., & Mann, M. (2000). Attention-deficit/hyperactivity disorder, predominantly inattentive type. *Child and Adolescent Psychiatric Clinics of North America, 9*(3), 499–510.

Castellanos, F. (2001). Neuroimaging studies of ADHD. In M. Solanto, A. Arnstein, & F. Castellanos (Eds.), *Stimulant drugs and ADHD: Basic and clinical neuroscience* (pp. 243–258). New York: Oxford University Press.

Comings, D. (2000). Attention-deficit/hyperactivity disorder with Tourette syndrome. In T. Brown (Ed.), *Attention-deficit disorders and comorbidities in children, adolescents, and adults* (pp. 363–391). Washington, DC: American Psychiatric Press.

Cox, D., Merkel, R. L., Penberthy, J., Kovatchev, B., & Hankin, C. (2004). Impact of Methylphenidate delivery profiles on driving performance of adolescents with attention-deficit/hyperactivity disorder: A pilot study. *Journal of the American Academy of Child & Adolescent Psychiatry, 43*(3), 269–275.

Davila, R., Williams, M., & MacDonalt, J. (September, 1991). *Clarification of policy to address the needs of children with attention deficit disorders within the general and/or special education*. Washington, DC: U.S. Department of Education, Office of Special Education and Rehabilitation Services.

DuPaul, G., & Stoner, G. (2003). *ADHD in the schools: Assessment and intervention strategies*. New York: The Guilford Press.

Eli Lily. (2002). *Strattera*. Indianapolis, IN: Eli Lilly & Co.

Fletcher, J., Aram, D., Shaywitz, S., & Shaywitz, B. (2000). Learning, language, and attention disorders in children: Comorbidity, assessment, and intervention. In P. Accardo, T. Blondis, B. Whitman, & M. Stein (Eds.), *Attention deficits in children and adults: Diagnosis, treatment, and management* (pp. 241–256). New York: Marcel Dekker.

Fletcher, J., Shaywitz, S., & Shaywitz, B. (1999). Comorbidity of learning and attention disorders: Separate but equal. *The Pediatric Clinics of North America, 46*(5), 885–897.

Greenhill, L. (1998). Diagnosing attention-deficit hyperactivity disorder in children. *Journal of Clinical Psychiatry*, 59(Suppl. 7), 31–41.

Greenhill, L. (2001). Clinical effects of stimulant medication in ADHD. In M. Solanto, A. Arnsten, & F.X.

Castellanos (Eds.), *Stimulant drugs and ADHD: Basic and clinical neuroscience* (pp. 31–72). New York: Oxford University Press.

Guevara, J., Lozano, P., Wickizer, T., Mell, L., & Gephart, H. (2002). Psychotrophic medication use in a population of children who have attention-deficit/hyperactivity disorder. *Pediatrics, 109*(5), 733–739.

Guyer, B. (2000). *ADHD: Achieving success in school and in life*. Boston: Allyn & Bacon.

Hallahan, D., & Keogh. (2001). *Research and global perspectives in learning disabilities*. Mahwah, NJ: Lawrence Erlbaum Associates.

Hechtman, L. (2000a). Assess and diagnosis of attention-deficit/hyperactivity disorder. *Child and Adolescent Psychiatric Clinics of North America, 9*(3), 481–498.

Hechtman, L. (2000b). Subgroups of adult outcomes of attention-deficit/hyperactivity disorder. In T. Brown (Ed.), *Attention-deficit disorders and comorbidities in children, adolescents and adults* (pp. 437–453). Washington, DC: American Psychiatric Press.

Individuals with Disabilities Education Act (IDEA). (1997). PL 105-17. Sections 601 and 602 [20 USC 1400].

Jensen, P., Arnold, L., Richters, J., et al. (1999). 14 month randomized clinical trial of treatment strategies for attention deficit hyperactivity disorder. *Archives of General Psychiatry, 56*, 1073–1086.

MacMillan, D., Gresham, F., & Bocian, K. (1998). Discrepancy between definitions of learning disabilities and school practices: An empirical investigation. *Journal of Learning Disabilities, 31*(4), 314–326.

Mannuzza, S., & Klein, R. (2000). Long-term prognosis in attention-deficit/ hyperactivity disorder. *Child and Adolescent Psychiatric Clinics of North America, 9*(3), 711–726.

Mather, N., & Goldstein, S. (2001). *Learning disabilities and challenging behaviors: A guide to intervention and classroom management*. Baltimore: Paul H. Brooke.

McBurnett, K., Pfiffner, L., & Ottolini, Y. (2000). Types of ADHD in DSM-IV. In P. Accardo, T. Blondis, B. Whitman, & M. Stein. *Attention deficits in children and adults: Diagnosis, treatment and management* (pp. 229–240). New York: Marcel Dekker.

Montgomery, D. (2003). *Gifted and talented children with special educational needs*. London: David Rulton.

MTA Cooperative Group. (2004). National Institute of Health Multimodal Treatment Study of ADHD Follow-up: 24-month outcomes of treatment strategies for attention-deficit/hyperactivity disorder. *Pediatrics, 113*(4), 754–761.

National Center for Learning Disabilities (NCLD). (2002). *About LD: LD fast facts*. Retrieved August 6, 2002 from http://www.ncld.org/info/fastfacts.cfrr.

National Institutes of Health (NIH). (November, 1998). *Consensus statement: Diagnosis and treatment of attention deficit hyperactivity disorder*. Bethesda, MD: NIH.

National Joint Committee on Learning Disabilities (NJCLD). (February, 1997). *Operationalizing the NJCLD definition of learning disabilities for ongoing assessment in schools*. Retrieved September 10, 2005 from http://www.ldonline.org/njcld/operationalizing.html

Pastor, P., & Reuben, C. (May, 2002). *Attention deficit disorder and learning disability: United States, 1997–1998*. National Center for Health Statistics. Vital and Health Statistics, 10(206). Hyattsville, MD: Department of Health and Human Services, Centers for Disease Control and Prevention.

Pelham, W., Gnagy, E., Burrows-Maclean, L., et al. (2001). Once a day Concerta methylphenidate versus three-times-daily methylphenidate—in laboratory and natural settings. Pediatrics, 107*(6), e105*.

Pliszka, S. (2000). Patterns of psychiatric co-morbidity of attention-deficit/hyperactivity disorder. *Child and Adolescent Psychiatric Clinics of North America, 9*(3), 525–540.

Pliszka, S., Carlson, C., & Swanson, J. (1999). *ADHD with comorbid disorders: clinical assessment and management*. New York: The Guildford Press.

Popper, C. (2000). Pharmacologic alternatives to psychostimulants for the treatment of attention-deficit/hyperactivity disorder. *Child and Adolescent Psychiatric Clinics of North America, 9*(3), 605–646.

Scahill L., & Schwab-Stone, M. (2000). Epidemiology of ADHD in school-age children. *Child and Adolescent Psychiatric Clinics of North America, 9*(3), 541–555.

Selekman, J. (2002a). Attention-deficit/hyperactivity disorder. *The Journal of School Nursing, 18*(5), 270–276.

Selekman, J. (2002b). Learning disabilities: A diagnosis ignored by nurses. *Pediatric Nursing, 28*(6), 630–632.

Selekman, J., & Moore, C. (2004). Primary care of the child with attention deficit hyperactivity disorder. In P. Jackson & J. Vessey (Eds.), *Primary care of the child with a chronic condition* (pp. 198–216). St. Louis: C. V. Mosby.

Silver, L. (1999). *ADHD: A clinical guide to diagnosis and treatment for health and mental health professionals*. Washington, DC: Psychiatric Press.

Smith, S. (2002). What do parents of children with learning disabilities, ADHD, and related disorders deal with? *Pediatric Nursing, 22*(3), 254–257.

Solanto, M. (2001). Attention-deficit/hyperactivity disorder: Clinical features. In M. Solanto, A. Arnsten, & F. Castellanos (Eds.), *Stimulant drugs and ADHD: Basic and clinical neuroscience* (pp. 3–30). New York: Oxford University Press.

Sousa, D. (2001). *How the special brain learns*. Thousand Oaks, CA: Corwin Press.

Spencer, T., Biederman, J., & Wilens, T. (2002). Attention-deficit/hyperactivity disorder. In S. Kutcher (Ed.), *Practical child and adolescent psychopharmacology* (pp. 230–264). Cambridge, UK: Cambridge University Press.

Stubbe, D. (2000). Attention-deficit/hyperactivity disorder overview: Historical perspective, current controversies, and future directions. *Child and Adolescent Psychiatric Clinics of North America, 9*(3), 469–479.

Thapar, A. (2003). Attention deficit hyperactivity disorder: New genetic findings, new directions. In R. Plomin, J. DeFries, I. Craig, & P. McGuffin, *Behavioral genomics in the postgenomic era* (pp. 445–462). Washington, DC: American Psychiatric Association.

Trapani, C. (2000). Psychoeducational assessment of children and adolescents with Attention Deficit Hyperactivity Disorder. In P. Accardo, T. Blondis, B. Whitman, & M. Stein (Eds.), *Attention deficits in children and Adults: Diagnosis, treatment and management* (pp. 197–214). New York: Marcel Dekker.

Turkington, C., & Harris, J. (2002). *The encyclopedia of learning disabilities*. New York: Facts on File, Inc.

U.S. Department of Health and Human Services (USDHHS). (October, 2002). Summary Health Statistics for U.S. Children. Health Interview Survey 1998. *Vital and Health Statistics*, Series 10, Number 208.

U.S. Food and Drug Administration. (September 29, 2005). FDA issues public health advisory on Strattera (Atomoxetine) for attention deficit disorder. Accessed November 10, 2005 from www.fda.gov/bbs/topics/news/2005/new01237.html

Ward, J., & Guyer, K. (2000). Medical management of ADHD. In B. Guyer (Ed.), *ADHD: Achieving success in school and in life* (pp. 38–54). Boston: Allyn & Bacon.

Wender, P. (2000). *ADHD: Attention-deficit hyperactivity disorder in children and adults*. New York: Oxford University Press.

Weyandt, L. (2001). *An ADHD primer*. Boston: Allyn & Bacon.

Whitman, B. (2000a). The genetic roots of organicity. In P. Accardo, T. Blondis, B. Whitman, & M. Stein (Eds.), *Attention deficits and hyperactivity in children and adults: Diagnosis, treatment, management* (pp. 119–140). New York: Marcel Dekker.

Whitman, B. (2000b). Living with a child with ADHD: Principles of family living, behavior management, and family support. In P. Accardo, T. Blondis, B. Whitman, & M. Stein (Eds.), *Attention deficits in children and adults: Diagnosis, treatment and management* (pp. 441–460). New York: Marcel Dekker.

Wilens, T., Faraone, S., Biederman, J., & Gunawardene, S. (2003). Does stimulant therapy of attention-deficit/hyperactivity disorder beget later substance abuse? A meta-analytic review of the literature. *Pediatrics, 111*(1), 179–185.

Wilens, T., & Spencer, T. (2000). Stimulants and attention-deficit/hyperactivity disorder. *Child and Adolescent Psychiatric Clinics of North America, 9*(3), 573–604.

Wilens, T., Spencer, T., & Biederman, J. (2000). Attention-deficit/hyperactivity disorder with substance use disorders. In T. Brown (Ed.), Attention-deficit disorders and comorbidities in children, adolescents, and adults (pp. 319–339). Washington, DC: American Psychiatric Press.

Willcutt, E., DeFries, J., Pennington, B., Smith, S., Cardon, L., & Olson, R. (2003). Genetic etiology of comorbid reading difficulties and attention deficit hyperactivity disorder. In R. Plomin, J. DeFries, I. Craig, & P. McGuffin (Eds.), *Behavioral genomics in the postgenomic era* (pp. 227–246). Washington, DC: American Psychiatric Association.

Chapter 31

Cerebral Palsy

KATHLEEN RYAN KUNTZ

Chapter Outline

INTRODUCTION

Cerebral palsy (CP) is an umbrella-like term used to describe a group of chronic disorders in which damage occurs to the developing brain, impairing control of movement and posture. The disorder is not caused by problems in the muscles or nerves, but rather by the disruption in the brain's ability to adequately communicate motor tasks. While the damage to the brain is nonprogressive, dependent on treatment, or lack thereof, complications of the disorder, such as muscle atrophy and joint contractures, can worsen, contributing to increased disability. In addition to motor impairments, children and adults with CP may also exhibit other symptoms related to damage to the brain, including cognitive deficits (i.e., learning disability, mental retardation), seizure activity, visual and auditory deficits, communication disorders, and/or behavior problems.

A child may sustain an injury to the brain before birth, during the birthing process, or during the childhood years. Damage to the brain early in life may result in the development of abnormal movements and posture at a young age. A previously healthy older child, however, may experience brain injury from infection, trauma (i.e., fall, accident, child abuse), poisoning, or a cerebral vascular accident, and demonstrate symptoms of CP as a result. In both instances, damage occurs to the child's brain before it has fully matured (at approximately age 16), although most cases involve an event prior to 3 years of age (Hays, 1997).

PREVALENCE AND ETIOLOGY

CP is identified as the leading cause of childhood disability, with a reported incidence in the United States of approximately two or three per 1000 live births, varying with geographical location and availability of prenatal care (Reddihough & Collins, 2003). The incidence is highest in infants, but occurs in later childhood years as well, adding to this estimate. Despite the fact that prenatal and perinatal care has dramatically improved, the prevalence of CP has remained relatively stable. While observers attribute this to the higher survival rates of smaller, more immature infants with ongoing advances in medicine and technology, Clark and Hankins (2003) refute this, instead stating, "except in rare instances, cerebral palsy is a developmental event that is unpreventable given our current state of technology" (p. 628).

William Jon Little, a London-based orthopedic surgeon in 1861, is credited with being the first to describe CP as a condition with a wide array of clinical symptoms, including tonal and developmental abnormalities. Many of the children he observed had been born to mothers with a history of prolonged labor, or preterm or breech delivery, and demonstrated depressed neurological function or seizures in the first days of life. Because of the frequency of these perinatal problems, Dr. Little postulated that they were the direct result of difficulties in the birth process. Critics of this theory speculated that these perinatal circumstances, as well as the subsequent neuromuscular symptoms observed, were the result of preexisting congenital abnormalities of the fetus.

The question of which came first, brain damage or problems in labor and delivery, was eventually addressed in a study performed by the National Collaborative Perinatal Project (NCPP). In this study, almost 38,000 infants born between 1959 and 1966 were followed for a period of 7 years to determine the incidence and risk factors contributing to the development of CP. As a result, an association was found between CP, low birth weight, and severe birth asphyxia. The risk of CP was 20 times greater for infants weighing 1,500 grams or less, and 250 times greater in infants of normal weight who had sustained severe asphyxia (defined as an Apgar score of 3 or less at 20 minutes). Many of these infants were also noted to have congenital brain anomalies. Asphyxia alone accounted for fewer than 10% of all cases (Nelson & Ellenberg, 1986; Van Eerden & Bernstein, 2003). Despite identification of high-risk circumstances, the most common cause of CP is idiopathic (Clark & Hankins, 2003; Reddihough & Collins, 2003; Rosenbaum, 2003).

Prenatal Factors

Noetzel and Miller (1998) determined that 75% to 90% of cases of CP occur between conception and delivery. Only 25% of full-term infants with CP had an Apgar score below 7 at 5 minutes (Nelson & Ellenberg, 1986). Other studies have suggested that prenatal events not evident at birth may be responsible, such as maternal disorders that interfere with normal fetal nutrition and oxygenation (i.e., uterine bleeding, placental dysfunction or maternal seizures).

Brain and skull deformities have been found in children with CP in the absence of birth trauma. These conditions have been associated with vascular or ischemic events (i.e., coagulation disorders or stroke) occurring during fetal brain development, contributing to a lack of developing brain tissue, or hypoxia. "Prematurity-related CP is most often caused by injury to the white matter of the brain as a result of periventricular leukomalacia or intraventricular hemorrhage" (Pellegrino, 2002, p. 444). Biochemical abnormalities, such as Rh incompatibility and hypoglycemia, can also contribute to the development of CP.

While CP is not referred to as a genetic condition, certain autosomal recessive disorders or inborn errors of metabolism are associated with a risk for developing symptoms that mimic CP. German measles (rubella) contracted by a pregnant woman can cause damage to the developing nervous system of the fetus, although the incidence of this has significantly decreased; exposure to other infections including cytomegalovirus and toxoplasmosis continues to be a threat. More recent studies have also identified chorioamnionitis as a risk factor in the development of CP (Yoon, 2000). Environmental toxins have been identified as factors contributing to damage to the central nervous system of a developing fetus, including radiation exposure, and methylmercury ingestion (from contaminated foods). Maternal ingestion of drugs of abuse may also affect the developing fetus.

Perinatal Factors

The risk of CP increases with a lower birth weight. Data from the NCPP study (Nelson & Ellenberg, 1986) show the risk to be 3.4 per 1,000 in infants 2,500 grams and over (5.51 pounds or more), 13.9 per 1,000 in infants 1,501 grams (3.3 pounds) to 2,500 grams (considered low birth weight), and 90.4 per 1000 in infants less than or equal to 1,500 grams (considered very low birth weight). A study conducted by Croen, Grether, Curry, and Nelson (2001) determined that congenital abnormalities play less of a role in the etiology of CP among children with birth weights less than 2,500 grams (5.51 pounds). Han, Bang, Lim, Yoon, and Kim (2002) suggest that the criterion determining "very low birth weight" be increased to 2,000 grams (4.4 pounds) as a significant risk for developing CP.

A strong relationship exists between children with CP and those with a history of hypoxic–ischemic-induced periventricular leukomalacia, although this influence is more difficult to identify in full-term infants. In the NCPP study, low Apgar score at 5 minutes, meconium passage, toxemia, or the use of middle and high forceps were also associated with an increased risk of CP. More recently, a task force on neonatal encephalopathy and CP sponsored by the American College of Obstetricians and Gynecologists (ACOG) and the American Academy of Pediatrics (AAP) established more specific criteria to suggest an intrapartum event (within 0 to 48 hours of delivery) as the cause of CP to include hypoxia immediately before or during labor; sudden and sustained fetal bradycardia or the absence of fetal heart rate variability in the presence of persistent, late, or variable decelerations; Apgar scores less than or equal to 3 beyond 5 minutes; and onset of multisystem involvement within 72 hours of birth (Van Eerden & Bernstein, 2003).

Additional risk factors that increase the possibility of an infant developing CP include breech presentation, multiple births, complicated labor and delivery, maternal hyperthyroidism, or seizures in the newborn. Bilirubin encephalopathy, or kernicterus, had been noted in the past to precipitate brain damage causing CP; however, with advances in medicine to include Rh immunization and treatment of severe bilirubinemia with phototherapy and exchange transfusion, these cases have become increasingly rare.

Postnatal Factors

Events following birth account for a much smaller percentage of cases of CP. Identified causes include viral and bacterial infections affecting the central nervous system (i.e., herpesvirus, beta streptococcus, meningitis, encephalitis), damage to the developing brain from vascular disturbances (i.e., intraventricular hemorrhage, stroke), introduction of chemical toxins (i.e., poisoning), and trauma (i.e., fall, motor vehicle accidents, traumatic brain injury, abuse, shaken-baby syndrome, assault).

CHARACTERISTICS

CP is a nonprogressive motor deficit. Many children with CP fail to reach developmental milestones; therefore, assessment of motor development is essential, including muscle tone, reflexes, and posture. CP is not generally diagnosed until 18 months to 2 years of age "because early muscle and motor tone abnormalities may signify another neurodevelopmental problem" (Nehring, 2004, p. 329) or just slower development related to prematurity.

Many classification systems have been proposed to identify CP, although no one system has been universally accepted. While each addresses the neuropathology and clinical features of related disorders, none has been able to clearly articulate the distinctions between subtypes without becoming unwieldy. One reason for this is that, unlike the adult brain, which demonstrates a direct correlation between an area of damage and clinical symptoms, the developing brain retains a degree of plasticity, or moldability, in assignment of functions. In general, CP is classified according to motor disorders and the most involved parts of the body identifying three main types: spastic (pyramidal), dyskinetic/athetoid (extrapyramidal), and mixed (Crothers & Paine, 1959).

The most common form, spastic CP (70% to 80%), involves abnormalities of the pyramidal tract, exhibited as increased deep tendon reflexes and increased tone. A more recent term for this type of CP is "upper motor neuron syndrome" (Nehring, 2004). Spasticity is identified as having an increased and exaggerated stretch reflex, in which there is resistance to movement; stimulus (noise, touch) is followed by a spasm, sometimes involving the entire body. Spasticity is often associated with clonus, an extensor plantar response, and persistent primitive reflexes or movement patterns, such as a positive Babinski reflex or asymmetrical tonic neck reflex. "In mild cases, the condition may not be recognized until the child is school-aged" (Nehring, 2004, p. 327). Red flags that would indicate the need for further assessment include toe walking, altered gait, or uncoordinated or involuntary movements. Scissoring is the most common gait disturbance; it occurs as a result of increased tone in the muscles that control adduction and internal rotation of the hips (Pellegrino, 2002). While any voluntary muscle group can be affected, the most common patterns of spastic CP are classified according to the extremities involved (Table 31.1).

Dyskinetic CP (10% to 15%) is most often exhibited as choreoathetosis with variable tone or rigidity, involving abnormalities of the extrapyramidal tract (Nehring, 2004). Abnormal involuntary movements are most notable when the individual initiates an action, as there is an inability to regulate the muscle tone and coordination. When the individual is at rest, usually full range of motion is possible with decreased tone and no changes in deep tendon reflexes. There are two main types of dyskinetic movement. The first is dystonia, in which abnormal shifts of muscle tone precipitate twisting of the trunk and extremities, causing abnormal posturing. The second is choreoathetoid, in which the initiation of movement in one extremity leads to movement of other muscle groups, causing a slow writhing movement (athetoid) in combination with abrupt, irregular, jerky movements (chorea) (Nehring, 2004).

Other forms of extrapyramidal CP are called rigid, atonic, and ataxic (5% to 10%). These forms do

Table 31.1 ■

CLASSIFICATION OF SPASTIC CEREBRAL PALSY

Monoplegia—one extremity
Hemiplegia—upper and lower extremity of one side
Diplegia—both upper and lower extremities, with lower extremities more severely affected
Triplegia—one upper extremity and both lower extremities
Quadriplegia (tetraplegia)—all four extremities and trunk, oral structures may be affected
Double hemiplegia—upper and lower extremities of both sides of body with upper extremities more severely involved.

not exhibit the choreoathetoid movements previously described. Rigid CP is notable for "lead pipe" rigidity in muscle tone in resistance to movement; atonic CP is characterized by floppy muscle tone throughout; and ataxic CP is exhibited by a disturbance in the coordination of voluntary movements caused by muscle dyssynergia, usually the result of cerebellar dysfunction. "Children with ataxia walk with an unstable, wide-based gait and have some difficulty trying to move a hand or arm voluntarily or timing such movement" (Nehring, 2004, p. 328).

Individuals with mixed CP (10%) display elements of spasticity and dyskinesia. In these cases, damage to the brain is more global, and affects all four extremities.

ASSOCIATED PROBLEMS AND TREATMENT

Impaired Motor Function

Alterations in muscle tone affect a wide range of functions necessary for mobility. Without the ability to independently roll over, or the muscle control to reach for or crawl to an item wanted, the child's ability to explore the environment is limited to what another person introduces. Increased flexor or extensor tone interferes with the child's ability to stand and walk. In addition to increased adduction and internal rotation (scissoring), gait disturbances can be due to increased flexor tone in the hips and knees (crouching), and increased extensor tone in the ankles (toe walking). Poor muscle tone may lead to hip dislocation and contractures. Multiple medical and surgical interventions are available for the treatment of motor problems related to CP.

Physical therapy generally addresses strength, range of motion, and motor planning, as they relate to posture and gross motor activities, including sitting, transfers, ambulation, and wheelchair mobility. In the education setting, the physical therapist will provide exercises to facilitate movement, improve gait and balance, and increase endurance. Adaptations, or the use of assistive devices, may be recommended to compensate for movements such as bending, squatting, kneeling, lifting, carrying, and climbing. Goals of treatment may be identified in relation to navigating hallways during change of class, maintaining balance while carrying books or a food tray, accessing desks and lockers, and support of mobility with assistive devices.

Occupational therapy interventions are generally focused on strength and range of motion as they relate to fine motor activities, activities of daily living, visual–perceptual tasks, and oromotor function (i.e., feeding). In the education setting, the occupational therapist will promote activities and compensatory strategies to enhance performance of skills such as reading, writing, note copying, keyboarding, fingering/manipulating coins and bills, sorting papers and materials, using switches, and to foster independence in activities of daily living such as basic hygiene, dressing, cooking, and household maintenance. Adaptations, or the use of assistive devices, may be recommended to compensate for movements such as reaching, pushing, pulling, and lifting. Goals of treatment may be identified related to writing, typing, note taking, operating vending machines, completing job applications, and performing tasks involved with various types of activities including those related to employment. Multiple approaches for physical and occupational therapy are available, although for many, empiric evidence to support their efficacy with children with CP is lacking (TABLE 31.2).

Other interventions for those with CP include oral medications, inhibitory bracing/splinting, the use of positioning devices and ambulation/mobility aides, motor point block injections, and surgical interventions to increase mobility and decrease spasticity and deformities (TABLES 31.3 and 31.4).

In addition to the motor and posture problems common to CP, it is very common to see comorbid conditions associated with it.

Table 31.2 ■

APPROACHES FOR PHYSICAL AND OCCUPATIONAL THERAPY WITH CEREBRAL PALSY

1. Neurodevelopmental treatment (NDT)—an approach to physical, occupational, and speech designed to provide sensorimotor experiences that enhance the development of positive movement patterns utilizing an individualized program of positioning, therapeutic handling, and exercise/play directed toward normalization of tone and control of movement during functional activities integrated into the child's daily routine (Pellegrino, 2002).
2. Adeli method of therapeutic intervention—uses an Adeli therapeutic suit (Therasuit®), based on research from the Russian space program. The suit creates a virtual muscular framework through the use of lines and pulleys, normalizing posture and stabilizing the trunk and extremities. Exercise and movement are facilitated to achieve optimal natural physiological responses and suppress pathological synergies in an effort to establish normalized reflex sequences. It is believed that these movements provide a therapeutic effect on the structures of the central nervous system responsible for motor activity and speech.
3. Functional electrical stimulation—electrical pulses administered to stimulate muscle response during specific movement patterns as part of a therapeutic regimen.
4. Therapeutic electrical stimulation—low-level electrical pulses, often administered at night, to stimulate sensory feedback to lesser used muscles, while providing an energized environment which has been shown to increase muscle fiber.
5. Biofeedback—conscious control of muscle responses utilizing electronic measurement or other system of feedback from activity to reinforce appropriate positioning and movement patterns (Dursun, Dursun, & Alican, 2004).
6. Constraint induced movement therapy (CI)—an experimental approach to physical and occupational therapeutic intervention in which the less impaired upper extremity is immobilized, and intensive therapy is provided for several hours each day over a period of 3 to 4 weeks (Taub, Ramey, DeLuca, & Echols, 2004).
7. Sensory integration—the organizing and processing of sensory information from various sensory channels, and the ability to have an adaptive response. A disturbance in response to sensory stimuli is thought to interfere with the individual's ability to appropriately react. Therapeutic intervention is based on providing controlled sensory stimulation (including tactile and vestibular input) while facilitating appropriate responses in functional tasks.
8. Hyperbaric oxygen therapy—a pressurized oxygen-enriched environment is provided in conjunction with therapeutic intervention with the belief that brain cells will be more receptive to appropriate movements and assume the function (Collet et al., 2001).
9. Myofascial release—in which the skin is manipulated at "trigger" points throughout the body so as to release the hold of the fascia layer of tissue in order to increase freedom of movement.
10. Aquatherapy—a program of exercise or movement performed in a warmer than average pool of water, stimulating circulation and providing a soothing environment, while utilizing the buoyancy of water to counteract the effects of gravity, thereby permitting increased movement.
11. Hippotherapy—a program of exercise performed on horseback, utilizing the warmth and movement of the horse to stimulate muscle responses to the pelvis and trunk, which mimic natural movement during ambulation.
12. Conductive education—a method of facilitating movement training and independence in an educational setting. Specific training of therapists and the use of specialized equipment are required.

Learning Disabilities and Mental Retardation

Approximately two-thirds of children with CP will have some level of mental retardation or a learning disability. Many with normal intelligence may still have perceptual impairments that place them at risk for learning disabilities. Some children and adolescents with CP demonstrate a superior level of intelligence, however. Cognitive ability somewhat correlates with topography of the disorder. Those with hemiplegia demonstrate the best intelligence

Table 31.3 ■
NONINVASIVE MEDICAL TREATMENT FOR CEREBRAL PALSY

1. Antispasmodics
   a. Diazepam (Valium)
   b. Dantrolene (Dantrium)
   c. Baclofen (Lioresal)

Often the effective dose causes a high degree of sedation, interfering with functional abilities. In some cases, Lioresal has also been shown to negatively affect the seizure threshold in individuals with a seizure disorder. It must be tapered when stopping the medication to prevent side effects such as hallucinations (Pellegrino, 2002).

---

2. Inhibitory bracing/splinting
   a. MAFOs—molded ankle foot orthoses worn inside the shoe to prevent shortening of the heel cords
   b. DAFOs—dynamic ankle–foot orthoses made with materials responsive to natural stepping action
   c. KAFOs—knee–ankle–foot orthoses offering support to the entire length of the lower extremity
   d. TLSO—thoracic–lumbar–sacral orthosis providing postural support of the trunk

Casts or molded orthotics fabricated to prevent excessive flexion and/or extension, facilitate a neutral position and enhance function in the upper extremities (finger, wrist, hand/arm splints) and lower extremities (shoe inserts)

---

3. Positioning devices
   a. Side-lyer
   b. Corner seat
   c. Positioning chair
   d. Adaptive wheelchair
   e. Prone or supine stander
   f. Wedges

Cushions or devices are used to maintain posture and prevent skin breakdown and contractures

---

4. Ambulation/mobility aids
   a. Single-point or quadruped canes
   b. Forearm crutches
   c. Forward or reverse walkers (with or without wheels)
   d. Tricycles
   e. Gait trainers
   f. Power wheelchairs (accessible by joystick, head array, or other switches)

Promote independence and encourage play and social interaction.

Source: Pellegrino (2002).

outcome, with 60% in the average or above average range. Conversely, fewer than 30% of those with spastic quadriplegia or mixed CP have average intelligence.

Among those with CP and mental retardation, 15% are in the mild range, 35% are in the moderate range, and 50% are in the severe range. It is noted, however, that precise cognitive testing in this population is difficult as most standardized tests are not directly applicable to individuals with disabilities. Typical intelligence tests for young children rely on visual and motor responses, while tests for older children consider speech and motor input, often resulting in inaccurate results. Evaluations by multiple healthcare disciplines may help delineate strengths and deficits and provide suggestions for compensatory strategies as well as treatment and education programs (Eicher, 1993, Hays, 1997; Pellegrino, 2002).

Visual Deficit

Vision requires the use of eye muscles, which are also affected in CP, resulting in visual disturbances. Visual impairments are common to individuals with

Table 31.4 ■

INVASIVE MEDICAL TREATMENT FOR CEREBRAL PALSY

a. Motor point block injections—Injections of botulinum toxin A (Botox) or phenyl and alcohol blocks, temporarily anesthetize nerve roots (for a period of 3 to 6 months), thereby facilitating therapeutic intervention to increase strength and range of motion (Edgar, 2001; Graham, 2000).
b. Surgical interventions
    i. Selective dorsal root rhizotomy to sever afferent nerve rootlets contributing to spasticity (McLaughlin et al., 2002)
    ii. Implanted medication delivery pump providing continual infusion of antispasmodic agent intrathecally to the nerve roots (Albright, 1997; Butler & Campbell, 2000) is inserted under the skin of the abdomen, with a catheter tunneled into the intrathecal space of the spine.
    iii. Tendon lengthening to release a fixed joint contracture
    iv. Tendon transfer to increase tension in one area, while diminishing tension in another, in an effort to normalize position and function
    v. Osteotomy to provide improved alignment of bone structures
    vi. Spinal fusion with implantation of a rod to arrest curvature and provide spinal stability
    vii. Additional experimental surgical techniques include chronic cerebellar stimulation and stereotaxic thalamotomy for control of spasticity

CP, and vary according to the type of brain injury sustained. The visual disturbance can originate with altered control of the muscles that move the eyes in a conjugate gaze (i.e., strabismus, nystagmus), can include deficits in acuity or field accommodation, or more significantly can affect the processing of visual input (cortical impairment). They can include refractive errors, field deficits, amblyopia, and cortical blindness. Strabismus is present in approximately 50% of children with CP. Preterm infants with retinopathy of prematurity (ROP) can exhibit a range of disorders from myopia to blindness. Individuals with hemiplegia may demonstrate a homonymous hemianopia in which there is blindness or defective vision in the right or left halves of the visual fields of both eyes. Each of these requires evaluation, monitoring, and intervention by an ophthalmologist specializing in neuromuscular disorders.

Treatment of muscle control of the eye may include the use of patches; the application of eye drops; or the use of vision lenses, prisms, or filters (vision therapy). Treatment of acuity, refractive, and accommodation errors generally involve the use of corrective lenses, many times requiring a double correction, or bifocal. Treatment of field cuts and cortical impairments (now more accurately called neurological visual impairments) require the use of additional therapeutic intervention to promote visual stimulation, learning about the environment, and the position of the self within that environment. In addition, the use of low-vision aids, such as closed circuit video systems (CCTV), speech recognition software, mylar guide templates, and Braille, can be introduced to assist the individual toward increased independence.

Hearing Deficit

Hearing impairments are present in fewer than 10% of children with CP, and are most often related to cases of a prenatal/postnatal infection of the central nervous system (i.e., congenital rubella), hyperbilirubinemia, or extensive treatment with antibiotics causing ototoxicity. Many hearing deficits related to CP are a result of anatomical abnormalities and/or frequent otitis media (Nehring, 2004; Pellegrino, 2002).

Treatment for hearing loss includes the use of hearing aids that facilitate the transmission of sound to the brain. Various types of ear molds can be utilized for children to facilitate wearing compliance (see Chapter 27). An assistive device that is used widely in the educational setting is a personal FM system, which is comprised of a wireless receiver worn by the individual, and a microphone worn by the teacher. Such a system overcomes the effects of background noise, reverberation, and distance from the speaker. An individual with profound hearing impairment in both ears may be a candidate for a cochlear implant (surgical implantation of an electronic device that stimulates the acoustic nerve). Additional environmental assistance with communication can be achieved through the use of closed captioning (CC), teletypewriters (TTY), and telecommunication devices for the deaf (TTD), which have become more widely available in the community as a result of the Americans with Disabilities Act of 1990 (see Chapter 14).

Communication Deficits

Communication impairments can be related to speech motor deficits or difficulties in central processing (i.e., expressive and receptive language). Dysarthria (imperfect articulation of speech resulting from disturbances of muscular control) is common among individuals with extrapyramidal damage, in which expressive and receptive disorders are associated with damage to other areas of the brain. Those with dysarthria may need to use some form of augmentative communication to assist in making their needs known, as well as to facilitate independent participation in social interactions.

Often those with higher-level cognitive function and functional fine motor ability can benefit from the integration of sign language early in development. Children with expressive difficulties, or those with an artificial airway, impairing verbal speech, can utilize signs to convey messages while further developing skill and ability to verbalize. In these instances, the Signing Exact English (SEE) system is preferred over the traditional American Sign Language (ASL) as grammatical structure and syntax are preserved (rather than the use of phrases), facilitating continued learning of the English language. It should be noted, however, that parents often see the use of sign language as a step backward, feeling that the therapist has given up on helping the child speak. In reality, it provides the child with a way to communicate meaningfully with others, preventing the child from developing frustrations and negative behaviors. Therefore, parents, siblings, teachers, and the school nurse should learn basic signing. As verbal or assisted communication becomes easier, the use of sign language fades.

Speech therapy generally provides support toward the development of speech and language ability. In the education setting, the speech therapist will support the ability to convey a message, participate in social interactions, and understand concepts. Goals of treatment may be related to speech production and articulation, the use of augmentative devices to adequately interact and communicate with others, and appropriate socialization skills (i.e., listening, turn taking, etc.).

Augmentative and alternative communication systems can be utilized to assist individuals to communicate their needs and participate in social interaction. These systems can be as simple as picture or symbol/word charts, or as complex as computerized devices with a speech synthesizer. The use of a system is generally recommended by the speech therapist, its design highly individualized to meet the communication needs of the individual, considering his or her cognitive and fine motor abilities. Often, the occupational therapist is consulted to assist in identifying an optimal means to access a device (i.e., pointer with wrist strap, head pointer, head array, eye gaze selection, etc.). To support the child's developing independence, it is important for the parents, teachers, therapists, and the school nurse to understand how the augmentative communication device operates, and to integrate its use into all activities throughout the day. It is important to identify a system of communication that will be utilized as a "back-up" in the event that the device requires updating or service, so as to not keep the child from interacting with others.

Additional items that can be considered cognitive or communication prosthetics include the use of a small recorder to record important information, such as the route one took to arrive at a destination, or the location to return to the correct bus. If the student is later unable to recall this information, the recorder can be played as a reminder, or to communicate to someone assisting the individual. A Data Link watch can be programmed with alerts at specific times denoting appointments or the need to take medication. It can also be programmed with important telephone numbers, so that when a selection is made, it will emit the appropriate tone into the telephone receiver to dial the number. A memory book, or personal digital assistant (PDA), can be utilized to assist in recalling or communicating essential information. With advances in technology, electronic devices and computers can also be utilized for this purpose, incorporating photographs to enhance identification of this information.

Seizures

Seizures occur in approximately one third of cases of children with CP and can present as any type (see Chapter 37) (Kwong, Wong, & So, 1998; Singhi, Jagirdar, Khandelwal & Malhi, 2003), although the frequency varies by the type of CP. Researchers have noted seizure disorders in 43% to 90% of those with quadriparesis, 34% to 66% of those with hemiplegia, 16% to 27% of those with diplegia, and 23% to 26% of those with extrapyramidal CP (Aicardi, 1990; Singhi et al., 2003). Most seizure disorders are apparent by 2 years of age, but can surface during puberty with alterations in metabolic processes and hormonal levels. The most frequent types of seizure exhibited include generalized tonic–clonic and partial complex (see Chapter 37). They are often severe and difficult to control, particularly in individuals with mental retardation (Hays, 1999; Singhi et al., 2003).

At times, seizures can be accompanied by symptoms of migraine headache, which may actually become more disabling than the seizure itself. The primary treatment for both of these conditions is the use of pharmacological agents. The treatment of seizures will usually involve the use of oral anticonvulsant medications (i.e., phenobarbital, carbamazepine, phenytoin, valproic acid), or benzodiazepines (i.e., diazepam, clonazepam, lorazepam, and clorazepate). Medications are taken regularly to maintain therapeutic blood levels, requiring adjustment in dose related to growth and changes in metabolism. The goal of pharmacological treatment is to attain a level of seizure control without undue sedation. Often, more than one anticonvulsant agent is utilized.

A degree of success in treating seizures has also been demonstrated by providing a diet high in fats and low in carbohydrates (ketogenic diet); in the absence of carbohydrates, the body will break down fats, leading to a state of ketosis. This regimen is unpalatable and difficult to administer consistently. If not maintained, seizures will return. During this therapy, supplemental vitamins and minerals must be provided.

More recently, the use of implanted vagal nerve stimulators has been utilized to control seizures that have a focal origin. Other surgical procedures that may be employed in cases in which more conservative treatment has failed include the focal excision of the area of origin in the brain, corpus callosotomy, or hemispherectomy. Each of these has significant risk factors and the potential for altered function and ability (see Chapter 37).

Feeding and Eating Problems

Feeding problems related to oromotor difficulties may be evident at an early age. Brain damage may result in hypotonia with a weak suck, poor coordination of swallow and inability to protect the airway, persistent tonic bite reflex or tongue thrust, hyperactive gag, and intolerance of textures in addition to an inability to communicate hunger and independently access food (Reilly, Skuse, & Poblete, 1996). The child may also be resistant to feeding in response to noxious stimuli surrounding the mouth and face at an early age, pain associated with untreated gastroesophageal reflux, or a diminished desire to eat related to constipation. An additional consideration of altered nutrition includes the energy expenditure resulting from involuntary muscle spasms or the increased effort necessary to perform various functions, which also contributes to fatigue and a further reduction in caloric intake (Stallings, Zemel, Davies, Cronk, & Charney, 1996; Sullivan et al., 2000). In these instances, nutritional supplements are frequently required.

All children have periods during which their nutrition is less than optimal or is high in fat or calories. Children with CP are at particular risk of this, as the ingestion of high-fat, high-calorie foods may have been overly emphasized during their younger years to facilitate weight gain and growth.

Care must be taken to avoid the possibility of aspiration. For some students who are severely affected, it may be necessary to provide external assistance with one's hand to keep the jaw closed during feeding (Nehring, 2004). Excessive drooling of food and fluids may occur, resulting in skin irritation. The nutritionist and occupational therapist can be of great assistance if feeding problems are present.

When the amount of nutrition taken orally is not sufficient to support the caloric needs of the child to facilitate growth and general health, enteral feedings will be recommended. These feedings can be delivered via a nasogastric or gastrostomy tube. As a nasogastric tube passes through the cardiac sphincter into the stomach, the risk of gastroesophageal reflux is increased. Should the tube slip out of place unobserved, formula being delivered could be aspirated into the airway. Many of those who need enteral feedings have a gastrostomy tube surgically placed percutaneously, directly into the stomach.

Bowel and Bladder Problems

Many individuals with CP are continent for urine and bowel, although altered tone and decreased mobility may precipitate lifelong problems with constipation. Care must be taken to provide sufficient hydration and dietary fiber to prevent fecal impaction and bowel obstruction. In addition, these same factors, coupled with the potential for bone demineralization, can predispose one to incidences of urinary calculi or stones. In instances in which continence is maintained but independent mobility or self-care abilities are lacking, a program of timed voids or bowel evacuation may be useful to assist the individual in remaining clean and dry.

Urinary incontinence may be associated with a neurogenic bladder, in which normal function of the bladder cannot be achieved because of neurological dysfunction at the level of the brain, brainstem, or spinal cord. The frontal lobe of the brain provides signals to the detrusor muscle to prevent the bladder from emptying (contracting) until a socially acceptable time and place is available. Injury to this area will cause the bladder to empty reflexively when fullness is reached, as in an infant. This is the most common cause of urinary incontinence associated with CP.

Urinary retention can also occur, risking pyelonephritis and kidney damage. Careful evaluation through urodynamic testing is necessary to identify this type of pattern, although frequent urinary tract infections may be an initial indicator. "A combination of incomplete bladder emptying, infrequent voiding, severe fluid restriction, and urinary reflux increase the likelihood of frequent urinary tract infections, as do chronic constipation, improper perineal hygiene, and motor impairments. Overall, children with CP are three times as likely to have urinary tract infections as the general population" (Nehring, 2004, p. 335). Treatment will include the use of antibiotics and the need for intermittent catheterization to empty the bladder.

Skin Problems

Careful assessment of the skin is an important element of ongoing care of individuals with CP. External causes of altered skin integrity include the following:

1. The use and wearing of braces, splints and casts, as well as the use of positioning devices and wheelchairs that provide pressure against bony prominences if ill fitting, applied incorrectly, or insufficiently padded, and those that trap moisture against the surface of the skin
2. The use of incontinence products precipitating skin breakdown owing to the pressure of folds and wadded padding, as well as exposure to skin damaging elements of urine and feces
3. Decreased oromotor control causing saliva to pool and drool over the face and neck precipitating chaffing
4. Moisture from sweat production in areas where skin folds are held tight because of joint contractures (i.e., neck, underarms, groin), precipitating moisture build-up, skin sloughing, and possible fungal infection
5. The presence of an ostomy, or opening to the body, as with a tracheostomy or gastrostomy, posing an added risk of skin irritation from mucus or stomach contents draining from the site
6. The risk for bumps and falls is markedly increased over the general student population, and combined with the student's lack of awareness or communication of an injury can lead to worsening sores and infections.

Factors related to altered nutrition can also contribute to delayed healing of wounds once they occur.

Safety Problems

Children and adolescents with altered mobility are at a greater risk for bumps and falls than the general student population. Accessibility in the environment must include not only ramps and elevators, but also measures to permit the student to safely get to a class, and obtain lunch in the cafeteria. Issues must be addressed related to congestion in the halls during change of class, obstacles such as book bags or debris on floors, and negotiating uneven or disrupted surfaces both indoors and outdoors. Changes in weather can pose additional risks for injury to the student with motor difficulties, requiring careful snow and ice removal and vigilant attention to wet floor surfaces indoors. Additional safety interventions may include the use of protective helmets and safety-proofing classrooms. The school nurse should recognize potential areas in which specific strategies are necessary to ensure a safe environment for students with CP, providing this input to individualized education programs and helping teachers to be more cognizant of their needs.

The presence of a cognitive impairment adds to the potential for injury, particularly if the student lacks safety awareness and judgment in potentially harmful situations. Often school systems will implement a "buddy" system to address emergency situations (i.e., fire drill, need to evacuate), but fail to recognize the risks that are posed on a daily basis.

Careful consideration of the student's individual needs is necessary, and should be addressed in the Individualized Education Program (IEP). Safety factors should be addressed related to the medical needs of the student (i.e., side effects of medications, seizure precautions), as well as the correct application and use of adaptive and assistive equipment (i.e., braces, splints, crutches, walkers, and wheelchairs). Adequate supervision and support is required for students who are unable to identify dangers or respond to the physical threats of others.

EFFECT OF CP ON THE GENERAL HEALTH OF STUDENTS

Respiratory Status

While respiratory difficulty is not typically a primary condition associated with CP, it can often be a complication. Altered respiratory function related to bronchopulmonary dysplasia and tracheomalacia can result from prematurity and low birth weight, and may have required the use of positive pressure ventilation or an artificial airway in infancy. These may have precipitated the development of scar tissue, affecting the pulmonary status of those with CP and leaving them at risk for reactive airway disease (asthma). Poor oromotor control and the inability to protect the airway from aspiration of saliva, food, and other foreign bodies pose the risk for pneumonia and chronic scarring, contributing to the development of restrictive lung disease. Decreased muscle tone will also affect the student's ability to accomplish full ventilation and lung expansion, thereby requiring him or her to take more frequent, shallow breaths. Sustaining this type of breathing pattern requires increased energy expenditure, contributing to decreased endurance and increased fatigue.

Children and adolescents with severe motor impairment may not be able to sufficiently support their own respiratory effort without a form of mechanical ventilatory support. These supports can be provided noninvasively in the form of negative pressure ventilation utilizing an externally worn poncho system, or by continuous positive airway pressure (CPAP) delivered via nasal cannula or face mask. However, the student may need positive pressure ventilation, which will require the placement of a tracheostomy tube and/or the use of a portable ventilator. Direct care for a child with a tracheostomy and/or ventilator assistance includes periodic chest physiotherapy and suctioning to mobilize secretions, as well as ongoing assessment to ensure the safety and well-being of the child. Many children who are ventilator-assisted are able to attend school with the support of a licensed nurse caregiver in attendance. Federal legislation requires this level of support to be provided by the school system; however, medical insurers frequently provide the necessary coverage to foster inclusion of these students in school.

Cardiovascular Status

Aside from the risk factors of cardiovascular disease that cannot be altered (i.e., age, sex, family history of cardiovascular disease, comorbid diabetes mellitus), students with CP face additional risk factors (i.e., physical inactivity; caloric imbalance leading to obesity; nutritional intake high in saturated fats, cholesterol, and salt). These may set the stage for future hypertension and coronary artery disease. Decreased mobility may also pose risks associated with venous stasis, precipitating the development of a deep vein thrombosis.

Activity/Rest Patterns

Children and adolescents with CP face many challenges in development when seeking to be included with their same-age peers. Often, they do not have the physical abilities or endurance to join in school activities and extracurricular events with other students. Participating in a full day of classes can precipitate fatigue requiring rest periods in the school nurse's office. Separation from the group, as with education and therapeutic support services, limits their ability to develop close friendships. As years pass, they share fewer and fewer common interests with others of the same age. Many activities are available to children and adolescents with motor and cognitive impairments, including adapted sports leagues. These organizations offer opportunities for students to learn new skills, participate in activities to their own level, develop a sense of "team," and gain a sense of accomplishment. Often their "peer" group develops from their participation in special education classes, or adapted activities and camps, matching them with others of various ages and developmental levels.

Comfort

Chronic and severe pain is a serious secondary problem for many individuals with CP. Despite the frequency of pain symptoms experienced, the available evidence suggests that CP-related pain is under-evaluated and undertreated (Jensen, Engel, Hoffman, & Schwartz, 2004). Limitations in mobility, difficulty with positioning, occurrences of muscle spasm, and the use of assistive and adaptive equipment may all precipitate situations of discomfort for children. It is important to recognize the risk factors for pain, as well as the manner in which the child typically exhibits pain symptoms. When the school nurse works closely with parents, teachers, and therapists, the student is best protected from experiencing unnecessary pain. A careful history of pain symptoms and treatments should be obtained.

While the student's self-report of pain is the most important factor in assessment, this can be difficult to ascertain, depending on his or her cognitive level and ability to communicate. Often one must be attentive to behavioral clues offered (i.e., crying, facial expression, or self-injurious actions). Developmental levels must be carefully considered in the use of tools that yield a subjective, quantitative measure of pain intensity, such as the FACES Pain Rating Scale. Once recognized, pain symptoms can be accurately addressed. Effective treatments can include over-the-counter analgesics (i.e., acetaminophen, ibuprofen), prescription antispasmodics, range-of-motion exercises, massage, warm compresses, whirlpool, ultrasound, and transcutaneous electrical stimulation (TENS). A plan for addressing pain symptoms in the school setting should be included in the IEP.

Students with lower cognitive ability can develop self-injurious behaviors in response to pain, discomfort, an inability to communicate their needs, or in an effort to exert control over their environment. Many children respond to behavior management techniques in which the negative behavior is ignored, and thereby extinguished, while the positive behavior is rewarded (see Chapter 38).

THE STUDENT WITH CP IN THE SCHOOL

The school nurse is an integral component in ensuring success for the student in the educational environment. It is essential for the nurse to know the following about the student:

- The student's medical history related to his or her CP (age at diagnosis, surgeries, age at which developmental milestones were met)
- The cause of the CP, if known
- The type of CP and how it manifests itself (spasticity/athetosis; which body parts are affected; scissoring, reflexes)
- The degree of motor involvement (gross and fine motor; activity tolerance)
- The presence of any associated problems (mental retardation, seizures, feeding problems, elimination problems, hearing and vision problems, communication, etc.)
- Medical treatment or interventions needed
- Accommodations needed to achieve success in the classroom
- Safety concerns
- Degree of self-care
- Self-concept

Depending on the findings from the above, the school nurse needs to develop an Individualized Health Plan and an Emergency Action Plan and then use these to assist in the development of the IEP. The family can be very helpful in assisting the school nurse to learn how to meet the needs of their child. Should the student require splints, braces, feeding devices, or other mechanical devices, it is important for the nurse to develop a list of resource people he or she can contact to assist in the use of, and troubleshooting for, this equipment.

Providing a safe environment should be the first priority. Accessibility in the home, school, and community involves more than simply adjusting the physical structure of a building or environment to permit safe entry/egress, or providing technology to enable the use of communication devices. Federal legislation mandates that children at risk of developmental delay receive support services from birth to age 3, and those with physical and cognitive disabilities must receive a free and appropriate public education from age 3 through 21 (see Chapters 14 and 27). In addition, requirements for public areas regarding parking, ramping, and door openings, as well as dimensions of doorways, hallways, and restroom stalls to accommodate wheelchairs are mandated. Systems must be in place to accommodate the needs of an individual to ascend and descend levels (i.e., elevators), as well as to accurately locate specific areas by directional signs.

The manifestations of CP may have an effect on the growth and development of the student. Physical growth parameters serve as a guideline for monitoring the health status of students; however, these are almost universally insufficient for those with CP. Difficulty in obtaining accurate measurement is common in the case of individuals with scoliosis or joint contractures. The development of more accurate measurement and evaluation tools is being investigated through multisite research studies that consider segmental length, anthropometric measurement of skin folds, bone density, and measurement of metabolic processes. The associated problems common to CP also make it difficult to screen accurately for hearing, vision, and posture.

Self-Care Ability

Activities of daily living include feeding, toileting, hygiene, transfers, and dressing/grooming. Instrumental activities of daily living further identify tasks involved in living independently, including use of the telephone, use of transportation, grocery shopping, meal preparation, household maintenance, laundry, taking medications/health management, and money management. Children and adolescents with CP may face obstacles to independence in several of these areas. Therapeutic intervention and the use of assistive/adaptive devices are key toward the development of these life skills and increased independence of the individual. School programs that focus exclusively on academic achievement without assessing and addressing abilities in self-care do little to support the child's transition to adulthood, and his or her future success within society. These issues are ideally addressed by the school nurse through identification of self-care and transition goals and interventions in the student's IEP.

Peer Relationships/ Sexuality/Self-Concept

Individuals with CP are dependent on others for many aspects of their care, and develop less independence than their same-age peers. Students with CP strive to be like their peers in every way, with their primary mission during this period to "fit in." Those with physical and cognitive disabilities hold the very same goals for acceptance as other children, many times being painfully aware of their differences. These students often become the subject of teasing and ridicule, irrespective of their levels of ability, because of their "differences." In addition, they can be victimized, physically, mentally, or financially, by individuals who would take advantage of their dependent status. It is important for them to develop friendships and peer relationships.

The school nurse should support an understanding of these concerns among staff, teachers, and therapists interacting with students with CP. In addition, concurrent to the development of support systems in the school for students with disabilities, the school nurse can facilitate efforts to provide instruction and interactive experiences to the general student body to increase their awareness, sensitivity, and acceptance of others' differences, including race, religion, ethnicity, sexual orientation, and level of ability as a foundation for mature social behavior in our society.

It is also important for children and adolescents with disabilities to develop a realistic self-concept, while establishing a healthy level of self-esteem. Too often parents and professionals overemphasize their accomplishments, making them feel as though they can do things as well as their same-age peers. As they proceed with that perspective, others may treat them differently, precipitating feelings of inferiority. Parents, teachers, and health professionals can better assist these children by helping them to identify and promote the areas in which they have strengths, as well as those in which they may require assistance. It is important that they recognize their limitations, and develop a level of comfort in asking for help when needed. Along with this is the ability to identify trustworthy individuals, and those in whom they can confide.

Developmental tasks addressing industry/inferiority, identity/role confusion, and intimacy/isolation are each addressed during their years in primary and secondary education settings, despite altered levels of physical and cognitive ability. An inability to navigate these levels successfully may precipitate depression, emotional lability, low self-esteem, or behavior difficulties. These may respond to psychological counseling or pharmacological management. Attention must be paid to the development of their sexuality and peer relationships in addition to acquisition of vocation and social skills.

A sound sense of self is integral to a child's developing sexuality. To the degree that they can understand, children with disabilities must learn the social expectations of personal hygiene, personal space and privacy, bodily functions, and socially appropriate behavior, including public displays of affection. Children with disabilities may wonder about things they see and hear, but be unsure how to articulate their questions, or whom they can ask. As adolescents, they may wish to participate in dating and other social activities with students of the opposite sex, just as their same-age peers. It is important for a trusted adult to provide them with a supportive open relationship in which sensitive issues can be discussed clearly and at a level they will understand.

COPING: INDIVIDUAL/FAMILY

Involvement of family members in an ongoing manner is essential in the care of children and adolescents with CP. Beyond the infant period, during which children are typically fully dependent, children with motor and cognitive impairments require continued assistance with many, or all, aspects of their care, often placing a heavy day-to-day responsibility on the family. The ability to send the child to school not only benefits the student, but also provides respite for the family members, allowing them to meet their own needs.

A higher degree of communication and support is often provided to parents of children with disabilities during preschool and elementary levels of instruction, which begins to wane as the child enters middle school. While typically developing children are able to take on more responsibility and develop a level of independence at this phase, those with physical and/or cognitive impairments continue to require the close support of family caregivers. Ongoing communication with the school nurse, teachers, and therapists will support the coordination of goals and enhance the efforts of each.

Families are often overwhelmed with the number of specialists their children see and the multiple problems identified. A memory book, planner, or personal digital assistant can be used to identify the many providers involved, their focus or specialty, treatment recommendations, and essential contact information. It can also be used to note the

Medical Condition – Seizures with Migraine Headache

When:
1-2 each month, usually in the afternoon or evening, or when I don't get enough sleep

What to Look For:
I will get a strange feeling and my vision gets blurry. Sometimes I see colored spots

What to Do:
- □ I need to relax and try to tell someone what is happening.
- □ I need to sit down on a chair or the floor away from the crowd, or else I might fall.
- □ If possible I will ask someone to time how long the seizure lasts.
- □ Once the seizure slows down, I need to take migraine medication.
- □ If the seizure is different in any way, I need to ask someone to tell the nurse.
- □ I need to record the seizure and how long it lasted on my calendar to tell my doctor.
- □ My next neurology appointment is scheduled for May 2nd.

Who to Call:
School Nurse – Ms. Black, x9876
Parents – Mr. and Mrs. Brown, (456) 123-6543
Neurologist – Dr. Smith, (123) 456-7890

Figure 31.1 ■ Healthcare checklist example.

frequency of physician and therapy visits and appointments made. The school nurse can assist the student to develop checklists to identify signs and symptoms of illness and suggested treatments, with notations of when to call the doctor and how to handle an emergency situation (FIGURE 31.1). The family, and later the student, should be instructed to maintain a journal of physical symptoms and health-related information in order to accurately convey them when needed. The school nurse and teachers can assist in the development of a journal to be incorporated as a life skill and part of a daily routine. Such a journal is easiest to maintain in a calendar format in a binder or a weekly or monthly planner, with room to write notes (FIGURE 31.2).

Monday	Busy day, up late doing homework
Tuesday	Tired all day, seizure after dinner (4 minutes) Headache lasting 2 hours (took three pills) No nausea
Wednesday	Feeling better, went to bed early
Thursday	Feeling better
Friday	Dr. Smith, 3 p.m.
Saturday	
Sunday	

Figure 31.2 ■ Healthcare journal example.

Careful consideration by the parents is necessary regarding the disabled individual's ability to make medical decisions as he or she enters adolescence and adulthood (i.e., consent to a surgical procedure, an advance directive, or organ donation) with the support of involved health professionals. Often steps toward full or limited guardianship should be taken during the student's adolescence.

It is important to recognize that siblings of students with disabilities also have specialized needs that are often overlooked. The school nurse is in a unique position to support the family and to provide information related to available resources that consider the needs of each member. This type of support can be offered through the development of a resource listing sent home to parents via the student or given at the time of the IEP meeting. Individual support can also be offered at the time a student is seen because of illness or accident, or if parents contact the school nurse with questions. Some resources are identified at the end of this chapter.

HEALTH MAINTENANCE

Physical, occupational, and speech therapists; nutritionists; and social workers are often essential healthcare providers in providing comprehensive care to students with CP. Children and adolescents with CP require the input of many specialists and educators to facilitate optimal development and function in the school setting. The IEP team is crucial in facilitating health-related service delivery and educational enrichment. The medical oversight is generally provided by the primary care provider, who prevents disease through screenings and immunizations, manages day-to-day health problems, and institutes treatments toward the prevention of complications. Additional support is received by specialists in physical medicine and rehabilitation, orthopedics, neurology, neurosurgery, ophthalmology, gastroenterology, and pulmonology, depending on the student's individual needs. Special attention should be made to support dental health, particularly if medications affect the health of teeth and gums, or if oromotor function is such that oral care is difficult. The school nurse can serve as the case manager to coordinate all services within the school and to be a liaison with the healthcare provider.

Therapeutic intervention is generally required to support the development of skills and abilities during early childhood years, and through various phases of growth. Therapeutic support services in the disciplines of physical, occupational, and speech therapy are provided by the school system as needed to facilitate the educational process. Additional rehabilitation may be required periodically to support recovery and enhanced function following medical or surgical intervention. Psychological supports may be needed for treatment of emotional or behavioral disturbances, but are also provided by the school system in order to monitor and evaluate cognitive abilities and provide input toward instructional strategies to meet educational goals. Social work and case management services are generally required to assist the child and family to navigate the complex healthcare and education systems.

TRANSITION PLANNING

Integration of transition planning into school programs and adding these to the IEP for adolescents beginning at age 14 is required in order to meet the student's goals for additional education or to prepare him or her to enter the workforce. Often transition planning focuses on independent living skills, such as personal care and the activities of daily living; these include use of the telephone, use of transportation, grocery shopping, nutrition and meal preparation, household maintenance, and money management. Frequently, it is the occupational therapist who will likely be involved in the development of a transition plan for adolescents, providing evaluation of potential job or school sites with recommendations for accommodations.

Independence in personal health management can easily be overlooked, but should be emphasized, as it is a lifelong need of the individual with CP, including the need for primary care. Adult rehabilitation services are not typically structured in the same integrated manner, leaving the individual and his or her family left to pull the pieces together. The use of support services, such as case management, should be explored to assist in the coordination of care.

Studies of adults with CP suggest that 33% can identify a desired vocation, and 25% are working. This appears to parallel findings that suggest that one third of the population with CP has average or above-average intelligence. Hays (1997) identified three factors that correlate with the employability of individuals with CP: independent mobility, intelligibility of speech, and normal intelligence. He found little correlation between employability and independence in activities of daily living, or the presence of visual and hearing impairments, and identified that 75% of those employed have a spastic motor impairment, while 14% have a dyskinetic impairment, and fewer than 5% demonstrate either ataxic or mixed motor disabilities.

When students approach the development of vocational skills in the school system, it is important to assess the individual's work values, interests, physical abilities, and awareness of occupational requirements. Additional studies have identified that parental attitudes during the early years, and the degree of social contact with other students during school years, are the greatest factors influencing successful employment of adults with CP.

CONCLUSION

CP can appear in many different forms. The needs of children and adolescents with this condition can range from minimal or supportive in nature to very complex. Treatments for the various health concerns related to CP continue to evolve with advances in medicine, technology, and therapeutic interventions. Needs and necessary treatments must be carefully considered on an individual basis, and should be incorporated into the student's IEP to facilitate communication among school professionals and collaboration with parents and others involved in the student's care. Goals should focus on the coordination of efforts to achieve the greatest level of ability and independence possible in preparation for the individual's adult role in society.

The school nurse, teachers, and health professionals working with these children and adolescents are in a position to advocate for the ongoing changes that continue to be necessary for them to succeed. All school nurses, teachers, and health professionals can influence the level of understanding and acceptance of the general student population toward others with differences, furthering the development of mature social behavior in our society. The school nurse is in a key position to work with the education team, as well as to interface with other professionals to ensure the many facets of CP are reviewed and addressed, thereby promoting the student's ultimate success.

Resources

ABLEDATA—Premiere Source for Information on Assistive Technology
National Institute on Disability and Rehabilitation Research
U.S. Department of Education
8630 Fenton Street, Suite 930
Silver Spring, MD 20910
800-227-0216
http://www.abledata.com

Administration on Developmental Disabilities
Administration for Children and Families
U.S. Department of Health and Human Services
Mail Stop: HHH 405-D
370 L'Enfant Promenade, S.W.
Washington, DC 20447
202-690-6590
http://www.acf.dhhs.gov/programs/add

American Academy for Cerebral Palsy and Developmental Medicine
6300 North River Road, Suite 727
Rosemont, IL 60018
847-698-1635
http://www.aacpdm.org

American Academy of Neurology
1080 Montreal Avenue
Saint Paul, MN 55116
800-879-1960 or 651-695-2717
http://www.aan.com

American Academy of Pediatrics
141 Northwest Point Boulevard
Elk Grove Village, IL 60007-1098
847-434-4000
http://www.aap.org

American Association on Mental Retardation
444 North Capitol Street, NW, Suite 846
Washington, DC 20001-1512
800-424-3688; 202-387-1968
http://www.aamr.org

American Occupational Therapy Association, Inc.
4720 Montgomery Lane
PO Box 31220
Bethesda, MD 20824-1220
301-652-2682
http://www.aota.org

American Physical Therapy Association
1111 North Fairfax Street
Alexandria, VA 22314-1488
800-999-APTA (2782); 703-684-APTA (2782)
http://www.apta.org

American Speech-Language-Hearing Association
10801 Rockville Pike
Rockville, MD 20852
800-638-8255
http://www.asha.org

Association of University Centers on Disabilities (formerly American Association of University Affiliated Programs)
1010 Wayne Avenue, Suite 920
Silver Spring, MD 20910
301-588-8252
http://www.aucd.org

Best Buddies
100 SE Second Street, #1990
Miami, FL 33131
800-89-BUDDY; 305-374-2233
http://www.bestbuddies.org

Brain Injury Association of America
8201 Greensboro Dr., Suite 611
McLean, VA 22102
703-761-0750
http://www.biausa.org

Cerebral Institute of Discovery
335 Valley Hill Rd
Stockbridge, GA 30281
http://www.cerebral.org

Easter Seals Project Action—Accessible Community Transportation in our Nation
700 13th St., NW Suite 200
Washington, DC 20005
800-659-6428; 202-347-3066
http://projectaction.easterseals.com

Grown Up Camps
6421 N. Congress Avenue, Suite 200
Boca Raton, FL 33487
877-242-9330; 561-443-2924
http://www.grownupcamps.com

Information on Human Neurological Diseases
Neuroscience on the Internet
http://www.neuroguide.com

Kids Camps
6421 N. Congress Avenue, Suite 200
Boca Raton, FL 33487
877-242-9330; 561-443-2924
http://www.kidscamps.com

Little League International Baseball and Softball—Challenger Division
539 US Route 15 Hwy
P.O. Box 3485
Williamsport, PA 17701-0485
570-326-1921
http://www.littleleague.org/divisions/challenger.asp

National Easter Seal Society
230 W. Monroe, Suite 1800
Chicago, IL 60606
800-221-6827; 312-726-6200
http://www.easter-seals.org

National Institute of Child Health and Human Development
P.O. Box 3006
Rockville, MD 20847
800-370-2943
http://www.nichd.nih.gov

National Institute on Disability and Rehabilitation Research
400 Maryland Avenue, S.W.
Washington, DC 20202-7100
202-245-7640
http://www.ed.gov/about/offices/list/osers/nidrr

National Institutes of Health
National Institute of Neurological Disorders and Stroke
PO Box 5801
Bethesda, MD 20824
800-352-9424; 301-496-5751
http://www.ninds.nih.gov

National Rehabilitation Information Center
4200 Forbes Boulevard, Suite 202
Lanham, MD 20706

800-346-2742; 301-459-5900
http://www.naric.com/

Neurodevelopmental Treatment Association
1540 S. Coast Hwy, Suite 203
Laguna Beach, CA 92651
800-869-9295
http://www.ndta.org

Parents Helping Parents
3041 Olcott Street
Santa Clara, CA 95054
408-727-5775
http://www.php.com

Pediatric Development and Behavior
631 6th Avenue South
St. Petersburg, FL 33701
727-502-8035
http://www.dbpeds.org

Sensory Integration International
PO Box 5339
Torrance, CA 90510-5339
310-787-8805
http://home.earthlink.net/~sensoryint/

Sibling Support Project of the Arc of the United States
6512 23rd Ave NW, No. 213
Seattle, WA 98117
206-297-6368
http://www.thearc.org/siblingsupport

Special Olympics
1325 G Street, N.W., Suite 500
Washington, DC 20005
202-628-3630
http://www.specialolympics.org

The Arc of the United States
1010 Wayne Avenue, Suite 650
Silver Spring, MD 20910
301-565-3842
http://www.thearc.org

The Council for Exceptional Children
1110 North Glebe Road, Suite 300
Arlington, VA 22201
703-620-3660
http://www.cec.sped.org

The Family Village—A Global Community for Disability Related Resources
Waisman Center, University of Wisconsin-Madison
1500 Highland Avenue
Madison, WI 53705-2280
http://www.familyvillage.wisc.edu

The National Information Center for Children and Youth with Disabilities
P.O. Box 1492
Washington, DC 20013
(800) 695-0285
http://www.nichcy.org

The United States Department of Health & Human Services
200 Independence Avenue, S.W.
Washington, DC 20201
877-696-6775; 202-619-0257
http://www.os.dhhs.gov

United Cerebral Palsy National
1660 L. Street NW, Suite 700
Washington, DC 20036
800-872-5827; 202-776-0406
http://www.ucp.org

References

Aicardi, J. (1990). Epilepsy in brain-injured children. *Developmental Medicine in Childhood Neurology, 31*, 191–202.

Albright, L. (1997). Intrathecal baclofen therapy for severe spasticity. *Exceptional Parent, 27*(9), 79–82.

Butler, C., & Campbell, S. (2000). Evidence of the effects of intrathecal Baclofen for spastic and dystonic cerebral palsy. *Developmental Medicine and Child Neurology, 42*, 634–645.

Clark, S., & Hankins, G. (2003). Temporal and demographic trends in cerebral palsy: Fact and fiction. *American Journal of Obstetrics and Gynecology, 188*(3), 828–833.

Collet, J., Vanasse, M., Marois, P., Amar, M., Goldberg, J., & Lambert, J. (2001). Hyperbaric oxygen for children with cerebral palsy: A randomized multicentre trial. *Lancet, 357*, 582–586.

Croen, L., Grether, J., Curry, C., & Nelson, K. (2001). Congenital abnormalities among children with cerebral palsy: More evidence for prenatal antecedents. *Journal of Pediatrics, 138*(6), 804–810.

Crothers, B., & Paine, R. (1959). The natural history of cerebral palsy. In R. Mitchell (Ed.), *Classics in developmental medicine* (Vol. 2, p. 38). Philadelphia: Lippincott.

Dursun, E., Dursun, N., & Alican, D. (2004). Effects of biofeedback treatment on gait in children with cerebral palsy. *Disability and Rehabilitation, 26*(2), 116–120.

Edgar, T. (2001). Clinical utility of botulinum toxin in the treatment of cerebral palsy: A comprehensive review. *Journal of Child Neurology, 16*, 37–46.

Eicher, P. (1993). Cerebral palsy. *The Pediatric Clinics of North America, 40*(3), 537–551.

Graham, H. (2000). Botulinum toxin A in cerebral palsy: Functional outcomes. *Journal of Pediatrics, 137*(3), 300–303.

Han, T., Bang, M., Lim, J., Yoon, B., & Kim, I. (2002). Risk factors of cerebral palsy in preterm infants. *American Journal of Physical Medicine & Rehabilitation, 81*(4), 297–303.

Hays, R. (1997). Cerebral palsy and employability. In Univerity of Washington *Medical aspects of disabilities for rehabilitation counselors*. Retrieved April 15, 2004 from http://wata.org/medaspects/reading6-1.htm

Hays, S. (1999). Management of central nervous system impairment. In P. Edwards, D. Hertzberg, S. Hays, & N. Youngblood (Eds.), *Pediatric rehabilitation nursing* (pp. 317–336). Philadelphia: W. B. Saunders.

Jensen, M., Engel, J., Hoffman, A., & Schwartz, L. (2004). Natural history of chronic pain and pain treatment in adults with cerebral palsy. *American Journal of Physical Medicine and Rehabilitation, 83*(6), 439–445.

Kwong, K., Wong, S., & So, K. (1998). Epilepsy in children with cerebral palsy. *Pediatric Neurology, 19*, 31–36.

McLaughlin, J., Bjornson, K., Temkin, N., Steinbok, P., Wright, V., Reiner, A., Roberts, T., Drake, J., O'Donnell, M., Rosenbaum, P., Barber, J., & Ferrel, A. (2002).

Selective dorsal rhizotomy: Meta-analysis of three randomized controlled trials. *Developmental Medicine and Child Neurology, 44*, 17–25.

Nehring, W. (2004). Cerebral palsy. In P. Jackson Allen & J. Vessey (Eds.), *Primary care of the child with a chronic condition* (pp. 327–346). St. Louis: C. V. Mosby

Nelson, K., & Ellenberg, J. (1986). Antecedents of cerebral palsy: Multivariate analysis of risk. *New England Journal of Medicine, 315*, 81–86.

Noetzel, M., & Miller, G. (1998). Traumatic brain injury as a cause of cerebral palsy. In G. Miller & J. Clark (Eds.), *The cerebral palsies: Causes, consequences, and management*. Boston: Butterworth-Heinemann.

Pellegrino, L. (2002). Cerebral palsy. In M. Barshaw (Ed.), *Children with disabilities* (pp. 443–466). Baltimore: Paul H. Brookes.

Reddihough, D., & Collins, K. (2003). The epidemiology and causes of cerebral palsy. *Australian Journal of Physiotherapy, 49* (1), 7–12.

Reilly, S., Skuse, D., & Poblete, X. (1996). Prevalence of feeding problems and oral motor dysfunction in children with cerebral palsy: A community survey. *Journal of Pediatrics, 129*, 877–882.

Rosenbaum, P. (2003). Cerebral palsy: What parents and doctors want to know. *British Medical Journal, 326*, 970–974.

Singhi, P., Jagirdar, S., Khandelwal, N., & Malhi, P. (2003). Epilepsy in children with cerebral palsy. *Journal of Child Neurology, 18* (3), 174–179.

Stallings, V., Zemel, B., Davies, J., Cronk, C., & Charney, E. (1996). Energy expenditure of children and adolescents with severe disabilities: A cerebral palsy model. *American Journal of Clinical Nutrition, 64* (4), 627–634.

Sullivan, P., Lambert, B., Rose, M., Ford-Adams, M., Johnson, A., & Griffiths, P. (2000). Prevalence and severity of feeding and nutritional problems in children with neurological impairment: Oxford feeding study. *Developmental Medicine and Child Neurology, 42*, 674–680.

Taub, E., Ramey, S., DeLuca, S., & Echols, K. (2004). Constraint-induced movement therapy improves motor control in children with cerebral palsy. *Pediatrics, 113*(2), 305–312.

Van Eerden, P., & Bernstein, P. (2003). Summary of the publication, "Neonatal encephalopathy and cerebral palsy: Defining the pathogenesis and pathophysiology," by the ACOG task force on neonatal encephalopathy and cerebral palsy. *Medscape OB/GYN & Women's Health, 8* (2). Retrieved April 15, 2004 from http://www.medscape.com/viewarticle/457882

Yoon, B. (2000). Fetal exposure to an intra-amniotic inflammation and the development of cerebral palsy at the age of three years. *American Journal of Obstetrics and Gynecology, 182*(3), 675–681.

Chapter 32

Cystic Fibrosis

CAROLE E. MOORE

Chapter Outline

INTRODUCTION

Care of students with cystic fibrosis (CF) in school is especially relevant to school nurses, as it is one of the most common genetic disorders in children. This chapter reviews the diagnostic process for CF, how CF affects the systems of the body, and treatments commonly used in CF management. Prognosis-related factors discussed include transplantation and gene therapy research currently underway.

Management of CF in the school setting is discussed in terms of the school nurse's many roles, including direct care provider, liaison to the CF care team, educator, resource provider, coordinator of practical aspects of school life, and supporter of the parent/caregiver. Resources available to school nurses, as well as to students and families coping with CF, are highlighted.

OVERVIEW OF CF

CF is the most common life-shortening genetic disease in the United States (Hay, Hayward, Levin, & Sondheimer, 2001), affecting primarily Caucasians (one in 3,000 to 3,300). Hispanic individuals account for approximately 6% of those with CF (one in 8,000); approximately 3% of people with CF are African American (one in 17,000). Approximately 30,000 children and adults are affected (McMullen & Bryson, 2004). The median life expectancy of individuals with CF is 33 years, up from 18 years in 1980. Almost 40% of individuals with CF in the United States are 18 or older (Cystic Fibrosis Foundation [CFF], 2003). CF is an autosomal recessive genetic disorder; to have CF, a person must inherit one defective copy of the CF gene from each parent (CFF, 2003). One in 22 Americans is a symptom-less carrier of the abnormal gene (Hay et al., 2001), a figure that represents approximately 10 million people in the United States (CFF, 2003).

CF is an exocrine system disorder, affecting multiple body organs that secrete to the outside of the body, for example, gastrointestinal (including hepatic), pancreatic, pulmonary, and reproductive systems, as well as salt loss through sweat glands. Although CF causes dysfunction in the hepatic, gastrointestinal, and male reproductive systems, the major cause of mortality and morbidity is lung disease (Hay et al., 2001). Close monitoring is needed because CF is a chronic, progressive disease. Generally, children who experience progression of the disease, reflected in repeated infections, hospitalizations, and impaired growth at an early age, are at greater risk for poor outcomes as they get older (Emerson, Rosenfeld, McNamara, Ramsey, & Gibson, 2002).

Contributions to the improvement in prognosis include aggressive use of antibiotics, more effective management of malabsorption, and the development of more than 117 CF care centers in the United States (Hay et al., 2001). Care of students with CF at these centers is multidisciplinary, involving a team of physicians, nurses, advanced practice nurses, social workers, nutritionists, physical therapists, respiratory therapists, and pharmacists. Treatment is intensive, time consuming, and costly. With modern therapies improving survival rates, children living with CF attend and usually graduate from school. Half will live into their 30s and beyond (CFF, 2001). School nurses acting as liaisons between the school and medical facility can be instrumental in promoting positive health and educational outcomes for children and adolescents coping with CF.

DIAGNOSIS

About 1,000 new cases of CF diagnosed each year. Diagnosis is made after a positive pilocarpine iontophoresis sweat test, which determines the amount of sodium and chloride in the sweat. Although individuals with CF do not sweat more than nonaffected individuals, they do have an increased amount of sodium and chloride in the sweat. Sweat chloride concentrations greater than 60 mmol/L collected on two separate occasions are consistent with the diagnosis of CF (CFF, 2003). Diagnosis can also be made with evidence of a genotype consistent with CF (Hay et al., 2001). Using these genetic markers, carrier status can also be determined with some degree of accuracy, as the tests can detect more than 85% of the mutant CF genes in North America (McMullen & Bryson, 2004).

The disease is diagnosed by the age of 1 year in 60% of patients; 85% of patients are diagnosed by age 5 (Durie, 2000). However, 8% of diagnoses are made in individuals older than 17 years of age (CFF, 2001). Clinical conditions raising suspicion of CF early in life include meconium ileus at birth, failure to thrive during infancy, and recurrent respiratory infections.

PATHOPHYSIOLOGY AND TREATMENT

CF is caused by a mutation in a gene on the long arm of human chromosome 7, which encodes a protein termed cystic fibrosis transmembrane conductance regulator (CFTR) (Wilmoth, Walters, Tomlin, & McCray, 2001). More than 900 mutations of the CFTR gene have been identified. The most common is *delta F508*. The numerous differences in genotype help explain the variability in the clinical course of CF in terms of onset, pattern of symptoms, and the rate of disease progression (Hay et al., 2001). Treatment of CF depends on which organs are involved, as well as the stage of the disease.

CFTR is found in epithelial cells of the sinuses, bronchial mucosa, pancreas, salivary glands, biliary tract, reproductive tract, and intestines. CFTR helps regulate the flow of sodium, chloride, and bicarbonate ions across the epithelial cell surfaces. Abnormal CFTR alters the ion permeability of the cell membrane, which results in thick, sticky secretions in multiple organs (Wilmoth et al., 2001). As a result, CF patients have abnormalities affecting the entire exocrine system.

Respiratory Symptoms and Treatment

Respiratory symptoms include persistent coughing, wheezing, and frequent infections of the upper and lower respiratory tracts caused by thick, viscous secretions. The dehydrated mucus impairs mucociliary clearance (McMullen & Bryson, 2004). A cycle of inflammation, obstruction, and infection is typical. Inflammation from infections increases mucus secretion even more, which causes further obstruction and encourages the growth of more infection-causing bacteria. Chronic infection leads to gradual destruction of lung tissue. Over time, irreversible damage to the airway occurs, leading to bronchiectasis and obstructive lung disease. In advanced states, hypoxia and cor pulmonale may be present (Hay et al., 2001).

A powerful prognostic predictor for individuals with CF is lung function, as measured by the percent predicted forced expiratory volume in 1 second (FEV1) (Smyth, 2002) in children older than 6 years of age and adults. Pulmonary function may be measured in infants and very young children through the use of a special vest. While the child is sedated, the lungs are inflated to normal capacity, and then the vest covering the child's chest is rapidly pressurized to help the child blow out air; measurements are taken. Typically there is a decline in FEV1 in children older than 6 years of age and in adults with

CF between 1.4% and 4% per year. Most of the 400 deaths from the disease each year are attributed to respiratory failure (Weiner, 2002).

Many children with CF have frequent respiratory exacerbations with increased sputum production, decreased exercise tolerance, and difficulty breathing, leading to hospitalization. Respiratory infection is a continuing concern. The most common organisms responsible are *Staphylococcus aureus, Pseudomonas aeruginosa, Haemophilus influenzae, Burkholderia cepacia*, and *Aspergillus fumigatus* (Ellmers & Criddle, 2002). These may cause the mucus to be yellow or greenish in color. Sinusitis is common, as is the presence of nasal polyps, which may result in headaches.

There is increasing evidence of individuals with CF being infected with methicillin-resistant *Staphylococcus aureus* (MRSA). In fact, 4.2% of individuals with CF in the United States were recently found to be carrying MRSA (Weiner, 2002). Proper identification of organisms from sputum and accurate drug sensitivity testing in the laboratory are crucial to the successful treatment of respiratory infections for those with CF (Weiner, 2002). Most children with CF acquire *Staphylococcus aureus* and *Haemophilus influenzae* during infancy and early childhood. By adolescence, most acquire *Pseudomonas aeruginosa* (Weiner, 2002). Early acquisition of *Pseudomonas aeruginosa* contributes to a worse prognosis (Emerson et al., 2002). Chronic infection caused by *Pseudomonas aeruginosa* is well recognized as the leading cause of morbidity and mortality among individuals with CF (Emerson et al., 2002). FEV1 is approximately 10% lower in individuals with CF carrying *Pseudomonas aeruginosa* than in those of the same age who are not infected with this organism (Conway, 2002).

Approximately 3.3% of patients with CF in the United States are colonized with *B. cepacia*, which is highly resistant to many antibiotics and difficult to treat. Approximately 20% of the individuals with *B. cepacia* experience rapid decline; another 20% have more rapid than expected decline in pulmonary function, especially after the first year of colonization. Because of this, many CF centers segregate patients colonized with *B. cepacia* to some degree (Weiner, 2002). For children with CF at school, this may have implications for classroom assignments. Students with CF are not contagious to classmates with normal immune function.

The coughing associated with CF is often considered disruptive in the classroom. Teachers frequently suggest that the student leave the class to go to the nurse or to get water. Neither of these is necessary unless the student feels as though he or she is in respiratory distress. It may be appropriate for these students to sit near a door so that if they have heavy coughing, they can move into the hall so as not to disrupt the class. However, they should never be made to feel self-conscious about their coughing or try to suppress it. Coughing is the body's way of clearing secretions. Since the mucus is continuously being made and thicker than for most individuals, it is harder to clear, but must be cleared to enhance breathing. If a student is unable to expectorate the mucus, he or she can swallow it without harm, although the student may complain of stomach discomfort or the stools may be greasier. Tissues should be readily available in all classrooms.

Treatment is focused on controlling infection, reducing obstruction, and decreasing inflammation. Guiding the choice of antibiotics are sputum culture results and drug sensitivity testing. A variety of oral or intravenous antibiotics commonly administered to reduce or control infection includes aminoglycosides (usually tobramycin), cephalosporins, ciprofloxacin, dicloxacillin, tetracycline, and sulfamethoxazole/trimethoprim. Higher than normal dosing and longer duration of treatment are not unusual in the person with CF. Individuals with CF are often given antibiotics with more frequent dosing schedules, as well, owing to increased clearance of many antibiotics (Weiner, 2002). Inhaled antibiotic therapy allows for high concentrations of drugs with lower risk of systemic toxicities. Most widely used is inhaled tobramycin (TOBI), given twice daily in 28 days on/28 days off cycles. This intermittent schedule has been shown to result in improved lung function and decreased need for intravenous antibiotics and hospitalization (Weiner, 2002). TOBI is administered by inhalation using a special jet nebulizer, the PARI LC PLUS, because of its aerosol particle size. Unlike the situation in most infections, the goal of therapy is not necessarily to rid the body of the organism, but rather to decrease its levels.

Another mainstay of CF treatment is daily airway clearance therapy, designed to loosen secretions and enhance the student's ability to expectorate them. This can be achieved through chest physical therapy techniques such as postural drainage and percussion, positive expiratory pressure (PEP) therapy, or devices such as the Flutter or the Vest. PEP therapy promotes mucus clearance by increasing collateral ventilation and preventing airway closure. This is achieved by breathing through a mask that has only a small hole to allow air to escape, creating backpressure in the lungs. The Flutter is a device designed to promote the upward movement of mucus through the airways using positive airway pressure, airway oscillations, and airflow acceleration. The Vest system uses high-frequency chest wall oscillation (HFCWO) technology. The Vest is attached to an air-pulse generator that rapidly inflates and deflates the vest, applying gentle pressure to the chest wall. This helps loosen and thin secretions, moving them to larger airways where they can be cleared through coughing or suctioning. Most airway clearance therapies are required twice daily for maintenance therapy and three to four times daily for those with severe disease or during acute exacerbations (Ellmers & Criddle, 2002). Breathing exercises may also be recommended to help move respiratory secretions.

If a student needs percussion and postural drainage during the school day, it is the responsibility of the school nurse to perform this treatment in the school building; it takes 20 to 30 minutes and then the student can return to class. If it is known that a student has CF, the school nurse can contact the Advanced Practice Nurse in the CF clinic, or someone equally qualified, in order to update the school nurse's skills regarding these treatments.

Mucolytic and bronchodilator treatments usually precede airway clearance techniques in order to promote productive coughing and expectoration of mucus. Mucolytic agents include *N*-acetylcysteine (Mucomyst) and dornase alfa (Pulmozyme). Dornase alfa (recombinant human DNase) lyses extracellular DNA into smaller pieces, thinning secretions and enhancing expectoration. Long-term dornase alfa treatment slows loss of lung function and reduces the frequency of infectious exacerbations (Conway, 2002). Bronchodilator agents such as albuterol improve pulmonary function in patients with reactive airways (Hay et al., 2001). Oxygen is required to treat hypoxemia, which may occur during acute exacerbations and which becomes a chronic need during end stages of the disease (Sprague, Graff, & Tobias, 2000). Anti-inflammatory agents aid in treating the chronic inflammatory response in lung tissue associated with CF (Hay et al., 2001), and may include corticosteroids as well as nonsteroidal anti-inflammatory drugs (NSAIDs). Cytokine inhibitors, antiproteases, and antioxidants (Ellmers & Criddle, 2002) are still being explored for their anti-inflammatory benefits.

Exercise continues to be included as an important tool used in the management of CF. Positive benefits from regular physical activity in the CF population include reduction of breathlessness, increased exercise capacity, improved pulmonary function, enhanced sputum clearance, and improved body image. Exercise programs are tailored to individual needs, considering variable fitness levels, preferences, and level of lung disease, and ideally include both endurance and upper and lower body strength-training exercises (Prasad & Cerny, 2002). Some students with CF may require alternate physical education classes or may have activity restrictions, but unless they are experiencing dyspnea, they can participate fully with their peers. If exercise results in increased expectoration of mucus or a need for increased rest periods, these needs should be accommodated.

Gene therapy trials are currently being conducted. In addition, bilateral lung and liver transplants are considered a treatment option for some individuals with end-stage CF. More than 100 lung transplants are performed each year for adolescents and young adults with CF (Weiner, 2002); CF is the second leading indication for lung transplantation (Liou et al., 2001). Although transplantation does not provide a cure, it can provide some relief of respiratory symptoms and prolongation of life for people with CF. The survival rate for lung transplant recipients with CF is currently 81.4% at 1 year and 62% at 3 years (Organ Procurement and Transplantation Network, 2005). Several parameters are considered for lung transplant candidates who have CF, including oxygen requirements, rate of deterioration, frequency of intravenous antibiotic use, and lung function. A baseline FEV1 of less than 30% of the predicted value is also used in qualifying CF patients for lung transplantation (Ellmers & Criddle, 2002). Individuals who are transplant recipients require lifelong immunosuppression therapy and require careful monitoring for adverse side effects such as hypertension, renal failure, diabetes, and susceptibility to infection. They are among those who must be notified if a varicella outbreak occurs.

Gastrointestinal and Nutrition Issues and Treatment

Gastrointestinal and nutrition issues in individuals with CF center around pancreatic insufficiency and malabsorption. Pancreatic ducts are blocked by thick mucus plugs that prevent secretion of digestive enzymes into the intestine (Ellmers & Criddle, 2002). The result is stool that is foul smelling, frequent, foamy, and fatty (steatorrhea), and has undigested food in it. The pancreas, over time, is destroyed and becomes fibrotic. Eighty-five percent of those with CF have pancreatic insufficiency and a loss of exocrine function of the pancreas resulting in decreased ability to digest nutrients (Durie, 2000). This results in malabsorption of nutrients, especially protein, fats, and the fat-soluble vitamins A, D, E, and K.

Untreated CF patients usually have steatorrhea and poor growth. They may have osteoporosis and/or osteopenia as a result of poor absorption of calcium and vitamin D. Malnutrition in people with CF is a result of increased expenditure of energy, decreased consumption of energy-producing nutrients, and malabsorption of nutrients caused by pancreatic insufficiency and chronic inflammation. Malnutrition is a major factor determining pulmonary function, nutritional status, and outcomes for children with CF (Hankard, Munck, & Navarro, 2002). There is a significant positive correlation between a child's weight and pulmonary function, with those who weigh more and gain weight at an appropriate rate-for-age having a better FEV1 trajectory (Peterson, Jacobs, & Milla, 2003). Students with CF may have ravenous appetites but still exhibit poor weight gain.

For these reasons, it is essential to monitor the student's height and weight at least twice a year. Eighteen percent of children with CF are below the 5th percentile for weight and 16% are below the 5th percentile for height on standard growth charts (Peterson et al., 2003). In addition, malabsorption may result in an increased need to go to the bathroom. Students with CF should never be stopped from using the bathroom; consider giving them free restroom privileges, perhaps with an agreed-on hand signal or a permanent hall pass.

Treatment includes pancreatic enzyme supplementation (amylase, lipase, protease) with each meal and each snack. Some brands of pancreatic enzymes are Creon, PANCRECARB, Ultrase, Pancrease, and Viokase. Enzymes need to be taken *immediately* before all meals, snacks, milk, or nutritional supplements. Foods and drinks that usually do not require enzymes are fruits, juices, soft drinks, sports drinks, hard candy, popsicles, fruit snacks, and jelly beans. Enzyme dose is based on weight, amount of food eaten, bowel movement consistency, growth, and weight gain. Enzyme capsules must not be crushed or chewed. If swallowing a capsule is difficult, the capsule may be opened and the contents sprinkled on a small amount of soft food, then swallowed. Young children need assistance at each meal and snack in taking their enzymes. Enzymes should not be refrigerated and, if sprinkled, should be eaten immediately, rather than prepared in advance.

Occasionally antacids are added (Hay et al., 2001) to lower the acidity in the stomach and increase the bioavailability of the enzymes (Ellmers & Criddle, 2002). The fat-soluble vitamins A, D, E, and K are given at doses two times normal with the hope that at least one dose will be absorbed; typical doses are 8,000 IU of vitamin A, 800 IU of vitamin D, and 100 to 200 mg of vitamin E (Valentine, Griffin, & Abrams, 2003).

These supplements are available in drops or tablets, which can be chewed, halved, crushed, or swallowed. Medications to combat osteoporosis or osteopenia may be added, such as alendronate sodium. Increased water intake helps prevent dehydration. Diets high in fats, calories, and carbohydrates are usually recommended to achieve normal height and weight as long as enzymes are taken. While low-fat diets were recommended for years, the trend now is to eliminate restrictions on their diet and to cover any increased fat intake with additional enzymes. Studies demonstrate that diets higher in fat with sufficient enzyme coverage increase life expectancy by 50% (Valentine et al., 2003).

Children and teens with CF need 120% to 150% of the recommended dietary calorie intake compared to others of the same age (Valentine et al., 2003); most do not achieve this level of intake (Peterson et al., 2003). Young children with CF 4 through 7 years of age need approximately 2800 calories daily, so more calories should be added to the diet. This can be achieved through adding whole milk products and snacks, such as crackers with peanut butter, ice cream, and bagels with cream cheese. Teens with CF typically need 3,000 to 5,000 calories daily, usually achieved through a balanced diet high in fat and protein. Salt can be added through including pretzels and potato chips. Snacks may include nuts, pie with ice cream, cheese, crackers, and high-calorie sports snack bars.

If a student's weight drops significantly below normal, high-calorie supplements or formulas, such as Polycose, are often added to the diet (Hay et al., 2001). Feeding via nasogastric or gastrostomy tube is utilized for some patients who do not respond to oral supplements (Hay et al., 2001), or for those who are below the 5th percentile for weight for a period of time.

Other GI-related diseases associated with CF include gastroesophageal reflux disease (GERD), hiatal hernia, intussusception, colonic strictures in children taking high doses of pancreatic enzymes, and cystic-fibrosis-related diabetes (CFRD) (Hay et al., 2001; McMullen & Bryson, 2004). CFRD has clinical features of type 1 diabetes as well as type 2 diabetes (Hardin, LeBlanc, Para, & Seilheimer, 1999).

Hepatic Issues

Hepatobiliary disease is common in individuals with CF who have pancreatic insufficiency, although jaundice is uncommon. Biliary and hepatic cirrhosis develops as thick secretions block the biliary tract (Ellmers & Criddle, 2002). A small percentage of affected individuals develop portal hypertension; others may develop esophageal varices that may cause gastrointestinal bleeding or hypersplenism (Hay et al., 2001). School nurses should assess for increased liver size if the student complains of abdominal pain. Liver disease is the fourth most common cause of death in CF patients (CFF, 2001) and, when indicated, evaluations for liver transplantation are done. In addition, adults with CF are at increased risk of cholelithiasis and cholecystitis (Hay et al., 2001).

Electrolyte Issues

Since students with CF secrete increased amounts of salt in sweat, the school nurse should ensure that they drink increased amounts of water and/or sports drinks before, during, and after vigorous exercise, particularly in hot weather. They should be encouraged to put salt on their food or to eat salty foods in hot weather.

Reproductive Issues

Nearly 95% of males with CF are infertile as a result of failure of development of the vas deferens (Hay et al., 2001); pubertal changes in males are often delayed 2 to 4 years. In women, pubertal changes and menarche are delayed, with a mean age at menarche of 14.5 years; amenorrhea is common (Ellmers & Criddle, 2002; McMullen & Bryson, 2004), but in general, women with CF are fertile, although the thick mucus in the cervical area may make conception more difficult (Hay et al., 2001). The school nurse should consider these issues while teaching about puberty in sex education classes involving students with CF. This is also a good time to talk about genetics and the fact that *all* of the children born to women with CF will be carriers of the CF gene.

PROGNOSIS

Most people with CF reach adulthood, but some do die during the school-age years. The prime factor determining survival is the rate of progression of lung disease (Hay et al., 2001). With the median survival age in 2000 being 32.5 years (McMullen & Bryson, 2004), many individuals with CF graduate from school, go on to secondary education, participate in professions, and marry and have families, although sometimes by alternative modalities.

THE SCHOOL NURSE'S ROLE

The school nurse can focus on several strategies to assist the student with CF to optimize learning opportunities and manage health-related challenges. Strategies include those described in the following subsections.

Provide Direct Care as Needed

- Medication administration, including oral, inhaled, or intravenous antibiotics, enzymes, mucolytics, bronchodilators
  - Maintain supplies of all medications and ask the family to notify the school nurse of medication and dose changes.
  - Develop a system with the student that allows him or her to take pancreatic enzymes with meals, snacks, or school eating events.
  - Ensure that these students do not take medication that suppresses their cough or dries their secretions, such as antihistamines.
- Diabetes care, if needed, including blood glucose testing and insulin administration
- Care of implanted venous access devices
- Enteral feedings, via gastrostomy, nasogastric, or jejunostomy tubes
- Total parental nutrition (TPN) administration
- Performance of spirometry or pulse oximetry
- Assistance with airway clearance techniques
- Provision of oxygen or other ventilatory support

Attend to Routine Screening

- High-frequency hearing loss may occur after numerous courses of some antibiotics; ensure careful hearing screening.
- Careful assessment of height and weight

Act as a Liaison to the CF Care Team

Exchange of information with the CF treatment team is critical, so written permission from parents of students with CF to communicate with the treatment team is essential. Clear, regular communication between the school nurse and the treatment team will enhance care of the student with CF during the school day as well as ensure appropriate accommodations are made for the student. Clarifying information for the student about the disease or treatment regimen is crucial for students with chronic conditions, for whom compliance is essential to maintain life (Hinton, Watson, Chesson, & Mathers, 2002). The school nurse can be the liaison between the treatment team and the school when the student is hospitalized or as the student transitions back to school.

Serve as Educator and Resource for School Staff

This may include education about CF, diabetes, nutritional needs, diet and snacks, enzymes, exercise needs and limitations, and explanation of the common occurrence of frequent coughing that is beyond the control of the student and does not require the student to leave class and see the nurse unless he or she is in distress. The school nurse may also assist in obtaining grief counseling for students and staff surrounding the death of a student with CF, particularly siblings or others in the school who may have CF.

Coordinate Practical Aspects of Life at School

The school nurse should assist in ensuring extra bathroom privileges for children with CF. At times they may have stomach pain, loose or urgent stools, or foul-smelling gas. Students should also have tissues at their desks or backpacks for expectorating mucus, as well as a plastic bag for the tissues, and an excuse to leave the room to cough so as not to disturb others. Separation of multiple students with CF into different classrooms may be necessary and requested by the CF treatment team, depending on the organisms with which the students are colonized.

A plan should be developed for the student with CF by parents, teachers, administrators, and the school nurse that addresses issues such as plan of care during illnesses, hospitalizations, frequent absences due to illness or doctor visits, and homebound instruction.

Serve as Support to Parent Caregivers and Siblings

Nurses are often the first persons who parent/caregivers turn to with concerns or for interpretation of medical information. Identifying stressors and supporting positive coping strategies can assist in maintaining healthy family functioning and also improve the physical health of the student living with CF (Hodgkinson & Lester, 2002). It may be helpful to keep extra medications at school for the student. The stress of caring for a child with CF is often overwhelming to the parents and siblings (Carpenter & Narsavage, 2004). Siblings in the school setting also need attention and support, as they may feel unappreciated and feel that all of the family's attention, energies, and finances are going toward the child with CF.

Through keeping their knowledge base current regarding advances in CF research and treatment, school nurses can help the student and family hold hope for the future. The school nurse can serve as a bridge builder between the CF care center and the school, and between school and home, and may need to initiate the contact. Continuity of care for the student with CF can be promoted by the school nurse. To optimize care of the student coping with CF, it is beneficial to look beyond the immediate care needs of the student to the needs of the family and adopt these roles, as appropriate, promoting the health of the student (Hodgkinson & Lester, 2002). Multiple organizations and resources are available to assist the family and school staff in anticipating and dealing with issues related to the student with CF (Table 32.1).

Table 32.1 ■
AVAILABLE RESOURCES ON CYSTIC FIBROSIS

TYPE OF RESOURCE	DESCRIPTION	INTENDED AUDIENCE	PUBLICATION INFORMATION
Teacher's guide to cystic fibrosis	Fact sheet	Teachers, school nurses	Cystic Fibrosis Foundation, 2003 http://www.cff.org/living_with_cf/teachers_guide.cfm
Cystic fibrosis in the classroom	19-page booklet by Tara Brascia and Kathleen Flynn	Teachers, school nurses	Cystic Fibrosis Research, Inc., 2001 http://www.cfri.org http://www.digestivecare.com

(continued)

Table 32.1 ■ *(Continued)*

TYPE OF RESOURCE	DESCRIPTION	INTENDED AUDIENCE	PUBLICATION INFORMATION
CF and your tomorrow: A guide to surviving and thriving with cystic fibrosis	33-page booklet by Dierdre Ann Croal	Adolescents with CF	Solvay Pharmaceuticals, Inc., 1994
Can we talk? My sibling has CF	22-page booklet by Dierdre, Kendra, and Andrea Croal	Siblings of students with CF	Solvay Pharmaceuticals, Inc., 1996
Taking cystic fibrosis to school	Book by Cynthia S. Henry and Tom Dineen	Children with CF, teachers, classmates	JayJo Books, 2000
Cystic fibrosis: A guide for patient and family (3rd ed.)	Book by David Orenstein, M.D.	Students with CF, family	Lippincott, Williams, & Wilkins, 2003
Living and coping with cystic fibrosis: A book for parents	Book	Parents	CF Family Education Project Baylor College of Medicine and Texas Children's Hospital, 1994
Managing lung problems in cystic fibrosis: A book for parents	Book	Parents	CF Family Education Project Baylor College of Medicine and Texas Children's Hospital, 1994
Managing nutrition and malabsorption in cystic fibrosis	Book	Parents	CF Family Education Project Baylor College of Medicine and Texas Children's Hospital, 1989
Cystic Fibrosis Foundation	Foundation	Individuals with CF, families	6931 Arlington Road, Bethesda, MD 20814 800-344-4823 http://www.cff.org

SPECIAL ISSUES

The school nurse should work within the school community to be proactive with regard to bullying. Bullying often arises if the child is thin, coughing, and producing large amounts of sputum, or taking many medications at school. Building self-esteem in these young people is essential. Providing creative ways to handle mucus and expectorating is important to their emotional well-being. They may be sensitive about their barrel chests or digital clubbing caused by chronic lung disease, their thinness, or their delayed puberty. Focus on their strengths and their health.

School nurses can also be instrumental in promoting student adaptation within the school environment after prolonged school absences, such as hospitalizations for pulmonary compromise or for lung and/or liver transplantation, through early intervention and serving as a liaison among the family, CF care team, and school. Significant numbers of children who undergo transplants experience difficulties at school, including underachievement, behavior problems, as well as academic and adjustment difficulties (Wray, Long, Radley-Smith, & Yacoub, 2001). The average length of time between transplant and returning to school is 6 months; children with CF sometimes have longer periods of absence than young transplant patients with other diagnoses, and may require home instruction. There appears to be a significant correlation between the length of absence from school after transplantation and the occurrence of underachievement. However, in one study, although students with CF were absent from school longer, their adjustment back into the school environment was better than that of students with other diagnoses who had undergone transplantation, because they were accustomed to frequent hospitalizations, medications, and disrupted school attendance (Wray et al., 2001).

CONCLUSION

Students with CF are common among the school population. They often have significant health needs that involve multiple body systems. Children and adolescents with CF do have a chronic condition that will shorten their lives. However, they should be treated as healthy normal children with goals and hopes for the future, since the vast majority will complete high school and participate in society.

References

Carpenter, D., & Narsavage, G. (2004). One breath at a time: Living with cystic fibrosis. *Journal of Pediatric Nursing, 19*(1), 25–32.

Conway, S. P. (2002). Evidence-based medicine in cystic fibrosis: How should practice change? *Pediatric Pulmonology, 34*(3), 242–247.

Cystic Fibrosis Foundation (CFF). (2001). *Facts about CF*. Bethesda, MD: Author.

Cystic Fibrosis Foundation (CFF). (2003). Cystic fibrosis foundation patient registry annual data report 2002. Retrieved April, 2005 from http://www.cff.org

Cystic Fibrosis Foundation (CFF). (2003). *What is CF?* Retrieved September 1, 2003 from http://www.cff.org/about_cf/what_is_cf.cfm

Durie, P. R. (2000). Pancreatic aspects of cystic fibrosis and other inherited causes of pancreatic dysfunction. *Medical Clinics of North America, 84*(3), 609–620.

Ellmers, K., & Criddle, L. M. (2002). A new age for childhood diseases. Cystic fibrosis. *RN, 65*(9), 60–66.

Emerson, J., Rosenfeld, M., McNamara, S., Ramsey, B., & Gibson, R. (2002). *Pseudomonas aeruginosa* and other predictors of mortality and morbidity in young children with cystic fibrosis. *Pediatric Pulmonology, 34*(2), 91–100.

Hankard, R., Munck, A., & Navarro, J. (2002). Nutrition and growth in cystic fibrosis. *Hormone Research, 58* (Suppl. 1), 16–20.

Hardin, D., LeBlanc, A., Para, L., & Seilheimer, D. (1999). Substrate utilization in cystic fibrosis. *Diabetes, 48*(5), 1082–1087.

Hay, W., Hayward, A., Levin, M., & Sondheimer, J. (2001). *Current pediatric diagnosis and treatment* (15th ed.) New York: Lange Medical Books/McGraw-Hill.

Hinton, S., Watson, S., Chesson, R., & Mathers, S. (2002). Information needs of young people with cystic fibrosis. *Paediatric Nursing, 14*(6), 18–21.

Hodgkinson, R., & Lester, H. (2002). Stresses and coping strategies of mothers living with a child with cystic fibrosis: Implications for nursing professionals. *Journal of Advanced Nursing, 39*(4), 377–383.

Liou, T., Adler, F., Cahill, B., Fitzsimmons, S., Huang, D., Hibbs, J., et al. (2001). Survival effect of lung transplantation among patients with cystic fibrosis. *Journal of the American Medical Association, 286*(21), 2683–2689.

McMullen, A., & Bryson, E. (2004). Cystic fibrosis. In P. Jackson-Allen & J. Vessey (Eds.), *Primary care of the child with a chronic condition* (pp. 404–425). St. Louis: C. V. Mosby.

Organ Procurement and Transplantation Network. (2005). *Lung Kaplan–Meier patient survival rates for transplants performed: 1995–2002*. Retrieved September 1, 2003, from http://www.optn.org

Peterson, M., Jacobs, D., & Milla, C. (2003). Longitudinal changes in growth parameters are correlated with changes in pulmonary function in children with cystic fibrosis. *Pediatrics, 112*(3), 588–592.

Prasad, S. A., & Cerny, F. J. (2002). Factors that influence adherence to exercise and their effectiveness: Application to cystic fibrosis. *Pediatric Pulmonology, 34*(1), 66–72.

Smyth, A. (2002). Treatment of children with cystic fibrosis: Central, local of both? *Acta Paediatrics, 91*(9), 894–895.

Sprague, K., Graff, G., & Tobias, J. D. (2000). Noninvasive ventilation in respiratory failure due to cystic fibrosis. *Southern Medical Journal, 93*(10), 954–961.

Valentine, C., Griffin, I., & Abrams, S. (2003). Nutritional support in children. In F. Bonner (Ed.), *Nutritional aspects and clinical management of chronic disorders and diseases* (pp. 1–22). Boca Raton, FL: CRC Press.

Weiner, D. (2002). Respiratory tract infections in cystic fibrosis. *Pediatric Annals, 31*(2), 116–123.

Wilmoth, D., Walters, P., Tomlin, R., & McCray, S. (2001). Caring for adults with cystic fibrosis. *Critical Care Nurse, 21*(3), 34–44.

Wray, J., Long, T., Radley-Smith, R., & Yacoub, M. (2001). Returning to school after heart or heart-lung transplantation: How well do children adjust? *Transplantation, 72*(1), 100–106.

Chapter 33

Diabetes Management in the School Setting

JAYNE CHATTERTON ▪ TARA KAUP ▪ MARY A. SWANSON

Chapter Outline

INTRODUCTION

Diabetes is one of the oldest conditions known to man, having been identified in 1500 B.C. (Lipman, 2002). Yet, even with all of the present-day scientific advances, one form of diabetes (type 2) is quickly becoming epidemic in American society among children and adolescents. Although a number of different types of diabetes exist, type 1 and type 2 are most common in the student body, and thus are the focus of this chapter. Both types have the potential to result in serious morbidity and early death if not controlled. The goals of this chapter are to provide school nurses with a better understanding of diabetes and its treatment options as well as to facilitate a continuum of self-management education in the school setting. To understand the impact of diabetes on school students, it is first necessary to understand the scope of the problem and to differentiate the two types of diabetes as they present in children and adolescents.

INCIDENCE

The incidence of diabetes mellitus (DM) is increasing in the school-age population, primarily because of the explosion in cases of type 2. Approximately 151,000 people younger than the age of 20 have a diagnosis of either type 1 or type 2 diabetes, with more than 13,000 children diagnosed with type 1 diabetes each year (U.S. Department of Health and Human Services [DHHS], 2003). Type 1 diabetes accounts for approximately 10% of all individuals who have been diagnosed with diabetes, but about 60% to 80% of children and adolescents with the disorder (National Institute of Diabetes and Digestive and Kidney Diseases [NIDDK], 2000). Approximately one in 400 to 500 children and adolescents have type 1 diabetes. Although the exact number of young people with type 2 diabetes is not known, it is estimated that type 2 accounts for 30% to 45% of those diagnosed with DM, compared to only 2% to 4% a decade ago (Quarry-Horn, Evans, &

Kerrigan, 2003). Type 2 accounts for 90% of the diabetes seen in adults.

NORMAL ENERGY METABOLISM: THE FUNCTION OF INSULIN

To survive, the cells of the body need energy from food. When food is consumed, it is broken down into a simple sugar called glucose. Carbohydrates are the principal precursor compounds but glucose can also be obtained through the breakdown of protein and fat. Glucose is absorbed from the gastrointestinal tract into the blood stream. Food intake stimulates the pancreas to release a hormone called insulin, which is made by beta cells. Insulin is needed to transport glucose from the blood stream into the cells for energy. When insulin is not available, the glucose builds up in the blood stream and cannot be used by body cells; the increasing need for glucose causes the body to break down fat and muscle for energy (Ratner, 2001).

WHAT IS DIABETES?

Diabetes is the most common endocrine disease in children (Lipman, 2002). It is a condition governed by insulin, which may be absent, deficient, or the body may be resistant to it. Regardless of the cause, glucose levels build up in the blood (hyperglycemia) because insulin is not available to move the glucose into the cells so that it can be used for energy. When the glucose level reaches approximately 200 mg/dL, the renal tubules have difficulty absorbing all of the sugar and it is spilled into the urine (glycosuria). Because sugar functions as an osmotic agent (diuretic), fluid and electrolytes are excreted, resulting in frequent urination (polyuria) and thirst (polydipsia).

Meanwhile, the cells are starving, since the glucose cannot enter. The body gives out signals that it is hungry, resulting in increased food intake (polyphagia). However, the breakdown of protein and fat that is ultimately used for fuel and the dehydration result in weight loss.

At the same time, the liver converts triglycerides to fatty acids that, in turn, change to ketone bodies. These are also used for energy, although their supply is limited. The ketones are excreted through the kidneys. Since ketones contain large amounts of free hydrogen ions, their resulting buildup results in metabolic acidosis and a lower serum pH. In the body's attempt to regain acid–base homeostasis, there is an increase in the rate and depth of respirations (the extreme of which is called Kussmaul breathing).

Another symptom may be temporary blurry vision, caused by excess glucose accumulation in the eyes. This usually resolves after treatment begins and is not related to diabetic retinopathy, which is a long-term complication of diabetes (Zombek, 2003). Fatigue, behavior changes, and decreased attention span may also be indicators of hyperglycemia.

DIAGNOSTIC CRITERIA FOR DIABETES

Specific criteria have been established by the American Diabetes Association (ADA, 2002a) to diagnose diabetes. These are: (1) two fasting plasma glucose levels greater than 126 mg/dL in someone who is asymptomatic, or (2) two random plasma glucose levels of greater than 200 mg/dL in someone who is asymptomatic, or (3) one high plasma glucose level at any time in someone who has symptoms of diabetes, or (4) an oral glucose tolerance test that shows a two-hour postprandial result of greater than 200 mg/dL.

Individuals who have symptoms of diabetes but do not meet the criteria stated above are classified as having *glucose intolerance*. They would benefit from education regarding nutrition and exercise interventions that can prevent or delay the onset of diabetes (Zombek, 2003).

The classification of diabetes has evolved over the past decade. Until recently, the main criterion for identifying the type of diabetes was based on the age of the individual at diagnosis. Research on the etiology of diabetes has helped to more accurately decipher the type of diabetes that a person may have. The American Diabetes Association's Report of the Expert Committee on the Diagnosis and Classification of Diabetes Mellitus (2002a) is the recognized standard for diabetes classification. While the causes of types 1 and 2 differ significantly, ultimately the same pathology occurs leading to the same potential sequelae.

TYPE 1 DIABETES

Type 1 was previously called juvenile diabetes or insulin-dependent diabetes mellitus. The primary defect in type 1 diabetes mellitus is destruction of beta cells of the pancreas, resulting in the cessation of insulin production (ADA, 1998a). Insufficient insulin secretion affects the body's ability to maintain normal plasma glucose, which leads to the abnormalities in carbohydrate, fat, and protein metabolism that are characteristic of diabetes (ADA, 1998a). Individuals with type 1 diabetes must take daily injectable insulin for life.

Etiology

Factors associated with the development of type 1 diabetes relate to immunological involvement, genetics, and environmental triggers (Rennert & Francis, 1999). Type 1 diabetes is primarily the result of a cell-mediated autoimmune destruction of the beta cells by T cells, resulting in permanent insulin deficiency (Rennert & Francis, 1999). Antibodies against the beta cells (also called islet cells) may be present up to 9 years before the onset of clinical symptoms (Lipman, 2002).

Genetic markers currently being researched that may predispose someone to develop type 1 diabetes are the human leukocyte antigens (HLA) of B8, B15, DR3, and DR4 (Boland & Grey, 2004). Only 20% of those with type 1 diabetes have a close relative with the disorder (Zombek, 2003), so the genetic link is not strong. The incidence in monozygotic twins is 30% to 50%, whereas in first-degree family members it is only 4% to 7% (Lipman, 2002). Viruses, especially enteroviruses, have been suggested as an environmental cause of type 1 diabetes, especially coxsakie B4 infection. However, because the antibodies were probably present for years, it is now thought that the virus may be the "last straw" that results in the appearance of symptoms of diabetes.

The peak age group in which type 1 diabetes occurs is 10- to 14-year-olds (Boland & Grey, 2004). However, it can occur at any age. It presents with an acute onset with the symptoms mentioned earlier.

TYPE 2 DIABETES MELLITUS

In the past, type 2 diabetes was called adult-onset diabetes, because until recently, this type of diabetes was diagnosed only in the adult population. Type 2 diabetes generally accounts for between 80% and 90% of the population with diabetes (ADA, 2002a). The past decade has seen a significant increase in type 2 in children of all ages, especially adolescents. It is strongly correlated with childhood obesity (see Chapter 36) and decreased physical activity. The rise in obesity levels in youth has led to an increased number of children and adolescents, average age of 13 years old, being diagnosed with type 2 diabetes (Brosnan, Upchurch, & Schreiner, 2001). It has been reported that 8% to 45% of new cases of type 2 diabetes are among the pediatric population in urban areas (Kaufman, 2002).

Etiology

It is speculated that, as in adults, the development of type 2 diabetes in children is a result of both genetic and environmental factors (Boland & Grey, 2004). Type 2 diabetes is defined by the American Diabetes Association as a type of diabetes that occurs primarily as a result of insulin resistance along with some insulin deficiency. Type 2 diabetes is characterized by diminished liver, muscle, and adipose tissue sensitivity to insulin, also known as insulin resistance, and impaired beta-cell function resulting in a deficiency in the amount of insulin produced (ADA, 1998b; Quarry-Horn et al., 2003). "Excessive body weight appears to contribute to a reduction in the number of receptor sites on the outside of the cell wall, thereby causing the cells to become resistant to the action of insulin" (Quarry-Horn et al., p. 197). It is not caused by an immune process as in type 1 and the pancreas continues to make insulin, but it is not enough to compensate for the insulin resistance. Basal insulin concentration is normal or increased until late in the disease course.

Genetic influences are much stronger with type 2 than with type 1 diabetes. Between 50% and 80% of children with type 2 have at least one parent with a family history of diabetes, and 75% to 100% have a relative with type 2 diabetes (Rosenbloom & Silverstein, 2003).

Although genetic susceptibility is present with type 2 diabetes, it is thought that environmental factors such as obesity, physical inactivity, and diets high in fat and refined carbohydrates are the main factors contributing to the development of this disease (Boland & Grey, 2004).

Type 2 diabetes is becoming more common among specific ethnic groups and adolescents. In addition, certain ethnic groups tend to have higher rates of obesity. Epidemiological data support higher insulin resistance in African American, Native Americans, and in Asian and Hispanic children and adolescents along with lower insulin sensitivity compared with Caucasian youth (Ruiz, Robertson, & Boyd, 2001). "African American children between the ages of 10 and 19 experienced a 10-fold increase over a decade in the incidence of type 2 DM" (Quarry-Horn et al., 2003, p. 196). Diagnosis of type 2 diabetes tends to occur at a higher rate in females and during mid-puberty, most likely related to the temporary evolution of insulin resistance during this developmental phase, accounting for approximately a 30% reduction in insulin action compared with prepubertal children or adults and increased demand for insulin during this growth phase (Libman & Arslanian, 1999).

In addition to the symptoms of diabetes mentioned earlier, acanthosis nigricans, a thickening and hyperpigmentation of the skin at the neck and flexural areas, typically signifies insulin resistance, and can be a marker for type 2 diabetes, although it occurs long before a diagnosis of diabetes is made. Up to 60% to 90% of youth who develop acanthosis nigricans develop type 2 diabetes (Kaufman, 2002). It may have a velvety appearance, or look like dirty dark patches around the neck and skin folds, and can easily be identified by the school nurse.

LONG-TERM COMPLICATIONS OF DIABETES

The goal of treatment and management of diabetes in young people is to prevent the myriad of complications that can occur in adulthood, primarily heart disease, stroke, vision loss, amputation, and kidney disease. Autoimmunity, tissue ischemia and hypoxia, glycosylation of cellular proteins, coagulation defects and insulin resistance are some of the pathophysiological mechanisms that have been hypothesized to contribute to the development of the microvascular and macrovascular complications in both type 1 and type 2 diabetes (Andrus, Leggett-Frazier, & Pfeifer, 2001). For most children diagnosed with type 1 diabetes, complications tend to develop after puberty (Andrus et al., 2001).

Cardiac disease is caused by atherosclerosis of the large blood vessels. Twenty-five percent of the deaths of those with onset of diabetes before age 2 will be due to cardiac disease (ADA, 2004). Blindness due to diabetic retinopathy develops more rapidly in males, especially if they were diagnosed with diabetes during their youth. Diabetic nephropathy occurs in 10% to 21% of those with early-onset diabetes and is the leading cause of end-stage renal disease, ultimately resulting in dialysis or kidney transplantation. "Diabetic ketoacidosis (DKA) is one of the most serious outcomes of poorly controlled diabetes, and primarily occurs in type 1 individuals.... DKA is responsible for about 10% of diabetes-related deaths in individuals with diabetes under age 45" (ADA, 2004). The Diabetes Control and Complications Trial Research [DCCT] (1991) has shown that improving blood sugar control will help prevent or prolong the onset of complications. Education and monitoring of other risk factors such as hypertension, hyperlipidemia, and smoking cessation are recommended (Andrus et al., 2001).

Research related to the development of complications of students with type 2 diabetes is limited. Many students who are diagnosed with type 2 diabetes also have other chronic conditions such as hypertension, hyperlipidemia, sleep apnea, and depression (Fagot-Campagna et al., 2000). Screening for comorbidities at the time of diagnosis will be essential for these young people. Education regarding decreasing other risk factors related to complications will be challenging. Because most of those diagnosed with type 2 diabetes are adolescents, making lifestyle changes to improve blood sugar control can be difficult (Fagot-Campagna et al., 2000). Monitoring and controlling blood sugar and blood pressure and following up with their health care team are essential in controlling the long-term complications of diabetes.

MANAGEMENT OF DIABETES

Diabetes is one of the few diseases in which the goal of self-management is initiated from the moment of diagnosis. Diabetes management requires an individualized approach; the goal is to achieve blood glucose control and allow the person with diabetes to live a normal life. The components of blood glucose balance are nutrition (food), medication, and exercise (FIGURE 33.1).

The management strategies used to achieve blood sugar goals are individualized for each student; the type of diabetes and the student's age and developmental level are examples of variables that may affect the treatment strategies in place for each student. The management of diabetes is rapidly changing. Technological advances have provided more options and therefore more individuality in diabetes management.

Type 2 diabetes in youth is challenging for many reasons. It is difficult for older children and adolescents to adhere to lifestyle modifications and medical treatment because of socioeconomic conditions and limited availability of resources for management. The challenge also lies in adolescents' perceptions regarding health along with their lack

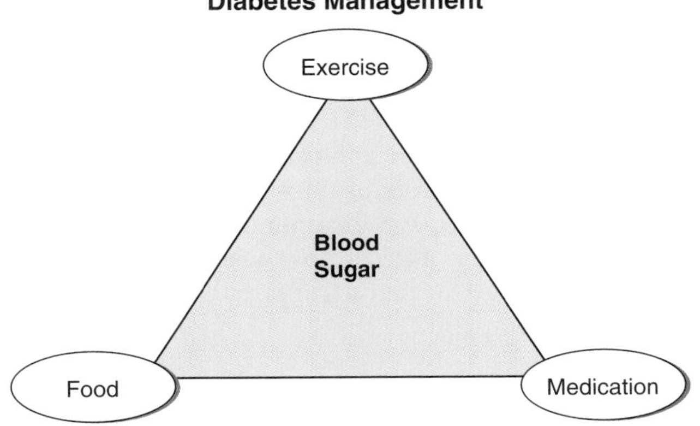

Figure 33.1 ■ Diabetes management.

of concern for the long-term complications of this disease. Peer pressure is a major factor that can prohibit students from participating in activities and following through on the prescribed plan of care (Rosenbloom & Silverstein, 2003).

One way to monitor the degree of compliance or control of blood sugar is by testing the HgA1c or the glycosylated hemoglobin. This blood test measures the average blood sugar control over a 3-month period of time. Students with diabetes need to try to maintain their optimal blood sugar range. Because glucose attaches to the circulating hemoglobin molecule and because red blood cells live for 120 days, a measure of the glucose attached to hemoglobin will be an average of the circulating glucose levels during that period of time. Normally, the glycosylated hemoglobin is 3% to 6% of the total hemoglobin. Those with diabetes try to keep their HgA1c around 7%. Values higher than that indicate increasing incidents of hyperglycemia (Boland & Grey, 2004).

Nutrition

A balance of food, medication, and exercise is needed to achieve target blood glucose levels. For youth with type 1 diabetes, caloric intake that is adequate to ensure normal growth and development is essential. The meal plan does not restrict calories but is intended to ensure reasonable consistent food intake and a nutritionally balanced eating pattern. Insulin needs to be adjusted to cover the amount of food consumed (Franz, 2001). However, for youth with type 2 diabetes, achieving and maintaining a healthy weight through healthy eating habits and exercise can help control blood glucose levels and delay the progression of the chronic complications of diabetes (Franz, 2001). Nutrition education is an important and ongoing part of diabetes management, but also the most challenging. An individualized meal plan should address personal preferences, cultural aspects, and the need/willingness to change one's lifestyle or adapt to a meal plan.

Principles for Meal Planning

Meal planning focuses on the carbohydrate content of food choices. Carbohydrate is the body's major source of energy. All carbohydrate consumed is converted into blood glucose. Protein and fat metabolism have little effect on blood glucose levels. A prescribed carbohydrate meal plan, an exchange plan, or a carbohydrate counting meal plan may be used; examples of each are described below. Dietary sources of carbohydrate are fruit, milk, breads, cereal, grains, and some vegetables such as corn and peas. Prepared foods with added sugars will increase the carbohydrate content and have an effect on blood sugar.

The principles for meal planning include the following:

- *Eat a well balanced diet.* This is good advice for everyone; it is particularly important to support growth in children.
- *Eat meals and snacks at the same time each day (this may vary depending on food and insulin regimen prescribed).* This is important for people who are using relatively constant insulin doses and are following a consistent carbohydrate or exchange program.
- *Be aware of insulin actions; time meals and snacks accordingly.* This is especially important in the school setting when schedules change. Meal times or physical education times that change throughout the school year may require an adjustment in meal planning to prevent hypoglycemia.
- *Use snacks to prevent insulin reactions.* For unplanned or extended activity, add snacks of extra carbohydrates to prevent low blood sugar.
- *Balance carbohydrate intake and insulin carefully.* The rise in blood sugar after eating is dependent on the total amount of carbohydrate eaten, not the form of carbohydrate. A carbohydrate is a carbohydrate.
- *Avoid overtreating low blood sugars.* This is one of the factors found in the Diabetes Control and Complications Trial (1991) to relate to better blood glucose control. This can be difficult because of the powerful response of feeling "ravenously hungry" that often occurs with low blood sugar.
- *Reduce cholesterol and saturated fat intake.* Blood cholesterol and triglyceride levels can be high if blood sugar levels are too high, which can lead to cardiovascular complications. Blood cholesterol levels should be monitored annually.
- *Monitor height and weight.* This will provide guidance regarding proper nutritional intake.
- *Avoid foods high in salt* (adapted from Chase, 2002).

In a **prescribed carbohydrate meal** plan, the number of carbohydrate (carb or CHO) choices is kept about the same for each meal and for snacks for each day. Although the type of carbohydrate can vary, consistency in the number of choices is important. One carbohydrate choice is 15 grams of carbohydrate. More carbohydrates may be needed for increased activity. An example of a prescribed carbohydrate meal plan is:

Breakfast	AM snack	Lunch
3 carbs	1 carb	3 carbs

Afternoon Snack	Dinner	Bedtime
2 carbs	3-4 carbs	2 carbs

In the **exchange meal plan**, foods are grouped into one of six food lists (meat, bread, fat, vegetable, fruit, and milk). A meal plan is developed that outlines the number of choices from each of the six food groups for meals and for snacks. This type of program may be helpful if weight control is an issue. An example of an exchange meal plan is:

Breakfast	Lunch	Dinner
Meat 1	Meat 2	Meat 3
Bread 2	Bread 3	Bread 3
Fat 0	Fat 1	Fat 1
Fruit 2	Fruit 2	Fruit 1
Vegetable 0	Vegetable 1–3	Vegetable 1–3
Milk 1	Milk 1	Milk 1

Snacks: am = 1 bread + 1 fruit;
afternoon = 2 bread + 1 fruit;
bedtime = 1 bread + 1 meat

The **carbohydrate counting meal plan involves counting the grams of carbohydrate and giving a corresponding dose of insulin**. It emphasizes carbohydrate intake while keeping protein and fat relatively constant. The variability of carbohydrate intake and insulin provide more flexibility and reduce the risk of hypoglycemia. The insulin used at meals and snacks for those with type 1 diabetes is rapid acting and requires use of a longer-acting background insulin (i.e., glargine, NPH, Lente, Ultralente, or insulin pump use). An example of a carbohydrate counting meal plan is listed below.

INSULIN DOSE 1 UNIT/CARB CHOICE OR 15 GRAMS OF CARBOHYDRATE

Breakfast	AM snack	Lunch
4 carbs	None	Missed lunch
4 U insulin	No insulin	No insulin

Afternoon Snack	Dinner	Bedtime
2 carbs	7 carbs	2 carbs
2 U insulin	7 U insulin	2 U insulin

Important points to remember in meal planning are as follows:

- There is no difference in the effect of a simple sugar compared with starch in raising the blood sugar level.
- A person with diabetes can eat almost any food in moderation if it is worked into the meal plan.
- A person with diabetes can eat foods with simple sugars in them. However, simple sugar should be eaten at a time when adequate insulin is present.
- Nutritious carbohydrate choices should be encouraged.
- Frequent blood glucose testing (2 hours after eating various foods) is encouraged to determine the effects of a given food.
- Blood sugar testing when an insulin reaction occurs is important in avoiding overtreatment of low blood sugars.

Meal Planning at School

To support students with diabetes in the school setting, the school nurse may need to include school nutrition services in the health plan for students. Issues related to food choice availability may be identified and the nurse may need to advocate for students.

SAMPLE INDIVIDUAL HEALTHCARE PLAN FORMAT for the STUDENT with DIABETES

Name__________________ **DOB**________________ **Grade**____________________ **Teacher**________________ **Date**________________

Nursing Diagnosis #1: Potential for physiological injury due to development of acute complications related to hypoglycemia or ketoacidosis

Student Outcome Goals:

1. Student does not experience signs/symptoms of hyperglycemia or severe hypoglycemia
2. Student maintains target blood sugar ________.
3. HbA1c within normal limits

Student Outcome: Blood Sugar Maintenance

Interventions:

- Set up schedule with student for blood testing and insulin injection.
- Have student sit near teacher if he/she is having frequent reactions.
- Treat for hypoglycemia as described on emergency care plan.
- Keep designated source of carbohydrate readily available in the classroom.
- Check blood glucose if hyperglycemia is suspected.
- Modify food and insulin plan with parent for activities such as gym and recess.
- Plan with teacher for the possible need for mid-morning and mid-afternoon snacks.
- Coordinate snack and meal times with peak action time of insulin.
- In-service school staff to recognize signs/symptoms of hypoglycemia and to intervene appropriately.

Delegation:

- Instruct an additional staff member to initiate the emergency plan in the absence of a professional.
- Review the procedure every few months.

Multidisciplinary Care Conference:

- Instruct staff that cognitive functioning does not return completely for 20 minutes after hypoglycemia episodes. Functioning may even take longer to return to optimal levels.
- Report any changes or problems to team members as appropriate.
- Report to parents and healthcare providers regularly.
- Review progress toward attainment of student outcome of goals regularly.

Nursing Diagnosis #2: Potential for knowledge deficit related to the need to balance glucose monitoring, insulin injection, diet, and exercise

Student Outcome Goals:

1. Student will increase his or her understanding of diabetes.
2. Student can monitor his or her blood glucose.
3. Student can administer his or her insulin.
4. Student understands his or her designated meal plan.
5. Student incorporates exercise into the school day.
6. Student can identify his or her symptoms of hypoglycemia.
7. Student can identify the effects of stress on his or her diabetes management.

Outcome: Age-Appropriate Self-Management

Interventions:

- Assess student's knowledge of diabetes, insulin administration, blood glucose monitoring, effects of diet and exercise, awareness of infection and proper skin care, signs/symptoms of hyper or hypoglycemia and appropriate treatment, and the effect of stress (physical or mental) on his or her diabetes.
- Provide appropriate assistance in diabetes management tasks.
- Discuss the health plan with physician and other health professionals involved in student's care.
- Have appropriate and current reference materials readily available.

Nursing Diagnosis #3: Self-esteem disturbances due to lifestyle changes demanded by diabetes and its management

Student Outcome Goal:

1. Student demonstrates comfort in discussing diabetes with peers and asking for help when needed.

Outcome: Adaptation to Diabetes

Interventions:

- Aim to increase self-care.
- Involve the child in the decision-making process.
- Stress the child's strengths.
- Provide support and assistance in problem solving.
- Encourage wellness behaviors, not a "sick" role.
- Refer to appropriate support groups.

*School Nurse*____

*Parent/Student signature*____________________________________

Figure 33.2 ■ Sample Individual Health Plan format for the student with diabetes. (Adapted from Blum, M. [2002].)

Access to nutritional information, primarily carbohydrate content of school menu items, is important. For all students, but particularly those students following a carbohydrate counting meal plan, accurate carbohydrate information is essential to minimize "guessing" and ensure a proper insulin/carbohydrate ratio for dosing. Many prepared menu items combine different foods and will require the support of school nutrition services staff to provide the correct content information. The popularity of ala carte choices, offering a wide variety of food options in many of the secondary schools, provides an additional challenge because accurate carbohydrate information may not be readily available. Food labels are an option but often are listed on the outside packaging of items and not on each individual item, so ready access to this information may be a problem for some students. The school nurse in partnership with school nutrition services can be helpful in obtaining this information for students.

Class Parties

Class parties and special events are a very important aspect of the overall school experience, and students with diabetes should participate fully. Discussing these events at the time the health plan is developed is the best way to address possible options. These may include:

- Student will eat the treat.
- Parents will provide a replacement alternative.
- Treat will be placed in a bag and sent home to be eaten as part of a scheduled snack.
- Other modifications, such as removing frosting or decreasing snack size, are student- and parent-specific, and the plan should be discussed as part of the student's individual school health plan (FIGURE 33.2). Send a note home in the beginning of the year or in preparation for class celebrations reminding families of the special food-related needs of students in the class.

Extended Field Trips

As students get older, there is often more opportunity for extended field trips. The school nurse should work closely with school staff and parents to provide adequate preparation and communication to ensure student safety. Planning for extended field trips should include the following items:

- A copy of the Emergency Action Plan (EAP), including emergency information and phone numbers (FIGURE 33.3). Staff training in procedures for recognition and treatment of hypoglycemia (also included in the individual school health plan) (Figure 33.2).
- Supplies for blood glucose monitoring
- Supplies for insulin administration
- Provisions to ensure proper storage of insulin
- Supply of meal/snack items
- For intensely active field trips, parents should send extra snacks to be eaten during increased activity and may elect to reduce the insulin dose to prevent hypoglycemia.
- Fast-acting carbohydrate in case of hypoglycemia

Diabetes Medications

Students with diabetes require careful balancing of the factors that affect blood sugar levels. Medication, food intake, and exercise are factors that require daily attention to meet blood sugar target goals. Medication and insulin regimens for managing diabetes change as scientific advances are made. The school nurse must keep current with the science related to diabetic medications.

Insulin Therapy

All students who have type 1 diabetes must take daily insulin. The findings of the Diabetes Control and Complications Trial (1991) demonstrated the benefits of intensive therapy for the management of type 1 diabetes. Intensive therapy using multiple insulin injections or an insulin pump is the therapy method that best mimics, as nearly as possible, the physiological profile of insulin secretion. The advent of new insulin analogs has provided many more choices and greater flexibility in diabetes management strategies. Current methods of insulin delivery may involve the use of a syringe and needle, an insulin pen, or an insulin pump.

For a newly diagnosed individual with type 1 diabetes, once exogenous insulin has been initiated, the beta cells in the pancreas may start to produce small amounts of insulin again (ADA, 2002a). This phenomenon is called the honeymoon phase. The pancreas begins producing insulin on its own and allows many people to decrease the amount of insulin they are taking. The honeymoon phase is very individualized. Some individuals with newly diagnosed type 1 diabetes never have a honeymoon phase, whereas for others it may last several months (ADA, 2002a). Some will misinterpret the honeymoon phase as

Sample EMERGENCY ACTION PLAN

For a Student with Diabetes

Name: ______ DOB: ______ Grade: ______ Date: ______
School: ______ Bus Number: ______

Emergency Contact Information:
Parent/guardian: ______ Work phone: ______ Home phone: ______
Parent/guardian: ______ Work phone: ______ Home phone: ______
Emergency contact: ______ Phone: ______
Healthcare provider: ______ Phone: ______ Hospital: ______
Location of Diabetic Supplies: Snacks: ______ Glucose meter: ______ Glucagon: ______

Signs and Symptoms of Low Blood Sugar, which can impair the student's level of consciousness:

- The student complains about feeling "low"
- The student exhibits some or all of the following symptoms:

☐ Hungry ☐ Shaky ☐ Unable to concentrate ☐ Lethargic ☐ Irritable
☐ Sleepy ☐ Sweaty ☐ Confused or disoriented ☐ Weak ☐ Pale
☐ Combative ☐ Dizzy ☐ Poor coordination ☐ Other ______

- The student is having a seizure or convulsion, is unconscious, unwilling or unable to swallow.
- A hypoglycemic emergency would most likely occur before lunch, after strenuous exercise or ______.
- Exercise lowers blood glucose. If exercise is more strenuous or longer than usual, it could result in low blood glucose. Extra snacks may be needed. If blood glucose is below ____ or above ____ at time of exercise, the student should not participate.
- PE teacher and playground supervisor should keep a fast-acting source of sugar with him/her at all times during exercise (like hard candy or glucose tablets). If symptoms of low blood glucose occur, fast-acting sugar should be given and contact the school nurse.

How to Treat Low Blood Sugar:
If the student complains about feeling "low" or exhibits symptoms of hypoglycemia but is conscious, cooperative, and can swallow:

- Give 15 grams of fast-acting carbohydrate such as ____ glucose tablets or ____ tube of gel, ____ ounces of non-diet soda, or ______.
- Contact the school nurse. Do not leave the student alone or send to the office alone.
- Check blood glucose in 15 minutes. If below ____ repeat 15 grams of carbohydrate.

If the student is unresponsive, having a seizure, or unable to swallow, contact the school nurse or trained diabetes personnel who will give glucagon as ordered in the medical management plan.

- Turn the student on his or her side and keep the airway open.
- Call 911 and the parent
- Give sugar water or non-diet soda (7UP) to drink when the student awakens and is able to swallow.

Signs and Symptoms of High Blood Sugar that can impair the student's cognitive abilities:

- The student with hyperglycemia will exhibit the following symptoms:

☐ Excessive thirst ☐ Frequent urination ☐ Personality/behavior change ☐ Nausea
☐ Blurry vision ☐ Fatigue ☐ Inability to concentrate ☐ Other ______

If the student exhibits any of the symptoms listed above, check the student's blood glucose and treat for hyperglycemia if blood glucose is higher than ___.

How to Treat High Blood Sugar:
If the student has any of the signs and symptoms above:

- Allow free use of the bathroom.
- Encourage the student to drink water or other sugar-free liquid.
- Contact the school nurse or trained diabetes personnel to check for urine ketones and to administer insulin as ordered in the medical management plan.
- If the student is vomiting or lethargic, ___ Call the parent or ___ call for medical assistance if the parent cannot be reached.

School Nurse:
______ Phone: ______

Figure 33.3 ■ Sample Emergency Action Plan.

either having been misdiagnosed or being cured. This may result in decreased attention to diet or to monitoring blood sugars. It needs to be reinforced that the honeymoon phase occurs only once and may last for weeks or for up to 2 years (Boland & Grey, 2004).

Individualized management plans for students are best developed when there is an understanding of the types of insulin each student is using and developing a plan to meet the needs of the student. There are several different types of insulin. Insulin is generally classified according to the onset, peak, and duration of action (White, Campbell, & Yarborough, 2001). The currently available rapid-acting insulins are Lispro and Aspart, the short-acting insulin is Regular, the

Table 33.1 ■
AVERAGE TIMES OF INSULIN ACTION

TYPE OF INSULIN	ONSET OF ACTION	PEAK ACTION (HOURS)	EFFECTIVE DURATION OF ACTION (HOURS)	MAXIMUM DURATION OF ACTION (HOURS)	VISUAL CHARACTERISTICS
Rapid-acting					
Lispro or Aspart (Humalog/Novolog)	10–15 minutes	30–90 minutes	3–4 hours	4–6 hours	Clear
Fast-acting					
Regular	30–60 minutes	2–3 hours	3–6 hours	6–9 hours	Clear
Intermediate-acting					
NPH	2–4 hours	6–10 hours	10–16 hours	14–18 hours	Cloudy
Lente	3–4 hours	6–12 hours	12–18 hours	16–20 hours	Cloudy
Long-acting					
Ultralente	6–10 hours	10–16 hours	18–20 hours	20–24 hours	Clear
Glargine (Lantus)	1–2 hours	none	24 hours	24+ hours	Clear
Combinations					
70/30 NPH/Regular	30–60 minutes	Dual	10–16 hours	14–18 hours	Cloudy
75/25 NPH/Humalog	10–15 minutes	Dual	10–16 hours	14–18 hours	Cloudy

Source: Adapted from M. Franz, K. Kulkarni, W. Polonsky, P. Yarborough, & V. Zamudio (Eds.), *A CORE Curriculum for Diabetes Education* (4th ed.). Chicago: American Association of Diabetes Educators.

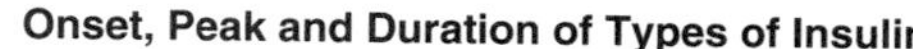

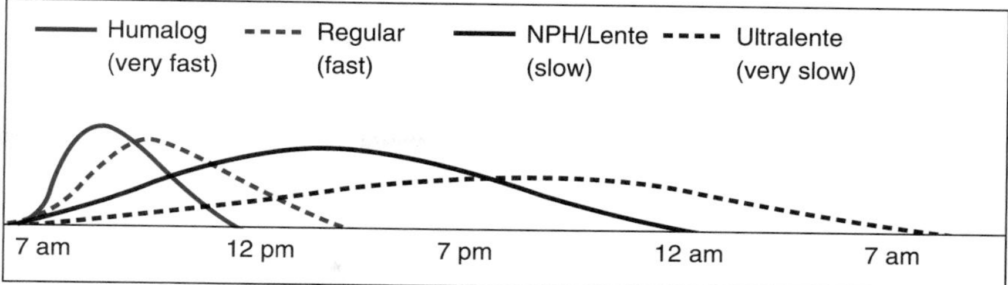

Figure 33.4 ■ Onset, peak, and duration of types of insulin. (Joslin Diabetes Center. (2005). Insulin Action. Accessed from Joslin.org/education/library/insulin_action.shtml)

intermediate-acting insulins are NPH and Lente, and the long-acting insulin is Ultralente. In addition, a true "peakless" long-acting insulin analog Glargine is now available (White et al., 2001). TABLE 33.1 compares the actions of these insulins while FIGURES 33.4, 33.5, AND 33.6 show how multiple injected insulins work together to achieve blood glucose control.

The site of the injection and exercise may influence insulin action (Chase, 2002). For example, if a student injects in the leg and exercises soon after there may be some enhanced absorption of the insulin. There may also be some variability from person to person and from one day to the next (Chase, 2002).

Insulin Dosing

Insulin is a medication; therefore, physician authorization and parent authorization are required for administration in the school setting. The variability and individuality of diabetes add to the complexity of insulin dosing. From the time of diagnosis, patients and families are taught to recognize blood glucose trends and adjust insulin to balance blood glucose, food, and exercise. This philosophy leads to variable insulin doses. Insulin dose parameters at school need to outline these factors and allow the student and parents to adjust doses to regulate blood sugar.

Insulin orders need to include the following information:

- The insulin type: Brand and type
- Administration times
- Device by which insulin is to be administered: syringe, pen, pump
- Dose to be determined by:
    - Standard dose: number of units
        - Example: Humalog insulin 3 units each day before noon meal
    - Dose based on blood sugar: sliding scale
        - Example: Blood sugar 100 to 200 mg/dL requires 3 units of Humalog
        - Blood sugar 201 to 300 mg/dL requires 4 units of Humalog
        - Blood sugar 301 to 400 mg/dL requires 5 units of Humalog
    - The dose is based on insulin-to-carbohydrate ratio.
        - Example: 4 carbohydrate choices = 4 units of Humalog (note the insulin dose will be different for each student. Some may use .5, 1, 1.5, or even 2 units/carbohydrate choice).
- Dose may include a "correction dose" for hyperglycemia.
    - The correction dose is calculated by number of points over target
        - Example: In addition to meal dose, give 1 unit of Humalog for every 50 points of blood glucose over 150. Ex: Blood sugar = 265

          Meal dose = 4 units

          Correction dose = 2 units

          Total dose = 6 units
- Dose may be decreased for low blood sugar or increased activity.

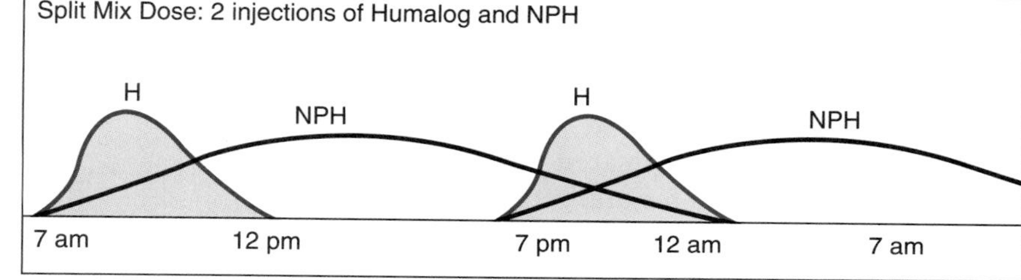

Figure 33.5 ■ Two injections per day. (Joslin Diabetes Center. (2005). Insulin Action. Accessed from Joslin.org/education/library/insulin_action.shtml)

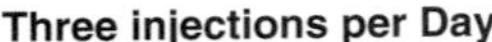

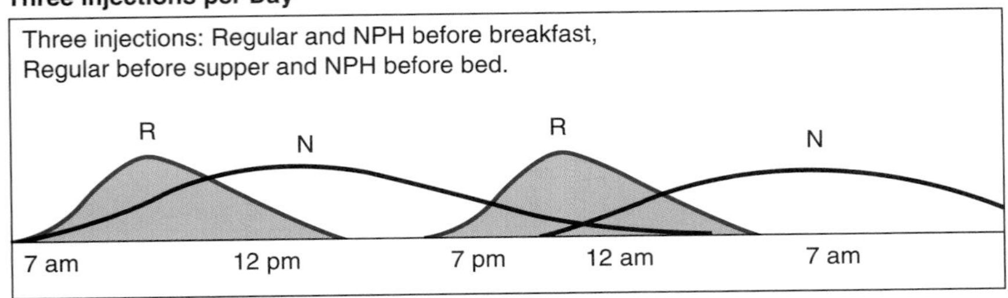

Figure 33.6 ■ Three injections per day. (Joslin Diabetes Center. (2005). Insulin Action. Accessed from Joslin.org/education/library/insulin_action.shtml)

- Decrease dose by ___% if anticipate increased, extended activity (Adapted from Zombek, 2002)

Insulin Storage Guidelines

- Insulin is affected by temperature extremes. Unopened vials should be stored in the refrigerator and are good through the manufacturer's expiration date.
- Opened vials may be stored at room temperature, between 59 and 86 degrees Fahrenheit, and used for one month.
- Storage guidelines for insulin pens and penfill cartridges vary. NPH pens last for 14 days and Humalog or Regular insulin pens are good for 30 days.
- Insulin vials should be visually inspected for sediment before an insulin dose is drawn. If sediment is seen, the insulin should be discarded.

Insulin Delivery Equipment

The task of taking multiple insulin injections can be overwhelming for many students and families. Technology has made many new devices available for the delivery of insulin. These pens, pumps, and auto-injectors make the delivery of multiple injections more convenient. Improved convenience and ease of use may, in many cases, improve patient compliance to the prescribed regimen.

Depending on the insulin regimen used, some students may require an insulin shot at school. In addition to the traditional method with vial and syringe, the insulin pen is either pre-filled or uses an insulin cartridge. Pens are available that are able to dose in whole and half-unit doses. Whenever it is available, an insulin pen should be used for insulin doses at school. The dialed dose option with a pen removes the need to draw the insulin into a syringe. In the school setting, where assisting a student with this task may be a delegated skill, if state law allows, the use of a pen for dialing may improve ease of training staff to help students with this task. It may be easier to look at a dialed number than to read the lines on a syringe when verifying the dose for accuracy.

Insulin Pump Therapy

Insulin pump therapy, or continuous subcutaneous insulin infusion (CSII), is a method of insulin delivery that uses a small mechanical pump to deliver a preset dose of short or rapid acting insulin. The insulin is delivered through small plastic tubing that is connected to a subcutaneously placed catheter in the child's abdomen or upper buttocks. This is called the infusion set. The insulin pump, which delivers the insulin, attaches to the infusion set. Students often wear the pump on the waist of their pants. It may look like a "pager" or "cell phone" to school staff. It is best to notify school staff that a student is wearing an insulin pump to prevent any confusion about the device. Students also have a disconnect mechanism that allows them to remove the pump while still leaving the catheter in place so that they can swim or bathe or engage in sports (Boland & Grey, 2004).

Insulin is dosed using a basal rate and a bolus dose. The basal insulin is the amount of insulin delivered in small amounts every few minutes, programmed to match pancreatic insulin release patterns. Bolus insulin doses are given to cover food intake or to correct a high blood glucose level.

Pump therapy holds many of the following advantages for people with diabetes:

- Insulin dosing with an insulin pump can be precise to within one tenth of a unit. This is a benefit, especially for small children who require smaller insulin doses.
- Differences in absorption from various sites are reduced.
- Continuous delivery improves insulin absorption.
- The dawn phenomenon (early morning rise in blood sugar levels) is easier to manage.
- The incidence of nocturnal hypoglycemia is reduced.

- Adjustments for illness are easier.
- Lifestyle flexibility is enhanced with more customized meal/snack schedules.

Limitations of pump therapy include the following:

- A learning curve is associated with pump therapy. Successful adaptation may take months.
- Technical failure is a possibility.
- The student may forget or neglect to bolus for meals/snacks. For students who used to receive NPH in the morning, the task to remember to cover the noon meal may lead to higher blood sugar levels.
- There is an increased risk of ketosis when only short- or rapid-acting insulin is used.
- There is an added expense for pump purchase and supplies.
- Weight gain can occur with increased food consumption and insulin use.
- Skin infections or skin irritation can occur. This can usually be minimized by more frequent site changes (Brooks, 2001).

Insulin Pump Therapy at School

Most students using an insulin pump at school will be educated and proficient in the use of the pump. There may be times when, for a variety of reasons, a very young child may be using an insulin pump. Students who receive insulin via an insulin pump and are not able to manage the pump may require supervision and/or pump operation by either a school nurse or other school personnel who have received training. The school nurse must complete an assessment of needs and develop an Individualized Health Plan (IHP) that outlines the needs and interventions. The school must be notified prior to the student attending so training can occur. For students who are able to self-manage their insulin pump dosing, school personnel should be trained in how to suspend the pump in times of hypoglycemia. This training should occur as part of a hypoglycemia emergency plan.

An example of an insulin pump school checklist is as follows:

- Extra pump supplies should be kept at school, including insulin, syringes, infusion sets and inserter, tape, and batteries.

Table 33.2 ■
ORAL DIABETES MEDICATIONS BY CLASSIFICATION AND ACTION

DRUG NAME	DRUG CLASSIFICATION	DOSE RANGE	SIDE EFFECTS	COMMENTS
Metformin (glucophage)	Biguanides—insulin sensitizer	500–850 mg tid or 1,000 mg bid	Dose start low and titrate up; gastrointestinal side effects, sweating, headache	Used alone is not associated with hypoglycemia
Glucotrol, Glucotrol XL, (glipizide) Amaryl (glimepiride)	Sulfonylurea—insulin secretagogue	Glucotrol 2.5–20 mg, single or divided doses; Amaryl 1–4 mg single dose	Hypoglycemia, weight gain, skin rash	
Actos (pioglitazone), Avandia (rosiglitazone)	Thiazolidinediones (TZDs)—insulin sensitizer	Actos 15-, 30-, 45-mg doses; Avandia 2-, 4-, 8-mg doses	Elevated hepatic enzymes, edema	Reduce insulin resistance. Used alone will not cause hypoglycemia

Source: Adapted from White (2001).

- Ketostix should be kept at school. These would be used in the event of an interrupted insulin dose. Ketones may quickly develop if insulin delivery is stopped or the student becomes ill.
- Pump reference cards and resource phone numbers should be available for school staff for use in troubleshooting pump problems.

Pulmonary Insulin

Recent technological advances have made it feasible to deliver insulin to the alveolar space, where it is rapidly absorbed into the alveolar capillaries and distributed throughout the systemic circulation (White et al., 2001). Several clinical trials have demonstrated the effectiveness, safety, and acceptability of inhaled insulin. As this book goes to press, inhaled insulin is going through the FDA approval process.

Oral Diabetes Medications

If type 2 diabetes cannot be controlled with diet and exercise, the student will need medication. Metformin (Glucophage), which decreases glucose production by the liver, is the oral medication typically used to treat children and adolescents with type 2 diabetes (Ruiz et al., 2001). Glucophage is the only oral diabetes medication approved by the FDA for the treatment of type 2 diabetes in children. To achieve target blood sugar goals, medications may be used in combination with insulin. TABLE 33.2 compares oral diabetes medications used in managing type 2 diabetes, keeping in mind that they are not approved for or tested in children, except for metformin.

Exercise

Exercise is an important component in the treatment plan for diabetes management. Exercising typically will lower blood sugar, but this effect is very individualized. The lowering blood sugar effect that occurs with exercise for an individual with diabetes can be attributed to a decreased need for or better utilization of insulin (Mullooly, 2001). Hypoglycemia is one of the main concerns with exercising and it is important to test one's blood sugar before exercise. If the blood sugar is not within a student's goal range, it needs be tested again while the student is exercising. When the blood sugar is less than 100 mg/dL, it would be beneficial to have an extra carbohydrate prior to exercising (ADA, 2002b).

Extracurricular activities at school are an important part of any school-age child's or adolescent's education. Having diabetes should not prevent anyone from participating in extracurricular activities if blood sugar levels are under control. Planning for these extracurricular activities is important. Students need to be encouraged to have supplies for testing and treating low blood sugar. Coaches and teachers involved in these activities need to be educated about diabetes and how to identify, prevent, and treat problems with blood sugar control.

Unfortunately schools vary in the amount of physical activity that is incorporated into school curricula. Schools may offer physical education classes on a daily or rotating schedule. It is important for the school nurse to work with students, teachers, and parents to incorporate physical education classes into the student's IHP. This may mean that students with diabetes need extra snacks on days when they are more active or they may need to adjust insulin to account for days when more activities such as field trips and increased exercise are planned. School nurses need to help students learn how exercise affects their blood sugar levels and to plan appropriate interventions.

Students may be involved in school-sponsored after-school sports and activities. Working with coaches, teachers, students, parents, and the healthcare team will be advantageous in preventing problems with blood sugar. Educating school staff about the needs of students with diabetes to be allowed to test their blood sugar and treat symptoms appropriately will help prevent a student from having possible problems during these activities. School staff and coaches working with students with diabetes need to be educated regarding symptoms of high and low blood sugar and appropriate treatment. IHPs and Emergency Action Plans (EAPs) (Figures 33.2 and 33.3) should be in place that outline appropriate plans of care for a specific student.

Monitoring Blood Glucose

The blood glucose levels measure the effects of balancing food, exercise, and medication for people with diabetes. Generally most people with type 1 diabetes will monitor their blood sugar levels a minimum of four times per day. The technology for blood sugar monitoring is rapidly advancing. Blood glucose meters are compact, give fast results, and require a small sample of blood. Retractable lancets and wicking test strips have greatly minimized the risk of exposure to blood. Alternate site (forearm) testing is also available with many of the new blood glucose meters. In the school setting, students who have demonstrated proper technique and understanding of results should be allowed to test their blood in multiple settings, for example, classroom or locker.

Students requiring assistance with blood glucose testing or with interpreting the results should be provided assistance with testing. If unfamiliar with the equipment, the school nurse should reference written material from the meter company for proper testing steps. Reference material is available either from the parents or through the manufacturer's toll-free number. Another resource is the Advanced Practice Nurse in the diabetes center used by the student.

Typically blood sugar level is tested before meals. However, while evaluating effectiveness of different insulin regimens or in type 2 diabetes, postprandial testing may provide additional helpful information. If postprandial testing is needed, the blood glucose should be obtained 2 hours after a meal or insulin dose (Childs, Hinnen, Guthrie, & Guthrie, 1998). Target blood glucose levels are individually determined and should be included in the student's IHP. Recording blood glucose results and regular communication of results to parents or the healthcare provider is an important aspect of the student's IHP.

The Continuous Glucose Monitoring System (CGMS) by Minimed was approved by the FDA in 1999. The sensor system involves the insertion of a small plastic catheter into the subcutaneous tissue. The catheter is attached to a small computer (sensor) that samples and reads the blood sugar every 10 seconds and provides an average reading every 5 minutes. When the patient is wearing a sensor, he or she is required to keep accurate blood glucose, food, and insulin records. The sensor data is compared to patient records. Episodes of undetected hypoglycemia or hyperglycemia and blood sugar trends are identified by the sensor data. Patients often wear a sensor for 3 days and may be required to wear a sensor during the school day. The school nurse may be asked to observe the insertion site or assist the student with recording food, blood glucose readings, and activity levels if a student is wearing a glucose sensor.

Ketone Testing

Ketone testing is an important aspect in the management of hyperglycemia and/or illness. Access to equipment and tools for the monitoring of ketones should be incorporated into the student's IHP. Both urine and blood can be tested for ketones. There is a blood glucose meter, the PrecisionXtra, that has the ability to test blood ketones using a special test strip. Some students may use this type of meter. Other students will use urine to test for ketones. Urine ketone testing is done using a test strip that is dipped into the urine. The color change of the test strip, after exactly 15 seconds, will indicate the level of ketones. If ketones are present, the parent should be notified and a plan for the management of ketones and or illness should be initiated.

DIABETES EMERGENCIES

Hypoglycemia (Low Blood Sugar)

Hypoglycemia is one of the most immediate emergencies for a person who has diabetes. With the emphasis on intensive management and near normal blood glucose control, occurrences of severe hypoglycemia have increased (Hernandez, Bradish, Rodger, & Rybansky, 1999). Hypoglycemia is defined as blood sugar that is less than 70 mg/dL (Gonder-Frederick, 2001). Symptoms identified can vary and the blood sugar at which individuals feel these symptoms also varies (Hernandez et al., 1999; Ryan, Dulay, Suprasongsin, & Becker, 2002). Identifying each individual student's symptoms for hypoglycemia and the treatment they use is important. Individuals with diabetes often can identify symptoms they may have when their blood sugar level is mildly decreased, moderately decreased, and severely decreased (TABLE 33.3).

Some people with diabetes start to lose the ability to sense low blood sugar until it is dangerously low. This phenomenon is called hypoglycemia unawareness and is believed to be caused by changes in hormonal counterregulation systems, especially a decrease in the hormonal response of epinephrine (Gonder-Fredrick, 2001). For these particular students, it may be important to prevent episodes of hypoglycemia.

Causes of Hypoglycemia (Low Blood Sugar)

Hypoglycemia can occur when the individual with diabetes has too much insulin or an inadequate amount of food in the prescribed meal plan, has skipped or delayed meals or snacks, or has participated in an unusually large amount of exercise (Gonder-Fredrick, 2001). Exercise helps the muscle utilize sugar in the blood (ADA, 2002b) and can affect the blood sugar for up to 18 hours after exercising (ADA, 2002b). When a student has low blood sugar frequently after exercise or notices patterns of low blood sugar levels related to exercise, it would be important to discuss a change in this student's diabetes regimen to prevent these low blood sugar occurrences. Examples include decreasing the rapid-acting insulin dose prior to a meal that is eaten before exercising, taking extra carbohydrates before and during exercise, or decreasing intermediate-acting insulin that may peak during exercise.

Table 33.3 ■

REPORTED SYMPTOMS FOR HYPOGLYCEMIA

MILD HYPOGLY-CEMIA	MODERATE HYPOGLY-CEMIA (SYMP-TOMS OF MILD HYPO-GLYCEMIA PLUS)	SEVERE HYPOGLY-CEMIA
Hunger	Sleepiness	Unable to swallow
Irritable	Erratic behavior	Unresponsive
Shakiness	Poor coordi-nation	Unconscious
Weak	Confusion	Seizures
Sweaty	Slurred speech	Combative
Anxious	Slow thinking	
Dizziness	Numbness	
Headache		
Unable to concentrate		
Not feeling well		
Feeling funny		
Heart racing		
Tingling in extremities		

Taking more insulin than the body needs may cause low blood sugar. Students who calculate their insulin dose based on the carbohydrates they consume must follow through with their meal plan. Insulin-to-carbohydrate levels can change for some students as they go through growth spurts, puberty, or when they are ill. These incidences cause an increased secretion of specific growth and counter-regulatory hormones that are related to insulin resistance, and therefore require more insulin to metabolize carbohydrate intake. It is important to assess the student's ability to accurately calculate the amount of insulin based on his or her blood sugar level and carbohydrates as prescribed by their primary care provider.

Missing a meal or taking in less food than what was planned can cause low blood sugar. Students can be more flexible with meals and snacks with the newer rapid-acting insulin analogs available. With some of the short- and intermediate-acting insulins, a student may need to eat meals or snacks at a specific time to prevent a low blood sugar reaction. It is important for the school nurse to be knowledgeable about the type of insulin the student is taking and whether the student needs to strictly adhere to meal times or can be more flexible. When a student has difficulty following a strict meal schedule because of his or her insulin analogs, it may be beneficial to discuss changes in the insulin regimen with the student, parent, or guardian, and physician so that low blood sugar reactions are prevented and a student has more flexibility.

Treatment for Hypoglycemia or Low Blood Sugar

Treatment for low blood sugar will also be very individualized and it is important to know what symptoms, if any, a student has with low blood sugar reactions. The recommendation is to treat low blood sugar at the first indication of symptoms, even if meter testing is unavailable to verify a low blood sugar (ADA, 2002c; Gonder-Fredrick, 2001). A student and school nurse should have a fast-acting carbohydrate, such as fruit juice, glucose tablets or gel, or regular soda pop available at all times in case of low blood sugar. It is important that the school nurse educate teachers and other school personnel regarding symptoms of low blood sugar and its treatment. A student who is having symptoms of low blood sugar should never be left unattended in case his or her blood sugar declines to a dangerously low level and the student loses consciousness.

Students should be encouraged to keep a supply of fast-acting carbohydrates in the classroom and in the nurse's office. During an episode of hypoglycemia, the student should consume 15 grams of carbohydrate. Some examples of 15 grams of carbohydrate include 4 oz of juice, $^1/_2$ cup of regular soda pop, five or six hard candies (lifesavers) three glucose tablets, 8 oz. of skim or 1% milk, cake icing (1 small tube).

The student or school staff personnel need to repeat testing of the student's blood sugar after 15 minutes. If the blood sugar is still less than 70 mg/dL, the student should repeat treatment with another 15 grams of carbohydrate. If the blood sugar is above 70 mg/dL but the student will not be eating a meal for more than an hour, the student should have a snack that has carbohydrate and protein such as crackers with peanut butter or cheese, or a special diabetes snack bar, such as Glucerna snack bar or nite-bite snack bars.

A parent or guardian should be notified regarding low blood sugars. It is important to discuss the incident with the student so that he or she can learn about the symptoms of low blood sugar and prevent these episodes in the future.

When a student has a severe low blood sugar reaction, the EMS system should be called immediately and glucagon given if available. Turn the student on his or her side after the glucagon has been given since individuals often vomit after receiving this medication (Gonder-Frederick, 2001). The parent should always be contacted for a severe low blood sugar reaction.

Students who have had mild to moderate low blood sugar reactions in which the blood sugar result was lower than 50 mg/dL should wait at least 15 to 30 minutes before resuming normal activities (Gonder-Frederick, 2001). When blood sugar results are less than 40 mg/dL, mental and motor function may not return to normal for one or more hours. Students who have had frequent episodes of mild hypoglycemia are at a greater risk for having a severe low blood sugar reaction.

Hyperglycemia (High Blood Sugar)

Hyperglycemia, which is generally considered a blood sugar level greater than 240 mg/dL, can occur gradually or more rapidly. The benefit of blood sugar testing is the ability to monitor blood sugars to prevent dangerously high levels. Symptoms of high blood sugar, which were discussed earlier, are frequent urination, frequent thirst, blurred vision, fatigue, hunger, weight loss, abdominal pain, and numbness in extremities. Long periods of hyperglycemia can lead to damage of the blood vessels along with nerve endings and affect major organs in the body, such as the circulatory system, eyes, kidneys, and nervous system (Andrus et al., 2001).

Most school-age children are not concerned about the long-term effects of high blood sugar and often forget that high blood sugar can be an emergency. When a person with type 1 diabetes does not take enough insulin, glucose remains in the bloodstream and cannot be properly utilized for cellular energy. As the muscles need sugar for energy, the body responds by releasing stored fats and proteins for energy; ketones are formed that upset the pH balance, and results in acidosis. This is a serious condition called diabetic ketoacidosis (DKA) and can cause a coma as the result of dehydration, electrolyte imbalance, and the acidosis (Davidson & Swartz, 2001).

Profound insulin deficiency is the main cause of diabetic ketoacidosis but this condition is very complicated. The insulin deficiency that occurs with DKA causes impaired protein synthesis and excessive protein degradation. The breakdown of stored fat and triglycerides is a result of severe insulin deficiency and an increase in counterregulatory hormones that occur with DKA (Davidson & Swartz, 2001). Following an acute case of DKA, short-term memory impairment may exist for a month (Zombek, 2003).

People with type 2 diabetes will not develop ketoacidosis but may develop a condition called hyperosmolar hyperglycemic state (HHS) which is also related to decreased amounts of available insulin (Davidson & Swartz, 2001). The hyperosmolar hyperglycemic state typically happens in the elderly individual with type 2 diabetes and can be related to massive fluid loss from prolonged osmotic diuresis secondary to hyperglycemia, illness, particular medications such as thiazides, and severe diarrhea (Davidson & Swartz, 2001).

Causes of Hyperglycemia

Hyperglycemia can have many causes, including missed insulin doses or not taking enough insulin, or eating more food than planned or foods that are high in carbohydrates and not taking enough insulin. Illness and growth spurts may lead to hyperglycemia, along with some medications that may cause the blood sugar to become elevated. Some medications associated with hyperglycemia are corticosteroids, cyclosporine, diazoxide, diuretics, protease inhibitors, and thyroid products (White et al., 2001).

Treatment for Hyperglycemia

Guidelines for checking urine or blood ketones should be included in the IHP for students with type 1 diabetes. For most students, when a blood sugar is greater than 240 mg/dL or a student with type 1 diabetes is ill, the primary care provider may want to have the urine or blood checked for ketones (ADA, 2002c). Some newer blood glucose meters use a separate strip in the meter to test for blood ketones. It is important to remind students and parents that they need to have a supply of urine or blood ketone test strips at school at all times. Plans should be in place regarding what to do if ketones are present when the blood sugar is high. Some students may have specific medical orders to take extra insulin to cover high blood sugar levels with the presence of ketones. When ketones are present, the parent and or physician should be contacted. This may mean that the student needs more insulin, needs more fluids for hydration, or may be sick and need to see his or her healthcare provider. A student should not participate in any physical activities, such as gym class, if ketones are present because this may cause the blood sugar to increase and make ketosis worse (Mullooly, 2001).

When a student has a high blood sugar and no ketones are present, it may be helpful to determine what may have caused the high blood sugar. Problem solving with a student regarding possible causes of high blood sugar may help keep blood sugars within the goal range in the future. A student who has missed a dose of insulin may need to contact the parents regarding taking the insulin at school.

Interventions for hyperglycemia include drinking extra water, exercising moderately if no ketones are present, and taking extra insulin if this is part of the student's diabetes treatment plan. The student can return to the classroom if he or she is feeling better, but should be encouraged to return if symptoms reoccur. Emergency care is needed for a student who is unable to tolerate fluids by mouth, has persistent vomiting, weakness, has readings of moderate or large ketones, or has a change in mental status.

EFFECT OF BLOOD SUGAR ON LEARNING

Students with diabetes need to manage their illness to minimize the effect of diabetic symptoms on their learning capabilities. When a student has a high blood sugar level, he or she typically does not feel good and has symptoms of polyuria, polydipsia, fatigue, and hunger. This student will have difficulty concentrating and may miss out on learning opportunities, especially if he or she needs to leave the classroom frequently. When a student is not succeeding in school, it would be beneficial to review this student's blood sugar control to rule out fluctuations in blood sugar as a possible cause of poor academic performance.

Effective diabetes management in school is necessary for the safety and long-term health of the student with diabetes, maximizes the student's readiness for learning and participation in school activities, and minimizes the possibility of hypoglycemic and hyperglycemic emergencies in school. Additional benefits for the student include better attendance and improved alertness and physical stamina. Schools need to work together with parents, students, healthcare providers, and the community in a comprehensive and coordinated approach to ensure that students with diabetes have the same educational opportunities as do other students (National Diabetes Education Program, 2003).

A greater threat to the learning capabilities of students with diabetes is hypoglycemia. Two variables that affect memory capability include the age of onset of type 1 diabetes and the history of severe hypoglycemia (Hershey, Bhargava, Sadler, White, & Craft, 1999; Northam et al., 2001). Students who have low blood sugar, even mild low blood sugar, show impairment in regards to fine motor and motor speed activities of tasks (Hershey et al., 1999). Students who are having symptoms of mild hypoglycemia during the school day may not be able to comprehend instructions and do poorly in testing situations.

When students with diabetes are visiting the school nurse with symptoms of low blood sugar they should get treatment and have their mental status assessed. It is important to remember that a student's blood sugar may be back in the optimal range but this student may still exhibit periods of unclear thinking that may affect optimal learning. Frequent school absences may be an indicator of poor blood sugar control. It is important to convey to the parents and student that school attendance is important and the school nurse can safely support the student in the classroom and school activities.

PSYCHOSOCIAL ISSUES WITH DIABETES

Any student may have issues related to school, friends, the home environment, and fitting in at school. Children with diabetes have a higher rate of psychosocial issues related to low self-esteem; worsening metabolic control can escalate these psychosocial issues (Castiglia, 2001). They have more difficulty during preadolescence and adolescence in managing their diabetes because adolescents do not want to be different.

Diabetes is considered to have one of the most complicated treatment regimens of any chronic condition. The student with diabetes needs to carefully incorporate diet, exercise, medications, and blood glucose testing into their daily routine. Adolescents find it more challenging to fit in and also follow a diabetes management routine. Some parents feel

Table 33.4 ■
AGE-APPROPRIATE DIABETES TASKS WITH EDUCATIONAL CONSIDERATIONS

AGE	DEVELOPMENTAL ISSUES	DIABETES TASKS	EDUCATION CONSIDERATION
4 to 5	Knows likes and dislikes Identifies with "good" and "bad" Fear of intrusive procedures Magical thinking	Can pinch own skin. Collects urine for ketones. Turns on glucometer; helps with recording. May begin to identify symptoms of hypoglycemia and alert an adult.	Can use guided play, play therapy, artwork to express their concerns and learn.
6 to 7	Physically coordinated Concrete reasoning Able to share and cooperate	Can begin to identify carbohydrates in foods. Can help with injections. Can help with blood testing. Able to prick own finger. Able to activate bolus on pump with supervision. Able to connect and disconnect Insulin pump with assistance.	May need reminders and supervision.
8 to 10	Increased need for independence Does not want to be different Developing "scientific mind"; intrigued by tests. Feelings of sadness, anxiety, isolation, and friendlessness.	Able to participate in meal planning. Correctly able to identify foods that fit into meal plan. Increased independence with injections, blood and urine testing. Able to keep records.	Understands only immediate consequences of diabetes control, not long term. Finds support groups, camps, individual counseling useful. Learns most effectively when information presented in a fun and interesting way.
11 to 13	Begins puberty; hormonal and physical changes may occur for females. Dependent versus independent struggles between parent and child.	Can help plan meals and snacks along with starting carbohydrate counting. Able to recognize and treat hypoglycemia Able to measure and inject own insulin.	Peer pressure begins to influence decisions.

(continued)

Table 33.4 ■ *(Continued)*

AGE	DEVELOPMENTAL ISSUES	DIABETES TASKS	EDUCATION CONSIDERATION
	Aware of body image; concerned with not being different. More involved with peers than family.	Able to recognize patterns in blood sugars. May need help in assessing urine tests. Able to connect and disconnect insulin pump. Able to calculate insulin to food intake.	
14+	Begins puberty; hormonal and physical changes occur for males. Increased physical and social activities. Experimentation and risk-taking behaviors Conflict in relationships with parents. Strong peer pressure Values independence and self-image.	Able to identify appropriate portion sizes. Able to alter food intake in relation to blood glucose level. Able to anticipate and prevent hypoglycemia. Able to calculate insulin dose based on blood glucose level. Can independently administer insulin. Able to understand role of exercise in calculating insulin needs.	Still needs some parental supervision and review regarding insulin dosing. Knows consequences of poor diabetes control. More involved with risk-taking and experimentation. Finds assuming responsibility for self-management the most difficult task. At risk for eating disorders. Learns best when educational content is pertinent to adolescent issues. Able to learn problem solving with adults and negotiate treatment. Likes discussion and support groups among peers.

Source: Betschart (2001); Fredrickson & Graff (2000); Zombek (2003).

that as their teenager becomes more independent in managing their diabetes, they do not need the parent's guidance. A student may make decisions regarding diabetes management that are not always in the best interest of his or her health, yet these decisions help the student feel more like his or her peers. A student with diabetes may experiment with drugs, alcohol, cigarettes, and other risk-taking behaviors to fit in and not be fully aware of the life threatening consequences this brings. This risk-

Sample 504 Plan
School Year 2004-05

Student: Dan
School: ***Arlington Middle School***
Parents: Sheila and Dave
Phone: 123-456-7890
Date of meeting: 9-02-04

Date of Birth: 3-18-92
Grade: ***7th***

Case Manager: ***Nick Smith***

Date of initial 504 Plan: 9-01-03

1. Describe the nature of the concern:
Dan was diagnosed with type 1 diabetes mellitus in 5th grade.

2. Describe the basis for the determination of disability:
Type 1 diabetes is a physiological disorder that affects the endocrine system. The pancreas does not produce the insulin that is necessary to convert glucose (from sugar, starches, and other food) into energy. Dan must take insulin to control his blood glucose levels. Optimal diabetes control is a careful balance of food, exercise, and insulin.

3. Describe how the disability affects a major life activity:
Dan must check his blood glucose level during the day, and take actions (eat extra food, take insulin, or modify his activity level) to maintain his glucose level within a target range. Low and high blood glucose levels can be life threatening and must be treated. These fluctuations also can affect his ability to learn in the classroom.

4. Describe the reasonable accommodations that are necessary:
Dan can check his blood glucose level in the classroom. He carries his monitoring system in his backpack.

Dan can take glucose tabs or snacks in the classroom. (Located in his backpack).

Dan shall be permitted to have immediate access to water in the classroom.

Dan shall be permitted to use the bathroom without restriction.

Dan can leave class to see the nurse for diabetes-related issues. If he is having a low or high blood glucose level, he needs to be accompanied by another student/adult.

Dan will be permitted to participate in all field trips and extracurricular activities without restrictions and with all the accommodations and modifications set in this plan.

If Dan needs to take breaks to get water, use the bathroom, do a blood glucose test, or treat hypoglycemia or hyperglycemia, he will be given extra time to finish the test or assignment without penalty.

If Dan is affected by a high or low blood glucose level at the time of regular or standardized testing, he will be permitted to take the test at another time without penalty. High blood glucose is defined as over 220 mg/dl and low blood glucose as less than 80mg/dl.

Dan will not be penalized for absences or tardiness required for medical appointment, illness, visits to the nurse's office, or time necessary to maintain blood glucose control.

Review/Reassessment Date:
January 15, 2005

Participants (name and title):

CC: Student's Cumulative File
Attachment: Information regarding emergency care.

Figure 33.7 ■ Sample 504 Plan School Year 2004–05.

taking behavior can have variable effects on blood sugars.

School nurses understand the importance of assessing all students for issues related to psychosocial concerns. This assessment is significant for students with diabetes because it has been shown that students with diabetes have more problems with self-esteem and depression (Grey, Davidson, Boland, & Tamborlane, 2001). Issues with poor self-esteem and depression can lead to other risk-taking behaviors. Eating disorders among females with type 1 diabetes have been a major concern. Girls with diabetes more often than boys misuse insulin for weight reduction, leading to higher blood sugar levels (Neumark-Sztainer et al., 2002). Studies also showed that females who were more dissatisfied with their weight were more likely to use unhealthy weight control behaviors.

Family support is very important when assessing students' ability to manage their diabetes at school and when looking at psychosocial concerns. Studies have shown that continuing parental support and guidance appear to help adolescents achieve success in blood glucose control (Grey et al., 2001). Grey et al. (2001) also showed that students who had poorer glucose control and less guidance from parents might benefit from special interventions to help with diabetes management. In this study, the most significant predictor of the worsening of the impact of diabetes on quality of life was the youth's perception of the impact of diabetes on quality of life at baseline (Grey et al., 2001). This supports the need for school nurses to seek out and assist those students with type 1 diabetes who are depressed or withdrawn along with those who are in poor glucose control.

AGE APPROPRIATE TASKS FOR THE STUDENT WITH DIABETES

Students learn diabetes self-care tasks at variable rates depending on their psychomotor and intellectual development, experience with diabetes, and motivation to provide self-care. TABLE 33.4 provides general guidelines for expecting the student to participate in and learn self-care diabetes activities.

CONCLUSION

An IHP and an EAP should be developed for all students with diabetes (Figures 33-2 and 33-3). The EAP should be made available to bus drivers, lunchroom staff, coaches, playground/campus supervisors, and adult chaperones for field trips. Because they are considered to have a disability, federal law (Section 504 of the Rehabilitation Act of 1973) requires schools to provide whatever accommodations are needed for them to fully participate in school activities and to be in the classroom (see Chapters 9 and 14). A sample 504 Plan can be found in FIGURE 33.7. Additional resources on diabetes are available from the Web sites listed below.

Resources

American Academy of Family Physicians (AAFP)
http://www.aafp.org

American Academy of Pediatrics (AAP)
http://www.aap.org

American Association of Diabetes Educators (AADE)
http://www.aadenet.org

American Council on Exercise (ACE)
http://www.acefitness.org

American Diabetes Association (ADA)
http://www.diabetes.org

American Dietetic Association (ADA)
http://www.eatright.org

American School Health Association (ASHA)
http://www.ashaweb.org

Centers for Disease Control and Prevention (CDC)
http://www.cdc.gov

Division of Diabetes Translation
http://www.cdc.gov/diabetes

Division of Nutrition and Physical Activity
http://www.cdc.gov/nccdphp/dnpa

Division of Adolescent and School Health
http://www.cdc.gov/nccdphp/dash

Children with Diabetes
http://www.childrenwithdiabetes.com

Disability Rights Education and Defense Fund (DREDF)
http://www.dredf.org

Diabetes Exercise and Sports Association
http://www.diabetes-exercise.org

Education Resources Information Center (ERIC)
http://www.eric.ed.gov

Indian Health Service HIS National Diabetes Program
http://www.his.gov

Joslin Diabetes Center
http://www.joslin.harvard.edu

Juvenile Diabetes Research International (JDRFI)
http://www.jdrf.org

National Association of Elementary School Principals
http://www.naesp.org

National Association of School Nurses
http://www.nasn.org

National Center on Physical Activity and Disability
http://www.ncpad.org

National Diabetes Education Program (NDEP)
http://www.ndep.nih.gov

National Information Center for Children and Youth with Disabilities
http://www.nichey.org

National Institute of Diabetes and Digestive and Kidney Diseases NIDDK)
http://www.niddk.nih.gov

National Diabetes Information Clearinghouse (NDIC)
http://www.info.niddk.nih.gov

Pediatric Adolescent Diabetes Research Education (PADRE Foundation)
http://www.peds.ws

Pediatric Endocrinology Nursing Society (PENS)
http://www.pens.org

President's Council on Physical Fitness and Sports
http://www.fitness.gov

U.S. Department of Agriculture (USDA) Center for Nutrition Policy and Promotion
http://www.usda.gov/cnpp

Food and Nutrition Information Center
http://www.nal.usda.gov/fnic

Food and Nutrition Service
http://www.fns.usda.gov/fns

U.S. Department of Education
http://www.ed.gov

References

American Diabetes Association (ADA). (1998a). *Medical management of type 1 diabetes* (3rd ed., pp. 12–20). Canada: American Diabetes Association.

American Diabetes Association (ADA). (1998b). *Medical management of type 2 diabetes* (4th ed., pp. 21–33). Canada: American Diabetes Association.

American Diabetes Association (ADA). (2002a). Committee Report: Report of the expert committee on the diagnosis and classification of diabetes mellitus. *Diabetes Care, 25*(Suppl. 1), S5–S20.

American Diabetes Association (ADA). (2002b). Position statement: Diabetes and exercise. *Diabetes Care, 25*(Suppl. 1), 64S.

American Diabetes Association (ADA). (2002c). Standards of medical care for patients with diabetes mellitus. *Diabetes Care, 25*(1), 213–229.

American Diabetes Association (ADA). (2003). Committee Report: Report of the expert committee on the diagnosis and classification of diabetes mellitus. *Diabetes Care, 26*(Suppl. 1), S5–S20.

American Diabetes Association (ADA). (2004). *Diabetes statistics for youth*. Retrieved August 24, 2004 from http://www.diabetes.org/diabetes-statistics/children.jsp

Andrus, M., Leggett-Frazier, N., & Pfeifer, M. (2001). Chronic complications of diabetes: An overview. In M. Franz, K. Kulkarni, W. Polonsky, P. Yarborough, & V. Zamudio (Eds.), *A CORE curriculum for diabetes education* (4th ed., pp. 45–61). Chicago: American Association of Diabetes Educators.

Betschart, J. (2001). Diabetes during childhood and adolescence. In M. Franz, K. Kulkarni, W. Polonsky, P. Yarborough, & V. Zamudio (Eds.), *A CORE curriculum for diabetes education* (4th ed., pp. 3–25). Chicago: American Association of Diabetes Educators.

Blum, M. (2002). Are school nurses using the recommendations of the diabetes control and complications trial in the care of students with diabetes? *The Journal of School Nursing, 18*, 138–143.

Boland, E., & Grey, M. (2004). Diabetes mellitus (types 1 and 2). In P. Jackson Allen & J. Vessey (Eds.), *Primary care of the child with a chronic condition* (pp. 426–444). St. Louis: C. V. Mosby.

Brooks, A. M. (2001). Insulin pump therapy and carbohydrate counting for pump therapy. In M. Franz, K. Kulkarni, W. Polonsky, P. Yarborough, & V. Zamudio (Eds.), *A core curriculum for diabetes education* (pp. 203–231). Chicago: American Association of Diabetes Educators.

Brosnan, C. A., Upchurch, S., & Schreiner, B. (2001). Type 2 diabetes in children and adolescents: An emerging disease. *Journal of Pediatric Health Care, 15*, 187–193.

Castiglia, P. (2001). Issues and concerns about diabetes in children. *Journal of Pediatric Health Care, 15*, 304–307.

Chase, P. M. (2002). *Understanding diabetes*. Denver, CO: Children's Diabetes Foundation. Childs, B. P., Hinnen, D. A., Guthrie, D., & Guthrie, R. (1998). Pattern management of blood glucose. In M. Franz, K. Kulkarni, S. Polonsky, P. Yarborough, & V. Zamudio (Eds.), *A CORE curriculum for diabetes education* (4th ed., pp. 389–412). Chicago: American Association of Diabetes Educators.

Davidson, M., & Schwartz, S. (2001). Hyperglycemia. In M. Franz, K. Kulkarni, W. Polonsky, P. Yarborough, & V. Zamudio (Eds.), *A CORE curriculum for diabetes education* (4th ed., pp. 21–39). Chicago: American Association of Diabetes Educators.

Diabetes Control and Complications Trial Research Group (1991). Epidemiology of severe hypoglycemia in the diabetes control and complications trial. *Journal of the American Medical Association, 90*, 450–459.

Fagot-Campagna, A., Pettitt, D., Engelgau, M., Burrows, N., Geiss, L., Valdez, R., Beckels, G., Saaddine, J., Gregg, E., Williamson, D.,& Narayan, K. M. (2000). Type 2 diabetes among North American children and adolescents: An epidemiologic review and a public health perspective. *Journal of Pediatrics, 136*(5), 664–672.

Franz, M. J. (2001). Medical nutrition therapy for diabetes. In M. Franz, K. Kulkarni, W. Polonsky, P. Yarborough, & V. Zamudio (Eds.), *A CORE curriculum for diabetes education* (4th ed., pp. 203–231). Chicago: American Association of Diabetes Educators.

Fredrickson, L., & Graff, M. R., (2000). *Pumper in the school: Insulin pump guide for school nurses, school personnel and parents*. Sylmar: MiniMed Inc.

Gonder-Frederick, L. (2001). Hypoglycemia. In M. Franz, K. Kulkarni, W. Polonsky, P. Yarborough, & V. Zamudio (Eds.), *A CORE curriculum for diabetes education* (4th ed., pp. 231–257). Chicago: American Association of Diabetes Educators.

Grey, M., Davidson, M., Boland, E., & Tamborlane, W. (2001). Clinical and psychosocial factors associated with achievement of treatment goals in adolescents with diabetes mellitus. *Journal of Adolescent Health, 25*, 377–385.

Hernandez, C., Bradish, G., Rodger, N. W., & Rybansky, S. (1999). Self-awareness in diabetes: Using body cues, circumstances, and strategies. *The Diabetes Educator, 25*, 576–584.

Hershey, T., Bhargava, N., Sadler, M., White, N., & Craft, S. (1999). Conventional versus intensive diabetes therapy in children with type 1 diabetes. *Diabetes Care, 22*, 1318–1325.

Joslin Diabetes Center. (2005). Insulin action. Retrieved September 14, 2005 from Joslin.org/education/library/insulin_action.shtml

Kaufman, F. (2002). Type 2 diabetes in children and young adults: A "new epidemic." *Clinical Diabetes, 20*, 217–218.

Leonard, B., Jang, Y., Savik, K., Plumbo, P., & Christensen, R. (2002). Psychosocial factors associated with levels of metabolic control in youth with type 1 diabetes. *Journal of Pediatric Nursing, 17*, 28–37.

Libman, I., & Arslanian, S. (1999). Type II diabetes mellitus: No longer just adults. *Pediatric Annals, 28*(9), 589–593.

Lipman, T. (2002). Type 1 diabetes. In L. Hayman, M. Mahan, & J. R. Turner (Eds.), *Chronic illness in children: An evidence-based approach* (pp. 27–46). New York: Springer.

Mullooly, C. (2001). Exercise. In M. Franz, K. Kulkarni, W. Polonsky, P. Yarborough, & V. Zamudio (Eds.), *A CORE curriculum for diabetes education* (4th ed., pp. 55–88). Chicago: American Association of Diabetes Educators.

National Diabetes Education Program. (2003). *Helping the student with diabetes succeed: A guide for school personnel* (NIH Publication No. 03-5217, pp. 1–4).

Washington, DC: U.S. Department of Health and Human Services.

National Institute of Diabetes and Digestive and Kidney Diseases. (2000). National Diabetes Statistics. Retrieved January 25, 2003 from http://www.niddk.nih.gov/health/diabetes/pubs/dmstats/dmstats.htm

Neumark-Sztainer, D., Patterson, J., Mellin, A., Ackard, D., Utter, J., Story, M., & Sockalosky, J. (2002). Weight control practices and disordered eating behaviors among adolescent females and males with type 1 diabetes. *Diabetes Care, 25*, 1289–1297.

Northam, E., Anderson, P., Jacobs, R., Hughes, M., Warne, G., & Werther, G. (2001). Neuropsychological profiles of children with type 1 diabetes 6 years after disease onset. *Diabetes Care, 24*, 1541–1546.

Quarry-Horn, J., Evans, B., & Kerrigan, J. (2003). Type 2 diabetes mellitus in youth. *Journal of School Nursing, 19*(4), 195–203.

Ratner, R. (2001). Pathophysiology of the diabetes disease state. In M. Franz, K. Kulkarni, W. Polonsky, P. Yarborough, & V. Zamudio (Eds.), *A CORE curriculum for diabetes education* (4th ed., pp. 1–18). Chicago: American Association of Diabetes Educators.

Rennert, O., & Francis, G. (1999). Update on the genetics and pathophysiology of type 1 diabetes mellitus. *Pediatric Annals, 28*(9), 570–575.

Rosenbloom, A., Joe, J., Young, R., & Winter, W. (1999). Emerging epidemic of type 2 diabetes in youth. *Diabetes Care, 22*, 345–354.

Rosenbloom, A., & Silverstein, J. (2003). Type 2 diabetes in children and adolescents: A clinician's guide to diagnosis, epidemiology, pathogenesis, prevention, and treatment. New York: McGraw-Hill.

Ruiz, E., Robertson, C., & Boyd, L. (2001). Type 2 diabetes in children. *RN, 64*, 44–51.

Ryan, C., Dulay, D., Suprasongsin, C., & Becker, D. (2002). Detection of symptoms by adolescents and young adults with type 1 diabetes during experimental induction of mild hypoglycemia. *Diabetes Care, 21*, 852–858.

U.S. Department of Health and Human Services. (2003). *Helping the student with diabetes succeed: A guide for school personnel*. NIH Publication No. 03–5217.

White, J. R., Campbell, R. K., & Yarborough, P. C. (2001). Pharmacologic therapies. In M. Franz, K. Kulkarni, W. Polonsky, P. Yarborough, & V. Zamudio (Eds.), *A CORE curriculum for diabetes education* (4th ed., pp. 89–150). Chicago: American Association of Diabetes Educators.

Zombek, M. (2003). *Pediatric education for diabetes in schools: A resource manual for school nurses)*. Orange, CA: PADRE Foundation and NASN.

Chapter 34

Mental Health Concerns

GLORIA GELMANN ■ JANICE SELEKMAN

Chapter Outline

INTRODUCTION

In 1999 the Surgeon General of the United States, Dr. David Satcher, reported on the state of mental health in children (U.S. Department of Health and Human Services [USDHHS], 1999). The report included the message that mental health is fundamental to overall health and that the stigma attached to mental disorders must be addressed. In an attempt to ensure that the mental health needs of children received attention, a conference on children's mental health resulted in a national action agenda related to mental health in children (U.S. Public Health Service [USPHS], 2000). The goals included increased access to services, training clinicians, promoting public awareness, improving assessment and recognition of mental health needs, increasing research efforts, and closing the gap between research and practice.

The report indicates that "one in ten children and adolescents suffer from mental illness severe enough to cause some level of impairment" but that only one in five receives specialty medical services (USPHS, 2000, p. 13). More boys are identified with problems than girls and mental health problems increase with age. African American and Hispanic American children are identified and referred at the same rate as other children; however, they are less likely to receive assistance. These statistics make the role of the school nurse even more meaningful as the person who can interact with school-age children and adolescents regarding their mental health concerns.

Asarnow, Jaycox, and Anderson (2002) note that most youth receive mental health services through the schools rather than through their primary care providers. They note that for nearly half of all students with serious emotional disturbances, the school system was the sole provider of mental health services. The school nurse is an integral participant in the provision of these services.

School nurses are likely to see children who have mental health needs in their offices on a regular basis and can assist them in receiving the proper care they need. It is vital that schools have systems in place to address barriers to learning for all students, including those with mental health needs. There is a significant relationship between school performance and the mental health of children and adolescents (DeSocio & Hootman, 2004).

In their central role in the education and socialization of all children, schools often have the resources that help with the prevention, identification, and management of psychosocial problems in their students. School nurses are in a position to work with teachers to identify students who need special help, and refer and follow them appropriately. The school nurse can establish rapport with families and work with them to meet the mental health needs of their children. For these reasons, the National Association of School Nurses (2000) approved an Issue Brief supporting and articulating the role of the school nurse in responding to the mental health needs of students.

Often the school nurse is the first person contacted about a student's behavioral or emotional development difficulties. Young people with emotional or behavioral disorders are probably the most under-identified youngsters with disabilities in the public and private schools and certainly the most neglected in the mental health system. It is estimated that up to 80% of children and adolescents with mental health problems do not receive appropriate services (Silverthorn & Frick, 1999).

The most common serious mental health problems seen in the student population are anxiety disorders, mood disorders, oppositional defiant and conduct disorders, eating disorders, Tourette syndrome, and autism and other pervasive developmental disorders. In addition, ADHD (Chapter 30), behavior problems (Chapter 38), violence and bullying (Chapter 39), mental retardation (Chapter 35), and substance abuse (Chapter 40) are major issues in the schools and impact on the mental health of both the affected students and the entire student body and faculty. This chapter focuses on specific mental health problems, although all of the aforementioned issues are considered to be mental health concerns.

It should be noted that the vast majority of the school nurse's role is related, in some way, to mental health. The pat on the back implies "I know you can do it," and the warm smile says, "I care about you." The health office is a safe zone and the school nurse is often one of the most trusted individuals in the school. It is because of this that the school nurse is often the person who students come to when they have a problem; she or he is also the person whom staff approach when they need to discuss how to handle certain students, to express their concern about a student, or to share concerns related to their personal mental health.

When a student presents to the school nurse, the nurse normally does a health assessment and health history, the contents of which include both objective and subjective data. The nurse knows the importance of assessing the student's mood, general feelings (depression, irritability, etc.), any behavior changes, and somatic symptoms. It is also important to know what is going on in the student's family and in the academic arena. The nurse can then determine if the appropriate referral should be to a physician, a psychologist, or perhaps the school counseling department, always working with the student, the family, the teacher and anyone else actively involved with the student.

Screening tools are not used for diagnosis, but are useful in identifying students who may need further evaluation. They can also be used in developing programs for some students who may be at risk. Use of screening tools may require parental consent. The tools mentioned below can easily be adapted by the school nurse for use in individual, group, or schoolwide assessments. Detecting mental health problems and making appropriate referrals so that interventions can begin is one of the most important roles for school nurses.

A tool that may be helpful to the school nurse is the Pediatric Symptom Checklist (PSC) (FIGURE 34.1), a brief youth report and parent-completed questionnaire that was developed by Jellinek and Murphy in 1978 to screen for psychosocial dysfunction in pediatric patients in the United States. The PSC is one of the few mental health questionnaires to be validated in multiple settings. This parent-completed tool is designed to be used for children 4 to 16 years of age. Scoring is easily done and students with emotional and behavior problems can be identified and referred.

Another tool that may be helpful is the Multidimensional Anxiety Symptom Checklist (MASC) (March, 1999). The school nurse who believes a student can benefit from the MASC can refer the student to a psychologist who can administer the test. It can be used for students from 8 to 18 years of age. The MASC provides an overall severity score, as well as subscale descriptions and index scores that can help classify the nature of the anxiety disorder. The MASC is age and gender normed.

The nurse can educate students, family members, school staff, and the community at large about instructional, behavioral, social, and emotional problems seen in the school-age child and adolescent. The nurse, as a member of the multidisciplinary team, can consult with family members, teachers, and

(text continues on page 784)

Pediatric Symptom Checklist (PSC)

Emotional and physical health goes together in children. Because parents are often the first to notice a problem with their child's behavior, emotions or learning, you may help your child get the best care possible by answering these questions. Please indicate which statement best describes your child.

Please mark under the heading that best describe your child:

		Never	Sometimes	Often
1. Complains of aches and pains.				
2. Spends more time alone.				
3. Tires easily, has little energy.				
4. Fidgety, unable to sit still.				
5. Has trouble with teacher.				
6. Less interest in school.				
7. Acts as if driven by a motor.				
8. Daydreams too much.				
9. Distracted easily.				
10. Is afraid of new situations.				
11. Feels sad, unhappy.				
12. Is irritable, angry.				
13. Feels hopeless.				
14. Has trouble concentrating.				
15. Less interest in friends.				
16. Fights with other children.				
17. Absent from school.				
18. School grades dropping.				
19. Is down on him or herself.				
20. Visits the doctor, doctor finds nothing wrong.				
21. Has trouble sleeping.				
22. Worries a lot.				
23. Wants to be with you more than before.				
24. Feels he or she is bad.				
25. Takes unnecessary risks.				
26. Gets hurt frequently.				
27. Seems to be having less fun.				
28. Acts younger than children his or her age.				
29. Does not listen to rules.				
30. Does not show feelings.				
31. Does not understand other people's feelings.				
32. Teases other.				
33. Blames others for his or her troubles.				
34. Takes things that do not belong to him or her.				
35. Refuses to share.				

Total score ______________

Does your child have any emotional or behavioral problems for which she or he needs help?

☐ N ☐ Y

Are there any services that you would like your child to receive for these problems

☐ N ☐ Y

If yes, what services?

Figure 34.1 ■ Pediatric symptom checklist (PSC).

other school personnel to make certain the student receives the proper attention.

The nurse is fully cognizant of the laws regulating accommodations, Individualized Education Programs (IEPs), the Individuals with Disabilities Education Act (IDEA), Section 504 of the Rehabilitation Act, and other disability-related issues (Chapter 14). Mental health conditions are included in these. The nurse, with members of the multidisciplinary team, recommends accommodations that may be appropriate.

THE SCHOOL NURSE'S ROLE AS COUNSELOR

While many schools have professional school counselors who provide mental health services, it is often the school nurse who interacts with most students and is often the first one approached when the student is experiencing a problem. However, it is essential for the school nurse to know the roles of each member of the school team and to forge relationships to enhance communication, identify roles, and know when to make a referral.

The issues range from academic or social difficulties, to family problems, to personal concerns. The student may be having difficulty with a particular class and develop psychosomatic symptoms because of the stress, rather than seek help from the teacher. Bullying may be occurring (Chapter 39), causing the student to be fearful of going to a class. The student may be fearful of using the bathrooms and seek the health office as a way to go to the bathroom "safely." Family problems can range from abuse against the student (Chapter 39), witnessing domestic violence or neighborhood violence, experiencing divorce or family displacement, or grieving for a significant family member. There are those who come because of injuries incurred by fighting, those who come to ask questions that have concerned them regarding sexuality or other highly charged issues, and those who are sent by the teachers who are concerned about them.

The counseling role aims to assist the student in coping with the problems, accessing assistance if it is warranted, building self-esteem and self-confidence, learning conflict resolution, recognizing that he or she is normal or understanding what normal behavior is, and gaining knowledge in order to decrease stress. The ultimate goals are to ensure that students are safe, promote academic success, and provide skills that will enhance good mental health as they move onto the next developmental stage.

All nurses have had pre-licensure classes in psychiatric nursing and learned the basic skills of establishing a therapeutic relationship and engaging in therapeutic communication. In the counseling role, the school nurse will focus on the needs, experiences, feelings, and ideas of students and staff. The components of a therapeutic relationship encompass all that makes a good nurse: trust, genuine interest, empathy, good listening skills, acceptance, positive regard, being nonjudgmental and providing interventions that are developmentally appropriate for the student's age, cognitive level, and social level (Videbeck, 2004).

The most important goal in this role is to promote trust. If promises are made, they must be kept; there must be congruence between what is said and what is done; the messages must be consistent from one meeting to the next; and the school nurse must be honest.

Good interviewing and communication skills are vital. It is important to look at students and/or staff when they are speaking. Perhaps more important than what they say is their nonverbal behavior and whether there is congruence between the two; observe their body language, facial expressions, tone of voice, speed and hesitations of speech, and whether they make eye contact.

Help them identify the most important concern so that it becomes the focus of the interventions. Take care to avoid speaking from your own value system. Guide the student to share feelings with lines such as, "Tell me what it is like…" , "Tell me about…" and "How do you suppose someone feels when this happens to them?" Additional reflective techniques include asking students what three wishes they have, or what scares them the most, or even what they like best about their best friend. It is helpful to restate important lines, such as "So you don't like being with the girls at lunch." It might also be necessary to have students clarify their feelings, such as how they feel when they get very angry.

It is essential for the school nurse to know the laws of confidentiality. While the student's privacy can be respected, there are limitations. No promises can be made to keep information absolutely private if it involves danger to themselves or to others. Because the school nurse often does not have the time to do one-on-one counseling for any prolonged period of time, and if it appears that the student needs professional counseling, the school nurse might ask, "Can I share what you have said with someone in counseling?" This will allow a transition of care so that the student's needs can be addressed.

Interventions start with formulating goals with students—what would they like to see changed? Praise them for their determination; point out their strengths. Have them identify those interventions they have already tried. Give concrete plans based on what the student is willing to do. Then ask, "What happens next?" Help the student think through the issue by asking, "What might happen if…?" Anxiety can be lowered by asking, "What is the worst thing that could happen?" Many students need to make mental tapes of what they are going to do or say. If they cannot see any way to resolve the story, have them tell the story but insist on changing the ending. Make a plan for the student to report back to the school nurse on the outcomes of the plan.

Bereavement Counseling

Bereavement counseling is needed more than might be expected. Students experience the loss of pets, grandparents, parents, and siblings; they may need to deal with the death of a classmate or school staff member. Children handle the concept of death differently based on their age, cognitive development, and culture. To a preschooler, death is temporary, reversible, and magical; for them death should not be compared to sleeping, as the young child wants the person to wake up and continue as before. Young children need to keep their daily routines; they may experience aggression or regression. Art therapy and activities that allow the child to reminisce about death and their lost person are helpful.

Young school-age children still have some magical thinking about what happens when death occurs and may blame themselves for the death. They may develop fears, regress in their behaviors, become aggressive or possessive, have difficulty concentrating, or experience psychosomatic complaints. Preteens want factual information about death; they want to know the mechanics of what a person looks like. They also may have some of the above problems experienced by the younger child.

Teens understand the abstract. They may feel intense anger at the loss. Some will avoid discussions, while others may try to defy death with risk-taking behaviors. They may try to cope using drugs or alcohol. Their grief may lead to suicidal ideation. Any significant regression or aggression, physical self-abuse, or social withdrawal requires a referral. The goal is to help these individuals through their grief, not around it, and not to deny it.

Support can be provided in whatever way makes the student feel better and whole again. If possible, start before the death. Encourage the asking of questions and expression of feelings, including crying. Use nature to explain death (leaves fall, animals die); show that death is part of the process of living. Use children's literature or videos; *Charlotte's Web* and *The Lion King* allow young children to act out sadness in an appropriate way. Reinforce that you are available to them.

If you must inform students of a death, stay with them; provide touch and simple clear explanations. It is okay for students to see you grieve. Reassure them that they did not cause the death nor could they have prevented it. Have students share memories of the person who has died. Allow them to tell their stories over and over again as they continue their routines. Let them say the name of their dead loved one as many times as they want.

Activities that can be initiated include the following:

- Write the word life and the word death and draw pictures to depict each.
- Draw pictures of how each family member is grieving.
- Write a good-bye letter, draw a picture, or write a poem.
- Make a workbook or poster on feelings.
- Role play or use puppets to pretend.
- Make implements to express anger.
- Make a rainbow jar full of regrets; fill with sand and name each layer.
- Make paper lanterns; put feelings, thoughts, regrets on the lantern and let them sail away on a body of water.
- Talk about what the person did to make you happy.
- Make a memory collage of things the person did or enjoyed.
- Plant a tree.

Be sensitive to difficult days when the student may be moodier, or when the class is making Mother's Day or Father's Day gifts. The anniversary of the death is also a difficult time and may result in increased depression or engaging in high-risk or even suicidal activity. The book by Lewis and Lippman (2004) may be very helpful in assisting young people to cope.

SELECTED MENTAL HEALTH CONDITIONS

Selected conditions are discussed below. While application is made to the student, it should be noted that staff members can, and do, present with the same mental health conditions and require similar nursing interventions. In each of the presented disorders, referral for a complete diagnostic assessment is crucial to determine appropriate interventions for the school setting.

Anxiety Disorders

Anxiety is a common manifestation of stress in all individuals; intermittent acute anxiety before presenting in front of the class or before an exam or first date is normal. It is only when the anxiety interferes with one's ability to engage in daily activities and when it recurs frequently or lasts significantly longer than expected that it requires professional intervention. "Anxiety disorders are among the most common forms of psychopathology in children and adolescents" (Kendall, Aschenbrand, & Hudson, 2003, p. 81).

There are multiple types of anxiety disorders. These include separation anxiety disorder, generalized anxiety disorder, panic disorders, agoraphobia, specific phobias, posttraumatic stress disorder, and obsessive–compulsive disorder (American Psychiatric Association [APA], 2000).

The generalized symptoms of anxiety are similar, regardless of the cause. They include tachycardia and tachypnea; the student may complain of shortness of breath. Other somatic complaints include nausea, stomachache and headache, diaphoresis, and tremors. The student experiences recurring negative and unrealistic thoughts, often resulting in decreased participation in the normal activities for age and difficulty concentrating. Sleep problems are reported, including nightmares (Sink & Igelman, 2004). These symptoms negatively impact on the student's self-esteem and relationships with others—both peers and family members. School performance is affected and the student may be tempted to try drugs or alcohol to dull the sensations and fixated thoughts.

It is important to identify the cause of the anxiety and assess its severity in order to effectively work with the student and the family. The Multidimensional Anxiety Symptom Checklist (mentioned earlier) is one tool that can be administered by a psychologist. Once the nurse knows the severity of the disorder, she or he is better able to determine the best course of action.

Youth with an anxiety disorder are different from children who have the "normal" anxieties of growing up. Highly anxious youth do not master their worries and fears but rather they become more intense. Fidgetiness, forgetfulness, disorganization, poor social skills, and a lack of concentration that may lead to learning difficulties are seen. Adolescent anxiety disorders presage the development of comorbid depressive disorders in one-third to one-half of teenagers. When combined with major depression, anxiety disorders increase the risk of suicide attempts threefold (Pawlak, Pascuel-Sanchez, & Rae, 1999; Walsh, 2002).

Evaluating anxiety in children and adolescents requires data from parents, teachers, significant others, and the student. In addition, the school nurse should assess for comorbid psychiatric conditions. If not identified early, they can become chronic and even debilitating. Teachers should provide data on school attendance, performance, and socialization. A health history and physical exam are also important. The school nurse, teachers, and others associated with the young person cannot assume that somatic complaints are symptoms of an anxiety disorder without adequate evaluation. If the young person is on any medication for a medical problem, this must be assessed for its impact on anxiety symptoms. Medications that can induce anxiety symptoms include theophylline, bronchodilators, steroids, phenothiazine antiemetics, digitalis, and antihistamines (Walsh 2002). Questions concerning exercise, sleep, dietary habits, use of caffeine and nicotine, and substance abuse must be asked by the nurse if a student comes to the health office with persistent symptoms indicating anxiety. High use of nicotine (one pack or more of cigarettes daily) by adolescents or young adults may be a factor in the development of anxiety disorders, particularly generalized anxiety disorder and panic disorder (Johnson, Cohen, & Pine, 2000).

As mentioned earlier, the CSC or the MASC can be used as screening tools. Rating instruments for child and adolescent anxiety disorders have markedly improved in the last 10 years (Dierker et al., 2001) and the school nurse can work closely with the school or community psychologist to see that these are administered.

Multiple interventions for anxiety can be initiated in the school environment. The nurse can use age-appropriate methods to induce relaxation. For example, encourage diaphragmatic breathing. Have the student place both feet on the floor and hands on their lap, close his or her eyes, and take deep breaths through the nose and slowly let the air out through the mouth. The abdomen should move instead of the chest. "Breathing in through the nose helps to stop hyperventilating as nostrils are smaller than the mouth so it takes longer for the breath to fill her lungs. And breathing out through the mouth means that she has to concentrate on what she is doing, so it distracts her panicking mind" (Csoti, 2003, p. 151).

The nurse can also work with the school psychologist or other professionals to set up group counseling sessions for these students. The school nurse can then facilitate attendance at these sessions. The affected students can see that others are afflicted with the same feelings and then can begin to develop the social skills to cope with the problems.

Self-esteem is often low at times of stress. Given that adolescents are developmentally dealing with esteem and self-image issues, this makes them particularly at risk. School nurses can boost students' self-esteem by showing confidence in their ability to perform even when the outcome is unclear. They can engage students to help with projects in the health office to both distract their thoughts and to allow success in activities. Teachers can also utilize these techniques.

Separation Anxiety Disorder

Separation anxiety is common in young school-age children and is perhaps the first type of anxiety seen in young children, especially at the start of the school year. It is normal for young children to be hesitant to enter the classroom the first week without the parents by their side. However, the separation anxiety should ease over time and cease to be a problem under usual circumstances. The need for an accurate diagnosis of separation anxiety disorder (SepAD) is important. Reluctance to go to school is not sufficient data on which to make a diagnosis.

The school nurse often becomes aware of children with SepAD when the child persistently refuses or is reluctant to come to school to a degree that is inappropriate for age. These children have unrealistic or persistent fears of separation from their caregiver(s). The fears are developmentally inappropriate, excessive, and interfere with social and academic functioning. Children with SepAD worry that something may happen to their caregivers, such as an accident or illness, or that they may desert the child or that something, such as kidnapping or illness will happen to the child and, as a result, children will be separated from their caregivers. The fears must be present for at least 4 weeks to make a diagnosis of SepAD. The DSM-IV lists eight symptoms of SepAD, three of which are sufficient to make a diagnosis (APA, 2000):

- Recurrent excessive stress related to actual or anticipated separation
- Persistent worry about losing, or harm befalling, attachment figures
- Excessive worry that an untoward event (kidnapping, getting lost) will separate child from attachment figure
- Persistent reluctance or refusal to go to school or elsewhere because of separation fears
- Excessive fear or reluctance to be at home alone or without significant adults in other settings or to sleep away from home
- Refusal to go to sleep alone or without a significant other nearby
- Repeated nightmares involving the theme of separation
- Repeated complaints of physical symptoms (headaches, nausea, stomachaches, vomiting) related to actual or anticipated separation

While separation anxiety is common in preschoolers and those in kindergarten and first grade, separation anxiety disorder peaks at 7.5 years of age and decreases in incidence as children get older (Bernstein & Layne, 2004). Approximately 4% of youth meet criteria for SepAD and after 10 years of age, the annual prevalence decreases by 23% per year of age (Walsh, 2002). Those affected are more likely to come from single-parent homes (Bernstein & Layne, 2004).

The school nurse suspects SepAD when the student refuses or is reluctant to attend school regularly or to let go of the mother at the entrance to the school, or the parent consults the nurse about the child's refusal to sleep alone. Younger children with SepAD may have nightmares and, faced with impending separation, they often cry, throw tantrums, and exhibit psychosomatic complaints, particularly musculoskeletal complaints and stomachaches.

The course of this disorder is variable. It may be insidious or abrupt and may wax and wane. It may occur after a long school vacation, after the child has been out of school for a time due to illness, if a parent becomes ill, or after the child changes schools. The etiology is a combination of factors, including the temperament of the student, the child's attachment to the caregivers, parental anxiety, parenting style, and negative experiences (Bernstein & Layne, 2004).

It is important that school nurses guide the parents appropriately and support the student. Parents who allow prolonged school absences, buy the young child a pager or cell phone, and refuse to leave their child do not help these children. The parents must be assured that the child will not suffer from tantrums or panic attacks if left at school. It should also be pointed out that some children have legitimate fears about school safety or the fate of an ill parent.

Psychotherapy is the treatment of choice for students diagnosed with SepAD and should include both the parents and children. Younger children respond to treatment better than older ones (Walsh, 2002). The goal is to have the child return to school as soon as possible. Regardless of the cause, the longer the child is out of school, the higher the chance of treatment resistance, chronicity, and school failure. An intervention plan can be developed whereby the parent drops the child off quickly and the child is escorted to the classroom by the teacher, the nurse, or some other school personnel.

Some have even been "bribed" by offers to give them a favorite poster if they are able to enter the classroom without problems for 1 week.

Children with this disorder may visit the nurse's office frequently on return to school, usually with somatic complaints, such as stomachache, nausea, abdominal distress, headache, shortness of breath, sweating, crying, chills, and a general feeling of "I don't feel good." There may also be nonverbal clues, such as an increase or decrease in eating; regression; withdrawal or accelerated talking; or avoidance of certain places, people, or situations. The school nurse may have the student check into the office when classes change or at the beginning and end of the school day, just to let the student know that someone is looking out for them.

If it is necessary to have the child stay at home initially, they should follow a school-like schedule in which there is no time for fun activities. In this case, once their symptoms improve, they may return to school for increasingly longer periods. Once in school, some children may find the nurse's office more pleasant than the classroom because they receive special attention. It is the school nurse's responsibility to assess the child, speak with the teacher, and make certain that the child is well enough to return to the classroom. Teachers may need information on the disorder and its implications for the school setting. Parents may need assistance in handling acting out behaviors and setting limits.

These children may be hypersensitive to negative comments in the classroom; therefore, the staff must be very careful about what is said to them. Acknowledge the effort it took to come to school. Do not punish them for refusing to participate and do not make a joke about it. Call on them the first time they raise their hands and provide activities in which the students can be successful (Csoti, 2003).

No medication has been found effective for separation anxiety disorder. Selective serotonin reuptake inhibitors (SSRIs) may be helpful in some cases.

Generalized Anxiety Disorder

The main symptom of generalized anxiety disorder (GAD) is worry. Normal youth worry about all sorts of things, including how they look and whether peers will accept them; however, they can be distracted from their worry. Those with GAD worry about everything but cannot be distracted, and frequently seek reassurance from adults. They have been described as perfectionistic, always wanting to please, and mature beyond their years. They worry about future events years ahead of time and also about past events of which they cannot "let go," for example, a poor grade they received a year ago.

The DSM-IV criteria for GAD include the following:

- Excessive worry most days for at least 6 months about many events or activities, such as school performance
- Anxiety associated with one of the following symptoms: restlessness, easily fatigue, poor concentration, irritability, muscle tension, sleep disturbance
- Anxiety that is not caused by other physical or psychiatric disorders or due to the effects of drugs
- Anxiety, worry, or physical symptoms that cause clinically significant distress or impairment in functioning
- An inability to control the degree of worry (APA, 2000).

Generalized anxiety disorder is a difficult diagnosis, mainly because it may occur with so many other conditions, such as major depression. It can have either an acute or insidious beginning. Because students' worries are often not connected to current events and are excessive, they interfere with family and social relationships and school performance. They recognize that they are anxious and begin to anticipate situations, which causes them to worry more (Sink & Ingleman, 2004). GAD appears to worsen with age, and more females than males are afflicted (Bernstein & Layne, 2004).

Often these young people have somatic symptoms and come to the health office with complaints of a headache or stomachache. They need encouragement, reassurance, and support. SSRIs may be needed for short-term intervention.

Phobias/Fears

All children have fears. These fears cause anxiety and are considered perfectly normal. The nature of the fears changes with age. While toddlers fear strangers and separation from parents, preschoolers typically fear the dark, certain animals or imaginary creatures, storms, and injections and persons associated with pain. Older children may have fears related to death, body safety, animals, bullying, and being liked by others. Children learn to cope with their fears; this process is helped by knowledge, such as what causes lightning and which snakes are dangerous and which are not.

Specific fears can result in extreme anxiety in the student. They are considered phobias when they last at least 6 months and interfere with the student's normal routine or interactions with others. Phobias are excessive and unreasonable. Just the thought of the feared object may cause the student to exhibit the signs of anxiety. If the cause of the phobia presents itself, the student may cry, cling, or freeze in place (APA, 2000). The reaction to a phobia can progress into a panic attack.

The most common phobias in children and adolescents include social phobias, agoraphobia, and school phobia. **Social phobia** was previously referred to as Social Anxiety Disorder. It is more common in adolescents, and those afflicted are "terrified of various social situations in which they can be criticized, embarrassed, ridiculed, or judged by others" (Sink & Igelman, 2004, p. 176). Examples include occasions when students must present in front of peers, or even when they are forced to sit with others in the cafeteria. Youth with social phobias may experience a panic attack just anticipating being in a social situation; as a result they will avoid social situations if at all possible. Some will even avoid going to school. It should be noted that some young persons prefer to be alone; these youth may be called unsociable but may not have a social anxiety disorder.

Agoraphobia also is more common in adolescents. It is an intense fear of being in places or situations in which they would feel trapped and unable to escape. Their responses could range from extreme embarrassment to a panic attack (APA, 2000). This may translate into being afraid of being in large groups (in an auditorium) or being confined in a small space (in a school bus, elevator, or standing in line). Some students have such severe reactions that they are unable to come to school.

School phobias are usually due to a specific phobia in the school, such as agoraphobia, social phobia, or fear of failure. The student often fears embarrassment or scrutiny by teachers, peers, or family. It might also be due to other mental health problems. Before a label is attached to the student, it is necessary to assess if the fears can be substantiated. Examples include weapons in the school or having been bullied. By addressing the primary problem and promoting trust, the fears will be eased. The school nurse can help the parents, the student, and teachers understand the problem. Learning to relax when anxious is a first step in overcoming the anxiety.

Panic Disorder

Panic disorder (PD) in children and adolescents is a disabling and chronic condition, which is accompanied by psychosocial and academic difficulties well into adulthood (Diler, 2003). The school nurse knows that "shortness of breath is a key symptom of panic attacks, which may be misdiagnosed as, or comorbid with, asthma" (Walsh, 2002, p. 74).

Four somatic or cognitive symptoms must be present to meet the diagnostic criteria for panic attack. These include:

- Palpitations, pounding heart, or accelerated heart rate
- Sweating
- Trembling or shaking
- Shortness of breath or feeling of choking
- Chest pain or discomfort
- Nausea or abdominal distress
- Feeling dizzy, unsteady, lightheaded, or faint
- Depersonalization or derealization
- Fear of losing control, "going crazy," or dying
- Paresthesias
- Chills or hot flashes (APA, 2000, p. 432)

Psychoeducation and psychosocial treatments are recommended, and it appears that SSRIs are a safe and promising treatment for students with PD (Diler, 2003). The nurse can try various ways to calm the young person, such as relaxation techniques, distraction methods, such as drawing and writing, and speaking calmly with understanding. As with other disorders, referral for a complete diagnostic assessment is crucial to determine appropriate interventions.

Obsessive–Compulsive Disorder

Children with obsessive–compulsive disorder (OCD) are preoccupied with compulsions and obsessions that occupy a large percentage of their time. In fact, these children or adolescents have little time left for normal developmental tasks, school, and social life. Their obsessions often concern contamination with germs or dirt and their safety and that of their parents. Compulsions take the form of repeated hand washing, checking doors and locks, praying, counting, saying certain words, checking that electric appliances are turned off, and making sure that items are correctly placed. A few children have obsessions without compulsions. Trichotillomania or compulsive hair pulling is in the spectrum of OCD; however, other symptoms are not usually seen.

The etiology of OCD is unknown, although it may have numerous biological causes. Performance of the aforementioned rituals seems to provide relief for those affected. Families often accommodate to the child's behavior and symptoms are concealed. Months may pass before the child is brought for evaluation, as parents often seek care only when the behaviors significantly disrupt the structure of the child's or family's life. Teachers may ask the student to leave the classroom for extended periods of time.

Children with OCD may come to the health office because of the behavioral or physical consequences of their ritualistic behaviors.

The school nurse must elicit a complete history. The student should be asked to describe in his or her own words the urges or worries that accompany the rituals, and to provide details of how the symptoms are interfering in his or her life. An example is going to the restroom and spending an inordinate amount of time hand washing, and as a result missing a large amount of class time. The school nurse must obtain information from the parents, family members, and other teachers to identify the context and severity of the symptoms so that an appropriate referral can be made.

Cognitive–behavioral therapy and pharmacological management have been shown to have direct effects on these abnormalities and to have the best outcomes for youth with OCD (Cohen, 2003; Cohen, Berliner, & Mannarino, 2003; Donnelly, 2003). Exposure and response prevention is a cognitive–behavioral treatment that has been shown to be effective with OCD. In this treatment modality, obsessions are identified as intrusive and unwanted thoughts and images that cause anxiety and distress, and compulsions as behaviors or actions that serve to reduce anxiety (Albano, March, & Piacentini, 1999). The student is usually attending school during treatment. The school nurse should make teachers and family aware that the student will slowly become desensitized to the anxiety-provoking stimulus and will eventually be able to tolerate it without distress or performing a ritual. For exposure and response therapy to be successful, a student must be able to comprehend that a ritualistic behavior stems from a triggering worry or fear and be willing to experience temporary anxiety in exchange for future relief (Piacentini, 1999). This is not possible for young children who do not yet have the ability to think abstractly.

Posttraumatic Stress Disorder

Posttraumatic stress disorder (PTSD) is a form of anxiety in response to severe, life-threatening trauma and is a common cause of morbidity in children and adolescents (Donnelly, 2003). It can be a reaction to sustained or multiple incidents, such as child abuse or domestic violence, or one incident of extreme trauma, such as the aftermath of the attack on the Twin Towers in New York City in 2001 or the flooding of New Orleans in 2005. In all cases, extreme sensitivity by the school nurse is vital.

Children or adolescents who have experienced one incident of trauma are usually hypervigilant and irritable; lack concentration; are easily startled; experience dizziness, sweating, or difficulty breathing, and avoid any reminders of the event, although they do experience mental images of the trauma. Younger children engage in repetitive play, usually having the traumatic incident as the central theme. Youth have sleep difficulties and frequent nightmares and often believe that the future is dim. Young people who have experienced multiple incidents may, in addition to the above symptoms, also have denial, detachment, a numbing flat affect, or anger (Russoniello et al., 2002).

Not everyone who is exposed to trauma experiences PTSD. Children with a history of major depression or other anxiety disorders seem to have a disposition toward PTSD. The symptoms may evidence themselves immediately or several months after the initial incident. The rates of remission vary depending on the traits of the student, the severity of the trauma, the duration of the event, the effect on the family, and the quality of the student's social supports (Lonigan, Phillips, & Richey, 2003).

Treatment is most satisfactory when using cognitive–behavioral therapy or psychopharmacological medications (Cohen et al., 2003; Donnelly, 2003). Many treatment techniques may be combined, such as modeling, role-playing, relaxation, desensitization, and imagery. Parents and school personnel may be involved in some aspects; most techniques require that the facilitator be specially trained.

Mood Disorders: Depression, Dysthymia, and Suicide Attempt/Ideation

Depression among children and adolescents is common but frequently unrecognized. Until approximately 40 years ago, many professionals doubted the existence of major depressive disorders in children, probably because they did not believe children had the cognitive and psychological maturity to experience these problems. However, there is a growing body of evidence to support that children and adolescents do suffer from mood disorders and the morbidity and mortality associated with them. The major mood disorders are dysthymic disorder, major depressive disorder, and bipolar disorder.

All children and adolescents have periods of sadness during which they mope around, withdraw from others, and have periods of crying. However, after a few hours or a day, they return to their normal affect or can be distracted with other life events. Symptoms associated with the pathology of depression last longer and interfere with social functioning, concentration on academic work, and feelings about self.

Mood disorders lead to school failure, dropping out of school, and suicide (Weller, Weller, & Danielyan, 2004a). Yet, they remain underdiagnosed in young children, perhaps because of the decreased verbalization skills of younger children and the increased comorbidity with other mental health conditions.

The prevalence of depressive disorders in children and adolescents is difficult to determine. Each year, approximately 1.3 million teens between 15 and 19 are depressed. The prevalence is listed as 0.4% to 8.3% for adolescents (Weller et al., 2004b). Statistics show that 0.3% of preschoolers, 1% to 2% of school-aged children, and 5% to 8% of adolescents have depressive disorders, but these data have not been updated in more than a decade (Weller et al., 2004a). The gender ratio is approximately equivalent in prepubertal children and increases to a 2:1 female/male ratio in adolescents (Emslie, Mayes, Laptook, & Batt, 2003). Girls tend to report more sadness or feelings that they internalize, while boys describe more anger and acting out behaviors than girls, such as running away, theft, or substance abuse (Weller et al., 2004b).

Numerous causes have been suggested as the etiology of mood disorders, including genetic influences (between 40% and 70%); biochemical factors, especially related to neurotransmitters such as serotonin; and environmental factors, such as stress, loss, and a family history of depression (Weller et al., 2004a). There is evidence suggesting that alteration in the neuronal connections in the prefrontal–subcortical limbic regions of the brain results in disorders of affect, including modulating normal affective expression (Todd & Botteron, 2002).

Factors that exacerbate mood disorders include academic failure, substance abuse, cormorbid anxiety disorders, and uncertainty regarding sexual orientation (Burt, Krueger, McGue, & Iacono, 2003; Emslie et al., 2003; Harrison, 2003; Hauenstein, 2003). Children who are experiencing overwhelming stress, have experienced a loss, or have learning problems of any sort are also at high risk for depression (Emslie et al., 2003).

Adolescence is a particularly difficult time for individuals. The developmental and physical changes are puzzling to this age group. They are striving to separate themselves from their parents and establish their own identities. Their peers are important. Because of all these changes, the adolescent is particularly vulnerable to experience a greater sense of hopelessness.

Social isolation or withdrawal from family and friends are of concern. Quitting sports and other activities the individual enjoyed is significant, as this may indicate that the child or adolescent is increasingly depressed. Athletic participation is often viewed as a positive outlet for adolescents. Manuel and colleagues (2002) explored psychological distress caused by sports injury in adolescents and found that strong athletic identity and high stress levels predict increased depressive symptoms after injury and that better coping skills and social support diminish such symptoms. The school nurse can be alert to the possibility that when injury sidelines a youngster, he or she may be emotionally at risk. The nurse can work with coaches, the family, and teachers so that they are aware of the psychological sequelae and give the injured adolescent the support needed.

The school nurse may be the first to suspect a mood disorder, based on his or her assessments of the student who frequently appears in the health office for psychosomatic ailments. It is important to ask about what else is going on in the student's life to get a more comprehensive picture of the student's sources of stress and how he or she is coping with it. Interaction with faculty will provide a picture of whether a change in behavior and performance has been observed. The school nurse can ask the student questions such as: "What are some things that you worry about?" "What makes you sad?" "What do you do when you feel depressed?"

Twenty percent of adolescents with depression present with drug abuse (Weller et al., 2004b). While risk-taking behaviors are often developmentally appropriate in adolescence, extreme forms of this behavior should be examined closely. A pattern of low self-esteem, preoccupation with death, self-mutilation, and self-destructive behavior are of great concern. Children or adolescents who have unexplained superficial scratches, evidence of cutting on their wrists, attempts at inhalation of a substance, or attempted strangulation are displaying signs of distress. School nurses and anyone associated with the child or adolescent need to recognize pleas for help. The adolescent who continuously drives recklessly, takes drugs, or is sexually promiscuous may also be calling out for help.

Diagnosis can be confirmed by a psychiatrist, psychologist, or a psychiatric Advanced Practice Nurse. It is actually unclear if major depression is meaningfully different from dysthymia. Both disorders share many of the same symptoms but differ in acuity and severity. Goodman and colleagues (2000) report data from youth with major depressive disorder alone, dysthymia alone, and major depression with dysthymia. The three groups did not differ in terms of sociodemographic, clinical, or life-event variables.

Diagnosis is made more difficult by the significant amount of comorbid psychiatric conditions that frequently occur with mood disorder. In major depressive disorder, 40% to 70% of people have comorbid psychiatric disorders, whereas dysthymia has a 50% to 70% comorbidity rate (Birmaher et al., 1998).

The evidence-based literature on treatment of a major depressive disorder in children and adolescents is limited. Most of the available treatment strategies are based on extrapolation of data on studies done on adults (Son & Kirchner, 2000). A multidisciplinary approach, including psychotherapy, pharmacotherapy (TABLE 34.1), and education of the child and family are employed.

Treatment is long term, although many insurance plans limit therapy to the acute phase. Individual therapy is the primary intervention, with family therapy also typically provided (Jones, 2004). SSRIs are considered to be first-line treatment for mood disorders, if pharmacological therapy is also needed. SSRIs replace the tricyclic antidepressants, which were effective in 60% to 80% of cases but were associated with sudden death in adolescents (Weller et al., 2004a).

There is serious undertreatment of children with depression (Jones, Dodge, Foster, & Nix, 2002). Wu et al. (2002) found that depressed girls appeared to be somewhat more likely to receive professional help for depression than boys. However, among children who received professional help for depression, boys were more likely to receive antidepressants. One may come to the conclusion that gender influences treatment.

The school nurse can support the student by focusing on the positive elements of the youth's life and thereby boosting self-esteem. In the classroom, the teacher should keep to a structured routine, as students with mood disorders have difficulty adjusting to change (Jones, 2004). Promote organizational skills, develop positive social skills and make sure they connect with their peers, encourage appropriate expression of feeling, and build self-esteem and self-confidence.

The mean recovery time from major depression is 1 year; but many struggle with the symptoms for years. Only two-thirds reach a full resolution of the problem. Those who have only partial remission are at increased risk of having additional episodes. More than 60% of individuals with a single episode of major depressive disorder will eventually have a second episode (APA, 2000), one-third of which occur within 2 years and 72% within 5 years (Weller et al., 2004a). Those with dysthymic disorder prior to major depressive disorder are even more at risk for future exacerbations. In addition, "approximately 10%-15% of adolescents with recurrent Major Depressive Episodes will go on to develop Bipolar I Disorder" (APA, 2000, p. 385).

Dysthymic Disorder

Dysthymic disorder is the formal name for general depression (Jones, 2004). It is a "long-term, low-grade form of depression" and is "the most common mood disorder seen in children and adolescents" (Jones, 2004, p. 194). The depression is apparent on most days over a one-year period; it is not seasonal. The difference between children and adults with this disorder is that children may appear irritable rather than depressed (APA, 2000). They must have at least two of the following symptoms: poor appetite or overeating, insomnia or hypersomnia, low energy or fatigue, low self-esteem, poor concentration, and feelings of hopelessness (APA).

Personalization, in which the child or adolescent blames him- or herself for all negative outcomes, is due to a distorted view of cause and effect. These children cannot express anger outwardly because of the belief that they are personally at fault. Their self-esteem becomes affected as they see themselves as responsible for negative outcomes. Explanations that they are not to blame are met with ridicule. Because of the variability of symptoms, it is essential for teachers and the school nurse to observe for behavior changes in students over time and to communicate those changes to one another and to the family.

Dysthymic disorder is considered a "gateway" disorder because of its relatively early onset and increased risk of subsequent affective disorders (Masi, Favilla, Mucci, Poli, & Romano, 2001).

Major Depressive Disorder

Major depressive disorder can occur as a single episode or as a chronic recurrent condition. To qualify for this diagnosis, there cannot have been a previous manic episode and the person must have a depressed mood for most of almost every day during a 2-week period (APA, 2000). The symptoms of depression include sadness, irritability, decreased interest in activities that previously gave pleasure, eating changes resulting in weight loss or gain, insomnia or hypersomnia, decreased concentration, feeling worthless or guilty, and recurrent thoughts of death. More than 90% of young people who commit suicide have a psychiatric disorder, most of which were mood disorders. Twenty-five percent to fifty percent of patients attempt suicide, and as many as 40% of manic episodes may be characterized by overt acts of physical violence (Mohr, 2001). In addition, comorbid anxiety is very common (Weller et al., 2004b). However, 15% have atypical symptoms.

Preschoolers do not have the ability to express feelings of sadness in language. Overt behavior,

(text continues on page 794)

Table 34.1 ■

PSYCHOTROPIC MEDICATIONS GIVEN TO CHILDREN AND ADOLESCENTS*

Selective Serotonin Reuptake Inhibitors	Side Effects
Fluoxetine (Prozac) Paroxetine (Paxil) Sertraline (Zoloft) Fluvoxamine (Luvox) Citalopram (Celexa) Escitalopram oxalate (Lexapro)	Nausea, weight loss, Anxious/nervous, Insomnia or sedation, Diaphoresis
[MOST EFFECTIVE CLASS FOR ANXIETY AND MOOD DISORDERS] [MOST NOT APPROVED FOR CHILDREN] [CAUTION: MUST BE OBSERVED CLOSELY FOR CLINICAL WORSENING, SUICIDALITY, OR UNUSUAL CHANGES IN BEHAVIOR. MUST BE SEEN WEEKLY BY PROVIDER FOR FIRST 4 WEEKS OF TREATMENT AND THEN EVERY OTHER WEEK DUE TO INCREASED RISK OF TEEN SUICIDE]	
Tricyclic Antidepressants	
Imipramine (Tofranil) Nortripyline (Pamelor) Desipramine (Norpramin) Amitriptyline (Elavil) Clomipramine (Anafranil) Doxepin (Sinequan)	Fatigue, constipation, Dry mouth, blurred vision, Orthostatic hypotension, Risk of seizures
[CATEGORY NO LONGER RECOMMENDED DUE TO CHANCE OF SUDDEN CARDIAC ARREST]	
Anticonvulsants (See Chapter 37)	
Psychostimulants (See Chapter 30)	
Others	
Bupropion (Wellbutrin)	[safety in children is not established] Irritability, insomnia, risk of seizures
Clonidine (Catapres) Guanfacine (Tenex)	Fatigue, sedation, hypotension, dry mouth, depression
Lithium	Monitor renal, thyroid, calcium/phosphorus indices May affect cognitive abilities
Risperidone (Risperdal)	Sedation, headache, agitation, weight gain, sweating, tachycardia
Olanzapine (Zyprexa)	Weight gain, somnolence, dizziness, headache, agitation, hostility
Quetiapine (Seroquel)	Dizziness, headache, somnolence, hypotension, tachycardia
Ziprasidone (Geodon)	Somnolence, dizziness, agitation, hypothermia
Venlafaxine (Effexor) Nefazodone (Serzone)	May worsen depression and increase risk for suicide at start of medication therapy
Alprazolam (Xanax)	Drowsiness, lightheadedness, dry mouth
Hydroxyzine (Atarax)	Anxious, decreased cognitive function, depressed
Clonazepam (Klonopin)	Drowsy, ataxia, behavior changes
Buspirone (BuSpar)	Dizzy, drowsy, nausea, headache, insomnia

*No psychotropic medications exist for learning disabilities, mental retardation, or autism.
Sources: Biederman, Spencer, & Wilens (2004); Findling et al., (2002); Kline & Silver (2004); Trigoboff (2005); Weller et al. (2004a).

apathy, withdrawal from caregivers, regression of developmental milestones, and nonorganic failure to thrive are among the symptoms that must be observed for a diagnosis to be made (Son & Kirchner, 2000).

Bipolar Disorder

Bipolar disorder was previously called manic–depressive disorder. In this condition, the symptoms of depression are interspersed with mania, as evidenced by anger or rage. This range of behaviors "from depression to euphoria to normal to anger" can occur within the same day (Jones, 2004, p. 198). Characteristics of the manic phase include inflated self-esteem, sleeping less than 3 hours per night, talkativeness with a pressured speech that is difficult to interrupt, being easily distracted, and feeling as if one's thoughts are racing. In young children, a hallmark of childhood mania is intense rage; children may exhibit seemingly unprovoked rage episodes that can last up to 2 to 3 hours and the child or adolescent may be misdiagnosed as having a conduct disorder. Symptoms may resemble those of the hyperactive/impulsive child with attention deficit hyperactivity disorder (ADHD).

Suicide Ideation and Attempts

Suicide is rare in childhood and early adolescence, and becomes more frequent with advancing age. However, suicide remains the third leading cause of death among Americans between 10 and 19 years of age, resulting in 4,243 deaths (Centers for Disease Control and Prevention [CDC], 2004b). "Clear-cut suicides in children younger than age 10 years have almost always been labeled accidental deaths" because of the myth that children are not depressed and would not intentionally kill themselves (Weller et al., 2004a, p. 417). The mean worldwide annual rates of suicide per 100,000 were 0.5 for females and 0.9 for males among 5- to 14-year-olds, and 12.0 for females and 14.2 for males among 15- to 24-year-olds, respectively (Pelkonen & Marttunen, 2003).

The National Youth Risk Behavior Survey by the Centers for Disease Control and Prevention indicated that 16.9% of American 9th through 12th graders seriously considered suicide in 2003. This was down significantly since 1991, when 29% had indicated these thoughts. In 2003, over 16% had made a suicide plan and 8.5% had attempted suicide (CDC, 2004a). There was no significant change in these percentages over the past decade. "The most common method of suicide in this age group was by firearm (49%), followed by suffocation (mostly hanging) (38%) and poisoning (7%)" (CDC, 2004b, p. 471).

Fascination with death is a common behavior among school-age children. Suicidal behavior, however, is defined as "a preoccupation or act that intentionally aims to inflict injury or death on oneself" (Pfeffer, 2004, p. 891). Suicidal ideation involves recurrent thoughts of death, recurrent suicidal ideation without a plan, and developing a specific plan for committing suicide (Goldston, 2003). An awareness of the finality of death is not necessary for someone to be diagnosed as suicidal. However, "in assessing the level of risk, clinicians should evaluate the objective and perceived lethality of an intended suicidal act" (Pfeffer, 2004, p. 891).

Suicidal ideation has multiple causes, the most common of which is depression. "The basic etiological elements of suicidal behavior are thought to be genetic," with the focus being on the function of serotonin (Pfeffer, 2004, p. 897). A number of antidepressants have been associated with suicidal behaviors as well, especially during the initiation of treatment. Aggravating factors include the death of a parent, parental discord (family violence or divorce), drug and alcohol use, parental drinking, school failure, rejection by a peer of the opposite sex, having a family member with a mental illness, and lack of a close confiding relationship with an adult.

The school nurse is in an excellent position to recognize youth at risk for suicide. She or he needs to identify the potential suicide victim and be active in prevention. It is important that the school nurse, who may suspect depression or be the first person with whom the child or adolescent speaks, implements referral so that screening measures can be done to help identify students in need. Comments such as "I wish I was dead" or "My parents would be better off if I was dead" are red flags that mandate immediate action. Another red flag is a student who has engaged in cutting him- or herself. It is essential for the nurse to ask the student if he or she has a plan for ending his or her life and to ask if he or she has access to a weapon. If the student answers in the affirmative to either of these questions, it is essential to keep the student in the health office until the parents are contacted and the student is referred for appropriate assessment and intervention.

A great majority of youth who are contemplating suicide provide some clues or pleas for help before they make the attempt. Students who are depressed and say, "I'm at the end of my rope" or "I can't take it anymore" or indicate in some way that they are giving up hope and life is not worth living are giving clear signals that they are thinking of suicide and need help immediately! Students who have a preoccupation with self-harm or aim to inflict injury or death to themselves need help. Students who draw pictures that always show mutilation, hanging, or other such drawings that make the teacher suspicious of the intent should be further evaluated. Students may fixate on heroes or friends who have died and contemplate death on special anniversaries or significant dates. At these times, additional supervision, interventions, or precautions are warranted. The teacher can confer with the school nurse and the parents should be notified.

Although it is known that suicide is frequently a response to an inability to cope with one's problems, whether it is a cognitive distortion, a reaction to an event, or a manifestation of depression, it must be addressed before suicide is considered to be a solution to the problems. The normal impulsive behavior of adolescents can escalate into a situation in which the person who uses banned substances or who has access to firearms and believes no one can help him or her can resort to use of these as an answer to his or her difficulties.

The nurse can work with teachers to identify these students and work with the parents and other school personnel, such as the guidance counselor and the social worker, to help them, utilizing the services of the crisis team if the situation warrants it. The nurse can interact with the student, listen to what the youth identifies as stressors, and use mental health education to promote adequate coping mechanisms. The nurse's listening to the student and establishing a sense of trust can be of great advantage as the student is referred for further professional help.

More than 75 instruments have been developed to assess for suicide ideation and risk. The student will need a thorough medical and psychiatric evaluation. A number of medical disorders, such as infections and neurological and endocrine disorders, as well as medication responses and alcohol or drug abuse, can mimic depression and it is important to rule them out. The psychiatric evaluation should also be extensive and include a detailed history regarding the characteristics of the symptoms, the family and personal histories, as well as a thorough developmental history. This interview will vary according to the age and developmental status of the child. Neuropsychological testing is also an important component of the evaluation to help rule out neurological or learning disorders and assess the student's developmental capabilities.

Mental health education must be offered, either in formal or informal settings, so that all those involved in the welfare of children will be able to understand and cope with the myriad of conditions, lessen the stigma, and improve early identification and treatment. The school nurse can also hold in-service programs for teachers and other interested personnel to assist them in recognizing students at risk and the need for effective prevention and treatment. Another strategy that the nurse can use is to participate in Parent–Teacher Association meetings (PTA) and to make certain that the community is aware of the needs of the school-age population.

School-based skills training is advised to teach students about suicide and its early symptoms and encourage them to seek help if they believe they or their friends may have thoughts of suicide. The main target of effective prevention of youth suicide is to reduce suicide risk factors. A study (Sund & Wichstrom, 2002) demonstrated that insecure attachment to parents during early adolescence strongly predicts depressive symptoms a year later. It suggests the school nurse can try to help family members learn about the adolescent's feelings of rejection, improve their communication skills with their children, and express positive feelings to demonstrate caring and acceptance.

Treatment consists of a combination of interventions, including family education, family therapy, development of an Individualized Education Program (IEP), and referral to appropriate support groups. The school nurse can take an active role in many of these areas and can follow these students and make certain they receive treatment and are compliant. Individual psychotherapy may be helpful in aiding children to express their feelings and to develop coping mechanisms.

Tourette Syndrome

The prevalence of Gilles de la Tourette syndrome (TS) is higher than previously thought, and may be present in up to 2% of the population (Faridi & Suchowersky, 2003). Onset is often during the elementary school years. It is a complex condition with a variety of comorbid conditions, and affects more males than females. TS is characterized by the presence of tics (repeated, intermittent, unpredictable, and purposeless contractions of groups of muscles) that cause unintentional movements (motor tics) and unintentional sounds (phonic or vocal tics) (Table 34.2). Some occur in response to an intense urge that is relieved only by the motor activity (Evidente, 2000).

To be diagnosed with TS, a person must have both motor and vocal tics, which may be simple or complex. The tics must have been present for at least a year with no "tic-free" period greater than 3 months (APA, 2000). There is no specific test to identify TS.

At least 60% of the diagnosed cases are hereditary in nature and may be related to the obsessive–compulsive phenomenon (King & Leckman, 2004). The genes may affect the functioning of the

Table 34.2 ■
TYPES OF MOTOR AND VOCAL TICS

Motor Tics
Eyes: blinking or rolling
Facial: grimacing or contortions
Nose: twitching
Jerking of various body parts
Lips: smacking or licking
Tongue: thrusting
Hands: flexing, flailing, flapping, hitting self or others, clapping, pinching, tearing items
Foot: tapping, dragging, shaking, toe walking
Body: stooping, hopping, kicking, jumping, body slamming
Vocal Tics
Throat clearing
Grunting
Sniffing
Belching
Spitting
Snorting
Squeaking
Coughing
Humming
Whistling
Hissing
Screaming
Laughing
Barking
Moaning
Making clicking or "tsk" noises

Source: Tourette Syndrome Association (2005).

basal ganglia and the action of dopamine. The remaining cases of TS are acquired. The acquired symptoms (Tourettism) might be related to environmental, infectious, or psychological factors (Zinner, 2000). One hypothesis is that "aberrant autoimmune mechanisms triggered by group A B-streptococcal infections may produce a spectrum of disorders including tics and OCD" (King & Leckman, 2004, p. 717); this condition is referred to as "pediatric autoimmune neuropsychiatric disorders associated with streptococcal infection" or PANDAS. Tics are also a common side effect of stimulant medication prescribed for ADHD (Chapter 30); however, stimulant medications do not cause TS. Antiepileptic medications may cause tics; discontinuation of the offending drugs leads to an immediate remission of the symptoms (Evidente, 2000).

Symptoms of TS fall into a continuum from barely noticeable to blatant and debilitating. Those afflicted may tic only when they are anxious or tired or may tic as much as 30 to 100 times a minute (Murray, 1997). Students may manifest TS by multiple mannerisms (see Table 34.2). Typically, symptom exacerbations follow in the wake of stressful life-events. These events need not be adverse in character, as long as there is a high level of emotional excitement, for example, the start of school, impending holidays or birthdays, vacation, or school day-trips.

Tics have the greatest effect on a child's self-esteem and peer and family relationships from age 7 to 12 years, especially during periods of forceful motor tics and loud phonic tics that can go on for hours virtually nonstop (Leckman, 2002). There is a negative effect on peer acceptance, school performance, and self-esteem. However, tics often develop during the preschool years.

The school nurse is likely to be very involved with these students and must provide adequate support and referral. The students may come to the health office as a refuge from their peers. The nurse provides understanding and attempts to build up the self-esteem of the afflicted child. Students and their parents can be encouraged to relate their experiences, sadness, and disappointments. The experience of being understood is often reassuring (Leckman, 2002).

A number of conditions are often comorbid with TS: ADHD, OCD, anxiety and phobia disorders, learning disabilities, oppositional defiant disorder, mood disorders, conduct disorder, speech and language disorders, sleep disorders, bedwetting, bipolar disorders, self-injurious disorders, executive function disorders, personality disorders, lack of impulse control, and rage attacks (Budman, Rockmore, Stokes, & Sossin, 2003; Carter et al., 2000; Coffey et al., 2000; Zinner, 2000).

An important question to be asked in assessment of the student is the extent to which tics are interfering with the student's emotional, social, familial, and school experiences. To establish this fact, symptoms may be monitored over a few months to assess their severity and fluctuation, effect on the family, and adaptation of the student, the family, and peers to them. It is most important to clarify and address family issues.

The school nurse can assist by working with the teacher to assess school-performance problems. The student with TS needs careful evaluation of cognitive functioning and school achievement. Students with this disorder tend to have difficulties in attention, perseverance, and ability to keep their schoolwork organized. Many have poor penmanship.

Schoolwork can be interfered with by compulsions, such as the need to erase, scratch out words, or return to the beginning of a sentence (Leckman, 2002). These children are often referred by their primary healthcare provider to a specialist, such as a neurologist, who will clearly establish the diagnosis and suggest treatment.

Common treatment may involve education and reassurance, psychosocial and school interventions, and choice from an array of pharmacological agents. The clinician must decide if the tics are severe enough to warrant pharmacotherapy (Swain & Leckman, 2003).

The Tourette Syndrome Association (TSA) (see Resources) is a national, nonprofit organization that offers a variety of medical and public educational materials. They also support those afflicted with this disorder, their families, and other interested, concerned supporters.

Oppositional Defiant Disorder and Conduct Disorder

Although all children and adolescents have periods of oppositional behavior, they do learn that there are rules for different environments as well as rules for society. They may attempt to push the limits of these rules, but usually do so with the hope of not being "caught." When these behaviors become persistent without the accompanying moral development, they enter the realm of a pathological condition.

Oppositional defiant disorder (ODD) and conduct disorder (CD) are listed as two different disorders in the DSM-IV-TR; however, they may be part of the same continuum of altered behavior. Of the two, ODD is the milder.

Oppositional defiant disorder refers to a recurrent pattern of developmentally inappropriate levels of negativistic, defiant, disobedient, and hostile behavior toward authority figures. Conduct disorder is broader in its characteristics; it involves violation of the rights of others and violation of the rules of society. Research shows that youth with CD and ODD are at increased risk of delinquent behavior and problems with the legal system (Loeber et al., 2002).

For a diagnosis of ODD to be made, the behavior must persist for at least 6 months and be characterized by the frequent occurrence of at least four of the following behaviors: losing temper with adults, arguing with adults, actively defying or refusing to comply with the requests or rules of adults, deliberately doing things that will annoy other people, blaming others for his or her own mistakes or misbehavior, being touchy or easily annoyed by others, being angry or resentful, or being spiteful or vindictive (APA, 2000). The behavior must occur more frequently than developmentally expected and must interfere with normal functioning.

The symptoms include being argumentative and defiant, being easily annoyed by others, and frequently losing one's temper. Symptoms such as these can be easily identified as problematic at school age, since loss of temper is infrequent in the school setting and cooperation with rules and routines is expected and necessary. Thus, the presence of disruptive behaviors may be cause for clinical concern. During the preschool period, the distinction between normative and problematic behavior is less clear. Sophisticated verbal skills, self-awareness, motor dexterity, and goal-directed behavior begin to emerge and these factors contribute to a strong push for independence on the part of the child. At the same time, rules and limits are being applied by the parents and in some cases the school, and these simultaneous processes contribute to frequent clashes between the child's self-assertions and the limit setting, leading to frequent episodes of frustration and upset. Regardless of developmental stage, determination of abnormality rests on establishing that the behavior is causing "significant impairment in social…functioning" (APA, 2000, p. 102).

Conduct disorder is a pervasive disorder with clinically significant antisocial behaviors such as excessive noncompliance, aggression, stealing, lying, truancy, violence, destructiveness, cruelty, and sexually coercive behavior (APA, 2000). The behavioral characteristics of CD include aggression to people and animals (bullies and threatens others; initiates physical fights, uses weapons, is physically cruel to people and animals, steals, and rapes); destruction of property (destroyed property and intentional fire setting); deceitfulness or theft (breaks into cars or houses, lies and steals); and serious violations of rules (runs away from home, truant from school, stays out all night despite parental rules) (APA, 2000). At least three of these criteria must have occurred within the past year.

Many of the students with ODD and CD are in school settings and yet most receive ineffectual or no treatment, despite their behavior (Markward & Bride, 2001). A study was done on a large group of students with ODD in order to understand the diagnosis independent of its association with conduct disorder. It was found that oppositional defiant youth with or without conduct disorder had significantly higher rates of comorbid psychiatric disorders and significantly higher family and social dysfunction relative to psychiatric comparison subjects (Greene et al., 2002). The families had poorer cohesion and a high degree of conflict. The youth were significantly impacted in the area of social functioning with school, parents, siblings, and peers.

The causes of these conditions appear to be multifactorial. While there is a 50% genetic impact, environment, especially parenting, also affect the manifestations (Ostrander, 2004). Poor parental monitoring occurs in many cases; many of the parents are unaware of their child's actions. In addition to these factors, there is a high degree of comorbidity between CD and ODD and other mental health conditions, especially ADHD and substance abuse.

Some students may misbehave in response to what is happening in their home environment. It is therefore important to assess what is going on in the student's home and neighborhood, as well as reviewing parenting skills, before a student is referred.

Because of the multiple etiologies and symptomatology, family-centered, comprehensive interventions are needed. The school nurse can work with the school social worker, counselor, and other supportive personnel to develop family-centered programs and services found to be effective in preventing problems in the school setting (Markward & Kurtz, 1999). Some students are placed in alternative classrooms with small teacher-to-student ratios and structured settings. Students should be given positive reinforcement whenever possible. Parents should be taught to monitor their children; physical punishment should be avoided and misbehaviors should be ignored, if possible, or rewards should be withdrawn (Ostrander, 2004). These students need to know what the specific expectations are. They need to be trained in social skills and should be encouraged to feel that they are part of a community.

Outcomes are poor, as there is a strong connection between adolescent conduct problems and later mental health and social problems (Fergusson & Woodward, 2000). Conduct disorder is very difficult to treat and even intensive treatment has been unsuccessful. School can be influential during adolescence as programs motivate teenagers to learn and achieve educational goals and thereby increase their self-esteem. Teachers and school personnel, particularly the nurse, can help by giving the student support that may be lacking at home.

The school nurse, working with families and youth can use nursing skills: to establish a sense of trust; work with families on parenting methods, discipline, and the need to learn how to resolve impasses, manage their feelings, and reconnect with each other; make it easier for students to explain their feelings; and refer these students as necessary.

The school nurse can provide support when these students present to the health office, especially with a somatic complaint; the school nurse can model adult behavior and assist in establishing a sense of trust. The nurse is in a unique position to develop a partnership with the young person and the family and to promote good health, good parenting, and prevention, all interventions that have been found helpful in preventing future difficulties.

Some of these students engage in serious offenses that result in police involvement. Once engaged in the juvenile justice system, adolescents and their parents have not been very successful in extracting themselves from the continuing cycles of probation and incarceration of the adolescent (Woolfenden, Williams, & Peat, 2002).

Eating Disorders

Eating disorders are common in all ages, although they are usually associated with adolescents. Eating disorders include eating too much, which leads to obesity (Chapter 36), refusing food, restricting foods either by choice (e.g., vegetarian) or for some physiological reason, eating nonfood items (e.g., Pica), eliminating foods already eaten, or having objectionable mealtime behaviors. When eating disorders continue for a period of time, they can cause significant health concerns.

In young children younger than age 6, feeding disorders are manifested by persistent failure to eat adequately with significant failure to gain weight or significant loss of weight over at least one month; not due to an associated gastrointestinal or other general medical condition (e.g., esophageal reflux); and not better accounted for by another mental disorder or by a lack of available food (APA, 2000). Common in the preschool and early school-age population, they may present as food aversions to specific foods or to foods based on their texture, smell, or taste (Chatoor, 2004).

School nurses should work together with staff to identify these students. Their weights can be assessed periodically; behavioral interventions can be developed for tantrums or other behavioral issues that may arise regarding food; and they can also be assessed to determine if their aversion might be related to food allergies presenting as uncomfortable gastrointestinal symptoms (Chapter 28). Many early education teachers have a policy of "just try it." If a child gags or vomits after eating a particular food, it is recommended that the food not be given again for a while. Other interventions include presenting the food in a different form (cooked vs. raw; frozen vs. warm); ensuring that foods are only offered one at a time and not touching one another; and modeling eating the food by faculty and staff and by other students, since children and youth often want to do what their peers do. Regardless of what is eaten, the school nurse should work with the family to ensure that the student obtains his or her needed nutrients, either through the foods or food supplements.

Something is an eating disorder when the behavior or thoughts about eating and one's body interfere with one's life or if eating fills an emotional need rather than a physical one. However, when most professionals speak of eating disorders, they are usually referring to anorexia nervosa (AN) and bulimia nervosa (BN). There are some who view these conditions as being on a continuum and others who view them as two separate but overlapping conditions. Regardless, they can both be life-threatening (Cummings et al., 2001).

Anorexia nervosa involves extreme weight loss (or failure to grow as expected and weighing less than 85% of the expected normal weight), intense fear of becoming fat or gaining weight, body-image distortions, denial of the seriousness of the student's current low body weight, loss of menstruation, and refusal to eat sufficiently to maintain a normal body weight for one's age (APA, 2000). There are two types of AN: restricting and binge-eating/purging. While those in the restricting group will severely limit their food intake and increase their exercise, the binge/purge group will engage in these activities plus attempt to eliminate the food they have eaten, either by inducing vomiting after eating, or using laxatives, enemas, diuretics, or diet pills (Herzog, Beresin, & Charat, 2004).

Bulimia nervosa is characterized by frequent, recurrent episodes of binge eating (defined as eating more than most people would in a 2-hour period) followed by compensatory behavior to avoid weight gain, such as self-induced vomiting and use of laxatives or diuretics (APA, 2000). Those who engage in these binge–purge cycles feel as though they have no control over their eating during the episodes. The diagnostic criteria specify that the behavior should occur approximately two times a week for a 3-month period (APA, 2000). Some believe that BN is the progression or sequela of AN.

There is no known single etiological factor causing these eating disorders; generally they are considered to be the result of a combination of biological (genetic and neurochemical), developmental, cultural, personality, psychological, family, and environmental factors (Johnson, Cohen, Kasen and Brook, 2002; Linscheid & Butz, 2003). During the past 30 years, there has been intense pressure on young women and girls to accept the cultural norm of thinness as the key to success, health, and happiness (Packard & Krogstrand, 2002). Some females misinterpret the normal changes that occur during puberty as a negative body change that requires dieting (McCarthy, 2000). For many, this is when the problem begins. Although overweight is more acceptable in males, there appears to be growing influence in the media on male physique and size. Some postulate that this will follow the trends seen in females.

Dieting behavior is often a precursor to eating disorders; "by age 13, 80% of North American girls and 10% of North American boys have already begun a weight-loss program" (Thoburn & Hammond-Meyer, 2004, p. 143). Attempts at dieting and extreme exercise may cause girls to develop problems such as body image disturbance, eating disorders, nutritional inadequacies, medical and emotional problems, and the inappropriate use of medications (Packard & Krogstrand, 2002; Smolak, Levine, & Thompson, 2001; Stewart, Carter, Drinkwater, Hainsworth, & Fairburn, 2001).

There is a positive correlation between eating disorders and families that emphasize achievement, beauty, and appearance. There is also a higher rate of reported sexual abuse in females with eating disorders, especially BN (Linscheid & Butz, 2003; Thoburn & Hammond-Meyer, 2004). Still others have unreasonable fears of choking or vomiting or of eating contaminated or unhealthy food (Robin, 2003).

Once limited to adolescents and young adult females, AN and BN are now also seen in males and in younger children, although they still occur primarily in adolescent females. Ninety to 95% of those affected are female, although among prepubertal children the ratio is closer to 3:1 female to male (Sigman, 2003). The age at onset is thought to be from age 8 to the mid 30s with one peak at ages 13 to 14 and another at ages 17 to 18 (Herzog et al., 2004). There is an increased incidence in ballet dancers, gymnasts, ice skaters, and models. Both male and female long-distance runners and male wrestlers also have a higher incidence of eating disorders, perhaps because all of these activities focus on body size. Approximately 20% of males with eating disorders are homosexual (Robb & Dadson, 2002).

The incidence of AN ranges from 0.48% to 3.7% whereas the incidence of BN is 0.7% to 2.5% (Linscheid & Butz, 2003; Robin, 2003). "However, 4%-6% of the general population is diagnosed with an atypical eating disorder – that is, one that does not meet all criteria for a diagnosis of Anorexia or Bulimia but has most of the features" (Thoburn & Hammond-Meyer, 2004, p. 143).

Eating disorders result in short-term symptoms and long-term medical complications. Adolescents with eating disorders have been found to suffer from cold intolerance, growth retardation, peak bone mass reduction, pubertal delay or interruption, hair loss, dry skin, structural abnormalities of the brain, cardiac dysfunction due to electrolyte disturbances, hypokalemia, peripheral edema, reappearance of lanugo, esophageal tear, orthostatic blood pressure changes, dizziness, gastrointestinal difficulties (abdominal discomfort, bloating, and constipation), and endocrine conditions resulting from the body's adaptive response to malnutrition (Herzog et al., 2004; Levine, 2002). Because of the impact of starvation on the cardiovascular system, lethargy should warrant an evaluation by the school nurse with a possible referral.

Those who engage in vomiting often have a sore throat and damage to their teeth, loss of enamel, and increased tooth decay (McCarthy, 2000). The fingers used in inducing vomiting may also be irritated. There is a 5.9% to 15% mortality rate for those with AN and BN (Powers & Santana, 2002; Thoburn & Hammond-Meyer, 2004). Herzog et al. (2004, p. 684) state that the mortality rate "is more than 12 times as high as that expected for young women in the general population." When the problem becomes serious enough, hospitalization, usually in a psychiatric facility, may be needed.

Psychologically, students with AN or BN may feel guilty or feel ashamed about eating; they may deny hunger and state they feel full, even after eating just a small amount. They may avoid eating with others and when they do, they may play with their food by moving it around on the plate and ultimately throw it out (Sigman, 2003). Seeing a student make frequent trips to the bathroom after eating should raise "red flags" for the school nurse. These students have a distorted body image and often have poor self-esteem. They may be perfectionists and overachievers who are strong willed.

Manley and Leichner (2003) stated that adolescents struggling against anorexia nervosa or bulimia nervosa often experience self-punishing thoughts and behaviors, including self-mutilation and suicide ideation and attempts. These arise out of profound anguish and despair frequently experienced by these young people. Empathic listening and the development of a strong alliance with the adolescent are initial steps in stemming these conditions. The nurse is also in a position to act as a role model whom the student knows he or she can come to in times of need, and convey an atmosphere of trust.

The school nurse can assess the quality and quantity of food eaten in the school setting by a student by choosing to join a table that includes the identified student during lunch. Thus, the nurse can identify the eating pattern of the student and model appropriate eating behaviors.

Prevention and intervention programs for maladaptive eating behaviors and eating disorders should be implemented early and continue throughout the teen-age years; they need to encompass a holistic view of the individual. School nurses can work with the multidisciplinary team to develop programs that will assist students to understand and cope with the challenges of puberty. They also can assist in enhancing the students' self-esteem as they change their physical appearance. The nurse, along with the school social worker, psychologist, and perhaps the guidance counselor can be actively involved in setting up these programs and encourage the students to take the lead in obtaining speakers and facilitators.

The nurse can ensure that school-based health education incorporates the needs of young women who are at risk for AN and BN. Education programs can stress the benefits of nutritional intake; the concept of a basal metabolic rate and what is needed for the basic functioning of the body; the normal physiological changes that occur during puberty, the rationale for these changes, and the concept that additional nutrition is needed to accommodate the increased body growth; and the beauty of diversity in bodies. Emphasize body functioning rather than esthetics; represent all sizes of students when using images or pictures to demonstrate a point. Above all, ensure that students are protected from teasing because of their body size. This "no tolerance" rule must apply to staff as well. Anorexia and bulimia are not due to a failure on the part of the student or the family (Thoburn & Hammond-Meyer, 2004).

Children should be taught early about body image and the need for healthy eating and exercise. Foods should not be categorized as good or bad. School nurses can work with teachers, students, and parents regarding the need for mutual respect, especially related to body size and shape. They can help select, develop, or implement curricula that include information on societal expectations, body changes at different times, and sociocultural factors that influence responses to these changes. School nurses can also work with the community to institute programs that address this problem. They can be role models by adhering to a healthy diet, being nonjudgmental, and allowing students to share their thoughts and feelings freely.

Sports personnel must also be part of the team to ensure that proper nutrition is mandated for all participants before and after sports activities. They may actually be the first to identify the problem student. They are ideal role models to provide sports participants with accurate information about the relationship of body composition and performance. Sports personnel can deemphasize weight issues and focus on performance areas in which the athlete can work on improving, such as strength.

Those with AN and BN are often resistant to treatment that focuses on weight gain. Psychotherapy is usually helpful. While many interventions are available, none has been proven to be most effective (Herzog et al., 2004). Family involvement, which may include family counseling, is recommended. The goal is to change students' thoughts, feelings, and behaviors, so that ultimately they gain weight. Psychotherapeutic agents may be prescribed for the student with comorbidity, such as depression.

Confrontations related to eating are nonproductive and only lead to power struggles. The affected students must be assisted "in establishing internal locus of control by giving real choices, mediating student attributions toward internal control, providing opportunities for success, and recognizing and attributing success to the student's hard work" (Thoburn & Hammond-Meyer, 2004, p. 161).

The prognosis is variable. "Only one-third of individuals with anorexia are likely to resume normal eating 4-8 years following diagnosis, 36% may continue to suffer severe eating disturbances beyond 11 years, and another 11% will die during that time from factors related to dysfunctional eating" (Thoburn & Hammond-Meyer, 2004, p. 143).

The Autistic Spectrum/Pervasive Developmental Disorders

The psychiatric category of pervasive developmental disorders is a continuum that spans from the subcategories of autism (or autistic disorder), childhood disintegrative disorder, Rett disorder, and Asperger syndrome, to pervasive developmental disorders not otherwise specified. It is commonly referred to as the autistic spectrum. The symptoms are similar but occur at different times during childhood and to varying degrees; they are all listed under the DSM-IV category of Communication Disorders (APA, 2000).

Autism affects 5/10,000 individuals but pervasive developmental disorders are estimated to affect 11/10,000 (APA, 2000; Hagin, 2004). It is three to four times more prevalent in males but differences no longer exist by socioeconomic, racial, cultural, or education backgrounds, nor are there specific risk factors (Hudson & Dixon, 2003; Simpson, 2005). As the breadth of these conditions was recognized, the number of milder cases diagnosed increased 200% between 1991 and 1997 (Hagin, 2004). Some believe the prevalence is as high as one in every 750 children (Lovaas & Smith, 2003) and even 3.4/1000 (Yeargin-Allsop et al., 2003) and one in every 200 (Sheehan, 2004).

Pervasive developmental disorders (PDDs) are a group of conditions characterized by severe and pervasive impairment in reciprocal social interaction and communication skills, as well as restricted and repetitive behaviors (Koenig and Scahill, 2001). Cognitive and motor delays may accompany these conditions.

The **communication deficits** for autistic disorder include at least one of the following:

- A delay in or lack of development of spoken language (without having a compensatory mode of communication)
- Among those who can speak, difficulty initiating or sustaining a conversation with others
- Repeating words or phrases (echolalia)
- Lacking spontaneous make-believe play or social imitative play that is appropriate for age (APA, 2000).

It is estimated that 28% are mute and 35% to 40% fail to develop a functional language they can use in communication (Campbell, Morgan, & Jackson, 2004). Some are able to use language to express their needs and wishes but do "not engage in a reciprocal conversation" (Lovaas & Smith, 2003, p. 325). In Asperger's disorder, there is no delay in the development of language, but there is difficulty in social interactions, especially involving nonverbal communication.

Impaired social interaction in autism is manifested by at least two of the following:

- Difficulty in the use of nonverbal behaviors with others (e.g., eye-to-eye contact, facial expressions, body postures, and gestures)
- Failure to develop developmentally appropriate peer relationships
- A lack of spontaneously sharing of ideas and items of interest with others
- A lack of social or emotional reciprocity (APA, 2000).

Students' inability to communicate and interact with others results in the fact that they "refuse physical affection, avoid eye contact, wander away from caregivers in public, and make little effort to share enjoyment" (Lovaas & Smith, 2003, p. 325).

This impaired responsiveness to others may also present as an inconsistency in their response to other sensations. They may be hypersensitive to sounds; the ringing of the telephone or school bells may be terrifying to them (Hagin, 2004). They may also be hypersensitive to the touch of certain textures against their skin; this may also cause behaviors that approximate severe agitation.

The third of the characteristics most common to autism includes **behaviors that are narrow in their focus and repetitive**. These may include preoccupation with an interest that is abnormal either in its intensity or focus; having rigid routines and rituals and being inflexible to change, including the placement of furniture; demonstrating repetitive motor mannerisms, most notably hand or finger flapping; or being preoccupied by parts of objects (APA, 2000). Affected children may be preoccupied by items that involve circular movement, such as fans or wheeled toys. Attempts at "interrupting these behaviors or making requests may trigger tantrums or aggression" (Hagin, 2003, p. 325). Tolerance for monotony is a typical finding and may be exhibited by the child repetitively rolling a toy car back and forth or lining toys up rather than playing imaginatively with them. The interests of these children are obsessive and limited to specific topics; rather than be interested in modes of transportation, they may fixate on bus schedules (Hagin, 2004).

Cognitive functioning is often uneven in those with autism. Sixty percent have an IQ that is below 50; 20% have an IQ between 50 and 70; and only 20% have an IQ that is in the normal range (Campbell et al., 2004). It must be noted that intelligence testing has major limitations in accurately measuring the IQ of individuals with communication deficits; therefore, interpret the results with caution. However, children with autism often have corresponding delays in developing self-care skills, such as toileting or dressing.

A number of popular movies have related the stories of individuals with autistic disorder who were savants; these individuals have exceptional talents in one limited area, such as music. mathematical calculation, or rote memory, but are significantly impaired in the other areas typical of autism. It is estimated that perhaps up to 10% of those with autism are savants (Campbell et al., 2004).

Other comorbid conditions that may be seen in individuals with autism include sleep problems, seizure activity, attention deficit hyperactivity disorder, and abnormal fears (Tsai, 2004). Their mood may be labile, with episodes of crying without explanation and being inconsolable. They may not recognize real danger, yet be terrified of inanimate objects that cannot cause them harm. Occasionally, students with autism may engage in self-injurious behaviors.

A crucial step in the assessment process is to determine which symptoms are primary and which are features of a comorbid condition (Koenig & Scahill, 2001). For a child to have the diagnosis of PDD, the social impairment must be primary, and other difficulties, such as inattention, must be secondary. For example, if impaired social relationships are secondary to inattention and impulsive behavior, a primary diagnosis of ADHD is appropriate and social problems are secondary to the child's attending to the social environment. By contrast, a child with PDD may be hyperactive and inattentive, but the social disability is more profound and not explained by the core symptoms of ADHD (Koenig & Scahill, 2001).

Because of the continuum of conditions, it is sometimes difficult to differentiate them. Autism is often the condition identified during toddlerhood; initial parental concern occurs at around 19 months and professional assistance is sought by the second birthday. It can certainly be diagnosed before the age of 3 years (Tsai, 2004). Indications for developmental evaluation include no babbling, pointing, or use of other gestures by 12 months of age, no single words by 16 months of age, no two-word spontaneous phrases by 24 months of age, and loss of previously learned language or social skills at any age. However, in retrospect, some parents relay that their child's responses to greeting and cuddling were muted in infancy (Rapin, 2001), with many reporting very early deviation in the development of nonverbal interpersonal skills, including eye contact and facial expressiveness (Robertson, Tanguay, L'Ecuyer, Sims, & Waltrip, 1999).

Rett's disorder or Rett syndrome is rare, affecting fewer than 4,000 females in the United States. Those with Rett's disorder develop normally for the first 5 months of life and then begin to lose motor, social, and prelanguage skills. Those with childhood disintegrative disorder develop normally until age 2 and then experience a gradual loss of social skills, adaptive behaviors, bowel and bladder control, and some motor skills up to their 10th birthday (Hagin, 2004; Simpson, 2005).

Asperger syndrome is considered to be high-functioning autism, with the primary deficit being a lack of social awareness. Individuals have language skills, but "lack knowledge of and skills for initiating and responding in various social situations" (Myles, Gagnon, Moyer, & Trautman, 2004, p. 75). They are awkward in social situations, have difficulty understanding nonverbal cues and interpreting the facial expressions and tone of voice of others, and are socially isolated, although not socially withdrawn when in the presence of others. Cognitive abilities vary, and some children with AS have high intelligence (Gardner, 2001). They often succeed in school, but may have trouble with reading and written expression.

These children have an atypical understanding of and use of pragmatic language, behavior problems, and a restricted set of interests (Gardner, 2001). They may develop language precociously and as preschoolers may speak like "little adults" and use language that is formalistic in tone (Koenig & Scahill, 2001). Although children with AS may use language precociously, their comprehension of complex language is not commensurate with their expressive abilities. The advantage of early language skills is superseded by multiple difficulties socializing with other children.

Social reciprocity is notably impaired in Asperger syndrome. This is manifested by poor understanding of the rules for conversation and social interaction. Taking turns, sharing a focus during conversation, and listening and responding to what the other person says are skills a person with Asperger finds difficult (Klin & Volkmar, 1997). Eye contact is poor and some children with Asperger have ill-coordinated movements (Frazier, Doyle, Chiu & Coyle, 2002). Social reciprocity is further compromised by their unusual and restricted interests. They may focus obsessively on details, such as maps, weather, or historical details. In-depth information about these topics is lacking. For example, they may know a great many biographical details about a particular political figure but may not be able to describe the political positions of that figure. These peculiarities in conversation and restricted interests impede their ability to relate to peers effectively. Students with Asperger syndrome crave relationships but do not know how to establish them (Koenig & Scahill, 2001).

The etiology for pervasive developmental disorders is unknown, but it is generally accepted that the basis is organic, perhaps with a genetic connection (Tsai, 2004). There appears to be a recurrence rate for autism in subsequent siblings ranging from 3% to 7% (American Academy of Pediatrics [AAP], 2001). Many of the conditions were first described in the 1940s. With improved research techniques, it is now known that these conditions are not the result of poor parenting or of vaccines.

Early detection and intervention significantly improve outcomes, with about one-third of autistic persons achieving some degree of independent living (Prater & Zylstra, 2002). Given the growing number of preschool programs within schools, the school nurse is positioned to provide early identification of these children. The differential diagnoses include psychiatric disorders, deafness, fragile X syndrome, lead poisoning, and metabolic disorders (Prater & Zylstra, 2002). Forty percent of children with autism are identified in the school setting (Yeargin-Allsop et al., 2003).

There is no cure for the conditions within the autistic spectrum, but experts agree that the earlier a child is diagnosed and receives treatment, the more likely he or she is to lead a quality life (Howlin & Asgharian, 1999). However, because of the need to be exposed to social situations, individuals with Asperger syndrome are often not diagnosed until late childhood and early adolescence (Howlin & Asgharian, 1999).

The prognosis for those with autism is much better if they have meaningful speech before age 6 years (Campbell et al., 2004). This certainly speaks to the need for early intervention services. However, 75% "continue to function within the mental retardation range as adults, being generally unable to lead independent lives" (Campbell et al., 2004, p. 438). The long-term outcome for individuals with Asperger syndrome is generally more positive than for those with autism. For example, many individuals with Asperger syndrome go on to college and start their own families (Frazier et al., 2002).

Intervention strategies must involve a collaborative approach; they often incorporate speech, occupational, and/or physical therapy. Other important strategies may involve special education, behavioral interventions, and, on occasion, pharmacotherapy (Hudson & Dixon, 2003). One of the goals is "to alleviate troublesome symptoms so that a child with autism can profit from intensive targeted education" (Hagin, 2004, p. 68).

No single treatment is effective in all cases. Approaches include communication therapy, social skills development, behavior modification, and interventions to decrease the altered response to sensory input. Olney (2000) gives five recommendations that may be valuable to school nurses and other professionals as they plan for and work with individuals who have autism: (1) work with, rather than against interests and abilities; (2) introduce changes gradually and thoughtfully; (3) communicate clearly and directly; (4) provide appropriate feedback; and (5) plan for relaxation and physical activity.

One approach is social skills training and skill-based interventions. The skills taught relate to the specific needs of the students. Students need to have the rationale as to why a behavior is necessary; behavior modification may be useful here. Since generalization is difficult for these students, it is necessary to teach each task rather than expecting the student to transfer learned skills to different situations. Perhaps most important is providing a means for communication. This may be accomplished by using pictures. Cognitive interventions help individuals "monitor their own behaviors and performance and to ultimately reinforce appropriate responses and otherwise manage their own behavior" (Simpson, 2005, p. 127).

Interventions include the following:

- Keep the environment simple and highly structured.
- Develop predictable routines.
- Be consistent (to decrease stress between teachers and related to new activities).

- Use multimodal presentations.
- Model the desired behaviors.
- Decrease loud sounds (muffle telephones and school bells; whisper to them).
- Avoid sensory overload.
- Use realistic pictures or photographs (students with autism have difficulty integrating line drawings into complete pictures).
- Use written schedules or lists of tasks (including a homework checklist to decrease lost, incomplete, or late homework or signed forms that are needed).
- Use a graphic organizer that shows the relationship between facts and concepts (the teacher can provide outlines for the student that show these relationships).
- Develop a list of how to act in social situations.
- Use social stories to describe specific social situations (Hagin, 2004).
- Encourage peer mentoring.
- Give concrete positive reinforcement.
- Pet therapy may be effective.
- The use of computer technology may be helpful.

The school nurse knows that IDEA (Chapter 14) mandates that every student with a condition on the autistic spectrum is to receive an appropriate education, free of cost. The nurse can help parents negotiate the system by working with them to access the resources these children should receive, such as testing, placement, and appropriate interventions. Many public schools use the **T**reatment and **E**ducation of **A**utistic and related **C**ommunication handicapped **Ch**ildren (TEACCH) program developed by the Department of Psychiatry at the University of North Carolina at Chapel Hill (University of North Carolina at Chapel Hill. Division TEACCH: Treatment and Education of Autistic and related Communication handicapped Children. Available at http://www.teacch.com. The TEACCH approach focuses on building skills based on each student's particular strengths, interests, and level of functioning.

Behavior modification approaches may include both behavioral enhancement (choosing appropriate type, timing, duration, and frequency of rewards) and behavior reduction (extinction, time-out, and punishment (Campbell, Schopler, Cueva, & Hallin, 1996). Intensive behavior therapy, also known as applied behavioral analysis (ABA), had gained much attention (Pelios and Lund, 2001). Behavior therapy requires intervention during much of the child's waking hours and involves the participation of not only therapists but also parents and teachers. Here the school nurse can assist by learning some of the techniques and then reinforcing use of the interventions, especially with the parents and teachers. The school nurse can be a resource to parents.

Pharmacological intervention may be tried for some autistic students,, although none have demonstrated consistent efficacy. Medications such as stimulants, selective serotonin reuptake inhibitors (SSRIs), neuroleptics, and mood stabilizers may be used as appropriate to relieve troublesome symptoms that interfere with social and occupational functioning (Hudson & Dixon, 2003). Target symptoms may differ, depending on the patient's age. In early childhood, hyperactivity, irritability, and temper tantrums may be prominent, whereas aggressiveness and self-injurious behavior may characterize the older child. In adolescence and adulthood, particularly in high functioning patients, depression or obsessive–compulsive disorder may develop (Palfrey & Frazer, 2000).

As part of the multidisciplinary team, the nurse is in a position to educate and serve as a resource. He or she might help teachers and parents understand that due to severe communication problems, the affected child needs assistance in making his or her needs known. With members of the team, the nurse can help determine which augmentative communication system might be best for the individual, for example, sign language, a communication board, cue cards, or computer communication facilitation. The nurse can also help by relaying her concerns to team members so that the team will be aware that such things as food preferences, toileting, and drinking need to be built into the time schedule for the child.

In addition, the school nurse can assess the family's perspective and coping skills so that effective interventions will be accepted by the family. He or she can educate the parents, assist them in coping with the diagnosis, and guide them as they choose interventions and advocate for their child. The nurse as part of the team can serve as the liaison among parents, physicians, school personnel, and the community and can ensure that the student is treated with respect, is receiving good care, and is being educated so that he or she can attain optimal functioning.

Schizophrenia

Schizophrenia is a form of psychosis that results in the student having at least two of the following during a period of at least 6 months: delusions, hallucinations, disorganized speech, gross disorganization in thought processes, catatonic behavior, and a flat affect (APA, 2000). Despite the similarities between childhood-onset and adult-onset schizophrenia, a diagnosis of schizophrenia or schizoaffective disorder in children is met with resistance in the medical community (Schaeffer & Ross, 2002). The onset of schizophrenia typically occurs in the late teens or afterward, although some cases have been reported in pre-adolescent children (APA, 2000).

Students suspected of hearing voices or seeing things that do not exist need immediate referral. Drug use must be ruled out and psychiatric professionals will rule out conditions such as bipolar behaviors. Treatment may require an inpatient stay; the approach is multimodal, including psychotherapy, family therapy, and often medication.

When the student returns to the classroom, teachers need to refrain from pointing out behaviors in which the student engages, unless the student is a danger to himself or to others. Teachers should refrain from embarrassing the student in front of classmates. The student may want to sit away from the group and may become anxious if forced into a group activity. The student may need additional time to complete school work. Any unexpected behaviors need to be shared with parents. The school nurse can be an integral member of the team that evaluates students and monitors their progress.

CONCLUSION

Schools are becoming the primary site for identification and intervention for students with mental health concerns. There is growing evidence that "school mental health programs improve educational outcomes by decreasing absences, decreasing discipline referrals, and improving test scores" (DHHS, 2003, p. 62). The school nurse must assume an active role in this endeavor.

Resources

About Our Kids
http://www.aboutourkids.org

Academy of Eating Disorders
http://www.aedweb.org

American Academy of Child and Adolescent Psychiatry
http://www.aacap.org

American Academy of Pediatrics
http://www.aap.org/policy/re060018.html

American Foundation for Suicide Prevention
http://www.afsp.org

American Society for Adolescent Psychiatry
http://www.adolpsych.org

Anorexia Nervosa and Related Eating Disorders Inc.
http://www.anred.com

A.N.S.W.E.R. Adolescents Never Suicide When Everyone Responds
http://www.teenanswer.org

Association for Science in Autism Treatment
ASAT@autism-treatment.org

Autism Resources
http://www.autism-resources.com

Autism Society of America
http://www.autism-society.org

Caring for Every Child's Mental Health Campaign
http://www.mentalhealth.org/child/

CDC fact sheet on suicide
http://www.cdc.gov/ncipc/factsheets/suifacts.htm

Center for Mental Health Child Services
http://www.mentalhealth.org/cmhs/ChildrensCampaign/

Center for School Mental Health Assistance
http://csmha.umaryland.edu/csmha2001/main.php 3

Child & Adolescent Bipolar Foundation
http://www.cabf.org

The Child and Family WebGuide
http://www.cfw.tufts.edu

Depression and Bipolar Support Alliance
http://www.DBSAlliance.org

Depression and Related Affective Disorders Association
http://www.med.jhu.edu/drada

Eating Disorders Awareness and Prevention Inc.
http://www.edap.org

Eating Disorder Referral and Information Center
http://www.edreferral.com

Federation of Families for Children's Mental Health
http://www.ffcmh.org

Families for Effective Autism Treatment (FEAT)
http://www.feat.org
http://www.health.state.ny.us/nyadoh/eip/autism/index.htm

Medlineplus Mental Health
http://www.nim.nih.gov/medlineplus/mentalhealth.html

National Alliance for Autism Research
http://www.naar.org

National Alliance for the Mentally Ill
http://www.nami.org

National Alliance for the Mentally Ill
http://ocd.nami.org/youth/index.html

National Association of Anorexia Nervosa and Associated Disorders
http://www.anad.org

National Center on Education, Disability, and Juvenile Justice
http://www.edjj.org

National Institute of Mental Health
http://www.nimh.nih.gov/publicat/childmenu.cfm

NIMH fact sheet on depression
http://www.nimh.nih.gov/publicat/depchildresfact.cfm

Office of Special Education Programs (OSEP)
http://www.ed.gov/offices/OSERS/OSEP/index.html

OSEP Technical Assistance Center on Positive Behavior Interventions and Supports
http://www.pbis.org

School Mental Health Project
http://smhp.psych.ucla.edu/

SNAP (for Tourette Syndrome)
www.snapinfo.org

Special education resource site
seriweb.com

Tourette Syndrome Association
http://tsa.mgh.harvard.edu/

U.S. Department of Health and Human Services
http://www.hhs.gov

Website for depressed teenagers
http://www.depressedteens.com

References

Albano, A., March, J., & Piacentini, J. (1999). Cognitive behavioral treatment of obsessive-compulsive disorder. In R. Ammerman, M. Hersen, & C. Last (Eds.), *Handbook of prescriptive treatments for children and adolescents* (pp. 193–215). Boston, Allyn & Bacon.

American Academy of Pediatrics (AAP), Committee on Children with Disabilities. (2001). Technical report: The pediatrician's role in the diagnosis and management of autistic spectrum disorders in children. *Pediatrics, 107*(5), E85.

American Psychiatric Association (APA). (2000). *Diagnostic and statistical manual of mental disorders: 4th edition* (DSM-IV-TR). Washington, DC: American Psychiatric Association.

Asarnow, J., Jaycox, L., & Anderson M. (2002). Depression among youth in primary care: Models for delivering mental health services. *Child and Adolescent Psychiatric Clinics of North America, 11*(3), 477–497.

Bernstein, G., & Layne, A. (2004). Separation anxiety disorder and generalized anxiety disorder. In J. Wiener & M. Dulcan (Eds.), *Textbook of child and adolescent psychiatry* (pp. 557–573). Washington, DC: American Psychiatric Publishing.

Biederman, J., Spencer, T., & Wilens, T. (2004). Psychopharmacology. In J. Wiener & M. Dulcan (Eds.), *Textbook of child and adolescent psychiatry* (pp. 931–973). Washington, DC: American Psychiatric Publishing.

Birmaher, B., Brent, D., & Benson, R. S. (1998). Summary of practice parameters for the assessment and treatment of children and adolescents with depressive disorders. *Journal of the American Academy of Child and Adolescent Psychiatry, 37*(11), 1234–1238.

Budman, C. L., Rockmore, L., Stokes, J., & Sossin, M. (2003). Clinical phenomenology of episodic rage in children with Tourette syndrome. *Journal of Psychosomatic Research, 55*(1), 59–65.

Burt, S. A., Krueger, R. F., McGue, M., & Iacono, W. (2003). Parent-child conflict and the comorbidity among childhood externalizing disorders. *Archives of General Psychiatry, 60*(5), 505–513.

Campbell, J., Morgan, S., & Jackson, J. (2004). Autism spectrum disorders and mental retardation. In R. Brown (Ed.), *Handbook of pediatric psychology in school settings* (pp. 431–450). Mahwah, NJ: Laurence Erlbaum Associates.

Campbell, M., Schopler, E., Cueva, J. E., & Hallin, A. (1996). Treatment of autistic disorder. *Journal of the American Academy of Child and Adolescent Psychiatry, 35*, 134–143.

Carter, A., O'Donnell, D., Scahill, L., Schultz, R., Lechman, J., & Pauls, D. (2000). Social and emotional adjustment in children affected with Gilles de la Tourette's syndrome: Associations with ADHD and family functioning. *Journal of Child Psychology and Psychiatry, 41*, 215–223.

Centers for Disease Control and Prevention (CDC). (2004a). *National youth risk behavior survey: 2003*. Washington, DC: Department of Health and Human Services.

Centers for Disease Control and Prevention (CDC). (2004b). Methods of suicide among persons aged 10–19 years—United States, 1992–2001. *Morbidity and Mortality Weekly Reports, 53*(22), 471–474.

Chatoor, I. (2004). Feeding and eating disorders of infancy and early childhood. In J. Wiener & M. Dulcan (Eds.), *Textbook of child and adolescent psychiatry* (pp. 639–657). Washington, DC: American Psychiatric Publishing.

Coffey, B., Biederman, J., Geller, D., Spenser, T., Kim, G., Bellordre, C., Frazier, J., Cradock, K., & Magovcevic, M. (2000). Distinguishing illness severity from tic severity in children and adolescents with Tourette's disorder. *Journal of the American Academy of Child and Adolescent Psychiatry, 35*(5), 556–561.

Cohen, J. A. (2003). Treating acute posttraumatic reactions in children and adolescents. *Biological Psychiatry, 53*(9), 827–833.

Cohen, J. A., Berliner, L., & Mannarino, A. P. (2003). Psychosocial and pharmacological interventions for child crime victims. *Journal of Traumatic Stress, 16*(2), 175–186.

Csoti, M. (2003). *School phobia, panic attacks, and anxiety in children*. London: Jessica Kingsley.

Cummings, M. M., Waller, D., Johnson, C., Bradley, K., Leatherwood, D., & Guzzeta, C. (2001). Developing and implementing a comprehensive program for children and adolescents with eating disorders. *Journal of Child and Adolescent Psychiatric Nursing, 14*(4), 167–178.

DeSocio, J., & Hootman, J. (2004). Children's mental health and school success. *Journal of School Nursing, 20*(4), 189–195.

Dierker, L. C., Albano, A. M., Clarke, G. N., Heimberg, R. G., Kendall, P. C., Merikangas, K. R., Lewisohn, P. M., Offord, D. R., Kessler, P. C., & Kupfer, D. J. (2001). Screening for anxiety and depression in early adolescence. *Journal of the American Academy of Child and Adolescent Psychiatry, 40*, 929–936.

Diler, R. S. (2003). Panic disorder in children and adolescents. *Yonsei Medical Journal, 44*(1), 174–179.

Donnelly, C. L. (2003). Pharmacologic treatment approaches for children and adolescents with posttraumatic stress disorder. *Child and Adolescent Clinics of North America, 12*, 251–269.

Education for All Handicapped Children Act (1975). U.S. Public Law 94–142. Washington, DC.

Emslie, G. J., Mayes, T. L., Laptook, R. S., & Batt, M. (2003). Predictors of response to treatment in children and adolescents with mood disorders. *Psychiatric Clinics of North America, 26*(2), 435–456.

Evidente, V. (2000). Is it a tic or Tourette's? *Postgraduate Medicine, 108*(5), 175–182.

Family Educational Rights and Privacy Act (FERPA) (1974). Washington, DC: U.S. Department of Education.

Faridi, K., & Suchowersky, O. (2003). Gilles de la Tourette's syndrome. *Canadian Journal of Neuroscience, 30* (Suppl. 1), S64–S71.

Fergusson, D. M., & Woodward, L. J. (2000). Education, psychosocial, and sexual outcomes of girls with conduct problems in early adolescence. *Journal of Child Psychology and Psychiatry, 41*(6), 779–792.

Findling, R., Feeny, N., Stansbrey, R., DelPorto-Beditam, D., & Demeter, C. (2002). Somatic treatment for depressive illnesses in children and adolescents. *Child and Adolescent Psychiatric Clinics of North America, 11*(3), 555–578.

Frazier, J., Doyle, R., Chiu, S. & Coyle, J. (2002). Treating a child with Asperger's disorder and comorbid bipolar disorder. *American Journal of Psychiatry, 159*(1), 13–21.

Gardner, M. R. (2001). Understanding and caring for the child with Asperger syndrome. *Journal of School Nursing, 17*(4), 178–184.

Goldston, D. (2003). *Measuring suicidal behavior and risk in children and adolescents*. Washington, DC: American Psychological Association.

Goodman, S. N., Schwab-Stone, M., Lahey, B., Shaffer, D., & Jensen, P. S. (2000). Major depression and dysthymia in children and adolescents: Discriminant validity and differential consequences in a community study. *Journal of the American Academy of Child and Adolescent Psychiatry, 36*(6), 761–770.

Greene, R. W., Biederman, J., Zerwas, S., Monuteaux, M. C. Goring, J. C., & Faraone, S. V. (2002). Psychiatric comorbidity, family dysfunction, and social impairment in referred youth with oppositional defiant disorder. *American Journal of Psychiatry, 157*(7), 1214–1224.

Hagin, R. (2004). Autism and other severe pervasive developmental disorders. In F. Kline & L. Silver (Eds.), *The educator's guide to mental health issues in the classroom* (pp. 55–73). Baltimore: Paul H. Brookes.

Harrison, T. W. (2003). Adolescent homosexuality and concerns regarding disclosure. *Journal of School Health, 73*(3), 107–112.

Hauenstein, E. J. (2003). Depression in adolescence. *Journal of Obstetrical and Gynecological Neonatal Nursing, 32*(2), 239–248.

Herzog, D., Beresin, E., & Charat, V. (2004). Anorexia nervosa. In J. Wiener & M. Ulcan (Eds.), *Textbook of child and adolescent psychiatry* (pp. 671–689). Washington, DC: American Psychiatric Publishing.

Howlin, P., & Asgharian, A. (1999). The diagnosis of autism and Asperger syndrome: Findings from a survey of 770 families. *Developmental Medicine and Child Neurology, 41*, 834–839.

Hudson, G. T., & Dixon, D. (2003). Autism: Challenges in diagnosis and reatment. *Clinical Reviews, 13*(7), 46–51.

Individuals with Disabilities Education Act (1990). 20 U.S.C.A. No. 14 et seq., Washington, DC.

Jellinek, M. S., & Murphy, J. M. (1978). Screening for psychosocial disorders in pediatric practice. *American Journal of Diseases in Children, 112*, 1153–1157.

Johnson, J. G., Cohen, P., Kasen, S., & Brook, J. S. (2002). Childhood adversities associated with risk for eating disorders or weight problems during adolescence or early adulthood. *American Journal of Psychiatry, 159*, 394–400.

Johnson, J. G., Cohen, P., Pine, D. S., Klein, D., Kasen, S., & Brook, J. (2000). Association between cigarette smoking and anxiety disorders during adolescence and young adulthood. *Journal of the American Medical Association, 284*, 2348–2351.

Jones, J. (2004). Mood Disorders. In F. Kline & L. Silver (Eds.), *The educator's guide to mental health issues in the classroom* (pp. 193–209). Baltimore: Paul H. Brookes.

Jones, D., Dodge, K. A., Foster, E. M., & Nix, R. (2002). Early identification of children at risk for costly mental health service use. *Prevention Science, 3*(4), 247–256.

Kendall, P., Aschenbrand, S., & Hudson, J. (2003). Child-focused treatment of anxiety. In A. Kazdin & J. Weisz (Eds.), *Evidence-based psychotherapies for children and adolescents* (pp. 81–119). New York: The Guilford Press.

King, R., & Leckman, J. (2004). Tic disorders. In J. Wiener & M. Dulcan (Eds.), *Textbook of child and adolescent psychiatry* (pp. 709–726). Washington, DC: American Psychiatric Publishing.

Klin, A., & Volkmar, A. (1997). Asperger's syndrome. In D. Cohen & F. Volkmar (Eds.), *Handbook of autism and pervasive developmental disorders* (2nd ed., pp. 94–122). New York: John Wiley & Sons.

Kline, F., & Silver, L. (2004). *The educator's guide to mental health issues in the classroom*. Baltimore: Paul H. Brookes.

Koenig, K., & Scahill, L. (2001). Assessment of children with pervasive developmental disorders. *Journal of Child and Adolescent Psychiatric Nursing, 14*(4), 159–166.

Leckman, J. F. (2002). Tourette's syndrome. *The Lancet, 360*, 1577–1586.

Levine, R. L. (2002). Endocrine aspects of eating disorders in adolescents. *Adolescent Medicine, 13* (1), 129–143.

Lewis, P., & Lippman, J. (2004). *Helping children cope with the death of a parent: A guide for the first year*. Westport, CT: Praeger.

Linscheid, T., & Butz, C. (2003). Anorexia nervosa and bulimia nervosa. In M. Roberts (Ed.), *Handbook of pediatric psychology* (pp. 636–651). New York: The Guilford Press.

Loeber, R., Farrington, D. P., Stouthamer-Loeber, M., Moffitt, T. E., Caspi, A., & Lyman, D. (2002). Male mental health problems, psychopathology, and personality traits: Key findings from the first 14 years of the Pittsburgh Youth Study. *Clinical Child and Family Psychology Review, 4* (4), 273–297.

Lonigan, C. J., Phillips, B. M., & Richey, J. A. (2003). Posttraumatic stress disorder in children: Diagnosis, assessment, and associated features. *Child and Adolescent Psychiatric Clinics of North America, 12*(2), 171194.

Lovaas, O. I., & Smith, T. (2003). Early and intensive behavioral intervention in autism. In A. Kazdin & J. Weisz (Eds.), *Evidence-based psychotherapies for children and adolescents* (pp. 325–340). New York: The Guilford Press.

Manley, R. S., & Leichner, P. (2003). Anguish and despair in adolescents with eating disorders—helping to manage suicidal ideation and impulses. *Crisis, 24*(1), 32–36.

Manuel, J. C., Shilt, J. S., Curl, W. W., Smith, J. A., Durant, R. H., Lester, L., & Sical, S. H. (2002). Coping with sports injuries: An examination of the adolescent athlete. *American Journal of Adolescent Health, 31*, 391–393.

March, J. (1999). *MASC: Multidimensional anxiety scale for children*. North Tonawanda, NY: Multi-Health Systems, Inc.

Markward, M. J., & Bride, B. (2001). Oppositional defiant disorder and the need for family-centered practice in schools. *Children and Schools, 23*, 73–83.

Markward, M. J., & Kurtz, D. (1999). Social work and the transition of youth with disabilities. In S. deFur & J. Patton (Eds.), *Transition and school-based services: Interdisciplinary perspective on enhancing the transition process* (pp. 207–230). Austin, TX: Pro-Ed.

Masi, G., Favilla, L., Mucci, M., Poli, G., & Romano, A. (2001). Depressive symptoms in children and adolescents with dysthymic disorder. *Psychopathology, 34*(1), 29–35.

McCarthy, A. (2000). *Healthy teens: Facing the challenges of young lives*. Birmingham, MI: Bridge Communications, Inc.

Mental health: A report of the Surgeon General (1999). U.S. Department of Health and Human Services, Substance Abuse and Mental Health Services Administration, Center for Mental Health Services, National Institutes of Health, National Institute of Mental Health, Rockville, MD.

Mohr, W. K. (2001). Bipolar disorder in children. *Journal of Psychosocial Nursing, 39*(3), 12–23.

Murray, J. B. (1997). Psychophysiological aspects of Tourette's syndrome. *The Journal of Psychology, 131*(6), 615–626.

Myles, B., Gagnon, E., Moyer, S., & Trautman, M. (2004). Asperger Syndrome. In F. Kline & L. Silver (Eds.), *The educator's guide to mental health issues in the classroom* (pp. 75–100). Baltimore: Paul H. Brookes.

National Association of School Nurses (NASN). (2000). *Issue brief: Mental health and illness*. Retrieved September 14, 2005 from http://www.nasn.org/briefs/mentalhealth.htm

Olney, M. F. (2000). Working with autism and other social-communication disorders. *Journal of Rehabilitation, 66*(4), 51–56.

Ostrander, R. (2004). Oppositional defiant disorder and conduct disorder. In F. Kline & L. Silver (Eds.), *The educator's guide to mental health issues in the classroom* (pp. 267–286). Baltimore: Paul H. Brookes.

Packard, P., & Krogstrand, K. S. (2002). Half of rural girls aged 8 to 17 years report weight concerns and dietary changes, with both more prevalent with increased age. *Journal of the American Dietetic Association, 102*(5), 672–677.

Palfrey, J. S., & Frazer, C. H. (2000). Determining the etiology of developmental delay in very young children: What if we had a common internationally accepted protocol?! *Journal of Pediatrics, 136*, 569–570.

Pawlak, C., Pascuel-Sanchez, T., & Rae, P. (1999). Anxiety disorders, comorbidity, and suicide attempts in adolescence: A preliminary investigation. *European Psychiatry, 14*, 132–136.

Pelios, L. V., & Lund, S. K. (2001). A selective overview of issues on classification, causation, and early intensive behavioral intervention for autism. *Behavior Modification, 25*, 678–697.

Pelkonen, M., & Marttunen, M. (2003). Child and adolescent suicide: Epidemiology, risk factors, and approaches to prevention. *Pediatric Drugs, 5*(4), 243–265.

Pfeffer, C. (2004). Suicide and suicidality. In J. Wiener & M. Dulcan (Eds.), *Textbook of child and adolescent psychiatry* (pp. 2891–2902). Washington, DC: American Psychiatric Publishing.

Piacentini, J. (1999). Cognitive behavioral therapy of childhood OCD. *Child and Adolescent Clinics of North America, 8*, 599–616.

Powers, P. & Santana, C. (2002). Childhood and adolescent anorexia nervosa. *Child and Adolescent Psychiatric Clinics of North America, 11*(2), 219–235.

Prader, C. D., & Zylstra, R. G. (2002). Autism: A medical primer. *American Family Physician, 66*(9), 1667–1674.

Rapin, I. (2001). An eight year old boy with autism. *Journal of the American Medical Association, 285*(13), 1749–1757.

Rehabilatation Act (1973). P.L. 93–112. *U.S. Statutes at Large*, Washington, DC.

Rehabilitation Act Amendments (1983). P.L. 98–221. *U.S. Statutes at Large*, Washington, DC.

Rehabilitation Act Amendments (1986). PL 99–506. Title 29, U.S.C. 701 et seq.: *U.S. Statutes at Large, 100*, 1807–1846.

Rehabilitation Act Amendments (1998). *U.S. Statutes at Large*, S. 1579. Washington, DC.

Robb, A., & Dadson, M. (2002). Eating disorders in males. *Child and Adolescent Psychiatric Clinics of North America, 11*(2), 399–418.

Robertson, J. M., Tanguay, P. E., L'Ecuyer, S., Sims, A., & Waltrip, C. (1999). Domains of social communication handicap in autism spectrum disorder. *Journal of the American Academy of Child and Adolescent Psychiatry, 38*, 738–745.

Robin, A. (2003). Behavioral family systems therapy for adolescents with anorexia nervosa. In A. Kazdin & J. Weisz (Eds.), *Evidence-based psychotherapies for children and adolescents* (pp. 358–373). New York: The Guilford Press.

Russoniello, C. V., Shalko, T. K., O'Brien, K., McGhee, S. A., Bingham-Alexander, D., & Beatley, J. (2002). Childhood posttraumatic stress disorder and efforts to cope after Hurricane Floyd. *Behavioral Medicine, 28*(2), 61–71.

Satcher, D. (2001). Address to U.S. subcommittee on children and families. *Hearing on Teen and Young Adult Suicide*, Washington, DC.

Schaeffer, J. L., & Ross, R. G. (2002). Childhood-onset schizophrenia: Premorbid and prodromal diagnostic histories. *Journal of the American Academy of Child and Adolescent Psychiatry, 41*, 538–545.

Sheehan, M. (2004). Autism. In P. Jackson Allen & J. Vessey (Eds.), *Primary care of the child with a chronic condition* (pp. 217–238). St. Louis: C. V. Mosby.

Sigman, G. (2003). Eating disorders in children and adolescents. *The Pediatric Clinics of North America, 50*(5), 1139–1177.

Silverthorn, P., & Frick, P. (1999). Developmental pathways to anti-social behavior: The delayed-onset pathways in girls. *Development and Psychopathology, 11*, 101–126.

Simpson, R. (2005). *Autism spectrum disorders: Interventions and treatment for children and youth*. Thousand Oaks, CA: Corwin Press.

Sink, C., & Igelman, C. (2004). Anxiety disorders. In F. Kline & L. Silver (Eds.), *The educator's guide to mental health issues in the classroom* (pp. 171–191). Baltimore: Paul H. Brookes.

Smolak, L., Levine, M. P., & Thompson, J. K. (2001). The use of the sociocultural attitudes towards appearance questionnaire with middle school boys and girls.

International Journal of Eating Disorders, 29, 216–233.

Son, S. E., & Kirchner, J. T. (2000). Depression in children and adolescents. *American Family Physician, 62*, 2297–2308.

Stewart, D. A., Carter, J. C., Drinkwater, J., Hainsworth, J., & Fairburn, C. G. (2001). Modification of behavior and eating attitudes in adolescent girls: A controlled study. *International Journal of Eating Disorders, 29*, 107–117.

Sund, A. M., & Wichstrom, L. (2002). Insecure attachment as a risk factor for future depressive symptoms in early adolescence. *Journal of the American Academy of Child and Adolescent Psychiatry, 41*, 1478–1485.

Swain, J. E., & Leckman, J. F. (2003). Tourette's syndrome in children. *Current Treatment Options in Neurology, 5*(4), 299–308.

Thoburn, J., & Hammond-Meyer, A. (2004). Eating disorders. In F. Kline & L. Silver. *The educator's guide to mental health issues in the classroom* (pp. 141–170). Baltimore: Paul H. Brookes.

Todd, R., & Botteron, K. (2002). Etiology and genetics of early-onset mood disorders. *Child and Adolescent Psychiatric Clinics of North America, 11*(3), 499–518.

Tourette Syndrome Association (2005). *What is Tourette syndrome?* Retrieved September 14, 2005 from www.tsa-usa.org

Trigoboff, E. (2005). *Psychiatric drug guide*. Upper Saddle River, NJ: Prentice Hall.

Tsai, L. (2004). Autistic disorder. In J. Wiener & M. Dulcan (Eds.), *Textbook of child and adolescent psychiatry* (pp. 261–315). Washington, DC: American Psychiatric Publishing.

U.S. Department of Health and Human Services (USDHHS) (1999). *Mental health: A report of the surgeon general-executive summary*. Rockville, MD: U.S. Department of Health and Human Services, Substance Abuse and Mental Health Services, National Institutes of Health, National Institute of Mental Health.

U.S. Department of Health and Human Services (USDHHS). (2003). *Achieving the promise: Transforming mental health care in America*. Rockville, MD: USDHHS Pub. No. SMA-03-3832.

U.S. Public Health Service (USPHS). (2000). Report of the Surgeon General's Conference on Children's Mental Health: A National Action Agenda. Washington, DC: Department of Health and Human Services.

Videbeck, S. (2004). *Psychiatric mental health nursing*. Philadelphia: Lippincott Williams & Wilkins.

Walsh, K. H. (2002). Welcome advances in treating youth anxiety disorders. *Contemporary Pediatrics, 9*(66), 66–85.

Weller, E. Weller, R., & Danielyan, A. (2004a). Mood disorders in prepubertal children. In J. Wiener & M. Dulcan (Eds.), *Textbook of child and adolescent psychiatry* (pp. 411–435). Washington, DC: American Psychiatric Publishing.

Weller, E., Weller, R., & Danielyan, A. (2004b). Mood disorders in adolescents. In J. Wiener & M. Dulcan (Eds.), *Textbook of child and adolescent psychiatry* (pp. 437–481). Washington, DC: American Psychiatric Publishing.

Woolfenden, S. R., Williams, K., & Peat, J. K. (2002). Family and parenting interventions for conduct disorder and delinquency: A meta-analysis of randomised controlled trials. *Archives of Diseases in Children, 86*, 251–256.

Wu. P., Hoven, C., Cohen, P., Liu, X., Moore, R. E., Tiet, Q., Okezie, N., Wicks, J., & Bird, H. R. (2002). Factors associated with use of mental health services for depression by children and adolescents. *Psychiatric Services, 52*, 189–195.

Yeargin-Allsop, M., Rice, C., Karapurkar, T., Doernberg, N., Boyle, C., & Murphy, C. (2003). Prevalence of autism in a U.S. metropolitan area. *Journal of the American Medical Association, 289*(1), 49–85.

Zinner, S. H. (2000). Tourette disorder. *Pediatrics in Review, 21*(11), 372–375.

Chapter 35

Mental Retardation

JANICE SELEKMAN ▪ MICHAEL GAMEL-McCORMICK

Chapter Outline

INTRODUCTION

People with mental retardation (MR) have experienced a long history of prejudice and discrimination. In the past, those with the symptoms of MR were seen as dangerous and, in some cases, a menace to society and thus were institutionalized and even sterilized (Beirne-Smith, Ittenbach, & Patton, 2002). Laws enacted in the 1960s and 1970s led the way to provision of more community-based services and supports for this population. Even today, society struggles to provide full inclusion for those with MR into the community and school settings (Turnbull, Turnbull, Shank, Smith, & Leal, 2002).

While MR is often referred to as a "condition," it is actually a "symptom" of hundreds of different conditions. It is a state of functioning that is multidimensional. By combining multiple conditions under one label, it becomes even more difficult to define MR.

DEFINITION OF MENTAL RETARDATION

The American Association on Mental Retardation (AAMR) defines mental retardation as "a disability characterized by significant limitations both in intellectual functioning and in adaptive behavior as expressed in conceptual, social, and practical adaptive skills. This disability originates before age 18" (AAMR, 2002, p. 13). The important components of this definition are that MR is not solely a reflection of intellectual functioning, but that it also relies heavily on one's adaptive behavior. It is a dual disability of mental ability and the ability to function in society (Graziano, 2002).

Some view the term *mental retardation* as negatively charged and neither sensitive nor politically correct (Snow, 2003; The Arc, 2003b; Turnbull et al., 2002). Use of such terms as "developmentally delayed," "cognitively impaired" or "having a cognitive deficit," "cognitively disabled," "mentally challenged," "intellectually disabled," and "learning disabled" has been proposed by advocacy groups and persons with MR themselves. None of these terms has been accepted by all professional and consumer organizations. Although MR is a component of the term "developmental disability," hearing and vision deficits, speech and orthopedic problems, and autism and pervasive developmental disorders are also part of the condition (Fisher, 2004). Therefore, developmental disability is too broad a concept for the discussions within this chapter.

Five assumptions must be considered before making a diagnosis of MR. These include the following:

1. Limitations in present functioning must be considered within the context of community environments typical of the individual's age group peers and culture.
2. Valid assessment considers cultural and linguistic diversity as well as differences in communication, sensory, motor, and behavioral factors.
3. Within an individual, limitations often coexist with strengths.
4. An important purpose of describing limitations is to develop a profile of needed supports.
5. With appropriate personalized supports over a sustained period, the life functioning of the person with MR generally will improve (AAMR, 2002, p. 13).

MEASUREMENT OF INTELLIGENCE

Intelligence is often thought to be a unitary trait on a continuum from very limited to extremely gifted. It includes one's ability to learn, reason, plan, problem solve, think abstractly, learn from experience, remember, and comprehend complex ideas (AAMR, 2002). The measurement of intelligence began in 1905 with the development of a mental test to categorize military personnel into job categories. This test was modified and became the Stanford-Binet Intelligence Scale (Beirne-Smith et al., 2002). Another test is the Wechsler Intelligence Scale and its companion instrument, the Wechsler Preschool and Primary Intelligence Scale. The purpose of the tests is "to predict likelihood for success in traditional academic settings" (Bierne-Smith et al., 2002, p. 97). These tests are thought to average a person's cognitive abilities, yet "cognitive functioning is not always uniform across all neurodevelopmental domains" (Batshaw & Shapiro, 2002, p. 293). Therefore, while the average may be "below the line," the individual may have some strengths that are, indeed, perfectly "normal." The score that is obtained from these tests is often referred to as an Intelligence Quotient (IQ).

MR should not be determined only by a score on an IQ test, for it is actually an expression of the interaction between the person with limited intellectual functioning and the environment (AAMR, 2002). Beirne-Smith et al. (2002) state that approximately half of intelligence is inherited (nature) and the other half is attributable to environmental influences (nurture). Individual functioning is multidimensional and includes intellectual ability; adaptive behavior; participation, interactions, and social roles; health; and context.

"Adaptive behavior is the collection of conceptual, social, and practical skills that have been learned by people in order to function in their everyday lives" (AAMR, 2002, p. 14). It refers to a person's "ability to meet age-appropriate standards of independence and personal responsibility" (Bierne-Smith et al., 2002, p. 108) and can be measured using the Vineland Adaptive Behavior Scales. Adaptive skills include communication, self-care, social skills, and self-direction (Fisher, 2004).

LEVELS/DEGREES OF MR

There is considerable disagreement as to how to differentiate the levels or degrees of MR. What is agreed on is that there is a continuum from mild to more severe. The traditional way to determine severity of MR is by evaluating tests that measure intelligence. While the AAMR is now recommending that the category of mild MR be eliminated, the *Diagnostic and Statistical Manual of Mental Disorders* (American Psychiatric Association [APA], 2000) still differentiates the degree of severity based on an IQ score. Because there is a variance of approximately 5 points on repeated testing, the demarcations between categories are now less clear and are indicated by a range (Batshaw & Shapiro, 2002).

Considering the average IQ score to be 100 with a standard deviation of 15 to 16 for the various tests, it is estimated that greater than two standard deviations below the mean would constitute a diagnosis of MR, or a score of less than 70. Because of the variance stated earlier, an IQ score below 65 to 75 might be considered to represent MR, depending on the other component, adaptive behaviors. Proposed levels of functioning correspond to the IQ scores. According to the APA (2000, p. 42), MR is differentiated as noted in TABLE 35.1.

Eighty-five percent of all those who have MR are in the mild category; 10% have moderate MR; 3% to 4%, severe MR; and 1% to 2%, profound MR (APA, 2000).

Table 35.1 ■
DIFFERENTIATING MENTAL RETARDATION

LEVEL	DEFINED	DESCRIPTION
Mild MR	IQ of 50–55 to approximately 70	Mental age of 9–12 years: able to work and contribute to society; able to maintain good social relationships; experiences learning difficulties in school.
Moderate MR	IQ of 35–40 to 50–55	Mental age of 6–9 years: can achieve some degree of independence in self-care; acquires simple academic skills (add/subtract up to 10; read easy readers); achieves adequate communication skills; needs varying degrees of support after completing school.
Severe MR	IQ of 20–25 to 35–40	Mental age of 3–6 years: requires continuous support but can learn simple skills.
Profound MR	IQ below 20–25	Mental age below 3 years: severe limitations in self-care, communication, and mobility (APA, 2000; World Health Organization, 1993)

Source: American Association on Mental Retardation (2004).

Caution must be taken, however, when equating the classification of MR to a particular age level. While a teenager with moderate MR might be considered to have a mental age of 6 to 9 years, this does not mean that the teen cannot remember tasks, routines, or discrete knowledge that a 15- or even a 20-year-old would typically be capable of (Graziano, 2002; Turnbull et al., 2002). The mental age refers only to the intelligence test score. It does not describe the level and nature of the person's experience and functioning in aspects of community life (The Arc, 2003b). Physical development, including sexual development, may or may not proceed as is typical for the chronological age.

Other approaches to determine the cognitive level of a student with MR are based on the amount and patterns of support needed by the individual to accomplish typical daily tasks such as communicating, caring for oneself, and interacting socially. These approaches to estimating cognitive levels are much more subjective than the traditional approach of using intelligence assessment data.

ETIOLOGY

There are multiple causes of MR. More than one-third of all causes are genetic or chromosomal in origin; over 750 genetic etiologies have been identified that result in MR (Dykens, Hodapp, & Finucane, 2000). These conditions may be caused by trisomies due to faulty cell division (nondisjunction) at meiosis, translocation of genes, single gene transmission, gene deletions and breakages, or other anomalies (TABLE 35.2).

Inborn errors of metabolism are another major cause of MR. These involve flaws in genes or enzymes that assist in the degradation of products; brain damage can result if these enzymes are malfunctioning or not present or if the genes are faulty (Batshaw & Shapiro, 2002). In some, such as phenylketonuria (PKU), the MR can be prevented once a diagnosis is made, whereas in others, nothing can be done to prevent the neurological decay, such as in Tay-Sachs disease.

Another set of etiologies involves the perinatal experience. Maternal behaviors during the pregnancy, such as drug, alcohol, and tobacco use; maternal infections during pregnancy, such as rubella, cytomegalovirus, or toxoplasmosis; maternal malnutrition; and lack of prenatal care resulting in delayed interventions for placental damage, hemorrhage, or hypertension and premature birth are all high-risk factors for the development of MR in the child. Intraventricular hemorrhage, common in premature and low-birth-weight infants, and hypoxia during the perinatal period can lead to brain damage and MR, as can untreated hyper-

Table 35.2 ■

SELECTED CAUSES OF MENTAL RETARDATION (IN ADDITION TO THOSE COVERED IN THE CHAPTER)

Genetic and Chromosomal Conditions

- Angelman syndrome—Same gene as Prader-Willi (15q11–q13), but passed by mother. Understands more than can express; generally happy disposition with bouts of inappropriate laughter
- Cri Du Chat syndrome—High pitched cat-like cry; growth retardation; hyperteliorism; downward slanting eyelids; lag in speech/language; moderate MR
- Klinefelter syndrome—47 chromosomes (extra chromosome on the 23rd pair) XXY; only in males. Gonadal dysgenesis; sterile; small testes; no secondary sex characteristics; gynecomastia due to presence of estrogen; very tall, slim, with long limbs; mild to moderate MR or learning disabilities
- Tay-Sachs—Inborn error of metabolism (IEM) for lipids/fats resulting in the development of both physical and mental retardation, blindness, and seizures; often dead by age 4.
- Phenylketonuria (PKU)—IEM for amino acids that prevents body from metabolizing phenylalanine
- Galactosemia—Inborn error of metabolism for carbohydrates
- Lesch-Nyhan—X-linked IEM with a buildup of uric acid; engages in self injury

Injuries/Abuse/Neglect

- Head injuries—Anoxia, hypoxia, bleeds
- Shaken baby syndrome—Child abuse resulting in shearing of the vessels in the brain
- Malnutrition in early infancy, especially of the essential fatty acids

Environmental

- Lead poisoning—A neurotoxin that can result in seizures (in pipes [and therefore in the water], batteries, paint, soil)
- Infection—Meningitis, encephalitis; in utero infections (CMV, toxoplasmosis, rubella)

Other Causes

- Extreme prematurity and intraventricular hemorrhage
- Other neurological insults—Untreated hydrocephalus; brain tumor; lack of brain development
- Medications/drugs—Dilantin (hydantoin), warfarin (Coumadin), oral Accutane (isotretinoin); drugs/alcohol

bilirubinemia or hypothyroidism. Cerebral dysgenesis in utero, such as in microcephaly or untreated hydrocephalus, are other physiological causes.

Other causes of MR include brain damage from head trauma and asphyxia, which can occur throughout childhood; degenerative neurological disorders; infections affecting the central nervous system, such as encephalitis and meningitis; untreated lead poisoning; shaken baby syndrome; and poor nutritional intake (especially deficiency of the essential fatty acids) during the first year of life. Pseudoretardation may result from a child being raised in a less stimulating environment, and an increased incidence is associated with lower socioeconomic status (Batshaw & Shapiro, 2002); for this group, early intervention can reverse the condition. For a large number of cases, the cause of the MR is never known.

INCIDENCE/PREVALENCE

According to the U.S. Department of Education, in 2001, the number of students between the ages of 6 and 21 in public schools who had MR was 612,978. This accounted for 10.6% of all the students with disabilities served by the U.S. public schools in 2001 (U.S. Department of Education [USDOE], 2003). However, the prevalence of MR is completely dependent on which definition and what criteria are used. Using only IQ testing, it is estimated that 2.5% of the population will fall more than two standard deviations below the mean and thus have MR (Batshaw & Shapiro, 2002). In reality, the numbers are much lower.

Males are approximately twice as likely to have MR as females, thought to be due to one of the 95

X-linked genetic conditions identified thus far (Batshaw & Shapiro, 2002). Since cognitive abilities continue to develop until mid-adolescence, it is not surprising that the numbers of those diagnosed with MR peak at ages 10 to 14 and then decline.

Down syndrome, fragile X syndrome, and fetal alcohol syndrome account for almost one third of all identifiable cases of severe MR (Batshaw & Shapiro, 2002). Other common conditions include Williams syndrome and Prader-Willi syndrome. These five conditions are covered below. Whereas four of these are caused by genetic or chromosomal defects, fetal alcohol syndrome is an acquired condition.

SELECTED CONDITIONS RESULTING IN MR

Down Syndrome

Down syndrome was first described in 1838; the extra chromosome was identified as the cause in 1959, although the reason why it occurs is still unclear. It is the most prevalent cause of MR, but the incidence is decreasing, presumably because of advances in prenatal diagnosis and the options available for termination of affected pregnancies. The prevalence rates range from 1:650 to 1:1,000 births in the United States (Nehring, 2004). These rates vary based on the age of the mother. There is increased risk with increased maternal age: a 1:2,000 chance if the mother is 20 and a 1:20 chance if she is 45 (Roizen, 2002). Yet, 80% of those with Down syndrome are born to mothers younger than 35 years of age.

Ninety-five percent of the cases are caused by nondisjunction, in which the chromosome pairs fail to separate during meiosis, resulting in 47 chromosomes, or 3 chromosomes on the 21st "pair." Four percent of the cases are due to translocation, in which part of an extra 21st chromosome is attached to another chromosome. The remaining 1% is due to mosaicism, in which some cells have 46 and some have 47 chromosomes (Roizen, 2002). Most cases are caused by nondisjunction of the mother's chromosomes; only 5% to 10% are from the father (Hunter, 2001).

It is the 21st chromosome that has the genetic loci for leukemia, MR, heart disease, epicanthal folds, the shape of the hands, and the upslanting palpebral fissures that are so characteristic of Down syndrome (Roizen, 2002). The common physical signs are short stature, with the average adult height being 5 feet for males and 4.5 feet for females (Roizen, 2002); a flat, broad round face with small ears and nose; upward slanting of the eyes (palpebral fissures) with folds of skin (epicanthal folds) at the inside corner of the eye; Brushfield spots close to the iris margin; a small oral cavity and short palate, which may cause the tongue to protrude and contributes to articulation problems; short broad hands; a single crease across the palm and other dermatoglyphics; increased space between the first and second toes; and reduced muscle tone (hypotonia) with hyperflexibility of joints. It is thought that the hypotonia is the cause of the delayed milestones characteristic of this condition.

The hallmark characteristic of Down syndrome is MR. IQ scores generally range between 40 and 60, which is primarily in the moderate MR range, but they may decrease during adolescence (Roizen, 2002). This may be manifested by the development of behavior problems or a worsening of academic performance. These individuals typically have poor verbal short-term memory skills. They have better performance on visual–spatial tasks than on verbal or auditory tasks. The average mental age for someone with Down syndrome ranges from 5.5 to 8 years, which should give the school nurse some idea of the skills and mental processes possible for most of these individuals (Carr, 2002; Hunter, 2001). Those who have Down syndrome due to translocation and mosaicism generally have higher intellectual abilities and an overall higher level of functioning than those whose Down syndrome has a different etiology, and these individuals may not require as much community or educational services (Baroff & Olley, 1999).

Students with Down syndrome usually learn to manage their self-care activities, although these are delayed 1 to 2 years; they also enjoy participating in recreational activities and sports. However, their speech development is often significantly delayed, with short phrases not appearing until the preschool years. "Their receptive language is generally better than their expressive language" (Roizen, 2002, p. 314) and they often mix sound and gesture as they communicate. They are described as having pleasant and sociable personalities (AAMR, 2002).

Sexual development progresses normally, and the average age at menarche is 12.6 years. These individuals are at increased risk of sexual abuse. In terms of fertility, one source indicated that, "There remain fewer than 50 cases of documented fertility in women, and apparently only one in a non-mosaic man with Down syndrome" (Hunter, 2001, p. 116). Others believe the women with Down syndrome "have a slightly reduced fertility rate, but they can conceive and bear children. Roughly half of the children born to women with DS will also have the condition" (McGuire & Chicoine, 2002, p. 231).

Numerous conditions are associated with Down syndrome. Heart defects are found in about two-thirds of cases, with endocardial cushion defect being the most common. This is a defect in the center of the heart where the four chambers meet, resulting in abnormal communication between at least two chambers (Roizen, 2002). Other medical conditions commonly seen in students with Down syndrome include ophthalmic problems (60%), most of which are correctable with eyeglasses; hearing loss (66%); hypothyroidism (30% to 50%) and obesity (50% to 90%); periodontal disease or malocclusion (60% to 100%); various skin conditions (50%); subclinical atlantoaxial subluxation (partial dislocation of the upper spine) (15%); gastrointestinal malformations (5%); celiac disease (5%); seizures (6%); and leukemia (Roizen, 2002). The risk of leukemia is low (one in 150); however, this is significantly higher than seen in children without Down syndrome, which is 1 in 2,800 (Roizen, 2002). Children with Down syndrome are considered to have a mild immunological deficiency that puts them at risk for pneumonia, skin infections, and leukemia (Hunter, 2001).

The orthopedic problems may be due to loose ligaments, which may result in the atlantooccipital instability of the neck, as well as mobility difficulty and neck problems. Little or no growth occurs between ages 8 and 11; this is a lateral plateau (Baroff & Olley, 1999). Because the growth patterns of these children are so unique, separate growth charts are available for use in the annual screening done by the school nurse.

Nursing Interventions

Interventions provided by the school nurse that will be helpful and should be considered for inclusion in the Individualized Education Program (IEP) (see Chapter 9) are as follows. Many of these will be helpful with most students with MR, not only those with Down syndrome.

- Complete routine hearing and vision evaluations and follow-up on referrals to ensure that sensory deficits are not further impacting on the student's ability to learn.
- Ensure semiannual dental checks and good dental hygiene in school to prevent periodontal disease; be aware that antibiotic prophylaxis is required prior to dental care because of the frequent comorbid cardiac problems.
- Ensure that X-ray films are obtained for students involved in organized sports, such as the Special Olympics, before their participation to evaluate the status of the atlantoaxial subluxation; discourage high-risk activities such as climbing trees or jungle gyms.
- Be aware that, because of deficiencies in their immune systems, students should be immunized against pneumococcus and hepatitis, in addition to maintaining full coverage for the other preventable communicable diseases.
- Suggest physical therapy, occupational therapy, and speech therapy if appropriate; sign language for important concepts (i.e., hungry, pain, juice, toilet) may assist students with communication problems.
- Promote a healthy diet and an exercise program because of students' predisposition to constipation and obesity.
- Teach sex education and care of one's body during menses often and at the appropriate level to be understood. Be aware that barrier methods are often ineffective for these women "because of the limitations of the person to use them correctly each time" (McGuire & Chicoine, 2002, p. 232). Also teach students about how to protect themselves against sexual abuse.
- Teach self-help skills related to hygiene and toileting.
- Be attentive to signs of physical illness, as these students have an increased incidence of upper respiratory and ear infections.

Because their facial characteristics are so well recognized, some parents are opting for plastic surgery to "normalize" a child with Down syndrome to reshape the eyes and to take a wedge out of the tongue so that it better fits into the mouth. It is thought that this will decrease the stigma associated with the condition and help with the problems of a protruding tongue, such as drooling and difficulties in eating, breathing, and speech. Research has not yet supported the efficacy of this practice and no improvement in speech clarity has been found after surgery (Baroff & Olley, 1999). However, the school nurse can promote self-esteem in these students and promote acceptance of differences among the student's peers. Life expectancy is shorter than normal, with half of the individuals with MR surviving into their 50s; only 13.5% are still alive at age 68 (Roizen, 2002). Many individuals with Down syndrome are able to find employment, although often in low-wage positions; others work in sheltered workshops and reside in supervised living arrangements. As adults with Down syndrome reach their 30s, the incidence of Alzheimer disease increases. Some believe that virtually 100% of adults with Down syndrome "show the neuropathologic changes of Alzheimer disease by the age of

35–40 years" (Hunter, 2001, p. 114); the pathology is thought to actually begin in the second decade of life. Others believe that the incidence of Alzheimer disease is much lower (McGuire & Chicoine, 2002). Clinical dementia is seen in 9% by age 40 and in 55% by age 60 (Baroff & Olley, 1999). This information may be helpful in planning transitional services for the student. It may also be helpful to the parents as they plan for their child's future.

Fragile X Syndrome

The condition known as fragile X was first noted in 1943, but was formally recognized in 1969. It is the most common inherited form of MR (Crane, 2002), although Down syndrome is the most common clinical type of MR.

Fragile X results from a pinched off or broken section of the lower arm of the sex-linked X chromosome. This is known as the fragile site. The gene involved is the *FMR1* (the Fragile X Mental Retardation, 1) at Xq27.3, which is responsible for the production of a protein that is needed for brain and neurological development and function (Meyer & Batshaw, 2002).

Normally, on this area of the chromosome, there are anywhere from 6 to 50 repeats of the three nucleotides cytosine–guanine–guanine (CGG). However, a carrier of fragile X (referred to as a premutation) will have from 50 to 200 repeats of CGG and someone with a full mutation has from 200 to a few thousand repeats (Hagerman, 2001; Meyer & Batshaw, 2002). While carriers show no signs of the syndrome, "premutations are unstable and can expand further when passed down to the next generation" (Dykens et al., 2000, p. 140). DNA testing can now differentiate among normal, carrier state, and a full mutation.

It is estimated that the fragile X premutation or full mutation occurs in 1:1,500 males and 1:1,000 females (Beirne et al., 2002). However, the prevalence rate of fragile X associated with MR is approximately 1 in 4,000 males and 1 in 6,000 females in the general population in the United States (Meyer & Batshaw, 2002). Therefore, it is suggested that some who have learning disabilities (LDs) may actually have fragile X. One in 259 women in the general population may be a carrier and at risk for having an affected child (Hagerman, 2001). One in 700 males may also be a carrier.

When one has the full mutation, the gene becomes methylated and is inactivated and does not send out the message to make the protein. This results in the symptoms seen in the condition (Hagerman, 2001). Although seen in both sexes, the symptoms are more severe in males (Crane, 2002). Characteristic features include a long face with a high forehead, protruding ears, a prominent jaw, a high arched palate, and large testicles after puberty. The individuals may be short for age. Hyperactivity and impulsivity, as in attention deficit hyperactivity disorder (ADHD), are seen in 70% to 80% of males and 30% to 50% of females (Hagerman, 2001), whereas inattention is seen in almost all of those affected. About two-thirds of those with ADHD symptoms benefit from stimulant medication. Aggression and anxiety are also common (Meyer & Batshaw, 2002).

Eighty percent of males and 70% of females with fragile X have mild to moderate MR. The amount of the available protein is a "powerful predictor of IQ" (Dykens et al., 2000, p. 145). Females usually have less of a cognitive deficit, with a greater risk of inattention and LDs. The IQ in males with fragile X may decrease with age; this does not result in a loss of skills, but rather a slower acquisition of newer skills (Dykens et al., 2000). Even though affected children usually have delayed developmental milestones, the symptoms of fragile X are not normally obvious during infancy. Therefore, it is often during the preschool years that the child is diagnosed, with some being diagnosed well into elementary school; the average age at diagnosis is 32 months (Bailey, Skinner, & Sparkman, 2003).

The strengths of individuals with this condition include a delightful sense of humor and a good long-term memory, especially when a task is learned by seeing or doing. They can perform the activities of daily living and appear to learn more from their environment than would be expected based on their IQ (Hagerman & Hagerman, 2002). However, they also have a number of weaknesses. They have difficulty with short-term memory tasks, whether auditory or visual; this impedes sequential thinking. While they have a good vocabulary, they have weaker communication and socialization skills, engaging in echolalia and perseverative and poorly articulated speech (Meyer & Batshaw, 2002). Temper tantrums are common during times of transition and during increased sensory stimulation.

These individuals are usually healthy, with a normal life span and no comorbidities, although mitral valve prolapse and seizures are possible in up to 20% (Hagerman, 2001). Other common health concerns include strabismus and refractive errors in 25% to 56%; orthopedic problems, such as hypotonia, hyperextensible finger joints, flat feet, and scoliosis; dental crowding and malocclusion; and recurrent sinus infections and otitis media, which has the possibility of resulting in conductive hearing loss. Those symptoms not due to the *FMR1* gene are thought to be associated with a connective tissue disorder (Hagerman & Hagerman, 2002).

An association between fragile X and autism is seen in 5% to 46% (Beirne et al., 2002), especially since many of the symptoms are described as "autistic-like," such as hand flapping (present in 85%), gaze aversion (90%), and echolalia (Crane, 2002; Meyer & Batshaw, 2002). However, these children are more sociable and warmly attach to their parents and other providers (Dykens et al., 2000). In contrast, children with autism have fragile X in 7% to 15% of cases. It is recommended that all children diagnosed with autism be tested for fragile X syndrome (Meyer & Batshaw, 2002).

Interventions

A number of educational approaches can be used for those with fragile X, depending on the severity of their symptoms. While it may appear that many of these are only for the classroom teacher, this is not the case. The school nurse will have numerous occasions to teach these students, whether for a classroom presentation or in the health office related to a particular problem. They will need to follow the same directions as other students with regard to hearing, vision, and postural screening and will need to be prepared for these activities. The interventions include the following:

- Present all parts of a task at the same time, since these students learn best in this manner. (This is different than for those with other causes of MR.)
- Be aware that these students "perform better with integrative tasks that stress the overall meaning of the concept to be learned" (Dykens et al., 2000, p. 164). This means teaching numbers by counting out medication or counting the number of times one does an exercise.
- Provide a structured learning environment; these students do better in smaller classrooms with decreased noise levels and minimal changes.
- Know that these students have increased sensitivity to noise, so the use of headphones, either alone or attached to music, may help decrease stimulation (Hagerman, 2001).
- Decrease excessive sensory stimulation; sensory integration therapy by an occupational therapist may be helpful.
- Maintain a behavior chart; use positive reinforcement.
- Give clear concrete directions, with visual cues if possible.
- Be aware that for those with significant language problems, sign language may be helpful. Speech and language therapy may also be helpful.
- Routinely screen for potential cardiac, orthopedic, dental, and neurological problems.

Adults with fragile X syndrome live a normal life span, but most continue to need support indefinitely (Meyer & Batshaw, 2002). Fertility is normal, but the number of genetic nucleotide replications increases with each generation; thus genetic counseling is essential. This information may be helpful in teaching sex education and answering the student's questions related to his or her future.

Williams Syndrome

Williams syndrome is a genetic condition caused by the microdeletion of 7q11.23, which involves 16 to 20 genes. It was first identified in the 1960s and is not common. It is estimated that 1:20,000 to 1:50,000 individuals in the United States are affected (Semel & Rosner, 2003). The most comprehensive description of children with Williams syndrome is those "who test as though retarded, speak as though gifted, behave sometimes as though emotionally disturbed, and function like the learning disabled" (Semel & Rosner, 2003, p. 1).

The strengths of individuals with this condition include excellent vocabulary, auditory short-term memory, and facial recognition skills. They have a talent for story telling and for music memory as well as for playing musical instruments. Their limitations are in visual–spatial functioning (replicating what is seen), perceptual–motor planning, number knowledge, and fine-motor skills (writing, buttons).

They often have characteristic facies, including a "pixie-like" appearance with a broad forehead, bitemporal narrowing, short upturned nose, periorbital fullness, lacy starburst pattern on the iris, bulbous nasal tip, malar flattening, elongated space between the upper lip and the nose, full lips, wide mouth, full cheeks, small widely spaced teeth, small jaw, and prominent ears (Dykens et al., 2000; Morris, 2001; Semel & Rosner, 2003).

Children with Williams syndrome often have a developmental delay in skill development and in their growth. As older individuals, they often have short stature, but their growth hormones are normal and bone age is commensurate with height. Special growth curve charts are available to the school nurse from the specialty organizations.

One of approximately 20 genes deleted includes the one responsible for elastin, a protein that gives strength and elasticity to the walls of organs and blood vessels as well as to the skin. This accounts for the connective tissue abnormalities commonly seen in the condition (Morris, 2001). This may result in supravalvular aortic stenosis; a hoarse, deep voice; hernias; soft loose skin and premature aging of the skin; and joint laxity initially that can result in delayed walking and then the development of contractures that interfere with motor skills, such as walking down stairs, writing, getting dressed, or cutting food. More than half have strabismus and other vision problems.

The cognitive profile displays a wide range from low average to severe MR; most have mild or moderate MR with an average IQ score of 50 to 60, but 48% have normal vocabulary tests and 65% are normal on digit recall tests (Dykens et al., 2000; Morris, 2001). They use good sentence structure with a well-developed vocabulary, but usually with the reasoning of a preschooler (Semel & Rosner, 2003). They are highly distractible and have difficulty with attention and controlling impulsivity.

Their personality is described as being overly friendly yet they have an impaired social intelligence, such as having inappropriate greeting behaviors, and therefore have difficulty making and keeping friends. They are caring and enjoy people, but are vulnerable to exploitation. They do not tolerate teasing very well and they have a low frustration tolerance. They have a high rate of developing anxiety in unfamiliar situations or "when confronted with unanticipated change" (Semel & Rosner, 2003, p. 6).

In addition to the preceding, more than 90% have hyperacusis or hypersensitivity to sound (Udwin, 2002). There is no hearing deficiency, but these students react with an increased startle and cover their ears in reaction to loud noises. They are also at an increased risk for otitis media (Dykens et al., 2000). Fifteen percent have hypercalcemia in infancy (Morris, 2001), which may be associated with constipation and abdominal pain. Eighteen percent have renal problems, and frequency and enuresis are common (Dykens et al., 2000).

Interventions

Medical follow-up is important on a number of fronts. Because of the possibility of cardiac problems and the fact that 40% develop hypertension, they should be monitored by a cardiologist (Dykens et al., 2000). These students should be followed routinely by an ophthalmologist to ensure that visual problems are not the cause of the visual–spatial deficits. Routine dental care should also be provided, as the students often have delayed eruption, enamel hypoplasia, and malocclusion (Semel, & Rosner, 2003; Udwin, 2002). Occupational and physical therapy can be helpful in decreasing contractures and promoting fine motor activities, especially related to the activities of daily living.

In school, these students benefit from speech/language therapy. They should be taught "to use their verbal and auditory strengths to remember and process spatial information" (Morris, 2001, p. 523). Other educational and health-related interventions include:

- Using audiotape recorders instead of writing
- Using raised lined paper
- Keeping the example being copied on the same piece of paper
- Verbally describing what you want them to do; demonstration also helps
- Promoting self-instruction in which they verbalize what they are to do
- Minimizing distractions; helping to focus
- Decreasing noise levels and preparing them for when noise is expected, such as the bell at change of classes and fire drills
- Providing social skills training; rehearsal is effective
- Using music therapy; these students can also learn to sing or play music "by ear"
- Teaching content through music and song
- Providing increased supervision to stay on task
- Decreasing anxiety; reduce external pressures
- Providing positive reinforcement (Dykens et al., 2000; Semel & Rosner, 2003)

The symptoms persist into adulthood. Studies demonstrate that most of these students live at home with parents or in sheltered living arrangements. Few can tell time and even fewer can manage money. Almost all of them are "dependent on others for the preparation of food and domestic chores, such as cleaning, shopping and laundry" (Udwin, 2002, p. 303). These outcomes should be considered when developing the transition plan for these students (see Chapter 27).

Prader-Willi Syndrome

First described in 1956, Prader-Willi syndrome (P-W) results from the partial deletion of the long arm of chromosome 15. It is only seen in 1 in every 10,000 to 15,000 births. Seventy-five percent of the cases of microdeletion of affected genes come from the father (15q11–q13); the remainder occurs when the mother passes both chromosomes on the 15th pair to her offspring and the father gives none (Cassidy, 2001).

The symptoms of P-W change significantly from infancy to childhood. Initially, these infants are hypotonic and are poor feeders. However, the trademark feature of this condition is the impaired satiety, food-seeking behavior, and obesity. It is the leading genetic cause of obesity, with children sometimes reaching 300 to 400 pounds (Dykens et al., 2000). The "hyperphagia is due to a hypothalamic abnormality resulting in lack of satiety" (Cassidy, 2001, p. 303). These students have been reported to eat huge portions of anything, including pet food, frozen food, uncooked food, and spoiled food from the garbage (Baroff & Olley, 1999). Weight gain is especially characteristic during the first six years of life and the obesity is central in its body distribution. Appetite suppressants are not effective.

Individuals with P-W usually fall into the mildly mentally retarded category with an average IQ of 60 to 70 (Cassidy, 2001). This means that while some may have moderate MR, some will also test in the low normal range of intelligence. They are prone to temper tantrums and are described as stubborn, controlling, manipulative, impulsive, and, at times, aggressive (Cassidy, 2001). They are concrete thinkers and exercise poor judgment. They do have strengths in visual processing and an unusual skill with jigsaw puzzles. "Given their behavior problems, many of these children are educated in more restricted settings than suggested by their IQ scores alone" (Dykens et al., 2000, p. 200).

Characteristic features of their body include short stature (the average height is 155 cm for males and 148 cm for females), small hands and feet, narrow hands with a straight ulnar border, hypopigmentation or a fair complexion, and genital hypoplasia due to hypogonadism. Sixty percent had surgery for undescended testicles (Baroff & Olley, 1999). They have delayed secondary sex characteristics at puberty. "Sexual activity is uncommon and fertility is rare" (Cassidy, 2001, p. 303). If hormone replacement is used, it is important to watch for increased aggressive behavior. The patch has been found to be more effective than injections in reducing behavioral side effects.

Many have thick viscous saliva that contributes to both dental caries and speech articulation defects (Cassidy, 2001). It is not uncommon to only say a few words by age 3. Other physical characteristics may include temperature control problems, a very low incidence of vomiting, and a high pain threshold. This latter trait is often accompanied by a tendency to scratch and pick at their skin to the point of self-injury.

The hypotonia may result in scoliosis and/or kyphosis, so postural screenings are needed annually for these students. They may also have strabismus and other eye muscle problems, requiring routine ophthalmologic exams. Other characteristic facies are almond-shaped eyes and turned-down corners of the mouth. Individuals with P-W are friendly, talkative, cheerful, and good-natured, but can be quick to anger. Obsessive–compulsive disorders are common, and these students have been described as hoarders.

Interventions

Interventions must be consistent between the home and the school. The primary concern involves food. Food needs to be locked up and access to it controlled; this includes cabinets and refrigerators. This can be quite a challenge during classroom celebrations and birthday parties. The school nurse can advocate for a low-calorie well-balanced diet being provided at a specific time and place and ensure that an exercise program is in place. The school nurse can support families by being the liaison between the family and the school to ensure continuity. "Avoid punishing for taking food, because it is involuntary, or withdrawing food as a form of punishment, as it may lead only to increased upset" (Baroff & Olley, 1999, p. 119). Students should never be left alone with food or unescorted. They need close supervision.

While some interventions are directly initiated by the school nurse, others are ideas that the school nurse might recommend to the classroom teacher. These interventions include the following:

- Because they have an increased tendency for daytime somnolence (Nativio, 2002), avoid increased in-seat activities.
- Provide sex education; as students with P-W move into adolescence they need the same type of support and information about sex as all adolescents.
- Stress good dental hygiene and the use of mouthwash or toothpaste to increase the production of saliva.
- Provide structure and a predictable routine; these students are upset by change.
- Provide clear behavioral expectations and limits.
- Be consistent.

"Unchecked weight gain leads to early death as a result of non-insulin dependent diabetes mellitus or cardiopulmonary compromise" (Nativio, 2002,

p. 301). The school nurse should be aware of the possibility of diabetes when the student presents with related symptoms. The vast majority will ultimately need to live in supportive settings as adults. This information may be helpful to those providing transition planning services.

Fetal Alcohol Syndrome and Fetal Alcohol Effects

Fetal alcohol syndrome (FAS) was identified in 1973, but the effects of alcohol on the developing fetus have been recognized since biblical days. In 1996, the term alcohol-related neurodevelopmental disorder was coined to focus more on the CNS characteristics and less on the facial characteristics. Most school districts do not yet recognize FAS as a diagnosis and usually classify these students under one of the other mental health conditions. FAS is not included in the DSM-IV.

In 1996, the Institute of Medicine "estimated that between 0.5 and 3.0 of every 1,000 infants are born with some degree of FAS" (Streissguth, 1997, p. 8). That translates into approximately 5,000 infants born with FAS per year (Beirne-Smith et al., 2002), most of whom enter the school system. The prevalence is two times that of Down syndrome, making it the most common known cause of MR. "On some Indian reservations, where alcohol abuse is common among women, FAS has been reported in 1 in 100 children" (Streissguth, 1997, p. 8). While the recurrence risk in families with one child with severe MR is 3% to 9%, the recurrence rate for women who continue to drink during their pregnancies is 30% to 50% (Batshaw & Shapiro, 2002).

Alcohol is known to be teratogenic, but it is not known exactly how that process occurs and how much alcohol is needed to cause the anomalies or low birth weight (LBW). What is known is that "the brain is the organ…most vulnerable to the effects of prenatal alcohol" (Streissguth, 1997, p. 9). In addition, those who drink heavily are at risk for nutritional and vitamin deficiency, which can also impact the developing fetus.

Most children with FAS appear normal at birth. The three criteria for diagnosis include (1) decreased height and/or weight; (2) facial characteristics (which disappear as the child ages) that include short palpebral fissures (narrow eye lengths) and a thin upper lip with a smooth philtrum (no ridges running from the small upturned nose to the lips); and (3) some CNS damage. This last category may include MR, ADHD, LDs, seizures, or problems with fine or gross motor function (Baroff & Olley, 1999).

Because of the wide spectrum of symptoms, MR is not necessary for the diagnosis. The mean IQ for this population is 90; therefore only 25% with FAS and 10% with fetal alcohol effects can be classified with mild to moderate MR (Streissguth, 1997). Most do have difficulty with retention, abstract thinking, and math (Beirne-Smith et al., 2002), and performance skills are better than verbal skills in both groups. Perhaps most difficult is their inability to learn from past experiences. They have erratic mood swings and are not self reflective, especially related to their limitations, and have difficulty separating the acts from the incidents that provoke them. This makes them unaware of the consequences of their behavior, especially in the social realm.

Because the symptoms are difficult to identify and there is a wide spectrum of symptoms, the term fetal alcohol effects (FAE) or atypical FAS is used for the milder and subtler signs, such as LDs and attention problems. The list of characteristics is long and may include:

- "Flits about with butterfly-like movements" (Baroff & Olley, 1999, p. 165)
- Friendly to the extreme; likes to touch, fondle, pet, and kiss
- Hyperactive/impulsive and inattentive ADHD
- Lack of inhibition
- Poor fine and gross motor skills
- Developmental delay in motor, social, and language skills
- Poor state regulation
- Possible gait coordination
- Central auditory processing problems and the possibility of sensorineural hearing loss
- Visual problems
- "May violate personal space conventions (e.g., stand too close, touch too much) and use inappropriate and ineffectual methods of trying to establish relationships (e.g., "will you sleep with me"?)" (Streissguth, 1997, p. 140).

Because there are no clinical lab tests and no validated checklists, a diagnosis is made only on the basis of a clinical examination. More than 50% of these students are adopted or in foster care, making it difficult to get a prenatal and birth history (Clarren & Astley, 2001). Without the facial characteristics, it is difficult to differentiate FAS and FAE from conditions such as ADHD with comorbid conditions (see Chapter 30) or other mental or behavioral problems. "Students with FAS/FAE are not all alike: they are not all retarded or learning disabled nor do they all have behavior problems. They are spread throughout the schools in both general and special education classrooms" (Streissguth, 1997, p. 211).

The long-term outlook for these young people is usually not positive. Ninety-four percent will have mental health problems (especially depression); 43% will drop out of school, many already having been suspended or expelled, and 42% will have trouble with the law. Inappropriate sexual behavior has been identified in 16% to 18%, with sexual touching and promiscuity the main behaviors (Streissguth, 1997). There are also difficulties with the ability to make and keep friends because of their inattention, immaturity, and difficulty in cooperation.

Interventions

Interventions that may be helpful in the school setting include the following:

- Make referrals for hearing and vision evaluation, if needed.
- "Careful supervision is warranted for these children; they may lack appropriate fearfulness, have a tendency to wander, and be unresponsive to verbal restrictions" (Baroff & Olley, 1999, p. 165).
- Encourage verbalization of their needs; teach to ask for help.
- Give frequent reminders, as they have difficulty following through on tasks.
- Keep instructions calm, clear, and short.
- Teach using both verbal and visual modalities.
- Help the child keep in control of a situation or task (have fewer toys available, provide a curtailed space).
- Decrease environmental stimuli.
- Provide close supervision when the student is with classmates; it is a fine line between encouraging friendships and ensuring the safety of the friends.
- Develop rules for appropriate behavior.
- Provide extra time to complete a task.
- Provide sex education, with rules and information on protection.

ISSUES

Labels

Because of the negative implications of having MR, there is an increasing trend to label those who have mild MR as LD, even though the official definition of LD is that the individual must have a normal level of intelligence (see Chapter 30). This trend is due to the negative stigma associated with the label MR. "The percentage of school-age students classified as having mental retardation has decreased enormously – 40% between the 1976–1977 school year and 1994–1995. At the same time, the percentage of students with learning disabilities during this period, greatly increased, some estimating an increase as high as 207%" (AAMR, 2002, p. 32). However, it should be noted that in Great Britain, an LD *is* synonymous with mild MR.

No matter the label classification, in the United States it is clear that even during the past decade there has been an enormous increase in students with MR. The latest report from the U.S. Department of Education indicates that there has been a 10% increase in the number of students with MR in the U.S. public schools from 1990 to 2000 (DOE, 2003).

There is a benefit to labels. Without them, students would not be eligible for services, benefits, or legal protections. The label also allows for reimbursement to school districts and assists in ensuring similar populations for research initiatives. Some, however, perceive them as a way for a student to get additional attention.

It is also possible that individuals are mislabeled. The test used must be appropriate to the individual's needs in order to appropriately measure the person's intelligence based on his or her ability to communicate. The problem with labels is that it could become a self-fulfilling prophecy. They lower one's expectations of the person. There have been many negative labels attached to MR that have resulted in prejudices, myths, and labels that are now considered offensive and insensitive. Terms such as idiot, imbecile, moron, feebleminded, and mentally defective were developed by the American Psychiatric Association and others to identify levels of MR. Other negative terms used include dumb, stupid, subnormal, and incompetent. If used in teasing, these terms becomes mean-spirited and offensive. For these reasons, in recent years there has been a change in some areas of the country from using the term mental retardation to terms such as "cognitive impairments," "cognitive delays," and "mental impairments" (Snow, 2003; The Arc, 2003b; Turnbull et al., 2002).

Comorbidity

MR is associated with a large number of neurological conditions, even though it is not the cause of nor caused by those conditions. These include "cerebral palsy, sensory impairments, seizure disorders, communication impairments, feeding difficulties, behavior/psychiatric disorders, and attention-deficit/

hyperactivity disorder (ADHD)" (Batshaw & Shapiro, 2002, p. 296). Other comorbid conditions include thyroid disease, obesity, and poor oral health (Fisher, 2004). Half of those with severe MR and 25% of those with mild MR have sensory impairments, with vision problems being the most common. Speech-language and feeding problems are also associated with MR, as are some psychiatric and mood disorders.

It is important that school personnel, and especially school nurses, help others to separate the assumption of comorbidity of MR with other chronic conditions or disabilities until clearly determined for the individual student. It was once thought that all or almost all children with autism also had MR, likewise with cerebral palsy (Batshaw & Shapiro, 2002). This is not the case. Even students with Down syndrome, if their genetic structure is mosaic, can approach typical or close to typical intellectual abilities (Oelwein, 1995).

Physical Inactivity

Individuals who have MR are often overweight because of the decreased structure and unstructured activity in their lives. Many have mobility problems that limit their ability to get around. This makes it more of a challenge to ensure that they have upper body exercise and engage in wheelchair activities; it also has significant implications for the modifications that may be needed in physical education class to ensure student participation. The Special Olympics have been especially effective in providing a forum for individuals with disabilities to compete and be rewarded for their efforts. This competition promotes participation that can often be a stimulus to exercise.

Exercise is also a social activity; it allows individuals to participate with others in a nonacademic setting. However, students with MR may actually have to be taught how to play. "It is a matter of indicating how toys and materials are intended to be used and teaching the social rules that govern group play" (Baroff & Olley, 1999, p. 292). Adults in the environment need to make sure that the activities in which students with MR engage build self-esteem, and promote skills that can be used throughout life, but do not demean or put them at risk of being embarrassed by their peers, such as cleaning trash and other janitorial positions.

Sexuality

Individuals with MR need repeated information and practice related to everyday hygiene, care of themselves during menses, and sex education. There are numerous reports of individuals with MR being sexually abused or raped (Baroff & Olley, 1999). This may be exacerbated by their need to be part of a social group and to be liked, their difficulty in problem solving, and their poor cognitive skills that make identifying their attacker more difficult. It is essential that sex education be provided often in a concrete way, including how conception occurs. They need to practice saying no and guidance as to what to do should someone try something. They also need to be helped with the distinction between public and private behaviors as well as appropriate ways to express affection.

In 1999, the American Academy of Pediatrics (AAP) issued a statement on the sterilization of minors with developmental disabilities. The AAP first recommend that the affected individual's capacity to make informed decisions be assessed. If such individuals can understand the facts and associated concepts and can make decisions, then they are able to give informed consent or refuse to do so. "The inconvenience of problems dealing with normal menstrual bleeding is generally an inappropriate indication for surgical sterilization" (AAP, 1999, p. 339). In addition, there is no evidence that castration of males will decrease aggressive behavior. Sterilization is not the answer to exploitation or prevention of sexually transmitted diseases (STDs). School nurses, as consultants to families and members of the school staff, may be called upon to address this topic when students reach adolescence.

Bullying, Abuse, and Neglect

School children can engage in bullying and teasing of those who are different. Children are often unaware of how deeply hurtful their comments and actions can be. These children and adolescents may also be physically or psychologically abused or neglected by their own families (see Chapter 39). This may be a factor in the increasing mental health concerns of those with MR as they move into adolescence and adulthood. While there have been great strides in creating an inclusive accepting atmosphere of differences (Coombs-Richardson & Meisgeier, 2001; Hester, 2002; Peterson & Skiba, 2001; Reinke & Herman, 2002), there has also been a history of bullying and abuse of individuals with disabilities, particularly those with MR (Cantu & Heumann, 2003; Fleitas, 2000). All school personnel should be working systematically to ensure that students with MR, as well as students with other differences, are considered part of the school population and treated with the same respect, dignity, and expectations as other students.

Problems with Financial, Medical, and Social Service Supports

Students with MR are in need of a case manager and an advocate (The Arc, 2003a). It is essential that a diagnosis be made by the time the student enters the school system. Many of the conditions described in the preceding are not diagnosed until the preschool or even the early elementary years. Once diagnosed, and the IEP team has met, the Individual Health Plan (IHP) must include ways to ensure that the multidisciplinary health care needs of the student are being addressed. Their need for screenings is more than for the average student. They may need twice-a-year growth measurements and annual vision and hearing tests. Much of this depends on the supports the child has outside of the school setting. One of the often neglected needs of children with special needs is their dental care. The school nurse can develop a list of dentists in the area able and willing to handle children with special needs.

While many students with cognitive deficits may see specialists, the school nurse can promote the necessity for routine primary care and health promotion. In addition, the families must engage in long-term planning, so that by the time the student enters adolescence, ideas have been discussed about the future. Planning is, indeed, a team effort. The comorbidities and sequelae of these conditions often result in increased medical costs and added stress for the family. Transition plans must be put into effect to assist the student in moving from pediatric healthcare to the adult healthcare system. This involves promoting responsibility for meeting one's own needs to the level of individual ability (see Chapter 27).

EDUCATION GOALS AND TECHNIQUES

The school nurse spends a good deal of his or her time in the role of health educator, whether in a structured environment or on a one-to-one basis. It is therefore essential that he or she be part of plans that address teaching approaches for students with special needs. Since the passage of the Education for All Handicapped Act in 1975, students with MR have been served in public schools throughout the United States. Prior to that time, students with MR were often turned away from schools (Hardman, Drew, & Egan, 2002). The assumption was that students with MR could not learn or could not learn in the typical school environment (Turnbull et al., 2002). Almost 30 years of research and practice have determined that with appropriate support, trained personnel, and adapted access to the general curriculum, students with MR can learn much more than once expected (Alper, 2003; Graziano, 2002; Lewis & Doorlag, 2003; Turnbull et al., 2002).

Because of the range of physical, social, and intellectual abilities of students with MR, assumptions about their possible academic achievements should not be made until individual assessments are completed and available instructional strategies are provided for the student. Even then, expectations should remain high for these students' academic achievement (Pugach & Warger, 2001). The focus should be on their functional age and not on their chronological age. Their cognitive strengths must be identified as should their areas of cognitive weaknesses. Other strengths of the student should be noted, even if it is just his or her smile.

Access to the General Curriculum

Young children with MR are often identified in early intervention programs. Therefore, they may already have an Individualized Family Service Plan (Chapters 9 and 27). This should facilitate transition to the preschool and kindergarten environment. Even after the passage of the Education for All Handicapped Children Act of 1975, students with MR and other types of disabilities did not have access to the same materials, books, and overall curricula that were provided for students without disabilities. Students with MR and their teachers often worked with limited numbers of books that were often out of date or with no materials at all. With the passage of the 1997 amendments to the Individuals with Disabilities Education Act (IDEA), the U.S. Congress required that all students have access to the general curriculum provided in public school districts and that only those students with the most severe cognitive impairments be instructed using non-academic curricula (IDEA, 1997).

This has meant that since 1997, most students with MR have access to the same curricula that is taught to students without disabilities and, in many cases, are included in the regular classroom; the law mandates that they should be taught in the least restrictive environment. Although there has been significant protest by a minority of families that the general curriculum is not appropriate for their children with MR, this change in policy has resulted in many more students with MR acquiring reading, writing, and mathematic skills far beyond the level that students of past generations have acquired. A consequence of the 1997 IDEA amendments and access to the general curriculum has made a drastic change in the goals for students' IEPs. Prior to 1997, it was common to find primarily developmental and functional objectives in a student's IEP. These objectives might have had some academic focus (e.g., writing one's name or recognizing common signs). After the passage of the 1997 amendments, teachers, family members, and other team members started to incorporate into IEPs state education standards that were being applied to students without disabilities (e.g., for a third-grade student, writing a three-paragraph essay). The expectations for students with MR have risen significantly with the results being that this category of students is achieving academic skills at a higher rate than at any time in the past (Turnbull et al., 2002). This also means that the majority of students with MR are now receiving their instruction in general education settings (Lewis & Doorlag, 2003).

Instructional Techniques

While most students now have access to the general education curriculum, special instructional techniques and strategies still must be tailored to the individual student. They will receive the same content instruction as students who do not have cognitive disabilities, including reading, mathematics, science, and social studies. Great care must be taken when identifying objectives and selecting teaching strategies to make the curriculum accessible for students with MR. Because cognitive disabilities can manifest themselves in many different ways and at many different levels, the implementation of instructional strategies truly must be individualized (Alper, 2003; Lewis & Doorlag, 2003; Turnbull et al., 2002). School nurses may be providing the instruction themselves, or may be providing guidance to the staff on appropriate interventions for students with MR.

Specific Instructional Techniques for Students with MR

To make the general curricula, including curricula related to health-related content, available and accessible to students with MR, a number of standard instructional strategies can be used by teachers and other school personnel. These strategies fall into three distinct categories: (1) teacher techniques, (2) social techniques, and (3) materials techniques (Table 35.3).

Table 35.3 ■

CATEGORIES OF INSTRUCTIONAL STRATEGIES FOR TEACHING STUDENTS WITH MENTAL RETARDATION

INSTRUCTIONAL CATEGORY	EXAMPLES OF SPECIFIC TECHNIQUES
Teacher strategies	Embedded instruction Task analysis Behavior-chain instruction Prompting
Social strategies	Peer-coaching Shadowing
Material and equipment strategies	Universal design Assistive technology

Teacher Strategies

Embedded Instruction

Embedded instruction is a strategy for teaching specific objectives to a student with MR within the general education curriculum. The teacher uses the general curriculum activities in a general education setting to allow the student with MR to learn and practice a specific skill or objective that may or may not be related to the general education activities taking place. For instance, a fifth grade student with MR who was working on telling time could learn this skill while participating in a typical mathematics word problem being presented to the general math class (Box 35.1).

Box 35.1 ■ ■ ■

AN EXAMPLE OF EMBEDDING A SKILL OBJECTIVE FOR A STUDENT WITH MENTAL RETARDATION IN THE GENERAL EDUCATION CURRICULUM

GENERAL CURRICULUM ACTIVITY

A small group (three or four students) solve a math word problem consisting of the following problem—A boy leaves his home at 1:00 p.m. He walks to his grandmother's house 10 miles away. He arrives at 4:30 p.m. the same day. How many miles per hour did the boy walk?

(Continued on the following page)

Box 35.1 ■■■

AN EXAMPLE OF EMBEDDING A SKILL OBJECTIVE FOR A STUDENT WITH MENTAL RETARDATION IN THE GENERAL EDUCATION CURRICULUM *(Continued)*

SKILL OBJECTIVE FOR STUDENT WITH MENTAL RETARDATION

To read time conventions and be able to verbally state them and depict them on a clock face.

EMBEDDED ACTIVITY

Teacher asks the student to draw two clock faces depicting the times the boy started and ended his journey and to state the times out loud to the group.

NOTE

This same activity could embed skill objectives for the student related to speaking in a small group, reading simple directions, working with a social group, and doing simple calculations.

Box 35.2 ■■■

AN EXAMPLE OF TASK ANALYSIS OF GREETING A FRIEND ON THE STREET

Step 1: Recognize the person from a distance.

Step 2: Decide to make a greeting gesture to the person.

Step 3: Decide whether to wave or smile.

Step 4: Wave.

Step 5: Walk closer to the person.

Step 6: Stop within an appropriate distance from the person (approximately 18–24 inches).

Step 7: Make eye contact with the person.

Step 8: Say "hello" or another opening greeting.

Step 9: Shake hands with the person.

Step 10: Ask "How are you?"

Task Analysis

Task analysis is a teaching strategy that takes complex tasks and breaks them into smaller, easier to learn units. Some skills, particularly social skills and self-care skills, are actually very complex in nature. The seemingly simple act of greeting people when you happen upon them on the street is not really a simple task. It includes at least 10 distinct steps (Box 35.2).

Task analysis divides specific skills into smaller components that a student may already know or that a student may be able to learn discreetly. Then the student, with assistance from a teacher or aide, can reconstruct the task by stringing the individual parts together. While this is often a teaching strategy for social and self-care skills, it is also common for math, reading, and science skills as well. A student may have many of the skills already. The critical instructional task becomes teaching the student how to use the skills in sequence.

Behavior-Chain Instruction

"Chain instruction" or "chaining" is a teaching strategy that is a variation of task analysis. Because task analysis can reveal that a specific skill or objective may have many parts, it is not unusual for a student to be unsuccessful in achieving a skill because of its complexity. Chaining starts with one part of the skill and slowly adds parts, all the while, making sure that as parts are added the student is successful.

Chaining of skills can occur in a forward or backward progression. Many teachers prefer backward chaining, because it reinforces the student with the outcome of the skill. For example, if the skill being taught is how to put on one's coat, a teacher may assist the student through all of the steps except for the last step of pulling up the zipper. In a backward chaining teaching strategy, the student would be expected to pull up the zipper independently. This allows the student to be successful and reinforces working on the task. Once pulling up the zipper can be accomplished independently, the next step would be inserting the two parts of the zipper together; the next step would be putting the student's second arm in the coat, and so on until the student is able to put on his or her own coat independently. Forward chaining reverses this process and starts with the first task in the task analysis list. Chaining, whether forward or backward, can be used for self-care skills, but also for skills as complex as algebra or the scientific inquiry method.

Prompts

For some students with MR, prompt systems are necessary for them to learn, accomplish, and/or maintain a skill. Prompts can be visual, auditory, physical, or some combination of all three. Prompts are used to help students focus on particular parts of a task or to remember steps in a task. If, for instance, a student has difficulty remembering the sequence of operations in an algebra problem, a visual prompt might be a series of colors at the bottom of the student's paper (for instance, red, green, blue). This sequence would be used in the operations in the algebra problem, with the teacher coloring the first operation to occur in red, the second in green, and the third in blue). This is a simple visual cue to help a student remember the sequence of operations. Physical prompts can be as simple as touching a student's elbow to begin a task such as cleaning up a work area. Auditory prompts can be as simple as a reminder from the teacher to a student to focus on the three steps in a paragraph of directions. Prompts are simple adaptations that can mean the difference between a student successfully completing a task and not knowing what to do.

Social Strategies

Peer-Coaching

Many of the instructional strategies developed for students with MR in inclusive classroom settings use the motivators and reinforcers of peer interaction as well as teacher interaction. Social interaction is often an important aspect in the lives of students with MR and the use of teaching strategies that rely on social interactions makes for effective teaching.

One of the most successful and frequently used social teaching strategies is peer-coaching. Since many students with MR in inclusive classrooms are motivated by their peers, systematically using other students as models, instructors, and reinforcers is a major teaching strategy. By using other students, either students with or without MR, as peer-coaches, teachers can capitalize on the social importance of peers.

Peer-coaching does not need to be overt or burdensome for the student peers in the classroom. Teachers can construct small working groups of the student with MR and students with strong skills in the task that is to be learned by the student with MR. Peer models are then provided. If the classroom is built on a collaborative learning system, student peers can assist the student with MR as he or she learns the new skill. Teacher support, through cues and prompts and specialized materials, also can aid the student with MR to learn the new skill within the social setting of a group of student peers (Cawley, Hayden, Cade, & Baker-Kroczynski, 2002).

Shadowing

Another strong social instructional strategy is shadowing the student with MR. A teacher, teacher's aide, family volunteer, or fellow student can "shadow" the student with MR through a new task. This is a version of "hand-over-hand" instruction in which a teacher walks the student through each part of the task, often doing many of the parts for the student. In shadowing, however, the teacher or other person is a social support for the student, reminding him or her of the steps, providing information when needed, and assisting the student to complete portions of the task that he or she has not yet mastered. As the student becomes more skilled at completing the task, the assistance is faded but the social reinforcement remains. Eventually, the social reinforcement is faded to being present only for brief periods of time during the task.

Materials and Equipment Strategies

Universal Design

Universal design refers to educational products designed to be used with and by students who have various different disabilities. Books that use universal design principles are created in multiple formats that allow all students to have access to their content. These would include books that are produced in traditional paper bound versions, audio-recorded versions, Web-based versions, Braille versions, and, most importantly, in digital versions where the page-background color can be changed, the font size can be adapted to the individual student's needs, and the text can be automatically scanned to produce spoken words (Turnbull et al., 2002).

Universal design is applied to all aspects of the curriculum so that all students, especially those with MR, can benefit from instruction. As with the textbook examples, the universal design of curricula means that multiple presentation strategies should be available to teachers and other school personnel, such as school nurses, when instructing any student. To support educators in the development of flexible, customizable curricula, researchers have begun to assemble ideas of how to instruct students with varying levels of cognitive abilities, sensory impairments, and physical disabilities (CAST, 1999; Orkwis & McLane, 1998). A research center dedicated to the development of such curricula also has been established; the Center for Applied Special

Technology's mission is to ensure that educational curricula are presentable in multiple methods (Kameenui & Simmons, 1999).

Assistive Technology

For many students with MR, assistive technology will allow them to benefit from the general curriculum. Assistive technology is any technology, teacher created or commercially purchased, that provides a student with access to information or provides the ability to respond and interact in school (Assistive Technology Act, 1988). Unlike universally designed products, assistive technology is an adaptation to an existing product or strategy of instruction. For example, a teacher who has always conducted a math lesson by showing the steps on the chalk board might use both the chalk board and an audiotape that only the student with MR uses so as to provide more information about the lesson as well as cues or other prompts to help him or her remember previous skills that have been learned that can be used for the new task. One of the concerns that teachers and other school personnel have had about assistive technology has been the cost. Although in some cases electronic assistive technology can run into the hundreds and even thousands of dollars, most assistive technology is relatively inexpensive in terms of financial costs.

Functional Curricula

Other students with MR have cognitive impairments that are significant enough to prevent access to the general curriculum through adaptations and teaching strategies. For these students, functional curricula are necessary. **Functional curricula** sets of objectives permit students to gain the skills they need to function on a day-to-day basis. These include functional reading skills (e.g., to be able to read road signs, menus, and simple instructions), use of money, balancing a check book, making decisions based on safety and health, cooking skills, and other daily living skills (Lewis & Doorlag, 2003). As of 2001, approximately 1% of the overall student population and less than 10% of the overall special education population are enrolled in functional curricula programs (USDOE, 2002).

No matter the measured cognitive level of a student, the curricula to be implemented should never underestimate the ability of a student to learn new information. Even for students enrolled in functional curricula programs, individualized programming should take place and general education goals should be included in the student's academic plan so that each student learns as much as possible, thus making him or her as prepared as possible for an independent life in the community.

Development and Coordination of a Student's IEP and IHP

Cognitive and health issues are intimately intertwined. It is therefore imperative that the student's individualized education plan (IEP) and the individualized health plan (IHP) be integrated as well. Although not explicitly mentioned in the reauthorization of IDEA (1997), school nurses should be a part of the student's IEP team from the point of assessment, through development of the IEP and on to implementation of services (National Association of School Nurses [NASN], 2002).

Since the IEP is the formal, contractual agreement between families and school districts, health services should be included in the document. To ensure that health services, including preventative, educational, acute care, and long-term care, are addressed appropriately, a school nurse should be a member of the IEP development team. His or her specific duties should include:

- Assisting in identification of students' needs
- Assessing students' physical health status (in collaboration with the student, parents, and other healthcare providers)
- Developing individualized health and emergency plans
- Assisting the IEP team in the development of specific goals and objectives
- Assisting parents and students to identify community resources
- Assisting parents and teachers in identifying and removing health-related barriers to learning
- Providing in-service training for teachers and other school personnel regarding students' health needs, including individualized needs of specific students
- Providing and/or supervising unlicensed assistive personnel to provide specialized healthcare services in school settings
- Evaluating the effectiveness of the health-related components of students' IEPs and serving as IEP team liaison to the medical community (NASN, 2002)
- Appropriately delegating tasks to those providing one-on-one care

The IEP can include information on billing for direct services under Medicaid for qualifying students (see Chapter 44).

STATE EDUCATION STANDARDS AND STANDARDS TESTING FOR STUDENTS WITH MR

General Education Standards Testing

The 1997 amendments to IDEA required states to ensure that *all* students with disabilities be included in the statewide testing that occurs to determine if students meet educational standards (IDEA, 1997). This includes students with MR or with other cognitive disabilities. Most students with cognitive disabilities participate in the general state testing programs, often with accommodations to the testing that include such modifications as no time limit, oral presentation of the test material, or how students make responses to the test questions (O'Neill, 2001). These accommodations are determined by the student's IEP team (including the student's parents or guardians and the student him-/herself if they are age appropriate) during the development of the student's IEP.

Alternate Standards Testing

For students with cognitive disabilities who have severe or profound MR (approximately 5% of the students with MR), an alternate standards assessment format must be implemented by the state to measure student progress (No Child Left Behind, 2002). These alternate assessments often take the form of portfolios that parallel the standards for students in the general education curriculum.

Whether the student with cognitive disabilities is participating in the general education standards testing or the alternate standards testing, testing periods can be significant times of stress and anxiety for students as well as their families. Many families feel that students with MR should not be included in the statewide standards testing. Parents report that this type of testing is a guarantee of failure for their children and that the testing is meaningless unless supported with significant academic instructional resources (Crocker, 2002). For those few students with severe cognitive disabilities, alternate assessment procedures are used to determine their academic and functional advancement (Burdett, 2001).

High School Graduation

With introduction of high-stakes testing and the inclusion of all students with disabilities in the testing process, including those with MR, there has been a reduction of students with MR graduating from high school. The standards tests that are now gatekeepers to graduation are resulting in students not passing and dropping out of school (Manset-Williamson & Washburn, 2002; O'Neill, 2001). Some states have instituted nonstandard diplomas or nonacademic diplomas for students who have met their IEP objectives but have not passed their respective state tests (Landford & Cary, 2000; O'Neill, 2002).

Transitioning to Community and Work

In addition to the changes in standards testing, access to the general curriculum and the push for inclusive settings, IDEA requires that school districts begin to plan with students with disabilities, including those with MR, for the students' transitions from school to the community. The regulations state that mandatory planning must begin at age 16 with a recommendation that the planning begin at age 14 (USDOE, 2003). This planning must include exploration of needs regarding housing, employment, socialization and recreation, and continued education. The purpose of this planning is to ensure that students have the knowledge and skills to be as independent as possible (Certo et al., 2003; Modell, & Valdez, 2002). Little mention is made, however, of students' needs for awareness of their health conditions and skills necessary to access and use health-care services.

As members of the IEP teams for students with MR, school nurses should work to include health-related issues in the transition plans of students with MR. Many of these students have significant health-related concerns that are often chronic in nature and may worsen with age. With the increased focus on self-determination and independence, students with MR should have as much information as possible about their health needs.

CONCLUSION

The school nurse is often an integral person for the support of students with MR, their families and other school personnel. Whether it is working with students with Down syndrome or a developmental delay, the school nurse can provide information about specific health issues. She also can act as a fellow school colleague who can use and reinforce the instructional strategies of teachers and other educators in the school. By fulfilling these multiple roles, the school nurse becomes a key person in the education of students with MR and a key support to students' families and teachers.

Resources

Council for Exceptional Children
1920 Association Drive
Reston, VA 20191
800-CEC-SPED
http://www.cec.sped.org

Developmental Disabilities Nurses Association
1733 H Street
Suite 330 PMB 1214
Blaine, WA 98230
320-332-9101
http://www.ddna.org

National Fragile X Foundation
P.O. Box 190488
San Francisco, CA 94119-0488
http://www.frax.org

National Organization of Rare Diseases (NORD)
55 Kenosia Avenue
P.O. Box 1968
Danbury, CT 06813
203-744-0100
http://www.rarediseases.org

National Organization on Fetal Alcohol Syndrome
1819 H Street N.W.
Suite 750
Washington, DC 20006
1-800-66NOFAS

Prader-Willi Syndrome Association
5700 Midnight Pass Road
Suite 6
Sarasota, FL 34242
http://www.pwsausa.org

The Arc of the United States (formerly the Association for Retarded Citizens of the US)
1010 Wayne Avenue, Suite 650
Silver Spring, MD 20852
301-565-3842
http://www.thearc.org

Williams Syndrome Association
P.O. Box 297
Clawson, MI 48017-0297
http://www.williams-syndrome.org

References

Alper, S. (2003). The relationship between inclusion and other trends in education. In D. Ryndak & S. Alper (Eds.), *Curriculum and instruction for students with significant disabilities in inclusive settings* (pp. 13–30). Boston: Allyn & Bacon.

American Academy of Pediatrics (AAP). (1999). Sterilization of minors with developmental disabilities. *Pediatrics, 104*(2), 337–340.

American Association on Mental Retardation (AAMR). (2002). *Mental retardation: Definition, classification, and systems of supports*. Washington, DC: American Association on Mental Retardation.

American Psychiatric Association (APA). (2000). *Diagnostic and statistical manual (DSM-IV-TR)*. Author.

Assistive Technology Act. (1988). Washington, DC: U.S. Government Printing Office.

Bailey, D., Skinner, D., & Sparkman, K. (2003). Discovering fragile X syndrome: Family experiences and perceptions. *Pediatrics, 111*(2), 407–416.

Baroff, G., & Olley, J. (1999). *Mental retardation: Nature, cause and management*. Philadelphia: Brunner/Mazel.

Batshaw, M., & Shapiro, B. (2002). Mental retardation. In M. Batshaw (Ed.), *Children with disabilities* (pp. 287–305). Baltimore: Paul H. Brookes.

Beirne-Smith, M., Ittenbach, R., & Patton, J. (2002). *Mental retardation*. Upper Saddle River, NJ: Merrill Prentice-Hall.

Burdett, P. (2001). Alternate assessment: Early highlights and pitfalls of reporting. *Assessment for Effective Intervention, 26*(2), 61–66.

Cantu, N., & Heumann, J. (2003). *Memorandum on harassment based on disability*. Washington, DC: U.S. Department of Education.

Carr, J. (2002). Down syndrome. In P. Howlin & O. Udwin (Eds.), *Outcomes in neurodevelopmental and genetic disorders* (pp. 169–197). Cambridge, UK: Cambridge University Press.

Cassidy, S. (2001). Prader-Willi syndrome. In S. Cassidy & J. Allanson (Eds.), *Management of genetic syndromes* (pp. 301–322). New York: Wiley-Liss.

Cawley, J., Hayden, S., Cade, E., & Baker-Kroczynski, S. (2002). Including students with disabilities into the general education science classroom. *Exceptional Children, 68*(4), 423–435.

Center for Applied Special Technology (CAST). (1999). *The National Center on Accessing the General Curriculum* [online]. Retrieved October 24, 2003 from http://www.cast.org/initiatives/national_center.html

Certo, N., Mautz, D., Pumpain, I., Sax, C., Smalley, K., Wade, H., Noyes, D., Luecking, R., Wechsler, J., & Batterman, N. (2003). A review and discussion of a model for seamless transition to adulthood. *Education and Training in Mental Retardation and Developmental Disabilities, 38*(1), 3–17.

Clarren, S., & Astley, S. (2001). Fetal alcohol syndrome. In S. Cassidy & J. Allanson (Eds.), *Management of genetic syndromes* (pp. 151–164). New York: Wiley-Liss.

Coombs-Richardson, R., & Meisgeier, C. (2001). *Discipline options: Establishing a positive school environment*. Norwood, MA: Christopher-Gordon.

Crane, L. (2002). *Mental retardation: A community integration approach*. Belmont, CA: Wadsworth/Thomson Learning.

Crocker, L. (2002). Stakeholders in comprehensive validation of standards-based assessments: A commentary. *Educational Measurement: Issues and Practice, 21*(1), 5–6.

Dykens, E., Hodapp, R., & Finucane, B. (2000). *Genetics and mental retardation syndromes: A new look at behavior and interventions*. Baltimore: Paul H. Brookes.

Fisher, K. (2004). Health disparities and mental retardation. *Journal of Nursing Scholarship, 36*(1), 48–53.

Fleitas, J. (2000). Sticks, stones, and the stigmata of childhood illness and disability. *Reclaiming Children and Youth, 9*(3), 146–150.

Graziano, A. (2002). *Developmental disabilities: Introduction to a diverse field*. Boston: Allyn & Bacon.

Hagerman, R. (2001). Fragile X syndrome. In S. Cassidy & J. Allanson (Eds.), *Management of genetic syndromes* (pp. 165–183). New York: Wiley-Liss.

Hagerman, R., & Hagerman, P. (2002). Fragile X syndrome. In P. Howlin & O. Udwin (Eds.), *Outcomes in neurodevelopmental and genetic disorders* (pp. 198–219). Cambridge, UK: Cambridge University Press.

Hardman, M., Drew, C., & Egan, M. (2002). *Human exceptionality: Society, school, and family* (7th ed.). Boston: Allyn & Bacon.

Hester, P. (2002). What schools can do to prevent behavior problems in schools. *Preventing School Failure, 47*(10), 33–38.

Hunter, A. (2001). Down syndrome. In S. Cassidy & J. Allanson (Eds.), *Management of genetic syndromes* (pp. 103–129). New York: Wiley-Liss.

Kameenui, E., & Simmons, D. (1999). *Toward successful inclusion of students with disabilities: The architecture of instruction*. Reston, VA: Council for Exceptional Children.

Kumin, L. (1994). *Communication skills in children with Down syndrome: A guide for parents*. Rockville, MD: Woodbin House.

Landford, A., & Cary, L. (2000). Graduation requirements for students with disabilities: Legal and practice considerations. *Remedial and Special Education, 21*(3), 152–160.

Lewis, R., & Doorlag, D. (2003). *Teaching special students in general education classrooms* (6th ed.). Upper Saddle River, NJ: Merrill Prentice-Hall.

Manset-Williamson, G., & Washburn, S. (2002). Administrators' perspectives of the impact of mandatory graduation qualifying examinations for students with hearing disabilities. *Journal of Special Education Leadership, 15*(2), 49–59.

McGuire D., & Chicoine, B. (2002). Life issues of adolescents and adults with Down syndrome. In W. Cohen, L. Nadel, & M. Madnick (Eds.), *Down syndrome: Visions for the 21st century* (pp. 221–236). New York: Wiley-Liss.

Meyer, G., & Batshaw, M. (2002). Fragile X syndrome. In M. Batshaw (Ed.), *Children with disabilities* (pp. 321–331). Baltimore: Paul H. Brookes.

Modell, S., & Valdez, L. (2002). Beyond bowling: Transition planning for students with disabilities. *Teaching Exceptional Children, 34*(6), 46–52.

Morris, C. (2001). Williams syndrome. In S. Cassidy & J. Allanson (Eds.), *Management of genetic syndromes* (pp. 517–533). New York: Wiley-Liss.

National Association of School Nurses (NASN). (2002). *School nurses and the individuals with Disabilities Education Act* [online]. Retrieved October 24, 2003 from http://www. nasn.org/briefs/idea.htm

Nativio, D. (2002). The genetics, diagnosis, and management of Prader-Willi syndrome. *Journal of Pediatric Health Care, 16*(6), 298–303.

Orkwis, R., & McLane, K. (1998). *A curriculum every student can use: Design principles for student access*. ERIC/OSEP Topical Brief. Reston, VA: ERIC/OSEP special project. Retrieved September 18, 2005 from http://www.cec.sped.org/osep/udesign.html

Nehring, W. (2004). Down syndrome. In P. Jackson Allen & J. Vessey (Eds.), *Primary care of the child with a chronic condition* (pp. 445–468). St. Louis: C. V. Mosby.

No Child Left Behind Act of 2001. (2002). Public Law 107-110. Retrieved September 18, 2005 from http://www.ed.gov/policy/elsec/leg/esea02/index.html

Oelwein, P. (1995). *Teaching reading to children with Down syndrome: A guide for parents and teachers*. Rockville, MD: Woodbin House.

O'Neill, P. (2001). Special education and high stakes testing: An analysis of current law and policy. *Journal of Law and Education, 30*(2), 185–222.

Peterson, R., & Skiba, R. (2001). Creating school climates that prevent school violence. *Social Studies, 92*(4), 167–175.

Pugach, M., & Warger, C. (2001). Curriculum matters: Raising expectations for students with disabilities. *Remedial and Special Education, 22*(4), 194–196.

Reinke, W., & Herman, K. (2002). Creating school environments that deter antisocial behaviors in youth. *Psychology in the Schools, 39*(5), 549–559.

Roizen, N. (2002). Down syndrome. In M. Batshaw (Eds.), *Children with disabilities* (pp. 307–320). Baltimore: Paul H. Brookes.

Semel, E., & Rosner, S. (2003). *Understanding Williams syndrome: Behavioral patterns and interventions*. Mahwah, NJ: Lawrence Erlbaum Associates.

Snow, C. (2003). *People first language: A commentary*. Retrieved October 22, 2003 from http://www.disabilityisnatural.com/peoplefirstlanguage.htm

Streissguth, A. (1997). *Fetal alcohol syndrome: A guide for families and communities*. Baltimore: Paul H. Brookes.

The Arc. (2003a). Individual service coordination for individuals with mental retardation. Retrieved October 23, 2003 from http://www.thearc.org/faqs/caseqa.html

The Arc. (2003b). *Introduction to mental retardation*. Retrieved October 22, 2003 from http://www.thearc.org/faqs/mrqa.html.

Turnbull, A., & Turnbull, R. (1997). *Parents, professionals, and exceptionality: A special partnership*. Upper Saddle River, NJ: Merrill Prentice-Hall.

Turnbull, R., Turnbull, A., Shank, M., Smith, S., & Leal, D. (2002). *Exceptional lives: Special education in today's schools* (3rd ed.). Upper Saddle River, NJ: Pearson.

Udwin, O. (2002). Williams and Smith-Magenis syndromes. In P. Howlin & O. Udwin (Eds.), *Outcomes in neurodevelopmental and genetic disorders* (pp. 299–325). Cambridge, UK: Cambridge University Press.

U.S. Department of Education (USDOE). (2003). *24th Annual Report to Congress on the Implementation of I.D.E.A.* Washington, DC: Author.

World Health Organization (WHO). (1993). *International statistical classification of diseases and related health problems* (10th revision). Geneva, Switzerland: WHO.

Chapter 36

Overweight Children: Making a Difference

NANCY W. MOSCA

Chapter Outline

INTRODUCTION

Overweight and obesity have become the fastest growing epidemics affecting Americans today. *Healthy People 2010*, the prevention agenda for the nation, has identified obesity as one of the top ten leading health indicators, underscoring the importance that obesity plays in negatively affecting the health status of Americans (U.S. Department of Health and Human Services [USDHHS], 2000).

The Surgeon General published *Call to action to prevent and decrease overweight and obesity* (USDHSS, 2001), making control of overweight and obesity a public health priority. This document called national attention to the obesity epidemic and identifies actions the nation can undertake to prevent and treat it.

Children have not been spared from this rising epidemic. The percentage of overweight children has increased, matching and surpassing that of the adult population. The percentage of young people who are overweight has more than doubled in the past 30 years. This is likely to result in earlier onset and increased prevalence of disease (U.S. Department of Agriculture, 2001). Schools have been identified as one of the contributing parties to the problem, as well as one of the hopes for a solution to curb overweight trends in the next generation of Americans. Because the school nurse is typically the only health professional in the school with daily student contact, it is logical that the school nurse's role would include assessment, prevention, and management of overweight children.

This chapter discusses the school nurse's role in prevention and management of overweight children from an individual student perspective, and a systems perspective.

DEFINITION

Obesity is an excess of adiposity, or body fat. It is "expressed either as the absolute fat mass (in units of kilograms) or alternatively, as the percentage of total body mass. Fat mass is highly correlated with body mass, while percent mass is relatively uncorrelated with body size" (Cole & Rolland-Cachera, 2002, p. 3).

With underwater weighing as the gold standard, there is currently no clinically practical method to measure body fat. Most methods rely on measurements of body weight as a surrogate for adiposity (Hoppin, 2004). Body Mass Index (BMI) has been established as a useful measure of overweight and obesity in adolescents and adults. Although not directly measuring body fat, BMI provides a reasonable estimate of adiposity (Dietz & Robinson, 1998). BMI is a calculated number using height and weight measurements (BMI = weight (kg)/height (m^2) or BMI = weight (lbs) × 703/height (in.)^2.

Childhood obesity is differentiated by the Centers for Disease Control and Prevention (CDC) into categories of "overweight" and "at risk for overweight" (Kuczmarski, Ogden, Grummer-Strawn et al., 2000). From the revised 2000 growth charts, "overweight" is defined as at or above the 95th percentile of body mass index (BMI) for age. "At risk for overweight" is defined as between the 85th and 94th percentile of BMI for age.

The 85th percentile on the CDC growth charts corresponds approximately to a BMI of 25 kg/m^2 by age 18 years, the definition of adult overweight. The 95th percentile on the CDC chart corresponds to about 30 kg/m^2 by age 18 years, the standard adult definition of obesity (Hoppin, 2004). Adult demarcations for obesity are further subdivided into obese (>30), moderately obese (>35), morbidly obese (>40), and super morbidly obese (>50) (Skelton, 2004). "The currently used cut points to categorize overweight and obesity in children, such as age- and gender-specific ≥85th and/or ≥95th percentile BMI or weight-for-height, are arbitrary statistical measures serving as reference values. They are not based on biological data linked to some estimate of adverse outcome" (Kimm & Obarzanek, 2002, p. 1005).

PREVALENCE OF THE PROBLEM

The increasing prevalence of childhood obesity in the United States has been well documented with national surveys and studies (Ogden, Flegal, Carroll, & Johnson, 2002; Strauss & Pollack, 2001). Since 1980, the prevalence of overweight has doubled for children 6 to 11 years of age and tripled for adolescents (Ogden et al., 2002). National data from the 1999–2000 National Health and Nutrition Examination Survey (NHANES) found the prevalence rate continuing to rise; 15.5% of adolescents 12 to 19 years of age were overweight; 15.3% of 6-through 11-year-olds were overweight; and more than 10% of 2- to 5-year-olds were overweight, as compared with 10.5%, 11.3%, and 7.2% prevalence, respectively, in 1988–1994 NHANES III data (Ogden et al., 2002). In 2005, CDC reported that 65% of adults are overweight and ≥ 16% of children 6-19 are overweight.

Some groups have a higher incidence of obesity than others. Non-Hispanic black and Mexican American teens, ages 12 to 19 years, had particularly high increases in overweight prevalence (greater than 10% since the NHANES III data). More than 21% of adolescents in these groups were overweight, significantly higher than the 12.7% for non-Hispanic white 12- to 19-year-olds; nearly 35% of African American teen girls and 30% of American Indian children are now overweight (CDC, 2005; Ogden et al., 2002; Strauss & Pollack, 2001).

ETIOLOGY

Although heredity does have a role in risk for overweight, the current rapid increase in the incidence of obesity cannot be attributed to genetic inheritance. The increase is occurring much too fast for genetic mutations to be implicated exclusively (Weinsier, Hunter, Heini, Goran, & Sell, 1998). Rather, interaction between biological, psychological, sociocultural, and environmental factors is the underpinning cause for childhood overweight (American Academy of Pediatrics [AAP] Committee on Nutrition, 2003). Modifiable risk factors for childhood overweight can be categorized into three groups: family, diet, and activity patterns.

Family Patterns

Genetic factors can explain 50% to 90% of the variation in BMI; however, in adoption studies, the genetic factors account for 20% to 60% of the variation. Therefore, it is thought that the impact of heredity on the obesity phenotype is between 30%

and 50% (Guillaume & Lissau, 2002). There is also empirical evidence that supports that genetics can impact on the success of diet programs for some individuals.

However, increased maternal BMI has also been shown to have a relationship with childhood overweight (Arluk, Branch, Swain, & Dowling, 2003). Nearly 75% of children with two obese parents will become obese themselves and 25% to 50% of children with one obese parent will become obese (Skelton, 2004). Parental obesity is a strong predictor up to age 3 years, when the child's own overweight status becomes an equal predictor for adult obesity. Between 6 and 10 years, the child's BMI begins to be a strong predictor for later overweight (Magarey, Daniels, Boulton, & Cockington, 2003; Whitaker, Wright, Pepe, Seidel, & Dietz, 1997). Low socioeconomic status coupled with maternal obesity has also been demonstrated as a predictor of overweight in children (Strauss & Knight, 1999).

Attitudes and behaviors of parents affect how children behave in relation to food and exercise. Children model their parents' habits. Parents' preferences for high-fat, high-calorie foods limit young children's acceptance of a variety of healthy foods (Birch & Fisher, 1998).

Diet Patterns

The American diet has undergone significant change in one generation's time, and today's children's nutritional intake is reflective of this change. "Over the past 20–30 years, the overall caloric intake has increased approximately 200 kilocalories per day....A positive energy balance of 120 kilocalories per day will produce a 50 kilogram increase in weight over 20 years" (Skelton, 2004, p. 9). (Note: As an example of calorie content, a 10-ounce glass of soda contains 120 calories.)

With the increase of one-parent families, two-parent working families, and busy family activity schedules, family mealtime and quality intake have suffered. The percentage of children and adolescents ages 9 to 14 eating daily dinner with their families ranges from 50% to 35%, with a decreasing pattern as the child ages (Gillman et al., 2000). However, children who eat meals with their families consume more fruits and vegetables, less carbonated soda, less fried foods, less saturated and trans-fat foods, and more fiber than those who do not (Gillman et al., 2000). "Ninety-one percent of children, ages 6 to 11 years, are not consuming the recommended 5 servings of fruit and vegetables per day, averaging 2.5 servings daily" (Copperman & Jacobson, 2004, p. 25).

The Youth Risk Behavior Survey findings show American adolescents are also drinking less milk and eating less than recommended amounts of fruits and vegetables (Centers for Disease Control and Prevention [CDC], 2004c). Only 17% of students reported drinking three or more glasses of milk per day during the seven days preceding the survey. Only 22% reported eating five or more servings of fruits and vegetables during the same time frame.

More families are relying on fast food meals and processed prepared food purchases to provide "quick" nourishment for families with little time to eat, or if parents have little time or energy available to cook a meal. Ready-made, convenience foods in grocery stores are higher in fat and sugar content. Food prepared away from home accounts for more than 40% of a family's food expenditure (U.S. Department of Labor [USDL], 2004). The proportion of foods that children consume from fast food establishments and restaurants has increased nearly 300% in less than one generation's time, with notable increases in soft drink consumption (St-Onge, Keller, & Heymsfield, 2003; Troiano, Briefel, Carroll, & Bialostosky, 2000). A typical child eating a fast food meal will consume more calories per gram of food, more total fat, more total carbohydrates, and less fiber that a child not eating fast food (Bowman, Gortmaker, Ebbleling, Pereira, & Ludwig, 2004). Portion size has increased, with the familiar "super-size" option becoming the norm (Nielsen & Popkin, 2003). Most students cannot even recognize what a normal portion size is. Most foods advertised to children and adolescents on television are high in fat and or salt. The schools are also at fault. "Nearly 93% of high schools have vending machines, stores, or snack bars, but only 21 percent sell low-fat yogurt, fruits, or vegetables" (Skelton, 2004, p. 9). In addition, lunch periods have been cut to as little as 20 minutes, impacting on the types of foods served and the development of slower eating practices with time to be aware of the sensations of hunger and satiety.

Finally, food is often used as a reward for good behavior. This practice is started early in the child's life and has often been incorporated into classroom activities (Kubik, Lytle, Hannan, Story, & Perry, 2002). Some families also engage in the practice of mandating that the vegetables or meat be eaten in order to get the "prize" of a dessert. This gives the wrong message regarding eating.

Activity Patterns

There has been a dramatic decline (up to 83%) in physical activity of American children between the ages of 9 and 19 years (CDC, 2004c; Kimm et al., 2002). CDC reports that only 38% of children ages 9 to 13 years participated in organized physical activity, and 77% of children engaged in free-time physical activity during nonschool hours (CDC, 2003b). Hispanic and black children were less likely to participate in organized physical activity compared to white, non-Hispanic children, as were children of parents with lower incomes and educational levels.

In 2003, one-third of high school students did not engage in the minimum recommended level of moderate or vigorous physical activity (CDC, 2004c). Male adolescents were more likely to engage in vigorous activity than females, and non-Hispanic white female adolescents were more active than black female adolescents. In addition, fewer than 8% of school-age children have daily physical education (Skelton, 2004), and many schools only require physical education for a few months of the academic year.

Several reasons contribute to the decreased physical activity of school-age children. Safe communities are one reason. With escalating crime rates, violence, and child abductions in the local news, parents have resorted to limiting their children's unsupervised outdoor playtime. Consequently, many children coming home after school are required to stay indoors until the parent(s) come home from work. Children turn to television viewing and computer gaming to occupy their time, both sedentary activities. TV watching is an activity that is also highly correlated with snacking.

Nationally, 38% of adolescents reported watching television for 3 or more hours per school day. Children with a TV in their bedroom watch approximately 38 minutes more per day than their peers (Skelton, 2004). The percentage of black female adolescents reporting watching 3 or more hours of television per school day was highest, at 70%. Overall, the prevalence of ≥ 3 hours/day of television viewing was higher among black (67%) and Hispanic (45%) than white (29%) students; higher among black female (70%) and Hispanic female (45%) than white female (26%) students; and higher among black male (64%) and Hispanic male (46%) than white male (31.7%) students (CDC, 2004c).

The relationship of obesity to sedentary activity of television and computer gaming is well documented (Crespo et al., 2001; Giammattei, Blix, Marshak, Wolitzer, & Pettitt, 2003; Robinson, 2001). By age 11, children watching 3 or more hours of television per day had significantly more body fat than children watching less than 2 hours per day (Proctor et al., 2003). In longitudinal data from the Framingham Children's Study, higher levels of physical activity during childhood led to less body fat acquisition by the time children turned 11 years old (Moore et al., 2003).

CONSEQUENCES OF AN OVERWEIGHT CHILDHOOD AND ADOLESCENCE

As illustrated in Figure 36.1, a student who has dietary and activity lifestyle risk factors leading to obesity begins a cycle of weight gain that contributes further to decreased physical activity and leads to other health complications. Chronic conditions once reserved for adults are now appearing with increased frequency in children and adolescents who are overweight. Using data from the Bogalusa Heart Study, Freedman and colleagues (1999) found that 60% of 5- to 10-year-olds who were overweight had at least one biochemical or clinical risk factor for cardiovascular disease, and 20% had two or more risk factors. Later analysis demonstrated the relationship of childhood obesity to heart disease as adults (Freedman, Khan, Dietz, Srinivasan, & Berenson, 2001).

Persistence of Obesity into Adulthood

The risk of obesity persisting into adult life is higher with more severe overweight and obesity in childhood and adolescence. About 40% of overweight children will continue to have increased weight during adolescence and 75% to 80% of obese adolescents become obese adults (Alemzadeh, Rising, Cedillo, & Lifshitz, 2003). In one study, "the most significant determinant of percentage of body fat at 10 years of age was percentage of body fat at 5 years of age" (Salbe, Weyer, Lindsay, Ravussin, & Tataranni, 2002, p. 299).

Hypertension

Hypertension is not a common finding in children. Although it is rare, increasing rates of hypertension have been noted in overweight children. As early as preschool, children who are overweight have been found to have higher blood pressure readings than their peers of normal weight (Hernandez, Uphold, Graham, & Singer, 1998). Overweight students are twice as likely to have elevated diastolic blood pressure readings and four times as likely to have elevated systolic blood pressure readings (Freedman et al., 1999). Prevalence of hypertension in children and adolescents has been shown to increase progressively as the BMI percentile increases (Sorof, Lai, Turner, Poffenbarger, & Portman, 2004).

The relationship between overweight in children and elevated systolic blood pressures was demonstrated regardless of parental history of hypertension (Nishina et al., 2003). Blood pressure elevations may not reach the point of hypertension

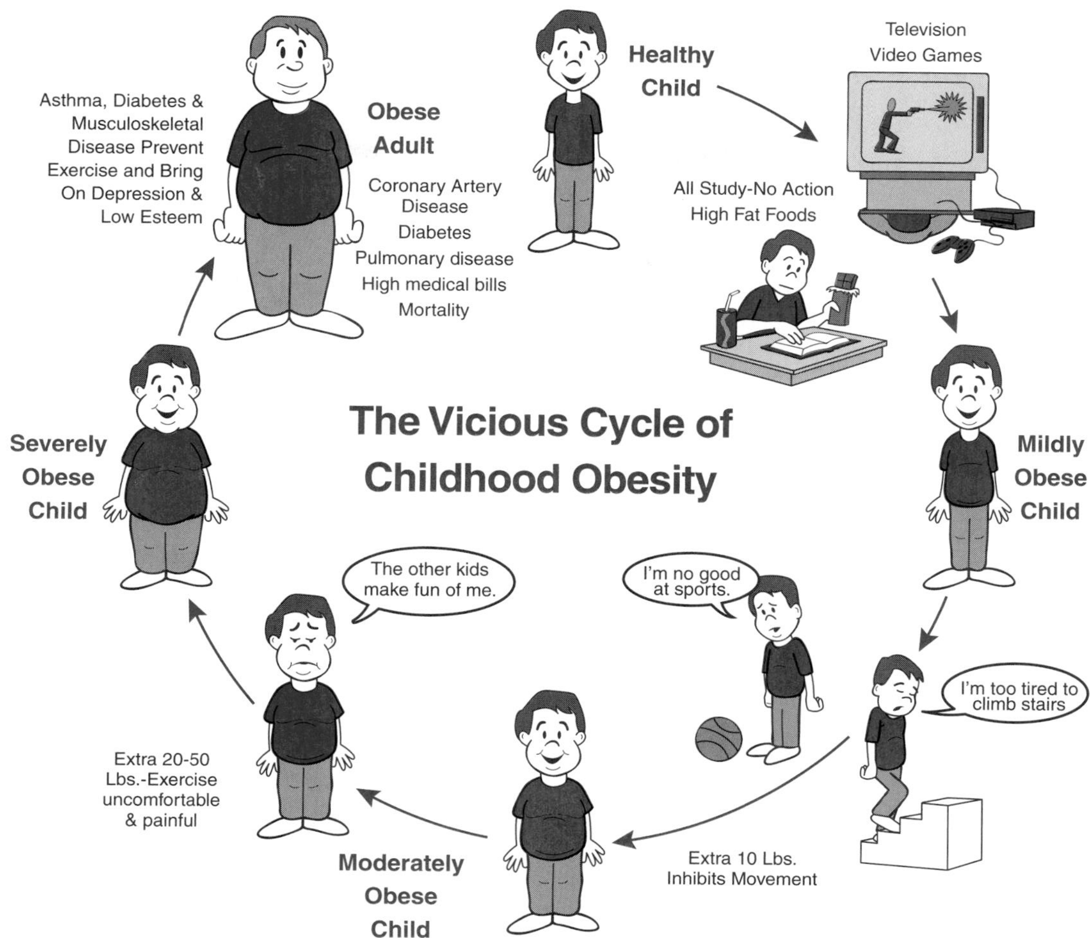

Figure 36.1 ■ The vicious cycle of childhood obesity. (Reprinted with permission from Sothern, M., von Almen, K., & Schumacher, H. [2001]. Trim Kids: The proven 12-week plan that has helped thousands of children achieve a healthier weight. HarperResource, at http://www.trimkids.com)

during childhood; however, it is clear that blood pressure of overweight children is moving in that direction. In one study, "children with BMI<85th percentile had a hypertension prevalence of only 2.6%. In comparison, children with BMI>95th percentile had a hypertension prevalence of 10.7%" (Sorof et al., 2004, p. 279).

Hyperlipidemia

Screening for hyperlipidemia was rarely considered for the typical child seen in a pediatric practice. Now elevated levels of cholesterol, triglycerides, and low-density lipoproteins coupled with low levels of high-density lipoproteins are seen with more regularity in overweight children and adolescents (Srinivasan, Myers, & Berenson, 2002a; Steinberger & Daniels, 2003). The incidence of children diagnosed with nonalcoholic fatty liver disease, a disease related to obesity, liver cell injury from free fatty acid toxicity, hyperinsulinemia, and insulin resistance is rising as the prevalence of overweight in children has risen (Roberts, 2003). These put young people at risk for cardiac disease as adults. Even though the symptoms may not be evident during childhood, it is recognized that atherosclerosis often begins during the childhood years (Alemzadeh et al., 2003).

Diabetes Mellitus, Type 2

Until recently, type 2 diabetes mellitus was rarely seen in children or adolescents. Type 2 diabetes mellitus is now a public health problem, representing up to 45% of all diabetes reported among children and adolescents (Aye & Levitsky, 2003). The incidence of type 2 diabetes mellitus among adolescents is increasing parallel to the national rise in overweight teens. Signs of insulin resistance and impaired glucose tolerance are now seen in children and adolescents who are overweight (Sinha et al., 2002). Overweight in children has been demonstrated to be a powerful predictor of the development of insulin resistance syndrome (Srinivasan, Myers, & Berenson, 2002b). One study demonstrated that 4% of obese adolescents referred to an obesity clinic had undiagnosed type 2 diabetes. This was in addition to the 21% of obese children and 25% of obese adolescents who already had impaired glucose tolerance (Estrada, 2004). This increased prevalence of school-age children and adolescents with diabetes increases the need for greater levels of school nursing services than in the past (see Chapter 33).

Asthma

A strong independent association between obesity and asthma has been observed in several studies of school-age children and adolescents (Gennuso, Epstein, Paluch, & Cerny, 1998; Luder, Melnik, & DiMaio, 1998; Rodriguez, Winkleby, Ahn, Sundquist, & Kraemer, 2002). An association of overweight and asthma was also identified in primary grade school girls (von Kries, Hermann, Grunert, & von Mutius, 2001) and school-age boys (Gilliland et al., 2003). Inner-city, overweight children used more medicine, wheezed more, and had more emergency room visits than their non-overweight counterparts (Belamarich et al., 2000). Increased frequency and severity of asthma symptoms have been associated with dietary fat intake (Spector & Surette, 2003).

The frequency and degree of bronchospasm in children with asthma are significantly greater in those who are also obese (Estrada, 2004). "The work of breathing is increased in obese individuals and larger body mass places increased demands for oxygen consumption and carbon dioxide elimination" (Alemzadeh et al., 2003, p. 824). While exercise may induce asthma symptoms, weight loss improves lung function in those with asthma.

Musculoskeletal Disorders

Overweight children carry a great deal more weight on their immature skeletons than leaner children, consequently requiring stronger bones at an earlier age. Yet, these children do not acquire greater bone mass, leaving them at risk for injury (Goulding, Taylor, Jones, Manning, & Williams, 2002). Obese adolescents are also at higher risk for slipped capital femoral epiphysis because of increased weight on the cartilaginous growth plate of the hip (Frelut & Flodmark, 2002).

Sleep Disorders

Poor sleep quality has been associated with childhood obesity. Obese adolescents sleep less than nonobese adolescents, and their sleep disturbance influences their daytime physical activity level (Gupta, Mueller, Chan, & Meininger, 2002). The occurrence of sleep-related breathing disorders in 6- to 11-year-old Hispanic and white children was associated with overweight as well as elevated blood pressure (Enright, Goodwin, Sherrill, Quan, & Quan, 2003). Sleep apnea occurs in approximately 7% of obese children and adolescents (Cooperberg & Faith, 2004).

Early Sexual Maturation

Obesity appears to have an impact on the development of sexual maturity, with opposite findings for boys and girls. Overweight girls experience early sexual maturation, while overweight boys are more likely to have delayed sexual maturation. Sexual maturation is associated with body fatness in females, and early-maturing females are more likely to be obese during adolescence and into adulthood than average and late-maturing females (Adair & Gordon-Larsen, 2001). Early-maturing boys have lower BMIs and tend to be taller than late-maturing counterparts (Wang, 2002).

With menarche occurring earlier, contraception use may also be initiated at an earlier age. Adolescent girls who are obese use contraceptive pills more often than other contraceptive devices. Since risk of complications from oral contraceptive use increases with the severity of obesity, these girls should be carefully evaluated and monitored, especially related to deep vein thrombosis (Frelut & Flodmark, 2002).

Psychosocial Issues

In many obese children and adolescents, the most common consequences of obesity are psychosocial. Stigmatization of obese children by other children has markedly increased. Children today are 40% more likely to stigmatize obese children than their peers of the 1960s (Latner & Stunkard, 2003). Five- and seven-year-old overweight girls reported lower self-concept with peer teasing and parent criticism (Davison & Birch, 2002). Overweight children have been characterized as more likely to be teased, bullied, and rejected by their peers (Frelut & Flodmark, 2002; MacNeil & Newell, 2004).

Overweight girls as young as 9 years old exhibit signs of decreased social acceptance, poor body image, and lower self-worth (Kimm et al., 2002a). Obese adolescents show lower levels of self-esteem by early adolescence, with females demonstrating lower self-esteem more often than males. Children and adolescents with decreasing levels of self-esteem demonstrate higher rates of sadness, loneliness, and nervousness, and are more likely to engage in high-risk behaviors such as smoking or consuming alcohol (Strauss, 2000).

Mental Health Issues

Adolescents with depression are at risk for obesity and those who are obese are at risk for depression. Goodman and Whitaker (2002) identified an association between depression and obesity in adolescents. Teens who were identified as depressed and overweight were significantly more likely to be obese 1 year later, compared with teens who were not depressed. They also found that normal weight teens who had depressive characteristics were more likely to become overweight a year later when compared with normal weight teens without depressive characteristics. Mustillo et al. (2003) demonstrated an association between obesity and psychiatric disorders in a trajectory from childhood into adolescence. Both oppositional defiant disorder and depression were associated with overweight children as they moved into adolescence.

School Performance Issues

An association has been made between obesity and low school performance, especially around the ages of 10 and 11 (Guillaume & Lissau, 2002). "Obese children and adolescents were also 4 times more likely than healthy children to report impaired school function" (Estrada, 2004, p. 22). If sleep apnea is present, the student may be tired and unable to concentrate. Many students who are obese engage in severe dieting, and go to school without breakfast. Those who fast or do not eat an adequate breakfast have demonstrated slower memory recall, increased errors, and slower stimulus discrimination (Lucas, 2004).

ASSESSING CHILDREN IN THE SCHOOL SETTING

When to Screen

In the past, school nurses monitored annual height and weight measures of students and plotted percentiles on growth charts; this routine screening has become less common throughout the United States. Ideally, growth screening should take place each year in a school child's life (AAP Committee on School Health, 2000). Universal school-based screening is supported by current research because of low identification rates by physicians of children at risk for overweight (Demerath et al., 2003). Because most school systems do not have school nurse-to-student ratios that would allow for this type of comprehensive school screening program or no longer require this screening, a compromise would be to conduct school screenings at critical times.

Kindergarten is one of the more common periods during which school nurses screen children for height and weight. This is certainly an excellent time to get baseline information on an incoming cohort of students. CDC recommends using the BMI-for-age charts and recording percentile or percentile ranges (Kuczmarski et al., 2000).

A second point in time to conduct growth screening in schools might be in the latency period of childhood, before the growth spurt. This would be around age 10 years, or grade 5 for most students. This period has been found to be a strong predictor of later obesity (Guo, Wu, Chumlea, & Roche, 2002). Kimm et al. (2002) demonstrated a doubling of obesity prevalence between the ages of 9 and 10 years through the adolescent years. Screening at this point would allow overweight and at-risk students to be identified before the adolescent period.

During a student's growth spurt, his or her caloric intake and energy expenditure may or may not worsen an "at-risk" or "overweight" state. With appropriate intervention at this time, a student who was at-risk or overweight prior to the growth spurt may have a BMI within the normal range at the end of the growth spurt.

Since adolescence represents the period of greatest risk for developing adult obesity (Magarey et al., 2003; Steinberger, Moran, Hong, Jacobs, & Sinaiko, 2001), at least one screening should take place during the teen years, preferably at the early high school level after the pubescent growth spurt. Ideally, this assessment should be coordinated to coincide with health education lessons on nutrition and physical activity as part of healthy weight management.

A series of measures over time are valuable in illustrating a student's pattern of growth. Growth is a fundamental characteristic of childhood and adolescence. Growth in children and adolescents is as unique as the individual student. Different degrees of increases in height and weight are expected at different ages. Deviations from the student's normal growth pattern may be early warning signs of some intrinsic illness/disease process or environmental insult. These deviations warrant referral. It should be noted that a student's height and weight may be measured on an individual basis at any time because of a concern for growth or general wellness.

Measures to Screen for Obesity

Multiple measures are available to attempt to identify those who are overweight, but they are either too expensive (i.e., the DEXA scan [dual-energy X-ray absorptiometry], computed tomography [CT] or magnetic resonance imaging [MRI]), impractical, or have poor reliability (skinfold thickness using calipers to measure subcutaneous fat and anthropometrics [waist to hip ratios]). Therefore BMI, which includes height and weight measurements, has been considered the best screening tool.

BMI is not an exact science related to children. It does not differentiate between body fat and lean body mass. It has a weaker correlation with body fat than skinfolds, but it has better reliability. The variables that can interfere with an accurate determination of BMI include the influences of puberty on body fat; increased muscle mass; ethnic differences in height and weight; and poor measurement technique (Skelton, 2004).

The Process

The protocol for completing weight screenings is similar for all screenings. Chapter 20 provides extensive detail on the screening process. As with all screening programs, it is first necessary to clarify if a legal or district mandate exists for screening and to have the support of the administration. A decision should be made as to which groups should be screened and whether permission from parents is needed. Even if permission is not required, it is helpful to send a letter home to parents to explain what will be done, why it is necessary, and when it will occur. Staff should be informed of what will occur, information about the obesity epidemic and the potential complications that arise from being overweight as a child or adolescent, and how they can assist in the process. Students should also be informed.

The most important component of an assessment is to ensure that the equipment is in a place that will guarantee privacy. Students who are already overweight may be very uncomfortable getting on a scale, especially in front of peers. Even if a private location is available, the school nurse needs to be sensitive to the student to ensure that the number is not stated out loud. Writing it down on a piece of paper and showing it to the student is sufficient and preserves confidentiality.

Once height and weights have been obtained, the BMI can be calculated. In 2000, BMI-for-age percentile charts were introduced for the first time with the publication of new growth charts from the CDC. There is now a normed reference tool for identifying children and adolescents as overweight or at risk for overweight. Determining a BMI-for-age is a three-step process. The first step is calculating the BMI value; step two is plotting the BMI value according to the student's age and gender to arrive at the BMI-for-age percentile; and the third step involves interpreting the BMI-for-age percentile finding.

Step One: Calculate the BMI.

Determining the student's BMI requires accurate height and weight measures (Table 36.1). The difference of an inch or more in height, or weight that is off by several pounds, may cause a student to be mislabeled. Standardized instructions for measuring height and weight and BMI can be found on the CDC Web site, http://www.cdc.gov/growthcharts.

The CDC tables can be used to determine the value (see Chapters 16 and 20). They can be accessed at http://www.cdc.gov/nccdphp/dnpa/bmi/00binaries/bmi-checkbook.pdf. These tables cross list height and weight measures in both metric and English units and do not require any mathematical calculations. Another method for determining a BMI value without calculation is by using a BMI wheel, which is approximately the size of a CD, and permits quick determination of a BMI value by aligning the height and weight measurements on the wheel. These wheels are inexpensive and can be purchased through most school nurse supply catalogs.

Another method to determine BMI is to use an online calculator such as the one on the CDC growth chart Web site at http://www.cdc.gov/nccdphp/dnpa/bmi/calc-bmi.htm. This calculator provides a BMI value after entering the height and weight measurements. Software programs for computerized health records typically have the capability to calculate BMI-for-age percentiles when the height, weight, age, and gender are entered.

Table 36.1 ■ BMI FORMULAS

Metric	weight (kg)/height (m^2)
English	weight (lbs.) × 703/height $(in)^2$

Source: Tools for Calculating Body Mass Index at http://www.cdc.gov/nccdphp/dnpa/growthcharts/bmi_tools.htm

Box 36.1 ■■■

BMI FOR AGE GROWTH CHARTS FOR BOYS AND GIRLS

Files can be downloaded for print quality at:

BMI-for-age percentiles 2 to 20 years: BOYS http://www.cdc.gov/nchs/data/nhanes/growthcharts/set1/all.pdf

BMI-for-age percentiles 2 to 20 years: GIRLS http://www.cdc.gov/nchs/data/nhanes/growthcharts/set1/all.pdf.

Step Two: Plot BMI Value to Determine BMI for Age Percentile.

Once the BMI is determined, the student's age and gender are used to select the appropriate growth chart. There are separate growth charts for girls and boys (Box 36.1). Using the gender-correct growth chart titled "BMI-for-Age," find the student's age on the horizontal axis and the BMI on the vertical axis. The point of intersection is the student's BMI-for-age percentile (Kuczmarski et al., 2000).

Step Three: Interpret BMI-for-Age Percentile Score (Table 36.2).

This is perhaps the most difficult portion of the process. For adults, it is easy to classify them according to their BMI number. However, knowing that the predictive value is not as solid for children as for adults, as well as knowing the factors that could intervene in the interpretation, the school nurse must be careful in how the findings are communicated.

While the International Task Force on Obesity recommends the BMI percentile for screening, it is recognized that evidence is lacking that a particular BMI in childhood is associated with significant morbidity as an adult (Skelton, 2004). Take, for example, an 11th grade football player who eats right, exercises regularly, and lifts weights to prepare for his role on the school team. He is 16.5 years of age, with a height of 69", and weighs 210 pounds. He has virtually no body fat, yet his BMI would be 30.1. His BMI percentile is above the 95th percentile and care must be taken to ensure that he is not mislabeled as obese.

It is also important for the school nurse to have checked to see if there had been any significant changes since the last measurements were done. There should be some consistency with measurements from previous screenings for this student. A significant percentile change should be rechecked for errors in measuring, recording, or graphing. Once a significant change is confirmed, the parents should be notified, with suggestions made that they share this information with their child's healthcare provider.

Table 36.2 ■
BMI-FOR-AGE PERCENTILE CATEGORIES

Overweight	BMI for age percentile $\geq$95th
At risk for overweight	BMI for age between 85th and 94th percentile
Normal range	BMI for age between 5th and 84th percentile
Underweight	BMI for age < 5th percentile

Source: CDC at http://www.cdc.gov/nccdphp/dnpa/bmi/bmi-for-age.htm

Reporting Results to the Family

Results should be reported to the family in a meaningful format. Avoid complicated graphs without clear explanation and avoid making a "judgment" about the weight issue. Information should be sent home in a way that ensures privacy. See Figure 36.2 for a sample parent letter.

PREVENTION APPROACHES IN THE SCHOOL SETTING

Opportunities to intervene at the individual student level with prevention measures occur daily for a school nurse. Messages about healthy eating and physical activity should be evident not only in the health office, but throughout the school. Bulletin boards, Web sites, school nurse columns in newsletters, and video messages can all be avenues to promote healthy eating and regular physical activity to prevent overweight. Health information provided to students and families should be accurate and developmentally appropriate. Professional sources should be consulted for information when writing newsletters, posting information on Web sites or displaying bulletin boards. The Resources section at the end of this chapter provides multiple Web sites that can be accessed for information and materials related to

ANYWHERE COMMUNITY SCHOOL DISTRICT
Health Services
Report of Height and Weight Screening

Dear Parent or Guardian:

Your child's growth is important because it is an indicator of overall health. A child's growth is determined by monitoring a child's height and weight over time. As part of our continuing effort to help ensure our students' health, we have measured your child's height and weight. The results are recorded below:

HEIGHT ______________ **WEIGHT** ______________
BMI-FOR-AGE PERCENTILE: ______________________

Body mass index (BMI) is a measure of body heaviness, and an indirect measure of body fat. According to the Centers for Disease Control and Prevention, a BMI-for-age greater than the 85th percentile or lower than the 5th percentile may be a health risk for your child. Your child's BMI-for-age was in the following percentile grouping:

________ At or above the 95th percentile (considered overweight)
________ 85th – 94th percentile (considered to be "at risk" for becoming overweight)
________ 5th – 84th percentile (considered average or typical, most children are in this group)
________ Below the 5th percentile (considered underweight)

If your child is at or above the 95th percentile, or below the 5th percentile, we recommend you contact your family doctor to discuss your child's health. If your child is between the 85th and 94th percentile, bring these findings to your family doctor's attention on your child's next scheduled visit.

Most children manage to reach a healthy weight range with daily physical activity and eating nutritious meals and snacks. Dieting to lose or gain weight is rarely needed for children, and should not be done without first discussing it with your doctor.

If you do not have a doctor or health insurance for your child, or need help finding health care, you can call the local health department at (area code)-123–4567.

If you have questions, would like information on available community resources, or would like to discuss these results with the school nurse, please call (area code)-555–5555.

______________________ ______________
(School Nurse) (Date)

Figure 36.2 ■ Sample letter to the parents.

healthy eating and exercise as well as current information on obesity and overweight in children and adolescents.

Role modeling is the ultimate prevention message to students in the school environment. However, one's own failing to engage in regular physical activity, or struggle with obesity, should not be a deterrent to advocating a healthy lifestyle for the next generation. Avoidance of the issue sends a message of its own. Healthy life choices do not come without some struggle, and for some, the struggle is daily. Recognizing this with students presents a realistic message.

Diet

Food remedies for minor ailments should be prescribed cognizant of the healthy eating behavior message they send. For example, the student who did not eat breakfast and comes to the school nurse for a stomachache will hear about the values of eating breakfast, but may also be provided with a serving of instant oatmeal versus a no- or low-fiber sweetened cereal choice. Diets rich in whole grain have been associated with greater insulin sensitivity and lower BMI's in adolescents (Steffen et al., 2003). Providing healthy food selections in the clinic should be a standard of care. Many nurses stock juice, crackers, cookies, cereals and the like for student needs. Choosing healthy food options that accomplish the same goal is a modification every school nurse can make. Displaying or distributing candy should be avoided, as it reinforces the negative message that sweets provide comfort.

American Heart Association guidelines for a healthy diet for children older than 2 years include total fat intake that averages no more than 30% of the total calories with saturated fat limited to 7% to 10% of total calories, and dietary cholesterol limited to no more than 300 mg daily. The dietary fiber intake guideline is "age plus 5" for children older than 2 years. For example, a 5-year-old should eat 5 + 5, or 10 grams of fiber per day. Once an adolescent's caloric intake approaches 1,500 calories or more, 25 grams of fiber should be consumed daily (Williams et al., 2002). Box 36.2 lists some helpful messages to give children and adolescents in schools.

Box 36.2 ■■■

HEALTHY EATING TIPS FOR STUDENTS IN SCHOOL

- Eat breakfast every morning before school.
- Choose healthy options from the school lunch choices and vending machines.
- Drink milk with lunch.
- Include fiber with every meal.
- Eat five servings of fruits and vegetables every day.
- Drink plenty of water.
- Eat a variety of different foods.

Physical Activity

Higher levels of physical activity during childhood lead to less body fat acquisition by adolescence (Moore et al., 2003). Promoting physical activity to every student is powerful prevention for later overweight. Physical activity is correlated with lower fasting insulin and greater insulin sensitivity in childhood, which, if consistently practiced over time, may reduce the incidence of type 2 diabetes in children and adolescents (Schmitz et al., 2002). Increasing time elementary students spend in physical education, by as little as one extra hour per week, has been demonstrated to reduce BMI-for-age percentiles for students overweight or at risk for overweight in kindergarten (Datar & Strum, 2004).

School nurses can recommend physical exercise as a remedy for stress-related complaints that students bring to the health office. A treadmill, stationary bike, or jogging trampoline in the health clinic can be a source of stress relief, and a positive health message as well. Equipment may be justified with increased numbers of insulin-dependent students who need opportunities to be physically active during the school day in concert with their diet and insulin regimen.

According to the American Heart Association, all children older than age 2 should engage in at least 30 minutes of fun, moderate-intensity activities every day (Williams et al., 2002). Elementary school age children should approach a minimum of 60 minutes of activity per day (Patrick, Spear, Holt, & Sofka, 2001). This 30 to 60 minutes can be broken down into 15-minute, or 10-minute sessions of vigorous activity, chosen for age, gender, and physical and emotional developmental level appropriateness.

Family Involvement

Anticipatory guidance throughout the school years can help parents prepare for the challenges of their child's behavior and provide them knowledge and strategies to guide their child with healthy choices (Gottesman, 2003). For example, messages to children to clean their plate should be discouraged, recognizing that children will stop eating when they are full. Using food for reward or withholding food as a punishment are control issues that parents need to understand can contribute to undesirable eating behaviors. Parents' negative comments about a child's appearance, weight, or athletic ability could also result in reinforcing negative behaviors (Story, Holt, & Sofka, 2002).

Parents should be complimented and provided with positive reinforcement for behavior they exhibit that is in their child's best interest. Any time a parent comes into school is an opportunity to compliment them on their child's health behaviors. However small the initiative, it should be noted. Parents are the most powerful role models for children, including in their nutritional and exercise behaviors. Box 36.3 lists helpful tips to give to parents related to diet and physical activity.

Box 36.3 ■ ■ ■

HEALTHY TIPS FOR PARENTS OF SCHOOL-AGE CHILDREN AND ADOLESCENTS

Help children to eat breakfast.

- Provide healthy foods that are fast and convenient: yogurt, cottage cheese, fruit, low-fat whole-grain bars, fresh fruit pieces.
- Help your child get organized so he or she has time to eat breakfast.
- Prepare the breakfast the night before. (If breakfast is prepared and ready in advance, the school-age child is more likely to eat, not having to wait for food to be prepared that morning. Examples are hard boiled eggs and whole wheat waffles, that now just need to be warmed up in the microwave in the morning, and oranges that are peeled the night before and ready to eat.)
- Offer food on the run, if your child is late, such as fruit, trail mix, or a whole grain breakfast bar.

Help children eat more fruits and vegetables.

- Keep a variety of fruits and vegetables on hand at home
- Have cleaned and cut-up fruits and vegetables available and in the refrigerator for snacking.
- Purchase only 100% juice products.
- Serve two or more vegetables with dinner.
- Serve salads that include a variety of vegetables, and even fruit pieces.

(Continued on the following page)

Box 36.3

HEALTHY TIPS FOR PARENTS OF SCHOOL-AGE CHILDREN AND ADOLESCENTS *(Continued)*

- Pack fruits or vegetables cut and ready to eat in your child's back pack to eat at school.
- Use plenty of vegetables in soups, casseroles, and sauces.
- Offer a variety of fruits and vegetables often as snacks.
- Be a role model for your child; eat more fruits and vegetables yourself.
- Plant a garden.

Help children get enough calcium in their diet.

- Serve low-fat or fat-free milk at every meal.
- Flavor milk with strawberry or chocolate syrup if necessary.
- Cut up cheese cubes, or have string cheese for snacking.
- Keep flavored yogurts and puddings made with low-fat or no-fat milk available.
- Cook with low-fat dairy products in soups and casseroles.
- Serve broccoli and collard and turnip greens, all high in calcium.

Eat healthy together as a family.

- Make grocery shopping and food preparation a family activity.
- Buy healthy ready-to-eat foods from the store.
- Choose healthy take-out foods.
- When eating together, turn the TV off, don't answer the phone, spend time talking about your day.
- Eat together at different times. For example eat lunch together one day, and breakfast or dinner another.

Encourage children to eat healthy foods.

- Serve new foods and regional and ethnic foods.
- Don't fight over food with your child/teenager.
- Keep a variety of healthy foods in the house.
- Limit the availability of high-fat and high-sugar foods.
- Keep a bowl of fruit on the kitchen table or counter.
- Be a role model; practice healthy eating behaviors yourself.

Help teens make healthy choices when away from home.

- Encourage your teenager to buy healthy foods at school, stores, restaurants, and vending machines.
- Look at menus with your teenager and discuss healthy food choices and appropriate portions. Find foods low in fat, sugar, and calories.
- Encourage your teenager to eat salads with low-calorie dressings, and broiled or baked meats.
- Encourage your teenager to avoid eating fried foods, or to reduce the serving size.
- Teach your teenager to ask for changes to make foods healthier, such as asking the waitress to "hold the mayonnaise."

Help children and teens be more active.

- Encourage active, spur of the moment physical activity, such as dancing to music.
- Limit the time your child watches television and plays computer games to 1 or 2 hours a day.
- For every hour your child reads, watches television, and plays computer games, encourage him or her to take a 10-minute physical activity break.
- Give your child household chores, such as shoveling snow, raking leaves, or walking the dog.
- Help your child find physical activities that are fun and not too difficult or embarrassing.
- Use the stairs instead of taking an elevator, walk instead of riding in a car whenever daily life allows.
- Enroll your child in planned physical activities such as swimming, martial arts, or dancing.
- Participate in physical activity together: play ball, go bowling, biking, and skating.
- Be a role model; participate in regular physical activity yourself. Children with active parents are active kids.

(Adapted with permission from Story, Holt, & Sofka (Eds.), [2002].: *Bright futures in practice: Nutrition* [2nd ed.]. Arlington, VA: National Center for Education in Maternal and Child Health.

School communities choosing strategies to prevent childhood overweight should ensure that goals for change in the school system are also in line with the *Healthy People 2010* goals. Many government funding streams require an explanation of how proposals are tied to the *Healthy People 2010* goals. Box 36.4 lists objectives from *Healthy People 2010* related to preventing overweight children and adolescents.

Box 36.4 ■ ■ ■

HEALTHY PEOPLE 2010 OBJECTIVES RELATED TO PREVENTING OVERWEIGHT CHILDREN AND ADOLESCENTS

OBESITY

- 19.4 Reduce the proportion of children and adolescents who are overweight (defined as at or above the gender and age specific 95th percentile of BMI based on revised CDC Growth Charts for the United States.)

NUTRITION

- 19.5 Increase the proportion of persons aged 2 years and older who consume at least two daily servings of fruit.
- 19.6 Increase the proportion of persons aged 2 years and older who consume at least three daily servings of vegetables, with at least one-third being dark green or orange vegetables.
- 19.7 Increase the proportion of persons aged 2 years and older who consume at least six daily servings of grain products, with at least three being whole grains.
- 19.8 Increase the proportion of persons aged 2 years and older who consume less than 10 percent of calories from saturated fat.
- 19.9 Increase the proportion of persons aged 2 years and older who consume no more than 30 percent of calories from total fat.
- 19.10 Increase the proportion of persons aged 2 years and older who consume 2,400 mg or less of sodium daily.
- 19.11 Increase the proportion of persons aged 2 years and older who meet dietary recommendations for calcium.
- 19.12 Reduce iron deficiency among young children and females of childbearing age.
- 19.15 Increase the proportion of children and adolescents aged 6 to 19 years whose intake of meals and snacks at schools contributes to good overall dietary quality.

PHYSICAL ACTIVITY

- 22.6 Increase the proportion of adolescents who engage in moderate physical activity for at least 30 minutes on 5 or more of the pervious 7 days.
- 22.7 Increase the proportion of adolescents who engage in vigorous physical activity that promotes cardio-respiratory fitness 3 or more days per week for 20 or more minutes per occasion.
- 22.8 Increase the proportion of the nation's public and private schools that require daily physical education for all students
- 22.9 Increase the proportion of adolescents who participate in daily school physical education.
- 22.10 Increase the proportion of adolescents who spend at least 50 percent of school physical education class time being physically active.
- 22.11 Increase the proportion of adolescents who view television 2 or fewer hours on a school day.
- 22.12 Increase the proportion of the nation's public and private schools that provide access to their physical activity spaces and facilities for all persons outside of normal school hours.

HEALTH EDUCATION

- 7.2 Increase the proportion of middle, junior high, and senior high schools that provide school health education to prevent health problems in the following areas: unintentional injury; violence; suicide; tobacco use and addiction; alcohol and other drug use; unintended pregnancy; HIV/AIDS; and STD infection; unhealthy dietary patterns; inadequate physical activity; and environmental health.

SCHOOL NURSING

- Increase the proportion of the nation's elementary, middle, junior high, and senior high schools that have a nurse-to-student ratio of at least 1:750.

(Retrieved from U.S. Department of Health and Human Services, *Healthy People 2010* at http://www.healthypeople.gov)

MANAGEMENT APPROACHES FOR OVERWEIGHT IN THE SCHOOL SETTING

Obesity, as a condition, has no effective pharmacological or surgical interventions for children, yet if untreated, can result in a great deal of morbidity (Copperman & Jacobson, 2004). Interventions related to diet management and weight control must be family centered and multidisciplinary. They must address nutrition, physical activity, and psychosocial issues. The goal is to achieve lifelong weight control, thus preventing health complications. Any change that is initiated must occur in the school as well as the home. Outcome measures can address a decrease in the incidence, the prevalence, and the morbidity of obesity.

Sponsored by the Maternal and Child Health Bureau, Health Resources and Services Administration, and the Department of Health and Human Services, expert committee recommendations were developed to guide the evaluation and treatment of overweight children (Barlow & Dietz, 1998). The first step in weight control for all overweight students older than 2 years of age is maintenance of baseline weight. Prolonged weight maintenance, which allows for a gradual decline in BMI as children grow in height, is a sufficient goal for many children (FIGURE 36.3). Families of children with secondary complications, such as elevated blood pressure or lipid levels, should be referred for medical evaluation.

The primary goal of a program to manage uncomplicated obesity is healthy eating and activity, not achievement of an ideal body weight. The committee outlined a nine-point approach to treatment. The following discussion summarizes the committee's treatment approach from a school nurse's perspective:

1. The intervention should begin early. Once children are in preschool or older, and identified as overweight, it is appropriate to initiate suggestions for healthy weight. Behavioral-based treatment programs can be started as early as preschool with success (Drohan, 2002; McGarvey et al., 2004).
2. The family must be ready for change. If a family is not ready to initiate change, then efforts should be toward referring the family to therapists who can address the family's readiness. Interventions to manage overweight children in the school setting need to begin with an understanding of the parents' perceptions of their child's overweight state, which are often contrary to the actual fact. Parents overwhelmingly underestimate their children's weight (Etelson, Brand, Patrick, & Shirali, 2003). Myers and Vargas (2000) found that more than one-third of parents did not believe their obese preschool child was overweight.
3. Families need to be educated about medical complications of obesity. School nurses should have developmentally appropriate, factual information to provide to students and their families on the complications and health risks of obesity, including hypertension, heart disease, and diabetes. Those families with a family history of these diseases may be more motivated to try to prevent the problems in their children.
4. Family and all caregivers should be involved in the treatment program. Once school nurses determine through their assessment that individual treatment in the school setting could be beneficial for a student, parents must be included in the development of an individual health plan. Without parental consent and cooperation, the plan is certain

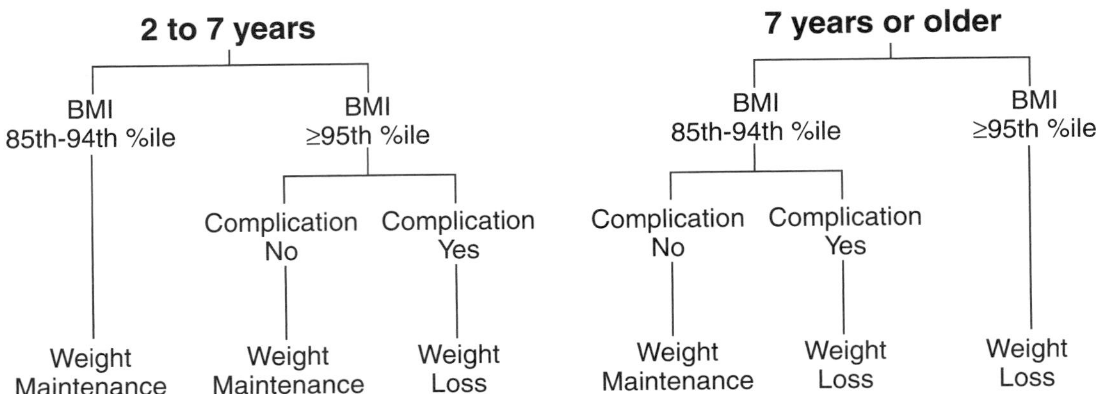

Figure 36.3 ■ Recommendations for weight management for children and adolescents 2 to 20 years old. (Reproduced with permission from *Pediatrics, 102*, e29, Figure 2, © 1998.)

to fail, and the student may feel caught in the middle between mixed messages from their parents and the school nurse. Since the school is also considered a caregiver for the student during school hours, teachers and other staff who interact with the student must be aware of the treatment plan, within the limits of confidentiality, and avoid choosing food-related activities that would jeopardize a student's success.

5. Treatment programs should focus on instituting permanent changes, not short-term diets or exercise programs aimed at rapid weight loss. Opportunities for the student to make healthy choices at school must be available. School nurses need to advocate for system changes in food and physical activity policies in the school so students have healthy choices acceptable for their developmental level.
6. Families need to learn to monitor eating and activity. This is a first step in independent problem solving. At school, the student needs to learn to make healthy choices. Periodic weight measurements, not more than once a week, may help the student stay focused and reinforce success. Frequent weighing can be detrimental to the end goal of behavior change, especially if the weight increases, if a lack of weight change leads to punitive attitudes from others, or if the student focuses more on body image and less on the goals of healthy eating and becoming more active.
7. Families should make small gradual changes. Two or three specific changes in diet or activity should be initiated at one time. Additional steps can be added after the child and family have accomplished the first changes to a point of mastery. Progress should be assessed every 1 or 2 weeks; even a brief visit will allow the school nurse to assess progress, evaluate the appropriateness of the recommended changes, measure weight, emphasize the school nurse's interest and concern, provide positive reinforcement, and encourage the student over the long term.
8. Clinicians should encourage and empathize, not criticize. School nurses promote continued efforts to improve healthy eating and activity when they empathize with the struggles of the students and their families. School nurses who are sensitive and not critical about "failure" are in a position to help the student and family try again.
9. A variety of experienced professionals can accomplish many aspects of a weight management program. A team approach may make best use of each. professional's expertise. School nurses are one such group of professionals. Group meetings for students may be efficient and effective ways for school nurses to intervene.

School nurses are ideal school staff members for implementing and managing school-based healthy weight programs. Neumark-Sztainer and Story (1997) found that overweight adolescents were interested in participating in school-based weight control programs provided they are conducted in a supportive manner, offer enjoyable activities, are informative, are sensitive to the needs of overweight youth, and do not conflict with other activities. Box 36.5 provides recommendations for developing school-based weight control programs.

Box 36.5 ■■■

TEN RECOMMENDATIONS FROM OVERWEIGHT YOUTH FOR SCHOOL-BASED WEIGHT CONTROL PROGRAMS

1. Have a leader who understands the difficulties faced by overweight teens. Try to have a leader or co-leader who is or has been overweight.
2. Provide a supportive, caring, and accepting environment for participants.
3. Have discussions on non-weight-related issues aimed at helping participants to feel better about themselves. Relate to participants as teens, not only as overweight teens.
4. Make the program fun! Avoid sitting around too much and have lots of physical activity.
5. Offer out-of-classroom and out-of-school activities such as walking in the park, going to the YMCA as a group, playing softball, jazzercise classes, shopping together, and healthy picnics.
6. Include activities aimed at increasing nutritional knowledge and skills including food tasting, food preparation, and identification of low-cost foods.

(Continued on the following page)

Box 36.5 ■■■

TEN RECOMMENDATIONS FROM OVERWEIGHT YOUTH FOR SCHOOL-BASED WEIGHT CONTROL PROGRAMS *(Continued)*

7. Be sensitive to the social stigma associated with being overweight in program recruitment and planning.
8. Try to reduce technical barriers to participating by offering the program at a convenient time, at low or no cost, and by providing transportation if necessary.
9. In program evaluation, assess improvements in self-perceptions, eating and exercise skills and behaviors, and perceived social support from the group, in addition to weight loss and maintenance.
10. Involve youth in all stages of planning prior to program implementation and throughout the program.

(From Neumark-Sztainer and Story [1997]. Recommendations from overweight youth regarding school based weight control programs. *Journal of School Health, 67*[10], 428–433.)

The practice of dieting is becoming commonplace for children and adolescents, although not all who engage in this activity need to be on a diet. One study indicated that 31% of fifth-grade girls had been on a diet. Another demonstrated that 45% of females and 20% of males in a large study of adolescents had dieted, with up to 62% of 12th graders having engaged in dieting. Yet another study of adolescents demonstrated that 30% of those who dieted were underweight or normal weight and only slightly more than half of those who were overweight were on diets. While most teens know what their ideal weight should be, 10% of adolescents prefer to be at a weight less than was is expected for age and height (Alemzadeh et al., 2003). Those who diet unnecessarily should also be provided with nutrition information that will allow them to make healthy food and exercise choices to maintain a healthy weight and body mass.

Individualized Health Plans (IHPs)

When a health problem is, or has the potential, to create a barrier to the student's education, or be a threat to the student's safety or well being, the school nurse is responsible for developing a health-care plan to manage the problem in the school setting (NASN, 2003). Once the school nurse assesses a student's health status and determines overweight exists, an Individualized Health Plan (IHP) can provide direction for management of the health problem during school (see Chapter 9).

Standardized IHPs have been developed for many chronic conditions commonly seen in the school setting. These templates allow for consistency in practice as well as efficient use of the school nurse's time. Table 36.3 lists potential nursing intervention (NIC) classification categories frequently

(text continues on page 851)

Table 36.3 ■

SELECTED NIC NURSING INTERVENTIONS AND THEIR DEFINITION FOR USE IN SCHOOLS WITH OVERWEIGHT OR AT-RISK FOR OVERWEIGHT CHILDREN AND ADOLESCENTS

NURSING INTERVENTION	DEFINITION
Active listening	Attending closely to and attaching significance to a student's verbal and nonverbal messages
Behavior management	Helping a student to manage negative behavior
Behavior modification	Promoting a behavior change.
Body image enhancement	Improving a student's conscious and unconscious perceptions and attitudes toward his/her body

(continued)

NURSING INTERVENTION	DEFINITION
Coping enhancement	Assisting a student to adapt to perceived stressors, changes, or threats that interfere with meeting life demands and roles
Counseling	Using an interactive helping process focusing on the needs, problems, or feelings of the student and significant others to enhance or support coping, problem solving, and interpersonal relationships
Decision-making support	Providing information and support for a student who is making a decision regarding health care
Developmental enhancement: Adolescent	Facilitating optimal physical, cognitive, social, and emotional growth of individuals during the transition from childhood to adulthood
Developmental enhancement: Child	Facilitating or teaching parents/caregivers to facilitate the optimal gross motor, fine motor, language, cognitive, social, and emotional growth of preschool and school-aged children
Emotional support	Providing reassurance, acceptance, and encouragement during times of stress
Energy management	Regulating energy use to treat or prevent fatigue and optimize function
Exercise promotion	Facilitating regular physical activity to maintain or advance to a higher level of fitness and health
Family involvement promotion	Facilitating family participation in the emotional and physical care of the student
Family mobilization	Utilizing family strengths to influence student's health in a positive direction
Family support	Promoting family values, interests, and goals
Health education	Developing and providing instruction and learning experiences to facilitate voluntary adaptation of behavior conducive to health in individuals, families, groups, or communities
Health screening	Detecting health risks or problems by means of history, examination, and other procedures
Impulse control training	Assisting the student to mediate impulsive behavior through application of problem-solving strategies to social and interpersonal situations
Learning facilitation	Promoting the ability to process and comprehend information
Mutual goal setting	Collaborating with student to identify and prioritize care goals, then developing a plan for achieving those goals

(continued)

Table 36.3 ■ *(Continued)*

NURSING INTERVENTION	DEFINITION
Nutrition management	Assisting with or providing a balanced dietary intake of foods and fluids
Nutritional counseling	Using an interactive helping process focusing on the need for diet modification
Nutritional monitoring	Collecting and analyzing patient data to prevent or minimize malnourishment
Parent education: Adolescent	Assisting parents to understand and help their adolescent children
Parent education: Childrearing family	Assisting parents to understand and promote the physical, psychological, and social growth and development of their toddler, preschool, or school-age child/children
Parenting promotion	Providing parenting information, support, and coordination of comprehensive services to high-risk families
Patient (student) contracting	Negotiating an agreement with an individual that reinforces a specific behavior change
Presence	Being with another, both physically and psychologically, during times of need
Referral	Arranging for services by another care provider or agency
Risk identification	Analyzing potential risk factors, determining of health risks, and prioritization of risk reduction strategies for an individual or group
Self-awareness enhancement	Assisting a student to explore and understand his or her thoughts, feelings, motivations, and behaviors
Self-esteem enhancement	Assisting a student to increase his or her personal judgment of self-worth
Self-modification assistance	Reinforcing of self-directed change initiated by the student to achieve personally important goals
Self-responsibility facilitation	Encouraging a student to assume more responsibility for own behavior
Socialization enhancement	Facilitating of another person's ability to interact with others
Support group	Using a group environment to provide emotional support and health-related information for members
Support system enhancement	Facilitating support to the student by family, friends, and community

(continued)

NURSING INTERVENTION	DEFINITION
Teaching: group	Developing, implementing, and evaluating a teaching program for a group of students experiencing the same health condition
Teaching: individual	Planning, implementing, and evaluation of a teaching program designed to address a student's particular needs.
Teaching: prescribed diet	Preparing a student to correctly follow a prescribed diet
Values clarification	Assisting another to clarify his or her own values in order to facilitate effective decision making
Weight management	Facilitating maintenance of optimal body weight and percentage body fat
Weight reduction assistance	Facilitating loss of weight and/or body fat

Source: From J. M. Dochterman & G. M. Bulechek (Eds.), *Nursing interventions classification (NIC)* (4th ed.), 2004, St. Louis: C. V. Mosby. Adapted with permission.

used in an IHP for a child/adolescent who is overweight or at-risk for overweight. Each plan, however, must be individualized to the student's particular needs and situation. An appropriate management plan for an overweight 6-year-old may not be effective or appropriate for an overweight 16-year-old.

Not every student in school with a BMI percentile indicating "at risk" or "overweight" will need an IHP developed. Considering the epidemic of overweight children and high school nurse-to-student ratios in many schools, it is impractical, and prioritization is essential. Consequently, when students are overweight, and their condition is compromising their well being, safety or ability to learn in school, and they and/or their family are committed to being involved in a treatment plan to remedy or manage the problem, *then* an IHP is warranted. Box 36.6 provides a sample IHP.

Support Groups

Students who are overweight may find a support group intervention beneficial. Support groups have been used in school settings with success in a variety of population groups to include elementary

(text continues on page 855)

Box 36.6 ■ ■ ■

SAMPLE INDIVIDUALIZED HEALTH PLAN

CASE STUDY

Sharena Jones is a 14-year-old girl who is new to the school district this year. During the "new student" interview and assessment with Sharena, the school nurse noted Sharena has a BMI percentile that identifies her as "overweight." When the school nurse asked Sharena to step on the scale for weight measurement, Sharena's eyes welled up with tears, and she moved with hesitation. Picking up on these cues the school nurse engaged Sharena in conversation and discovered that Sharena is very aware of her problem with being overweight and is very unhappy about how she looks. She says that at her old school, she had no friends, and the kids made fun of her size. She confides to the school nurse her desire to "fit in" at this new school, but she worries it will be more of the same.

In further questioning, the nurse finds that Sharena is the oldest of five children; her parents are divorced, and her mother works during the evenings until 8:30 p.m. Sharena is responsible for preparing most dinners during the week for herself

(Continued on the following page)

Box 36.6 ■■■

SAMPLE INDIVIDUALIZED HEALTH PLAN *(Continued)*

CASE STUDY *(cont'd)*

and her four other male siblings, ages 12, 10, and 8-year-old twins. Some evenings, her mother has dinner planned and started, and other evenings, everything is ready and just needs to be warmed up. Sharena tells the nurse that her mother is also overweight, and explains to the nurse that it runs in their family, and her mother said she (Sharena) will be overweight too, and needs to deal with it.

After reviewing the brief health history form, and screening Sharena for vision, hearing, growth, and blood pressure, the nurse decides to call Mrs. Jones to discuss Sharena's weight. Mrs. Jones confirms that she knows Sharena is bothered by her weight, but that the pediatrician has said there is nothing wrong with Sharena that diet and exercise can't fix. Mrs. Jones agrees to allow the school nurse to work with Sharena about her weight, and is willing to come in and meet with the nurse one day after school on her day off.

The school nurse prepares an individualized healthcare plan for Sharena, and reviews it with both Sharena and her mother.

BEAVER VALLEY LOCAL SCHOOL DISTRICT INDIVIDUAL HEALTH PLAN

IHP date: 11/23/05
Name: Sharena Jones
Parent/Guardian: Mrs. Brenda Jones
Primary Physician: Dr. Hazel
Date of Birth: 5/28/91
Home Phone: 555–4848
Office phone: 555–5757
Grade: 8
Work phone: 555–9898 (evenings)
Teacher: Mrs. Connell
Cell phone: 555–3433
Building: Williamson Middle

Health Concern Summary

New to the school system this fall, Sharena presents with behaviors indicative of low self-esteem, attributable (self-report) to her physical stature of being overweight for her age, gender, and height, as determined by BMI > 97th percentile. She was last seen at Dr. Hazel's office for a well child visit in August 2005. At that time, mother reports Dr. Hazel suggested Sharena get involved in some sport and to eliminate nonnutritive food availability in the home.

ASSESSMENT	NURSING DIAGNOSIS	GOAL	INTERVENTION	OUTCOME
Height 60 inches Weight 144 pounds BMI above 97th percentile	Growth and development, altered	Sharena will maintain or decrease body weight with good health habits: improving her rating from 2 to 3 within two months and from 3 to 4 by end of school year	Nutritional Counseling (NIC 5246) • Establish schedule of visits to clinic. • Determine Sharena's eating habits. • Discuss Sharena's food likes and dislikes. • Discuss her knowledge of basic food groups, food pyramid. • Teach how to maintain food diary.	Child development: adolescence (NOC 01909) Practices good health habits (NOC 010901) 1 never demonstrated 2 rarely demonstrated 3 sometimes demonstrated 4 often demonstrated

ASSESSMENT	NURSING DIAGNOSIS	GOAL	INTERVENTION	OUTCOME
			• Teach caloric value/energy expenditure relationship. • Discuss healthy food choices in the school cafeteria. • Establish realistic short- and long-term goals for changing diet habits. • Monitor Sharena's adherence to healthy eating weekly. Exercise Promotion (NIC 0200) • Explore Sharena's prior exercise/physical activity experiences. • Explore barriers to physical activity. • Help Sharena to schedule regular times for physical activity in her weekly routine. • Teach her about health benefits of physical activity. • Monitor Sharena's adherence to physical activity plan. Weight management (NIC 1260) • Weight recorded in clinic every week for first month, then bimonthly until end of school. • Encourage Sharena to consume adequate amounts of water each day. Family Involvement Promotion (NIC 7110) • Include the mother in planning physical activity opportunities. • Include the mother in plan for healthy food choices. • Follow up with the mother regarding Sharena's progress.	5 consistently demonstrated

(Continued on the following page)

Box 36.6 ■ ■ ■

SAMPLE INDIVIDUALIZED HEALTH PLAN *(Continued)*

ASSESSMENT	NURSING DIAGNOSIS	GOAL	INTERVENTION	OUTCOME
Reports past experiences of being made fun of by school children for "being fat". Reports she has no friends, expresses desire for friends Not involved in any clubs, sports, group activity in school or community Rarely makes eye contact, gazes downward when speaking to adult Posture slumped, with shoulders rounded Hair unkempt	Self-esteem disturbance	Sharena will demonstrate improved self-esteem (NOC 1205) improving her rating from 2 to 4 by the end of the school year	Self-esteem enhancement (NIC 5400) • Explore Sharena's previous achievements. • Encourage Sharena to identify personal strengths • Reinforce the strengths she identifies. • Explore opportunities at school Sharena would feel comfortable joining, where her strengths would be an asset. Family Involvement Promotion (NIC 7110) • Discuss with mother: - her capability for assisting in plan of care - her expectations for Sharena Weight management (NIC 1260) • Plan rewards for Sharena as she meets small short-term goals in diet or physical activity health behavior changes	Self-esteem (NOC1205) • Stands erect and makes eye contact. • Participates in organized social group, club, sport. • Describes successes in social groups. • Comes to school well groomed with good personal hygiene. • Describes successes in school work. • Expresses feelings of self worth. Self-esteem indicators measured by: 1, never positive 2, rarely positive 3, sometimes positive 4, often positive 5, consistently positive

This plan was prepared by ________________________ (school nurse) and will be shared as needed to promote the health of __________________________(student) while in school.
Reviewed by parent /legal guardian ____.
(Date)______________________
Reviewed by physician _________________________________
(Date)_____________________

school children with attention disorders, socially withdrawn girls, high school students "at risk" for depression and suicide, and chronic absentee middle school students (Frame, Kelly, & Bayley, 2003; Houck, Darnell, & Lussman, 2002; Houck, King, Tomlinson, Vrabel, & Wecks, 2002; Houck & Perri, 2002; Houck & Stember, 2002).

If changes in behaviors are desired for adolescents, intervention must occur within the adolescent's social context (Eggert, 2000). School-based support groups have been effective in reducing risk factors and enhancing personal strengths with adolescents (Eggert, 2000; Thompson, Eggert, Randell, & Pike, 2001). Skills training and emotional support provided through support groups at school can result in decreased stress and depression with high school students (Houck et al., 2002).

Support groups for middle school or high school overweight students may prove to be beneficial not only in changing student behavior regarding diet and physical activity, but also in improving a student's perception of self-worth, creating friendships and bonds with fellow students and the school nurse, and ultimately improving a student's connectivity and sense of belonging with the school. This is a prime research area for school nurse practice.

School nurses can teach stress reduction techniques, including the use of physical activity to students. Other helpful counseling suggestions may be where to shop for stylish large size clothes. Most important in any support group or counseling session is to promote respect for the person and build their self-esteem.

ASSESSING THE SCHOOL SYSTEM: A TEAM APPROACH

School Health Index

The *School Health Index* (SHI) is a self-assessment and planning tool for schools that was developed by the Centers for Disease Control and Prevention (CDC, 2004a, 2004b). The SHI takes a team approach to assessing the school system and developing a plan of action to improve nutrition, physical activity, tobacco abstinence, and injury prevention. The third edition, released in 2004, includes injury prevention, healthy eating, physical activity, and a tobacco-free lifestyle as the foci for the assessment. There are two versions: an elementary school and a middle/high school version. School nurses can obtain a free copy of either version of the SHI at http://www.cdc.gov/HealthyYouth/SHI.

The SHI has eight different modules, each corresponding to a component of the coordinated school health model (health education, physical education, health services, nutrition services, counseling, school environment, staff health promotion, and family/community involvement). A team is organized representing different groups within the school: parents, teachers, students, administrators, school nurses and other staff, and concerned community members. Team members complete a questionnaire for each module. Responses are scored and school strengths and weaknesses are identified. It can be completed in as little as 5 hours. The SHI also includes a planning section to assist the team in developing an action plan for improving healthy eating and physical activity in the school. Many of the improvements can be done with existing resources.

Changing the Scene: Improving the School Nutrition Environment

Changing the Scene is a packaged kit developed by the United States Department of Agriculture (USDA) to improve the nutrition environment in schools across the country (2001). *Changing the Scene* deals exclusively with nutrition: assessment, plan development, and implementation. School nurses can request a copy of the kit for use in their school at http://www.fns.usda.gov/tn. The kit guides the user to examine the school nutrition environment, develop a plan for improvement, and put the plan into action to make a difference. Handouts, a videotape, a power-point presentation, brochures, and a CD-ROM with presentation scripts and transparency masters are all provided in the kit.

This program takes a six-step approach to accomplishing an improved nutrition environment in the schools. Step one is to create a team and get buy-in. Step two involves conducting a needs assessment. The kit provides guidelines for the needs assessment, or the CDC's SHI assessment tool can be used. Step three guides the team through development of an action plan. Step four is putting the plan into action and assigning responsibilities to specific team members. Step five is an evaluation, to review progress and make necessary revisions. Finally, step six is communicating to the community and other interested stake holders the efforts of the process.

POLICY DEVELOPMENT

Policymaking is a way of creating official statements that guide the actions of those in the educational system, both students and staff. Policies also create accountability and offer legal protection in a variety of circumstances. School nurses should involve themselves whenever possible in the formation and

Growth Screening Policy for Beaver Local School District

Rationale for Policy: Whereas children are better able to learn when attending school in a healthy state, and whereas growth parameters of children are a fundamental index of health, and whereas, all children are recommended by the American Academy of Pediatrics to be screened annually for growth as part of school health assessments, Beaver Local School District (BLSD) recognizes the importance of providing this school health service for BLSD children.

Therefore,

Students of BLSD will be screened for growth in the following circumstances:

- Grades K, 2, 4, 6, 8, and 9.
- New students to the school district
- Students undergoing IEP initial assessment
- Other special health need students as individually identified

Program Implementation: The school nurse is responsible for implementation of this policy by conducting growth screenings with the student populations identified above. The school nurse will follow recommended procedures and protocols as identified by Centers for Disease Control and Prevention and National Association of School Nurses, demonstrating best practice models, and compliance with current standards of practice for school nurses. This procedure will include confidential individual student reports to parents of the screening results.

Definitions:

Growth screening—process by which students' heights and weights are measured, and Body Mass Index for age is determined

Body Mass Index for age—An anthropometric calculation determined by the students' height, weight, gender, and age, and represented in a percentile.

Overweight—A student with a BMI for age percentile > 95th percentile

At risk for overweight—A student with a BMI for age percentile between 85th and 94th percentile

Normal range—A student with a BMI for age percentile between 5th and 84th percentile

Underweight—A student with a BMI for age <5th percentile

Responsibility for the administration of this policy is at the building principal level, and will be reflected in the job performance evaluations of both building administrators, and school nurses.

Results from annual growth screenings will be reviewed by administration as aggregate group information. This aggregate evaluation will be used to determine program evaluation concerning nutrition and physical activity school policies as well as provide guidance for future policy needs.

Policy in effect as of: 9/01/2004

Signature ____________________

(Superintendent)

(Date)

To be reviewed by: 6/01/2006

Signature ____________________

(BLSD Board President)

(Date)

Figure 36.4 ■ Sample growth screening policy.

revision of school health policies, or policies that influence the health of students and staff. FIGURE 36.4 illustrates a sample policy for growth screening. School nurses would be wise to invest time and energy preventing and decreasing the prevalence of overweight school children through policies and actions focused on the school system.

Fit, Healthy, and Ready to Learn: A School Health Policy Guide was developed by the National Association of State Boards of Education (NASBE) and the National School Boards Association (NSBA) to address the policy issues of physical activity, healthy eating, and tobacco use in school systems (Bogden, 2000). The manual can be purchased through NASBE at their Web site: http://www.nasbe.org/merchant2/merchant.mvc. *Fit Healthy and Ready to Learn* does not go into detail about action plans; rather, it is designed to assist in policy development necessary before programs and plans can be implemented in the school. The manual is divided into five sections: the art of policymaking; general school health policies; policies to encourage healthy eating; policies to encourage physical activity; and policies to discourage tobacco use. Each section ends with a list of resources.

SURGEON GENERAL'S CALL TO ACTION

The surgeon general's report *Call to Action to Prevent and Decrease Overweight and Obesity* (2001) provides guidelines for selecting action at the local level. These guidelines can provide evidence and support for changing policies and initiating programs in school to help with obesity prevention. Recommendations for action are organized in a framework using the acronym "CARE": **C**ommunication, **A**ction, **R**esearch, and **E**valuation.

Communication: Provision of information and tools to motivate and empower decision-makers at the governmental, organizational, community, family, and individual levels who will create change toward the prevention and decrease of overweight and obesity.

Action: Interventions and activities that assist decision-makers in preventing and decreasing overweight and obesity, individually or collectively.

Research and Evaluation: Investigations to better understand the causes of overweight and obesity, to assess the effectiveness of interventions, and to develop new communication and action strategies.

The *Call to Action* (available at http://www.surgeongeneral.gov/topics/obesity/) identifies five settings where strategies should take place: families and communities, schools, health care, media and communication, and worksites. Schools are identified as a vital setting since children spend a large portion of their time in school. Within the school setting, the CARE framework outlines actions for preventing and decreasing the prevalence of overweight and obesity (BOX 36.7). School nurses can encourage

(text continues on page 858)

Box 36.7 ■ ■ ■

SURGEON GENERAL'S OPTIONS FOR SCHOOLS TO PREVENT AND DECREASE OVERWEIGHT CHILDREN

COMMUNICATION

- Build awareness among teachers, food service staff, coaches, nurses, and other school staff about the contribution of proper nutrition and physical activity to the maintenance of lifelong healthy weight.
- Educate teachers, staff, and parents about the importance of school physical activity and nutrition programs and policies.
- Educate parents, teachers, coaches, staff, and other adults in the community about the importance they hold as role models for children, and teach them how to be models for healthy eating and regular physical activity.
- Educate students, teachers, staff, and parents about the importance of body size acceptance and the dangers of unhealthy weight control practices.
- Develop sensitivity of staff to the problems encountered by the overweight child.

ACTION

- Provide age-appropriate and culturally sensitive instruction in health education that helps students develop the knowledge, attitudes, skills, and behaviors to adopt, maintain, and enjoy healthy eating habits and a physically active lifestyle.
- Ensure that meals offered through the school breakfast and lunch programs meet nutritional standards.
- Adopt policies ensuring that all foods and beverages available on school campuses and at school events contribute toward eating patterns that are consistent with the *Dietary guidelines for Americans*.
- Provide food options that are low in fat, calories, and added sugars, such as fruits, vegetables, whole grains, and low-fat or nonfat dairy foods.
- Ensure that healthy snacks and foods are provided in vending machines, school stores, and other venues within the school's control.
- Prohibit student access to vending machines, school stores, and other venues that compete with healthy school meals in elementary schools and restrict access in middle, junior, and high schools.
- Provide an adequate amount of time for students to eat school meals, and schedule lunch periods at reasonable hours around midday.
- Provide all children, from pre-kindergarten through grade 12, with quality daily physical education that helps develop the knowledge, attitudes, skills, behaviors, and confidence needed to be physically active for life.
- Provide daily recess periods for elementary school students, featuring time for unstructured but supervised play.
- Provide extracurricular physical activity programs, especially inclusive intramural programs and physical activity clubs.
- Encourage the use of school facilities for physical activity programs offered by the school and/or community-based organizations outside of school hours.

RESEARCH AND EVALUATION

- Conduct research on the relationship of healthy eating and physical activity to student health, learning, attendance, classroom behavior, violence, and other social outcomes.
- Evaluate school-based behavioral health interventions for the prevention of overweight in children.
- Develop an ongoing, systematic process to assess the school physical activity and nutrition environment, and plan, implement, and monitor improvements.
- Conduct research to study the effect of school policies such as food services and physical activity curricula on overweight in children and adolescents.
- Evaluate the financial and health impact of school contracts with vendors of high-calorie foods and beverages with minimal nutritional value.

(From U.S. Department of Health and Human Services, Public Health Service, Office of the Surgeon General. [2001]. *Surgeon general's call to action to prevent and decrease overweight and obesity 2001*, Rockville, MD.)

school administrators to adopt policies that would lead to achievement of identified actions.

The *Call to Action* report (USDHHS, 2001) identifies the following 15 activities as national priorities for immediate action (Box 36.8). Eleven of these actions relate directly to schools and students.

Policy Formation and the Coordinated School Health Model

Using the coordinated school health model as a framework for policy and action provides a familiar and organized approach to the problem (Chapter 3). In 2000, the CDC's Division of Adolescent and

Box 36.8 ■ ■ ■

SURGEON GENERAL'S NATIONAL PRIORITIES FOR IMMEDIATE ACTION

"The Nation must take an informed, sensitive approach to communicate with and educate the American people about health issues related to overweight and obesity. Everyone must work together to:

- Change the perception of overweight and obesity at all ages. The primary concern should be one of health and not appearance.
- Educate all expectant parents about the many benefits of breastfeeding.
  - Breastfed infants may be less likely to become overweight as they grow older.
  - Mothers who breastfeed may return to pre-pregnancy weight more quickly.
- Educate healthcare providers and health profession students in the prevention and treatment of overweight and obesity across the lifespan.
- Provide culturally appropriate education in schools and communities about healthy eating habits and regular physical activity, based on the *Dietary guidelines for Americans*, for people of all ages."

"The Nation must take action to assist Americans in balancing healthful eating with regular physical activity. Individuals and groups across all settings must work in concert to:

- Ensure daily, quality physical education in all school grades. Such education can develop the knowledge, attitudes, skills, behaviors, and confidence needed to be physically active for life.
- Reduce time spent watching television and in other similar sedentary behaviors.
- Build physical activity into regular routines and playtime for children and their families. Ensure that adults get at least 30 minutes of moderate physical activity on most days of the week. Children should aim for at least 60 minutes.
- Create more opportunities for physical activity at worksites, Encourage all employers to make facilities and opportunities available for physical activity for all employees.
- Make community facilities available and accessible for physical activity for all people, including the elderly.
- Promote healthier food choices, including at least five servings of fruits and vegetables each day and reasonable portion sizes at home, in schools, at worksites, and in communities.
- Ensure that schools provide healthful foods and beverages on school campuses and at school events by:
  - Enforcing existing U.S. Department of Agriculture regulations that prohibit serving foods of minimal nutritional value during mealtimes in school food service areas, including vending machines.
  - Adopting policies specifying that all foods and beverages available at school contribute toward eating patterns that are consistent with the *Dietary guidelines for Americans*.
  - Providing more food options that are low in fat, calories, and added sugars such as fruits, vegetables, whole grains, and low-fat or nonfat dairy foods.
  - Reducing access to foods high in fat, calories, and added sugars and to excessive portion sizes.
- Create mechanisms for appropriate reimbursement for the prevention and treatment of overweight and obesity."

"The Nation must invest in research that improves our understanding of the causes, prevention, and treatment of overweight and obesity. A concerted effort should be made to:

- Increase research on behavioral and environmental causes of overweight and obesity.
- Increase research and evaluation on prevention and treatment interventions for overweight and obesity, and develop and disseminate best practice guidelines.
- Increase research on disparities in the prevalence of overweight and obesity among racial and ethnic, gender, socioeconomic, and age groups, and use this research to identify effective and culturally appropriate interventions."

(From U.S. Department of Health and Human Services, Public Health Service, Office of the Surgeon General. [2001]. *Surgeon general's call to action to prevent and decrease overweight and obesity. Rockville, MD: USDHHS.)*

School Health conducted a nationwide school health policy study, organized around the coordinated school health model. The findings (Division of School Health, 2001) provide rationale and direction for schools and school nurses to make policy changes. Documented need for change is presented. When the eight components of the model are in concert, it can create a synergistic effect in preventing and controlling childhood obesity.

Fund Raising and Vending Machines: Giving the Wrong Message

There has been a tremendous amount of media coverage about how schools are undermining approaches to counter the obesity epidemic in their attempt to raise money. Candy drives, in which students are encouraged to sell candy and other sugar products, are promoted across the country. Students win prizes for selling the most. In addition, vending machines are in many high schools in the country. Most of what they offer is listed as "inappropriate" for those who are trying to make healthy choices. Schools argue that these are ways for the school to raise money. In addition, cafeterias often sell foods that are high in fat and low in vegetables and fruit. This is also the case at school sports activities. Policies must be developed to ensure consistency in the message being delivered to students and staff. These are identified as priorities for immediate action by the surgeon general.

In addition, school nurses and teachers should avoid providing low-nutritive food as a reward. Lunch needs to be served at reasonable times in the school day, with adequate time allowed for food consumption. At least 10 minutes to eat breakfast and 20 minutes for lunch, from the time students are seated, are recommended minimum amounts of time (CDC, 2003a).

School Environment

Opportunities should be created for school facilities (i.e., basketball courts, tennis courts, track, weight room) to be used by students as well as all community members outside of school hours.

Physical Education

The American Academy of Pediatrics (2003) advocates for significant changes in the opportunities for physical activity in schools, after school programs and other community settings. In a report by the National Governors Association Center for Best Practices (2003) titled "Preventing Obesity in Youth through School-Based Efforts," many recommendations are made for states. One recommendation includes strengthening school physical education requirements to meet national recommendations for physical activity for children and adolescents. Although this may seem directed at state boards of education, this recommendation can be cited as support for a local school district to take the lead and change physical education policies in their schools. The school nurse should be a member of a committee advocating for this change. If there is no such committee in the local district, the school nurse could call for the initiation of such a committee by presenting the issue to the local school board.

Health Education

The K–12 curriculum should adequately address nutrition and physical activity and their relation to healthy weight. Healthy lifestyle curriculum is an important component of a comprehensive school-based plan to help prevent and decrease overweight children (Weepie & McCarthy, 2002). School nurses have the expertise to educate students, faculty, and parents on the importance of role modeling, dietary guidelines that promote balanced meals, reading and interpreting food labels, relating dietary guidelines to food preparation, the need for daily physical exercise, and the negative influence of inactivity (NASN, 2002). Newly released healthy eating guidelines for all Americans, as well as a new food pyramid providing an individualized approach to nutrition (see http://www.mypyramid.gov) should be a central focus of curriculum revision at all K–12 schools.

Family and Community Involvement

Schools need to support programs for families to be physically active together, and to learn new and different healthy cooking and eating options. School nurses should look for connections that can be established with community businesses and agencies in the interest of providing services and programming for students and families. Such community entities may include local YMCA's, hospitals, private health clubs, food establishments, or grocery stores. The VERB campaign, sponsored by the CDC, is a national media campaign aimed at families, communities, and preteens to increase physical activity in the middle school age youth (http://www.cdc.gov/youthcampaign).

Staff Health Promotion

Obesity is an epidemic affecting adults as well as young people, and adults who work in schools are no exception. School staff serve as role models for students. School nurses can take the lead in promoting prevention policies for school staff. Weight management programs for staff can be organized during, after, or before school hours. Policies concerning refreshments at staff meetings and vending machine selections in staff lounges should be considered.

CONCLUSION

The epidemic of overweight children in America has drawn the attention of the Nation. Efforts from federal, state, and local government, and health-focused nonprofit agencies are all identifying ways to combat the problem and prevent its further spread. Schools are an integral site for assessment and prevention of overweight children as well as a focus for system change to manage the problem as it currently exists. The CDC (2005) recommends weight-related measures that "(1) include nutrition and physical activity components in combination, (2) allot additional time to physical activity during the school day, (3) include noncompetitive sports (e.g., dance), and reduce sedentary activities, especially television viewing" (p. 5). School nurses, as coordinators of health service programs in schools, must be skilled in assessment and management of overweight and obese students, and be proactive in assisting school systems to adopt policy changes and institute programming that will have a positive impact on the healthy weight of school children.

Resources

Organizations

American Academy of Pediatrics
http://www.aap.org

Prevention of Pediatric Overweight and Obesity Policy Statement
http://www.aap.org/policy/s100029.html
http://aappolicy.aappublications.org/cgi/content/full/pediatrics;112/2/424

American Cancer Society
http://www.cancer.org

Prevention and Detection Food and Fitness/Great American Weigh In
http://www.cancer.org/docroot/PED/PED_0.asp

American Diabetes Association
http://www.diabetes.org

American Heart Association
http://www.americanheart.org

Obesity and Overweight in Children: AHA Recommendation http://www.americanheart.org/presenter.jhtml?identifier=4670

American Obesity Association
http://www.obesity.org

Bright Futures
http://www.brightfutures.org/

Bright Futures in Practice: Nutrition
http://www.brightfutures.org/training/index.html#Nutrition

Bright Futures in Practice: Physical Activity
http://www.brightfutures.org/physicalactivity/about.htm

Center for Science in the Public Interest
http://www.cspinet.org

A Guide to Improving School Foods & Beverages.
http://www.cspinet.org/schoolfood

Commercial Alert
http://www.commercialalert.org

Child Obesity Overview
http://www.commercialalert.org/index.php/category_id/5/subcategory_id/72/article_id/176

Kids Source
http://www.kidsource.com

Child obesity
http://www.kidsource.com/kidsource/content2/obesity.html

National Association of School Nurses
http://www.nasn.org

Overweight Children and Adolescents Position Statement
http://www.nasn.org/positions/2002psoverweight.htm

National Association of School Psychologists.
www.nasponline.org

National Association for Sport and Physical Education.
http://www.aahperd.org/naspe/

National Association of State Boards of Education.
http://www.nasbe.org

Fit, Healthy, and Ready to Learn
http://www.nasbe.org/HealthySchools/fithealthy.mgi

Government Sites

Center for Disease Control and Prevention
http://www.cdc.gov

Guidelines for Community and School Programs to Promote Lifelong Physical Activity among Young People
http://www.cdc.gov/mmwr/preview/mmwrhtml/00046823.htm

Guidelines for School Health Programs to Promote Lifelong Healthy Eating
ftp://ftp.cdc.gov/pub/Publications/mmwr/rr/rr4509.pdf

National Center For Health Statistics 2000 Growth Charts
http://www.cdc.gov/growthcharts/

Youth Media Campaign—VERB
http://www.cdc.gov/youthcampaign/

National Center for Chronic Disease Prevention and Health Promotion (NCCDPHP)
http://www.cdc.gov/nccdphp

Division of Adolescent and School Health
http://www.cdc.gov/HealthyYouth/index.htm

School Health Policies and Programs Study
http://www.cdc.gov/nccdphp/dash/shpps/index.htm

School Health Index
http://www.cdc.gov/nccdphp/dash/SHI/

Youth Risk Behavior Surveillance System (YRBSS)
http://www.cdc.gov/nccdphp/dash/yrbs/

Division of Nutrition and Physical Activity
http://www.cdc.gov/nccdphp/dnpa/index.htm

CDC Growth Chart Training Modules
http://www.cdc.gov/nccdphp/dnpa/growthcharts/training/modules/index.htm

Overweight and Obesity.
http://www.cdc.gov/nccdphp/dnpa/obesity/index.htm

National Institutes of Health
http://www.nih.gov

National Heart, Lung, and Blood Institute
http://www.nhlbi.nih.gov

Hearts N' Parks Community Mobilization Guide
http://www.nhlbi.nih.gov/health/prof/heart/obesity/hrt_n_pk/hnp_resg.htm

Jump Start Program
http://www.nhlbi.nih.gov/health/prof/heart/other/jump-strt.htm

National Institute of Diabetes and Digestive and Kidney Diseases Weight Loss and Control.
http://www.niddk.nih.gov/health/nutrit/nutrit.htm

Office of the President & U.S. Department of Health and Human Services. Healthier US.Gov Initiative
http://www.healthierus.gov

Nutrition
http://www.healthierus.gov/nutrition.html

Exercise
http://www.healthierus.gov/exercise.html

U.S. Department of Agriculture
http://www.usda.gov

Food and Nutrition Information Center.
http://www.nal.usda.gov/fnic

Food Guide Pyramid.
http://www.mypyramid.gov/

Food and Nutrition Service.
http://www.fns.usda.gov

School Breakfast Program Home Page.
http://www.fns.usda.gov/cnd/Breakfast/default.htm

School Lunch Program Home Page.
http://www.fns.usda.gov/cnd/Lunch/default.htm

Changing the Scene
http://www.fns.usda.gov/tn/Healthy/changing.html

References

Adair, L. S., & Gordon-Larsen, P. (2001). Maturational timing and overweight prevalence in U.S. adolescent girls. *American Journal of Public Health, 91*, 642–644.

Alemzadeh, R., Rising, R., Cedillo, M., & Lifshitz, F. (2003). Obesity in Children. In F. Lifshitz (Ed.), *Pediatric endocrinology* (pp. 823–858). New York: Marcel Dekker.

American Academy of Pediatrics (AAP), Committee on Nutrition. (2003). Prevention of pediatric overweight and obesity. *Pediatrics, 112* (2), 424–430.

American Academy of Pediatrics (AAP), Committee on School Health. (2000). School health assessments. *Pediatrics, 105*(4), 875–877.

Arluk, S. L., Branch, J. D., Swain, D. P., & Dowling, E. A. (2003). Childhood obesity's relationship to time spent in sedentary behavior. *Military Medicine, 168*(7), 583–586.

Aye, T., & Levitsky, L. L. (2003). Type 2 diabetes: An epidemic in childhood. *Current Opinion in Pediatrics, 15*(4), 411–415.

Barlow, S. E., & Dietz, W. H. (1998). *Obesity evaluation and treatment: Expert committee recommendations. Pediatrics, 102* (3), Retrieved January 30, 2004 from http://www.pediatrics.org/cgi/content/full/102/3/e29 .

Belamarich, P. F., Luder, E., Kattan, M., Mitchell, H., Islam, S., Lynn, H., & Crain, F. (2000). Do obese inner-city children with asthma have more symptoms than nonobese children with asthma? *Pediatrics, 106*(6), 1436–1441.

Birch, L. L., & Fisher, J. O. (1998). Development of eating behaviors among children and adolescents. *Pediatrics, 101*(Suppl.), 539–549.

Bogden, J. F. (2000). *Fit, healthy, and ready to learn: A school health policy guide*. Alexandria, VA: National Association of State Boards of Education.

Bowman, S. A., Gortmaker, S. L., Ebbeling, C. B., Pereira, M. A., & Ludwig, D. S. (2004). Effects of fast-food consumption on energy intake and diet quality among children in a national household survey. *Pediatrics, 113*(1), 112–118.

Centers for Disease Control and Prevention (CDC). (2003a). *Ten strategies for promoting physical activity, healthy eating, and a tobacco-free lifestyle through school health programs*. Retrieved September 18, 2004 from http://www.cdc.gov/HealthyYouth/publications/pdf/ten_strategies.pdf.

Centers for Disease Control and Prevention (CDC). (2003b). Physical activity levels among children aged 9–3 years—United States, 2002. *Morbidity and Mortality Weekly Report, 52*(33), 785–788.

Centers for Disease Control and Prevention (CDC). (2004a). *School health index: A self-assessment and planning guide. Elementary school version*. Atlanta, GA.

Centers for Disease Control and Prevention (CDC). (2004b). *School health index: A Self-assessment and planning guide. Middle school/high school version*. Atlanta, GA.

Centers for Disease Control and Prevention (CDC). (2004c). Youth risk behavior surveillance—United States 2003. *Morbidity and Mortality Weekly Report, 53* (surveillance summary-2), 1–96.

Centers for Disease Control and Prevention (CDC). (2005). Public health strategies for preventing and controlling overweight and obesity in school and worksite settings. *Morbidity and Mortality Weekly Report, 54* (RR-10), 1–12.

Cole, T., & Rolland-Cachera, M. F. (2002). Measurement and definition. In W. Burniat, T. Cole, I. Lissau, & E. Poskitt (Eds.), *Child and adolescent obesity* (pp. 3–27), Cambridge, UK: Cambridge University Press.

Cooperberg, J., & Faith, M. (2004) Treatment of obesity II: Childhood and adolescent obesity. In J. K. Thompson (Eds.), *Handbook of eating disorders and obesity* (pp. 443–460). Hoboken, NJ: John Wiley & Sons.

Copperman, N., & Jacobson, M. (2004). Interventions for the prevention and treatment of pediatric overweight. *Consensus in Pediatrics: Childhood Obesity, 1*(4), 25–36.

Crespo, C. J., Smit, E., Troiano, R. P., Bartlett, S. J., Macera, A., & Andersen R. E. (2001). Television watching, energy intake and obesity in US children. *Archives of Pediatric Adolescent Medicine, 155*, 360–365.

Datar, A., & Sturm, R. (2004). Physical education in elementary school and body mass index: Evidence from the early childhood longitudinal study. *American Journal of Public Health, 94*(9), 1501–1506.

Davison, K. K., & Birch, L. L. (2002). Processes linking weight status and self concept among girls from ages five to seven years. *Developmental Psychology, 38*(5), 735–748.

Demerath, E., Muratova, V., Spangler, E., Li, J., Minor, V. E., & Neal, W. A. (2003). School-based obesity screening in rural Appalachia. *Preventive Medicine, 37*(6), 553–560.

Dietz, W. H., & Robinson, T. N. (1998). Use of the body mass index (BMI) as a measure of overweight in children and adolescents. *Journal of Pediatrics, 32*, 191–193.

Division of School Health, CDC. (2001). School health policies and programs study (SHPPS) 2000: Summary report. *Journal of School Health, 71*(7), 249–350.

Dochterman, J. M., & Bulechek, G. M. (2004). *Nursing interventions classification*. St. Louis: Mosby.

Drohan, S. H. (2002). Managing early childhood obesity in the primary care setting: A behavior modification approach. *Pediatric Nursing, 28*(6), 599–610.

Eggert, L. L. (2000). Science based prevention approaches to promoting healthy adolescent behaviors. *Communicating Nursing Research, 34*, 59–75.

Enright, P. L., Goodwin, J. L., Sherrill, D. L., Quan, J. R., & Quan, S. F. (2003). Blood pressure elevation associated with sleep-related breathing disorder in a community sample of white and Hispanic children: The Tucson children's assessment of sleep apnea study. *Archives of Pediatrics and Adolescent Medicine, 157*(9), 901–904.

Estrada, E. (2004). Childhood obesity: Complications. *Consensus in Pediatrics: Childhood Obesity, 1*(4), 13–24.

Etelson, D., Brand, D. A., Patrick, P. A., & Shirali, A. (2003). Childhood obesity: Do parents recognize this health risk? *Obesity Research, 11*(11), 1362–1368.

Frame, K., Kelly, L., & Bayley, E. (2003). Increasing perceptions of self-worth in preadolescents diagnosed with ADHD. *Journal of Nursing Scholarship, 35*(3), 225–229.

Freedman, D. S., Dietz, W. H., Srinivasan, S. R., & Berenson, G. S. (1999). The relation of overweight to cardiovascular risk factors among children and adolescents: The Bogalusa heart study. *Pediatrics, 103*, 1175–1182.

Freedman, D. S., Khan, L. K., Dietz, W. H., Srinivasan, S. R., & Berenson, G. S. (2001). Relationship of childhood obesity to coronary heart disease risk factors in adulthood: The Bogalusa heart study. *Pediatrics, 108*, 712–718.

Frelut, M. L., & Flodmark, C. E. (2002). The obese adolescent. In W. Burniat, T. Cole, I. Lissau, & E. Poskitt (Eds.), *Child and adolescent obesity* (pp. 154–170). Cambridge, UK: Cambridge University Press.

Gennuso, J., Epstein, L. H., Paluch, R. A., & Cerny, F. (1998). The relationship between asthma and obesity in urban minority children and adolescents. *Archives of Pediatric Adolescent Medicine*, 152, 1197–2000.

Giammattei, J., Blix, G., Marshak, H. H., Wolitzer, A. O., & Pettitt, D. J. (2003). Television watching and soft drink consumption: Associations with obesity in 11- to 13-year-old school children. *Archives of Pediatric and Adolescent Medicine, 157*(9), 882–886.

Gilliland, F. D., Berhane, K., Islam, T., McConnell, R., Gauderman, W. J., Gilliland, S. S., Avol, E., & Peters, J. M. (2003). Obesity and the risk of newly diagnosed asthma in school-age children. *American Journal of Epidemiology, 158*(5), 406–415.

Gillman, M. W., Rifas-Shiman, S. L., Frazier, A. L., Rockett, H. R., Camargo, C. A., Field, A. E., Berkey, C. S., & Colditz, G. A. (2000). Family dinner and diet quality among older children and adolescents. *Archives of Family Medicine, 9*, 235–240.

Goodman, E., & Whitaker, R. C. (2002). A prospective study of the role of depression in the development and persistence of adolescent obesity. *Pediatrics, 110*(3), 497–504.

Gottesman, M. M. (2003). Healthy eating and activity together (HEAT): Weapons against obesity. *Journal of Pediatric Health Care, 17*(4), 210–215.

Goulding, A., Taylor, R. W., Jones, I. E., Manning, P. J., & Williams, S. M. (2002). Spinal overload: A concern for obese children and adolescents? *Osteoporosis International, 13*, 835–840.

Guillaume, M., & Lissau, I. (2002). Epidemiology. In W. Burniat, T. Cole, I. Lissau, & E Poskitt (Eds.), *Child and adolescent obesity* (pp. 28–47). Cambridge, UK: Cambridge University Press.

Guo, S., Wu, W., Chumlea, W., & Roche, A. (2002). Predicting overweight and obesity in adulthood from body mass index values in childhood and adolescence. *American Journal of Clinical Nutrition, 76*, 653–658.

Gupta, N. K., Mueller, W. H., Chan, W., & Meininger, J. C. (2002). Is obesity associated with poor sleep quality in adolescents? *American Journal of Human Biology, 14*(6), 762–768.

Hernandez, B., Uphold, C. R., Graham, M. V., & Singer, L. (1998). Prevalence and correlates of obesity in preschool children. *Journal of Pediatric Nursing, 13*(2), 68–76.

Hoppin, A. G. (2004). *Assessment and management of childhood and adolescent obesity*. Retrieved July 7, 2004 at http://www.medscape.com/viewprogram/3221_pnt.

Houck, G. M., Darnell, S., & Lussman, S. (2002). A support group intervention for at-risk female high school students. *Journal of School Nursing, 18*(2), 212–218.

Houck, G. M., King, M. C., Tomlinson, B., Vrabel, A., & Wecks, K. (2002). Small group intervention for children with attention disorders. *Journal of School Nursing, 18*(2), 196–200.

Houck, G. M., & Perri, C. (2002). A support group for absentee middle school students. *Journal of School Nursing, 18*(2), 201–205.

Houck, G. M., & Stember, L. (2002). Small group experience for socially withdrawn girls. *Journal of School Nursing, 18*(2), 206–211.

Kimm, S., Barton, B., Berhane, K., Ross, J., Payne, G., & Schreiber, G. (1997). Self-esteem and adiposity in black and white girls: The NHLBI growth and health study. *Annals of Epidemiology, 7*(8), 550–560.

Kimm, S. Y., Barton, B. B., Obarzanek, E., McMahon, R. P., Kronsberg, S. S., Waclawiw, M. A., Morrison, J. A., Schreiber, G. B., Sabry, S. I., & Daniels S. R. (2002a). Obesity development during adolescence in a biracial cohort: The NHLBI growth and health study. *Pediatrics, 110*(5), e54.

Kimm, S. Y., Glynn, N. W., Kriska, A. M., Barton, B. A., Kronsberg, S. S., Daniels, S. R., Crawford, P. B., Sabry, Z. I., & Liu, K. (2002b). Decline in physical activity in black girls and white girls during adolescence. *New England Journal of Medicine, 347*(10), 709–715.

Kimm, S., & Obarzanek, E. (2002). Childhood obesity: A new pandemic of the new millennium. *Pediatrics, 110*(5), 1003–1007.

Kubik, M. Y., Lytle, L. A., Hannan, P. J., Story, M., & Perry, C. L. (2002). Food-related beliefs, eating behavior, and classroom food practices of middle school teachers. *Journal of School Health, 72* (8), 339–345.

Kuczmarski, R. J., Ogden, C. L., Grummer-Strawn, L. M., et al. (2000). CDC growth charts: United States. *Advance data from Vital and Health Statistics*. No. 314. Hyattsville: National Center for Health Statistics.

Kuczmarski, R. J., Ogden, C. L., Guo, S. S., et al. (2002). 2000 CDC growth charts for the United States: methods and development. *Vital and Health Statistics*. No. 246. Hyattsville, MD: National Center for Health Statistics.

Latner, J. D., & Stunkard, A. J. (2003). Getting worse: the stigmatization of obese children. *Obesity Research, 11*(3), 452–456.

Lin, B. F., Frazao, E., & Guthrie, J. (1999). Away from home foods increasingly important to quality of American diet. *Agriculture Information Bulletin* 749. Washington, DC: U.S Department of Agriculture.

Lucas, B. (2004). Normal nutrition from infancy through adolescence. In P. Smour, K. Helm, & C. Lang (Eds.),. *Handbook of Pediatric Nutrition* (pp. 99–120). Boston: Jones & Bartlett.

Luder, E., Melnik, T. A., & DiMaio, M. (1998). Association of being overweight with greater asthma symptoms in inner city black and Hispanic children. *Journal of Pediatrics, 132*, 699–703.

MacNeil, G. A., & Newell, J. M. (2004). School bullying: Who, why, and what to do. *Prevention Researcher, 11*(3), 15–17.

Magarey, A. M., Daniels, L. A., Boulton, T. J., & Cockington, R. A. (2003). Predicting obesity in early adulthood from childhood and parental obesity. *International Journal of Obesity and Related Metabolic Disorders, 27*(4), 505–513.

McGarvey, E., Keller, A. Forrester, M., Williams, E., Seward, D., & Suttle, D. E. (2004). Feasibility and benefits of a parent-focused preschool child obesity intervention. *American Journal of Public Health, 94*(9), 1490–1495.

Moore, L. L., Gao, D., Bradlee, M. L., Cupples, L. A., Sundarajan-Ramamurti, A., Proctor, M. H., Hood, M. Y., Singer, M. R., & Ellison, R. C. (2003). Does early physical activity predict body fat change throughout childhood? *Preventive Medicine, 37*(1), 10–17.

Mustillo, S., Worthman, C., Erkanli, A., Keeler, G., Angold, A., & Costello, E. J. (2003). Obesity and psychiatric disorder: Developmental trajectories. *Pediatrics, 111* (4 Part 1), 851–859.

Myers, S., & Vargas, Z. (2000). Parental perceptions of the preschool obese child. *Pediatric Nursing, 26*(1), 23–30.

National Association of School Nurses (NASN). (2002). *Position statement: Overweight children and adolescents*. Available at http://www.nasn.org/positions/overweight.htm.

National Association of School Nurses (NASN). (2003). *Position statement: Individualized Health Care Plans*. Available at http://www.nasn.org/positions/careplans.htm.

National Governors Association Center for Best Practices. (2003). *Issue brief: Preventing obesity in youth through school-based efforts*. Retrieved February 1, 2004 from http://www.nga.org/center/divisions/1,1188,C_ISSUE_BRIEF^D_5109,00.html

Neumark-Sztainer, D., & Story, M. (1997). Recommendations from overweight youth regarding school-based weight control programs. *Journal of School Health, 67* (10), 428–433.

Nielsen, S. J., & Popkin, B. M. (2003). Patterns and trends in food portion sizes, 1977–1998. *Journal of the American Medical Association, 289*, 450–453.

Nishina, M., Kikuchi, T., Yamazaki, H., Kameda, K., Hiura, M., & Uchiyama, M. (2003). Relationship among systolic blood pressure, serum insulin and leptin, and visceral fat accumulation in obese children. *Hypertension Research, 26*(4), 281–288.

Ogden, C. L., Flegal, K. M., Carroll, M. D., & Johnson, C. L. (2002). Prevalence and trends in overweight among US children and adolescents, 1999–2000. *Journal of the American Medical Association, 288*, 1728–1732.

Patrick, K., Spear, B., Holt, K., & Sofka, D. (Eds.). (2001). *Bright futures in practice: physical activity*. Arlington, VA: National Center for Education in Maternal and Child Health.

Proctor, M. H., Moore, L. L., Gao, D., Cupples, L. A., Bradlee, M. L., Hood, M. Y., & Elison, R. C. (2003).

Television viewing and change in body fat from preschool to early adolescence: The Framingham children's study. *International Journal of Obesity and Related Metabolic Disorders, 27*(7), 827–833.

Roberts, E. A. (2003). Nonalcoholic steatohepatitis in children. *Current Gastroenterology Reports, 5*(3), 253–259.

Robinson, T. N. (2001). Television viewing and childhood obesity. *Pediatric Clinics of North America, 48*(4), 1017–1725.

Rodriguez, M. A., Winkleby, M. A., Ahn, D., Sundquist, J., & Kraemer, H. C. (2002). Identification of population subgroups of children and adolescents with high asthma prevalence: Findings from the third national health and nutrition examination survey. *Archives of Pediatrics and Adolescent Medicine, 156*(3), 269–275.

Salbe, A., Weyer, C., Lindsay, R., Ravussin, E., & Tataranni, P. A. (2002). Assessing risk factors for obesity between childhood and adolescence: I. Birth weight, childhood adiposity, parental obesity, insulin, and leptin. *Pediatrics, 110*(2), 299–306.

Schmitz, K. H., Jacobs, D. R., Hong, C-P., Steinberger, J., Moran, A., & Sinaiko, A. R. (2002). Association of physical activity with insulin sensitivity in children. *International Journal of Obesity and Related Metabolic Disorders, 26*(10), 1310–1316.

Sinha, R., Fisch, G., Teague, B., Tamborlane, W., Banyas, B., Allen, K., Savoye, M., Rieger, V., Taksali, S., Barbetta, G., Sherwin, R. S., & Caprio S. (2002). Prevalence of impaired glucose tolerance among children and adolescents with marked obesity. *New England Journal of Medicine, 346*, 802–810.

Skelton, J. (2004). Childhood obesity: Overview. *Consensus in Pediatrics: Childhood Obesity, 1*(4), 1–12.

Sorof, J., Lai, D., Turner, J., Poffenbarger, T., & Portman, R. (2004). Overweight, ethnicity, and the prevalence of hypertension in school-aged children. *Pediatrics, 113*(3), 475–482.

Spector, S. L., & Surette, M. E. (2003). Diet and asthma: Has the role of dietary lipids been overlooked in the management of asthma? *Annals of Allergy and Asthma Immunology, 90*(4), 371–377.

Srinivasan, S. R., Myers, L., & Berenson, G. S. (2002). Distribution and correlates of non-high-density lipoprotein cholesterol in children: The Bogalusa heart study. *Pediatrics, 110*(3), e29.

Srinivasan, S. R., Myers, L., & Berenson, G. S. (2002). Predictability of childhood adiposity and insulin for developing insulin resistance syndrome (syndrome x) in young adulthood. *Diabetes, 51*(1), 204–209.

Steffen, L. M., Jacobs, D. R., Jr., Murtaugh, M. A., Moran, A., Steinberger, J., Hong, C-P., & Sinaiko, A. R. (2003). Whole grain intake is associated with lower body mass and greater insulin sensitivity among adolescents. *American Journal of Epidemiology, 158*(3), 243–250.

Steinberger, J., & Daniels, S. R. (2003). Obesity, insulin resistance, diabetes, and cardiovascular risk in children: An American health association scientific statement from the atherosclerosis, hypertension, and obesity in the young committee. *Circulation, 107*, 1448–1453.

Steinberger, J., Moran, A., Hong, C. P., Jacobs, D. R., Jr., & Sinaiko, A. R. (2001). Adiposity in childhood predicts obesity and insulin resistance in young adulthood. *Journal of Pediatrics, 138*(4), 469–473.

St-Onge, M. P., Keller, K. L., & Heymsfield, S. B. (2003). Changes in childhood food consumption patterns: A cause for concern in light of increasing body weights. *American Journal of Clinical Nutrition, 78*(6), 1068–1073.

Story, M., Holt, K., & Sofka, D. (Eds.). (2002). *Bright futures in practice: Nutrition* (2nd ed.). Arlington, VA: National Center for Education in Maternal and Child Health.

Strauss, R. S. (2000). Childhood obesity and self-esteem. *Pediatrics, 105*(1), e15.

Strauss, R. S., & Knight, J. (1999). Influence of the home environment on the development of obesity in children. *Pediatrics, 103*(6). Retrieved January 30, 2004, from http://pediatrics.org/cgi/content/full/103/6/e85 .

Strauss, R. S., & Pollack, H. (2001). Epidemic increase in childhood overweight, 1986–1993. *Journal of the American Medical Association, 286*, 2845–2848.

Taras, H. L., & Gage, M. (1995). Advertised foods on children's television. *Archives of Pediatric Adolescent Medicine, 149*, 649–652.

Thompson, E. A., Eggert, L. L., Randell, B. P., & Pike, K. C. (2001). Evaluation of indicated suicide risk prevention approaches for potential high school dropouts. *American Journal of Public Health, 91*(5), 742–752.

Troiano, R. P., Briefel, R. R., Carroll, M. D., & Bialostosky, K. (2000). Energy and fat intakes of children and adolescents in the united states: Data from the national health and nutrition examination surveys. *American Journal of Clinical Nutrition, 72*(5 Suppl.), 1343s–1353s.

U.S. Department of Agriculture (USDA). (2001). *Changing the scene: Improving the school nutrition environment*. Washington, DC: U.S. Government Printing Office.

U.S. Department of Health and Human Services (USDHHS). (2000). *Healthy People 2010*. Washington, DC: U.S. Government Printing Office.

U.S. Department of Health and Human Services (USDHHS), Public Health Service, Office of the Surgeon General (2001). *The surgeon general's call to action to prevent and decrease overweight and obesity 2001*. Rockville, MD: Author.

U.S. Department of Labor. (2004). Consumer expenditures in 2003. *News: Bureau of Labor Statistics*. Accessed 4/05 at http://www.stats.bls.gov/news.release/cesan. toc.htm

Von Kries, R., Hermann, M., Grunert, V. P., & von Mutius, E. (2001). Is obesity a risk factor for childhood asthma? *Allergy, 56*, 318–322.

Wang, Y. (2002). Is obesity associated with early sexual maturation? A comparison of the association in American boys versus girls. *Pediatrics, 110*(5), 903–910.

Weepie, A. K., & McCarthy, A. M. (2002). A healthy lifestyle program: Promoting child health in schools. *Journal of School Nursing, 18*(6), 322–328.

Weinsier, R. L., Hunter G. R., Heini, A. F., Goran, M. I., & Sell, S. M. (1998). Etiology of obesity: Relative contribution of metabolic factors, diet, and physical activity. *American Journal of Medicine, 105*(2), 145–150.

Whitaker, R. C., Wright, J. A., Pepe, M. S., Seidel, K. D., & Dietz, W. H. (1997). Predicting obesity in young adulthood from childhood and parental obesity. *New England Journal of Medicine, 37*(13), 869–873.

Williams, L. C., Hayman, L., Daniels, S. R., Robinson, T. N., Steinberger, J., Paridon, S., & Bazzarre, T. (2002). Cardiovascular health in childhood. *Circulation, 106*(1), 143–160.

Chapter 37

Seizure Disorder

JULIE HENDERSON

Chapter Outline

INTRODUCTION

Seizures are the result of the misfiring, or abnormal discharges of neuronal activity in the brain. Normally, brain cells communicate with each other via electrical impulses. When a person has a seizure, the normal pattern of electrical impulses is interrupted by a surge of electrical activity that results in a temporary change in consciousness, sensation, motor activity, or behavior (Devinsky, 2002). A seizure can occur once in a person's life as a result of life events such as a high fever or an electrolyte imbalance, or they can occur with some frequency. The signs and symptoms depend on the cause and the location in the brain where the problem arose. There may be a single symptom unilaterally, or a group of symptoms affecting the whole body; there may be a staring spell lasting seconds or total body involvement lasting for minutes.

Seizure is a generic term. A seizure is a symptom of another problem; it is not a disease unto itself. Epilepsy, or seizure disorder, is a chronic condition that occurs when unprovoked seizures occur repeatedly, separated by more than 24 hours but not due to a current single trauma or illness event (Hauser, 2001; Pruitt, 2000). According to the Epilepsy Foundation (2003), seizures and epilepsy are not the same and the terms are not interchangeable. Seizures are a symptom of epilepsy. The terms *convulsion* and *fit* are no longer appropriate to describe either seizures or epilepsy; the medical terminology for seizure is *ictus*.

INCIDENCE

More than 2.5 million people in the United States have seizure disorders; of these, 300,000 are children from birth through age 14 (Epilepsy Foundation, 2003). The incidence is highest during infancy, and then decreases through childhood. While 40% of all those who seek medical attention each year because of new seizure activity are children or adolescents, the reason for most visits is a febrile seizure. Between 20,000 and 45,000 children and adolescents are diagnosed with epilepsy each year, with 5 to 6 years of age being the median age at seizure onset (Shinnar & Pellock, 2002).

CLASSIFICATION OF SEIZURES

The classification of seizures was developed by the International League Against Epilepsy, last modified in 1989 (Commission of Classification and Terminology of the International League Against Epilepsy, 1989). Seizures are classified as *partial* or *primary generalized* based on how the abnormal brain signals begin (see FIGURE 37.1). Seizures with a focal onset are called partial seizures, whereas seizures with a generalized onset are called primary generalized (Mayo Clinic, 2005). There are also seizures that do not fit into the any of these categories.

Partial seizures are classified as three types: simple partial, complex partial, or partial seizures that evolve into secondarily generalized seizures. Simple partial seizures begin in a localized area of the brain and do *not* result in a loss of consciousness. They may present with motor, somatosensory, autonomic, or psychic symptoms. For example, they may cause uncontrollable shaking of an arm, leg, or any other part of the body; a change in the way things look, smell, feel, taste, or sound; a speech disturbance; or altered emotions (Mayo Clinic, 2005).

Complex partial seizures, previously known as psychomotor or temporal lobe seizures, also begin from a localized area of the brain. They result in the same symptoms as simple partial seizures, except that there is an alteration in consciousness. This may present as staring spells and may include nonpurposeful movements, called automatisms, such as repeated hand rubbing, lip smacking, posturing of the arm, vocalization, or swallowing. The child may appear to be sleepwalking or intoxicated, and some children experience fear as a part of the seizure and may try to run away. After the seizure, the child may be confused and sleep for a few minutes and on awakening may be unaware of having had the seizure. The temporal lobe is the most common focus of these seizures (Mayo Clinic, 2005).

I. Partial seizures—focal origin
  A. Simple partial—originate in localized area of one hemisphere
    - No loss of consciousness
    - Motor symptoms: nonpurposeful movements
    - Autonomic symptoms: pallor, sweating, flushing, papillary dilation
    - Somatosensory symptoms: altered sensations
    - Psychic symptoms: altered emotions
  B. Complex partial seizures—originate in localized area of one hemisphere; temporal lobe is most common area.
    - Same symptoms as above, plus:
    - Aura—sensation of fear, epigastric discomfort, odd smell or taste
    - Impaired consciousness
    - Automatisms
  C. Secondary generalized seizures—partial seizures with secondary generalization; begin as a partial seizure and spread to both sides of the brain or the entire brain
    - Staring
    - Nonpurposeful movements
    - Tonic–clonic movements, extremity stiffening

II. Primary generalized seizures—originate in both hemispheres
  A. Absence seizures—previously known as petit mal seizures
    - Staring
    - Automatisms
    - Brief lapses of awareness
    - Mild loss of muscle tone
  B. Myoclonic seizures—unilateral or bilateral jerking movements
    - Sudden jerks of extremities
    - Brief
    - No loss of consciousness
  C. Atonic seizures—also known as astatic; sudden loss of muscle tone
    - Sudden collapse
    - Brief loss of muscle tone
    - Brief period of altered consciousness
  D. Generalized tonic–clonic seizures previously called grand mal—affect muscles and functions of the entire body
    - Aura-premonition that seizure is coming
    - Loss of consciousness
    - Tonic component: stiffening of entire body
    - Clonic component: spasm of muscle groups
    - Incontinence of urine and stool
    - Drooling
    - Brief hypoxia
    - Biting of tongue, clenching teeth
    - Eyes roll back
    - Postictal state of several minutes to several hours—period of confusion followed by sleep

Figure 37.1 ■ Seizure classification. (From Epilepsy Foundation [2003]; Gilbert, K. [1999].)

Secondarily generalized seizures, also called partial seizures with secondary generalization, occur when simple or complex partial seizures spread to the entire brain. They begin as simple partial or complex partial seizures with staring and nonpurposeful movements, and become more intense, leading to a generalized seizure characterized by stiffening (tonic) and/or shaking (clonic) of the extremities and the trunk.

A possible sequela of a complex partial or secondarily generalized seizure is a Todd paralysis. "This is a weakness (associated with the affected region of the brain) of a part or whole side of the body that can last from minutes to hours after a seizure" (Blair & Selekman, 2004, p. 474).

There are multiple types of primary generalized seizures. These include absence seizures, previously known as petit mal seizures; myoclonic seizures; atonic seizures, also known as drop attacks; clonic or tonic seizures; and generalized tonic–clonic seizures, also known as grand mal seizures (Blair & Selekman, 2004). Absence seizures are characterized by staring, subtle body movements (automatisms), and brief lapses of awareness and responsiveness for up to 20 seconds. They are brief and usually no confusion or sleepiness occurs when the seizure is over. Myoclonic seizures appear as sudden jerks of the arms and legs that are usually unilateral. They last from less than a second to a few seconds and involve quick muscle jerks. Atonic or akinetic seizures, also called drop attacks, cause the student to suddenly collapse or fall down with a brief loss of muscle tone. After a few seconds, the student regains consciousness and is able to stand and walk. Some individuals can bring on an atonic seizure by hyperventilating (Devinsky, 2002).

Generalized tonic–clonic seizures are the most intense of all types of seizures. They may be preceded by an aura, a change in behavior, or a sensation that is a premonition of the seizure; this is a preictal sensation. Some believe that the aura is a simple partial seizure. Particular smells or tastes, perceptual visual changes, or heightened hearing may signal the onset of seizure activity by minutes. The tonic component is usually first, starting with an utterance that might sound like a cry, but is actually "air being forced through the contracting vocal cords" (Devinsky, 2002, p. 26). In the tonic phase, all of the muscles tighten and stiffen, including the clamping down of the jaw. It is possible for a student to bite the tongue when this occurs. This phase is followed by the longer clonic phase, in which there is jerking of the arms and legs. Loss of consciousness occurs, and during the 1 to 3 minutes of the ictal phase, the student may have excessive saliva production and incontinence. Rarely, there is bowel incontinence, brief or prolonged color change due to hypoxia, and rolling back of the eyes during the seizure. In generalized tonic–clonic seizures, a period of confusion and sleepiness is often present in the postictal state, lasting a few minutes to a few hours (Mayo Clinic, 2005).

In addition to epilepsy, there are a number of medical syndromes for which seizure activity is a component. Seizure disorder may be a sequelae of a brain infection, such as viral meningitis; hypoxic brain trauma, such as near drowning; surgical adhesions resulting from tumor removal surgery; or brain damage resulting from vascular disorders such as stroke or aneurysm (Epilepsy Foundation, 2003). Some cases of epilepsy are mild and may resolve by adolescence; others result in significant developmental delay and cognitive impairment, with hundreds of seizures each day (Blair & Selekman, 2004).

A number of conditions may resemble seizure activity, but do not have the electroencephalographic (EEG) changes typical of the various seizure types. These include psychogenic seizures, migraine headache syndromes, narcolepsy, sleepwalking, night terrors, staring spells, complex tics, breath-holding spells, and syncope spells. Psychogenic seizures, or pseudoseizures, are symptoms of psychiatric conditions such as conversion disorder or dissociation disorder (American Epilepsy Society [AES], 2004). They result from "subconscious mental activity (not abnormal brain electrical activity)" (Devinsky, 2002, p. 90). They are more common in adolescent females than in other groups and often occur in students who also have true epileptic seizures (Paolicchi, 2002). These students need to have an EEG done during the event.

Migraine headache syndromes can mimic seizures. They can be characterized by severe headache, focal neurological deficits, photophobia and phonophobia, and loss of awareness (Pruitt, 2000). According to Prensky (2001), children with narcolepsy fall asleep suddenly during the day with accompanying temporary loss of muscle tone and may also have sleep paralysis, an inability to move on awakening. Sleepwalking can mimic complex partial seizures because the child's eyes are open as he or she walks around the house mumbling and can become agitated if restrained during the episode. Tics can be simple and involve one or two muscle groups, such as eye blinking, shoulder shrugging, head turning, tongue thrust, or sniffing. Complex tics involve a number of muscle groups and produce complex repetitive movements, but no loss of consciousness (Prensky, 2001). Night terrors occur during stages 3 or 4 of slow-wave sleep and are characterized by the child sitting up in bed screaming inconsolably and appearing terrified with dilated pupils and diaphoresis. They can last up to 15 minutes or more and the child falls back to sleep with no recollection of the event (Prensky, 2001).

Breath-holding spells occur in children younger than 8 years of age as a result of fear, frustration, injury, or crying and can result in cyanosis and loss of consciousness for 1 to 2 minutes. Syncope can be confused with epilepsy owing to the loss of consciousness and tonic or tonic–clonic movements that occur during the event (AES, 2004). The prodromal symptoms such as lightheadedness, blurred vision, visual dimming, pallor, and diaphoresis resemble a seizure aura. However, none of these are considered seizures or epilepsy.

STATUS EPILEPTICUS

In the event that seizure activity lasts more than 30 minutes without the student regaining consciousness, the student is considered to be in status epilepticus; this is a medical emergency requiring immediate attention with EMS intervention. Results of a status epilepticus event may include stroke, cerebral infarct, aspiration, hypoxia, high fever, hypotension, and death (Hay, Hayward, Levy, & Sondheimer, 2003). "Status epilepticus is classified as convulsive (tonic–clonic, 90%) or nonconvulsive (characterized by altered mental status or behavior with subtle or absent motor components, 10%)" (Hay et al., 2003, p. 729). Absence status and rarely, partial complex status epilepticus, are examples of the nonconvulsive type. From 25% to 75% of children experience status epilepticus with their first seizure. Infection or metabolic disorders are the most common causes of status epilepticus in children, and it occurs most commonly (85%) in children 5 years and younger (Hay et al., 2003).

To facilitate a rapid emergency response, it is helpful for the parent and school nurse to register the child experiencing seizures with the local fire department and emergency medical service (EMS) so that they will be able to respond with the type of equipment most helpful to the student with seizures, particularly if the student often has hypoxic episodes and requires oxygen therapy. In addition, the Seizure Action Plan developed by the school nurse will also facilitate care and transport. (The Seizure Action Plan is discussed below.)

Since the development of the diazepam (Valium) rectal gel, Diastat, emergency room visits associated with status epilepticus have decreased (Shafer, 1999). The ability to administer Diastat gives parents and caregivers in the school the reassurance that treatment can begin immediately and the sequelae of delayed treatment can be avoided. Diastat is a single-dose diazepam (Valium) gel within a prefilled rectal delivery system. It is well absorbed following rectal administration, with peak plasma concentrations reached in 1.5 hours (*Physician's Desk Reference* [PDR], 2004). Approved by the FDA in 1997 and used primarily in inpatient settings, Diastat is now prescribed more often for use in the school setting. Parents and caregivers can administer Diastat in the event that a student experiences refractory seizures or a seizure cluster, if school policy allows. Circumstances under which the Diastat will be administered are clearly outlined in the physician's order and include assessments to be made for 4 hours after the drug is given. The main side effect is central nervous system (CNS) depression and somnolence.

Nursing considerations in the school setting include the provision of privacy in the administration of a rectal drug. Seizures can occur in any school location, and it may be necessary to administer medication on the playground, in a stairwell, or in the computer lab. School nurses can utilize several drapes and furniture screens, as well as modest positioning to protect the student's dignity when Diastat is administered. After the administration of Diastat in the school setting, the child needs frequent assessment of vital signs (every 5 to 15 minutes) and possible transport to an emergency room. Pulse oximetry measurement is helpful to assess the need for oxygen therapy. The manufacturer recommends that Diastat be used to treat no more than five episodes a month and no more than one episode every 5 days. If a second dose is ordered for a single episode, it may be given 4 to 12 hours after the first dose (PDR, 2004).

FEBRILE SEIZURES

Febrile seizures are the most common cause of seizures seen in children, with approximately 3% experiencing a febrile seizure at least once (Shinnar & Glauser, 2002). They are most commonly seen before the age of 7 years and occur when the fever reaches a rectal temperature greater than 102°F. A tonic–clonic seizure usually occurs shortly after the fever starts and while the fever is on a rapid increase; it can last anywhere from a few seconds to 2 minutes (Devinsky, 2002; Febrile Seizures, 2001).

"The vast majority of febrile seizures are harmless" (National Institute of Neurological Disorders and Stroke [NINDS], 2001). They do not cause brain damage and rarely result in continued seizure activity and epilepsy. Hospitalization is not required, unless a student has injured him or herself during the seizure or if it lasts longer than 10 minutes (Febrile Seizures, 2001). Antiepileptic medications are also not recommended, unless other conditions exist that warrant it. While there is some increase in incidence if a family member has a history of a febrile seizure, in general, "the older a child is when the first seizure occurs, the lower the risk that more seizures will follow" (Febrile Seizures, 2001).

ETIOLOGY

For the medical team to plan care, it is important for the etiology of the child's seizures to be determined, perhaps by the process of exclusion. The most common causes include a prior insult to the brain, which might be from episodes of asphyxia before, during or after birth, or at any point during the life cycle; neurological bleeding, whether caused by trauma, premature birth, or vascular lesions; lesions caused by infection, such as meningitis; electrolyte disorders; and degenerative encephalopathies. Seizure disorders are classified as symptomatic when the cause is identified or presumed, idiopathic when the cause is unknown or presumed to be genetic, or cryptogenic when the cause is unknown but is thought to have a pathological component. The younger the child, the more likely it is the cause can be identified. Epilepsy due to genetic causes most often appears between ages 4 and 16 (Hay et al., 2003).

A history of any of the above scenarios will help to explain the possible etiology of the seizure activity. Complications with the pregnancy or childbirth that may have resulted in a hypoxic episode or maternal drug use, neurological infections, exposure to lead or other heavy metals or carbon monoxide poisoning, or episodes of severe electrolyte disturbance may be some of the causes of a seizure disorder (Hingley, 1999). A history of head trauma with subarachnoid hemorrhage or depressed skull fracture can infrequently cause seizures within months to years, but emboli and cortical vein thrombosis are more likely to result in seizures in young adults (Pruitt, 2000). There may also be a family history of seizures, perhaps caused by a genetic structural abnormality or a dysfunction of the ion channels (Blair & Selekman, 2004).

HOW A DIAGNOSIS IS MADE FOLLOWING THE FIRST SEIZURE

School nurses should be familiar with the extent of diagnostic testing that is involved when the student is referred to a neurologist after the first seizure. School nurses will then be able to assist the child and family to understand the treatment plan and to work with the interdisciplinary team. To rule out CNS infection, a lumbar puncture and CBC with differential may be performed. A chemistry profile, including a serum calcium measurement, is performed to rule out hypocalcemia, electrolyte imbalances, and renal failure. Liver function tests are performed to rule out hepatic failure, and alcohol and drug levels are performed if alterations in the levels are suspected. An EKG is obtained to ascertain the presence of an arrhythmia or heart block. Magnetic resonance imaging (MRI) or computed tomography (CT) scan is performed if a tumor, cerebral hemorrhage, or trauma is thought to be a cause of the seizures. CT scans are utilized to identify bleeding and gross structural abnormalities such as subdural fluid collections, congenital abnormalities, and cerebral infarcts. MRIs are more sensitive and evaluate for abnormalities in the brain parenchyma and structure such as small tumors, scarring, neural migration disorders, and slow bleeding (Gilbert, 1999).

The magnetoencephalogram (MEG) is a newer tool used to measure the magnetic signals in the brain. The MEG is useful because it can detect normal and abnormal signals from deeper in the brain without the use of electrodes (National Institutes of Health [NIH] Medline Plus, 2003). In addition, positive emission tomography (PET scan) is used in some centers to identify areas of the brain producing seizures (Epilepsy Foundation, 2003).

The electroencephalogram (EEG) is a standard diagnostic tool for new onset seizures. It is rare that a seizure will be recorded during an EEG, but generalized types of seizures will produce abnormalities of general spike and wave activity or generalized slowing on routine EEG recordings. On the other hand, interictal EEG abnormalities that are either focal or generalized do not necessarily signal seizure activity. Epileptiform abnormalities that are recorded interictally can assist in localizing the focal area of the seizure activities (Gilbert, 1999).

In some cases a video EEG can be done, although this can involve a hospital admission of several days, during which the child is sleep-deprived in order to trigger seizure activity that can be recorded simultaneously by an EEG and video monitoring system. Laboratories also use photic stimulation and hyperventilation during video EEG. Kotagal (2001) found that sleep deprivation is known to influence not only the occurrence but also the symptomatology of seizures. Gilbert, DeRoos, and Bare (2004) studied the practice of encouraging partial or complete sleep deprivation in order to elicit seizure activity on EEG and found that use of sleep deprived EEG does not necessarily increase the odds of finding interictal epileptiform discharges. Sleep architecture and daytime alertness are influenced by seizures and antiepileptic medications. Seizures occur extensively during sleep or on awakening in a substantial portion of individuals with epilepsy and can be captured with this technology.

THE SCHOOL NURSE'S ROLE IN ASSESSMENT AND PLANNING

The school nurse is responsible for developing an Individualized Health Plan (IHP) for these students (Table 37.1). When interviewing the student with a history of seizures and his or her parents, the nurse needs to elicit an accurate description of the child's seizures from both the student's and parents'

(text continues on page 872)

Table 37.1 ■
INDIVIDUALIZED STUDENT HEALTH PLAN

School Year ______________
Student ______________________________ Date of Birth ______________ Grade __________
Homeroom ____________________
Medical Diagnosis ______________ Medications ______________________________
Medical Home ________________ Parent/Guardian ______________

NURSING DIAGNOSIS	GOALS	NURSING INTERVENTIONS	EXPECTED STUDENT OUTCOMES
Potential for injury related to uncontrolled movements of seizure activity	Student will not be injured during a seizure.	Protect child before, during, and after the seizure: Helmet if head-banging, seat belts used on school bus and in wheelchair; when possible, use carpeted area of classroom for a place to go if feeling a seizure is coming. Encourage teacher to assign double buddies for the child with seizures, if appropriate: one to stay with the child to allay fears and one to run or call for assistance. Administer antiepileptic medications as prescribed and document child's responses. Establish appropriate activity restrictions in cooperation with physician orders and parents. Gym may be modified based on seizure types. (Reassess each semester.) Document seizure activity which occurs during school hours in detail and communicate to parents and healthcare providers. Provide emergency care: have oxygen and/or suction available, wheelchair accessible, and possibly elevator key for transport where available. First aid for seizures to be reviewed with staff and assistive personnel.	Student will not experience injury during seizures. Student will have seizure activity controlled with medications, diet, treatments as prescribed. Staff and administration will demonstrate understanding of the Emergency Action Plan. School staff will respond promptly to a seizure emergency according to the plan.

(continued)

NURSING DIAGNOSIS	GOALS	NURSING INTERVENTIONS	EXPECTED STUDENT OUTCOMES
Potential for aspiration related to seizure activity	Student will not aspirate during a seizure.	Demonstrate effective positioning on side and clearing secretions from child's mouth to prevent aspiration.	Student will not aspirate during a seizure.
Potential for impaired social interactions related to chronic condition	Student will receive support and encouragement toward successful social interactions.	Give classmates roles to play during an emergency, such as clearing area, calling to office, noting the time and remaining in their seats. Assist student to disclose disability to peers and friends within compliance with HIPAA confidentiality laws and as needed. Provide support for development and maintenance of social skills. Assist parents and student to become involved in scouting programs, clubs and non-contact sports.	Peers accept classmate as an equal with full inclusion.
Potential self-esteem disturbance related to chronic condition	Student will have positive self-esteem. Student will experience school success proportionate to ability rather than disability.	Coach student to do a class presentation about seizure disorder. Praise for measures taken to prevent a seizure from occurring or diminish the possibility of injury (taking medications, VNS, moving to a safe area)	Student shares feelings about how he/she views self. Student assumes role-related responsibilities. Student demonstrates confidence in ability to succeed despite disability.
Fear related to recurrent seizures unresponsive to treatment	The source of the child's fear will be identified. The child will have less fear of the unknown results of treatment.	Provide emotional support to students and staff. Assess factors contributing to fear; reduce or eliminate contributing factors through education and referral to health care provider	Student verbalizes and identifies sources of fear, reports increased sense of comfort. Student verbalizes less anxiety about fear of the unknown and about loss of control.
Altered health maintenance related to knowledge deficit of benefit of compliance to prescribed regimen	The child and family will verbalize the importance and benefits of treatment.	Support parents to seek Child Study Team/Special Education classification as having a chronic condition, which will justify absences and provide intermittent home instruction and other services.	Student describes his/her condition, causes and factors contributing to symptoms and procedures for disease and symptom control.

(continued)

Table 37.1 ■ *(Continued)*

NURSING DIAGNOSIS	GOALS	NURSING INTERVENTIONS	EXPECTED STUDENT OUTCOMES
		Make referral to counseling as needed related to loss issues. Collaborate with staff of medical home regarding compliance with medical regimen and/or ketogenic diet, seizure log, appointments, medication effectiveness and side effects. Reduce or eliminate barriers to learning. Provide instruction in area of knowledge deficit. Provide self-care education to student related to seizures, medications, safety issues and diagnostic testing. Refer student and family to community agencies in order to facilitate participation in a support group, or to ensure child receives specialty care.	Student understands and complies with medication and the medical treatment plan. Student participates in classroom and extracurricular activities as tolerated. Student will use less medication to control seizures after ketogenic diet induction. Student actively participates in health behaviors prescribed or desired in collaboration with neurology specialist team.

Source: Gerber, M. (1999). Seizures. In M. Haas (Ed.), *The school nurse's source book of individualized healthcare plans* (pp. 385–402). North Branch, MN: Sunrise River Press.

perspective and description of typical and atypical events that occur before, during, and after the seizure. The description may include the presence of an aura, or warning prior to the seizure. The aura may include sensory symptoms such as an unusual scent or taste or visual disturbance, or may be characterized by a headache or muscle weakness. For example, complex partial seizures that originate in the temporal lobe are often preceded by a gastric sensation (Gilbert, 1999). Seizures may be characterized by incontinence, falls resulting in injury, or tongue-biting. The school nurse needs to note when and how often seizures occur, how they start, what part or parts of the body are affected and how seizures are manifested, as well as changes in consciousness and behavior during the seizure. The events of the postictal period may include confusion, weakness of one or both sides, severe headache, and the need to sleep.

Document the frequency, duration, and characteristic behaviors of any past seizures and the presence of any predisposing factors that may trigger seizure activity such as illness, injury, or emotional factors; others might include flashing lights or hyperventilation. The physical examination is usually normal and unremarkable between periods of seizure activity, but there may be signs that seizure activity has occurred such as the tongue or cheek bitten on one side, leg and arm bruises, or weakness (Gilbert, 1999). Neurological signs such as unilateral weakness, memory changes, or changes in reflexes may be residual from prior seizure activity.

For a student with a history of seizures, it is helpful to know how old the student was at the diagnosis of the seizure problem, whether hospitalizations have ever been needed, and how long it has been since the last seizure. It is essential to know how the seizure is generally managed during the seizure and between seizures (i.e., medications, safety helmets, identification tags, or activity restrictions), and how the diagnosis has affected the family. If there was no past history prior to the current seizure, exploring the history of head trauma in the past month, whether chemicals or medications were taken within the previous 24 hours, dietary intake for the past 24 hours, and other health conditions may assist the nurse and family in understanding the cause of the problem (Hootman, 2004).

Baseline height and weight measurements will be helpful in assessing whether the medications given for treatment are affecting the student's growth. A developmental assessment can also be used as baseline for future evaluations

A Seizure Action Plan (see FIGURE 37.2) should be developed as part of the student's healthcare plan. In school districts in which there is not a nurse assigned to each building, the seizure action plan designates particular staff with preassigned roles to respond to the seizure incident. When a student with a history of seizures is admitted to a school, the administration has the obligation to work with the parents to develop an appropriate action plan and to have the needed equipment on hand. It should be stipulated how the student will be transported to the nurse's office for care in the event of a seizure if the school does not have an elevator or the fact that the student would not be transported to the hospital for routine seizure activity. If oxygen might be needed, it would need to be ordered by the student's physician. A portable pulse oximeter is useful to assess the need for oxygen therapy and to assess the student's response to the therapy. If transport in an ambulance is needed, the school nurse or school personnel designated by the principal should accompany the student and bring a copy of the seizure history and medication regimen.

The Seizure Action Plan should be given to the main office, classroom teacher/s, physical education teacher, custodial staff, and security officers with information about the student with seizures in the building, the type of seizures, and first aid to be given by the first responder. The main office needs to have several ways to contact the parent or guardian during the school day.

The nurse should be aware that fever associated with any immune response may result in an increase in seizure activity; therefore, more attention will be paid to the student with a history of seizures who is febrile. Standing orders should be on hand to provide antipyretics at the first sign of fever.

School nurses evaluating immunization records need to know that the American Academy of Pediatrics (AAP) has made recommendations regarding the administration of the new attenuated pertussis vaccine to children with a history of seizures. The recommendation states that children with neurological

Seizure Action Plan

Date: __________ Student: __________ Room/Teacher __________
Date of Birth __________ Bus Student? Y N
School/Route# __________

Parent name __________ Address __________
Home phone __________ Cell phone __________
Work location, phone __________
Emergency contact name __________ Phone __________

Local primary care provider __________ Phone __________ FAX __________
Address __________
Neurologist/ specialty center __________
Address __________
Phone __________ FAX __________

Seizure type(s) __________ Frequency __________
Aura/type __________ Duration __________
Medication regimen:
____
____

Child uses Diastat rectal suppositories for status epilepticus or refractory seizures Y N
(See physician orders)
Diet: __________
Respiratory distress/treatment __________
History of cyanotic seizures? Y N Oxygen orders? __________
Incontinent: Urine __________ Stool __________ Postictal state: __________
Equipment needed: (circle) Wheelchair Oxygen tank Elevator Blanket/pillows
In the event of a seizure emergency, caretakers are instructed to take the following steps:
Child is evacuated first in the event of an emergency evacuation
____
____
____
____
____
____

Figure 37.2 ■ Seizure action plan.

impairments, particularly seizures, need to be assessed individually to determine if the potential value of pertussis vaccine outweighs the risk of increasing seizure activity. Children with well-controlled seizures can be immunized for pertussis (Centers for Disease Control and Prevention [CDC], National Immunization Program, 2005).

MEDICAL MANAGEMENT

Treatments for seizure disorders are varied; some students need only a safe environment, whereas others take antiepileptic drugs (AEDs), have surgical procedures, or use special diets.

Pharmacological Interventions

The ideal pharmacological treatment for recurrent seizures is monotherapy, the administration of a single antiepileptic drug according to the seizure type diagnosed. Generalized seizures respond best to treatment; full seizure control is possible using one drug for as many as 60% to 80% of patients with seizures (Mayo Clinic, 2005). The drug is used in doses sufficient to control the seizures as fully as possible with minimal side effects. If side effects of the drug become intolerable, the drug is replaced with another one until it is clear that the seizures cannot be controlled on a single drug. When a drug is no longer effective and needs to be replaced, physicians generally will add a second drug to the regimen rather than to substitute a second drug for the first. This will provide some seizure protection while the serum concentration of the second drug is rising. In this way, the first drug can then be tapered before being discontinued to offer continuous protection. A combination regimen of two or three antiepileptic drugs can control another 15% to 20% of patients with seizures (Pruitt, 2000). For the remaining patients, surgery or experimental drug therapy is an option.

Some of the AEDs (Table 37.2) block the sustained repetitive firing; these include carbamazepine (Tegretol) and phenytoin (Dilantin). Others, such as phenobarbital, valproic acid (Depakene, Depakote), and the benzodiazepines (Diastat), block the sustained firing and enhance gamma-aminobutyric acid (GABA) inhibitory transmission (Pruitt, 2000). GABA is an inhibitory neurotransmitter that limits or prevents transmission of an electrical stimulus, while glutamate is excitatory and increases them. Some effective anticonvulsants work by increasing the activity of GABA or decreasing the activity of glutamate.

Electrolyte channel conduction of sodium, calcium, and chloride ions is involved in seizure discharges. "Sodium and calcium conduction is important in the initiation and maintenance of seizure discharge, and chloride is linked to decreased neuronal firing rate and membrane hyperpolarization" (Noviasky, Porsteinsson, & Lee, 2001, p. 104). Many of the second-generation anticonvulsants decrease sodium and calcium channel conductance or increase chloride channel conductance. Different medications work on the different types of seizure activity.

Some AEDs, such as phenytoin and phenobarbital, have been used for decades, with demonstrated efficacy against various types of seizures, especially partial, secondarily generalized, and tonic–clonic seizures. However, all AEDs have side effects (Table 37.2), especially drowsiness, fatigue, nausea, and dizziness. More serious side effects include bone marrow depression for many and gingival hyperplasia specific to phenytoin (Pruitt, 2000). Many new AEDs developed over the past decade are becoming quite popular. Gabapentin (Neurontin), lamotrigine (Lamictal), topiramate (Topamax), and oxcarbazepine (Trileptal) are now utilized to treat partial and secondarily generalized tonic–clonic seizures (Pruitt, 2000). Felbamate was approved in 1993, but in 1994 was relabeled to warn against development of aplastic anemia and liver problems in some patients (Hingley, 1999). Newer drugs, however, are generally more costly and availability in some areas varies.

Antiepileptic medications can decrease the effectiveness of hormonal contraception methods. Teens who use AEDs may need to use a higher estrogen dose oral contraceptive (Gilbert, 1999). Many of the antiepileptic drugs, such as phenytoin, carbamazepine, and valproic acid, are teratogenic if used during the first trimester of gestation. Phenytoin can cause digital and craniofacial abnormalities and cardiac defects. Both valproic acid and carbamazepine can cause neural tube defects and carbamazepine can also cause facial abnormalities (Pruitt, 2000). The American Academy of Neurology (AAN) recommends that women of childbearing age be treated with monotherapy whenever possible to decrease the risk of teratogenesis (Pruitt, 2000). Healthcare providers will prescribe folic acid supplements and monitor folic acid levels in pregnant teens to decrease the risk of neural tube birth defects (Penovich, 2000).

Women taking phenytoin have a 94% chance of having a completely normal pregnancy outcome (NINDS, 2003). Pregnancy has no effect on the severity of seizures for about half of patients, but one-fourth of them experience worsening of their seizures during pregnancy (Pruitt, 2000). One sixth of women have a decrease in seizure activity during pregnancy (Klein & Herzog, 2000). Students with

(text continues on page 879)

Table 37.2 ■

ANTIEPILEPTIC DRUGS

DRUG	DOSAGE RANGE	SIDE EFFECTS	HALF-LIFE/ PEAK EFFECT	DRUG LEVELS (μG/ML)	COMMENTS
Phenobarbital (Luminal)	60–250 mg/day PO in single or divided dose	Drowsiness (tolerance develops), difficulties with memory and cognition, exacerbates depression	Half-life: 46–136 hours Peak: 20–60 minutes after oral dose	10–40 (levels take 3–4 weeks to stabilize)	Cannot be stopped suddenly, needs to be tapered. Used in simple, complex partial, and generalized tonic–clonic seizures.
Phenytoin (Dilantin)	300–600 mg daily	Gingival hyperplasia, mild sedation, rash, nausea, vomiting, lethargy, nystagmus, ataxia with high doses, difficulty with concentration and memory	Half-life: 10–34 hours PO, 10–15 hours IV Peak: 4–12 hours	10–20 (levels stay therapeutic 7–10 days after discontinuing)	Used in complex partial and generalized tonic–clonic seizures. IV preparation used to treat status epilepticus. Levels need to be drawn more often if patient also taking valproic acid. Degree of nystagmus guides dosing.
Carbamazepine (Tegretol)	600–1,200 mg daily in divided doses	Drowsiness, dizziness, nausea, vomiting which decrease over time. Titration started slowly to minimize side effects. Bone marrow suppression is major concern	Half-life: 12–17 hours Peak: 4–5 hours	4–12	Used in simple and complex partial seizures, but not for absence seizures. Take with food. Generic preparations associated with breakthrough seizures.

(continued)

Table 37.2 ■ *(Continued)*

DRUG	DOSAGE RANGE	SIDE EFFECTS	HALF-LIFE/ PEAK EFFECT	DRUG LEVELS (μG/ML)	COMMENTS
Primidone (Mysoline)	Dosage titrated slowly by 125 mg until 250–500 mg tid is reached	Ataxia, vertigo and drowsiness may occur but decrease over time or with dose reduction	Half-life: 16–18 hours	5–12	Used in complex partial, generalized tonic–clonic, and simple partial seizures. Metabolizes to phenobarbital, phenobarbital levels need to be monitored.
Valproic acid (Depakote sprinkles, Depakene)	15–60 mg/kg/day to maximum of 3,500–4,000 mg/day	Nausea, vomiting, tremor, possible weight gain, hair loss, platelet dysfunction, liver dysfunction, neural tube defects in developing fetuses	Half-life: 6–16 hours Peak: 1–4 hours	50–100, over 100 may be tolerated by some patients if well controlled.	Used in complex partial and primary generalized seizures such as absence and myoclonic.
Lamotrigine (Lamictal)	5–15 mg/kg/day bid 1–5 mg/kg/day bid with valproic acid	Dizziness, nausea, somnolence, psychomotor slowing, mood disturbances, weight loss, thrombocytopenia, rash, Stevens–Johnson Syndrome, toxic epidermal necrolysis	Half-life: 18–30 hours Peak: Within 2 hours	4–20: dosage titrated according to effectiveness, not a blood level	Used with valproate for partial seizures and for primary generalized seizures. Increase daily total fluid intake. Used to treat seizures associated with Lennox–Gastaut Syndrome. Risk of serious dermatological side effects greater if taken with valproic acid. Avoid sunlight (Photosensitivity)

Gabapentin (Neurontin)	900–1,800 mg/day; titrated to 300 mg tid then increased by 300 mg increments.	Somnolence, dizziness, ataxia, fatigue; Side effects are short-lived; Reduced interactions if taken as adjunct therapy with other AEDs	Half-life: 5–9 hours Peak: 2–3 hours	2–20; Because drug is not metabolized completely, significance of levels is uncertain.	Used in simple partial, complex partial, and generalized tonic–clonic seizures. To be taken at least 2 hours after Maalox to avoid changes in bioavailability.
Topiramate (Topamax)	200–600 mg/day bid; titrated slowly at 25 mg weekly increments	Somnolence, dizziness, psychomotor slowing, speech hesitancy, mood disturbances, weight loss related to nausea, diplopia, renal calculi.	Half-life: 18–30 hours Peak: Within 2 hours	Because drug is not metabolized completely, significance of levels is uncertain.	Used as adjunct therapy in partial seizures in adults, but for myoclonic and primary generalized seizures and Lennox–Gastaut syndrome in children. Cognitive effects need to be monitored, especially speech disturbances, confusion and anger/hostility Increase total daily fluid intake to minimize risk of renal stone formation. Tablets have bitter taste–do not break.
Tiagabine (Gabitril)	32–56 mg/day; Titrated by 4 mg/week	Somnolence, headache, mild memory impairment, hand tremors, abdominal pain.	Half-life: 5–9 hours Peak: 0.5–1 hour	Levels not established.	Used as adjunct therapy in simple and complex partial and generalized tonic–clonic seizures. Take with food.

(continued)

Table 37.2 ■ *(Continued)*

DRUG	DOSAGE RANGE	SIDE EFFECTS	HALF-LIFE/ PEAK EFFECT	DRUG LEVELS (μG/ML)	COMMENTS
Felbamate (Felbatol)	600–3,600 mg/ day	Insomnia, anorexia, headache, nausea, and vomiting. **Manufacturer warning of aplastic anemia and hepatic failure**	Half-life: 20–23 hours	Levels of adjunct therapy affect titration.	Used in complex partial, absence and generalized tonic–clonic seizures and an adjunct therapy for Lennox–Gastaut Syndrome and uncontrolled seizures. Avoid sunlight (photosensitivity). CBC and LFT's monitored frequently. Assess for signs of infection, signs of bleeding, and signs of anemia. Assess for signs of hepatic insufficiency–bruising, nausea, weight loss, jaundice.
Zonisamide (Zonegran)	2–4 mg/kg/day titrated to 12 mg/kg/day qd to tid	**Manufacturer warning of aplastic anemia and agranulocytosis** Risk of serious dermatological side effects: Stevens–Johnson syndrome and toxic epidermal necrolysis. Oligohydrosis, decreased ability or inability to sweat. Drowsiness		15–40	Used in infantile spasms. Sulfonamide base, should not be used in patients allergic to sulfa drugs. CBC and LFTs monitored frequently. Assess for signs of infection, signs of bleeding, and signs of anemia. Monitor for increased temperature and ability to reduce temperature with sweating.

Source: Data from Noviasky, J., Porsteinsson, A., & Lee, Y. (2001). Second-generation anticonvulsant medications. Their use in children. *Journal of School Nursing, 17*(2), 103–111; Physician Desk Reference (2004); Blair, J., & Selekman, J. (2004). Epilepsy. In P. Jackson & J. Vessey, *Primary care of the child with a chronic condition* (p. 482). St. Louis: C. V. Mosby; Gilber, K. (1999), Seizure disorder. In Buttaro, T., Trybulski, J., Bailey, P., & Sandberg-Cook, J. *Primary care: A collaborative practice*. St. Louis, C. V. Mosby.

seizures who inform the school nurse that they are sexually active should be encouraged to speak to their healthcare providers to make sure that they understand the risks associated with pregnancy to them and their developing fetus and to ensure that contraceptives are available, if appropriate.

Ketogenic Diet

Developed more than 80 years ago, the ketogenic diet is still used today as an adjunct to medications in the treatment of frequent seizures. One-third of children will become seizure free after using the diet for 1 to 3 months (Epilepsy Foundation, 2003). Some parents say that the diet makes the child more alert.

During a state of fasting, the body has a 24-hour backup supply of glucose to use for energy. When that supply is used, the body begins to break down fat stores for energy. The products of fat breakdown are ketones. For reasons unknown to researchers, being in a state of ketosis stops or decreases seizures dramatically in about half of those who comply with the diet.

The diet has a ratio of 3 to 5 grams of fat to 1 gram of carbohydrate and protein at each meal, and the total calories are reduced (Epilepsy Foundation, 2003). By keeping the caloric amount low and the fat content high, the process of ketosis is maintained and the antiepileptic effect is achieved. The diet contains small amounts of fruits and vegetables, which are the carbohydrate source; a small amount of meat, fish or poultry to meet the protein requirement; and a large amount of fat, such as mayonnaise, eggs, butter, and cream. The most important aspect of the diet is the exclusion of sugars, even those in small amounts as in sweeteners added to syrup medications, toothpaste, and sugar sprinkles (Epilepsy Foundation, 2003).

Some students on the ketogenic diet test their urine daily for the maintenance of a ketotic state, and most test weekly for hematuria. Hematuria can develop as a result of kidney stones, which are a side effect of the diet (Epilepsy Foundation, 2003). The diet is initiated when the child is an inpatient in the hospital with a 24- to 72-hour fast; the child may have only water during this time, with no solid foods. The child may become lethargic during this switch from glucose to fat as an energy source and monitoring of strict compliance is necessary. After the initial fast, foods on the diet are introduced slowly and the parents are taught how to prepare and measure the small meals. Side effects of the diet include dehydration and constipation, complications of gall and kidney stones, menstrual irregularities in teens and adults, pancreatitis, decreased bone density, and high serum cholesterol and triglyceride levels (Epilepsy Foundation, 2003). Follow-up studies indicate that serum cholesterol and triglyceride levels will return to normal levels when the child has been off the diet for 2 years.

Patients are advised that if the diet proves successful, they can plan to taper or discontinue anticonvulsants within 2 years. Gilbert, Pyzik, Vining, and Freeman (1999) studied the medication cost reduction associated with the ketogenic diet, and found that of the 57% of children who stayed on the diet for a year, medications were reduced in 74%. Forty-eight percent of the children who stayed on the diet were on no medications at their 12-month follow-up. Daily medication costs were reduced by 70%.

Children who are using the ketogenic diet as adjunct treatment for their seizures need to be followed by the nutritionist at their neurology clinic. The nutritionist will provide the school nurse with a detailed diet plan. The safest way to ensure compliance with the diet and to avoid errors is to have the parent pack the child's lunch and to supply the school nurse with additional powdered drink mix and packaged snacks for alternative birthday party snacks. It is vital for the classroom teacher to be educated about the diet so that it can be reinforced with the student. Children in the lower elementary grades need daily monitoring of their food intake in the classroom and cafeteria, and on field trips. School nurses need to inform the teaching assistants, bus and lunch aides, and classroom teachers of the child's diet provisions, which should be incorporated into the Individualized Health Plan (IHP) as a part of the student's health record. It is helpful to note the child's flavoring preferences, as the bland fatty food on the diet can be flavored to appeal to the child. With the parent's and child's permission, the school nurse can work with the classroom teacher to explain the child's diet to the class. School nurses can obtain additional information about the ketogenic diet through the Epilepsy Foundation or the Stanford University Division of Neurology Ketogenic Diet Parental Reference Web site: http://www.stanford.edu/group/ketodiet. FIGURE 37.3 provides a sample ketogenic diet menu.

School nutritionists and the school lunch programs should be aware that a student is on the diet so that appropriate foods and beverages can be ordered. The school nurse can chart the student's urine ketone results and send them home weekly. School celebrations such as the child's birthday, when the parent may wish to send in a snack for the class, can be challenging. The student on the ketogenic diet can have milkshakes, cheesecake, quiche, and omelets on hand for the parties. On hot days, extra vigilance is needed to replace fluids lost

Sample Menu on Ketogenic Diet

Breakfast	Lunch	Dinner
Two eggs cooked in two tbsp butter	Two cups shredded squash with two tbsp parmesan cheese and two tbsp butter	Two sliced hot dogs with sugar-free catsup
Eight ounces heavy cream diluted in half with water	One cup torn leaf lettuce with three tbsp mayonnaise dressing	One cup asparagus cooked with two tbsp butter
Four ounces of unsweetened orange juice	Eight ounces orange diet soda with one half cup whipped cream added	One cup torn leaf lettuce with three tbsp mayonnaise dressing
		Sugar-free vanilla cream popsicle

Some children use a formula with MCT oil, such as Alimentum, as part of their diet.

TIPS:

Steaming vegetables preserves their vitamins.

Use a smaller plate and separate/arrange foods to give the illusion of a larger amount of food.

Offer chicken, tuna, and egg salads often at school—they are less unusual foods.

Figure 37.3 ■ Sample menu for ketogenic diet. (From Ketogenic Diet Support Group, Division of Pediatric Neurology, Packard Children's Hospital, Stanford University. http://www.stanford.edu/group/ketodiet)

through evaporation and perspiration. Fluids are restricted on the diet, but the student can have saccharin-sweetened water or cream popsicles made with ketogenic ingredients. These fluids are also used to replace those lost during illness and the accompanying vomiting and diarrhea.

Vagus Nerve Stimulation

Seizures are electrical short circuits within the human brain. The implantation of a stimulation device under the skin on the upper left side of the chest area with lead wires to the left vagus nerve is used to control the number and severity of seizures for many individuals for whom medication is not effective. FDA approval was granted in 1997 for use of the device for refractory partial onset seizures for patients older than 12 years of age (Kennedy & Schallert, 2001), but it has been used in much younger children. The stimulator uses regular pulses of electrical energy to prevent or interrupt electrical disturbances in the brain.

Electrical signals to the vagus nerve come from a thin round pulse generator, or battery, which is about 2 to 3 inches in diameter. The surgery to insert the battery takes 1 to 4 hours. There are two small incision sites, the left side of the neck and below the collar bone on the left in the chest or the armpit. Reported side effects range from hoarseness and a tickling sensation in the throat to a cough and changes in the voice tone during the administration of the stimulation dose (Devinsky, 2002).

The device is programmed to deliver stimulation 24 hours a day. The typical dose is 30 seconds on, 5 minutes off. The titanium battery lasts about 4 to 10 years and is used because there is less chance of immune system rejection of the titanium. Patients are followed up every 2 weeks until stable, then every 6 months. The device is reprogrammed using a computer and software with a programming wand.

The vagus stimulator implant also has a magnet tool so that students and their families can control the device externally. The magnet tool is worn as a watch or on a belt like a pager. The magnet triggers the device to deliver extra electrical stimulation between cycles when a seizure occurs. The student or trained caregiver passes the magnet over the device. Some patients have reported that using the magnet during the aura of a seizure can stop the seizure, shorten it, make it less severe, or reduce the recovery time afterward (Devinsky, 2002).

The magnet can also be used to stop stimulation by taping it in place over the device. There are various reasons to stop stimulation. If the student needs to speak or sing in public when a change in the voice tone is undesirable, as would occur during stimulation, or if there is a preexisting condition that makes swallowing difficult, the magnet could be used to stop stimulation during eating. The magnet could be used to stop stimulation if the student is having pain during the stimulation phase.

With parental permission to adhere to confidentiality laws, students, teachers, and school staff can be taught about the magnet. All involved should be cautioned that it needs to be stored or placed no closer than 10 inches away from credit cards, televisions, computers, computer disks, and microwave ovens. Students are taught to carry the magnet with them at all times. The student who uses the magnet needs to be seated away from these devices in the classrooms and other rooms such as the library, home economics room, or computer lab (Cyberonics, Inc. 2004).

It is interesting to note that the vagus stimulator is not affected by ultrasound or X-rays, but special arrangements need to be made for the patient to safely undergo an MRI due to magnetic sensors. The manufacturer, Cyberonics, Inc., has a toll-free clinical technical support number for health professionals.

RESPONSE TO SEIZURE ACTIVITY IN THE SCHOOL SETTING

Most students who have seizures while in the school setting have them in the presence of school staff and their peers. As the health expert on staff, the school nurse should have already developed a seizure action plan (see Figure 37.2) and, with the permission of the parents, discussed it with the student's teachers and relevant staff. With the plan, the entire school staff is able to respond to the needs of the affected child and then to contact the parent or guardian.

When a seizure occurs, the adult supervising the student must stay with the student. Other students can be sent to notify the nurse directly or the main office of the school so that the designated person can respond. Depending on the type of seizures the child has, the nurse or designee needs to respond to the call with a treatment bag. The treatment bag is used by the nurse and perhaps the EMS responders and should contain some or all of the following items: paper and pen, napkins or tissues, stethoscope, blood pressure monitoring equipment, and airway maintenance supplies such as portable suction, portable pulse oximeter, oxygen tank, and mask/cannula and may contain other items listed on the seizure action plan (Box 37.1).

Box 37.1 ■ ■ ■

SCHOOL FIRST AID FOR SEIZURES

- Students assume positions sitting in desks silently or performing emergency roles (runner, timekeeper, etc.), if age appropriate. Adults remain calm and reassure students.
- Assist student to lie on the floor (preferably a carpeted area); position side-lying with knees bent to assist with breathing and airway clearance.
- Place folded blanket, towel, or jacket under the student's head to prevent injury. Keep the body in alignment.
- Clear the area around the student of furniture and any hard or sharp objects to prevent injury during the event.
- Note time seizure began and any precipitating events or aura observed. Assess airway patency, respiratory status, location of movements, and other symptoms.
- Do not place objects such as rulers or tongue blades into the student's mouth that may cause aspiration or broken teeth and bitten tongue.
- Do not attempt to hold down or restrain the student's movements, which may cause fractures or bruising.
- An adult needs to stay with the student until help arrives and the seizure event is finished.
- Do not attempt to make the student swallow, eat, drink, or take medication during the seizure.
- Reassure and reorient the student when the seizure activity is over, and reassure his or her classmates when the student regains consciousness.
- Allow the student to continue to rest for at least 30 minutes after the last seizure in a safe, supervised setting.
- Notify parents and the student's physician of the event, especially if the seizure required use of Diastat or oxygen, if the event was atypical, or if EMS involvement and ER transport was necessary.
- Seizures lasting $>$ 15 to 30 minutes with or without cyanosis require immediate medical attention with EMS deployment and ER follow-up at the nearest hospital, unless other standing medical orders are in effect.

The first two priorities during a seizure are airway patency and safety. While assuring that the student's airway is open and that the student is breathing, the nurse should also be positioning the student in a comfortable and safe place, usually the floor. For tonic–clonic activity, place the student on their side. Loosen clothing at the neck and waist; remove eyeglasses. It is important not to restrain the limbs of a student having tonic-clonic movements, as bruising or fractures may result. Blow-by oxygen administered by mask or open tubing may be utilized for cyanotic seizures according to the physician's orders. No objects, such as tongue blades or spoons, are to be inserted into the mouth of the student having a seizure, as teeth can be knocked out or the tongue may be pushed further back and occlude the airway. A folded piece of clothing or blanket under the child's head and neck may help to keep proper alignment and prevent injury; if nothing is available, use your arms or lap.

Creating a safe environment for the student requires the nurse to direct others to move objects or furniture with which the student may come in contact that might result in injury. Other adults such as the teacher can encourage the onlookers to leave the site or can walk their class down the hall. Throughout this period, the nurse will be timing the seizure activity and noting the type of seizure activities being demonstrated. The nurse needs to assess the events of the seizure, including loss of consciousness, the types of movements that occur and the body parts affected, the length of the movements, the presence of cyanosis, incontinence of urine or stool, vomiting, and the events of the postictal period. Generalized seizures often result in a recognizable postictal state characterized by a brief awakening with grogginess followed by sleep that may last from a few minutes to several hours. It is appropriate to transfer the student to the health office in a wheelchair during the period of brief awakening.

Vital signs need to be measured when the tonic–clonic movements have stopped and every 5 to 15 minutes thereafter until the student is alert and oriented. EMS should be called (1) if the seizure has lasted longer than 5 minutes; (2) if two or more consecutive seizures have occurred; (3) if the student has a respiratory or cardiac arrest; (4) if there is no previous history of seizures; or (5) if the student has not returned to his or her baseline level of consciousness within 30 to 60 minutes (Hootman, 2004). Other reasons to contact EMS may be if an injury occurred during the seizure.

The student who has experienced seizure activity may be aware that a seizure has occurred and be embarrassed or frightened. The school nurse should reorient the student to time and place and tell him or her what occurred during the seizure; these actions may be reassuring. The student may need to change clothing if there was incontinence, and may appreciate being able to wash his or her face and hands and rinse out his or her mouth if vomiting was part of the event. Ask the student what comfort measures would be most helpful and allow the child to eat or sleep. Once stable, and with the parent's approval, have the student return to class as soon as possible to maintain a normal routine (Hootman, 2004). The school nurse needs to then record all observations made related to the seizure on a Seizure Activity Log (TABLE 37.3).

The student's classroom teacher will reassure the class that the returning student has recovered from the incident. The school nurse can assist the classroom teacher by reviewing the incident at the student's level of understanding and giving positive feedback to a class who supports the student through helpful behavior and by fulfilling the roles assigned to them. It is understood that the teacher

Table 37.3 ■
SEIZURE ACTIVITY LOG

Student Name: ______________________ Date of Birth: ______________

Grade/Room/Teacher: ______________________

DATE	TIME START	TIME END	AURA/ TYPE	ACTIVITY OBSERVED	POSTICTAL STATE	COMMENTS

and nurse take care to maintain the child's medical confidentiality and that the debriefing session is age-appropriate. The school nurse's affect gives students in the class the message that seizures do occur, and that they are frightening to witness, but their classmate may not remember the seizure and will recover.

WORKING WITH THE MEDICAL TEAM

School nurses are the vital link for students with seizure disorders between their healthcare providers and their schools. School nurses, through their collaboration with the primary care provider and the specialty neurology center team, work to normalize the student's school experience. After a seizure disorder is diagnosed, the school nurse works to ensure that the medical regimen being prescribed can be implemented by the family and the school. Whether reinforcing information to the child and family about medications and possible side effects, informing the physician about side effects the student is experiencing, or arranging for home instruction if necessary, the school nurse helps the student to continue to attend school and live a normal life. The school nurse who informs the medical team of a student who appears not to be compliant with the medication regimen prescribed is able to make them aware that the dosage adjustment is not the issue. Social service assistance referral for the family can ensure that prescriptions are affordable and can be filled, while a visiting nurse service can assess the child and family as they implement the plan. Through the use of Internet resources such as the Answerplace by Audience, a section of the Epilepsy Foundation Web site (http://www.epilepsyfoundation.org), and information provided by the neurology team, the school nurse informs the teachers, support staff, and parents of their role in helping the student with seizures to participate fully in school activities. The school nurse supports the student and family, setting the tone for acceptance of the medical needs and treatments.

On admission of the child to the school or the return of a student who has had a first seizure, the school nurse begins to build the bridges between the home, healthcare, and education settings. Meeting with the classroom and specialty area teachers, the nurse reviews the role they each play in maintaining normalcy, ensuring safety in the student's environment, responding to emergency situations, and assisting in the social and emotional adjustment of the student with a seizure disorder. The physical education teacher needs to know the prescribed activity limitations for the student. However, HIPAA laws require that the parent give specific written permission for release of health information to particular individuals in the school. The school nurse can have the parent sign and date such a provision in the child's IHP, which is very specific in its list of the student's potential contacts who need this information. Some healthcare providers require that their form be signed by the parent before they can release any information to the school.

THE SCHOOL NURSE'S ROLES

With a holistic approach to the child and family as clients, the school nurse assumes the roles of teacher, advocate, collaborator, counselor, and provider. The school nurse needs to promote a positive social and emotional climate for the student with seizures, attending to self-image, fear, knowledge, safety issues, family acceptance of a chronic condition, and changes in the child's developmental and educational needs. Because of a specialized understanding of the medical and emotional challenges of a seizure disorder, the school nurse is in a position to provide educational programs for staff and students, and to oversee the healthcare planning for the student.

Buelow (2001) conducted a study that provides insight into the perceptions of people with epilepsy and how the nurse might help them to live well with their disorder by addressing self-management issues and appropriate management techniques. She suggests that nurses need to assist patients to first find a way to fit their medical treatment into their lives. Treatment failure due to noncompliance is a common problem for adolescents, but assisting them to make adjustments in treatments in order to attend the prom could be the key to their adherence to the ketogenic diet, for example. Buelow stresses that nurses need to address patients' fears of the consequences of seizures, which are embarrassing and potentially dangerous. Adolescents may need to be debriefed about seizure events in order to participate fully in their plan of care.

In their study of family experiences with seizures and their needs for information and support, Aytch, Hammond, and White (2001) found that children and families coping with early-onset, poorly controlled seizures and accompanying developmental delay have a great need for services based on the effects on educational achievement, family life, future employment, and transition to adulthood. Their study revealed that in the presence of high-quality medical care, families also needed multidisciplinary, comprehensive information, support, and resources provided by nurses and other health team members in a center that could refer to developmental pediatric care, early intervention professionals, and social resources. Hightower, Carmon, and Minick (2002) studied children's personal experiences with and perceptions of epilepsy and suggested developmentally appropriate, comprehensive methods to assist these children to cope with the disorder, such as positive reinforcement for compliance with medications and encouraging supportive friendships in order to build self-esteem and confidence.

Comprehensive periodic visits to the neurology specialty center can be intimidating to families because so much information is exchanged. Often the family leaves a visit with folders and binders full of information to absorb. They usually have questions about the long- and short-term consequences of the diagnosis and the school and community implications of the seizure disorder for their child. School nurses who nurture an ongoing rapport with the family can be instrumental in decoding this information for families and assisting them to develop questions for future encounters, as well as to organize the printed materials they receive into workable units. In addition, nurses can open the channels of communications for families by informing the medical care team of recent changes related to school, providing copies of the School Seizure Log to the family in preparation for the medical appointment (Table 37.2), assisting the family to prepare the questions they have to take to the medical appointment, and reinforcing the plan of care.

Classification as a Student with a Chronic Health Condition

Students with a newly diagnosed or established seizure disorder need to be considered for Special Education Classification for the purpose of identifying their specific educational needs and accommodations. Most children with seizures have an idiopathic seizure disorder uncomplicated by other medical problems and fit easily into the criteria for classification as chronically medically disabled under the Individuals with Disabilities Education Act (see Chapter 14). While most students need very few modifications to their school activities, those who are more severely affected may need special services within the school system, such as, but not limited to, intermittent home instruction, enrichment programs, mentoring, after-school programs, medical day care, special accommodations, and respite care. Application for Special Education Classification includes a letter of medical recommendation/justification from the health care provider. Frequent school absences may require the need for home instruction so the student can keep up with classmates.

Children who have a seizure disorder complicated by other medical and emotional problems may indeed need classification as behaviorally disturbed, emotionally disturbed, or learning disabled and the resources of a child study team to plan for the comprehensive needs of this student in their Individualized Educational Program. Children with uncontrolled seizures and normal intelligence should not be placed in self-contained classroom environments in which academic progress is not required; such placement does little for their self-esteem and ambition. The school nurse is often a member of the team that develops the Individualized Educational Program (Chapters 14 and 27) and provides information to the team regarding the needs of students with seizure activity. Students with chronic health problems necessitating episodic absences of several days to weeks qualify for intermittent home instruction services in some school districts. Intermittent home instruction is ordered by the pediatrician and provides rapid tutor deployment in cases of repeated hospitalization or illness. It is a useful tool because it protects the child from retention in a grade level due to absences and regression in class performance caused by missed instruction, both of which can have a significant influence on the development of independence.

Safety in the Classroom and Building

Before a student with seizures enters the school, the school nurse needs to evaluate the environment to ensure the student's safety and well-being. Because the nurse is aware of the potential for injury during a seizure, safety measures are built into the Individualized Health Plan (Table 37.1). The process begins with choosing the student's classroom; considerations may be a first floor or ground floor carpeted classroom with wide-wheelchair accessible doorway, sufficient room so that furniture is spaced far apart and flexibility so that the student with seizures does not have to sit near hazards such as electric cords or radiators. Two-piece desks are best, as the child with seizures in a one-piece desk and chair unit could potentially become entangled and trapped during a generalized seizure. The ideal classroom will be near the hallway rest room and have a two-way intercom so that students can call the Main Office to ask for assistance while the teacher attends to the student; these call stations will also need to be located in the rest rooms.

If the student's seizures are precipitated by flashing lights or loud sounds, attention should be paid to computer screens and programs, the noise level in the classroom, and the flashing lights attached to some fire alarms. If this is the case, evacuate the child with seizures first in the event of an emergency and before the alarm sounds for fire drills. Many classrooms have a carpeted area or corner that is designated as a reading center and may already be equipped with pillows, blankets, and stuffed animals for comfort. Such an area can be a safe haven for the child with seizures to seek out when an aura signals an impending seizure. If a first floor classroom is unavailable, the designated first responders to an emergency should have an elevator key and access to a wheelchair to transport the student.

With the parents' approval, the Seizure Action Plan and the IEP may need to identify two children as buddies for the child with seizures. These buddies need to be trained by the school nurse to recognize an aura or seizure activity and how to signal for adult help. Utilizing print materials from the Epilepsy Foundation and perhaps video, as well as the experience of witnessing the affected child's seizures at school, the school nurse can begin to expose the buddies to seizure activity and the assistance they are expected to render during the episodes. Role playing the possible scenarios is a helpful way for children to internalize the behaviors needed to respond. The student with seizures should travel within the building or on the school bus with two buddies at all times. One of the buddies is designated to stay with the child if a seizure occurs, note the time, and if age appropriate, taught to turn the child onto his or her side and provide reassurance. The second buddy is then able to leave and notify an adult. This system is particularly helpful for the use of the boys' rest room or athletic locker room when the teacher is female and vice versa.

The Epilepsy Foundation recommends that children with generalized and drop seizures be fitted with a helmet with a face guard to protect against head and facial injuries (Epilepsy Foundation, 2003). They also recommend that children with a history of seizures have one-to-one adult supervision in and around water, and that they wear a life vest when near water, especially pools. Lifeguards who are CPR certified should always be at poolside and should be informed of the disorder to facilitate the student's placement in the pool near the guard, to increase vigilant observation, and to ensure early rescue in the event of a seizure. The student with a seizure history needs to avoid the top bunk bed on school camping trips. Medical Alert jewelry is very helpful for the school-age child who may be treated at an emergency room before a parent or guardian arrives to share information. Medical Alert jewelry can be purchased with a phone number on it that can be called by the emergency medical team to give them access to a data bank containing the child's health information such as current medications and treatment plan.

Emotional Support

Although well-meaning, parents and adults in the life of a child with seizures may tend to overprotect the child by limiting his or her participation in usual childhood activities. They may fear that a seizure may occur during the activity or that the physical exertion will somehow trigger a seizure. The Epilepsy Foundation (2003) cautions against this for two reasons. First, vigorous physical activity is not associated with a greater number of seizures, and some studies suggest that fewer seizures will occur when the average child is active. Second, the student is excluded from experiences that would help to develop social skills and self-confidence. They also suggest that the student who is made to feel different because of not being able to do what others are doing can remain dependent and socially immature. The school experience offers the student the unique opportunity to break the pattern of overprotection and isolation.

School nurses need to be advocates for the student with seizures. Using evidence-based practice, the school nurse is able to create policies and procedures to protect the student, while promoting that they be educated in the least restrictive setting. Through staff education programs and effective role modeling, the nurse is able to set the tone in the school for acceptance and tolerance of the disability. Fear and misunderstanding can lead to the student becoming isolated and treated differently by staff and peers. Advocating for the student with seizures to participate in a variety of activities boosts self-esteem and self-confidence.

The Epilepsy Foundation also recommends that, whenever possible, the student with seizures be encouraged to take part in all school activities with minimal modifications. For example, modifications may have to be made in shop class to include the teacher operating the power equipment for the student and allowing the student to use hand tools with one-to-one adult supervision. In the physical education class, requirements need to be modified for the student with seizures to coincide with the recommendation that children with epilepsy should not engage in contact sports, climb on equipment, or provide safety assistance to other students such as holding a tow line for rock-wall climbing.

Some children may need minor accommodations in their school day depending on the seizure type they have most often. Making adjustments in the timing and location of the child's recess period can protect the child from injury while ensuring that the child has fresh air, exercise, and a rest period from academics. Assigning the child to recess when the child's medication is near the peak and not near a trough in blood levels is helpful. If the child finds outdoor recess too stimulating, an alternate time to read quietly or play in a smaller group may be helpful. Allowing extra time for eating lunch can help relieve medication side effects in some cases.

In addition, the parent needs to know that the child with seizures wants and needs to have behavioral limits set like any other child in order to feel loved. Parents need to be encouraged to comply with and support the school's disciplinary policy, but to encourage modifications in the consequences if necessary. For example, the student who verbally assaults another student needs to receive discipline, but the recommended consequence of staying after school to help lift heavy objects may need to be modified.

Staff Preparation

Teachers, coaches, bus drivers, and lunch workers who supervise children with seizures need to be trained in the recognition of an aura and seizure activity, and be familiar with the system to get help and the child's care in the first few minutes of the seizure. It should be emphasized that a known seizure disorder is not considered an emergency, but that certain assessments and interventions are warranted at the time of the seizure. The Epilepsy Foundation Web site has downloadable forms for teachers and school personnel regarding the recognition and early treatment of seizures at http://www.epilepsyfoundation.org/answerplace. Review of these steps during an inservice can instill staff members with the confidence necessary to calmly handle a seizure emergency until medical help arrives. Steps to be followed can be posted in the classroom and on the school bus.

The Epilepsy Foundation Web site has a teacher education section regarding emergency management that states that an average convulsive seizure in a child with a known seizure disorder is not a medical emergency and usually resolves without problems. They recommend that immediate medical attention is not required *unless* the child having a seizure does not have a history of seizures, consciousness does not return after the seizure ends, a second seizure begins shortly after the first without the child regaining consciousness in between, or the seizure shows no signs of ending after 5 minutes (Epilepsy Foundation, 2003, Emergency Management). The Epilepsy Foundation also recommends that medical attention be sought immediately if the child strikes his or her head with force either before or during the seizure, is difficult to arouse after 20 minutes, is vomiting, complains of difficulty with vision, has a persistent headache after a short rest period, has unconsciousness with failure to respond, or if the pupils are unequal in size or dilated.

PSYCHOSOCIAL ISSUES

Taking care of a student with seizures involves not only managing the physical manifestations, but also resolving the psychosocial and social issues that are important to the student's well-being and continued development. The school, along with specialty neurological treatment centers and the child's primary care provider, can assist the family in managing the child's needs.

Children need to feel normal, to feel that despite having a chronic condition, they are like every other student in the class. Seizures affect the brain, and students may believe that they are not like others because they act differently when they have a seizure. Students also may think that having seizures is their fault or the fault of their parents. This belief may manifest itself in poor self-esteem or feeling unworthy of having friends. The lack of control students may feel over the frequency and severity of their seizures can make them feel isolated, and frequent absences and hospitalizations can compound these feelings (Hightower et al., 2002).

Medications taken for seizures may stimulate curiosity among one's classmates, particularly when the student has breakthrough seizures despite taking medication. Classmates may feel that the student with seizures in the class is receiving special attention from the teacher and staff, misperceiving that it is acceptable if this student does not always pay attention in class or appears to be daydreaming or very sleepy. The child with seizures may be viewed as spending a great deal of time in the nurse's office for reasons that are not clear, sometimes even getting to go home early. If the student with seizures has activity restrictions, it adds to the list of things that make him or her different at school. If the child has protective gear, such as a helmet, other children may view him or her as fragile or overprotected, and not include him or her in the games at recess. Children in the class may believe that their classmate with seizures can control the abnormal movements and speech that occur during a seizure and the sleepiness after the seizure and that he or she is just being lazy or trying to get attention.

Children's and adolescents' feelings and fears are best dealt with directly. When a student in school has a seizure disorder, it is helpful for the school nurse to assist the affected student to provide information about his or her disability to classmates, with the approval of the parent and the affected student. Information demystifies the disorder for the classmates. The student with seizures can be coached to present a program to his or her class about his seizures, his feelings, medications, treatments, and care. Part of a student's task in accepting the chronic condition is to be able to verbalize his needs to others. Information coming directly from the student demystifies the seizures and reassures the classmates that their peer with seizures is normal. Role-playing a seizure emergency in various situations in the school with the class can instill the confidence the children need to handle a seizure episode in gym, library, or recess.

ADOLESCENT ISSUES

Adolescents dealing with a chronic disorder present unique challenges. Although able to understand the medical plan, the importance of medications to control seizures, and the importance of avoiding situations that can trigger seizure activity, adolescents may rebel against the best advice. As they establish themselves as individuals separate from their parents, adolescents accept some aspects of their parents' lifestyle and reject others. Many of the accommodations that are necessary to maintaining health are burdensome to teens; they are developing their self-image and complicated, time-consuming medical routines may be rejected if they interfere with this perception. Teens may begin to take risks, to "try out" the consequences of risky behavior, in order to assert their independence. The risk-taking behavior for a teen with a seizure disorder may mean trying to attend a sleepover without taking their prescribed AEDs in order that friends not know about their disorder or see them taking medication and begin to ask questions.

The school nurse can assist teens by helping them to get as much information about their condition, treatment, and prognosis as possible, and to encourage teens to ask questions and become involved participants at follow-up appointments. Teens who have frequent seizures or frequent hospitalizations need to feel a sense of control over some aspect of their care and can have this by making some of the minor decisions independently. If they remain in reasonable compliance with necessary safety measures, teens should be able to negotiate accommodations in sports, after-school activities, and social interaction.

Consult the local branch of the state motor vehicle agency for information about driving regulations for those with a seizure disorder in your area. Regulations vary, but generally, there are provisions that driving is restricted for weeks to months after the last seizure and reapplication for licensing needs to be accompanied by a physician's certification that the person has their seizures controlled. The teen who does not have driving privileges is necessarily dependent on others. Developing a sense of autonomy and independence needs to be fostered in other areas for the teen to meet this developmental need. Encouraging the teen to become team captain or yearbook editor helps to foster independence and a sense of accomplishment in the transition to adulthood.

PROGNOSIS

The majority of children will become seizure free within a few years of diagnosis and treatment with AEDs and some can even discontinue treatment after a period of time. "About 70% of individuals with epilepsy achieve long-term remission, leaving approximately 30% continuing to be refractory to treatment" (Blair & Selekman, 2004, p. 485).

CONCLUSION

Epilepsy is a chronic medical condition that can be successfully treated in childhood and through adulthood. However, with 22,000 to 42,000 deaths annually from status epilepticus (Epilepsy Foundation, 2003), vigilance in caring for children and adolescents with seizures is a priority for school nurses. Changes in the delivery of acute health care mean that students are discharged from hospitals within a few days after admission for seizures and return to the least restrictive school environment. In partnership with parents and the community, school nurses can assist the student to live successfully with seizures. School nurses have multiple roles to play in working with students and their families. As educators, researchers, and care providers, nurses are in a unique position to encourage feelings of normalcy, acceptance, and competence in students who have seizures. Using the students' own insights into how they and their families cope with a chronic condition, the school nurse uses the nursing process to provide leadership in planning and implementing comprehensive age-appropriate health care plans.

References

American Academy of Pediatrics (AAP). (2000). *2000 Red book: Report of the Committee on Infectious Diseases*. Elk Grove Village, IL: Author.

American Epilepsy Society (AES). (2004). *Basic mechanisms underlying seizures and epilepsy*. Retrieved September 25, 2005 from http://www.aesnet.org/visitors/professionaldevelopment/meded/newppt/clinical/clinical33–36.pdf

Aytch, S., Hammond, R., & White, C. (2001). Seizures in infants and young children: An exploratory study of family experiences and needs for information and support. *Journal of Neuroscience Nursing, 33*(5), 278–285.

Blair, J., & Selekman, J. (2004). Epilepsy. In P. Jackson Allen & J. Vessey (Eds.), *Primary care of the child with a chronic condition* (pp. 469–497). St. Louis: C. V. Mosby.

Buelow, J. (2001). Epilepsy management issues and techniques. *Journal of Neuroscience Nursing, 33*(5), 260–269.

Centers for Disease Control and Prevention (CDC), National Immunization Program. (2005). *Contraindications to vaccine chart*. Retrieved September 25, 2005 from http://www.cdc.gov/nip/recs/contraindications_vacc.htm

Commission on Classification and Terminology of the International League Against Epilepsy. (1989). Proposal for revised classification of epilepsy and epileptic syndromes. *Epilepsia, 30*(4), 389–399.

Cyberonics, Inc. (2004). *Epilepsy patient's manual for vagus nerve stimulation*. Houston, TX. Retrieved March 2005 from http://www.vnstherapy.com

Devinsky, O. (2002). *Epilepsy: Patient & family guide*. Phildelphia: F. A. Davis.

Epilepsy Foundation. (2003). *Epilepsy in childhood*. Retrieved September 8, 2004 from http://www.epilepsyfoundation.org/answerpace/Life/children/

Febrile Seizures. (2001). *Postgraduate Medicine online, 110* (2). Retrieved September 25, 2005 from http:// www.postgradmed.com/issues/2001/08_01/pn_seizure.htm

Gerber, M. (1999). Seizures. In M. Haas (Ed.), *The school nurse's source book of individualized healthcare plans* (pp. 385–402). North Branch, MN: Sunrise River Press.

Gilbert D., DeRoos, S., & Bare, M. (2004). Does sleep or sleep deprivation increase epileptiform discharges in pediatric electroencephalograms? *Pediatrics, 114*(3), 658–662.

Gilbert, D., Pyzik, P., Vining, E., & Freeman, J. (1999). Medication cost reduction in children on the ketogenic diet: Data from a prospective study. *Journal of Child Neurology, 14*, 469–471.

Gilbert, K. (1999). Seizure disorder. In T. Buttaro, J. Trybulski, P. Bailey, & J. Sandberg-Cook (Eds.), *Primary care: A collaborative practice* (pp. 842–849). St. Louis: C. V. Mosby.

Hauser, W. (2001). Epidemiology of epilepsy in children. In J. Pellock, W. Dodson, & B. Bourgeois (Eds.), *Pediatric epilepsy: Diagnosis and therapy* (pp. 81–96). New York: Demos.

Hay, W., Hayward, A., Levy, M., & Sondheimer, J. (2003). *Current pediatric diagnosis and treatment* (16th ed). New York: McGraw-Hill.

Hightower, S., Carmon, M., & Minick, P. (2002). A qualitative descriptive study of the lived experiences of school-aged children with epilepsy. *Journal of Pediatric Health Care, 16*(3), 131–137.

Hingley, A. (1999). *Epilepsy: Taming the seizures, dispelling the myths*. Retrieved September 24, 2005 from http://www.fda.gov/fdac/features/1999/199_epil.html

Hootman, J. (2004). *Quality nursing interventions in the school setting*. Scarborough, ME: National Association of School Nurses

Kennedy, P., & Schallert, G. (2001). Practical issues and concepts in vagus nerve stimulation: A nursing review. *Journal of Neuroscience Nursing, 33*(2), 105–112.

Klein, P. & Herzog, A. (2000). Hormones and epilepsy. In D. Schmidt & S. Schachter (Eds.), *Epilepsy: Problem solving in clinical practice* (pp. 413–433). London: Martin Dunitz.

Kotagal, P. (2001). The relationship between sleep and epilepsy. *Seminars in Pediatric Neurology, 8*(4), 241–250.

Mayo Clinic Brain and Nervous System Center. (2005). *Epilepsy*. Retrieved September 23, 2005 from http://www.mayoclinic.com/

National Institute of Neurological Disorders and Stroke (NINDS). (2001). *NINDS Febrile Seizures Information Page*. Retrieved September 11, 2004 from http://www.ninds.nih.gov/health_and_medical/disorders/febrile_seizures.htm

National Institute of Neurological Disorders and Stroke (NINDS). (2003). *Epilepsy*. Retrieved from http://www.nim.nih.gov/medlineplus.druginformation

National Institutes of Health (NIH) Medline Plus. (2003). *Antiepileptic meds*. Available at http://www.nlm.nih.gov/medlineplus.druginformation

Noviasky, J., Porsteinsson, A., & Lee, Y. (2001). Second generation anticonvulsant medications: Their use in children. *Journal of School Nursing, 17*(2), 103–111.

Paolicchi, J. (2002). The spectrum of nonepileptic events in children. *Epilepsia 43* (Suppl. 3), 60–64.

Penovich, P. (2000). The effects of epilepsy and its treatment on sexual reproductive function. *Epilepsia, 41*(Suppl 2), S53–S61.

Physician's desk reference (PDR). (2004). Montvale, NJ: Thomson PDR.

Prensky, A. (2001). An approach to the child with paroxysmal phenomenon with emphasis on nonepileptic disorders. In J. Pellock, W. Dodson, & B. Burgeois (Eds.), *Pediatric epilepsy: Diagnosis and therapy* (pp. 97–116). New York: Demos.

Pruitt, A. (2000). Approach to the patient with a seizure. In A. Goroll & A. Mulley (Eds.), *Primary care medicine* (pp. 962–969). Philadelphia: Lippincott Williams & Wilkins.

Shafer, P. (1999). New therapies in the management of acute or cluster seizures and seizure emergencies. *Journal of Neuroscience Nursing,* 31(4), 224–230.

Shinnar, S., & Glauser, T. (2002). Febrile seizures. *Journal of Child Neurology, 17*(Suppl. 1), S44–S52.

Shinnar, S., & Pellock, J. (2002). Update of the epidemiology and prognosis of pediatric epilepsy. *Journal of Child Neurology, 17*(Suppl. 1), S4–S17.

PART VII

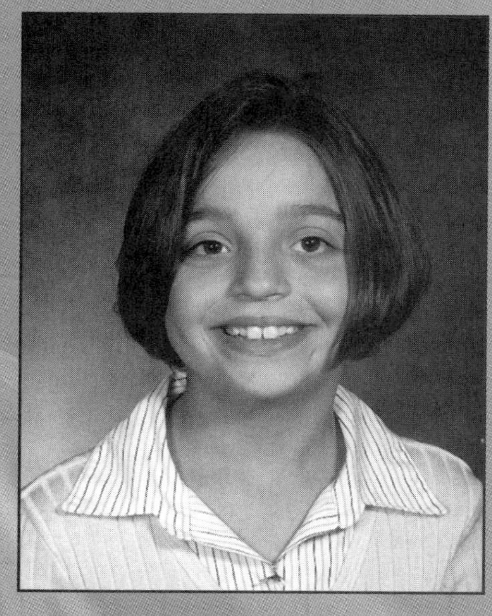

Acting Out and High-Risk Behaviors

Chapter 38

Behavior Assessment and Management in School

ANN MARIE MCCARTHY ▪ JILL ASPREY ▪ SUSAN ADAMS

Chapter Outline

INTRODUCTION

Children and adolescents in school settings display a variety of behaviors, some of which are viewed as problematic by those around them. Behavior problems in children are classified into two major groups: externalizing and internalizing (Achenbach & Ruffle, 2000; Shapiro & Kratochwill, 2000a). Externalizing behaviors are displayed outwardly by the student, such as noncompliant, oppositional, inattentive, hyperactive, or aggressive behaviors (MacDonald, 2003). Internalizing behaviors are focused inwardly by the individual and manifest as anxiety, depression, or withdrawal. Frequently, children and adolescents who display externalizing behaviors while in school are identified as having a behavior problem because their behaviors are disruptive to others. Because students with internalizing problems may not be disruptive to the adults in their environment, they often are not recognized as having a problem. Depression and suicide, commonly associated with internalizing difficulties, are discussed in Chapter 34.

This chapter discusses students with troublesome, externalizing behavior problems. Many children and adolescents act out at some point during their years in school. Externalizing behavior problems range from minor acts of misbehavior to more persistent disruptive activities to violent, potentially dangerous behaviors. The milder, more common forms of externalizing behavior are the focus of this chapter. Some more extreme externalizing behaviors, specifically bullying and violence, are discussed in Chapter 39. However, some of the behavioral assessment and management approaches discussed in this chapter may be effectively incorporated into assessment and treatment plans for children with more severe externalizing behavior problems as well as those with internalizing problems.

When behaviors are seen as disruptive to the adults in the environment, the student may be labeled as having a behavior problem that needs some type of intervention. Disruptive behavior may be behavior that is typical of a particular student's developmental stage but is viewed as occurring more frequently or more intensely than might be expected and is therefore annoying to others in the environment (Campbell, 2002). Alternately, the disruptive behavior may be a behavior more appropriate to a developmental stage younger or older than the student's current developmental stage. The behavior may be an ongoing problem, or of recent onset. The harmful behaviors and unusual behaviors are all clinically significant. Behaviors that are harmful to the student or others, such as kicking or biting, require immediate intervention by an adult. Extreme, unusual behaviors may be clear signals that the student needs further evaluation and a possible mental health referral. For example, cruelty to animals, violent temper tantrums, and eating problems warrant further investigation (Being Alert to Indicators of Psychosocial and Mental Health Problems, 2002).

When a child or adolescent in school displays inappropriate behaviors, the school nurse may be approached by parents or teachers to screen the student, assist in assessment, and provide recommendations regarding the development of a behavior management plan or need for further evaluation. In addition, school nurses are often asked to assist in the ongoing monitoring of behavior management interventions for students during the school day. This chapter discusses behavior theory, provides guidelines for assessing students with behavior problems, and offers basic strategies for behavioral interventions. Cases are presented to illustrate assessment and intervention approaches.

BACKGROUND ON BEHAVIOR PROBLEMS

Behavior is a result of both biological (nature) and environmental (nurture) factors (Campbell, 2002). In students who display disruptive behaviors, the factors that are associated with the development of behavior problems are a complex combination of child characteristics, family interactions, and social context including the school environment. Between 12% and 25% of school-age children and adolescents are considered to have a diagnosed behavioral and/or emotional problem (Albrecht, Dore, & Naugle, 2003).

Child characteristics that may contribute to problem behavior include difficult temperament, cognitive difficulties, and social skills deficits (Christophersen & Mortweet, 2002; Cook, Greenberg, & Kusche, 1994). When thinking about students who display concerning behaviors in school, it is important to rule out possible medical problems that may be causing or contributing to the behavior. Health problems may actually present as behavior problems. For example, a student with new-onset diabetes may initially be seen as disrupting class with frequent requests to go to the bathroom and get a drink of water (Box 38.1); a student with undiagnosed absence seizures may be viewed as intentionally not paying attention; and a student with verbal outbursts may have undiagnosed Tourette's syndrome. In addition, students with substance abuse problems or psychiatric diagnoses often display a range of problem behaviors.

Box 38.1 ■ ■ ■

HEALTH IMPACTING A STUDENT'S BEHAVIOR: ANNA

Mr. K. stopped by the nurse's office late one afternoon. He was concerned about one of his third-grade students, a girl named Anna. Anna had always been a good student, but lately she was having trouble. The change had started gradually over the last month or two. Anna was always thinking of reasons to leave her desk and even when she was there, she did not seem to be able to concentrate. Her frequent requests to go to the bathroom or get a drink disrupted the class. She was not getting her homework completed and often did not complete her assignments during class. "I thought it would pass but now it's been at least a month and she isn't improving." The school nurse could tell that Mr. K. was genuinely concerned and that this was becoming a problem for Anna, whose work was suffering, and for Mr. K. and the other students.

After Mr. K. left, the school nurse reviewed Anna's academic and medical files. There was nothing remarkable. Anna was a good student with no previous medical problems. The nurse decided to contact Anna's mother to see if she could shed some light on the situation.

Anna's mother, Mrs. L., was aware of the situation. Mr. K. had talked with her at the last conference and since then, she was "watching" Anna more closely. She said Anna was not going outside as much to play, preferring to watch TV. She reported that Anna's appetite was better than usual, but she had noticed that she was not sleeping well. "Anna says nothing is wrong. I don't know. Maybe it's her age."

After talking with Mrs. L., the school nurse concluded that circumstances at home were not a factor in Anna's behavior change. Anna's mother seemed appropriately but not overly concerned, and did not seem to blame the school or the teacher for Anna's problems. She also seemed puzzled by Anna's behavior.

The nurse decided to have a visit with Anna. She had known Anna since kindergarten and felt comfortable with her. They talked about the latest news, the spring carnival, and a few other recent events before they "got down to business." Anna said she knew Mr. K. was not happy that she was not getting her work done but it was not her fault because the work was too hard. The nurse asked her if she thought Mr. K. was unfair. She thought a minute and said, "Oh, not really, he's pretty fun most of the time." While she was talking, the nurse was observing Anna. Anna had been screened several months earlier for height, weight, and vision. There were no observable differences now, but the nurse did a quick physical assessment: no swollen glands, no pallor, pulse and BP normal, and no fever. One finding did stand out, however, and that was a 7 pound weight loss since her weight had been checked 3 months ago. That is unusual for an 8-year-old. The weight loss, combined with the frequent trips to the bathroom and water fountain, were concerning. A new thought occurred to the nurse. She called Anna's mother and recommended Anna have a physical exam and suggested that mom alert the doctor to the need for a blood sugar check, "just to be on the safe side."

A few days later, Mrs. L. called back with the results. The blood sugar was very high, and the diagnosis was type 1 diabetes. Anna and her mother headed over to the diabetes clinic for teaching. She thanked the school nurse for suggesting the check-up, and asked if she would handle things at school. The nurse informed the teacher and began preparations for Anna's return to school, developing the protocol for glucose monitoring and insulin injections and providing in-service education for the staff.

Parental characteristics, such as emotional unavailability, limited social stimulation, over control, lax control, strict physical punishment, and/ or inappropriate developmental expectations have been associated with child behavior problems. Family factors such as single-parenting, marital discord, parents who disagree in their childrearing approaches, and parents experiencing psychosocial problems such as substance abuse or mental health problems may contribute to child behavior problems. In addition, social factors, such as unemployment, limited financial resources, few social supports, family stress, inadequate child care services, limited education, cultural differences, and disadvantaged neighborhoods, may further impact on the development of these problems (Campbell, 2002).

School factors, such as type of instruction, curriculum, physical environment, and learning abilities, may also contribute to behavior problems. For example, learning problems in some students go unrecognized and result in the student displaying behaviors to try to escape from academic demands; for other children the strict structure of the typical school environment is too demanding and similarly results in behaviors that disrupt the class (Grier, Morris, & Taylor, 2001). Peers can provide a powerful influence on children, both positive and negative.

The etiology of disruptive behavior problems and the factors that contribute to them can be quite complex. To provide a framework for assessing and managing disruptive behaviors in school, the ABC Behavior Model and Functional Behavioral Assessment (FBA) are presented. Behavioral approaches focus on environmental factors that contribute to behavior problems. While multiple factors contribute to behavior problems, behavioral approaches are frequently used in the schools because the environment is often the only aspect of the problem that school personnel can alter directly. However, the school nurse needs to provide the school team with a broader view of the student's problem by including a range of assessment approaches, such as reviewing existing records and interviewing the student, family, and teachers.

The ABC Behavior Model

To understand problem behaviors and develop behavior-based interventions, the antecedents and consequences that influence the development and maintenance of the behavior must be considered. The ABC Model describes the relationships among behaviors, antecedent stimuli, and consequences (Albrecht et al., 2003; Shapiro & Kratochwill, 2000a). This model can be depicted as:

Antecedent Stimuli → Behavior ↔ Consequences
A B C

Antecedent stimuli are factors that occur prior to a behavior that trigger the occurrence of the behavior (Conroy & Stichter, 2003; Smith & Iawata, 1997). For example, a word, situation, person, or request may be a stimulus that triggers a specific behavioral response in a student. Consequences occur after the behavior and impact whether the behavior will occur again (Alberto & Troutman, 2003). Consequences are either reinforcing or punishing. Consequences that are reinforcing increase the likelihood of the behavior occurring again. Reinforcement can be either positive or negative. Positive reinforcement occurs when a reward is provided following a behavior, such as praise or a sticker; as a result, the occurrence of the behavior increases. For example, a kindergarten teacher wants her students to use "polite words," such as "please," "thank you," and "excuse me." Each time a child uses one of these words (the behavior), she praises the child (provides something). The children like being praised so they start to use the "polite words" more frequently. Positive reinforcement may also increase an undesired behavior. For example, Sally is very vocal in class, constantly raising her hand and demanding the teacher call on her to answer every question (the behavior). The teacher is annoyed by this behavior, but finds himself always calling on Sally first so that he can move on to other children (provides something). Sally gets the attention that she wants so she continues to disrupt the class.

Negative reinforcement occurs when something is removed or withdrawn following a behavior, such as withdrawing a command or withdrawing disapproval; as a result, the occurrence of the behavior increases (MacDonald, 2003). For example, students in a class who turn in all their homework (the behavior) in a term do not have to complete one written assignment (removing something). This increases the desired behavior (completing their homework). However, negative reinforcement may also increase an undesired behavior. For example, Emily is on the playground and wants to use a swing that another child is using. She screams and yells at the child (the behavior), so the child gets off the swing (something removed) and lets Emily have the swing. In the future, Emily will again use screaming and yelling to obtain the swing (Coucouvanis & McCarthy, 2000).

Punishing consequences decrease the likelihood of the behavior occurring again. Punishment can be an aversive event, such as a reprimand, or the removal of something positive, such as losing a privilege (MacDonald, 2003). Extinction occurs when consequences that have maintained or reinforced a behavior are discontinued, the environment no longer reinforces the behavior, and the behavior eventually stops occurring (Alberto & Troutman, 2003; Christophersen, 1995). There are two problems with extinction when used to manage disruptive behavior. First, extinction is a slow and gradual process, and may be discouraging for those who would prefer quick changes in the student's behavior. Second, when a reinforcer is initially removed, the behavior tends to increase as the student tries to produce the expected reinforcing response. However, over time, because the reinforcing event no longer occurs, the behavior eventually stops.

The ABC Behavioral Model provides a valuable tool for understanding, assessing, and treating problem behaviors in school. When obtaining a description of the disruptive behavior, factors that trigger the behavior and the reactions of others need to be explored. When developing a behavior management plan to decrease the occurrence of the behavior, environmental factors, specifically antecedents and consequences, can be manipulated in an effort to alter the disruptive behavior. This behavior management plan can be developed by an individual, such as the school nurse or teacher, or by a team, depending on the situation.

Functional Behavioral Assessment/Analysis (FBA)

Disruptive behavior serves a purpose or a function for the student who carries out the behavior. In behavioral terms, the student carries out the behavior to change something in the environment. If the behavior gets the desired change, the student is likely to repeat or maintain that behavior. This is an example of a reinforcing consequence. The same behavior in two children may serve two different functions. Two categories of functions are escape functions and gain functions. Escape functions include behaviors that assist the student in escaping from a demand made by others; escaping undesired social interaction or attention; or escaping an activity, object, or event. For individuals who have limited ability to communicate, their behavior may reflect a desire to escape from something painful, such as physical discomfort, that they cannot communicate. Gain functions include behaviors that assist the student to gain attention from adults or peers; gaining an activity, object, or event; or gaining a sensory stimulation. Consequences that are positive reinforcements tend to maintain behaviors that have a gain function, and consequences that are negative reinforcements tend to maintain behaviors that have an escape function (Alberto & Troutman, 2003).

Behavioral processes used to clarify environmental factors that impact on behavior include functional assessment and functional analysis. A functional behavioral assessment (FBA) involves gathering information through interviews, questionnaires, or direct observation and using the ABC framework to identify the purpose of the behavior (Roberts, Marshall, Nelson, & Albers, 2001). After the assessment is completed, the clinician states what he or she thinks, or hypothesizes the reason for why the student displays the problem behavior. This process often occurs within a multidisciplinary school team. As stated earlier, typical reasons may be to escape from something or to gain something. FBA is viewed by many as the best empirical approach within the school setting for developing classroom behavioral interventions, and is required under certain conditions by the Individuals with Disabilities Education Act (Myers & Holland, 2000).

A functional behavioral analysis involves manipulating the student's environment, specifically the consequences thought to be maintaining the behavior, to evaluate the effect on the student's behavior (Alberto & Troutman, 2003; Shapiro & Kratochwill, 2000a). The functional analysis allows the clinician to evaluate whether or not the hypothesized reason is actually maintaining the problem behavior. Understanding the function or purpose of a behavior for a student can assist in developing a management plan. If the function of the behavior is identified, then the consequences can be manipulated.

A teacher can carry out a functional analysis in the classroom setting to test the hypothesized function. The behavior of concern, or target behavior, needs to be clearly defined and a system for measuring it established. For example, if the behavior is off-task behavior that includes the student frequently jumping out of his chair without permission, then it may be measured as the number of times the student gets out of his chair in a certain time period. The teacher may hypothesize that the reason the student engages in this behavior is to avoid academic tasks that the teacher wants the student to complete. The teacher could create multiple conditions in which the student's behavior is observed. For example, the student could be given an academic demand situation such as a math worksheet (a task from which the child would want to escape), an attention condition such as assisting the teacher with errands (an activity that gains the child desired attention), and a free playtime condition. The number of times the off task behavior occurs under each condition can then be compared. The function of the behavior can be identified by the condition in which the behavior most frequently occurs. Once the function is identified, a management plan can be developed.

ASSESSMENT

The school nurse is often consulted when a student is displaying a behavior problem in school. The student's teacher(s), parent(s), or the students themselves may ask the school nurse for his or her opinion of a situation. Sometimes the school nurse is the person to identify a student with a behavior problem. For example, a student may be a frequent visitor to the school nurse's office, resulting in the school nurse questioning why the student needs to come to the office so often. Patterns of visits to the health office may provide important information. For example, a student may go to the office at the same time each day in order to avoid a certain class or teacher. If a student consistently leaves a class at the same time every day, the teacher involved may recognize this pattern. However, other visit patterns may only be noted by the school nurse (Box 38.2). For example, a student may go to the health office daily, but at different times, so that teachers in high school, where students rotate through various classes and teachers, may not be aware the student is having a problem.

Box 38.2 ▪▪▪

ENVIRONMENT IMPACTING A STUDENT'S BEHAVIOR: JUSTIN

The school nurse stopped in at the teacher's lounge. The topic of discussion was Justin, a seventh grader who apparently was spending about as much time in the principal's office for in-school suspension as he was in some of his classes. Ms. F., the English teacher, was insisting that Justin was just looking for attention. "He's loud and obnoxious and if his parents would give him a little attention at home he wouldn't be like this." Mr. K., the science teacher, wasn't so sure. "You know, he always seems pretty quiet in my room; in fact, I don't even notice him much." The nurse left the lounge puzzled. Three teachers had constant trouble with Justin and three did not. She was

(Continued on the following page)

Box 38.2 ■■■

ENVIRONMENT IMPACTING A STUDENT'S BEHAVIOR: JUSTIN *(Continued)*

not so sure it was attention seeking. Why would it just be happening for the same three teachers? She thought back to what she knew about behavior management. According to the ABC model, there were antecedent stimuli that triggered behaviors and the consequences that maintained the behavior, or reinforced the child doing the behavior because they liked the consequence that occurred. The consequence was being sent to the office each day. He was not getting any attention there. In fact, he had to sit in a cubicle by himself, and could not eat lunch with his friends. That did not seem a very positive reinforcement if he wanted attention. Therefore, the school nurse concluded that there might be something from which Justin wanted to escape.

The nurse decided to do a little investigating. She started by talking with several of the teachers privately. No one seemed to really know why Justin acted out. There did not seem to be any provoking incidents; he just started behaving rudely, talking back to the teacher, and occasionally even shoving another student. The nurse then decided to talk with Justin. One day when he was in the office, she began a conversation with him. They covered many different topics until one finally seemed to hit a nerve. When discussing several new students who had recently entered the school, Justin became upset. The nurse recommended that the counselor, Mr. C., explore this issue further with Justin.

A week later, Mr. C. let the nurse know that he talked with Justin and, indeed, there had been some problems with one of the new students. Justin had been the victim of bullying and had been dealing with it by getting into trouble and escaping from the classes that had the other student in them. The nurse recognized that the antecedent stimuli in this case were the classes with the child who bullied Justin, and the consequence was being removed from the class, an escape-motivated behavior. Mr. C. was able to intervene, and expected that Justin would be spending a little less time in the principal's office.

When the school nurse is asked to assess a student with a behavior problem, the nurse should obtain information from multiple sources, including teachers, parents, and the student. Information may be obtained through existing records, interviews, structured questionnaires, and direct observation of the student's behavior. How data are obtained may vary depending on the individual situation. In the initial screening of a student with difficult behaviors, the school nurse is often trying to decide if the student has an underlying health problem, a learning disability, a social problem, an emotional problem, an independent behavior problem, or a combination of these. In assessing the student, remember that the student may have comorbidities, either multiple psychosocial and/or health problems. For example, a student with attention deficit/hyperactivity disorder (ADHD) may also be depressed; a student with encopresis may also have a specific learning disability.

Existing Records

It is often helpful to begin the assessment by reviewing the student's past school and medical records. The school nurse is looking for any incidents or experiences that may contribute to the student's current behavior. In reviewing the student's academic records, identify if behavioral concerns were noted in the past. Has the student had similar problems, and if so, how was the behavior managed? Explore whether the student has a history of academic difficulties. Has the student had previous testing? Does the student have an Individualized Educational Program (IEP)? Review the student's attendance record, looking for the number and patterns of school absences. If the student has attended multiple schools, obtain records from each school and clarify the reasons for any moves, such as a divorce. Identify previous behavior problems that may contribute to the student's current behavior. Review the student's academic grades to detect if there is a pattern. Did the student have good grades followed by a sudden marked drop in grades? Students in the middle grades may also have a sudden drop as they begin to experiment with risky behaviors outside school, or in response to family events.

Review medical records to see if the student has any health-related concerns that may impact on behavior. For example, a child who has fragile X syndrome or ADHD may have associated behavioral concerns (Hatton et al., 2002; Roberts, 2003). Students with common chronic conditions, such as diabetes, may have adjustment difficulties that are demonstrated in behavior problems in school (Glazebrook, Hollos, Goodman, & Coates, 2003; Grey, Cameron, Lipman, & Thurber, 1995). Students who have experienced traumatic brain injury (TBI) often have altered behaviors, particularly when compared to their earlier behavior (Roberts, 2003). Awareness of the health condition may influence how the behavior is addressed within the school setting.

Interviews

The school nurse will want to obtain a history of the problem by interviewing those involved. This typically includes talking with the teacher(s), the child, and the parent(s). Questions that the school nurse might ask are included in Box 38.3. Remember to include questions that have an ABC focus; specifically include questions that clarify what precedes or precipitates the occurrence of the disruptive behavior (antecedents) and what follows the behavior that might be encouraging the student to continue the disruptive behavior (consequences).

Teacher Interviews

The goals of the nurse–teacher interview are to obtain the teacher's description of the behavior in question, to assess the student's overall academic and social performance, and to assess the teacher–student and teacher–parent relationships. When asking for a detailed description of the problem behavior, obtain information on what triggers the behavior, and what the consequences of the behavior have been. Ask what strategies the teacher has tried in addressing the student's behavior, and what data have been collected on the occurrence of the behavior or the results of any interventions implemented.

Box 38.3 ■ ■ ■

INTERVIEW QUESTIONS FOR ASSESSING A STUDENT WITH A BEHAVIOR PROBLEM

QUESTIONS FOR THE TEACHER

Obtain the teacher's description of the behavior in question:

1. What is the specific behavior of concern, the target behavior?
2. When did it begin?
3. When does it occur (time of day, in relationship to a class or activity)?
4. How frequently does the behavior occur?
5. What precedes the behavior (antecedent stimuli)?
6. In what type of setting does it occur (large group/small group interactions, playground, cafeteria)?
7. What occurs immediately following the behavior (consequences)?
8. What strategies have you tried to change the behavior? What has worked?
9. Why do you think this behavior is occurring (function)?

Assess the student's academic and social performance:

1. How is the student performing academically? What are the student's grades? Are there specific areas of difficulty? Are there patterns to the student's grades, such as a sudden drop in grades?
2. Is there an increase in school absences?
3. How is the student doing socially? Does the student have friends?
4. How does his behavior compare to the other students his age? (Is it age appropriate and just excessive or totally inappropriate?)
5. Is the student a target of bullies?
6. How is the student's behavior on the playground and in the cafeteria?

Assess the teacher–student and the teacher–parent relationships:

1. Does the student's behavior affect the teacher's ability to teach?
2. How does it affect the other students?
3. Why do you think the behavior is occurring?
4. Did the student have similar behavior problems in previous grades? If not, what has changed in his life? (Is the only thing that has changed the teacher or did something else happen in his life?)
5. Has the teacher talked with the student's parents? What was their response?

(Continued on the following page)

Box 38.3 ■■■

INTERVIEW QUESTIONS FOR ASSESSING A STUDENT WITH A BEHAVIOR PROBLEM *(Continued)*

QUESTIONS FOR THE STUDENT

Assess the student's perception of his academic and social activities and home environment:

1. How does the student feel he is doing in school?
2. Who are the student's friends?
3. In what activities is he involved? What is his favorite/least favorite class or activity and why?
4. What do adults or peers do that help or hinder the student's ability to control the behavior?

Obtain the student's description of the behavior in question:

1. Is the student aware of the problem?
2. If so, what does he think causes the problem?
3. According to him, what does the student think precedes the behavior and possibly triggers the problem (antecedent stimuli)?
4. What does the student report occurs immediately following the behavior (consequences)?
5. According to the student, what do others think causes the problem?
6. What has he done to alleviate the problem (or make it worse)?
7. What does he think would help?
8. How does he feel about what is happening?

QUESTIONS FOR THE PARENT

Obtain the parents' descriptions of the behavior in question:

1. Are the parents aware of the behavior that is concerning to school personnel (target behavior)?
2. Do they see similar behaviors at home? In other social situations, such as scouts or church?
3. Has the student had the behavior before or is it new?
4. If they have seen the behavior, what do they report occurs just before the behavior to trigger the occurrence of the behavior (antecedent stimuli)?
5. If they have seen the behavior, what occurs immediately after the behavior (consequences)?
6. If they have seen the behavior, what strategies have they tried to change the behavior? Have any of the strategies they have tried been effective?
7. Is the student under a healthcare provider's care or on medication?
8. Is anything different going on in the home?
9. Why do the parents think the student is behaving this way?
10. Do the parents have any additional information that would be helpful?

Assess the parenting skills and home environment:

1. If the behavior occurs at home, what have the parents tried to do to cope with the problem behavior? Has anything they tried been effective?
2. How do other adults in the home handle this?
3. How are the other children in the family doing? Do they have similar behavior problems? How do they handle this child's behavior problem?
4. Have other family members had similar problems?

Evaluate the teacher–parent relationship:

1. What has the student told his parents about what is happening at school?
2. Have the parents talked with the teacher about this?
3. What did he say? What has he tried?

In responding, the teacher may realize that nothing proactive has actually been tried yet, or that a range of interventions had been carried out, but none consistently. Ask about the student's cognitive performance, since frustration with undetected learning problems may present as a behavior problem. In addition, gifted students who are bored and unchallenged may act out behaviorally. Ask the teacher if bullying or teasing from other students might be contributing to the child's behavior (see Chapter 39), although unfortunately teachers are not always aware of this type of behavior occurring in the school (Selekman & Vessey, 2004).

It is important for school nurses to recognize that the student's behavior difficulties may be the result of a teacher–student mismatch. For example, a teacher with a controlling, structured approach may be uncomfortable with an overly energetic, creative student. Some teachers have unrealistic expectations of what an individual student can accomplish. Explore the teacher's expectations of the student's behavior, deciding if they are age, gender, and developmentally appropriate. When assessing teacher–student interactions, watch for the use of emotional or judgmental descriptions. Is there any frustration on the part of the teacher that may be affecting the student's behavior? For example, does the teacher say "I get a headache everyday and can't get anything done" versus "I have less time to teach because of his disruptive behavior"? Does the teacher describe the student as "lazy" or "spoiled" as opposed to "he is frustrated because he's behind"? Find out if the behavior is new this school year or has occurred in previous grades. If it is only this year, assess whether it is a conflict between the teacher and student, if the new academic demands are too challenging for the student, or if something else has changed in the student's life. When asking about teacher–parent interactions, listen to see if there is a positive working relationship or a negative hostile relationship (Pianta, 1999).

It may be necessary to talk to more than just the student's primary classroom teacher. In elementary school, playground and cafeteria monitors and teachers of classes such as physical education, art, or music may have a unique perspective on the student's behavior. In junior and senior high school, the multiple teachers with whom the student interacts as he or she moves from class to class and the coaches and other adult supervisors of the student's extracurricular activities may have important observations to contribute. Find out if the problem behavior occurs across school settings or only within a specific class. This information can help in understanding the possible stimulus for the behavior, such as academic demands or possibly a student–teacher conflict, and can help in developing a behavioral intervention, such as using a preferred activity as reinforcement for appropriate behavior in the classroom.

Student Interviews

Students, regardless of age, should be interviewed to assess their perceptions of themselves and obtain their understanding of the problem. School nurses communicate with students under many conditions. Discussions may be informal, occurring on a daily basis. For example, during a typical day, one student may come to the school nurse complaining of a headache, another student may see the school nurse for her daily medication, and another student may stop by to tell the school nurse about a great cross country meet. However, if a school nurse plans a more formal interview with a student specifically focused on assessment of his disruptive behavior or health issues, the school nurse may want to notify the student's parents/guardians of plans to talk with their child and, depending on individual school system policies, parental permission may need to be obtained. The school nurse may be able to obtain additional information from the student that the student has not shared with anyone else. This is likely to occur if the school nurse has built a trusting relationship with the student over time. In all interviews, confidentiality is a concern. The school nurse needs to be honest about what will happen with the information discussed in the interview. It is important that students, particularly adolescents, understand that if they indicate that they may harm themselves or others, this information must be disclosed and appropriate action taken. A student who discloses this type of information is often seeking help (see Chapter 34). Students and parents often recognize that school nurses are advocates for students.

A challenge for the school nurse may be finding an appropriate place to interview the student (Shapiro & Kratochwill, 2000a). Some children may respond better in a quiet, private setting, such as a separate office, whereas this type of setting may intimidate others. Taking a walk with the student or having a snack together in the cafeteria may be less threatening. It may be easier to begin to talk with the student about unrelated issues. Talk about positive areas, such as things that are going well or what he or she enjoys, before moving into areas of concern. Rather than just asking a series of questions, allow the student to talk. Use open-ended questions, with active listening. As the student talks, listen and watch for verbal and nonverbal clues. Letting the student talk usually uncovers areas of concern that can be pursued for further clarification. For example, ask the student if there is a favorite class or one that is more difficult than another. Ask what activities the student is involved in outside of school, such as sports, music, scouts, and employment. Explore if there are factors disrupting normal sleeping and eating patterns, such as poor supervision or family disruptions. With older students, assess whether they are working too many hours or involved in too many extracurricular activities.

When discussing the specific behavior problem, most students will be aware of the behavior that is causing concern and disruption. However, the student, like the adults involved, may not understand why the problem is occurring or what to do to resolve the problem. Again, remember the ABC model and identify factors that occur prior to the behavior and what occurs as a result of the behavior. Are there certain activities, individuals, or situations that seem to trigger the behavior? Is the response of others actually reinforcing the occurrence of the behavior? For example, is the student always disruptive in algebra class and often asked to leave the class, thus escaping from a class the student dislikes?

For some students, the school nurse may need to be more directive in asking questions, since the student may not recognize that there is a problem or, if aware of the problem, may be reluctant to discuss it. The student who does not realize there is a problem may see the situation as the teacher's or someone else's problem, and not understand that the behaviors he displays trigger the teacher's concerned response. If the student recognizes there is a problem, ask the student if he has done anything to alleviate the problem. Discussing what the student has done and what the student thinks might improve the situation recognizes the student's efforts and role in improving the situation. Teachers may not be aware that children and adolescents may believe they have already tried to solve the problem. Ask how the student feels about the problem, since behavior problems in children often make students feel that they are "bad" or "stupid" and that others "hate" them. Let the student know that you respect his or her views, take the student's comments seriously, and understand his or her feelings. It can be helpful to tell the student about your own experiences or those of other students (unnamed) to normalize the situation and encourage sharing. Most students are comforted by statements such as "Other students have told me..." or "It's common for students your age to..." Allow the student to talk and digress while you listen. As the discussion comes to an end, review what was discussed, clarify what information will be shared with others, and end with a plan that includes what you will do with the information (Talking with Kids, 2002).

Parent Interviews

Parents should be interviewed to obtain their perspectives on the current problem and relevant history (Shapiro & Kratochwill, 2000a). In speaking with the parents, the school nurse wants to review the child's medical history, obtain the parent's description of the behavior in question, assess parenting skills and the home environment, and evaluate the parent–teacher relationship. Parents should be asked about any health problems and treatments that their child might be experiencing. For example, a new medication may have a side effect that is contributing to the behavior problem.

It is important to find out if the behavior of concern is occurring in other settings or just at school. The student who is only acting out in school has a situational problem that requires more intense assessment of the school setting. A student with a problem behavior across multiple settings will need a treatment plan that can be carried out by adults in all settings. Ask if other family members have similar behavior problems. It is not uncommon for parents to say the child is "just like his father" or another family member. Some families may view the behavior as normal and not understand the teacher's concerns; some parents may view the problem as resting with the school staff and not them. Consider cultural differences, as behaviors accepted in one culture may not be acceptable in another.

For those families who are aware of the child's problem, taking an empathetic and nonjudgmental approach to parents may encourage them to share more of their concerns. Asking the parents how they are doing and acknowledging their difficulty helps to build an alliance. Have the parents describe the disruptive behavior, including their perceptions of factors that may precipitate the behavior and the responses of others to the behavior. If both parents and other adults care for the child, find out if they agree on whether or not a problem exists, what the problem is, factors that occur prior to and following the behavior, and how the problem should be treated. Disagreements among family members can exacerbate the child's problem and obstruct treatment plans.

Inquire about the home situation and any recent changes in the family, such as a new sibling or a separation, that may contribute to the child's acting out behavior. Consider and rule out any abuse or an unstable home situation (Iowa Department of Human Services, 2001). Encopresis, urinary incontinence, other bathroom problems, frequent stomachaches, or other somatic complaints may be associated with problems in the home (van Zanten, 2003). Obtain the parent's perspective on any interactions that have occurred between the parent and school personnel. Poor communications or misunderstandings that may have occurred over time may have impacted on the family–school relationship.

Structured Questionnaires

Behavior rating checklists and questionnaires are often helpful in assessing a student's behavior problem (Achenbach & Ruffle, 2000; Glascoe, 2000; Perrin & Stancin, 2002). Behavior checklists and questionnaires are instruments that have been "normed," which means data have been collected on a large number of children to determine the typical behavior for children of various ages. Using normative behavior checklists allows comparisons of a child's behavior with other children and, if completed by multiple caregivers, comparisons across settings (i.e., school and home). The instruments are typically available in several versions that allow the child, a parent, and a teacher to complete comparable versions of the instrument.

A rigorous process is used in the development of behavior rating checklists and questionnaires. Manuals for questionnaires include data on validity, which refers to the ability of the instrument to measure what it says it measures, and data on reliability, which refers to the consistency of results provided by the instrument. Items are often grouped into subscales, clusters of items that assess specific behavioral areas, such as anxiety, aggressiveness, and impulsivity. Many questionnaires allow comparison of the student's raw score to standardized scores, providing the ability to interpret how much the student's behavior differs from behavior norms for age.

Questionnaires are considered indirect measures because they assess perceptions of behavior rather than a first-hand, direct assessment of the student's behavior (Shapiro & Kratochwill, 2000b). Indirect measures are helpful because they allow the clinician to see the student's behavior through the student's self-perceptions or through the view of someone who regularly interacts with the student. However, there is a limitation regarding the use of indirect assessment measures. They reflect the interpretation of the person completing the form and may not necessarily be a true reflection of the behavior. For example, the same child may be scored differently by two individuals with different experiences and expectations.

Examples of checklists and rating scales include general behavior checklists such as the Child Behavior Checklist (CBCL) and the Behavior Assessment System for Children (BASC). Information for these and other selected instruments used by behavioral assessment teams in schools or clinics are included in Tables 38.1 and 38.2. Some instruments are copyrighted and have an associated cost and some require

(text continues on page 903)

Table 38.1 ■

LIST OF BEHAVIORAL CHECKLISTS, RATING SCALES, QUESTIONNAIRES, AND SELECTED BEHAVIORAL SCREENING INSTRUMENTS USED IN THE PEDIATRIC AND ADOLESCENT POPULATION

INSTRUMENT	AGE RANGE	DESCRIPTION	ITEMS AND SUBSCALES	TIME FRAME
Pediatric Symptom Checklist (PSC) and Youth Pediatric Symptom Checklist (Y-PSC)	4–16 yrs.	Parent and youth report forms. A brief screening questionnaire that is used by pediatricians and other health professionals to improve the recognition and treatment of psychosocial problems in children. Forms can be downloaded and used free of charge. Other translations available.	35 short statements of problem behaviors rated as never, sometimes, or often present and scored 0, 1, 2, respectively. Includes both externalizing (conduct) and internalizing (depression, anxiety and adjustment) statements. Cut off score suggests need for further evaluation by a qualified health or mental health professional.	About 5 minutes

(continued)

Table 38.1 ■ *(Continued)*

INSTRUMENT	AGE RANGE	DESCRIPTION	ITEMS AND SUBSCALES	TIME FRAME
Eyberg Child Behavior Inventory (ECBI) & Sutter-Eyberg Student Behavior Inventory-Revised (SESBI-R)	2–16 years	Parent and teacher report forms. Comprehensive, behaviorally specific rating scales that assess the current frequency and severity of disruptive behaviors in the home and school settings, as well as the extent to which parents and/or teachers find the behavior troublesome.	36 items for the ECBI and 38 items for the SESBI-R. Single refer/non refer score for externalizing problems (e.g., conduct, attention, aggression). Does not address internalizing behaviors.	About 5 minutes to adm., 5 minutes to score
Child Behavior Checklist (CBCL) • Child Behavior Checklist 1/2–5 (CBCL/1/2–5) • Child Behavior Checklist for ages 6–18 (CBCL/6-18) • Caregiver-Teacher Report Form (C-TRF) • Teacher's Report Form for ages 6–18 (TRF) • Youth Self Report Form for ages 11–18 (YSR)	1–18 years	Parent, teacher, caregiver, and youth report forms. Teacher report and child self-report measure. Multidimensional and multiple informant evaluations. Provides a profile of behavior deviancy and social competence. Standard T scores provide norm-based comparisons by age and gender. Available in other languages. Based on CBCL. Forms now available for completion by child care providers or preschool teachers for children 2–5 years of age	C-TRF and CBCL/1/2–5 have 99 items plus descriptions of problems, disabilities, what concerns the respondent most about the child, and the best things about the child. The CBCL/6-18 and TRF have 118 problems. The TRF and C-TRF have 138 items. Requires a 5th grade reading level.	20–25 minutes to adm. Complex scoring-computer scoring recomended
Behavior Assessment System for Children (BASC)	2–18 years	A comprehensive set of rating scales and forms including the Teacher Rating Scales (TRS), Parent Rating Scales (PRS), Self-Report of Personality (SRP), Student Observation System (SOS),	126–148 items. 20 scales and subscales. Subscales include externalizing, internalizing, school, other problems (atypicality, withdrawal) and adaptive skills.	TRS, PRS: 10–20 minutes

(continued)

INSTRUMENT	AGE RANGE	DESCRIPTION	ITEMS AND SUBSCALES	TIME FRAME
		and Structured Developmental History (SDH) to assess children's and adolescents' emotions and behaviors. Multidimensional and multiple informant evaluations. Spanish version available.	Norms available by age and gender.	SRP: 30–45 minutes
Preschool and Kindergarten Behavior Scales, 2nd ed. (PKBS-2)	3–6 years	Provides an integrated and functional appraisal of the social skills and problem behaviors of young children.	76 items on two different scales	12 minutes
Revised Behavior Problem Checklist-PAR Edition (RBPC)	5–18 years	Used to rate problem behaviors observed in adolescents and young children. Can be used to screen for behavior disorders in schools.	89 items. 6 subscales.	20 minutes to adm., 10 minutes for scoring and profiling.
School Social Behavior Scales, 2nd ed. (SSBS-2) and Home and Community Social Behavior Scales (HCSBS)	5–18 years	Screening and assessing social competence and antisocial behavior of children and youth. Also designed for identification and classification, intervention planning, monitoring intervention progress and evaluation intervention outcomes. SSBS-2 is completed by teachers and other school personnel, the HCSBS is completed by parents, group home supervisors and other home or community-based raters.	32 social competence items with 3 subscales and 32 antisocial behavior items with 3 subscales	5–10 minutes

a psychologist or mental health professional to score and interpret the results. Although the school nurse might not initiate the use of more complex instruments, the school nurse can be of assistance to the evaluation teams by facilitating the distribution of the instrument to the parents or teachers and encouraging parents to complete and return them to the clinicians or specialists for their review.

An example of a screening instrument that may be appropriate for school nurses to use in the school setting is the Pediatric Symptom Checklist (PSC) (Jellinek et al., 1988, 1999). Both a parent and child version of the PSC are available. (Figures 38.1, 38.2, and 38.3 provide the parent PSC, the child PSC and scoring information, respectively.) The tool is a one-

(text continues on page 906)

Table 38.2

LIST OF BEHAVIORAL CHECKLISTS, RATING SCALES, QUESTIONNAIRES, AND CONTACT INFORMATION FOR INDIVIDUAL INSTRUMENTS

TITLE	AUTHOR	ADDRESS	TELEPHONE NO.	E-MAIL ADDRESS/ WEB SITE
Pediatric Symptom Checklist (PSC) and Youth Pediatric Symptom Checklist (Y-PSC)	Michael Jellinek, MD	Child Psychiatry , Massachussetts General Hospital, 351 Bullfinch, Boston, MA 02114	617-724-3163	http://www.mgh.harvard.edu/children/psc/psc_order.htm
Eyberg Child Behavior Inventory (ECBI)	Sheila Eyberg, PhD	Psychological Assessment Resources, 16204 N. Florida Ave., Lutz, FL 33549	813-968-3003 or 800-331-8378	http://www.parinc.com
Child Behavior Checklist (CBCL)	Thomas M. Achenbach, PhD	ASEBA, Room 6436, 1 South Prospect St., Burlington, VT 05401-3456	802-656-8313 or 802-656-2608	http://www.ASEBA.org or http://ASEBA.uvm.edu
Behavior Assessment System for Children (BASC)	Cecil R. Reynolds, PhD and Randy W. Kamphaus, PhD	AGS Publishing, 4201 Woodland Road, Circle Pines, MN 55014-1796	800-328-2560	http://www.agsnet.com
Preschool and Kindergarten Behavior Scales, 2nd ed. (PKBS-2)	Kenneth W. Merrell, PhD	Pro-Ed, Inc. 8700 Shoal Creek Blvd., Austin, TX 78757-6897	800-897-3202	http://www.proedinc.com
Revised Behavior Problem Checklist-PAR Edition (RBPC)	Herbert C. Quay, PhD and Donald R. Peterson, PhD	Psychological Assessment Resources, Inc., 16204 N. Florida Ave., Lutz, FL 33549	813-968-3003 or 800-331-8378	http://www.parinc.com
School Social Behavior Scales, 2nd ed. (SSBS-2)	Kenneth Merrell, PhD	Assessment Intervention Resources, 2285 Elysium Avenue, Eugene, OR 97401	541-338-8736	http://www.assessment-intervention.com

Pediatric Symptom Checklist - Parent Report

Child's Name ______________________ Record Number ______________________
Today's Date ______________________ Filled out by ______________________
Date of Birth ______________________

Please mark under the heading that best fits your child:

	Never	**Sometimes**	**Often**
1. Complains of aches/pains	☐	☐	☐
2. Spends more time alone	☐	☐	☐
3. Tires easily, little energy	☐	☐	☐
4. Fidgety, unable to sit still	☐	☐	☐
5. Has trouble with a teacher	☐	☐	☐
6. Less interested in school	☐	☐	☐
7. Acts as if driven by a motor	☐	☐	☐
8. Daydreams too much	☐	☐	☐
9. Distracted easily	☐	☐	☐
10. Is afraid of new situations	☐	☐	☐
11. Feels sad, unhappy	☐	☐	☐
12. Is irritable, angry	☐	☐	☐
13. Feels hopeless	☐	☐	☐
14. Has trouble concentrating	☐	☐	☐
15. Less interest in friends	☐	☐	☐
16. Fights with others	☐	☐	☐
17. Absent from school	☐	☐	☐
18. School grades dropping	☐	☐	☐
19. Is down on him or herself	☐	☐	☐
20. Visits doctor, doctor finds nothing wrong	☐	☐	☐
21. Has trouble sleeping	☐	☐	☐
22. Worries a lot	☐	☐	☐
23. Wants to be with you more than before	☐	☐	☐
24. Feels he or she is bad	☐	☐	☐
25. Takes unnecessary risks	☐	☐	☐
26. Gets hurt frequently	☐	☐	☐
27. Seems to be having less fun	☐	☐	☐
28. Acts younger than children his or her age	☐	☐	☐
29. Does not listen to rules	☐	☐	☐
30. Does not show feelings	☐	☐	☐
31. Does not understand other people's feelings	☐	☐	☐
32. Teases others	☐	☐	☐
33. Blames others for his or her troubles	☐	☐	☐
34. Takes things that do not belong to him or her	☐	☐	☐
35. Refuses to share	☐	☐	☐

Other comments:

Total Score:_____

Figure 38.1 ■ The Pediatric Symptom Checklist: Parent.

Pediatric Symptom Checklist - Youth Report (Y-PSC)

Please mark under the heading that best fits you:

	Never	Sometimes	Often
1. Complain of aches or pains	☐	☐	☐
2. Spend more time alone	☐	☐	☐
3. Tire easily, little energy	☐	☐	☐
4. Fidgety, unable to sit still	☐	☐	☐
5. Have trouble with teacher	☐	☐	☐
6. Less interested in school	☐	☐	☐
7. Act as if driven by motor	☐	☐	☐
8. Daydream too much	☐	☐	☐
9. Distract easily	☐	☐	☐
10. Are afraid of new situations	☐	☐	☐
11. Feel sad, unhappy	☐	☐	☐
12. Are irritable, angry	☐	☐	☐
13. Feel hopeless	☐	☐	☐
14. Have trouble concentrating	☐	☐	☐
15. Less interested in friends	☐	☐	☐
16. Fight with other children	☐	☐	☐
17. Absent from school	☐	☐	☐
18. School grades dropping	☐	☐	☐
19. Down on yourself	☐	☐	☐
20. Visit doctor, doctor finds nothing wrong	☐	☐	☐
21. Have trouble sleeping	☐	☐	☐
22. Worry a lot	☐	☐	☐
23. Want to be with parent more than before	☐	☐	☐
24. Feel that you are bad	☐	☐	☐
25. Take unnecessary risks	☐	☐	☐
26. Get hurt frequently	☐	☐	☐
27. Seem to be having less fun	☐	☐	☐
28. Act younger than children your age	☐	☐	☐
29. Do not listen to rules	☐	☐	☐
30. Do not show feelings	☐	☐	☐
31. Do not understand other people's feelings	☐	☐	☐
32. Tease others	☐	☐	☐
33. Blame others for your troubles	☐	☐	☐
34. Take things that do not belong to you	☐	☐	☐
35. Refuse to share	☐	☐	☐

Total Score: ____

Figure 38.2 ■ The Pediatric Symptom Checklist: Youth Report.

page, 35-item screening questionnaire completed by parents or youth and designed to help clinicians in outpatient practice identify school-age children with difficulties in psychosocial functioning. The instrument has been validated in general pediatric office settings, a variety of subspecialty clinics, schools, and low-income and minority settings. The Web site provides information on the reliability and validity of the PSC (see Table 38.2). For example, the specificity of the PSC is 0.68, meaning that 68% of children who receive a score above the cut off level are found to have problems when further evaluated. Sensitivity of the PSC is 0.95, meaning that 95% of children who receive scores below the cutoff level

Instructions for Scoring the Parent PSC: Item scores are summed and the total score is recorded into a dichotomous variable indicating psychosocial impairment. For children ages 6 through 16, the cut-off score is 28 or higher. For 4- and 5-year-old children, the PSC cut-off is 24 or higher. Items that are left blank are simply ignored (score=0). If four or more items are left blank, the questionnaire is considered invalid. A score higher than the cut-off suggests the need for further evaluation.

Instructions for Scoring the Youth PSC: The youth self-report can be administered to adolescents 11 years of age and older. Item scores are summed and the total score is recorded into a dichotomous variable indicating psychosocial impairment. The cutoff score for the Y-PSC is 30 or higher. Items that are left blank are simply ignored (score=0). If four or more items are left blank, the questionnaire is considered invalid. A score higher than the cut-off suggests the need for further evaluation.

Figure 38.3 ■ The Pediatric Symptom Checklist: Scoring.

are normal on further assessment. An overall score is determined and a cutoff score for consideration of referral is provided. This instrument is free and can be printed off the Web site provided in Table 38.2.

The PSC has been included in the Bright Futures curriculum, a national health promotion and disease prevention initiative launched in 1990, with the support of the Maternal and Child Health Bureau, Health Resources and Service Administration, and the Medicaid Bureau, Health Care Financing Administration. Bright Futures is dedicated to developing educational materials for health and education professionals and families. The latest publication in the Bright Futures in Practice series is Bright Futures in Practice: Mental Health, a guide that provides information on healthy emotional, behavioral, and cognitive development in children, and on early recognition and intervention for mental health problems (Bright Futures, 2002). The consensus guidelines were developed by more than 150 external reviewers and are supported by more than 50 national organizations. The Bright Futures website provides PDF files of many assessment instruments and clinician and parent educational materials from Bright Futures in Practice: Mental Health.

Direct Observation

Direct observation requires the school nurse or school personnel to observe the student and record behaviors or events. It provides a measure of clearly specified behaviors that occur within a specific environment and within a given time period. It can provide reliable and valid data that can assist in making educational decisions and in developing practical interventions. The direct link between assessment procedures, such as FBA, and interventions is one of the most important strengths of behavioral theory (Shapiro & Kratochwill, 2000a).

An FBA observation system first requires clearly defining the target behavior. The behavior of concern or target behavior needs to be clearly defined in a way that is observable, measurable, and repeatable (Alberto & Troutman, 2003). How the behavior is quantified and within what time frame must be decided, such as the number of occurrences in a class period or percentage of time the behavior occurs in 10 minutes. In addition, factors that occur prior to the target behavior, possible triggers, and the responses of others need to be documented. As described earlier, in a functional behavioral analysis various conditions may be presented to the student and the student's behavioral responses observed to assist in identifying the underlying function or purpose that the behavior serves for the child.

An example of a direct assessment in which school nurses often participate is recording attention to a task or on-task behavior (Shapiro & Kratochwill, 2000b). Typically, on-task behavior is the amount of time a student is actually engaged in a specific learning activity, with various operational definitions used depending on the child and the task (Alberto & Troutman, 2003). On-task behavior is often recorded in number of minutes the student is on or off-task, and is compared to a typical classmate's behavior. School nurses are sometimes asked to conduct these observations and to provide information to the school psychologist or assessment team. To observe on- and off-task behavior, the behavior must be defined. There are multiple definitions of on-task behavior in the literature, such as working on an assigned task for seven consecutive seconds, or looking at the assigned work and holding a pencil in a writing or erasing position (Alberto & Troutman, 2003). A coding sheet needs to be used that allows the observer, in this case the school nurse, to sit in the classroom and note the occurrence of the defined behavior in the identified student.

Direct observation within the classroom setting can allow the school nurse to gather specific information about the student and the behavior that could not be accomplished to the same degree in another way. For example, when the school nurse is in a classroom environment, he or she can get a sense of the behavioral context in the classroom setting and may also be able to identify other health-related concerns that non-health personnel may not identify, such as absence seizures or tic behavior. A limitation of direct observation is that the presence of an observer may alter the behavior of the student, teacher, and class, and the behaviors of concern may not occur during the observation session (Box 38.4).

Box 38.4 ■■■

USE OF DIRECT OBSERVATION: JOHNNY

A school nurse worked at an alternative high school in an urban area that served students who had not previously been successful in the traditional high school setting and also offered a daycare center for the children of the high school students to enable the teen parents to continue working toward a high school diploma while parenting a young child. Professional daycare providers as well as the young parenting teens themselves, on a rotating basis, staffed the center. The daycare director contacted the school nurse to discuss a serious problem the daycare was having with biting and requested that she help develop a plan to remedy the problem. One of the children, Johnny, had recently had three episodes of biting another child in his class. The parent of the biter, the family of the students who had been bitten, and the daycare center staff were very concerned because of the risk of blood-borne pathogen exposure, scarring, and emotional distress of the child victims.

The school nurse visited the daycare center and began by checking the immunization status of all of the enrolled children to make sure that their immunizations, including hepatitis B, were up to date. She then developed and presented an in-service for the young parents and staff regarding normal growth and development, reasons children bite, appropriate management of the biting wounds, as well as appropriate behavioral management of the child biter with a focus on prevention and teaching new behaviors. The parents and staff participated in the in-service, and gained knowledge about biting behaviors and confidence in its management. At the culmination of the in-service and discussion, they agreed to be more consistent in how they handled these situations.

The nurse's next step was to meet with those specifically involved with Johnny. Interviews provided some information on what might be the factors precipitating the biting (antecedents) and maintaining the biting (consequences). It appeared to the nurse that Johnny had more immature expressive language skills than his classmates and out of frustration at not being understood would bite the other child. The response of the adults was a lot of attention for both Johnny and the other child. The group decided to do two things. First, a biting chart was created to further assess Johnny's biting behavior and to test her hypothesis. The biting chart focused on direct observation, and included details about who, what, when and where the biting incident occurred. The chart also included a note of why the caregiver thought the biting occurred, specifically what happened before (antecedents) and after (consequences) the biting incident. Second, the staff made a plan for how the staff should respond if Johnny tried to bite. Staff were instructed to provide an immediate response using their voice and facial expressions to show that biting was unacceptable by speaking firmly and to have eye-to-eye contact with Johnny. Following the next incident, the nurse again met with the staff. They discussed how they would work with Johnny to learn to use words when possible or an alternative way to communicate his needs if necessary so that he would not become so frustrated and aggressive.

Other Assessments

After reviewing the above information, the school nurse may suggest further evaluation of the student. In some school systems, depending on the type of assessment that the school nurse determines is needed, the evaluation may be conducted by either the school or an outside agency. Depending on the individual school district's guidelines, written permission from parents may be needed to initiate a formal referral. If an outside professional is consulted, having the parents sign a two-way release of information for the school nurse to provide information to and receive information from the agency is not only helpful in facilitating communication, but is required by federal and state laws (see Chapters 13 and 14). Examples of referrals that the school nurse might suggest include requests for an evaluation by a speech therapist if there are speech problems or by a school psychologist if there are possible learning problems.

If there is a question that a medical condition might be the underlying problem, the school nurse should suggest that the family obtain a medical evaluation. Before the visit, and with parental written permission, the healthcare provider should receive copies of any pertinent psychological or academic testing carried out by the school and an objective, chronological report of the child's behavior. It is also advisable to send a letter with the parents that describe the concerns and questions of school personnel. Does the child need a neurological exam or a psychiatric referral? Is there a need for hearing or speech evaluations? If possible, sending the child to a pediatrician who specializes in behavior problems is ideal. When referring a student to a healthcare provider, it is important to specify the school personnel's specific concerns; otherwise, the student may return with a cursory exam declaring him or her in "good physical health."

A final assessment that the school nurse might want to consider in assessing a student's behavior problem is a home visit. A home visit is helpful in providing information related to the home environment, the student's behavior at home, and parental expectations of the child and the school. However, the school nurse's availability for making a home visit will vary depending on the model of school nursing utilized in each school district. For safety reasons, it is advisable to make a home visit with another individual, such as the school social worker or principal. The school nurse should have a cell phone for his or her safety and to expedite obtaining services if a crisis is found in the home setting.

INTERVENTIONS

In the school setting, behavioral interventions can be implemented with individual students or groups of students, such as a class or an entire school. These interventions incorporate approaches based on multiple theories, including behavioral and social learning theory. For students who experience behavior problems, behavioral intervention plans are developed to teach and reinforce appropriate behaviors and discourage inappropriate behaviors. Using the ABC model, interventions focus on the antecedents that trigger behaviors and the consequences that maintain behaviors. If a functional analysis is carried out and the function of the behavior identified, the intervention can address the identified function, such as escape or gain.

Development of individual behavior plans requires the participation of many parties, including the student, the teacher, other appropriate school personnel, and the family. In particular, students need to know what behaviors are expected of them and what the implications are for appropriate or inappropriate behavior. For a behavioral intervention plan to be effective, all of the adults in the student's environment need to be consistent in their interactions with the student, implementing the management plan across settings in the school and at home. This may be difficult; often a plan is undermined and ineffective because of inconsistent implementation.

When planning interventions, it is important to remember that students bring their own temperament, personalities, and experiences to the school setting. While school personnel may need to alter the environment to teach students appropriate behaviors that will allow them to succeed in school, a student's basic temperament is unlikely to change. A shy child can be helped to be more comfortable in social situations, but will probably never be the most outgoing child in the class. The adolescent with ADHD can be taught to think before acting, but will still tend to be impulsive. School personnel need to take the individual student's unique characteristics into consideration, and as much as possible, make accommodations for the student. One student might need a structured environment, another might need frequent praise, and still another might need quiet alone time to perform optimally. The same environment and the same intervention plan are not necessarily supportive for all students.

Individual Interventions: Altering Antecedents

There are multiple stimuli in the school environment, such as instruction style, curriculum, and environment that can trigger disruptive behaviors in students and, if identified, may need to be altered (Conroy & Stichter, 2003; Grier et al., 2001). An unstructured, chaotic classroom may confuse and overstimulate some children, particularly children with decreased impulse control. An inflexible, overly structured classroom may be too rigid for some students to control their behavior for long periods. A curriculum that does not match an individual student's abilities may be stressful and result in behavior problems, such as a high school student in an advanced math class who does not have the needed basic skills. Some need a more hands-on approach to learning than is routinely provided. Specific aspects of the environment that may trigger disruptive behaviors in certain children include seating placements that provide distractions to the child, such as next to a window, a door, or in the back of the class. A class with a number of students with acting-out behaviors may trigger similar behaviors in other children. The multiple environments of school, such as classrooms, bus rides, cafeteria, music room, playground, and physical education, and the different demands of each setting, can be confusing for some students, thereby resulting in problem behaviors (Gunter, Coutinho, & Cade, 2002).

As noted earlier, teacher–student mismatches are important to identify. School personnel should carefully plan the appropriate placements for children with behavioral difficulties, trying to match a student's temperament and learning style with a teacher's style. If a teacher–student mismatch does occur, consideration should be given to moving the student to a class with a teacher who is more experienced or skilled with this type of student. Alternatively, the teacher may be advised to seek assistance from the school administrator, counselor, or an experienced teacher to assist the teacher in developing an appropriate management plan for this student.

How teachers communicate with students can impact on students' behavior (Blum, Williams, Friman, & Christophersen, 1995; Gunter et al., 2002). Rules and directions are more likely to be followed if they are clearly presented, either verbally or in writing, and are stated positively, with expectations of appropriate behavior. For example "Don't run in the hall." is a negative directive and does not tell the student what is the expected behavior. This type of directive often triggers a noncompliant behavioral response in the student. The preferred statement would be "The rule is—walk in the hall" which can be presented neutrally and tells the student what he should be doing (Carns & Carns, 1994).

Peers may provoke disruptive behaviors in some students. Bullying, teasing, and simple encouragement from other children may result in behavioral outbursts or withdrawal in the targeted student. This type of student interaction can affect the learning environment for the entire class. School personnel should be vigilant in identifying these situations. School nurses are often the first adults aware of teasing or bullying since the victim may use the health office as a safe refuge from this stressful situation. If the school nurse is aware of such a situation, she needs to be an advocate for the victim, quickly communicating with the teacher, principal, and parents, and insuring appropriate consequences for the bully (see Chapter 39).

Physical symptoms, such as hunger, fatigue, and pain, can contribute to a student's behavioral response (Conroy & Stichter, 2003). The child or adolescent who is hungry, tired, or experiencing exaggerated or heightened responses from a headache, stomachache, menstrual cramps, or allergies may respond with inappropriate behaviors. Unfortunately, these symptoms may be unknown to the child's teacher and, as a result, the teacher may respond to the behavior and not to the trigger. For some students, the school nurse is aware of social situations or physical problems that may contribute to behavioral difficulties. School nurses should alert teachers to these potential difficulties within the limits of maintaining confidentiality.

In summary, it is important for school personnel to identify antecedent stimuli and alter them. Often, simple changes, such as structuring the environment, monitoring other children's behaviors, or alleviating physical discomfort, can decrease at least some inappropriate behaviors.

Individual Interventions: Altering Consequences

Based on the ABC assessment and/or the FBA, consequences thought to be maintaining the disruptive behavior need to be changed. This is typically accomplished by replacing inappropriate consequences with appropriately placed positive reinforcements in the student's behavior management plan. Two examples of positive reinforcement that are frequently incorporated into school behavioral management plans are token systems and contracts. Punishing consequences, which tell a student which behaviors are not acceptable, can also be used in schools, but if used, they are typically combined with positive reinforcement approaches that teach expected appropriate behaviors.

Reinforcing Consequences/ Positive Reinforcement

As noted earlier, positive reinforcement occurs when something is provided following an appropriate behavior, such as praise or stickers; as a result, the occurrence of the behavior increases (MacDonald, 2003). An event or object is said to be reinforcing if the child will work to obtain access to it (Christophersen, 1995). A reinforcing consequence is often referred to as a reward.

Adults are sometimes uncomfortable using positive reinforcement. They may believe that the child should act appropriately without a reward. Explaining that using rewards accelerates behavioral changes and that reinforcers occur routinely in our daily lives, may be helpful. For example, adults receive paychecks contingent upon completing their work, yet parents may perceive reinforcement as a form of bribery. The difference between bribery and reinforcement should be addressed. Bribery, frequently used "after the fact," may stop a negative behavior that is already in progress. However, bribery places the child in control and does not teach the child appropriate behavior (Coucouvanis & McCarthy, 2000). For example, a student who continually acts out in class and stops only when the teacher gives him what he wants is responding to a bribe. A reinforcement program that is planned in advance keeps the adult in control and teaches acceptable behavior. The teacher might say the following to teach acceptable behavior, "If you raise your hand and wait your turn, you can earn extra time on the computer."

Positive reinforcement is often used in the school environment. A student does a desired behavior that is reinforced or immediately rewarded by the teacher. For example, a student may be encouraged to raise her hand to be called on, instead of shouting out in class or jumping out of her seat. In order to shape the more appropriate behavior, the teacher may quickly call on the student and praise the student for raising her hand instead of shouting or leaving her seat. If this praise makes the student feel pleased, it is more likely that the student will again raise her hand to be called on. Positive reinforcement is frequently used in schools to teach the use of appropriate communication, often referred to as functional communication training, a part of social skills training. In other cases, a student may be informed that involvement in a desired activity is contingent upon the student completing a less desired activity. For example, "When you finish your math problems, you can go out to recess" uses a behavior that is highly desirable to reinforce and increases the occurrence of a behavior that is less likely to occur on its own. It is important when using positive reinforcement that the student knows what the expected behaviors are and what the consequences are for both doing the behavior and not doing the behavior.

Token Systems

A token economy system is a form of positive reinforcement used to shape desired, appropriate behaviors (Christophersen & Mortweet, 2002; MacDonald, 2003). In our society, receiving money for working, which can then be exchanged for desired goods, is a classic example of a token economic system. In schools, token systems are used to encourage preferred behaviors in students with behavior problems or can be adapted for the same purpose with groups of children. Simple token economies can be useful for children as young as 3 to 5 years of age, while more sophisticated systems can be developed for teenagers.

The success of a token economy depends on how consistently it is used and the variety of reinforcing activities available to the student (Christophersen, 1995). Token economy systems include both tokens and backup reinforcers/rewards. Depending on the age of the child and the preference of the participants, tokens can be stickers, poker chips, points, play money, cards, or stamps. Tokens have no value by themselves but are reinforcing when they can be exchanged for backup rewards, items, or activities that are desired by the child. It is critical that the rewards be desirable to students involved in the token system (Box 38.5). For some children, more recess time may be rewarding; for others, time on the computer may be the desired reward. Therefore, the student often has input into the rewards and a menu or list of rewards may be developed. Some students

Box 38.5 ■ ■ ■

BEHAVIORAL INTERVENTION, USE OF A TOKEN ECONOMY: TONY

It was well known around the school that Mrs. W., the second grade teacher, had been having trouble with Tony. She had been asking for ideas on how to handle his disruptive behavior. He had been evaluated by the school nurse, and did not seem to have any medical problems. At the nurse's suggestion, Mrs. W. established a token economy for Tony.

Tony would need to earn some type of token that could be traded in for a reward that he would value enough to want to earn. The first step was to identify a reward (reinforcer) that Tony could earn. "Oh, that's easy," replied Mrs. W., "He loves basketball. That's all he talks about. He idolizes the high school boys on the team." That gave the nurse an idea. What if Tony could earn points toward watching a practice, or serving as an "assistant" during a game and sitting on the bench? The basketball coach was agreeable to giving it a try.

The next step was to set up a series of desired behaviors Tony could successfully accomplish. She decided to start by having Tony raise his hand before speaking out in class and waiting to be called. She discussed this with Tony and explained that if he waited until he was called, he would earn a sticker on a card she would keep at her desk. When the whole row was filled, the basketball coach had agreed to let Tony watch part of the practice. At first, Mrs. W. called on Tony quickly to give him confidence in his ability to succeed. After his first basketball practice, she made him wait just a little longer to be called upon. She gradually added other tasks after discussing her expectations with Tony. The rewards also became larger. Tony's greatest achievement came after several weeks of reaching his goals, which were becoming increasingly difficult. He had been rewarded with going to practices, and now would be allowed to sit with the team at a game. He was thrilled, his mother was excited, and the boys on the team enjoyed having Tony there.

lose interest in the reward quickly; therefore changes in the rewards may need to occur over time. The format for documenting that the student has carried out the appropriate behavior and earned the tokens varies with different systems. For younger children, charts with fun pictures that can be colored to document behavior may be used. For older children, a list of specific behaviors and a place for a check mark, date, and time may be more appropriate.

In setting up a token system, the rules need to be clear to the participating student (Garrick-Duhaney, 2003; Salend, 2001). The specific behaviors for which the child will earn tokens need to be delineated, and the rules for earning or losing tokens must be explained. It is helpful to set initial behavioral expectations low, such as raising one's hand before leaving the class, so that the child can be successful, earn the tokens and the rewards, and experience success. The behaviors expected of the child may then be increased in order to attain the desired reward. In addition, the delay between earning the tokens and exchanging them for the reward should be realistic for the child's age. Very young children may need to be able to make exchanges on a daily basis, while older children can delay receiving their reward to once a week. School staff are often unrealistic about what they expect of a student, setting up token systems that are too complicated or difficult thereby resulting in student failure.

When token systems are developed for an individual student in a class, fairness to other students must be considered. Older classmates often understand the need for an individualized approach for a classmate with behavioral difficulties. However, younger children may not understand, and a teacher may choose to develop a token economy for appropriate behavior for all students in the class. Schools have limited budgets, so a decision about who funds the rewards must be made. In some situations, school systems fund the rewards; in other situations, families may contribute rewards. Unfortunately teachers often pay for the rewards for individual token systems—or entire class token programs—out of their own pockets. In these instances, it may be necessary to decrease using tangibles as rewards and incorporate rewards that are attention-focused. Students may be able to earn time with others, such as lunch with a favored teacher, or the privilege of a desired activity, such as to be an office assistant.

Contracts

For some students, a formal, written contract may be helpful in eliciting the desired behavior from the child. Contingency contracts are similar to token economies. A contract states the relationship between the desired behavior of the student and the reinforcing consequences that the child will receive when those behaviors occur (Carns & Carns, 1994; Garrick-Duhaney, 2003). Ideally, the student, teacher, and parents participate in the development and signing of the written contract. The first step in developing a contract is to define the desired behavior, preferably in positive terms (Carns & Carns, 1994). Like token economies, it is important to set behavioral expectations at a level that allows the child to succeed. For example, the first week, the student may be expected to raise his hand to answer a question instead of yelling out in class, at least three times a day in order to obtain the reward. Over the following weeks, the student may have to increase the occurrence of raising her hand in order to obtain the reward until eventually the reward is earned only for raising her hand consistently throughout the day. Because contracts are written and incorporate both positive rewards and punishment as the consequences, they are typically used for older students (Box 38.6). For example, a junior

Box 38.6 ■ ■ ■

BEHAVIORAL INTERVENTION, CONTRACTS: KATIE

While checking the absentee list, the school nurse noticed that Katie's name appeared again. She looked back over the past month and saw that Katie had been absent several times, especially on Mondays. The excuse was always the same. "Katie isn't feeling well today." The nurse recalled that Katie had frequently been in the nurse's office with one complaint or another when she was younger. Since she had started high school, her visits have been infrequent. However, it did seem a little unusual that she was missing so much school, especially since it was always on Monday.

She decided to talk with a few of the teachers. Mr. K, the science teacher, assured her that Katie was doing fine in school, except for missing so much schoolwork. "She's smart enough, but if you miss enough homework you get behind." The English teacher, Mrs. B, agreed, "She is doing ok, but I think it's just her personality-you know, her dad is a little different; she doesn't like people, and she stays at home a lot. I think she's a little different and the kids notice it. I think her parents might be having some trouble; I heard rumors of a divorce." The school nurse tried to associate Katie's office visit complaints of stomachaches and headaches with what might be happening in the family environment. She decided to call Katie in for a visit.

The next day, the school nurse met with Katie and told her about her concerns that Katie's grades might be affected by her absences, and reminded Katie about what a good student she was. Katie had no explanation, just that she didn't feel good. Then, without prompting, she began to talk openly about her parents' separation and divorce, not appearing upset. Yes, she had been to the doctor, and they didn't know what was wrong. The doctor said they would have to do more tests if she didn't feel better. "I think it is just migraines" Katie said cheerfully.

The school nurse asked the school psychologist whether he thought the problems at home might have prompted Katie to want to stay home. The psychologist agreed that Katie might be feeling more comfortable at home. "It might be a good idea to be proactive and intervene now while it is a minor problem. We can find out what she really enjoys and develop a contract with Katie. If she makes it in on Mondays, she gets a positive reinforcement-something that makes it worth her while to come in. The key is to find out what Katie really wants."

A meeting was set up with Katie the following day. The psychologist explained that the absences were a little concerning. "We know you may not be feeling the best, but we think you need to make an extra effort to come every day. One thing that might help is to find something that you like, even when you may not be feeling well. Do you have any ideas of what really helps make you feel better?" Katie immediately replied, "Oh what I really love is working in the library as an aide. I can do that even with a headache!" The psychologist suggested they draw up a contract. "Since we know you seem to have headaches on Mondays, what if you used your study hall on Monday afternoon to work in the library. The deal is, if you come to school each day, you can work in the library during your afternoon study hall." "It's a deal!" Katie replied happily.

Several weeks later, the school nurse noticed that Katie's name had not appeared on the absentee list. She saw the psychologist later in the hall and commented on Katie's perfect attendance. "Well, that really was a win–win situation," he said. "Katie is here every day, so her grades are good. And actually, she's a great aide in the library!"

high student with diabetes who is reluctant to routinely test blood sugars or a high school student who wants to quit smoking might each benefit from a contract.

Punishing Consequences

Consequences that are punishing decrease the likelihood of the behavior occurring again. Punishment can be the introduction of an aversive event, such as a reprimand, or the removal of something positive, such as losing a privilege (Alberto & Troutman, 2003). Punishing consequences may be used to decrease the frequency of a disruptive behavior, such as hitting other children. Punishment may be incorporated into a behavior management plan that focuses primarily on the use of reinforcing appropriate behaviors. However, punishment should be used cautiously. There are five commonly used punishing consequences: extinction, verbal reprimand, natural consequences, response cost, and time out.

Extinction

With extinction, no reward or attention follows the behavior; the behavior is simply ignored (Alberto & Troutman, 2003; Shapiro & Kratochwill, 2000a). Ignoring inappropriate behaviors is difficult to carry out, particularly in the busy school setting. Ignoring requires that the adult not respond to the inappropriate behavior and maintain a neutral appearance, look away from the student, or not speak to or touch the child. When the child is not given attention for an inappropriate behavior, the behavior should occur less frequently and eventually stop occurring. Changing behaviors through extinction is a slow process. Parents and teachers should be warned that ignored behaviors often increase in frequency initially, as the child tries to illicit the desired consequences that used to occur. Eventually, without the reinforcing consequence, the inappropriate behavior will gradually stop (Christophersen, 1995). This approach is helpful for gain-motivated or attention-seeking children, but may not be helpful for escape-motivated children or children engaged in self-stimulating behavior.

Reprimand

A verbal reprimand given after an inappropriate behavior can decrease the recurrence of that behavior. A verbal reprimand includes eye contact between the student and the adult, the use of a stern voice, a statement conveying disapproval, and a command that is clear, direct, and specific (Barkley, 1987). The reprimand should be unambiguous, delivered immediately following the behavior, and address the behavior; it should not be directed at the child (Garrick-Duhaney, 2003). The adult using a reprimand should be calm rather than overly emotional, and should not demean the child. Examples of verbal reprimands are "No swearing!" and "No pushing!" If necessary, a reprimand may include potential consequences that may occur if the child does not comply with the command given. Reprimands set limits on behaviors and identify inappropriate behaviors. However, a concern with the use of reprimands is that while they tell a child what they should not do, they do not teach the child what the appropriate, alternative behavior should be. Many prefer to use statements such as "No running, walk" or "No yelling, quiet voice," thereby coupling the reprimand with a reminder of the appropriate behavior.

Natural Consequences

Natural consequences are events that naturally follow a behavior unless someone does something to prevent them. These occur frequently in the school setting. For example, getting an incomplete on a homework assignment is a natural consequence to not completing the homework; failing a test is the consequence of not studying for an exam; and not being able to practice is the consequence of forgetting one's soccer shin guards. The use of natural consequences is thought to improve behavior when students are allowed to experience the naturally occurring negative consequences that follow the inappropriate behavior. Parents often try to protect their children from negative consequences by completing homework assignments for the child or driving a child to school who missed the bus. School personnel may need to explain to parents the importance of allowing their child to learn responsibility by experiencing natural consequences.

Response Cost

Response cost refers to the loss of something viewed as a reinforcer, like a privilege, as a result of an inappropriate behavior (Alberto & Troutman, 2003; Garrick-Duhaney, 2003). A concern with response cost is that if used alone, it does not teach or shape the expected, appropriate behaviors. Response cost is often part of a token economy. Some token economies include both the child earning tokens for appropriate behaviors and losing acquired tokens for inappropriate behaviors. The loss of the token is referred to as the "response cost." Systems that include response cost components should clearly define the behaviors for which the child can earn tokens as well as the behaviors that result in a loss of tokens. For example, in a school-based token system, a student might earn two points for raising his hand to ask a question, but lose one point for yelling out in class. Token economies that incorporate response cost may be complex and therefore more appropriate for older students.

Time Out

Time out is actually time out from positive reinforcement. With time out, the child is removed from a situation that is reinforcing the problem behavior to one that is not at all reinforcing (MacDonald, 2003). Time out is often used to decrease the occurrence of a behavior that cannot be ignored, such as hitting or acting out (Turner & Watson, 1999). It is appropriate for preschool or school age children, and for one to two specific, targeted behaviors. Typically in time out, the child is removed from the reinforcing setting to an area that does not provide any reinforcers such as television, toys, people, or books. In schools, the setting may be a corner of a room or a separate room. Time out is usually brief, lasting from 1 to 10 minutes; the younger the child, the shorter the timeout (Coucouvanis & McCarthy, 2000). If time out is part of a behavior plan, the rules of time out need to be explained to the child before it is implemented. When the child misbehaves, time out is immediately applied. The child should be told, in a neutral way, what behavior he or she has done that is resulting in the time out. For example, "You just hit Johnny. Time out." To be most effective, time out should be used after each episode of the specific behaviors.

It is important to remember that time out is most effective for behaviors that are gain functions; that is, behaviors that children display in order to obtain attention or specific objects or activities. However, for children whose behavior is a means to escape, being put into time out may allow them to escape from an undesirable activity or interaction. In these instances, time out becomes highly reinforcing and the child may act out to avoid a task (Coucouvanis, 1997). For some children, time out may be the only time that they receive attention, and therefore time out is actually reinforcing. To avoid this, it is crucial to make sure the child receives attention when behaving appropriately. A number of parenting manuals (Christophersen & Mortweet, 2003) and references (Christophersen & Mortweet, 2002; Coucouvanis & McCarthy, 2000; MacDonald, 2003) provide an in-depth discussion on the implementation of time out, including use of time out in the classroom (Turner & Watson, 1999).

Group Interventions: Creating a Positive School Climate

Although this chapter focuses on students with disruptive behavior problems and the assessment and interventions for individual students, there are also some general approaches used in schools to foster positive behaviors within the student body and prevent problem behaviors from occurring (Rones & Hoagwood, 2000). These approaches generally involve the school developing a continuum of positive behavior support (PBS) that focuses on universal prevention/early intervention as well as individualized student support systems for those who display chronic problem behaviors. These programs typically incorporate providing clearly defined behaviors or a common set of rules, strategies for staff to teach the expected behaviors, strategies to encourage students to practice appropriate behavior, and consistency within and across school systems. Several studies in the literature demonstrate the effectiveness of school-wide systems of PBS to reduce behavior problems (Colvin, Sugai, Good, & Lee, 1997; Nakasato, 2000; Scott, 2001; Taylor-Greene et al., 1997; Taylor-Greene & Kartub, 2000). Some studies have also focused specifically on building systems of support in non-classroom settings such as the cafeteria, hallway, and playground (Colvin et al., 1997; Kartub, Taylor-Greene, March, & Horner, 2000; Lewis, Powers, Kelk, & Newcomer, 2002; Lewis, Sugai, & Colvin, 1998). These approaches may be most beneficial for at-risk students who have not learned or observed positive skills modeled at home. When programs are fully integrated within the curriculum, they provide numerous skill-building opportunities throughout the day and ultimately may serve to decrease the number of behavior problems within the school. This is based on the theory that frequent reinforcement of expected appropriate behavior results in the desired behaviors occurring.

Some school programs focus on the power of a smaller group of peers to positively impact individual behavior more than on adults in the environment (Garrick-Duhaney, 2003). One example of this is the “Circle of Friends” approach used by some school districts. This process involves identifying a target student with behavioral or social problems whom school staff determines would benefit from a handful of peers to serve as positive role models and supportive peers for the identified student. This “Circle of Friends” may have some of the same classes, may eat lunch together, or may even arrange activities outside of the regular school day. This group allows the target student to experience positive interactions and mentoring from same age peers. As the target student is able to develop positive social and behavioral skills within the safe small group, there can be many positive outcomes. The target student, peer mentors, and greater student body experience benefits as the behavior problems diminish.

The school nurse, as an integral part of the school team, can assist with providing positive behavioral support for individual students, as well as groups of students and the entire student body. She or he may be able to help identify students who would benefit from special mentoring opportunities, or may even function as a mentor for a particular student. He or she can also help to create a positive school environment by focusing on positive proactive behavioral strategies rather than punitive strategies. The school nurse can also hold students accountable for the school-wide initiatives when they are in the school health office.

CONCLUSION

Students with disruptive, problem behaviors are frequently a concern for school personnel. School nurses are often instrumental in the assessment of and interventions for children with these difficulties. School nurses bring a unique health-centered perspective on behavior problems, with a holistic view of the individual that is valuable to the staff as they assess and develop an approach to the student’s problems. For the child and family, the school nurse is an advocate who provides support and services as needed. The goal for all involved is to develop interventions that result in a student obtaining a state of optimal health, ready to learn and succeed.

References

Achenbach, T. M., & Ruffle, T. M. (2000). The Child Behavior Checklist and related forms of assessing behavioral/emotional problems and competencies. *Pediatrics in Review, 21*(1), 265–271.

Alberto, P. A., & Troutman, A.C. (2003). *Applied behavior analysis for teachers* (6th ed.). Upper Saddle River, NJ: Merrill, Prentice-Hall.

Albrecht, S. J., Dore, D. J., & Naugle, A. E. (2003). Common behavioral dilemmas of the school-aged child. *Pediatric Clinics of North America, 50*, 841–857.

Barkley, R. A. (1987). *Defiant children: A clinician’s manual for parent training*. New York: The Guilford Press.

Being Alert to Indicators of Psychosocial and Mental Health Problems. (2002). *Resource materials and assistance*. Center for Mental Health in Schools at UCLA, Los Angeles, CA. Retrieved June 6, 2003 from http://smhp.psych.ucla.edu/qf/assess&screen_qt/beingalert.pdf

Blum, N. J., Williams, G. E., Friman, P. C., & Christophersen, E. R. (1995). Disciplining young children: The role of verbal instructions and reasoning. *Pediatrics, 96*, 336–341. Bright Futures in Practice. (2002). Georgetown University. Washington, DC: U.S. Department of Health and Human Services Administration, Maternal and Child Health Bureau.

Campbell, S. B. (2002). *Behavior problems in preschool children: Clinical and developmental issues* (2nd ed.). New York: The Guilford Press.

Carns, A. W., & Carns, M. R. (1994). On the scene: Making behavioral contracts successful. *The School Counselor, 42*, 155–160.

Christophersen, E. R. (1995). Behavioral management: Theory and practice. In S. Parker & B. Zuckerman (Eds.), *Behavioral and developmental pediatrics*. New York: Little, Brown and Company.

Christophersen, E. R., & Mortweet, S. L. (2002). *Treatments that work with children*. Washington, DC: American Psychological Association.

Christophersen, E. R., & Mortweet, S. L. (2003). *Parenting that works*. Washington, DC: American Psychological Association.

Colvin, G., Sugai, G., Good, R. H. III, & Lee, Y (1997). Using active supervision and precorrection to improve transition behaviors in an elementary school. *School Psychology Quarterly, 12*, 344–363.

Conroy, M. A., & Stichter, J. P. (2003). The application of antecedents in the functional assessment process. *Journal of Special Education, 37*(1), 15–26.

Cook, E. T., Greenberg, M. T., & Kusche, C.A. (1994). The relations between emotional understanding, intellectual functioning, and disruptive behavior problems in elementary-school-aged children. *Journal of Abnormal Child Psychology, 22*(2), 205–220.

Coucouvanis, J. A. (1997). Behavioral intervention for children with autism. *Journal of Child and Adolescent Psychiatric Nursing, 10*(1), 37–44.

Coucouvanis, J. A., & McCarthy, A. M. (2000). Behavior Modification. In M. J. Craft & J. A. Denehy (Eds.), *Nursing interventions for infants and children* (2nd ed.). Philadelphia: W. B. Saunders.

Garrick-Duhaney, L. M. (2003). A practical approach to managing the behavior of students with ADD. *Interventions in School & Clinic, 38*(5), 267–280.

Glascoe, F. P. (2000). Early detection of development and behavioral problems. *Pediatrics in Review, 21*(8), 272–278.

Glazebrook, C., Hollos, C., Goodman, H., & Coates, L. (2003). Detecting emotional and behavioural problems in paediatric clinics. *Child; Care, Health, & Development, 29*(20), 141–149.

Grey, M., Cameron, M. E., Lipman, T. H., & Thurber, F. W. (1995). Psychosocial status of children with diabetes in the first 2 years after diagnosis. *Diabetes Care, 18*(10), 1330–1336.

Grier, R., Morris, L., & Taylor, L. (2001). Assessment strategies for school-based mental health counseling. *Journal of School Health, 71*(9), 467–469.

Gunter, P. L., Coutinho, M. J., & Cade, T. (2002). Classroom factors linked with academic gains among students with emotional and behavioral problems. *Preventing School Failure, 46*(3), 126–132.

Hatton, D. D., Hooper, S. R., Bailey, D. B., Skinner, M. L., Sullivan, K. M., & Wheeler, A. (2002). Problem behavior in boys with fragile X syndrome. *American Journal of Medical Genetics, 108*, 105–116.

Iowa Department of Human Services. (2001). *Child abuse: A guide for mandatory reporters*. Retrieved June 9, 2003 from http://www.dhs.state.ia.us/

Jellinek, M. S., Murphy, J. M., Robinson, J., Feins, A., Lamb, S., & Fenton, T. (1988). Pediatric symptom checklist: Screening school-age children for psychosocial dysfunction. *The Journal of Pediatrics, 112*, 201–209.

Jellinek, M. S., Murphy, J. M., Little, M., Pagano, M. E., Comer, D. M., & Kelleher, K. J. (1999). Use of the Pediatric Symptom Checklist to screen for psychosocial problems in pediatric primary care. *Archives of Pediatric and Adolescent Medicine, 153*, 254–260.

Kartub, D. T., Taylor-Greene, S., March R. E., & Horner, R. H. (2000). Reducing hallway noise: A systems approach. *Journal of Positive Behavioral Interventions, 2*, 179–182.

Lewis, T. J., Powers, L. J., Kelk, M. J., & Newcomer, L. L. (2002). Reducing problem behaviors on the playground: An investigation of the application of schoolwide positive behavior supports. *Psychology in the Schools, 39*(2),181–190.

Lewis, T. J., Sugai, G., & Colvin, G. (1998). Reducing problem behavior through a school-wide system of effective behavioral support: Investigation of a school-wide social skills training program and contextual interventions. *School Psychology Review, 27*, 446–459.

MacDonald, E. K. (2003). Principles of behavioral assessment and management. *Pediatric Clinics of North America, 50*, 801–816.

Myers, C. L., & Holland, K. L. (2000). Classroom behavioral interventions: Do teachers consider the function of the behavior? *Psychology in the Schools, 37* (3), 271–280.

Nakasato, J. (2000). Data-based decision making in Hawaii's behavior support effort. *Journal of Positive Behavioral Interventions, 2*, 247–251.

Perrin, E. C., & Stancin, T. (2002). A continuing dilemma: Whether and how to screen for concerns about children's behaviors. *Pediatrics in Review, 23*(8), 264–275.

Pianta, C. (1999). *Enhancing relationships between children and teachers*. Washington, DC: American Psychological Association.

Roberts, M. C. (Ed.). (2003). *Handbook of pediatric psychology* (3rd ed.). New York: The Guilford Press.

Roberts, M. L., Marshall, J., Nelson, J. R., & Albers, C. A. (2001). Curriculum-based procedures embedded within functional behavioral assessments: Identifying escape-motivated behaviors in general education classroom. *School Psychology Review, 30*(2), 264–278.

Rones, M., & Hoagwood, K. (2000). School-based mental health services: A research review. *Clinical Child and Family Psychology Review, 3*(4), 223–241.

Salend, S. J. (2001). *Creating inclusive classrooms: Effective and reflective practices* (4th ed.). Upper Saddle River, NJ: Prentice-Hall.

Scott, T. M. (2001). A school-wide example of positive behavioral support. *Journal of Positive Behavioral Interventions, 3*, 88–94.

Selekman, J., & Vessey, J. (2004). Bullying: It isn't what it used to be. *Pediatric Nursing, 30*(3), 246–249.

Shapiro, E. S., & Kratochwill, T. K. (Eds.). (2000a). *Conducting school-based assessments of child and adolescent behavior*. New York: The Guilford Press.

Shapiro, E. S., & Kratochwill, T. K. (Eds.). (2000b). *Behavioral assessment in schools* (2nd ed.). New York: The Guilford Press.

Smith, R. G., & Iawata, B. A. (1997). Antecedent influences on behavior disorders. *Journal of Applied Behavior Analysis, 30*, 343–375.

Talking with Kids (2002). *Center quick training aid: Re-engaging students in learning*. Center for Mental

Health in Schools at UCLA, Los Angeles, CA: Author. Retrieved June 6, 2003 from http://smhp.psych.ucla.edu.

Taylor-Greene, S., Brown, D., Nelson, L., Longton, J., Gassman, T., Cohen, J., Swartz, J., Horner, R. H., Sugai, G., & Hall, S. (1997). School wide behavioral support: Starting the year off right. *Journal of Behavioral Education, 7*, 99–112.

Taylor-Green, S. J., & Kartub, D. T. (2000). Durable implementation of school-wide behavior support: The high five program. *Journal of Positive Behavioral Interventions, 2*, 233–235.

Turner, H. S., & Watson, T. S. (1999). Consultant's guide for the use of time-out in the preschool and elementary classroom. *Psychology in the Schools, 36*(2), 135–148.

van Zanten, S. V. (2003). Diagnosing irritable bowel syndrome. *Review of Gastroenterological Disorders, 3* (Suppl. 2), S12–S17.

Chapter 39

Violence in Schools

JANICE SELEKMAN ■ SUSAN G. PRAEGER

Chapter Outline

INTRODUCTION

Violence has become a common problem for today's children. It occurs in the home, the school, and the community, and is shown in the media; it occurs between children, and between adults and children on small and large scales. Violence can also be self-inflicted. It crosses sociopolitical, economic, racial, ethnic, and cultural boundaries. Regardless of its cause, "violence, or the threat of it, is also highly disruptive to the school environment and interferes significantly with the teaching–learning process" (Walker, Ramsey, & Gresham, 2004, p. 351). The purpose of this chapter is to provide a broad overview of the scope of the problem of violence facing children and a description of the roles of the school nurse in addressing this problem.

The World Health Organization defines violence as "the intentional use of physical force or power, threatened or actual, against oneself, another person, or against a group or community, that either results in or has a high likelihood of resulting in injury, death, psychological harm, maldevelopment, or deprivation" (2002, p. 2). School violence is defined as "any behavior that violates a school's educational mission or climate of respect or jeopardizes the intent of the school to be free of aggression against persons or property, drugs, weapons, disruptions, and disorder" (U.S. Department of Health and Human Services [USDHHS], 2001). Violence is a public health problem. It can have physical and emotional sequelae that can affect individuals for life. However, violence is a learned behavior; it is preventable and its impact can be reduced.

Violence affects everyone—from students and their classmates to playground supervisors, bus drivers, classroom teachers, families, and all school staff. National and local agencies are dedicated to the eradication of violence in society. Administrators, law enforcement officers, legislators, and community officials, as well as teachers, parents, healthcare providers, and students themselves need to work together to address this issue to make schools a safe place for all.

Arrest rates for violent crimes committed by youth increased 70% from the early 1980s, with a peak in 1993 (Youth Violence, 2001). Of the 104,000 arrests of youth under age 18 in 1999, 1,400 were for homicides. However, the Surgeon General's report on youth violence found that since 1994, the number of homicide arrests has decreased and the use of firearms has been declining. While the number of homicides has decreased, arrests for nonfatal aggravated assault, many of which involve use of weapons, have increased (Youth Violence, 2001). Involvement in gangs remains a significant problem.

While children can be victims of violence from infancy, the initiation of violent behavior can occur before puberty. Those who begin younger generally commit more serious crimes that may last into adulthood (Youth Violence, 2001). However, the vast majority of violent behavior in youth begins and ends during adolescence. Approximately 15% to 30% of female youth and 30% to 40% of male youth report having committed a serious violent offense by age 17 (Youth Violence, 2001).

Violence is manifested on a wide spectrum, although there is great overlap. At the lower end are teasing, bullying, and harassment. This is followed by an escalation of activities that can result in arrest, such as physical aggression, assault, and child abuse. At the other end of the spectrum is violence that is life-threatening, such as homicide and suicide. It should be noted that violence at the "milder" end of the spectrum can progress to severe violence. This does *not* imply, however, that less severe violence results in less severe psychological sequelae, as this is not the case. Seventy-five percent of school shootings during the past decade have been related to bullying and the perpetrator feeling persecuted, threatened, attacked, or injured prior to the incident (Fox, Elliott, Kerlikowske, Newman, & Christeson, 2003).

TEASING

All children and adults have engaged in teasing or playing pranks on their peers or have been the brunt of these behaviors. Teasing often results in laughter and positive feelings. It is defined as "verbal and/or nonverbal behaviors among peers that are generally humorous and playful" (Vessey, Swanson, & Hagedorn, 1995). It can be used as a way to show interest in another or to send messages to the person; when both individuals find the incident funny, it can help build interpersonal relationships. Within this description, it would not be considered appropriate in a chapter on violence.

However, it is difficult to determine how individuals will respond to teasing. Their response depends on their relationship with the instigator, what else is going on in their environment, and how they interpret the teasing. If they do not see the humor or are embarrassed by sensitive material, they will not see the situation as funny and may feel threatened, especially if the teasing is persistent. Therefore, teasing can be interpreted as or deteriorate into bullying and harassment, even if that was not the intent of the initiator. It is therefore important for the school nurse and other school personnel to be able to differentiate between benign teasing and bullying and to ask students how they feel about the teasing. Other suggestions are provided in the section on bullying that follows.

BULLYING

Teasing can be a gateway behavior to bullying and "most school violence begins with bullying" (Garrett, 2003, p. 1). Any definition of bullying has three important components: (1) the behavior identified is aggressive and involves intentional "harm doing" by one person or a group; (2) the behaviors are carried out repeatedly and over time; and (3) there is a power imbalance between the bully and the victim (Nansel et al., 2001). The National Association of School Nurses (NASN) defines bullying among peers as "dynamic and repetitive persistent patterns of verbal and/or non-verbal behaviors directed by one or more children on another child that are intended to deliberately inflict physical, verbal, or emotional abuse in the presence of a real or perceived power differential" (NASN, 2003). Bullying is sometimes referred to as "mobbing," peer abuse, or peer harassment (Harris & Petrie, 2003). Bullying by any definition is a form of violence.

Bullying Behaviors

Bullying is a learned behavior. Bullying behaviors can be physical, verbal, or nonverbal. Table 39.1 identifies these behaviors. There is also emotional bullying, in which classmates are defamed, humiliated, blackmailed, or ostracized. Sexual bullying involves propositioning, exhibitionism, voyeurism, and abuse (Walker et al., 2004). Regardless of the form, all of these behaviors have a psychological impact. In addition, there are situations in which one bully gets others to do his bullying for him or her. This is referred to as "bully by proxy" (Thompson, Arora, & Sharp, 2002). An example may be the hazing that occurs in sorority and fraternity pledging rituals or when seniors initiate new students into the school or initiate juniors who are

Table 39.1 ■
BULLYING BEHAVIORS

PHYSICAL ACTS	VERBAL/NONVERBAL ACTS
Physical injury (hit, punch, kick, trip)	Threaten.
Damage belongings of others.	Insult, call names, humiliate.
Take belongings of others (money, lunch, homework).	Spread rumors about person or family.
Embarrass by snapping bra, lifting skirt, pulling down pants.	Shun or exclude.
	Make gestures.
	Engage in extortion.

Source: Selekman & Vessey (2004).

about to be seniors, having been encouraged to do so by their peer leadership. New to the bullying repertoire is "online bullying" in which students spread rumors and pictures for all to see. These can be quite vicious, as students may feel less accountable when they are not face to face with the victim. "Regardless of the form, it must be recognized that all bullying is aggression, although not all aggression is bullying, and aggression is a form of violence" (Selekman & Vessey, 2004, p. 247).

It must be remembered that enacting any of these behaviors once does not make one a bully, for the definition indicates these behaviors are repeated over time. However, knowing that the behavior occurs even once is an indication that action should be taken to prevent it from becoming a pattern of behavior.

Red flags of suspicion would include the student who comes to the nurse's office with unexplained injuries or a change in behavior. Reports of students repeatedly not eating lunch because they "lost it" or "lost their money" might be another warning sign. When there is damage to the school or to personal property or accusations of one student copying from another's paper, the school staff should suspect bullying.

Where Bullying Occurs

Students of all ages are careful to engage in bullying away from the eyes and ears of adults. The most common places include the route to and from school, on the bus, in the cafeteria, in the hallways, at the lockers, in the gym locker room, on the playground, and even in the classroom (Drake, Price, Telljohann, & Funk, 2003). It may also occur in front of adults who have not taken any action to stop the behaviors in the past (Garrett, 2003).

Incidence of Bullying

Almost all children throughout the world have engaged in bullying behavior or been the victims of that behavior at some point during their childhood. However, unless it is persistent, it does not get counted in statistics regarding bullying. Approximately 30% of students are either bullies or victims; some are both (Fox et al., 2003). This translates into almost 7 million students involved with bullying.

There is no difference in the incidence of bullying by gender, but males tend to be more physical and direct, while females more frequently use the psychosocial indirect route (Garrett, 2003). There is also no difference in the incidence of bullying in urban, suburban, or rural schools or by race or socioeconomic status (Thompson et al., 2002). One study on an elementary school playground found that bullying behaviors occurred every 7 minutes; of these events, adults intervened in 4%, peers intervened in 11%, and there was no intervention for the remaining 85% of incidents (Garrett, 2003).

Bullying behaviors can be seen in the preschool years, but they are not considered bullying until the child reaches "a certain level of awareness and understanding" of the intent to harm another person (Thompson et al., 2002, p. 18). Early signs of bullying seen in the elementary years include physical acts of causing injury or taking possessions, followed by taking pleasure in the victim's reaction and appearing unconcerned when disciplined for the action (Selekman & Vessey, 2004).

There are two peak ages for bullying behaviors. The first is around ages 7 and 8 and again around ages 11 to 14 (NASN, 2003). While the incidence decreases somewhat in high school, its occurrence at that time may have more serious consequences on the victim. These result in reports of students bringing guns to school, often with disastrous results. Bullying behaviors that continue into adulthood are often referred to as harassment. Harassment is defined as an illegal act of verbal or nonverbal taunting or demeaning someone on the basis of certain attributes, such as their sex, race, religion, appearance, or sexual orientation (Walker et al., 2004).

Bullying behaviors are influenced by parental attitudes and behaviors, including how or if it is punished, the degree of supervision, and the modeling of aggressive behaviors as a way to attain a goal (Garrett, 2003). The violence in the media and in videogames as well as the behaviors of role models also affect a student's tendency to engage in these behaviors. The incidence of bullying behaviors increases when parents and teachers take no action when they see or hear about bullying; this failure to intervene condones the bully's behaviors.

The Bully, the Victim, and the Watchers

Bullying is often an indication of insecurity and a need for attention on the part of the bully. By dominating another, there is a false sense of being "tough" and having power and control. Bullying is a social activity; rarely is it just one bully to one victim. The bully often has a group of peers who fear the bully but support him by their presence. Because the bystanders or watchers often fail to prevent the bully from taking action, they are supporting his or her actions and assisting him or her in building a false sense of bravado.

Extensive research has been conducted to identify risk factors for becoming a bully. This information has been compiled by the National Youth Violence Prevention Resource Center (NYVPRC, 2003) and indicates some of the characteristics of bullies (Box 39.1). Most of those involved in bullying are considered to be underachievers (Elliott, 2002).

The victim is often perceived by the bully as "different." Sometimes the differences are obvious, such as height, weight (Lunner et al., 2000; MacBrayer, Smith, McCarthy, Demos, & Simmons, 2001), glasses or braces, disabilities, restricted mobility (Prellwitz & Tamm, 2000), mannerisms, clothing, or lack of coordination. Sometimes the difference is not as apparent, such as religious beliefs, sexual orientation, or having gay or lesbian parents (Ahmann, 1999); sometimes a student is just described as being "weird." The victim may already be insecure and have a low self-esteem, with less tolerance for teasing by classmates (Vessey, 1999). Other characteristics can be found in Box 39.2. Victims do not usually seek adult help because they believe it will not make the situation better but will just lead to increased harassment from the bully (Garrett, 2003).

The watchers have been referred to as "bully-assistants" or reinforcers. They want to be accepted by the bully and his group. They get caught up in

Box 39.1 ■■■

CHARACTERISTICS OF BULLIES

- Show artificially high self-esteem and artificial confidence (actually has a poor self-concept).
- Feel relatively unloved and unnoticed by significant others.
- Generally physically aggressive.
- May have experienced family violence; may have been abused verbally, physically, or emotionally in the home.
- Unable to channel their anger and frustration in acceptable ways.
- Do not accept responsibility for their actions.
- Strong need to dominate others; use others to get what they want.
- Egocentic: want to satisfy their own needs and pleasures; have a sense of entitlement.
- Little empathy for their targets; unwilling to accept others' ideas or to negotiate during play or to view something from a different perspective.
- Male often physically bigger and stronger than peers.
- Lack parental supervision.
- Role models use adversarial problem-solving skills.
- Excessively harsh parental approach to discipline.

(Coloroso, 2003; MacNeil & Newell, 2004)

Box 39.2 ■ ■ ■

CHARACTERISTICS OF VICTIMS OF BULLYING

- More anxious and insecure.
- Suffer from low self-esteem.
- Rarely defend or retaliate when confronted by bullies.
- Socially isolated; less popular.
- Lack social skills in relation to peers, in general.
- Often don't "fit in."
- Males tend to be physically weaker than their peers.
- Refuses to go to school or takes an unusual route to school.
- Has frequent psychosomatic complaints related to particular classes or activities.
- Has disheveled, torn, or missing clothing.
- Is hungry after school, claiming he lost his lunch money.

(Coloroso, 2003; MacNeil & Newell, 2004)

the "power trip" of the situation and feel both protected and restricted by a code of silence. In this environment, they may not see the target as a person and not consider the consequences of their actions or those of the bully (Elliott, 2003). Their reasons for not intervening include fear that the bully will turn on them, believing that it is none of their business, that they would not be successful if they tried, or even in the bully's logic that the victim "deserved" it (Selekman & Vessey, 2004). This group, above all, underestimates their true power to make change.

Effects of Bullying

"Bullying affects the school climate and the learning environment of every classroom" (Garrett, 2003, p. 9). Both victims and perpetrators of bullying are at risk for serious health and social consequences. Bullying behavior may be the first sign of serious antisocial behavior later in life (Fox et al., 2003). Bullies are seven times more likely to carry a weapon to school than non-bullies. Long-term studies indicate that approximately 60% of those identified as being bullies in middle school had been convicted of at least one crime by the age of 24 (Garrett, 2003). "Bullies are more likely to manifest defiant behavior and negative attitudes toward school and use drugs" (Juvonen, Graham, & Schuster, 2003, p. 1231). Bullying in childhood may be a precursor to peer dating violence in adolescence; it does appear to be "an antecedent of more serious harassing and antisocial behavior" (Garrett, 2003, p. 17).

The short-term effects of being a victim are usually psychological in nature, resulting in nightmares and sleep disturbances, psychosomatic complaints (abdominal pain, headaches, chest pain), increased incidence of illness (related to chronic stress), impaired concentration, stress behaviors (i.e., nail biting, comfort measures, and enuresis), and depression (Hawker & Boulton, 2000). Nansel, Overpeck, Haynie, Ruan, and Scheidt (2003) identified a positive relationship between the presence of health symptoms and frequency of bullying with problems related to sleeping, feelings of sadness, occasional headaches, and stomach aches in 2.4% to 3.6% of students.

Victims may become fearful of coming to school and so may be truant (Garrett, 2003); the National Center for Education Statistics estimated that 160,000 students across America in 2002 missed school each day because of bullying. They may fear going to particular classes, and thus may visit the school nurse often, or with a pattern. The results are decreased class time, decreased school performance, and decreased participation in certain school activities. Poor concentration, school avoidance, tension, anxiety, lowered self-esteem, and impaired feelings of self-worth are reported as consequences of bullying (NYVPRC, 2003).

Bullying is both a school and a social problem. As a school problem, bullying affects attendance and participation. Victims fear being excluded and ridiculed by their classmates; they may feel lonely and without friends or emotional support. This may further lower their self-esteem and increase their depression and anxiety. They do not talk about the bullying at home or at school because they "fear retaliation from the bully, are afraid they will not be believed, or perceive their situation in the long run as normal" (van der Wal, de Wit, & Hirasing, 2003, p. 1315).

Students who are bullied are five times more likely to be depressed than those who were not (Fox et al., 2003). Suicidal thoughts may result; bullied girls are eight times more likely to be suicidal and bullied boys are four times more likely to be suicidal than those who were not bullied (Fox et al., 2003; van der Wal et al., 2003). Committing suicide because of the impact of bullying has been referred to as "bullycide" (Elliott, 2003). The psychological impact of indirect bullying is much more than for direct physical bullying. Indirect bullying is more difficult to detect and consequently often goes unnoticed by adults for longer periods of time. Long-term problems in adults bullied as children include higher levels of depression and poorer self-esteem than among other adults (NYVPRC, 2003).

Often, when victims have "had enough," they become bullies themselves; they have the most serious sequelae, especially conduct, school, and peer relationship problems (Juvonen, Graham, & Schuster, 2003). "It is not physical abuse by peers but inability to cope with social ridicule and personal rejection that can fuel extreme outbursts of violence" (Juvonen et al., 2003, p. 1231). Bullying is a factor in more than two-thirds of school shootings, as the victim takes revenge on the bully and those who supported him (Harris & Petrie, 2003).

Interventions that Do NOT Work

Inappropriate responses by adults can make the situation worse for the victim. Comments such as, "These experiences build character," "It will help toughen you up for life," "Just ignore them," or "They are just being kids" may make the victim feel that he or she is at fault and that nothing can be done; they are neither helpful nor supportive. Doing nothing, especially after being told that there is a problem, is the worst thing of all.

Misinterpretation of bullying as anger is equally ineffective. It does not work to have them try to "stay away" from the bully or to pound out their feelings on a pillow. School strategies of peer mediation are inappropriate with bullying because of all of the dynamics involved and the need for adult intervention. Zero tolerance policies are also ineffective, as they do not address the behaviors nor do they give direction of how to change them.

Interventions for the School and the School Nurse

The problem of bullying in schools is broad, complex, and multidimensional. Because it is a systems problem that involves the school, the community, the families, and the students, it requires "a multifaceted, systematic approach that includes all community stakeholders" (Garrett, 2003, p. 17). School-wide programs that are initiated generally decrease bullying behaviors by 50% (Garrett, 2003). This includes inservice programs for staff to provide them with both whole-school and classroom-based bullying prevention activities to promote a culture that does not accept bullying behaviors (Drake et al., 2003).

Solutions are rarely found in one intervention alone. The first intervention is to identify the key "players" in the school related to bullying. These will always include the students, the staff, and the parents. These are the people who must develop a definition of bullying and identify the behaviors. School staff must acknowledge that indirect psychological bullying is a form of aggression and it must be included in any definition of bullying.

Discussions can be held in classrooms or in student groups of why people bully, why people watch bullies and don't act, how it feels to be bullied or to bully others, and the effects that bullying has. This is difficult for some teachers, since some teachers may shy away from discussing feelings. These discussions can be in history classes to explore bullying and prejudice throughout history; civics classes to discuss the law and violence and what society would be like if bullying was acceptable; and psychology classes to discuss the moral dilemmas faced with bullying and the possible solutions. Many elementary schools now use school counselors to engage in these discussions with students.

The questions asked and the responses given may give the school some insight into the types of incidents occurring and the concerns students have about coming forward when bullying takes place. Suggested questions are shown in Box 39.3.

It is essential that schools promote a trusting environment. Students must be able to trust the staff and, especially, the school nurse. They want to trust that something will be done but they fear that the adults will over-react. Adults must be positive role models in managing relationships and emphasize sharing, caring, and helping. It is essential to listen to what students are saying and to be supportive. Let them know that they will now have support.

Teachers can ensure that students do not choose their own teams or partners, so that those who are not often included will be paired with supportive classmates. It should be assured that the bully and the victim are not together. They should have no contact, direct or indirect. Desks should be placed in such a way that the victim is in the midst of supportive classmates. Victims should be observed during lunchtime to ensure that they have their lunch or their lunch money and that they are supported by peers.

Teachers must reinforce positive behaviors (including sensitivity and kindness toward others), build self-concept for the victim and for the bully in more positive areas, and identify school hot spots for

Box 39.3 ■ ■ ■

QUESTIONS THAT CAN BE ASKED IN CLASS DISCUSSIONS ABOUT BULLYING

1. Why do students say or do "mean" things to other students?
2. What makes one group of students think they are better than others?
3. What types of people or groups make you feel angry or hurt or not think well of yourself?
4. Would I want that said or done to me? How would I feel? How would it affect me?
5. If you saw a student being picked on or made fun of, what would affect whether you stepped in to help or stepped out of the way?
6. What happens when students report incidents to teachers/parents?
7. Do you feel safe in the school (playground, locker area, busses, bathrooms, etc.)?

bullying behaviors. Staff must implement a plan to infiltrate these hot spots. Differences, similarities, and uniqueness should be celebrated.

If bullying behaviors are seen, interventions should occur immediately. By saying, "We don't do that here," the staff is stating clear expectations and creating a safe zone. It is important to point out to students engaging in bullying behaviors that what they did was wrong. Staff should not allow students to use excuses, such as "I just..." or "I only..." in their attempt to justify or lessen their offense. Another approach is to try to get the offending student to take another point of view by asking, "What would your classmates say you did wrong?"

Perhaps most effective is to discuss the power of the bystanders. Explain their responsibility in promoting and preventing these behaviors. They need to be empowered to band together and protect their classmates; to be buffers to the student being bullied; and to distract the bully so that the victim can escape. Thompson et al. (2002) call them the "befrienders." Reinforce to all students that telling an adult is not tattling, since all students have a right to be safe. In establishing empathy, students must be helped to realize the following:

> Everything I say or do to another person matters.
>
> Everything I say or do to him leaves its mark on me too.
>
> People will remember me by how I made them feel (Elliott, 2003).

It is also essential for all students to sign an agreement about the ethical use of the Internet every year. It is important that the school's definition of bullying "include actions that are either on or off campus, in writing or in person" (Selekman & Vessey, 2004, p. 249).

Multiple programs are available to assist school personnel in ensuring a safe school environment and one that promotes respect for others. The United States Department of Health and Human Services, the Health Resources and Services Administration, and the Maternal Child Health Bureau have developed a bullying prevention effort that includes a media campaign. Their materials are specifically geared to 9- to 13-year-old students, as well as their parents and other interested adults. All materials are free and are available at: http://www.StopBullyingNow.hrsa.gov. *Bully Busters* (Horne, Bartolomucci, & Newman-Carlson, 2003), geared to elementary-age students, and *Don't laugh at me*, geared to students in grades 6 to 8 (Yarrow, 2000), are examples of programs that provide teachers with specific exercises to do with their students to promote acceptance of and respect for others and to decrease bullying behaviors.

The school nurse can be there to support the victims (as well as the bullies). Provide an opportunity for open communication. Having the victims keep diaries of the events may help them stay calmer during the attacks so that they can make mental notes of who said and did what. Rehearsal scripts may help the student become more assertive and know how to respond. Give him or her ideas on how to dress and stand in order to be less vulnerable; be a role model.

The school nurse is in a prime position to increase the self-esteem of students. One school nurse told of an elementary student who had been the victim of bullies. The student often visited the school health office for a myriad of minor complaints. The school nurse acknowledged her smile and asked her to stop by each morning just to "start my day off with a smile." This gave the young girl a measure of importance and a place to start her day safely (and to be assessed by the school nurse) before she went off to class.

Bullying must be tackled at the group level, rather than one on one. It is a school issue and affects every area of the school environment, including the time spent traveling, starting when students leave their home to when they return at the end of the day. "Bullying is abuse and abuse is not tolerated" (Selekman & Vessey, 2004, p. 249). Schools are legally responsible for the safety of their students. They must take complaints seriously and take action.

FIGHTING/VIOLENCE IN SCHOOLS

Fighting is seen among children and adolescents of all ages in all settings. It may be fighting with words, fists, or weapons. It may occur one-on-one between two individuals of similar age and abilities, or it could involve gangs of youngsters in this aggression. Regardless of how it occurs, it is intentional and harmful.

There were almost 700,000 violent crimes in American schools in 2000 (CNN, 2003) and 1.87 million crimes reported in 2001 committed by youth ages 12 to 20 (Centers for Disease Control and Prevention [CDC], 2004b). In 2000, 9% of murders in the United States were committed by youth under the age of 18; this age group accounted for 15% of violent crime arrests in 2001 (NYVPRC, 2003). There are four types of violent criminal acts: murder, felony assault, rape, and robbery (Walker et al., 2004). However, in the school setting, any type of physical aggression and assault is considered to be violence, as is vandalism (damage to school property or the property of others), carrying a weapon, and threatening others with violence. The spectrum of violence starts with offensive touching, which is a misdemeanor with a minimum, non-injury-causing impact, such as a push or a shove. The lowest level of assault involves physical violence with minimum resultant physical injury. The next level of assault involves serious physical injury, such as broken bones or missing teeth. Finally, the most violent level of assault results in serious injury associated with the use of a weapon. As the degree of violence increases, more individuals need to be contacted, including the police.

Threats of violence should always be taken seriously. Adolescents have been found with "hit" lists or "take-out" lists of those they wish to harm. Fifty-five percent of juvenile homicides involved friends or acquaintances (Walker et al., 2004). Adolescent boys are more likely to be injured in school or another public place, whereas adolescent girls are more likely to be injured in their home or another residence (Moskowitz, Griffith, DiScala, & Sege, 2001). Girls were more likely to be stabbed and boys were more likely to be shot.

According to the Children's Defense Fund (CDF, 2002b), the incidence of crime and violence by youth is declining. There has been a 23% drop in arrests for violent crime by juveniles since 1996. However, children and adolescents are 12% of the victims of crime, including 71% of all sex crimes and 38% of all kidnapping victims (CDF, 2002a). The homicide rate for those younger than age 19 is 10% higher than the average homicide rate for all Americans (CDF, 2002a); 13% of all adolescent deaths are due to homicide and 10% are due to suicide (CDC, 2001).

While accidents remain the number one cause of death of adolescents, death caused by use of a firearm is second. Homicide and suicide are the causes of one-fourth of all deaths in young people between 10 and 23 years of age (CDC, 2004a). These rates are significantly higher than for any other industrialized nation. Use of firearms causes the death of between 3,000 and 4,000 American children and adolescents each year. That equates to one in 1,056 young people who will be killed each year by gunshot before they reach the age of 20. Sixty percent of these are murdered, 32% use firearms to commit suicide, and the rest die from accidental shootings (CDF, 2002a).

The Centers for Disease Control and Prevention (CDC) (2004a) report that during 2003, approximately 6.1% of students at regular high schools carried a weapon to school, such as a gun, knife, or club. However, 18.3% admit to carrying a weapon off of school property. This number has decreased from the high of 26.1% a decade before. Even higher numbers are seen in alternative high schools, where the rate of weapon carrying was 32.9% (Escobar-Chaves, Tortolero, Markham, Kelder, & Kapadia, 2002).

One-third of high school students have engaged in physical fighting (down from 42.5% in 1991), with only 12.8% having engaged in a physical fight on school property (CDC, 2004a). The incidence of physical aggression is also higher in those who attend alternative high schools (Escobar-Chaves et al., 2002). What is becoming a major concern to schools is that 5.4% of high school students indicate that there were times that they did not go to school just because they were concerned about their safety. This has increased from 4.4% in 1993 (CDC, 2004a).

The behaviors considered to be precursors to violent behavior in adolescents include "alienation, an unusual interest in sensational violence, manipulation of others, anger and other forms of disturbing conduct, an obsession with guns and violence, excessive Internet use, and verbal threats" (Velsor-Friedrich, 2001, p. 127). Additional risk factors for juvenile violence include "low socioeconomic status, inadequate parental supervision, harsh and erratic discipline, and delinquent peers" (CDC, 2004b, p. 2).

There may also be problems with drug abuse, mental illness, or school performance.

Schools use a variety of modalities to increase safety in the schools. These include having students pass through metal detectors as they enter the school, having full-time police officers in the school, installing mounted cameras to monitor the halls and school property, and locking down the building after the start of school. Schools must have a plan in place to deal with violent acts or threats. School nurses should be intimately involved in the development of this plan, as they may have to initiate the process when caring for the victims of violence.

Regardless of one's stand on gun control, most would agree that it is essential to keep guns out of the hands of children and adolescents. Some states have mandated gun locks be placed on weapons to prevent discharge; all schools ban the presence of weapons on school property. Many elementary schools have implemented gun safety programs for young children; these include instructing children that when they see a gun, they should not touch it, but need to run away from it, and tell an adult. When a gun is found on school property, the first action is to move students away from the scene to a more secure site. The police will be called to remove the weapon.

While homicide of children and adolescents is a major concern, fewer than 1% of all homicides among school-aged children (5 to 19 years of age) occur in or around school grounds or on the way to and from school. Of the victims fatally wounded in school-associated violence, 65% were students, 11% were teachers or other staff members, and 23% were community members who were killed on school property (CDC, 2003).

Most experts in areas of criminal justice and psychology agree that incarceration and boot camps are not effective in decreasing the amount of violence among teens (Walker et al., 2004). All agree that the earlier these behaviors are identified and interventions occur, the better the outcomes.

Conflict resolution involves (1) stopping the violence and separating the parties, (2) maintaining some semblance of calm, (3) using active listening to hear what each party is saying, (4) avoiding making assumptions, and (5) jointly developing a plan. In developing the plan, generate multiple solutions, looking at the pros and cons of each; find a solution that both parties can live with, even though it may not please either; try the intervention for a specified period of time; and evaluate the effectiveness of the plan (Cheldelin & Lucas, 2004). Remember, the first goal is safety. Conflict resolution does not mean that all parties are happy at its conclusion. Policies in place may guide the possible end results.

The National Youth Violence Prevention Resource Center (NYVPRC) was established by the Federal Working Group on Youth Violence and the Centers for Disease Control and Prevention (CDC, 2003) to provide parents, teenagers, healthcare providers, law enforcement officials, other professionals, and concerned citizens a single, user-friendly point of access to critical information regarding youth violence and effective strategies to control and prevent such violence. The Web site is http://www.safeyouth.org. Although an international issue, national resources in the United States have been put to use to collaboratively address the problem of youth violence. "Facts About Violence Among Youth and Violence in Schools" (CDC, 2003) is a document available thorough CDC's National Center for Injury Prevention and Control (NCIPC) in conjunction with CDC's National Center for Chronic Disease Prevention and Health, the U.S. Department of Education, Department of Justice, and the National School Safety Center.

GANGS

Gangs are no longer just an inner-city problem. They appear in urban, suburban, and rural areas, although membership in rural areas is more racially and ethnically mixed than is traditionally assumed in large urban areas (NYVPRC, 2003). Youth gangs can be found in every state and represent a pervasive and increasing problem of young people identifying with and following the lead of each other, often to the detriment of social and legal norms (NYVPRC, 2003). There are approximately 4,800 known gangs in the United States (Gillig & Cingel, 2004).

There is no official definition of what constitutes a gang. Youth hanging out together on a street corner are not necessarily a gang, nor are their behaviors to be considered "gang activity." Some of the characteristics of gangs are that they usually have "membership"; they have territoriality; they engage in illegal activities; they may have unique symbols, such as dress or tattoos; and they frequently involve those children, adolescents, and adults who are or have placed themselves on the fringes of society or are marginalized. These young people are not fully included and are often left out of activities of their peers. "Alienated or marginalized youth are more likely to join gangs than are young people who fully participate in school and work" (Duffy, 2004, p. 4).

Membership in a gang tends to be transient, with more than half leaving by the end of 1 year. The range of ages for members tends to be from 12 to 24 years, with the majority older than 18 years of age.

Younger members involved in gangs are at risk for engaging in high-risk behaviors as a result of the influence of older and experienced gang members who may engage in more serious and violent crimes (NYVPRC, 2003). The risk for school-age students being involved in gangs and violent gang behavior is a real concern for the school community.

Reports about gang membership by gender vary. While males are more likely to be members in a gang and engage in more violent behavior, female gang members tend to be younger, are found more in the heavily populated urban areas, and engage in less lethal behavior (NYVPRC, 2003). "Law enforcement agency surveys estimate that about 8 to 11 percent of all gang members are female, while the proportion of self-identified gang members who were female ranged from 8 to 38 percent" (Gillig & Cingel, 2004, p. 217).

The implications for gang violence in schools cannot be overlooked. Schools with gangs have higher rates of serious problems at both the elementary and secondary levels than communities without gang activity. These problems include weapon carrying, property destruction, drugs, and violent victimization in schools. Studies reporting the incidence of intentional injuries in schools do not always indicate if those injuries were related to gang membership activity. What is known is that "schools are heavy recruiting sites for new gang members" (Walker et al., 2004, p. 376).

Singer and Flannery (2000) indicate that students who threatened others with interpersonal violence were more likely to engage in violent behavior, including retaliation, than students who did not report threatening behavior. Therefore, it is important of take threats of violence as seriously as one would take threats of suicide. Singer and Flannery stress the importance of helping students understand the need to report threatening behavior in order to protect other students and the school community from harm.

Although not reported in relation to gang violence, the incidence of intentional injuries in schools is alarming enough to warrant both individual and school-wide assessment of why and how intentional injuries are occurring and if there is the presence of violent gang behavior. While unintentional injuries at school far exceed intentional injuries (at a rate of 1.34 per 100 students to 0.29 per 100 students), the majority of intentional injuries in elementary, middle, and high schools are related to physical fighting, beating, or assaulting other students. The areas surrounding the school grounds and those places that are less supervised tend to be areas of greater violence (Limbos & Peek-Asa, 2003).

It is important for the school nurse to be aware of the types of gangs and gang activities in the community. This includes an awareness of gang symbols, tattoos, or clothing style. Especially at risk are those with access to firearms, those who engage in drug and alcohol use, those with self-esteem issues, and those who have been truant or engaged in school delinquency.

Screening questions might include:

Do you feel safe in your neighborhood/school?

What would you do if you needed protection?

Do you have access to a handgun?

What is the significance of your tattoo/style of clothing?

Do you have friends or siblings who are involved in a gang?

Once the players are known, it would be a good idea to initiate programs to prevent younger siblings from being involved and to keep high-risk students involved in supervised school activities. Promote inclusion of students in school activities and provide after-school supervised recreation and leisure activities. Develop a reasonable and enforceable dress code. Have strong role models available in the school setting.

Programs for parents can alert them to abrupt changes in friends and dress (i.e., wearing the same color combination all the time), gang symbols on books or clothing, and secretiveness about activities. Parents should be empowered to check on their children to make sure that they are doing what they say they are doing and to get to know the parents of their children's friends.

CHILD ABUSE: VIOLENCE IN THE HOME

Child abuse is often referred to as "nonaccidental trauma" and is a very common occurrence in society. It is estimated that an American child is reported abused or neglected every 11 seconds (Children's Defense Fund, 2002b); this results in approximately 1,300 deaths per year (Lindsey, 2004). While it usually occurs outside of the school environment, children who have been abused are often identified by school personnel who have daily contact with them; this includes the school nurse who may also have the responsibility for reporting the suspected abuse to the state agency. Therefore it is essential for school nurses to understand their state laws regarding reporting protocols. In every state, the school nurse is mandated by law to report suspected abuse and neglect, lest the nurse be considered an "accessory to a crime" (see Chapter 13).

Child abuse is defined by the Child Abuse Prevention and Treatment Act of 1996 as: "any recent act or failure to act resulting in imminent risk of serious harm, death, serious physical or emotional harm, sexual abuse, or exploitation of a child (a person under the age of 18) by a parent or caretaker (including any employee of a residential facility or any staff person providing out-of-home care) who is responsible for the child's welfare" (Section 111, 42 U.S.C. 5106g). It includes physical, emotional/ psychological, or sexual abuse (acts of commission) or neglect (acts of omission) by a parent or caretaker. That caretaker might also be defined to include school personnel who are responsible for the safety of the student during the school day. Intent is not considered when charging someone with abuse or neglect. Thus, maltreatment of children can be either active or passive behaviors on the part of an adult.

The unique entity of child abuse, previously named battered child syndrome, was not officially described until the 1960s. Prior to that time, if children needed to be protected, they were covered under the laws that prevented abuse to animals. Yet even today, newer forms of abuse have surfaced. These include Munchausen syndrome by proxy, child pornography, and child exploitation on the Internet. Munchausen syndrome by proxy, first described in 1977, involves a parent or caregiver who falsifies physical and/or psychological signs and symptoms in the child, implying that the child is ill and requires care. The resulting invasive diagnostic tests or treatment modalities cause a form of "abuse" to the child. The parent is often seen as overprotective and caring and thrives on the attention garnered from health-care professionals. In some cases, the parent may be poisoning or otherwise harming the child in order to produce the symptoms. In actuality, there are two diagnoses: one for the child and one for the parent (Schreier, 2002; Thomas, K., 2003)

How Children Are Abused and Neglected

TABLE 39.2 identifies the common ways in which the various forms of abuse and maltreatment are inflicted. Physical abuse refers to "actions that cause or permit significant physical injury to the body of a child" (Ellis, Dulmus, & Wodarski, 2003, p. 22). This injury is nonaccidental and is perpetrated by an adult caretaker (Crosson-Tower, 2003). Emotional abuse involves the sustained and repetitive inappropriate emotional response to a child's needs or behaviors. Neglect "involves the failure to provide adequate resources to protect a child from harm, to provide a reasonable assurance of health, to receive an adequate education, or to promote adequate emo-

(text continues on page 931)

Table 39.2 ■
COMMON FORMS OF CHILD ABUSE

TYPE OF ABUSE	METHODS BY WHICH ABUSE IS INFLICTED
Physical abuse	• Hit/punch/beat with hands or an object/slap/kick. • Burn/scald/stab/cut. • Poison. • Asphyxiate/crush. • Shake/throw the child/throw objects at the child. • Scratch/pinch/twist/squeeze/grab. • Keep in a cage or bound. • Engaging in acts that result in physical illness or lie about symptoms that result in invasive medical treatments of the child (Munchausen syndrome by proxy).

(continued)

Table 39.2 ■ *(Continued)*

TYPE OF ABUSE	METHODS BY WHICH ABUSE IS INFLICTED
Emotional/psychological abuse	• Verbally telling a child he or she is not loved, not worth anything, not important, not wanted, ugly. • Constantly harshly criticizing, ridiculing. • Ignoring the child/no communication with child/rejection • Withdrawing affection/lack of warmth and contact • Telling others of child's shortcomings. • Ignoring the child's accomplishments. • Blaming the child for everything • Threatening harm; terrorizing • Forcing the child to engage in illegal activities (selling drugs) • Making the child beg (for money or necessities)
Sexual abuse	• Intercourse (vaginal or anal) • Oral sex • Penetrating with objects or animals • Masturbating in the child's presence or having the child assist • Manually stimulating/fondling of genitals • Sexual comment or conversation • Touching/fondling/kissing in a sexual manner/engaging in indecent exposure • Soliciting a minor over the Internet • Forcing the child to participate in video or photography of sexual acts • Forcing the child into child prostitution
Neglect	• Failing to provide adequate or appropriate food, clothing, warmth, shelter, or health care (including primary care and dental prophylaxis) • Failing to wash/bathe child or brush teeth • Providing an unsafe environment • Failing to provide adequate supervision • Abandoning the child • Failing to developmentally stimulate a child (failing to interact with the child, provide objects for play, or expose to books) • Failing to ensure that the child attends school and arrives ready to learn

Sources: Crosson-Tower (2003); Ellis et al. (2003); Kay (2003).

tional development" (Ellis et al., 2003, p. 23). It is an act of omission.

Sexual abuse involves activities that are sexual in nature and that are imposed on a young person by someone of a more advanced developmental age who uses the child for his or her own gratification. It involves power and control. More recently, the Internet has played a role in sexual abuse with the increase in exposure to and participation in pornography and sexual solicitation. It is estimated that "one in five children has received sexual solicitation over the Internet" each year (Finkelhor, Mitchell, & Wolak, 2000, p. 49) and that 1 in 30 is aggressively solicited with money or plans for a rendezvous. Pornography gives children a distorted view of sexuality. "It is often used by perpetrators to desensitize children to sexuality and groom them for being sexually abused. Further, this glimpse into adult sexual practices may over-stimulate children to the point that they choose to act out their fantasies" (Crosson-Tower, 2003, p. 47).

Another cause of sexual abuse involves caretakers and significant others of single parents. "Statistically, children of reconstituted families have been exposed to a greater number of men if their mother dated before her remarriage" (Crosson-Tower, 2003, p. 20). The rate of sexual abuse is higher among families with stepfathers. Three-fourths of perpetrators are known to the child, with the ages of 8 to 12 being the most vulnerable time (Crosson-Tower, 2003).

According to the NASN position statement on Child Abuse and Neglect (2002), approximately 54% of substantiated reported cases involved neglect, 11.5% involved sexual abuse, and 23% involved physical abuse. However, multiple types of abuse and neglect might be imposed on children and adolescents at the same time.

Why Child Abuse Occurs

There are numerous theories of why adults abuse children. Those who abuse come from all walks of life; approximately three-fourths of perpetrators are the parents (NASN, 2002); others include individuals known to the child. These may also be adults in trusted positions, such as coaches, clergy, or teachers. There are theories that focus on the individual, family functioning, and sociological issues. Some of these factors are listed in Box 39.4. Yet even with lists of factors that place someone at high risk for being an abuser or being abused, it must be emphasized that not all individuals with many of these risk factors become child abusers. Therefore, school personnel should withhold prejudging individuals based on their meeting these criteria.

Box 39.4 ■ ■ ■

CHARACTERISTICS OF ADULTS WHO ABUSE CHILDREN

- Abused when they were children.
- Had poor role models of adults during their childhoods.
- Have unrealistic expectations of their children—whether a result of their own unmet needs or a lack of education as to what is appropriate and an inability to recognize their child's needs.
- Have mental or physical health problems or a history of drug or alcohol abuse.
- Have a need to completely control their child.
- Had an unwanted pregnancy or having a child who does not have the anticipated characteristics (e.g., wrong sex or not being well coordinated).
- Has had an unstable relationship with his or her partner.
- Has poor self-esteem and a limited social support network.
- May be isolated from the larger community and its resources (inadequate income/unemployment/lack of education).

(Kay, 2003)

Recognizing Abuse and Neglect

It is imperative for the school nurse to identify possible signs of abuse and neglect. One need only to observe students arriving at school to identify those who are dressed inappropriately for the weather, or to watch students in the cafeteria to see who is not eating or what students eat for that meal. Any student seen in the health office can easily be assessed for malnutrition, body hygiene, and suspicious injuries. One of the hallmarks of abuse is that the stories often do not match the degree of healing or the placement of injuries. All bruises should be questioned. It is important to know the normal healing pattern of a bruise (Table 39.3) and to have students relate how they got their bruises. However, while superficial bruises may discolor the skin soon after the trauma, deep bruising may take days to appear. While red has no bearing on the age of the

Table 39.3 ■

THE HEALING SEQUENCE FOR BRUISES

TIME SINCE INJURY	APPROXIMATE COLOR OF THE INJURED AREA*
Immediate to 1 day	Red
1–4 days	Blue, purple
5–7 days	Green, yellow
8–10 days	Yellow, brown
1–3 weeks	Cleared

*These colors may differ with various skin coloring.
Source: Schwartz & Ricci (1996).

bruise, a bruise that is yellow must be older than 18 hours (Schwartz & Ricci, 1996).

Common signs of potential abuse include bruises, cuts, burns (especially those caused by cigarettes, hot implements, or scalding), missing patches of hair, blackened eyes, loss of or damage to teeth, and guarding of extremities or the abdomen. The skin may even show the outline of the hand or object used to hit the child, such as a strap, a cord, a hanger, teeth marks, or rope burns on the wrists and ankles. The quantity of the marks as well as the pattern of inflicted injuries and the age of the injuries are important to note. Each must be fully described, within the scope of the school nurse's assessment and without further traumatizing the student. Each school nurse must follow mandated steps for the assessment and reporting of potential abuse and neglect.

Failure to grow, failure to receive needed medical care or follow up on referrals, poor dental hygiene, persistent hunger or fatigue, and inappropriate clothing for the weather may be signs of neglect or may indicate a need for social service intervention to provide the family with resources or education. Difficulty sitting or walking, pain during urination, itching or discomfort in the genital area, or pregnancy may be signs of sexual abuse (Kay, 2003). To maintain their secret, students may refuse to change clothes for gym, fearing that someone could detect the abuse just by seeing them (Crosson-Tower, 2003). "A child who is sexually abused is a child who is more needy and has a poorer self concept than his or her peers" (Crosson-Tower, 2003, p. 24).

Emotional abuse or the emotional results of abuse of other forms are much more difficult to identify, as the presenting signs and symptoms are similar to those seen with many other causes. These may include withdrawal from peers or aggression toward them; acting out in the classroom or regressing in their behaviors; decreased performance in classes; increased truancy; clinging to another adult; demonstrating inappropriate responses to physical affection; or engaging in self-mutilation (Crosson-Tower, 2003; Kay, 2003). On the other hand, a student may describe what appears to be excessive punishment, in which case the situation should be evaluated by the authorities to whom the report is made. Regardless of the cause of the abuse, long-term outcomes for at least half of those who are abused include aggression, depression, anxiety, and anger (Gushurst, 2003).

The school nurse should be able to communicate effectively with the student to determine if the student (or the witness) is credible, if the act described constitutes a behavior described in the child abuse laws of that state, and what visible evidence is present. School nurses are then mandated to report the alleged abuse to social service agencies, as per the state protocol. Listening to what the student has to say has always been a strength of school nurses; spending a little time with the student to clarify the concerns and what he or she is experiencing will assist the school team in knowing how to proceed. It is the responsibility of social services or law enforcement to conduct the investigation to determine whether abuse exists.

To do proper assessments, the school nurse must have the necessary space, equipment, and resources. The space needs to be private to ensure confidentiality. The equipment includes adequate lighting and measuring tapes, if needed for documentation. The resources include the support for privacy so that the school nurse is not interrupted during the assessment and assurance that the other students are being supervised.

Usually a parent is called when a student appears with an injury or a health need. Should child abuse or neglect be suspected, the school nurse needs to note the response of the parent on the phone or when he or she picks up the child. Parents may deny knowledge of the injury or how it occurred, they may trivialize the problem, or they may delay seeking medical assistance. It is never the responsibility of the school nurse to inform parents that they are suspected of abusing their child. However, school policy will dictate who needs to be informed. It is also essential for the school nurse to have access to privacy when making any telephone calls.

School personnel may be the initial individual to suspect abuse. This is especially true when students submit papers and drawings that are indicative that abuse might have occurred.

It is essential that the school nurse *never* promise a student that he or she will not tell someone about the abuse. The standard line regarding confidentiality (see Chapter 13) is to say that you must report anything that poses harm to the student or to others. What you can promise is that you will be there when the student wants to come and talk or if he or she needs a safety zone. Multiple issues arise when dealing with abuse. Two are described in Box 39.5 along with recommended interventions.

Interventions

The first and most appropriate intervention in a case of suspected child abuse is to treat the presenting problem, especially any bleeding or wounds, with appropriate first aid, such as ice for areas of swelling, or emotional support as needed. Once these actions have been initiated and an assessment completed, the school nurse should notify only those individuals identified by the school district and the state who need to be informed. "It is important to remember that a school employee's or volunteer's obligation is fulfilled by making the initial factual report; it then becomes the responsibility of the department of family services and/or law enforcement agencies to initiate and complete the investigation" (NASN, 2002). The National Child Abuse Hotline is 1-800-422-4453. Issues regarding where the record of the report is kept that indicates who made the report and whether parents would have access to this report under FERPA laws (see Chapter 13) are often of concern. The Family Policy Compliance Office of the U.S. Department of Education, which is responsible for the FERPA regulations, "has determined that parents have a right to examine the report of suspected abuse but that school administrators may copy the record and delete the name of the reporter from the copy" (American Academy of Pediatrics [AAP], 2004, p. 95).

Students who have been abused need experiences that build positive self-esteem; they may believe that the abuse they experienced was deserved. They may need to learn positive social skills and to build a sense of trust with adults. Students can be taught to recognize their own needs and feelings identify individuals in whom they can confide, and understand that they have the right to food, shelter, safety, love, and affection. If they believe they are abused, they need to be taught to keep telling people until something is done.

Multiple programs exist for educating children and adolescents about personal body safety and protecting themselves against abuse, which hopefully will decrease their risk for abuse. It is always best to be proactive rather than reactive. Encouraging children and adolescents to believe that "My body is mine and no one can touch it without my permission" may begin to empower them to say "no." Programs for young children, such as "Good Touch–Bad Touch" encourage children to be aware that if the touch "feels wrong" it probably is wrong. Kidscape Good Sense Defense program includes the following: how to avoid being tricked by adults; how to fight if abduction or assault is taking place; that it is OK to break rules to protect yourself; their right to personal privacy during toileting or bathing; normal sleeping behaviors; empowerment to never go with strangers; and interventions to build self-confidence and self-esteem.

Parenting seminars might be provided by the school on topics related to managing behavior problems, knowing what to expect of children of specific ages, and what they can do if they think they might abuse their child (e.g., walking away from the situation, exercise, deep breathing, etc.). Some teachers have parents sign contracts that they agree to send their children to school rested, fed, with their homework completed, and ready to learn. In many states, school employees are mandatory reporters. Therefore, it is crucial that school employees be informed about child abuse, what to look for, and what to do if they suspect abuse. The school nurse may be the one asked to provide this information to staff. This is especially true when students submit papers and drawings that are indicative that abuse might have

Box 39.5 ■ ■ ■

ISSUES RELATED TO CHILD ABUSE

Problem 1: The child is removed from the home or from the custody of one parent and now is in school. The noncustodial parent arrives at the school. *Solution: A plan should already be in place. Keep the noncustodial parent in a safe area and contact the police.*
Problem 2: The child acts out abuse on other children or in doll play or in pictures or stories; the child may innocently do to others what is done to him or her, as he or she may assume it is normal behavior. *Solution: Do not label or criticize. Refer to the school psychologist or counselor. These children should not be expelled from school; they need the protective and educational environment of the school to learn how to react and survive.*

occurred. The school nurse can be the link to the community resources that are available to assist the victims and their families.

Computers in the home and school should be placed in public areas. Blocks or filters can be placed on the computers to prevent access. These can either be end-user blocks, which are installed on individual computers (e.g., Surfwatch, Net Shepherd, Cyber Snoop, CYBERsitter, NetNanny, and Cyber Patrol) or they can be placed on a server to block access from the entire network (e.g., Net-filter, I-Gear, AME®, GuardiaNet, WeSENSE, EdView, and X-Stop's Shadow). Within the school setting, students must be taught online safety, preferably during health education classes. They need to know that perpetrators lie, flatter them, and play on their emotions for the purpose of eventually soliciting sex. Additional resources include the National Center for Missing and Exploited Children (http://www.ncmec.org) and The National Clearinghouse on Child Abuse and Neglect Information (http://www.nccanch.acf.hhs.gov).

VIOLENCE IN THE HOME THAT AFFECTS CHILDREN AND ADOLESCENTS

Children may be exposed to domestic violence in the home in a number of ways. They may see it, hear it from another room (i.e., parents fighting), observe its outcomes (i.e., the bruises on mom or broken furniture), or hear about it. The events may occur only once, or frequently. There is also a strong co-occurrence (approximately 40%) of child abuse and domestic violence (Graham-Bermann & Edleson, 2001).

"Children who witness violence between their parents suffer from fear, depression, delays in development, acute anxiety, and violent acting out against others as well as hyperactivity, defiance, and delinquency" (Crosson-Tower, 2003, p. 39). They may also suffer from posttraumatic stress disorder (Rossman, 2001). These stressors can have a direct impact on students and their ability to learn, how they express emotions, how they deal with interpersonal relationships, and how they use information (Rossman, 2001). With the high incidence of domestic violence, it is no surprise that children of abused women are more likely to have behavior problems and decreased attention to processing information; they also are at a higher risk for suicide than are children of nonabused women. While the school nurse can provide emotional support for the student, additional supports from a social worker or mental health professional may be needed to assist the student to report the abuse to authorities.

DATING VIOLENCE

Issues related to dating violence are more specific to the adolescent population and social conventions of the community. The reports on dating violence indicate that physical and sexual dating violence among high school students ranges from 10% to 60%, although this number increases when verbal threats and emotional abuse are considered (Ely, 2004). Approximately "9.8% of female high-school students and about 9.1% of male students said they had been hit, slapped, or physically hurt on purpose by their boyfriend or girlfriend in the past year" (CDC, 2002). While females are more likely to report sexual abuse than males, both report being victims of physical abuse in dating relationships, with many instances of mutual physical abuse, although girls report more serious injuries and more feelings of being terrified than boys do.

Roberts and Klein (2003) reported that boys and girls do not differ significantly in frequency of intimate partner abuse, which included being insulted in public, swearing, being threatened with violence, being pushed, and having an object thrown at them that could cause an injury. However, in terms of involvement in risk behaviors, when there was a history of abuse by an intimate partner, the intimate partners of girls were more likely to be involved in substance use and abuse than the partners of boys. Boys who reported intimate partner abuse were more likely to report antisocial, violent behavior, and depressed moods, while girls engaged in suicidal thoughts and substance use (Roberts & Klein, 2003).

It is not clear which comes first, the dating behavior or the violent behavior; however, the associated risks relative to dating violence are significant and increase when both physical and sexual violence have been experienced. These risks are:

- Alcohol, tobacco, and cocaine use
- Unhealthy weight control activities
- First intercourse before the age of 15 years
- Multiple sexual partners
- Pregnancy
- Seriously considered or attempted suicide
- A need for power or control
- Demonstration of threats, verbal abuse, and aggression
- Violence in the home
- Owning a weapon (Ely, 2004; NYVPRC, 2003).

When assessing whether a student was a victim of dating violence, avoid emotionally charged terms such as rape or abuse. Focus on the specific behaviors that occurred and their impact on the student rather than labeling the behavior. Speak with adolescents privately. Observe for physical signs of injury and question about abdominal and pelvic pain. Provide whatever first aid is needed. Communicate support to the victim, using phrases such as, "I'm sorry this happened to you," and "This is not your fault." Access medical or mental health services should the student need these.

Most importantly, ensure that the student is safe. Question about the possibility of danger from future attacks and whether the perpetrator has weapons. If there is any potential for danger, the school nurse must notify the appropriate authorities. This may be the police, or the school social worker or the principal, depending on state law and school policies. Students who have been victimized should be made aware of legal resources, such as legal advocacy groups, and assisted in obtaining restraining orders or contacting the police to make an arrest. Provide information about community services, such as support groups. Documentation is important, including what the student reported, what behaviors and injuries were observed, and what actions were taken.

Preventive interventions include communication skills and elimination of the risk factors. Informing students about the existence of and potential harm associated with dating violence must be combined with reinforcing that this behavior is criminal behavior. Discussion should include the types of behaviors that are expected in intimate relationships, including how to demonstrate caring and show respect. Students should be encouraged to develop a specific safety plan for themselves. The content can be reinforced with the use of posters or classroom discussions.

EXPOSURE TO VIOLENCE IN THE MEDIA

Rising concern about the impact of exposure to violence through vicarious experiences, especially in the form of media, recreation, and play activities has raised the consciousness of both the public and the media about the importance of social responsibility through mass communication. Although children and adolescents are in school between 6 and 7 hours each day, their potential for being exposed to violence during their waking nonschool hours in an unsupervised (or supervised) home can match or exceed the number of hours in school. While recent studies indicate a decrease in portrayal of serious violence on television, especially on network broadcasts and premium cable stations, it has increased on the basic cable stations, as well as on video games and in the words to music to which young people are exposed. The number of top grossing movies containing violence remained about the same from 1998 to 2000 (NYVPRC, 2003).

A study published in 1998 (Smith and Donnerstein, 1998) demonstrated the following regarding television and violence:

- Sixty-one percent of television programs contain some violence, and only 4% with violent content feature an "anti-violence" theme.
- Forty-four percent of the violent interactions on television involve perpetrators who have some attractive qualities worthy of emulation.
- Forty-three percent of violent scenes involve humor either directed at the violence or used by characters involved with violence.
- Nearly 75% of violent scenes on television feature no immediate punishment for or condemnation of violence.
- Forty percent of programs feature "bad" characters who are never or rarely punished for their aggressive actions.
- Of all violent behavioral interactions on television, 58% depict no pain, 47% depict no harm, and 40% depict harm unrealistically.
- Of all violent scenes on television, 86% feature no blood or gore.
- Only 16% of violent programs feature the long-term, realistic consequences of violence.

Although there is less spectacular press surrounding violence in video games, almost 74% of households with school-age children have video games and their children spend close to an average of 1 hour a day with much less parental supervision than is used for television viewing (Woodard & Gridina, 2000). A 2001 review of the 70 top-selling video games found that 89% contained some kind of violence. Almost half of all games (49%) contained serious violence, while 40% contained comic violence. In 41% of the games, violence was necessary for the protagonists to achieve their goals. In 17% of the games, violence was the primary focus of the game itself (Children Now, 2001). According to the USDHHS (2001), violence in video games can teach children aggressive strategies as children learn to imitate and identify with characters.

VIOLENCE AGAINST SELF: SELF-ABUSIVE AND SUICIDAL BEHAVIORS

Self-inflicted violence is intentional and harmful behaviors directed at oneself, for which suicide represents the fatal outcome. Other types include attempts to commit suicide and behaviors where the intent is self-destructive, but not lethal (e.g., self-mutilation).

Self-Injury

Students may intentionally engage in physical injury to their own bodies. This may include self-tattooing or piercing of body parts (although most see this as a process of enhancing the beauty of their bodies. See Chapter 40). Elementary and middle school students have been seen using pencil erasers so hard on their skin that abrasions are caused. Cutting one's own skin, usually on the arms, is another way for youth to harm themselves. They often cut more than once and wear long sleeves to cover the scars. Eating disorders, including starving oneself or bingeing and purging, are other forms of self injury (see Chapter 34). These activities may be an attempt by students to draw attention to themselves or an internal anger or disappointment with themselves. In most cases, these students will need professional assistance and should be referred for counseling.

Suicide

Suicide is often considered to be the ultimate act of violence. However, it could be understood in a number of ways depending on the perspective of the person completing the act and those left behind. Some research suggests that while statistically the U.S. government lists suicide as a violent death, it can also be seen as a part of the symptomatology of depression, co-morbid chemical dependency, and in various affective disorders. Because the vast majority of cases are caused by mental health concerns, especially depression, this behavior is covered in Chapter 34.

The problem of accurately recognizing suicidal ideation in students is complicated by the developmental tasks of adolescence and the propensity to engage in risky behavior that can result in loss of life, whether intentional or unintentional. In many cases it is difficult to know the suicidal intent of those who have killed themselves unless there was a clear message or indication in their behavior. For instance, how does one know the intent of the adolescent who dies after hitting a tree in a motor vehicle crash? Adolescents who are moving from concrete to abstract thinking may still not understand the consequences of risk-taking behavior, including contemplating suicide. They might not understand that it is a permanent solution to what are often temporary problems of adolescence. The impact of suicide on survivors, those who are left behind to try to understand, can be profound and long lasting. The role of the school nurse when suicide involves a student or staff member is discussed in Chapter 34. The following statistics from NYVPRC (2003) related to suicide continue to be staggering:

- It is the third leading cause of death for 10- to 19-year-olds.
- More teenagers die from suicide than from cancer, heart disease, AIDS, birth defects, stroke, pneumonia and influenza, and chronic lung disease combined.
- Suicide rates for 10- to 14-year-olds have increased by 70% since 1981.
- Suicide attempt rates far exceed completion rates.
- Girls attempt suicide more often than boys.
- Boys complete suicide more often than girls, using more lethal approaches.
- Nineteen percent of high school students reported seriously considering attempting suicide.
- Fifteen percent reported having made plans to attempt suicide.
- Nine percent reported having attempted suicide during the previous year.

Although white males have the highest rate of suicide, Native American males have a disproportionately high rate of suicide and there has been an increase in the number of African American males who are attempting and completing suicide. All school and community members need to be aware of the potential for disappointment, despair, and/or hopelessness that may precede suicidal behavior (NYVPRC, 2003).

Risk factors for suicide include (1) previous suicide attempts; (2) depression and/or alcohol or substance abuse; (3) a family history of mental disorders, substance abuse, or suicide; (4) a stressful situation or loss, including getting into trouble at school or with the police, and fighting or breaking up with a boyfriend or a girlfriend; (5) easy access to guns; (6) exposure to other youth who have died by suicide; (7) a history of physical and/or sexual abuse; (8) poor communication with parents; and (9) lack of access or unwillingness to seek mental health treatment (NYVPRC, 2003). Strategies for preventing youth suicide are provided in Chapter 34.

RISK AND PROTECTIVE FACTORS FOR YOUTH VIOLENCE

Students function within a complex network of family, community, and environmental contexts that impact on their capacity to deal with the consequences of risky behavior. These must all be considered when identifying approaches to prevent or intervene in any of the behaviors involving violence. Jessor (1993) described the value of considering both risk and protective factors within the ecological context when working with youth to understand the consequences of youth behavior.

Just because a student lives in a violent world does not mean that the child will become violent. How to explain this apparent contradiction has been the work of numerous researchers in trying to predict who is at risk for engaging in risky behaviors. It is important to consider the presence of risk and protective factors: are the protective factors in place strong enough to counter the risk factors? In other words, are there sufficient supports at all levels in a youth's life to overcome the risk factors? S. P. Thomas (2003) points out that academic failure, truancy, not feeling connected to school, dropping out of school, hating school, and feeling that they are disliked by classmates puts students at risk for engaging in violent behaviors. However, strengthening a feeling of school connectedness through good classroom management, small school size, participation in school-related activities, and disciplinary procedures that are balanced can be protective factors that may help balance some of the risk factors.

Students who were held back in school were more likely to be involved in violent activity, including weapon carrying in school. When there was a strong sense of school community and emotional well-being along with family support, the risk factors of being held back were balanced by those protective factors (Borowsky, Ireland, & Resnick, 2002). School nurses can asses risk and protective factors in the community, school, families, and individual students when determining the propensity for serious consequences of behavior and strategies to increase protective factors at all levels of a student's life.

TABLE 39.4 summarizes the risk and protective factors often related to violent behavior by juveniles.

Table 39.4 ■
AN ECOLOGICAL MODEL FOR UNDERSTANDING RISK FOR VIOLENT BEHAVIOR

RISK FACTORS	PROTECTIVE FACTORS
Environmental factors consider larger issues such as social values and the impact of media, policy or legal decisions.	
Poverty	National, state, and local policies that support child and youth-oriented programs
Unemployment	Adult understanding and commitment to working with and engaging young people
Media exposure to violence	Caring, supportive relationships
Adults' disregard and mistrust of young people	Commitment of resources to programs that support meaningful opportunities for adult/youth interaction
Lack of connection from mainstream society	
Community factors consider physical environment, available economic and recreational opportunities, existing social supports and other issues that have an impact on the successful functioning of the residents.	
Availability of drugs and firearms	Strong community infrastructure
Community deterioration	Opportunities for youth participation in activities where they have choices, decision-making power, and shared responsibility
Limited economic opportunities	Opportunities to develop new skills, increase self-confidence, and offer a chance to make a difference
Community disorganization	Access to quality education
High crime rates	Recreational opportunities
Gang activity	
Poor housing	
Lack of quality schools	
Lack of recreational facilities	

(continued)

Table 39.4 ■ (Continued)

RISK FACTORS	PROTECTIVE FACTORS
Family factors relate to a family's structure, support, culture, and functioning and ultimately affect the behavior of the individual members.	
Lack of parental interaction and involvement, particularly among males Failure to set clear expectations Inadequate supervision and monitoring Severe or inconsistent family discipline Child abuse and neglect Exposure to high levels of marital and family discord or conflict Antisocial or delinquent behavior by siblings and peers	Family members emphasize importance of education and offer support and affection Frequent, in-depth conversations and communication Non-kin support network Access to a variety of adult viewpoints and experiences Clear boundaries for behavior that enforce structure and rules within the home Reasonable disciplinary actions when rules are violated.
Individual-level factors affect one person's risk of, or resistance to, potentially engaging in violent behavior.	
Hyperactivity Concentration problems Restlessness Risk taking Mental health disorders, i.e., depression Aggressive behavior during childhood (from ages 6 to 13 among males) Early onset of violence and delinquency Substance use Stealing Destruction of property Poor academic achievement School failure Absenteeism during early adolescence Early school leaving (before age 15)	Sense of purpose Belief in a positive future Commitment to education and learning Ability to act independently Sense of control over own environment Adaptable and flexible Empathy and caring for others Ability to solve problems Plan for the future Resourceful in seeking out support Conflict resolution and critical thinking skills

Source: Adapted from NYVPRC (2003).

It is important to not inappropriately label or stigmatize individual students because they fit some of the above risk factors. It is also important to keep a developmental perspective as students learn to resolve conflicts and experiment. "Finally, it is necessary to remember that violent behavior is a product of multiple factors operating on many levels in the absence of protective factors and that individual youth are largely acting within the context of their environment and experiences" (NYVPRC, 2003). The ecological model may be helpful in reminding the school nurse to consider more than just the student or even the family when determining risk for the student. Protective factors may be absent from the home, but a community committed to caring for each of its children may be able to overcome some of the individual or family risk factors.

Making a decision about the severity and nature of a problem depends on numerous factors including the meaning of the problem to the students, their family, their school and community; the severity of the problem; and the potential for the problem to interfere with meeting the appropriate developmental tasks of the student. The school nurse should weigh the prevalence, severity, and frequency of both risk and protective factors as they impact on violent behavior. It is important to keep in mind that the school nurse could be working with either or both a victim of violence and a perpetrator of violence in the school setting.

NURSING INTERVENTIONS

Interventions can be individually directed to the student, the family, school, community, or environment at large. Interventions overlap in many situations but there are some specific strategies appropriate to different manifestations of violence. Successful strategies often depend on a knowledgeable school nurse, the support of informed school staff, parental reinforcement, and community buy-in. While school nurses need to address the immediate situation with the student, they also work in collaboration with other colleagues, the family, and community resources to promote the health of students. Guidelines are available at http://www.safeyouth.org for updated strategies and data related to preventing violence among youth.

The state violence prevention plan, if one exists, should serve as a guide for each school. School nurses need to be aware of school policies regarding the presence of violent behaviors in schools. If there are no written policies, then the school nurse needs to work with the school team to develop an awareness of the need for strategies and collaborate to develop these policies. Once the policies are in place, the school nurse can be instrumental in making sure that these policies are implemented by sharing them with parents and students, putting information about school safety and its relationship to health in health newsletters, on bulletin boards, in classroom presentations, and on the school nurse Web page. Keeping data about the incidence of intentional injuries as indicated by visits to the health office can help track changes in injury rates and the effectiveness of school safety programs. This information is required by the No Child Left Behind Act (U.S. Department of Education [USDOE], 2002) and helps schools, states, and the nation determine the need for changes in safe school interventions.

Collegiality is an essential behavior when dealing with violence in schools. School nurses need to know each of the team members and their roles, especially those on the designated crisis team who are committed to promoting safe schools. Working together can reduce duplication of efforts, increase productivity and present a unified and consistent front to the student body, the entire school staff, families, and the community. The school nurse should be knowledgeable about the school curriculum related to behavioral issues and serve as a member of the crisis and curriculum teams. Working with other school nurses helps to identify successful strategies that have been implemented in other schools as well as lessons learned from less successful ventures.

Recommendations to decrease the potential for violence include helping students feel "connected" to the school; establishing a climate that promotes and practices respect for others and for the property of others; providing caring and support to those who are the victims of violence; having unambiguous disciplinary policies that are communicated clearly to students, staff, and parents; ensuring that there are no weapons on school property, including school buses; and involving parents into all aspects of school life (CDC, 2001).

Perhaps one of the most challenging goals of the school nurse is helping students learn to trust enough to share information. In the case of bullying, date violence, gang violence, extortion, and other forms of harassment, students may have been threatened that if they tell, they or someone they care about will be hurt. Threats not to disclose the violence can hold a victim captive and unwilling to share that information. Helping students to divulge that they are the victims of violence is a challenge that requires considering school policy, state laws, and federal guidelines regarding the protection of confidential information. The school nurse needs to know when confidentiality can and cannot be respected and when he or she is obligated to share information.

Staff also may feel that they are in a crisis situation. The school nurse needs to be skilled in crisis intervention strategies that help de-escalate the crisis situation so that solutions can be identified. This can be done by maintaining a calm manner and using a calm tone of voice that avoids shouting. Avoid touching, challenging, or arguing with the person who is experiencing the crisis as this could be perceived as threatening. Let the person know that you understand his or her concerns without necessarily validating the concerns. Try to buy time until the person calms or until help arrives.

The Society of Pediatric Nurses (2000) has issued a position statement on children and violence, declaring that pediatric nurses are responsible for identifying children and families at risk; educating students, staff, families, and the community; being positive role models; participating in legislative activities that support safe environments for children; and promoting self esteem in children of all ages. The National Association of School Nurses has published both an Issue Brief on the role of school nursing services in school violence (NASN, 2000a) and a Position Statement (NASN, 2000b) on the role of the school nurse in violence prevention. These affirm that students and staff need to feel safe in school in order to concentrate on education and learning. Without question, violent acts are major barriers to learning.

Parents and the community need to know that students are safe and that the school community is acting to minimize violence. NASN recommends "zero tolerance" for weapons, as well as anger management strategies, counseling and peer mediation programs, and problem solving and conflict resolution skills (NASN, 2000a). Schools must be perceived as "safe zones" for children, adolescents, and staff.

CONCLUSION

Violence is a serious problem in society as well as in the school environment. "Schools have a responsibility to prevent injuries from occurring on school property and at school-sponsored events. In addition, schools can teach students the skills needed to promote safety and prevent unintentional injuries, violence, and suicide while at home, at work, at play, in the community, and throughout their lives" (CDC, 2001, p. 1). School nurses must work with other members of the school team to develop and implement plans so that students and staff feel safe in the school setting. Violence can result in lost classroom time. Many schools report numbers of students who are staying home from school because of fear of violence, yet many are also exposed to violence in the home. Building a climate of tolerance, safety, and respect for others requires a whole school effort. The school nurse can play an integral role in facilitating this process by identifying programs that can be used in the schools, by identifying children who are at risk for being victims of violence, and by role modeling positive behaviors in the schools.

References

Ahmann, E. (1999). Family matters. Working with families having parents who are gay or lesbian. *Pediatric Nursing, 25*(5), 531–535.

American Academy of Pediatrics (AAP). (2004). *School health policy & practice*. Elk Grove Village, IL: Author.

Borowsky, I. W., Ireland, M., & Resnick, M. D. (2002). Violence risk and protective factors among youth held back in school. *Ambulatory Pediatrics, 2*(6), 475–84.

Centers for Disease Control and Prevention (CDC). (2001). School health guidelines to prevent unintentional injuries and violence. *Morbidity and Mortality Weekly Report, 50* (RR–22), 1–73.

Centers for Disease Control and Prevention (CDC). (2002). Youth risk behavior surveillance—United States, 2001. In: CDC Surveillance Summaries, June 28, 2002. *Morbidity and Mortality Weekly Report, 51*(SS-4), as cited in The National Youth Violence Prevention Resource Center (NYVPRC, 2003). Retrieved May 23, 2003 from http://www.at www.safeyouth.org

Centers for Disease Control and Prevention (CDC). (2003). *Facts about violence among youth and violence in schools*. Retrieved May 16, 2003 from http://www.cdc.gov/ncipc/factsheets/schoolvi.htm

Centers for Disease Control and Prevention (CDC). (2004a).Violence-related behaviors among high school students—United States, 1991–2003. *Morbidity and Mortality Weekly Report, 53*(29), 651–655.

Centers for Disease Control and Prevention (CDC). (2004b). Therapeutic foster care for the prevention of violence. *Morbidity and Mortality Weekly Report, 53* (RR–10), 1–9.

Cheldelin, S., & Lucas, A. (2004). *Academic administrator's guide to conflict resolution*. San Francisco: John Wiley & Sons.

Children's Defense Fund (CDF). (2002a). *Facts on youths, violence, and crime*. Retrieved April 4, 2004 from http://www.childrensdefense.org.

Children's Defense Fund (CDF). (2002b). *The state of children in America's union: A 2002 action guide to leave no child behind*. Washington, DC: Author.

Children Now. (2001). *Fair play: Violence, gender, and race in video games* as cited in The National Youth Violence Prevention Resource Center (NYVPRC, 2003). Retrieved May 23, 2003 from http://www.at www.safeyouth.org

CNN.com. (September 25, 2003). *'Dangerous' school list irks some officials*. Retrieved October 7, 2003 from http://www.cnn.com/2003/EDUCATION/09/25/unsafe.schools.ap/inde…

Coloroso, B. (2003). *The bully, the bullied, and the bystander*. New York: HarperResource.

Crosson-Tower, C. (2003). *When children are abused: An educator's guide to intervention*. Upper Saddle River, NJ: Pearson Education.

Drake, J., Price, J., Telljohann, S., & Funk, J. (2003). Teacher perceptions and practices regarding school bullying prevention. *Journal of School Health, 73*(9), 347–355.

Duffy, M. (2004). Introduction: A global overview of the issues of and responses to teen gangs. In M. Duffy & S. Gillig (Eds.), *Teen gangs: A global view* (pp. 1–11). Westport, CT: Greenwood Press.

Elliott, G. (2003). *School mobbing and emotional abuse*. New York: Brunner-Routledge.

Elliott, M. (2002). *Bullying: A practical guide to coping for schools*. London: Pearson Education.

Ellis, R., Dulmus, C., & Wodarski, J. (2003). *Essentials of child welfare*. Hoboken, NJ: John Wiley & Sons.

Ely, G. (2004). Dating violence. In L. Rapp-Paglicci, C. Dulmus, & J. Wodarski (Eds.), *Handbook of preventive interventions for children and adolescents* (pp. 415–437). Hoboken, NJ: John Wiley & Sons.

Escobar-Chaves, S., Tortolero, S., Markham, C., Kelder, S., & Kapadia, A. (2002). Violent behavior among urban youth attending alternative schools. *Journal of School Health, 72*(9), 357–362.

Finkelhor, D., Mitchell, K., & Wolak, J. (2000). *Online victimization: A report on the nation's youth*. Arlington, VA: National Center for Missing and Exploited Youth.

Fox, J., Elliott, D., Kerlikowske, R. Newman, S., & Christeson, W. (2003). *Bullying prevention is crime prevention*. Washington, DC: Fight Crime: Invest in Kids.

Garrett, A. (2003). *Bullying in American schools*. Jefferson, NC: McFarland & Co., Inc.

Gillig, S., & Cingel, P. (2004). The United States. In M. Duffy & S. Gillig (Eds.), *Teen gangs: A global view* (pp. 215–223). Westport, CT: Greenwood Press.

Graham-Bermann, S., & Edleson, J. (2001). *Domestic violence in the lives of children*. Washington, DC: American Psychological Association.

Gushurst, C. (2003). Child abuse. Behavioral aspects and other associated problems. *Pediatric Clinics of North America, 50*(4), 919–938.

Harris, S., & Petrie, G. (2003). *Bullying: The bullies, the victims, the bystanders*. Lanham, England: A Scarecrow Education Book.

Hawker, S., & Boulton, M. (2000). Twenty years research on peer victimization and psychosocial adjustment: A meta-analytic review of cross sectional studies. *Journal of Child Psychology and Psychiatry, 41*, 441–455.

Horne, A., Bartolomucci, C., & Newman-Carlson, D. (2003). *Bully busters: A teacher's manual for helping bullies, victims, and bystanders*. Champaign, IL: Research Press.

Jessor, R. (1993). Successful adolescent development among youth in high-risk settings. *American Psychologist, 48*(2), 117–126.

Juvonen, J., Graham, S., & Schuster, M. (2003). Bullying among young adolescents: The strong, the weak, and the troubled. *Pediatrics, 112*(6), 1231–1237.

Kay, J. (2003). *Protecting children: A practical guide*. London: Continuum.

Limbos, M. A., & Peek-Asa, C. (2003). Comparing unintentional and intentional injuries in a school setting. *Journal of School Health, 773*(3), 101–106.

Lindsey, D. (2004). *The welfare of children*. New York: Oxford University Press.

Lunner K., Werthem, E. H., Thompson, J. K., Paxton, S. J., McDonald, F., & Halvaarson, K. S. (2000). A cross-cultural examination of weight-related teasing, body image, and eating disturbance in Swedish and Australian samples. *International Journal of Eating Disorders, 28*(4), 430–435.

MacBrayer, E. K., Smith, G. T., McCarthy, D. M., Demos, S., & Simmons, J. (2001). The role of family of origin food-related experiences in bulimic symptomatology. *International Journal of Eating Disorders, 30*(2), 149–160.

MacNeil, G., & Newell, J. (2004). School bullying: Who, why, and what to do. *The Prevention Researcher, 11*(3), 15–17.

Moskowitz, H., Griffith, J., DiScala, C., & Sege, R. (2001). Serious injuries and deaths of adolescent girls resulting from interpersonal violence. *Archives of Pediatric and Adolescent Medicine, 155*, 903–908.

Nansel, T. R., Overpeck, M., Pilla, R. S., Ruan, W. J., Simons-Morton, B., & Scheidt, P. (2001). Bullying behaviors among US youth. Prevalence and association with psychosocial adjustment. *Journal of the American Medical Association, 285*(16), 2094–2100.

Nansel, T. R., Overpeck, M. D., Haynie, D. L., Ruan, W. J., & Scheidt, P. C. (2003). Relationships between bullying and violence among US youth. *Archives of Pediatrics & Adolescent Medicine, 157*(4), 348–353.

National Association of School Nurses (NASN). (June 2000a). *Issue brief. School health nursing services role in health care: School violence*. Retrieved May 16, 2003 from http://www.nasn.org/briefs/violence.htm

National Association of School Nurses (NASN). (June 2000b). *Position statement: Role of the school nurse in violence prevention*. Retrieved May 16, 2003 from http://www.nasn.org/positions/violenceprev.htm

National Association of School Nurses (NASN). (2002). *Position statement: Child abuse and neglect*. Retrieved 12/03 from http://www.nasn.org/positions/childabuse.htm

National Association of School Nurses (NASN). (2003). *Peer bullying issue brief: School health nursing services role in health care*. Retrieved September 7, 2003 from http://www.nasn.org/briefs/bullying.htm

National Youth Violence Prevention Resource Center. (2003). *Youth violence*. Retrieved August 20, 2004 from www.safeyouth.org/scripts/news/statistics.asp

Prellwitz, M., & Tamm, M. (2000). How children with restricted mobility perceive their school environment. *Scandinavian Journal of Occupational Therapy, 7*(4), 165–173.

Roberts, T. A., & Klein, J. (2003). Intimate partner abuse and high-risk behavior in adolescents. *Archives of Pediatrics & Adolescent Medicine, 157*(4), 375–80.

Rossman, B. (2001). Longer term effects of children's exposure to domestic violence. In S. Graham-Bermann & J. Edleson (Eds.), *Domestic violence in the lives of children* (pp. 35–65). Washington, DC: American Psychological Association.

Schreier, H. (2002). Munchausen by proxy defined. *Pediatrics, 110*(5), 985–988.

Schwartz, A., & Ricci, L. (1996). How accurately can bruises be aged in abused children? Literature review and synthesis. *Pediatrics, 97*(2), 254–256.

Selekman, J., & Vessey, J. (2004). Bullying: It isn't what it used to be. *Pediatric Nursing, 30*(3), 246–249.

Singer, M. I., & Flannery, D. (2000). The relationship between children's threats of violence and violent behavior. *Archives of Pediatrics & Adolescent Medicine, 154*(8), 785–790.

Smith, S. L., & Donnerstein, E (1998). Harmful effects of exposure to media violence: Learning of aggression, emotional desensitization, and fear. In R. G. Green & E. Donnerstein (Eds.), *Human aggression: Theories, research, and implications for social policy* (pp. 167–202). New York: Academic Press. Cited in: U.S. Department of Health and Human Services. (2001). *Youth violence: A report of the surgeon general*, p. 88. Available from NYVPRC (2003). Retrieved May 17, 2003 from http://www.safeyouth.org

Society of Pediatric Nurses (SPN). (2000). *Position statement on children, violence, and resiliency*. Retrieved December 24, 2003 from http://www.pedsnurses.org/html/psviolence.htm

Thomas, K. (2003). Munchausen syndrome by proxy: Identification and diagnosis. *Journal of Pediatric Nursing, 18*(3), 174–180.

Thomas, S. P. (2003). Identifying and intervening with girls at risk for violence. *Journal of School Nursing, 19*(3), 130–139.

Thompson, D., Arora, T., & Sharp, S. (2002). *Bullying: Effective strategies for long term improvement*. London: Routledge/Falmer.

U.S. Department of Education (USDOE), Office of Elementary and Secondary Education. (2002). *No Child Left Behind: A desktop reference*. Washington, DC: U.S. Department of Education. Also retrieved May 27, 2003 from http://www.ed.gov/offices/OESE/reference.html

U.S. Department of Health and Human Services (USDHHS). (2001). *Youth violence: A report of the surgeon general*. Rockville, MD: U.S. Department of Health and Human Services. Retrieved May 17, 2003 from http:// www.at www.safeyouth.org

van der Wal, M, de Wit, C. & Hirasing, R. (2003). Psychosocial health among young victims and offenders of direct and indirect bullying. *Pediatrics, 111*(6), 1312–1317.

Velsor-Friedrich, B. (2001). Guns killing our children: A status report. *Journal of Pediatric Nursing, 16*(2), 127–128.

Vessey, J. (March, 1999). Bully-proof your child. *The Johns Hopkins Health Insider, 2* (4), 8.

Vessey, J., Swanson, M., & Hagedorn, M. (1995). Teasing: Who says names will never hurt you? *Pediatric Nursing, 21*, 297–300.

Walker, H., Ramsey, E., & Gresham, F. (2004). *Antisocial behavior in school*. Belmont, CA: Wadsworth/Thomson Learning.

Woodard, E. H., & Gridina, N. (2000). *Media in the home 2000, the fifth annual survey of parents and children*. Philadelphia, PA: The Annenberg Public Policy Center of the University of Pennsylvania as reported in NYVPRC (2003). Retrieved May 17, 2003 from http:// www.at www.safeyouth.org

World Health Organization (WHO). (2002). *World report on violence and health*. Geneva: World Health Organization.

Yarrow, P. (2000). Don't laugh at me. New York: Peter Yarrow Productions and Educators for Social Responsibility.

Youth Violence: A Report of the Surgeon General.(2001). Retrieved January 27, 2004 from http://www.surgeon-general.gov/library/youthviolence/summary.htm

Chapter 40

High-Risk Behaviors in Children and Adolescents

JANICE SELEKMAN

Chapter Outline

INTRODUCTION

High-risk behaviors have always been associated with adolescents. In the past, these behaviors were limited to engaging in sexual activity, drinking alcohol, using illegal drugs, smoking tobacco, and driving too fast or without a seat belt. The concept of risky behaviors has now expanded to include body modification, use of anabolic steroids, tanning, gambling, theft, and carrying weapons. These behaviors now also occur in the elementary schools, yet the research available involves primarily junior and senior high school students. While the common high-risk behaviors are covered in this chapter, content on violence is covered in Chapter 39.

Almost three-quarters of all teens have engaged in at least one high-risk behavior; 50.6% have engaged in more than one (Romer, 2003). This gives strong support for comprehensive education and prevention programs in the schools; curricula must look at the total picture of high-risk activity and not just selected behaviors. For example, the younger students are when they first get drunk, especially those who got drunk prior to age 13, the greater is the likelihood they will have unplanned and unprotected sex during their adolescence (Hingson, Heeren, Winter,

& Wechsler, 2003). In addition, these behaviors must also be discussed in the context of the family and the community.

It is beyond the scope of this text to discuss the societal components that increase risk, such as poverty, public policy related to welfare and health care, or food assistance, yet it is known that all of these issues ultimately affect the student and his or her ability and availability to learn.

INCIDENCE AND PREVALENCE

Since 1991, the Centers for Disease Control and Prevention (CDC) have supported biennial national surveys of high school students in grades 9 through 12 to gauge the status of youth risk behaviors. During 2003, more than 15,000 students were surveyed about their behaviors regarding alcohol and other drug use, injury prevention, tobacco use, sexual activity and unintentional pregnancy, nutrition, physical activity, obesity, knowledge and attitudes regarding sexually transmitted diseases and acquired immune deficiency disease (AIDS), attempted suicide, and violence-related behaviors. The Youth Risk Behavior Surveillance System monitors these behaviors, as they are leading causes of death, disability, and social problems among young people (CDC, 2004a).

Selected findings from the 2003 survey are presented in Table 40.1. During the past decade, improvement has been made in all categories except the use of marijuana and cocaine. However, since 2001, there have been no significant changes in the incidence of high-risk behaviors among high school students except for a decrease in cigarette use and an increase in condom use during sexual intercourse (CDC, 2004b). The only exception in these statistics is that there has been no significant change in the incidence of adolescent suicide since 1991.

Table 40.1 ■

YOUTH RISK BEHAVIOR SURVEILLANCE RESULTS: 2003

70.8% of all deaths in the 10- to 24-year-old range are from:
- Motor-vehicle crashes
- Other unintentional injuries
- Homicide
- Suicide

Within 30 days of the survey,
- 30.2% rode with a driver who had been drinking alcohol
- 17.1% carried a weapon
- 44.9% drank alcohol
- 22.4% used marijuana
- 4.1% used cocaine
- 21.9% had smoked a cigarette (6.7% use/chew smokeless tobacco)
- 13.5% were overweight

In the 12 months preceding the survey,
- 33% had been in a physical fight
- 8.5% had attempted suicide
- 8.2% rarely or never wear seatbelts

Ever:
- 74.9% ever used alcohol
- 58.4% ever smoked a cigarette
- 46.7% (high school students) had sexual intercourse
- 37% of those who engaged in sex had not used a condom at last intercourse
- 3.2% had injected an illegal drug

Source: CDC (2004b).

WHY DO ADOLESCENTS ENGAGE IN HIGH-RISK ACTIVITIES?

There are multiple theories about why adolescents engage in high-risk behaviors. It may be their need to test the limits of adulthood and childhood, to rebel against adult authority in order to develop their own identity, to cope with psychosocial issues, or a need for sensation and stimulation. Zuckerman's 1994 theory of sensation seeking defines it as "seeking of varied, novel, complex, and intense sensations and experiences, and the willingness to take physical, social, legal, and financial risks for the sake of such experience" (p. 27).

Risk implies taking a chance. This can be a positive characteristic, as when trying new experiences that lead to positive growth. However, risky behaviors usually refer to something that detrimentally exposes the young person to a potential threat to his or her health or well-being. Risk is balanced by resilience. "Resilience involves a healthy set of behaviors and coping mechanisms that are integrated into decision making and elicited in response to a threatening situation" (Neinstein, MacKenzie, & Morris, 2002, p. 1402). Some students are more resilient than others and can recover from, adapt to, or respond to risky situations better than others.

All individuals have a number of internal and external assets that promote or deter risky behavior and assist in their resiliency. External factors include the following:

- Family cohesion—how caring family members are to each other; the child feels loved and supported; the family is available; the family is accepting or rejecting of behavior.
- Family supervision—parental rules and monitoring of whereabouts exist; there is concern for the well-being of the child; consistent discipline exists.
- The safety of the environment/neighborhood risks—the presence of guns, violence, drugs, gambling, and so forth in the immediate environment of the child's home
- Peer pressure
- Role models
- Parental drug and alcohol use or sexual promiscuity
- Prevention education provided at home and at school
- Media advertising

Internal factors are those characteristics within individuals that affect how they respond to situations. These include:

- If the student feels bonded with/connected to the family
- If the student feels connected to the school (referred to as "connectedness")
- The degree of self-control over actions and impulses and internal locus of control
- The student's intelligence
- Academic success
- Self-confidence
- Social skills
- The ability to be empathic
- A sense of humor
- Genetic predisposition (family history)
- Temperament
- Comorbid psychiatric conditions that affect behavior and decision making (LeCroy & Mann, 2004; Neinstein et al., 2002; Sullivan & Farrell, 2002).

USE OF ALCOHOL

For many in the United States, drinking alcohol is a normal occurrence. It is a common part of a meal, it is used to celebrate occasions, and it is used in religious ceremonies. Alcohol is sold at sports events and restaurants and is found in most homes. Children frequently see their parents and other adults drinking and may even be allowed to taste alcohol, even at very young ages. Therefore, drinking behaviors are learned from the environment. The "reasons to drink, or not to drink, are shaped to some extent by observation of others around us, and especially by those we value most, e.g., parents, friends, and peers" (Roche, 2001, p. 2). Alcohol is perceived by adolescents as a positive experience and a symbol of adulthood. Perhaps because of this perception and all of the advertising that is present, "alcohol is the most commonly used drug among adolescents" (Millstein & Marcell, 2003, p. 114).

The law is clear that drinking alcohol is not allowed prior to age 21, except for religious reasons. Stores and restaurants may not sell or serve alcohol to minors; those who buy it for, sell it to, or serve it to minors can be arrested. Yet, 80% of high school students have consumed alcohol, 52% by the eighth grade and 18% by age 12 (Biglan, Brennan, Foster, & Holder, 2004; Millstein & Marcell, 2003). Girls now drink at the same rate as boys; the typical age students start to drink is between seventh and ninth grade (Millstein & Marcell, 2003). From 2001 to 2003, there has been a decrease in the percentage of high school students who have ever used alcohol, down to 74.9% in 2003 (CDC, 2004b).

Almost one-third of eighth graders, half of tenth graders, and 62% of high school seniors report having gotten drunk at least once. The majority of states have defined being drunk as having a blood alcohol level of ≥ 0.08 g/dL (Child Passenger Deaths, 2004). Binge drinking involves having four to five or more drinks in a row and occurs in 13.2% of eighth graders and 29.7% of twelfth graders (Biglan et al., 2004; Millstein & Marcell, 2003). For some, the aim of drinking is to get drunk (Roche, 2001). More than 5% of teens report drinking alcohol on school property (CDC, 2004b).

Alcohol "is responsible for more mortality and morbidity in this age group than are all other drugs combined...Among adolescents who drink, 38% to 62% report having had problems related to their drinking, such as interference with work, emotional and psychological health problems, the development of tolerance, and the inability to reduce use" (Millstein & Marcell, 2003, p. 114). In adults, increased use of alcohol is associated with cirrhosis, cancer, heart disease, stroke, injury, and depression. Alcohol use by pregnant women can have a significant impact on the developing brain of the fetus, with sequelae ranging from a slight lowering of the IQ to profound mental retardation to fetal alcohol syndrome, which includes disorders of the central nervous system (CNS), growth retardation, and facial malformations (Weber, Floyd, Riley, & Snider, 2002). (See Chapter 34.)

Some believe that the message should be to avoid alcohol altogether. Others believe that alcohol use is a rite of passage for many adolescents and the message should be to drink responsibly within safe limits. The Substance Abuse and Mental Health Services Administration (SAMHSA) provides free information for schools to decrease alcohol use. They stress the following:

- Drinking alcohol can cause a loss of coordination, poor judgment, slowed reflexes, distorted vision, memory lapses, and blackouts.
- Because alcohol depresses the CNS, it lowers inhibitions and impairs judgment, leading to increased sexual activity and the dangers that can result from that (human immunodeficiency virus [HIV], pregnancy, sexually transmitted diseases [STDs]).
- Alcohol can kill.
- One drink can cause you to fail a breath test.

SAMHSA and Scholastic, Inc. have developed a curriculum for fifth graders and their parents to prevent underage drinking. It includes in-class materials as well as materials to take home. It includes a science experiment to see the effects of pouring alcohol on an egg, and a unit on making healthy decisions by using critical-thinking skills and finding alternative activities to drinking. SAMHSA and the National Association for Children of Alcoholics have a Children's Program Kit to help children and adolescents of alcoholics make sense of what they have been experiencing, cope with the stresses of their families' problems, and strengthen their potential for resilience. It includes educational activities, a video, and a program manual.

Alcohol poisoning may result in emergency room visits and even death. One of the differential diagnoses of teens presenting to the school health office in the morning with complaints of headache is having been drunk the night before. Teens must be taught of these dangers, as well as the potential for interactions between alcohol and medications they may be taking.

SMOKING/TOBACCO

Smoking tobacco is one of the areas showing the most significant decrease in use, especially since 1999. The percentage of adolescents experimenting with tobacco, even one puff, has decreased from more than 70% in the 1990s to 58.4% in 2003. Only 21.9% had smoked a cigarette in the month before the Youth Risk Behavior Survey was administered; this included more than 17% of ninth graders (CDC, 2004b,c). One of the *Healthy People 2010* objectives is to decrease the prevalence of current cigarette use to less than 16%. However, 9.7% of adolescents had used at least 20 cigarettes in the month before the survey and 8% acknowledged smoking on school property. There is currently no difference in the smoking prevalence between males and females, and Caucasians smoke more than members of other racial groups (CDC, 2004c). Of interest, a 2002 study found that 13.3% of middle school students reported the current use of tobacco (CDC, 2003b).

In 2001, approximately 22.8% of adults in the United States were current smokers (CDC, 2003a). This implies that very few adults become smokers after the age of 18. It is estimated that every day in the United States, 4,400 youth between ages 12 and 17 try their first cigarette (CDC, 2003b). This includes cigarettes, cigars, smokeless tobacco that is chewed, pipes, leaf-wrapped flavored cigarettes from India called bidis, and clove cigarettes called kreteks (CDC, 2003b). In addition, students whose parents smoke or who work in facilities that do not have a ban on smoking in public places are exposed to secondhand smoke, which is known to exacerbate respiratory conditions and possibly cause cancer in adulthood.

Of those who become regular smokers, one-third will die of smoking-related illnesses (American Lung Association [ALA], 2004). Even smokeless tobacco (chewing tobacco or snuff) users face 50 times the risk of developing cancers in their cheeks and gums as those who do not chew. "The tar in the cigarette...exposes the user to high risks of lung cancer, emphysema, and bronchial disorders. The carbon monoxide in the smoke increases the chance of cardiovascular diseases" (Bellenir, 2002, p. 103).

"Nicotine is among the most addictive substances, and dependence is common after one smokes as few as 100 cigarettes" (Heyman, 2002, p. 377). It increases the release of neurotransmitters, which suppress the appetite, enhance pleasure, and assist in relaxation. Young females may use cigarettes as a way to lose weight or control weight. Youth who become addicted have as much difficulty quitting as do adults. Adolescents are often "dependent on nicotine, even before they become regular or daily smokers" (Mermelstein, 2003, p. 126). In one study of seventh graders, "smokers who reported symptoms of nicotine dependence were nine times more likely to smoke at school compared to those who did not report any symptoms of nicotine dependence (Soteriades, DiFranza, Savageau, &

Nicolaou, 2003, p. 157). Therefore the vast majority of students caught smoking on school property have a nicotine dependency.

Tobacco is considered to be a gateway drug, as it opens the door to reliance on a substance to change they way students feel. Students learn to be devious in how they obtain the tobacco, since it is illegal for them to buy it; they may need to lie about using it (such as using mouthwash before they see their parents to hide the odor); and they ignore the warning signs of habitual use and believe that they can stop any time they want (Heyman, 2002).

A "tobacco-free environment" is mandated in policies of at least half of the schools and of many states. Some indicate that there are legal repercussions if any cigarettes are even exposed in the school setting. The bathrooms are often places students go to sneak a cigarette. If anyone enters, they can quickly flush it down the toilet. This suggests that faculty and staff should routinely monitor the bathrooms between classes. The CDC's guidelines for school health programs recommend that tobacco use be prohibited in all school facilities and at all school events. Some states have banned smoking from any public facility.

The Hooked on Nicotine Checklist (Soteriades, DiFranz, Savageau, & Nicolaou, 2003) is one list of questions that can be used to assess for dependence on tobacco. The questions include the following:

1. Have you ever tried to quit, but couldn't?
2. Do you ever have strong cravings to smoke or felt like you really needed a cigarette?
3. When you try to stop or stop for a while, do you find it hard to concentrate, or feel more irritable or nervous?

"The unassisted quit rates among adolescents are surprisingly low primarily because of the long held assumption that adolescents "mature out" of smoking or easily quit on their own" (Mermelstein, 2003, p. 126). Very few will stop smoking without some type of external intervention. Multiple intervention programs are available to assist adolescents to stop smoking. The American Lung Association's Not on Tobacco (N-O-T) program is perhaps the most frequently used and tested program for 14- to 19-year-olds. It is user-friendly, youth-focused, and gender-sensitive, and can easily be used in the school setting. The program consists of 10 weekly sessions (50 minutes each) and 4 follow-up or "booster" sessions (at 2-week intervals) that are grounded in social–cognitive theory. Most groups are limited to only one gender with a leader of the same gender as the group. The state Lung Association will provide training to the school nurse or other group leader and provide materials for a successful program. Materials and training can be arranged by calling 1-800-586-4872 (800-LUNG-USA), which will connect the school nurse to his or her state lung association. The sessions include motivational issues, smoking history, stress management; nicotine addiction; physical, psychological, and social consequences of smoking; preparing to quit; dealing with urges and cravings; relapse prevention; dealing with family and peer pressure; recognizing social, cultural, and media ploys; increasing healthy lifestyle behaviors; and accessing resources and support. The quit rate 6 months after the program is approximately 22%, especially for girls, with another 65% decreasing the amount of cigarettes used (ALA, 2004). These rates compare to approximately 12% who were able to stop with the help of brief interventions in the school (Dino et al., 2001; Mermelstein, 2004).

Recruitment into smoking cessation programs is more successful if the programs are held during the school day rather than after school. School-based Wellness Centers are an ideal location for the program. Some states have used some of the tobacco settlement monies to sponsor youth groups committed to promoting the prevention and control of tobacco. Delaware's Kick Butts Generation has more than 4,000 youth involved. There are three chapters in the state and they communicate via a newsletter and a website (http://www.ysmoke.org). One school nurse mobilized her high school students to develop posters that were so successful that they were picked up by local advertisers and used on billboards along major highways. In one poster, football players sit on the bleachers in uniform but with their bare feet exposed. The right side of the poster has half-smoked cigarettes lying askew. The caption reads, "Both smell…only one kills." Another poster is of 13 Ashleys against tobacco, picturing 13 students named Ashley in the school (Mattey, 2003). The school nurse also conducted a study in the school and found that students perceive more students as smoking than actually do (Mattey, 2003).

The American Lung Association supports a teen mentoring program called Teens Against Tobacco Use. It helps teens develop leadership skills and influence younger children to not use tobacco. Tar Wars is another tobacco-free education program designed for fourth- and fifth-grade students by the American Academy of Family Physicians. This free program consists of a pre-activity exercise, a 1-hour classroom presentation by the school nurse, and a follow-up poster contest. Information can be accessed at http://www.tarwars.org. The Centers for Disease Control and Prevention (CDC, 2002) has developed a School Health Index, with one version for elementary school and another for middle and high school. It is a self-assessment and planning guide in the areas of physical activity, healthy eating, and a tobacco-free lifestyle. It relies on the Coordinated School Health model (Chapter 3) and assesses policies in the school related to these activities, the content related to tobacco use prevention, and ways to include the family and community. The materials are free and can be requested by e-mail at HealthyYouth@cdc.gov or by calling toll free at 888-231-6405.

DRUG USE

Illegal Street Drugs

In addition to the Youth Risk Behavior Surveillance System, the National Institute on Drug Abuse surveys eighth-, tenth-, and twelfth-grade students annually regarding their use of licit and illicit drugs. The results are available free at http://www.monitoringthefuture.org. There is great consistency between the findings of the two groups. In most cases, drugs are used as social tools, rather than as experiences in their own right. While they may initially be used singly, often users combine drugs or combine drugs with alcohol and tobacco.

Marijuana has been used by more than 40% of high school students, with 22.4% having used it within 30 days of the National Youth Risk Behavior Survey (CDC, 2004b). While there has been a slight decrease since 1997, there has been no statistically significant change in the use of marijuana since 1991. The average age for experimenting with marijuana in the U.S. is 14 (Gruber & Pope, 2002). Often called by its street names of pot, grass, weed, or mary jane, it is a greenish-gray mixture of the dried, shredded leaves, stems, seeds, and flowers of *Cannabis sativa*, the hemp plant (Bellenir, 2002). The tobacco-looking material is rolled into a cigarette called a joint, bone, or nail. When marijuana replaces the tobacco of a cigar (sometimes mixed with cocaine), it is called a blunt, and when it is smoked in a water pipe, it is referred to as a bong. It can be brewed as tea or mixed into foods.

While there are more than 400 chemicals in marijuana, the active ingredient is delta-9 tetrahydrocannabinol, or THC. The effects depend on the potency of the THC. It causes an increase in the dopamine levels to induce pleasure sensations, and distorted perceptions of time and visual sensations (Gruber & Pope, 2002). However, some may experience an anxiety reaction when using it. About half of those who use it experience tachycardia and hypertension; hunger increases, intraocular pressure decreases, and the drug exerts a mild antiemetic effect. There are no reports of death due to marijuana.

Cannabinoids are stored in fatty tissue, from which they are eliminated very slowly. With regular use of marijuana, “fatty tissue can become a reservoir resulting in the constant presence of cannabinoids in the brain” (Gruber & Pope, 2002, p. 390). Because of this slow release, it can be detected in the urine for more than a month in regular users.

The “high” that occurs with smoking marijuana occurs within minutes and lasts up to several hours. Marijuana negatively affects learning, remembering, concentrating, decision making, and reaction time. The drug’s suppressive effect on the hippocampus is what causes the short-term memory loss (Bellenir, 2002). Its use is associated with engaging in other high-risk activities, such as using alcohol and tobacco, having early unprotected sex, and driving while drinking or smoking.

“Of those who try marijuana more than once, approximately one third will subsequently use marijuana regularly for some period of time.... Marijuana use generally precedes the use of other illegal drugs, just as the use of tobacco and alcohol usually precede marijuana use” (Gruber & Pope, 2002, pp. 392–393).

Cocaine, whether in the form of a powder or “crack,” has been tried by 8.7% of adolescents, with 4.1% using it within 30 days of the survey (CDC, 2004b). While the numbers who tried it increased until 1999, there has been no significant change since that time. Cocaine is the active chemical in the coca plant, primarily grown in South America. It can be snorted intranasally through a straw or rolled up dollar bill, injected, or smoked (Cooper, 2002).

Smoking cocaine results in the quickest action (8 to 10 seconds), but it lasts only for 2 to 5 minutes; it has to be mixed with an alkali, boiled with a solvent, and dried to form a free base (crack) before it can be smoked. Because cocaine is water soluble, it can be strained and injected for a reaction that takes 30 to 60 seconds to work and lasts a short time. Intranasal snorting requires the user to first chop the cocaine and line it up on a table, often with a razor blade. This method takes 5 minutes to work and lasts 20 minutes to 2 hours (Cooper, 2002).

Cocaine is an extremely addictive drug. Addiction to it has been reported to control all aspects of a person’s life. Its actions include increasing all vital signs and interfering with the electrical system of the heart, leading to heart attacks, strokes, respiratory failure, seizures, and reduced immune function (Bellenir, 2002). It can also result in hallucinations, confusion, anxiety, and loss of touch with reality. “Cocaine may give users a temporary illusion of power and energy, but it often leaves them unable to function emotionally, physically, and sexually" (Bellenir, 2002, p. 163).

Inhalants include those substances that are sniffed (such as glue, nail polish remover, gasoline, solvents, or butane), or "huffed" and breathed in, such as the contents of aerosol spray cans or paints and sprays or the propellants used in commercial products, such as whipped cream dispensers, for the purpose of getting high. They may be sniffed directly from an open container or "huffed" from a rag soaked in the substance and held to the face or place the rag in a bag and let the vapors concentrate. More than 12% of high school students acknowledge trying this activity at least once. The incidence has steadily decreased since 1995 (CDC, 2004b). These products are cheap, legal, and available to younger children. In some areas of the country, they are viewed as "kids'" drugs and their use peaks during eighth grade (Bellenir, 2002; Johnston et al., 2004). It is sometimes referred to as "vapor abuse." Users may be identified by the odor of the product they inhaled or by remnants of the inhaled substance near their mouth or nose.

Inhalants cause an immediate high. The effects of inhalant intoxication resemble those of alcohol inebriation: loss of inhibition followed by depression, distorted perceptions of time and space, and decreased motor coordination. Chronic use of inhalants can cause permanent brain damage as well as cause localized damage to the lungs.

Amphetamines are stimulants that are often prescribed for some medical conditions, such as attention deficit hyperactivity disorder (ADHD). It should be noted that those individuals who take amphetamine drugs for their ADHD do *not* have the symptoms listed below and do not experience addiction to the drug (see Chapter 30). Amphetamines were initially abused by college students to stay awake all night for studying or for their anorexic effect on dieting.

One subclass of amphetamines is methamphetamine, which is called "speed" or "meth" on the street. One form of meth is crystal methamphetamine, or ice; "the chunks can be heated and the fumes inhaled, much like crack cocaine" (Johnston et al., 2004, p. 22). Methamphetamine is cheap and easy to make, with the directions available on the Internet. It is sometimes used to "cut" or add to other drugs. Amphetamines function by increasing the amount of dopamine released (Yudko, Hall, McPherson, & Twemlow, 2003). "At low doses, methamphetamine causes generally positive effects, such as increased alertness, energy, euphoria, elevated self-confidence, persistent activity and work, increased talkativeness, increased sexual pleasure and hypersexuality, a sense of well-being, increased strength, and a loss of appetite" (Hall, McPherson, Twemlow, & Yudko, 2003, p. 55). Higher doses increase the potential for violence and can result in motor symptoms, such as tremors, spasms, tics, athetoid movements, and teeth grinding. Other symptoms of abuse include slurred speech, agitation, hallucinations, and paranoia (Hall et al., 2003).

Heroin is an old drug that is a derivative of opium. It is usually injected, but recently it has been snorted and smoked (Johnston et al., 2004). It is processed from morphine, which is extracted from the Asian poppy plant. The effects of heroin include a "rush" of euphoria, dry mouth, warm flushed skin, and a state of drowsiness. The CNS is depressed (Bellenir, 2002). Its dangers include blood-borne infections contracted from contaminated needles as well as vascular infections and their sequelae.

Some students may be abusing **prescription drugs**. Oxycodone (OxyContin) and other opioids are commonly used, as are CNS depressants (barbiturates and benzodiazepines) that are used to treat anxiety and sleep disorders.

Club/Party/Designer Drugs

"Club drugs" is a general term that refers to a number of illicit drugs, primarily synthetic, that are most commonly encountered at nightclubs and "raves" (all-night dance parties with loud and repetitive electronic music). The drugs include MDMA (ecstasy), ketamine, GHB, rohypnol, LSD, PCP, methamphetamine, and, to a lesser extent, cocaine and psilocybine mushrooms (Table 40.2). The drugs have gained popularity as a result of the false perception that they are not as harmful, nor as addictive, as mainstream drugs, such as heroin.

Designer drugs are drugs manufactured in underground laboratories as modified versions of substances controlled by the U.S. Food and Drug Administration (FDA) in order to supply the black market economy with street drugs that technically are not illegal. The Drug Enforcement Administration refers to these drugs as Controlled Substance Analogs (CsA).

MDMA (methylenedioxymethamphetamine) is also called *ecstasy, X, XTC, adam, clarity,* and *lover's speed*. Approximately 11% of twelfth graders have tried it (Holland, 2001). Its use among adolescents peaked in 2002 and has just started to decline (Johnston et al., 2004). It was developed in the early 1900s as a chemical precursor in the synthesis of pharmaceuticals. In 1985, it was classified as a Schedule I drug ("a substance with high abuse

Table 40.2 ■
CLUB AND DESIGNER DRUGS

Hallucinogens: LSD Ecstasy Mescaline DMT DOM/STP Psilocybin
Stimulants: Amphetamine Cocaine
Sedatives/depressants: GHB Rohypnol
Analgesics: Opiates Opiate derivatives
Inhalants: Solvents Nitrous oxide
Miscellaneous: Ketamine Phencyclidine

potential, no accepted medical uses, and illegal to possess") (Koesters, Rogers, & Rajasingham, 2002, p. 416). Chemically, MDMA is similar to the stimulant amphetamine and the hallucinogen mescaline; it produces both stimulant and mild hallucinogenic effects, both of which are dose dependent (Yudko et al., 2003).

Its effects last 3 to 5 hours, but confusion, depression, sleep problems, anxiety, and paranoia have been reported to occur for weeks after taking it. Ecstasy increases the level of serotonin released by brain cells, producing "profound euphoria, heightened feelings of empathy, emotional warmth, and self-acceptance, prompting its nicknames of "hug drug" or "love drug" (Koesters et al., 2002, p. 418); however, as the brain is depleted of serotonin, processes that are regulated by it, that is, mood, sleep, appetite, and cognition, are affected. Adverse effects include diaphoresis, rapid and irregular heartbeats, hypertension, fatigue, muscle aches, involuntary muscle contraction, such as jaw-clenching, and insomnia. Many users suck pacifiers or lollipops to ease the tight jaw muscles.

At high doses, it can be deadly. It allows the user to dance for hours, resulting in dehydration, muscle breakdown, and liver and cardiovascular failure. This may lead to heart attacks, strokes, and seizures (Koesters et al., 2002). A significantly increased body temperature has also been reported. Because MDMA is neurotoxic, chronic use damages the neurons that release serotonin and result in long-term memory impairment (Malberg & Bonson, 2001). The price on the street is approximately $40 for 100 mg, a typical dose. An overdose is seen when more than 200 mg is ingested.

GHB is gamma-hydroxybutyrate and goes by the street names of *liquid ecstasy, soap, easy lay, Georgia home boy, grievous bodily harm, liquid X,* and *G*. It is a CNS depressant. GHB generates feelings of euphoria and intoxication; it also decreases inhibition, making sexual activity easier. Therefore, it is also used for date rapes. At lower doses, GHB causes drowsiness, dizziness, nausea, and visual disturbances; at higher doses, it results in loss of consciousness, seizures, severe respiratory depression, and coma. GHB starts working in 15 minutes and its effects last for 6 to 8 hours (Koesters et al., 2002). It is usually sold by the capful at $5 to $10 per cap.

Ketamine is an anesthetic drug used mostly by veterinarians. It causes reactions similar to PCP, a hallucinogen. It induces a dream-like state and visual hallucinations; it makes users feel separated from their body and mellow, and they have no pain. It does not depress respiratory function. It goes by the street names of *special K, K, vitamin K,* and *cat Valium*. The powdery substance is ingested orally or nasally or made into a liquid and snorted or injected. One dose is 50 to 100 mg and it costs $80/gram. Side effects include tachycardia, hypertension, and schizophrenic reactions (Koesters et al., 2002). Long term, it can result in impaired memory or attention and flashbacks.

Rohypnol (flunitrazepam) is related to the benzodiazepines. It is tasteless and odorless and dissolves easily in carbonated beverages. A dose as small as 1 mg can impair a victim for 8 to 12 hours and cause profound "anterograde amnesia." Because of this, it is often the drug used in sexual assaults (date rape). Its street names include *roofies, rophies, roche*, and the *forget-me pill*. Other adverse effects include hypotension, drowsiness, visual disturbances, dizziness, confusion, and urinary retention.

LSD (lysergic acid diethylamide) is a well-known hallucinogen that induces abnormalities in sensory perceptions. It is sold in tablet, capsule, and liquid forms and is also placed on blotter paper where it is licked off. Within 30 minutes, the pupils dilate, the body temperature increases, as does the heart rate and blood pressure, and diaphoresis occurs. Loss of appetite may progress to nausea, and numbness, weakness, or trembling may occur. Long term disorders associated with LSD include flashbacks (now called hallucinogen persisting perception disorder) and psychosis. More recently, teens are using Morning Glory seeds and a type of sage called *Salvia divinorum* for their hallucinogenic effects.

These drugs are made in underground laboratories that do not account for inconsistencies in dose or even what else is mixed into the drug. Many are adulterated or laced with other illegal drugs, so that users have no guarantee about what they are taking. In addition, many are synergistic with alcohol or marijuana, causing more serious reactions. Most cannot be detected in the urine after a few hours of use.

Other hallucinogens include **PCP**, known as angel dust, crystal, or hog, which is often sprayed on leaf material and smoked, and **psilocybin mushrooms**, which can be ingested or used to make tea.

Performance-Enhancing Drugs

Adolescents are acutely aware of the impact of muscle, speed, and endurance in attaining athletic prowess. Some are told that they have college potential, but that they need to be "bigger" or stronger, or will need to "bulk up." There are also those who believe that it is more attractive to the opposite sex to be more muscular. Substances that enhance performance are known as ergogenic drugs. They enhance the body's use of energy, often at the expense of various body systems. Included in this category are anabolic steroids, ephedra, and creatine.

Ergogenic products are often considered nutritional supplements and therefore do not fall under the FDA's regulations (Rogol, 2003). Because of this, there is no guaranteed consistency in the potency from one batch to another. They claim to increase lean body mass, decrease fat mass, and increase energy. They have increased in popularity since the late 1990s when the media made the public aware of the large numbers of professional athletes who were using them.

Research on their effects has not been conducted in individuals younger than 18. Many are effective in building muscle mass when combined with rigorous training. There is no evidence to support that these products aid in recovery from sports injuries.

Anabolic steroids are related to male sex hormones and stimulate the development of muscle and bone. Anabolic refers to the building of muscle. More than 6% of high school students have used them without a doctor's prescription, with the peak being in tenth grade (Bellenir, 2002; CDC, 2004b). "Anabolic steroids are taken orally or injected, typically in cycles of weeks or months (referred to as "cycling"), rather than continuously" (Bellenir, 2002, p. 149). When athletes refer to "stacking," they are indicating that they use multiple types of steroids in the hope of minimizing the negative side effects.

There are multiple potential consequences of taking anabolic steroids. These include liver involvement (resulting in tumors or jaundice); high blood pressure (possibly presenting as nose bleeds); increased levels of low-density lipoprotein (LDL) and decreased high-density lipoprotein (HDL); severe acne; decreased size of the testicles, resulting in a reduced sperm count and infertility; and mood changes, especially aggression and irritability. Uncontrolled outbursts of anger are referred to as "roid rages" (Bellenir, 2002). Females may experience increased facial hair and cessation of menses. Injectable anabolic steroids increase the risk of transmitting HIV or hepatitis B.

Two precursors to the androgenic hormones are often used by teens, believing that they are safer than the anabolic steroids. These include androstenedione (referred to as andro) and DHEA (dehydroepiandrosterone); both can be bought in health food stores. They can impact negatively on the levels of liver enzymes and cholesterol levels but there is no scientific evidence of their effectiveness in building muscle (Rogol, 2003).

Ephedra is a Chinese herb, also called mahuang, that was commonly added to dietary supplements or stimulants to increase the amount of time muscles can work before becoming exhausted. However, those taking ephedra had a higher risk for hypertension, tachycardia, cardiac arrhythmias, myocardial infarctions, and stroke (Rogol, 2003). Therefore, in 2004, the FDA banned the use of ephedra in the United States, although it is still advertised on the Web.

Creatine is "found almost exclusively in skeletal muscle, where it is one of the main energy sources available to fuel the energy bursts for explosive contractions, such as those in jumping and weight training" (Rogol, 2003, p. 919). While it increases the availability of ATP for energy within cells, it also has osmotic properties and causes weight gain, edema, muscle cramps, and gastrointestinal cramps (Rogel, 2003).

Other products are used to increase energy and perceived performance. **Caffeine**, usually via carbonated beverages, is consumed by 98% of all school-age students at least weekly (Pollak & Bright, 2003). It is often used to counteract the daytime sleepiness resulting from not getting enough sleep on school nights, although it is unknown if it also causes some of the late bedtimes. While there is no research to correlate caffeine intake to school performance, there is certainly a wealth of data to correlate lack of sleep with decreased school performance. **Beta-2 adrenergic *agonists***, commonly used by those with asthma, are often abused by athletes in a mistaken belief that they can increase the amount of oxygen they can get to the lungs. Some even inject these products, resulting in vasoconstriction and its multiple consequences.

Some schools have initiated urine testing for these products, although it can be costly. In addition, "designer" steroids are being developed, such as THG (tetrahydrogestrinone), which cannot be detected by current tests. The school nurse has an important role in working with the athletic trainers to teach potential athletes proper weight-training techniques combined with nutritional interventions that will best reduce body fat, increase muscle mass, and improve strength.

Drug Testing

Drug testing in the schools is an issue often debated as a way of decreasing use and abuse of drugs, although research does not support this association. Civil rights as well as cost to the school district are often reasons given for not engaging in this practice; costs range from $14 for testing of marijuana, tobacco, cocaine, heroin, opiates, amphetamines, barbiturates, and tranquilizers to more than $100 to test for steroid use (Yamaguchi, Johnston, & O'Malley, 2003). Athletic groups were the first to promote random drug testing as a way to ensure that teens were not using drugs that would affect their performance. The right of schools to require random drug testing has been upheld in the U.S. Supreme Court. Drug testing should only be half of the approach; there must be intervention programs available for the students should they test positive. The school nurse may be involved in both the drug testing process and the intervention programs.

A variety of modalities can be used to screen for drug use: urine and hair analyses for multiple drugs and breath and saliva tests for alcohol. Many kits are available for home or school use. However, teens have been known to dilute, "adulterate" (add bleach, hand soap, vinegar, etc.), or substitute urine samples collected from their peers or siblings. The detection period varies with the drug. The average is 72 hours post use; however, chronic users may have positive screens up to 4 weeks from their last use (Bellenir, 2002). Some appropriately used over-the-counter medications may throw off the results, and use of these products must be taken into consideration. Even secondhand marijuana smoke can result in positive results. Therefore, a history is essential before any penalty is given. A negative screen does not guarantee that the student has not tried drugs, nor does it imply that education is not needed. In addition, many drugs are not tested for in the drug-testing kits.

SEXUAL ACTIVITY

Sexual activity among adolescents was the first high-risk behavior addressed by the schools, starting in the 1960s. The incidence of intercourse among teens peaked in 1991 and then decreased significantly until 1997, since which time there has been little change. In 2003, 46.7% of high school students indicated that they had had intercourse, 34.3% within 3 months preceding the study (CDC, 2004b). More than 14% of adolescents acknowledge having four or more partners. Of those who were active, 63% used a condom and 17% used birth control pills. More than 25% of those who had intercourse used alcohol or drugs before having sex (CDC, 2004b). Sexual activity was higher among black (73.8%) and Hispanic (56.8%) males than black (60.9%) and Hispanic (46.4%) females.

For each year of high school, the incidence of sexual activity increased, averaging 32.8% in the ninth grade to 61.6% in the twelfth grade (CDC, 2004b). However, 7.4% indicated that they had experienced intercourse before age 13. Those who did engage in intercourse before age 13 included 31.8% of black males and 11.6% of Hispanic males. In 2003, Idaho and Wisconsin had the lowest rates of sexual activity among adolescents and Mississippi and Washington, DC had the highest rates (CDC, 2004b).

The total number of pregnancies has decreased 7% in the United States over the past decade. The decrease is even more significant for adolescent pregnancies. According to The Alan Guttmacher Institute (2004a), in 2000, there were 281,900 pregnancies among girls 15 to 17 years of age and 19,640 pregnancies among girls age 14 or younger. These pregnancies resulted in 157,209 births for the 15- to 17-year-olds and 8,519 for those 14 and younger. Of this total number of pregnancies, at least 42,480 were reported to have ended in miscarriage and 93,330 ended with an abortion (The Alan Guttmacher Institute, 2004a). These numbers continued to decrease in 2003. "However, the abortion ratio was highest for those <15 years (701 abortions per 1,000 live births)" (CDC, 2003c, p. 4).

There are many reasons why sexual activity is common among teenagers. Puberty occurs earlier, with breast development now considered normal in white girls from age 7 on and in black girls from age

6 on (Kaplowitz, Oberfield, & the Pediatric Endocrine Society, 1999). With puberty occurring earlier and marriages occurring later, there is increased time for sexual experimentation. Reasons adolescents give for having intercourse include the need to be loved or accepted by peers, conquest and power, the need to feel grown up, peer pressure, rebellion or revenge, a need for attention, bragging rights, curiosity, and because it is a pleasurable experience. Sexuality education, both at home and in school, must address these issues. Spencer, Zimet, Aalsma, and Orr (2002) found that "girls who scored low on the self esteem measure were 3 times more likely to subsequently initiate sexual intercourse [when questioned two years later]. Conversely, boys who scored high on the self-esteem measure were 2.4 times more likely to initiate coitus during the subsequent 22 month period" (p. 583). Alcohol and drug use are other antecedents to sexual activity.

Another fact to consider is that sexual awareness is very normal and part of the developmental process. Awareness of the body begins from the moment an infant is touched. Parents may touch the genitals differently than other body parts during bathing. During early childhood, it is normal for a child to look at and touch his or her body parts: the infant pulls his feet to his mouth, the toddler holds onto and fondles his genitals, and the school-age child may sit in front of a mirror trying to get a view of what it looks like between their legs. Young children play "house" and "doctor." They ask about their birth or "how they got in their mommy's tummy," they may view nude photos of themselves as infants, they are told to keep parts of their bodies covered when in public, and there is continuous interest in their voiding and defecation patterns.

Some parents label self-touch as "bad" when it involves the genitals. In addition, there is discomfort by adults to use the appropriate terms when identifying parts of the body associated with sexual development. It is essential for the school nurse to always use accurate terminology.

The media has a significant impact on the developing sexuality of children and adolescents. Children and adolescents are repeatedly exposed to sexual images in magazines, movies, and on TV; they hear graphic discussions of sexuality, intimacy, and abuse on TV or through their music; the news is filled with stories of rape, sexual abuse by clergy, adultery by politicians, and advertisements for Viagra and other drugs to enhance sexual performance.

The culture of the school and of the student's environment also has an impact on the developing sexuality. Whether the parents set limits on, punish for, or engage in sexual activities will impact on the student's acceptance of or guilt related to these behaviors. Children and adolescents learn rules for behavior; they learn what they can and cannot touch in public, what words they cannot use, especially in the presence of adults, and whether intercourse is considered taboo or a desired accomplishment of adolescence.

The behaviors that may indicate cause for concern include the frequency and duration of sexual behaviors, even when asked to stop, and engaging in play behaviors that include "inserting or attempting to insert into, or oral contact with, another child's genitals, a child putting his or her mouth on a doll's genital area, and a child asking to be touched in his or her genital area" (Hornor, 2004, p. 60). These may be indicators of sexual abuse and the child should be referred for an evaluation.

"To most teens, sexuality is not just about having intercourse. It's also about attractiveness, reputation, relationships, and finding love and intimacy" (Brown, Steele, & Walsh-Childers, 2002, p. 4). Attractiveness is evidenced by the way teens dress, the attention paid to their hair and skin, and even the way they walk and act. Dating behaviors are often dictated by the school or community culture: the age at which dating is allowed, whether dating implies an exclusive relationship with one person, and the activities that are included in dating behaviors (kissing, touching, or intercourse). These behaviors are often reinforced by teen magazines and television.

Sex Education/Sexuality Education

Sexuality education should be a celebration of the students, of who they are and who they will be. It should be about relationships, communication, and family. It should be about growing up and responsibility. Included within it is information on reproduction of all species and how species care for and tend to their young. It talks about needs and how to maturely meet those needs, based on the age of the student. Sexuality education includes cognitive, affective, and psychomotor components. It needs to build self-esteem of female students and incorporate "connectiveness" with the school and the family. The school nurse is an integral part of this education.

Recognizing the increase in sexual intercourse among adolescents, the *Healthy People 2010* objectives include increasing the proportion of adolescents who abstain from sexual intercourse and to increase the proportion of sexually active adolescents who use condoms (U.S. Department of Health and Human Services [USDHHS], 2000). Because of the significant number of children under the age of 14 who are engaging in sex, it is essential that content on human sexuality be started in the elementary grades. However, it is also essential that the school nurse know the policy of the school related to sexuality education

There is great debate, however, about sexuality and sex education programs. The Alan Guttmacher Institute (2004b) found that only 22 states and the District of Columbia mandate that public schools teach sex education; however, 38 states and the District of Columbia require that STD/HIV education be provided to students. It is virtually impossible to teach these subjects without students having a knowledge base related to sexual intercourse and other ways to transmit fluids.

A national poll by National Public Radio (NPR), the Kaiser Family Foundation, and the Kennedy School of Harvard University (2004) was conducted in 2003 regarding sex education in America. Ninety-three percent agreed that sex education should be taught in the schools. Only 15% believed that only abstinence from intercourse should be taught and that information on contraception, including condoms, should not be taught in schools. Forty-six percent wanted their children to be taught abstinence "plus," so that those teens who do not abstain can prevent the consequences of sexually transmitted diseases and pregnancy. Thirty-six percent believed that the focus should be on teaching teens how to make responsible decisions about sex. In comparing what American citizens want to what schools actually provide, the survey found that 30% of schools where sex education is taught teach abstinence only, 47% teach abstinence-"plus," and 20% taught responsible decision-making related to sexual intercourse. Of note, more middle schools taught abstinence only and more high schools taught the abstinence-"plus."

Abstinence should certainly be stressed as the only way to completely prevent pregnancy and some STDs. However, abstinence should not be defined in terms of virginity. This negates the students who were sexually active and now have decided to stop or abstain until they are older.

Those opposed to sex education programs believe that teaching the material condones and promotes early sexuality. This has never been documented by research. Sexual behaviors are just another high-risk behavior common among adolescents and younger children. Responses to those who object might include the following: "We teach safe driving, including the laws and what to do in the event of an accident, even though our hope is that they drive safely and responsibly; we teach about avoiding drugs, alcohol, and cigarettes even though these substances are illegal for teens, yet we never hear complaints that this will cause students to use; and we teach fire and gun safety, yet we do not hear complaints about increasing curiosity about matches and weapons." The goal of sex education is to provide the same knowledge and awareness of the issues so that students will be able to make responsible decisions whenever they decide to have intercourse.

The American Academy of Pediatrics (AAP, 2001) supports comprehensive sexuality education to children and adolescents. Proponents of comprehensive sex education programs believe that programs must include the facts about intercourse as well as sexual responsibility. They must address cultural and psychological components common to the school population. The biological component should include the components of puberty, intercourse, pregnancy, and sexually transmitted diseases, including HIV. The ethical and legal components should also be addressed. Students should feel free to explore why society views behaviors as right or wrong.

Multiple curricula are available related to comprehensive sex and sexuality education. The concepts can be started in early elementary school with respect for one's body and for the bodies and belongings of others. This approach not only begins the life-long process of self-caring, but also addresses the bullying problem that is so prevalent (see Chapter 39). It also includes not taking what is not yours, which not only addresses stealing, but also addresses rape in the older student. Table 40.3 addresses the components of a comprehensive sex education program and Table 40.4 provides strategies that can be used in teaching the sensitive nature of this content.

The National Campaign to Prevent Teen Pregnancy (2004) provides numerous sex education programs that are effective in delaying sexual intercourse and decreasing teen pregnancy. The Sexuality Information and Education Council of the United States (SIECUS) and Planned Parenthood of America also offer excellent resources related to sex education. In addition, the Centers for Disease Control and Prevention coordinated nine non-governmental organizations to develop a National Framework to Help Schools Become Partners in Preventing Teen Pregnancy (CDC, n.d.). This body recommends that schools:

- Provide HIV, STD, and pregnancy prevention programs to reduce reproductive risk behaviors.
- Include school-based policies and strategies for enhancing school connectedness as well as academic outcomes as important components of prevention initiatives.
- Foster a sense of purpose and a vision for the future.

Table 40.3 ■

COMPONENTS OF A COMPREHENSIVE SEX EDUCATION PROGRAM

1. Male and female reproductive anatomy and physiology
2. Body changes that occur during puberty; body differences
   a. Health and hygiene
   b. Menstruation
   c. Nocturnal emissions
3. Reproduction
   a. Pregnancy and childbirth
   b. Being a teen parent and its impact
   c. Preventing pregnancy
      i. Abstinence
      ii. Birth control
      iii. Responsibilities of both partners
4. Vaginal, oral, and anal sex
5. Sexually transmitted infections (including HIV and hepatitis)
6. Relationships
   a. Dating
   b. Sexual decision making
   c. Impact of drug and alcohol use on decision making
   d. Communication: verbal and nonverbal messages
   e. How to say "no"; respecting "no" (assertiveness training; refusal skills)
   f. How to express affection/caring without having intercourse
7. Feelings
   a. Desire/crush/love
8. Values clarification/cultural differences
   a. Cultural ideas of masculinity and feminity
   b. Religious values
9. Respect for others: their bodies, their decisions, their feelings, their belongings
10. Legal issues regarding sexuality (consenting, rape, obtaining birth control, obtaining pregnancy services)
11. Sexual abuse/domestic abuse

- Incorporate youth development principles and practices as foundations for prevention education initiatives.
- Engage supportive partners in state and community initiatives to prevent teen pregnancy.

While parents want the responsibility to teach sexuality to their children, they are often reluctant

Table 40.4 ■

APPROACHES TO TEACHING SENSITIVE CONTENT IN SEX EDUCATION (THESE CAN BE MODIFIED FOR ANY AGE STUDENT)

1. Have the students write or bring in "Dear Abby" letters related to sexual issues and let the students discuss and debate how to respond to the letter.
2. Play "What Happens Next." Start with a scenario of a girl who is dressed provocatively. Ask, 'What happens next?' and let the students think out the sequence of events. After each one, say, 'What happens next?' (boys are attracted – boys want to have sex with her – boy rapes her). The goal is to get them to think about their actions.
3. Role play what to say to set limits. Give responses or let them develop the responses in a group. Examples: "You would if you loved me!" "If you loved me you wouldn't put that pressure on me right now." (Make sure that boys and girls are together in the class for these role plays so that they see they are both getting the same message.)
4. Values clarification. Explain the various values related to the issues of sexuality and reproductive health from the perspective of multiple religious and cultural groups, making sure to provide the rationales so that students can see the reasons why rules and laws were developed. Discuss the values of relationships and the difference between manipulation and caring.
5. Delaying gratification. This can be taught by saving money or coupons for something desired later.
6. Have students ask their parents what they were taught about sex when they were in school.
7. Have young people who are teen parents talk about how it has changed their lives: socially, educationally, financially, and related to employment and baby caretaking.

[NOTE: The signing of virginity contracts or taking virginity oaths has had no effect on the incidence of sexually transmitted diseases. The incidence is the same for those who have signed these pledges and those who have not.]

and uncomfortable to do so. Programs for parents can be held in the school to share with them what will be taught to their children so that they can continue the conversations at home. This approach fosters communication between the school and the parents as well as between the parents and their children. TABLE 40.5 lists guidelines that can be provided to the parents when approaching the subject of sex and sexuality with their children. Programs for parents can also address the myths regarding sex education as well as helping them listen to and communicate with their children regarding this topic. They need to understand that most intercourse in teens occurs after school in homes where the parents are not home and the children are not supervised (Cohen, Farley, Taylor, Martin, & Schuster, 2002).

Teachers must be comfortable with the content to be taught and know how to respond appropriately to young children regarding these topics. Price, Dake, Kirchofer, and Telljohann (2003) surveyed fifth- and sixth-grade teachers to determine the types of sexual questions students ask. The most common questions involved information on HIV, puberty, STDs, sexual abuse, the function of reproductive organs, dating, love, and divorce. In high schools, the two topics that present the most difficulty for teachers to discuss are masturbation and homosexuality.

The United States has the highest teen pregnancy rate among industrialized nations. "In countries with lower teen pregnancy rates, contraceptive services are confidential, widely available, and very inexpensive or free....(In the U.S.), a sexually active teenage girl who does not use contraceptives has a 90% chance of becoming pregnant within one year" (McWhirter, McWhirter, McWhirter, & McWhirter, 2004, p. 138).

If schools only provide the message to not have sex, students will turn to the media and their friends for information, neither of which are usually accurate or comprehensive. "A well-educated population protects against uninformed mistakes but also is more cost-efficient to society as a whole. Sexuality education programs that stress abstinence, but also provide information on contraceptives, preventing sexually transmitted diseases, unintended pregnancies, and alternative lifestyles are proven effective at better informing adolescents in making decisions in reducing risky sexual behavior" (Eddington & Hecht, 2003, p. 14). The schools, including the school nurse, need to ensure that students are prepared for adulthood. There is no other time or place where this information will be presented to them.

Table 40.5 ■

GUIDELINES FOR PARENTS WHEN DISCUSSING SEXUALITY WITH THEIR CHILDREN

1. Be willing to answer any and all questions.
2. Be honest—don't lie.
3. Develop a rapport first: Show your child you are not afraid of or embarrassed by the material.
4. Tell your child how normal his or her questions are and that it is normal to be curious and to have a lack of knowledge about their own bodies.
5. It's O.K. to acknowledge that you don't know something. You and your child can look it up together or you can get the answer and have another 'session' with them, thus continuing the dialog.
6. Buy age-appropriate books with explanations and have them available on family bookshelves; when the books are missing from the shelf, then you know your child has a question and this is a good time to start a conversation.
7. Encourage pride in their bodies; there is no 'sin' involved and nothing about it is 'dirty'.
8. Dispel myths and fears.
9. When your child tells a 'dirty' joke, have him or her explain it (they may want you to really explain it to them!).
10. When your child uses words with a sexual context, have him or her define them.
11. Encourage children that they need to know about their bodies so that they can take good care of themselves in the future.
12. Enforce the idea that only THEY can touch their own bodies; that if someone wants them to do something and it "feels" wrong, then it is wrong.
13. Explain your values related to sex and sexuality and your rationale for those values.
14. When your child has a first period or wet dream, have a private celebration (e.g., a dinner out with adults only). Let your child know that it is exciting and special to grow up and that you are proud of them...but that this is the beginning of new responsibilities related to their bodies.
15. Teach them to respect the bodies (and belongings and reputation) of others.

BODY DECORATION/MODIFICATION

Body piercing and tattoos are now commonplace among high school students. These behaviors are now becoming riskier and expanding to include cutting, branding, scarring, and having permanent surgery to modify the body. Body decoration needs to be viewed on a continuum. On one end is body painting, including face painting of young children, body painting by football game fans, and temporary tattoos for children. The middle of the continuum includes body adornment. It is commonly practiced by the vast majority of individuals and includes all that is done to make ourselves more attractive. These include cutting, curling, coloring, shaving and removing hair, cutting and painting nails, wearing makeup, and wearing jewelry. Ear piercing is now considered normal for females and is becoming more common among males. It is just another way to wear jewelry. Body adornment might also include some behaviors that last for a few days or weeks, such as botox injections to remove wrinkles and henna decoration.

Body modification involves more permanent forms of body alteration. Body **piercing** is now commonly seen on every part of the body. The entire area of the ear has been pierced, as has the tongue, nose, lips, eyebrows, nipples, and navel. There are multiple piercings of the genitals as well as the newest trend to pierce flat areas of skin, such as along the forearm or on the back. Some are also "placing grommets (round metal eye-lets) or stretching tapers into already pierced and healed tissues (usually the earlobes) for the purpose of enlarging the hole to approximately 1/2 to 1 cm or more. Once these heal, the individual can either wear a curved barbell piece of jewelry in the grommet or attach chains through the grommet to ones placed in other parts of the body" (Selekman, 2003, p. 78).

Aftercare of piercings includes twice a day washing with mild antibacterial or antimicrobial soap, application of neomycin or bacitracin, and then patting it dry (Armstrong & Kelley, 2001). Alcohol and hydrogen peroxide are no longer used to clean piercings because they also cause tissue destruction and delay healing. For tongue piercing, the student should rinse with Listerine after meals. If the site becomes infected, it is essential to treat it as a puncture wound. Apply warm compresses and antibacterial wash but *do not remove the jewelry*; this will put the student at risk for developing an abscess. If it appears that the student is having an allergic reaction to the jewelry of the piercing, the jewelry must be removed. Healing time ranges from 4 to 10 weeks, with the navel taking up to 12 months to heal.

While piercings can be removed leaving little more than a scar, **tattoos** are much more permanent. They can be multiple sizes and colors and placed on any part of the body. Some teens use common household products to tattoo themselves. Using sewing needles, straight pins, forks, paper clips, and pens, they inject pigments, such as charcoal, soot, mascara, or carbon, into their skin (Montgomery & Parks, 2001). Most of the designs are a series of uneven dots in black or brown. The pigments used in professional tattooing are mostly from metallic salts (iron and titanium dioxide, India ink, synthetic organic dyes). The pigments are not regulated by the FDA.

Tattoos are applied using an electrically powered vertically vibrating instrument that injects pigment up to 3,000 times per minute into the dermis at a depth of 1 to 2 mm. There are multiple sizes of needles, but they are solid; therefore when they are sterilized, there is no chance of blood getting caught within them. Aftercare of a tattoo is similar to that of a burn. The bandage is kept on only for a few hours. The tattoo should be patted dry rather than rubbed and the student needs to avoid direct sunlight; both of these will result in losing the sharpness of the picture.

Tattoo removal is much more complicated than applying the tattoo. A laser is used to break up the tattoo into particles that can be eliminated through the normal skin cleansing process. Multiple treatments are usually required and it is much more expensive than having the tattoo applied initially. Some colors are easier to remove than others. If an allergic reaction occurs to one of the colors, the only treatment is to re-tattoo over the affected area with needles that have no dye on them in order to allow the color to ooze out of the skin.

Cutting, **branding**, and **scarification** are more risqué and permanent behaviors. Cutting into the tissue to leave scars may be a cry for help, but it also may be a way to make a design in the skin that will be unique to them. Those who are proud of their designs want people to see them; those who wear long sleeves even in hot weather may be cutting to hurt themselves and need to be referred for an evaluation. Branding and scarification result in second- and third-degree burns. Again, a design is burned into the skin with a hot implement, such as an Italian cookie iron or an electric wood burning kit. Extreme modification includes some common procedures, such as rhinoplasty and breast reduction or the insertion of breast implants. However, some have had Teflon inserts inserted under their skin into various parts of the body to give it a "bumpy" appearance or have had their tongue split.

Adolescents give multiple reasons why they engage in body modification. Some indicate that it is art and that the body is a canvas; others feel that it enhances their sexuality or enhances the pleasure of their partner. Other reasons are that it is a social bonding act—something that friends can do together; it is a way to get attention; it provides a sense of control and a sense of permanence; and it transmits messages. Recently, tattooing has been used to permanently commemorate the loss of a loved one. Occasionally, it is a cry for help and considered self-injury.

Complications of body modification includes scarring, disfigurement, rejection and migration of piercings, interference with the data obtained from magnetic resonance imaging (MRI), harm to others, infection, and embarrassment. The literature is replete with articles on damage to the teeth and gums as a result of to oral piercings. Those who have engaged in these procedures may not donate blood for 1 year, owing to the risk of hepatitis.

The school nurse has many opportunities to educate students both before and after they have engaged in these behaviors. This is an ideal time to ensure that they have had their updated tetanus and hepatitis immunizations. If they are on sports teams, they should be encouraged to wait until the season is over, in order to prevent damage to the area. Students should be informed about what to look for in a qualified piercer or tattoo artist. There is an Association of Professional Piercers (http://www.safepiercing.org). Tattoo artists should autoclave their instruments between patrons and must glove and use small individual containers for the various colors that are *not* put back into the large vat of color after the procedure.

Other cautions may include that certain professions will not allow these art forms in places where they can be seen. The Armed Forces has specific policies about how much of the body can be tattooed and where it is or is not allowed. Nipple piercing may interfere with the ability to breast feed and abdominal tattoos will be stretched by weight gain and pregnancy. In cold areas of the country, students are at higher risk of frostbite with metal piercings.

TANNING

There is significant concern that frequent use of indoor tanning booths and sunlamps, especially by Caucasian teen females, may result in a significant increase in the incidence of skin cancer at the expense of "looking tan and healthy." Teens remain unconcerned about the future leathery appearance of their skin after age 60 or the risk of malignant melanoma. It is estimated that between 13% and 34% of youth engage in this behavior; the incidence increases when the parent also engages in this activity (Cokkinides, Weinstock, O'Connell, & Thun, 2002). In addition, those who use tanning booths are less likely to use sun-screen when outside.

GAMBLING

Gambling is not often associated with adolescents, but more than 80% of adolescents have gambled in some form, whether it was cards, dice, board games, pool, or wagers on sports games. However, 4% to 8% of U.S. high school students are considered to be pathologic gamblers (Griffiths, 2003). This means they engage in persistent gambling that disrupts their personal or family pursuits; they keep betting more in an attempt to recoup their losses. The incidence increases if the parents or peers also engage in gambling, whether by lotteries, bingo, or illegal betting. Pathological gambling will impact on the student's academic performance and may result in stealing in order to have the money to place a bet. They often ask individuals over 18 to buy their lottery tickets for them. Some have even placed bets through bookies and owe thousands of dollars. This may result in some engaging in selling drugs in order to pay back gambling debts.

INTERVENTIONS

Programs related to high-risk behaviors either aim to prevent children and adolescents from initiating the activities or attempt to help them to change behaviors to decrease engaging in these activities. Intervention programs for high-risk behaviors fall into the same three community health approaches of primary, secondary and tertiary prevention. Primary prevention is universal prevention. It is directed to all youth, regardless of risk. Its aim is to educate and prevent initiation, decrease the precursors, resist the temptation to use, and establish norms against engaging in the high-risk behaviors. It is taught to large groups, such as the entire school or an entire grade level. Secondary prevention would be selective prevention for youth known to be at high risk or to have risk factors that make them likely candidates to engage in these behaviors. Selective prevention programs must be longer in duration and more intensive than Universal Prevention programs because the group is already at risk. They must be specific to the risk and the group of students. Tertiary prevention is indicated prevention, which is specified for those youth already engaging in these behaviors to decrease their use; programs must be comprehensive and include the family. Tertiary prevention programs are best led by qualified counselors or psychologists (LeCroy & Mann, 2004).

"Typically, school-based programs have reflected knowledge-only approaches, affective approaches that appeal to moral values and norms, social influence or skills training approaches as well as school climate change or mentoring approaches" (LeCroy & Mann, 2004, p. 213). It is well documented that didactic information alone is not sufficient to deter students from engaging in high-risk behaviors. It is also clear that no single treatment or intervention program is appropriate or effective with all individuals. All addictions have a psychological component. Most also have legal, physical, social, and educational implications as well. Intervention programs must include continuous monitoring as well as support. The family is a primary source of support, but they may need education and support as well. Success in abstaining from drugs or other addictions is a long-term process and may require frequent episodes of treatment, as relapses are common.

One approach is the social influence approach, which includes normative education and resistance-skills training. Normative education promotes the concept that most students do *not* engage in this activity; the norm is not to do it. Resistance skills assist students to practice what to say and to avoid being pressured into engaging in the behavior. The social influence approach is better geared toward those who have not yet begun engaging in the behaviors. The competence-enhancement approach can be used with the social influence approach. Its aim is to assist students to increase their competence in decreasing high-risk behaviors, and thus increase their self-esteem.

Motivational interviewing is another approach used to help students make positive behavior changes and explore alternatives. It involves "using nondirective and self-directed counseling skills, eliciting self-motivating remarks, listening carefully to students, evaluating their desire to change and, at an opportune time, choosing the appropriate moment to explore motivation" (Taylor, 2004, p. 22). Other approaches include behavioral contracting, peer mediation, self-control training, and cognitive-behavioral training, where students learn to "increase self control of behavior through self monitoring, self-evaluation, and self reinforcement" and to compare their behaviors with those standards imposed by their peers related to the behavior (Taylor, 2004, p. 24).

Regardless of whether the intervention is for large or small groups or individualized counseling, programs must be culturally sensitive, reflect the problems of the local community, provide the same education to parents and teachers, and be interdisciplinary. Content can be continued in history, English, mathematics, and science classes and in the arts. In addition to content, interventions should address positive ways to use free time, how to handle stress (from family, peers, and the school), and legal implications.

In addition to structured class or auditorium presentations, the school nurse has multiple "teachable moments" when she is one-on-one with a student in the health office and can respond to specific questions, raise questions based on her assessment of suspicious signs the student presents, or identify that the student is concerned about something and needs prodding to "let it out." These teaching/counseling sessions promote trust and allow the student to obtain accurate information and appropriate guidance in a safe environment.

Drug and alcohol education must begin in elementary school; the age range of 9-12 is an ideal time to reinforce and expand on the earlier education (Taylor, 2004). Programs that begin in the elementary schools have been more effective in decreasing the drug and alcohol use during the middle school years (Taylor, 2004). However, outcome data for the most popular drug education program (Drug Abuse Resistance Education [D.A.R.E.]) indicates that it is not significantly effective in reducing substance abuse among students (LeCroy & Mann, 2004).

Regardless of the intervention chosen, the aim must be designed to reverse or decrease known risk factors to risky behaviors while at the same time, enhance protective processes. Programs must include refusal skills, communication skills, listening skills, and parent involvement. Parents may need the information and skills provided in a separate program. Long-term community-wide involvement is needed to decrease risk factors off of school property, to promote risk-free after-school activities, and to promote media announcements to promote healthy behaviors.

CONCLUSION

Engaging in high-risk behaviors must be viewed on a continuum: abstinence, experimenting with limited use, frequent use, and abuse. In addition to adolescents, the behaviors must also be anticipated among elementary school students. The goals of the school program and where on the continuum a program is focused must be determined to assist in evaluating the outcomes. If avoidance of risky behaviors is truly the goal, educational programs that promote behavior changes must begin with young children.

Resources

National Campaign to Prevent Teen Pregnancy
1776 Massachusetts Avenue, NW
Suite 200
Washington, DC 20036
http://www.teenpregnancy.org

Sexuality Information Education Council of the United States
130 West 42nd Street, Suite 350
New York, NY 10036-7802
212-819-9776
http://www.siecus.org

Substance Abuse and Mental Health Services Administration
Center for Substance Abuse Prevention
National Clearinghouse for Alcohol and Drug Information
U.S. Department of Health and Human Services
http://www.samhsa.gov and http://ncadi.samhsa.gov
800-729-6686

Bradley, L., Jarchow, E., & Robinson, B. (1999). *All about sex: The school counselor's guide to handling tough adolescent problems*. Thousand Oaks, CA: Corwin Press.

References

American Academy of Pediatrics (AAP). (2001). Sexuality education for children and adolescents. *Pediatrics, 108*(2), 498–502.

American Lung Association (ALA). (2004). *Not-On-Tobacco (N-O-T) Backgrounder. Retrieved November 16, 2004 from http://www.lungusa.org*

Armstrong, M., & Kelly, L. (2001). Tattooing, body piercing, and branding are on the rise: Perspectives for school nurses. *Journal of School Nursing, 17*(1), 12–23.

Bellenir, K. (2002). *Drug information for teens*. Detroit, MI: Omnigraphics

Biglan, A., Brennan, P., Foster, S., & Holder, H. (2004). *Helping adolescents at risk: Prevention of multiple problem behaviors*. New York: The Guilford Press.

Brown, J., Steele, J., & Walsh-Childers, K. (2002). *Sexual teens, sexual media: Investigating media's influence on adolescent sexuality*. Mahwah, NJ: Lawrence Erlbaum Associates.

Centers for Disease Control and Prevention (CDC). (2002). *School health index for physical activity, health eating, and a tobacco-free lifestyle: A self-assessment and planning guide*. Elementary school version. Atlanta, Georgia: CDC.

Centers for Disease Control and Prevention (CDC). (2003a). Cigarette smoking among adults—United States, 2001. *Morbidity and Mortality Weekly Report, 52*(40), 953–956.

Centers for Disease Control and Prevention (CDC). (2003b). Tobacco use among middle and high school students—United States, 2002. *Morbidity and Mortality Weekly Report, 52*(45), 1096–1098.

Centers for Disease Control and Prevention (CDC). (2003c). Abortion Surveillance —United States, 2000. *Morbidity and Mortality Weekly Report, 52*(SS-12). 1–32.

Centers for Disease Control and Prevention (CDC). (2004a). Methodology of the youth risk behavior surveillance system. *Mortality and Morbidity Weekly Report*, 53(RR-12), 1–13.

Centers for Disease Control and Prevention (CDC). (2004b). Youth risk behavior surveillance—United States, 2003. *Morbidity and Mortality Weekly Report, 53*f(SS-2), 1–96.

Centers for Disease Control and Prevention (CDC). (2004c). Cigarette use among high school students—United States, 1991–2003. *Morbidity and Mortality Weekly Report, 53*(23), 499–502.

Centers for Disease Control and Prevention (CDC). (n.d.). *A national framework to help schools become partners in preventing teen pregnancy*. Washington, DC: Department of Health and Human Services.

Child passenger deaths involving drinking drivers—United States, 1997–2002. (2004). *Morbidity and Mortality Weekly Report, 53*(4), 77–79.

Cohen, D., Farley, T., Taylor, S., Martin, D., & Schuster, M. (2002). When and where do youths have sex? The potential role of adult supervision. *Pediatrics, 110* (6). Retrieved September 25, 2005 from http://www.pediatrics.org/cgi/content/full/110/6/e66.

Cokkinides, V., Weinstock, M., O'Connell, M., & Thun, M. (2002). Use of indoor tanningsunlamps by US youth, ages 11–18 years, and by their parent or guardian caregivers: Prevalence and correlates. *Pediatrics, 109*(6), 1124–1130.

Cooper, E. (2002). *The emergence of crack cocaine abuse*. New York: Novinka Books.

Dino, G., Horn, K., Goldcamp, J., Fernandes, A., Kalsekar, I., & Massey, C. (2001). A 2-year efficacy study of Not On Tobacco in Florida: An overview of program successes in changing teen smoking behavior. *Preventive Medicine, 33*(6), 600–605.

Eddington, E., & Hecht, M. (2003). The legal foundations of adolescents' education. In R. Levesque (Ed.), *Sexuality education: What adolescents' rights require* (pp. 3–23). New York: Nova Science Publishers.

Griffiths, M. (2003). Adolescent gambling. In D. Romer (Ed.), *Reducing adolescent risk: Toward an integrated approach* (pp. 223–238). Thousand Oaks, CA: Sage.

Gruber, A., & Pope, H. (2002). Marijuana use among adolescents. *Pediatric Clinics of North America, 49*(2), 389–413.

Hall, H., McPherson, S., Twemlow, S. & Yudko, E. (2003). Diagnosis of methamphetamine use. In E. Yudko, H. Hall, & S. McPherson (Eds.), *Methamphetamine use: Clinical and forensic aspects* (pp. 55–63). Boca Raton, FL: CRC Press.

Heyman, R. (2002). Reducing tobacco use among youth. *The Pediatric Clinics of North America, 49* (2), 377–387.

Hingson, R., Heeren, T., Winter, M., & Wechsler, H. (2003). Early age of first drunkenness as a factor in college students' unplanned and unprotected sex attributable to drinking. *Pediatrics, 111*(1), 34–41.

Holland, J. (2001). *Ecstasy: The complete guide*. Rochester, VT: Park Street Press.

Hornor, G. (2004). Sexual behavior in children: Normal or not? *Journal of Pediatric* Health Care, 18(2), 57–64.

Johnston, L., O'Malley, P., Bachman, J., & Schulenberg, J. (2004). *Monitoring the future: National results on ado-*

lescent drug use. NIH Publication No. 04-5506. Bethesda, MD: National Institute on Drug Abuse.

Kaplowitz, P., Oberfield, S., & the Drug and Therapeutics and Executive Committees of the Lawson Wilkins Pediatric Endocrine Society. (1999). Reexamination of the age limit for defining when puberty is precocious in girls in the United States: Implications for evaluation and treatment. *Pediatrics, 104*(4), 936–941.

Koesters, S., Rogers, P., & Rajasingham, C. (2002). MDMA ('ecstasy') and other 'club drugs': The new epidemic. *The Pediatric Clinics of North America, 49*(2), 415–433.

LeCroy, C., & Mann, J. (2004). Substance Use. In L. Rapp-Paglicci, C. Dulmus, & J. Wodarski (Eds.), *Handbook of preventive interventions for children and adolescents* (pp. 198–226). Hoboken, NJ: John Wiley & Sons.

Malberg, J., & Bonson, K. (2001). How MDMA works in the brain. In J. Holland (Ed.), *Ecstasy: The complete guide* (pp. 29–38). Rochester, VT: Park Street Press.

Mattey, E. (2003). Knights against tobacco: Teens lead the charge to prevent tobacco use among adolescents. *Pediatric Nursing, 29*(5), 390–396.

McWhirter, J., McWhirter, B., McWhirter, E., & McWhirter, R. (2004). *At risk youth: A comprehensive response*. Belmont CA: Thompson Learning.

Mermelstein, R. (2003). Teen smoking cessation. *Tobacco Control, 12*(Suppl. 1), i25–i34.

Millstein, S., & Marcell, A. (2003). Screening and counseling for adolescent alcohol use among primary care physicians in the United States. *Pediatrics, 111*(1), 114–122.

Montgomery, D., & Parks, D. (2001). Tattoos: Counseling the adolescent. *Journal of Pediatric Health Care, 15*(1), 14–19.

Neinstein, L., MacKenzie, R., & Morris, R. (2002). High-risk and out-of-control behaviors. In L. Neinstein (Ed.), *Adolescent health care: A practical guide* (pp. 1402–1416). Philadelphia: Lippincott, Williams & Wilkins.

NPR, Kaiser Family, Kennedy School of Government. (2004). *Sex education in America*. Washington, DC: The Henry Kaiser Family Foundation.

Pollak, C., & Bright, D. (2003). Caffeine consumption and weekly sleep patterns in US seventh-, eighth-, and ninth-graders. *Pediatrics, 111*(1), 42–46.

Price, J., Dake, J., Kirchofer, G., & Telljohann, S. (2003). Elementary school teachers' techniques of responding to student questions regarding sexuality issues. *Journal of School Health, 73*(1), 9–14.

Roche, A. (2001). Drinking behavior: A multifaceted and multiphasic phenomenon. In E. Houghton & A. Roche (Eds.), *Learning about drinking* (pp. 1–33). Philadelphia: Brunner-Routledge.

Rogol, A. (2003). Dietary supplements to enhance athletic performance. In F. Lifshitz (Ed.), *Pediatric endocrinology* (pp. 917–922). New York: Marcel Dekker.

Romer, D. (2003). *Reducing adolescent risk: Toward an integrated approach*. Thousand Oaks, CA: Sage.

Selekman, J. (2003). A new era of body decoration: What are kids doing to their bodies? *Pediatric Nursing, 29*(1), 77–79.

Soteriades, E., DiFranza, J., Savageau, J., & Nicolaou, M. (2003). Symptoms of nicotine dependence and other predictors of student smoking at school: Implications for school smoking policy. *Journal of School Health, 73*(4), 154–158.

Spencer, J., Zimet, G., Aalsma, M., & Orr, D. (2002). Self-esteem as a predictor of initiation of coitus in early adolescents. *Pediatrics, 109*(4), 581–584.

Sullivan, T., & Farrell, A. (2002). Risk Factors. In C. Essau (Ed.), *Substance abuse and dependence in adolescence* (pp. 87–117). New York: Taylor & Francis.

Taylor, G. (2004). *Youths serving youths in drug education programs*. Lanham, MD: Scarecrow Education.

The Alan Guttmacher Institute. (2004a). *U.S. teenage pregnancy statistics with comparative statistics for women aged 20–24*. New York: Author.

The Alan Guttmacher Institute. (2004b). *State policies in brief: Sex and STD/HIV education*. New York. Retrieved December 2004 from http://www.guttmacher.org

The National Campaign To Prevent Teen Pregnancy. (2004). Putting what works to work. Retrieved December 2004 12/04 from http://www.teenpregnancy.org/works/default.asp

U.S. Department of Health and Human Services. (2000). *Healthy People 2010*. Washington, DC: Author.

Weber, M., Floyd, R. L., Riley, E., & Snider, D. (2002). National task force on fetal alcohol syndrome and fetal alcohol effect. *Morbidity and Mortality Weekly Report, 51* (RR-14), 9–12.

Yamaguchi, R., Johnston, L., & O'Malley, P. (2003). Relationship between student illicit drug use and school drug testing policies. *Journal of School Health, 73*(4), 159–164.

Yudko, E., Hall, H., McPherson, S., & Twemlow, S. (2003). Physiology. In E. Yudko, H. Hall, & S. McPherson (Eds.), *Methamphetamine use: Clinical and forensic aspects* (pp. 37–46). Boca Raton, FL: CRC Press.

Zuckerman, M. (1994). *Behavioral expressions and biosocial bases of sensation seeking*. New York: Cambridge University Press.

Chapter 41

Pregnant and Parenting Teens

MARILYN MARCONTEL-SHATTUCK

Chapter Outline

INTRODUCTION

Within the past 25 years, it has become commonplace for pregnant and parenting students to continue to attend high school. These students may have complex physical, social, and emotional problems requiring the assistance of the school nurse and other interdisciplinary team members such as school psychologists, social workers, and counselors to help them successfully complete high school. Nurses and other adults are also called on to assist pregnant and parenting students in middle and elementary schools.

Despite notable progress in reducing the number of teen pregnancies, approximately 10% of young women 15 to 19 years of age become pregnant each year and nearly 500,000 infants are born to these teens (Miller, Bayley, Christensen, Leavitt, & Coyl, 2003; Ventura, Matthews, & Hamilton, 2001). This is the highest birth rate among teenagers in Western industrialized countries (Ventura et al., 2001), with a staggering cost of more than 7 billion dollars annually related to direct and indirect costs for caring for these teens and their offspring (National Campaign to Prevent Teen Pregnancy, 2001; U.S. Department of Health and Human Services ([USDHHS], 2000). About 40% of American females (almost 900,000) become pregnant as teenagers. Of that group, about 30% have an abortion, 14% miscarry, and 56% give birth (Alan Guttmacher Institute, 1999a,b; Henshaw, 1999). The highest incidence of teen pregnancy occurs among the poor and young women of color, the fastest growing segments of the population (National Association of State Boards of Education [NASBE], 1998; USDHHS, 2000). Eighty percent of teen pregnancies are unintended and 80% of pregnant teens are not married (Miller et al., 2003).

National Vital Statistics Reports of 2000 show the birth rate for U.S. teenagers declined steadily throughout the 1990s, from 62.1 births per 1,000 teenagers 15 to 19 years of age in 1991 to 48.5 in the year 2000, a decrease of 22% (Figure 41.1). The rates

Table 1. Birth rates for teenagers aged 15–19 years, by age group and State and territory, and percent change by age: United States, 1991 and 2000

State	1991			2000			Percent change between 1991 and 2000		
	15–19 years	15–17 years	18–19 years	15–19 years	15–17 years	18–19 years	15–19 years	15–17 years	18–19 years
United States[1]	62.1	38.7	94.4	48.5	27.4	79.2	−21.9	−29.2	−16.1
Alabama	73.9	47.7	109.5	62.9	37.9	97.3	−14.9	−20.5	−11.1
Alaska	65.4	35.3	111.7	42.4	23.6	69.4	−35.2	−33.1	−37.9
Arizona	80.7	51.4	122.6	69.1	41.1	111.3	−14.4	−20.0	−9.2
Arkansas	79.8	49.4	122.8	68.5	36.7	114.1	−14.2	−25.7	−7.1
California	74.7	46.9	113.6	48.5	28.6	75.6	−35.1	−39.0	−33.5
Colorado	58.2	35.3	91.4	49.2	28.6	79.8	−15.5	−19.0	−12.7
Connecticut	40.4	26.3	59.4	31.9	16.9	56.3	−21.0	−35.7	**−5.2
Delaware	61.1	40.3	87.1	51.6	30.5	80.2	−15.5	−24.3	**−7.9
District of Columbia	114.4	102.8	125.5	80.7	60.7	101.8	−29.5	−41.0	−18.9
Florida	68.8	44.0	102.9	52.6	29.7	88.0	−23.5	−32.5	−14.5
Georgia	76.3	50.6	110.9	64.2	36.8	104.3	−15.9	−27.3	−6.0
Hawaii	58.7	34.7	91.5	45.1	24.7	70.5	−23.2	−28.8	−23.0
Idaho	53.9	29.3	90.8	43.1	21.3	72.8	−20.0	−27.3	−19.8
Illinois	64.8	40.6	99.1	49.5	28.5	81.1	−23.6	−29.8	−18.2
Indiana	60.5	35.2	95.2	50.3	26.2	85.9	−16.9	−25.6	−9.8
Iowa	42.6	22.8	71.5	34.7	17.4	60.3	−18.5	−23.7	−15.7
Kansas	55.4	29.4	94.1	45.3	22.4	78.5	−18.2	−23.8	−16.6
Kentucky	68.9	42.6	105.5	55.3	29.2	92.2	−19.7	−31.5	−12.6
Louisiana	76.1	51.1	111.4	62.1	36.3	97.1	−18.4	−29.0	−12.8
Maine	43.5	23.8	70.1	28.7	13.4	52.8	−34.0	−43.7	−24.7
Maryland	54.3	35.2	79.8	41.6	23.8	68.8	−23.4	−32.4	−13.8
Massachusetts	37.8	25.2	52.9	27.1	15.0	44.9	−28.3	−40.5	−15.1
Michigan	59.0	35.5	91.1	39.2	21.3	66.3	−33.6	−40.0	−27.2
Minnesota	37.3	20.7	61.4	29.6	15.6	51.0	−20.6	−24.6	−16.9
Mississippi	85.6	60.1	120.4	72.0	45.0	109.9	−15.9	−25.1	−8.7
Missouri	64.5	38.7	100.7	48.8	26.5	82.2	−24.3	−31.5	−18.4
Montana	46.7	23.6	83.0	35.8	19.1	60.8	−23.3	−19.1	−26.7
Nebraska	42.4	23.6	69.2	37.2	19.3	62.7	−12.3	−18.2	−9.4
Nevada	75.3	43.9	119.1	62.2	34.2	106.7	−17.4	−22.1	−10.4
New Hampshire	33.3	17.1	53.8	23.4	9.8	45.4	−29.7	−42.7	−15.6
New Jersey	41.6	26.3	62.9	31.7	17.0	54.9	−23.8	−35.4	−12.7
New Mexico	79.8	50.0	124.4	66.2	40.2	105.1	−17.0	−19.6	−15.5
New York	46.0	29.1	69.0	35.6	20.1	58.1	−22.6	−30.9	−15.8
North Carolina	70.5	46.2	101.7	59.9	32.8	101.4	−15.0	−29.0	**−0.3
North Dakota	35.6	18.1	62.4	28.2	12.5	51.4	−20.8	−30.9	−17.6
Ohio	60.5	36.2	93.8	45.6	24.1	77.2	−24.6	−33.4	−17.7
Oklahoma	72.1	41.7	115.6	60.1	32.9	99.8	−16.6	−21.1	−13.7
Oregon	54.9	31.3	90.7	43.2	23.5	72.8	−21.3	−24.9	−19.7
Pennsylvania	46.9	29.2	70.5	35.2	19.6	58.8	−24.9	−32.9	−16.6
Rhode Island	45.4	30.1	63.6	38.4	21.3	64.0	−15.4	−29.2	**0.6
South Carolina	72.9	48.0	105.4	60.6	36.7	92.9	−16.9	−23.5	−11.9
South Dakota	47.5	26.3	79.2	37.2	19.4	62.2	−21.7	−26.2	−21.5
Tennessee	75.2	47.8	112.1	61.5	34.2	101.6	−18.2	−28.5	−9.4
Texas	78.9	50.4	119.3	69.2	42.7	107.1	−12.3	−15.3	−10.2
Utah	48.2	27.0	79.8	40.0	22.0	62.7	−17.0	−18.5	−21.4
Vermont	39.2	21.3	62.0	24.1	10.6	44.5	−38.5	−50.2	−28.2
Virginia	53.5	31.8	81.2	40.8	21.7	66.9	−23.7	−31.8	−17.6
Washington	53.7	31.0	86.5	38.2	20.3	64.5	−28.9	−34.5	−25.4
West Virginia	57.8	32.4	93.2	46.4	22.8	79.8	−19.7	−29.6	−14.4
Wisconsin	43.7	24.8	71.2	34.5	18.3	58.8	−21.1	−26.2	−17.4
Wyoming	54.2	26.4	98.6	40.8	19.0	73.4	−24.7	−28.0	−25.6
Puerto Rico	72.4	50.8	105.9	71.5	49.1	103.8	**−1.2	**−3.3	**−2.0
Virgin Islands	77.9	48.6	124.0	51.9	29.2	86.6	−33.4	−39.9	−30.2
Guam	95.7	55.0	156.1	80.3	55.0	120.5	−16.0	**−0.0	−22.8
American Samoa	...	...	...	44.8	20.4	83.8	...	...	...
Northern Marianas	...	...	...	54.0	40.8	70.9	...	...	...

.... Data not available.

**Not significant at $p < 0.05$

[1]Excludes data for the territories.

NOTE: Birth rates by State shown in this table are based on population estimates provided by the U.S. Bureau of the Census, projected from the 1990 census; see reference 2. Therefore, the rates shown here may differ from rates computed on the basis of other population estimates.

Figure 41.1 ■ Birth rates for teenagers aged 15 to 19 years, by age group and state and territory.

in the year 2000 were at an all-time low (Ventura et al., 2002).

The rate of births for girls ages 10 to 14 years dropped from 1.4 births per 1,000 during 1989–1994 to 0.9 per 1,000 in 1999 and 2000 (FIGURE 41.2). This is the lowest level in more than 30 years (Ventura et al., 2001). The decline occurred despite the fact that the population of girls in this age group increased. The number of births to girls younger than 15 years dropped to 8,561 in 2000, 34% below the high of 12,901 in 1994 (Ventura et al., 2001).

Teenage birth rates vary substantially among states (Figure 41.1). In 2000, birth rates for teenagers 15 to 19 years old ranged from 23.4 to 72.0 births per 1,000 teens. Among teenagers 15 to 17 years old, the rates ranged from 9.8 to 49.1 births per 1,000 teens. Among older teenagers 18 to 19 years of age, the rates by state ranged from 44.5 to 114.1 births/1,000 teens (Ventura et al., 2002).

Birth rates in 2000 for teen mothers 15 to 19 years of age were significantly lower than in 1991 in every state (FIGURE 41.3). Generally, the year-to-year decline since 1991 in the state-specific rates echoed the national decline, but there was considerable variability among the states. Among teenagers 15 to 17 years of age, birth rates dropped in all states, with statistically significant declines ranging from 15% to 50% (Ventura et al., 2002).

The rate of second births to teenagers who already have one child declined by 21% in the 1990s. This finding is encouraging, as the outcomes for the mother and the child are often more adverse than with the first birth (Ventura, Martin, Curtin, Matthews & Park, 1998; Ventura, Matthews, & Curtin, 1998; Ventura et al., 2001).

WHY TEENS GET PREGNANT

Current pregnancy rates for adolescents are at their lowest level in 20 years, and teen birth rates are the lowest recorded in this country (Ventura, Mosher, Curtin, Abma, & Henshaw, 2001). Despite this good news, teen pregnancy and parenting continue to be viewed by many as major issues, particularly because of the intergenerational effects of early pregnancy and parenthood. The concerns are related to the medical, educational, psychological, and economic problems that often result from early and typically unintended pregnancy and the demands of parenting offspring while lacking emotional and fiscal resources for this task. The consequences affect primarily the teen mother and child and, to a lesser degree, the young father (Hockenberry, Wilson, Winkelstein, & Kline, 2003; Kirby, 2001).

Adolescents at every social, cultural, economic, and intellectual level are at risk of succumbing to internal and external pressures to have sex, which places them at risk for pregnancy. As the number of risk factors in a teen's life increase and protective factors decrease, the chance of the teen engaging in unprotected sex increases (Kirby, 2002). Some of the risk factors categorized as social disadvantages that are frequently associated with adolescent pregnancy include poverty, low educational attainment, family and residential instability, unemployment, limited career opportunities, and membership in a minority group (Kirby, 1997). The early onset of hormonal changes and physical maturity, earlier initiation of sexual activity, and abuse (either sexual or physical abuse and/or violence in the home) are also considered social disadvantages (Kirby, 1997). Behavioral,

Births and birth rates for teenagers by age: United States, 1991–2000

Number of births Birth rate

year	Number of births			Birth rate		
	10–14 years	15–17 years	18–19 years	10–14 years	15–17 years	18–19 years
2000	8,561	157,661	312,845	0.9	27.5	79.5
1999	9,054	163,588	312,462	0.9	28.7	80.3
1998	9,462	173,231	311,664	1.0	30.4	82.0
1997	10,121	180,154	303,066	1.1	32.1	83.6
1996	11,148	185,721	305,856	1.2	33.8	86.0
1995	11,242	192,508	307,365	1.3	36.0	89.1
1994	12,901	195,169	310,319	1.4	37.6	91.5
1993	12,554	190,535	310,558	1.4	37.8	92.1
1992	12,220	187,549	317,866	1.4	37.8	94.5
1991	12,014	188,226	331,351	1.4	38.7	94.4
Percent change 1991–2000	−28.7	−16.2	−5.6	−35.7	−28.9	−15.8

Note: Data for 2000 are preliminary.

Figure 41.2 ■ Births and birth rates for teenagers ages 10 to 19: United States, 1991–2000.

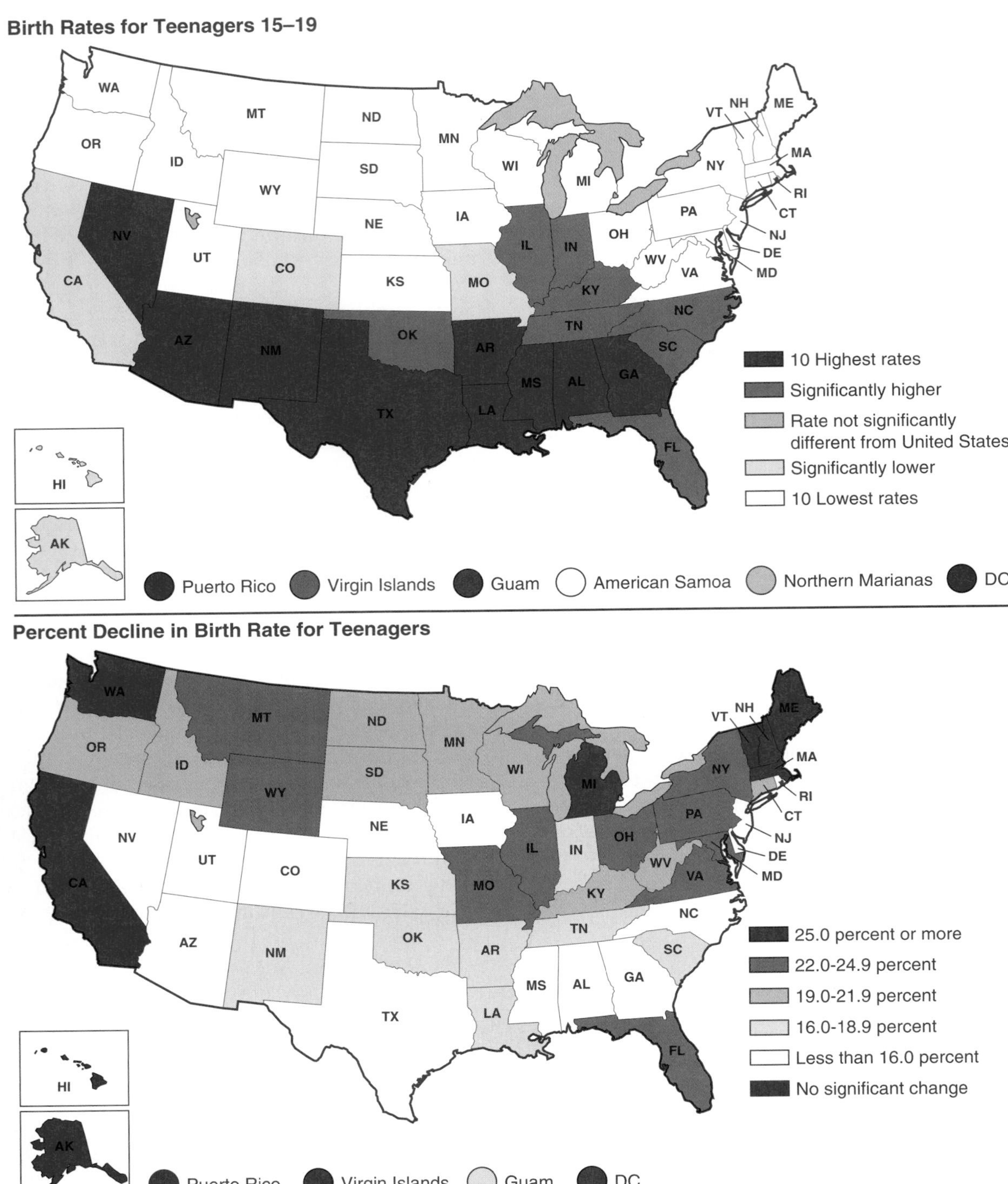

Figure 41.3 ■ Birth rates and percent decline in birth rates for teenagers 15 to 19 years by state, 2000.

developmental, and emotional factors that may lead to early sexual activity and pregnancy include desire of the adolescents for reassurance that they are "sexually normal" or "grown up," rebellion against their families, peer pressure, desire to belong to a group, feelings of being invulnerable, a low value on educational achievement, less religiosity, poverty, and lower intelligence level (Neinstein & Farmer, 2002).

Within the past three decades numerous social changes in this country have had an impact on adolescents and their families, some of which place them at greater risk of early parenthood. Women more frequently work outside of the home before and after marriage and return to work after childbirth. The high divorce rate continues, and the number of single-parent families has increased. Children and youth are frequently "on their own" after school until a parent returns home from work, placing the young people at risk for involvement in early sexual activity. These students are called "latchkey kids." Emphasis is frequently placed on sexuality and violence in advertisements, movies, television, and other entertainment. In addition, widespread use of "recreational drugs," such as marijuana, alcohol, cocaine, cigarette smoking, and other substances of abuse is common in teens and may contribute to impaired judgment and lowered inhibitions that contribute to sexual exploration and to sexual intercourse (MacKenzie & Kipke, 1998).

According to a report of the Youth Risk Behavior Surveillance (YRBS) 2001, a national survey that addresses adolescent health risk behaviors, by grade 9, 34.4% of adolescents have had sexual intercourse. This increases to 40.8% by the grade 10, 51.9% by grade 11, and 60.5% by grade 12 (Centers for Disease Control and Prevention [CDC], 2002b). This report noted that about one-third of high school students had sex in the 3-month period preceding the survey (CDC, 2002b).

Compared to their peers in other countries, sexually active teens in the United States are less likely to use any contraceptive method, and those who do are much less likely to use highly effective hormonal methods (primarily the birth control pill) (Alan Guttmacher Institute, 2002). In addition, U.S. teens are less likely to have an induced abortion. This trend is likely due to problems accessing abortion services, higher levels of antiabortion sentiment, and greater acceptance in this country of teen motherhood (Alan Guttmacher Institute, 2002).

Numerous studies have identified factors that influence teens to have sex. These include cultural issues; values; living in a family or community in which the female has an early initiation to sexual activity; experiencing physical and sexual abuse; and having a mother, sister, or peers who have had an out-of-wedlock pregnancy as a teen (Alan Guttmacher Institute, 2002). One study of sexually active non-pregnant African American females demonstrated a significant correlation between wanting to become pregnant and low family support and having a male partner at least 5 years older who desired pregnancy (Davies et al., 2003). A study by Esparza and Esperat (1996) examined the effects of childhood sexual abuse on minority adolescent mothers and identified that prior to pregnancy, these mothers were more likely to have had earlier sexual relations and to become pregnant. They also had poor psychosocial adjustments in many areas critical to developing into healthy adults.

The Young Father

There are fewer studies on the partners of pregnant teens and less is known about the impact of teen pregnancy on the young father (Mazza, 2002). This may be due in part to the fact that the father can more easily separate himself from the responsibility of parenthood, and because traditionally, the primary responsibility of taking care of the child has fallen on the female. Sometimes the young mother chooses not to tell her partner of the pregnancy. Some adolescent fathers, particularly those from lower socioeconomic and educational backgrounds, believe that impregnating a woman enhances their masculinity. These males may have multiple partners and do not use measures to prevent pregnancy (Olds, London, Ladewig, & Davidson, 2004).

On the other hand, many adolescent males are involved in a meaningful relationship with their partners. The couple may or may not live together, but they usually have similar socioeconomic backgrounds, common educational achievement levels, and are within 3 to 4 years of each other in age (Olds et al., 2004). The teen father is rarely a significant source of childcare or financial help, but may have strong emotional ties to the mother and the child and concern for their welfare (Juszczak, 1998).

The teenage father who does assume parental responsibility is faced with socioeconomic, cultural, and educational factors that may complicate his successful negotiation of the developmental tasks of adolescence (see Chapter 16). Initially, he may be no more knowledgeable about assuming the parenting role than the adolescent mother. In addition, he may face negative responses from his family, from her family, from his pregnant partner, and from others in the school and community who know of the pregnancy. He may feel isolated and alone, at a time in his life when peer relationships are of great importance. His need for adult counseling and support is evident. School personnel aware of the teen's concerns can offer him many of the same support services the pregnant teen receives. "Young men go through emotional and psychological changes as they prepare to become fathers" (Barr & Monserrat, 2002, p. 140). His concerns may be influenced by the amount of involvement he has with the young mother and the relationship he continues (or does not continue) with her. If he plans to be with her during the pregnancy and childbirth process, or if he plans to marry her and be a father to the child, the school nurse may encourage him to enroll in and complete childbirth classes. Generally these will be with the young mother. He may also be encouraged to participate in classes of child growth and development and child care. These school or community classes are designed for young parents and he will be able to meet and learn with other young fathers.

The parenting characteristics of adolescent fathers are not as well described in the literature as those of adolescent mothers. Involvement of the male with the adolescent mother during pregnancy and following childbirth appears to increase her sense of confidence and security as well as improve his sense of self-esteem. In addition, compared to children raised without fathers, involved adolescent fathers improve the child's sense of trust. After the birth of the child, the degree to which the adolescent male bonds with his baby is dependent on his relationship with the mother. This may be strong if the young family lives together. When the father lives separately, his bond with his child may be lessened or nonexistent (Barr & Monsarrat, 2002).

Recently several programs for young men, directed at teaching teen parenting skills to adolescent fathers as well as preparing those teens about to become fathers, have been developed and implemented in schools and community settings. The common themes in these programs are self-esteem, decreasing the pressure of male stereotyping, and increasing self-responsibility (Barr & Monsarrat, 2002). Additional information and Web sites regarding programs are listed in this chapter in the section on Providing Programs of Support and Services.

Legal efforts to establish paternity and child support for children of teenage mothers is receiving attention in many states. When paternity is established, many states require payment of child support for the first 18 years of the child's life (Barr & Monsarrat, 2002). The young father who initially wants to quit school to provide financial support may benefit from counseling before making this decision. This effort is frequently counterproductive in the long run because dropping out of school to provide for a family may limit his earning potential. Remaining in school or in a job training program is often more appropriate.

The Teenage Mother

For most teenage females, pregnancy is a crisis. Initial reactions may be shock, denial, fear, anger, disappointment, or embarrassment. As the physiological changes occur in the pregnant teen's body, her feeling of self-control is reduced and fear of the unknown may cause her to mask her feelings. She may become very quiet and reluctant to participate in social activities or act indifferent or "tough."

The developmental tasks of the adolescent female (see Chapter 16) are complicated by the developmental tasks of pregnancy and parenting. For instance, in normal development teenagers are very concerned with their changing body image. The preferred adolescent body image of "slender" will be replaced during pregnancy with an increase in size and weight that may cause feelings of embarrassment and dissatisfaction (Olds et al., 2004).

Many pregnant and parenting females drop out of school and do not return, despite laws in most states that require them to remain in school until they are 17 or older (Cohn, Gelfman, & Schwab 2001) (FIGURE 41.4). The day (and night time) care of the infant, additional financial burdens, family stress, and previous academic difficulties are reasons commonly cited for school interruption and/or failure to complete high school (Juszczak, 1998).

Impact on the Child

Children of young parents are at a greater risk than their peers for various health, social, and economic problems. According to Juszczak (1998), many of these children are from disadvantaged environments where a less stable family structure, larger family size, and less educational attainment are risk factors for their growth and development. Rates of illness, injury, and poor health are higher for infants of mothers younger than 17 years of age than for infants of older mothers. The ongoing negative consequence may include poor health, school problems, lower test scores on intelligence and cognitive tests, retention in a grade, and poor parental and teacher evaluation of the child's performance (Juszczak, 1998). Children of adolescent mothers are more at risk for academic and behavior problems in late childhood and adolescence than their peers (Klerman, 1993).

Adolescent mothers smile less and have less positive eye and physical contact with their infants than adult mothers, even when matched on socioeconomic and ethnic characteristics. As their infants grow, many teen mothers talk to them less, give more verbal commands, make more authoritarian statements, and make fewer descriptive, and articulate responses (Culp, Appelbaum, Osofsky, & Levy, 1988). The teens' lack of knowledge and skills in parenting may result in delayed growth and development patterns of their children. The amount of cognitive stimulation in a child's early home environment is associated with their level of cognitive attainment. If this stimulation is lacking or neglected, ongoing consequences of learning problems may be seen in the infant and young child (Hockenberry et al., 2003).

Title IX of the Education Amendments of 1972 is the primary federal statutory guarantee of equal educational opportunity for pregnant and parenting students. Title IX applies to a broad range of educational institutions including preschool, elementary, secondary and vocational schools, as well as institutions of higher education and professional schools. Title IX's coverage extends to most public and many private institutions as long as these institutions receive federal funding.

General Prohibition Against Discrimination (Section 106.31)

Sex Discrimination is prohibited in the treatment of students; provision of aid, benefits, or services; the application of rules of conduct and disciplinary measures or other sanctions; and the determination and assessment of fees, including residency requirements of attendance, admission, or tuition.

Discrimination Against Pregnant Students (Section 106.40)

- Schools are prohibited from discriminating against pregnant students based upon their marital status and cannot discriminate against a student because of childbirth, false pregnancy, or recovery from these conditions.
- A school is permitted to require a doctor's certificate from a pregnant student only if the school imposes the same requirement upon all other students with physical or emotional conditions requiring a physician's care.
- Participation in special schools or programs reserved or designed for pregnant or parenting students must be completely voluntary on the part of the student. Such programs or schools must be comparable to programs and schools offered to nonpregnant students.
- Schools must treat pregnancy as they treat other medical conditions. Health plans, medical benefits, and related services are to be provided to pregnant students in the same manner as services are provided to students with "other temporary disabilities."
- A pregnant student may be granted a leave of absence for as long as it is deemed medically necessary and at the conclusion of her leave must be allowed to resume the status she held when the leave began.

Schools May Not Discriminate on the Basis of Marital or Parental Status (Section 106.40)

- A school that excludes female students because of their marital or parental status but permits male students who are married or parents to continue their studies clearly violates this provision of the regulations.
- The statute may, in addition, serve as a vehicle to challenge facially neutral rules that disproportionately harm students of one gender. For example, a rule prohibiting parents from bringing children under the age of six onto school property may violate Title IX if it was created to prevent female student parents from bringing babies to school or if it disproportionately affects female rather than male students.

Discriminatory Courses and Programs Are Prohibited (Section 106.34)

- The Title IX's regulations forbid requiring a student to take a course or participate in a program on the basis of sex.
- Classes devoted to human sexuality may be conducted separately for males and females in elementary and secondary school classes.

Discriminatory Counseling and Use of Appraisal and Counseling Materials Are Prohibited (Section 106.36)

- Discriminatory counseling and materials that treat students differently on the basis of sex are prohibited.

Programs Not Run Directly by the School (Section 106.31 (d))

- The regulations prohibit discrimination in activities that are considered part of the school's education program even if they are not wholly operated by the school. Therefore, a student cannot be excluded from a program such as a student exchange program, foreign study and travel, or coursework offered in conjunction with other academic or nonacademic institution on any basis prohibited by Title IX.

Figure 41.4 ■ Title IX Education Amendments of 1972 Fact Sheet created by the Department of Education, State of California.

Are the Consequences Always Negative?

Some teenage mothers take good care of their infants and young children, continue and complete high school, and go on to college. Some teen fathers make every effort to complete their education, provide emotional and financial support for their family, and become good fathers (Newton, Adams, & Marcontel, 1997). Financial, childcare, and emotional support that comes from the family, the school, or community helps the young family to succeed. Perrin and Dorman (2003) collected personal life stories of 221 teen mothers who considered themselves successful mothers and who attained financial independence and educational prestige by completion of a master's or doctoral degree. Schultz (2001) examined the paradox of females without children who claimed they could succeed only if they managed to avoid pregnancy and young mothers in the same socioeconomic group who credited their success in their educational endeavors to their children and their perception that they must succeed in order to adequately care and provide for their child.

Early marriage and pregnancy were common in the United States until the middle of the 20th century. Since that time, the average age of both men and women when they marry has increased. In many cultures, early marriage and parenting are still acceptable norms. In Southeast Asian populations living in the United States, marriage and parenting among teens as young as 13 are considered desirable (Get Real About Teen Pregnancy, 2002). In the Latino culture, there is concern about hindering the teen parents' potential future and the child's future as well, but babies are usually welcomed into the family and community, and teen mothers are often showered with attention and affection. This may give a mixed message and confuse teens and their siblings about the desirability of early motherhood (Get Real About Teen Pregnancy, 2002).

It should be remembered that teenage parents vary in age, motivation for pregnancy, circumstances, and behavior. A comparison between a pregnant or parenting 13-year-old middle school student and a 19-year-old senior or high school graduate shows clearly how the age and maturity of the teen may result in significant differences in approaches to their parenting. Individuals who are 19 years old are beginning young adulthood and are more likely ready to accept adult responsibilities compared to their early adolescent counterparts. The older teen parent is not necessarily burdened with low academic achievement or a need to drop out of school.

In the Position Statement of the National Association of School Nurses on Adolescent Parents (NASN, 1997), school nurses are encouraged to "provide counseling and information regarding pregnancy to pregnant adolescents and their families" ...and to "take a leadership role in helping to encourage community involvement to establish day care services for children of students, permitting parenting adolescents to continue their education." These efforts by the nurse and school staff are a way to assist teen students to have a positive outcome in their pregnancy and parenting experience.

INITIAL COUNSELING, REFERRAL, AND OPTIONS

The school nurse is frequently the first adult the student and sometimes her partner contact for advice or for help when concerned about health issues for either a known or suspected pregnancy. The nurse needs to balance the student's right to confidential health care; the need for support, including emotional, moral, and financial challenges; and the potential desire or need of the teen's parents to know of the pregnancy. If the teen has not told her parent(s) of the pregnancy, the nurse, as she counsels the student, may offer to assist the teen in informing them. Parents may be requested to attend a nurse/parent conference in the school nurse's office, or the nurse may go with the student to her home, although in some states, the school nurse does not make home visits. The site for disclosure about the pregnancy will be determined by the nurse based on the teen's feelings about the reaction of the parents (Cohn et al., 2001). The advantage of hosting a meeting in the school environment is that help would be more readily available if the parent(s) become angry by the news of the pregnancy. It is important that the school nurse document the decision regarding informing the parent and also any referrals made for counseling or prenatal care. Often the law and school policy and procedures do not clearly define when the school nurse should notify or must notify the parent(s) about a possible pregnancy. The school nurse must be aware of federal laws about parental notice, as well as any specific state regulations and school policies, and proceed accordingly.

According to Cohn and colleagues, "the current standard of practice seems to confirm that unless there is a life-threatening emergency, pregnancy-related information will be kept confidential and not disclosed against the wishes of the minor, even to a parent unless there is a life threatening emergency" (2001, p. 243) if this is the desire of the student. In the past decade, pregnant students are generally less reluctant for others, including parents, to know of their pregnancy. With the student's permission, the information is shared with other school professionals who may have a legitimate need to know and who may be of help, such as the counselor, school social worker, substitute nurse, and physical education teacher. This information sharing should also be documented.

The teen and her partner will need to have medical confirmation of the pregnancy. The school nurse may assist the student in finding an appropriate medical resource for this important first step. Some school nurses perform pregnancy testing in the school health office or in school based clinics; others do not. Whether testing is allowed depends on approval by the School Board and administrative guidelines. Some teens will have purchased a pregnancy test kit and will tell the nurse their results of the test. The early diagnosis of pregnancy has become revolutionized by the development of sensitive and highly specific over-the-counter (OTC) tests for pregnancy (Polaneczky & O'Connor, 1999), many of which are relatively inexpensive. The OTC pregnancy tests are about 97% accurate if the instructions are followed. The school nurse should inform students that results may vary, depending on how the test was performed, and students should be encouraged to seek medical attention to confirm the pregnancy.

"Counseling the pregnant adolescent about her pregnancy options is perhaps the most important aspect of early pregnancy management" (Neinstein

& Farmer, 2002, p. 819). When the student has a confirmation of the pregnancy by a healthcare provider, it is essential that she and her partner receive expert counseling on the options available to her regarding terminating or continuing the pregnancy to term. As the pregnancy continues, the prospective parents also need assistance with adoption planning and placement or preparation for the parenting role. In addition, the pregnant teen needs to be encouraged to seek gynecological or obstetrical care as soon as the pregnancy is known because prenatal care is associated with improved labor and delivery outcomes. With adoption and abortion, pregnant teenagers need help to work through feelings of loss; when they plan to keep the baby, they must be prepared for coping with the demands of parenting and childcare. If providers of these early counseling services are judgmental, lacking in knowledge, or do not offer unbiased and unhurried counseling for the student, the teen should be helped to find another source of such services. Ideally, counseling would continue for several sessions, and if appropriate, throughout the pregnancy and early parenting. The school nurse can assist in providing guidance.

It is important for school personnel (generally the nurse) to refer the student and her partner to an agency or healthcare provider who can provide nondirective counseling to the teens in a manner that is safe, supportive, and adheres to confidentiality guidelines. Prior to making any referrals for pregnancy determination and counseling, the school nurse, school counselor, or social worker will want to talk with the agency personnel in an effort to become familiar with them, their philosophy, services provided, and the cost of these services.

The counselors in these clinics or agencies need to be able to establish rapport and assess the pregnant teen and her partner's developmental level and work with them at that level. The teens may need to be encouraged to express their negative and positive feelings. They may need time to explore and ask questions about each option. The counselor will need to explain prenatal care, abortion procedures, parenting, and adoption and foster care alternatives in such a way that the information can be part of the decision-making process. Follow-up counseling, if the issues are not resolved in an initial session, will need to be scheduled.

If the pregnant teen and her partner attend counseling together, it is important that the nurse assure the student that the decision for the pregnancy is hers and that, while the partner may help and support her, she needs to be the one who makes the final choice about the pregnancy and its resolution.

Relinquishment for Adoption

Placing infants for adoption is not a common practice in the United States (Chandra, Abma, & Bachrac, 1999). The incidence of adoption as an option for teenagers has decreased even more in recent decades (Strasburger & Brown, 1998). Among never-married African American women, 1.5% of infants were relinquished for adoption prior to 1973, 1.1% in the 1980s, and virtually none in the first half of the 1990s (Chandra et al., 1999). Approximately 2% to 3% of teen pregnancies that progress to delivery involve the mother opting for an adoption plan. Teens who choose to relinquish their child for adoption are more likely to be white, have a higher socioeconomic status, have educational aspirations, and live in suburban residences (Mosher & Bachrach, 1996). Unusually mature teens are more likely to consider relinquishing their infant for adoption, as are teenagers who were adopted, those who have friends who were adopted or friends who relinquished their infants through adoption, or have mothers who are supportive of adoption (Strasburger & Brown, 1998).

It is of interest to note that nearly every state permits minor parents to make the decision to relinquish their infant for adoption. This is explicit in state policy in 34 states and the District of Columbia, or in policy in 11 states by making no distinction between minor or adult parents. Only five states require parental involvement in a minor's decision to place an infant for adoption (Alan Guttmacher Institute, 2003a).

Abortion

Approximately 4 in 10 teen pregnancies (excluding those ending in miscarriage) are terminated by induced abortion (Henshaw, 1999). Since 1980, abortion rates among pregnant adolescents have declined. This is attributed to fewer teens becoming pregnant, the limited availability and accessibility of abortion providers because of restrictive abortion laws, decreased public funding for abortions, and fewer teens choosing this option. When a teen chooses to have an abortion, the reasons frequently given are a concern for how a baby would change her life, feeling she is not mature enough to have a child, and concerns about finances (Alan Guttmacher Institute, 1999a).

A majority of states have laws requiring parental involvement in a minor's decision to have an abortion (Alan Guttmacher Institute, 2003b). Case law has confirmed that the minor herself may decide whether to continue the pregnancy (Cohn et al., 2001). Two U.S. Supreme Court rulings have prohibited parents from having absolute veto over their teen's decision to have an abortion (Alan Guttmacher Institute, 2003b). Counselors who are providing this information to teenagers must be knowledgeable of the current legal considerations in order to accurately present this option to them.

Adolescents who decide to terminate their pregnancy should be encouraged to do so while in the early stages of pregnancy. Unfortunately many adolescents delay the decision. The reasons may be denial of the pregnancy, or financial problems, or that they do not fully understand the need to follow through with the abortion as quickly as possible (Neinstein & Farmer, 2002).

Parenting

If the choice is made to keep the child, the school nurse and appropriate others in the school or community should focus on referrals for prenatal health care, providing health education, involving the father, if feasible, encouraging the mother (and father) to complete their academic or vocational training, counseling to prevent subsequent unintended pregnancies, and teaching them how to use existing community resources that provide support and care to pregnant and parenting adolescents and their children.

Providing information and resources for classroom presentations in health, science, home and family living, human growth and development, and sexuality and other appropriate classes is also a school nurse responsibility and provides an opportunity for presenting medical and health information to large numbers of students.

Medicaid, a federally aided, state-operated program for providing medical care for low-income individuals, and Women Infants and Children (WIC) services, a supplementary food program, are available. In many large urban cities, the Healthy Start Program, a federal government program that provides ongoing counseling for parents and childcare for their children, is available for pregnant and parenting teens and their infants. The school nurse or social worker can often assist students in accessing these programs.

PHYSICAL HEALTH ISSUES

The majority of negative maternal health consequences associated with teenage pregnancy and childbearing are attributable to lower socioeconomic status, pre-pregnancy health, late entry into prenatal care, and limited knowledge about self-care and health behaviors (Neinstein & Farmer, 2002). The nursing interventions offered by the school nurse and assistance from other key healthcare professionals in the school and community will affect the course of the pregnancy and the birth outcome. In most cases, the school nurse will have more opportunity for contact with the pregnant teen during the prenatal period than will other healthcare providers. She will often be the person to whom the teen will bring her questions concerning her health and the health of the fetus. It is important for the nurse to understand health issues during pregnancy that indicate the need for a referral for care. It is also important for the nurse to frequently encourage the young teen to take good care of herself during pregnancy and to continue her education.

Prenatal Care

Early, comprehensive prenatal care is an important factor in a healthy outcome for the mother and the newborn regardless of the mother's age. Unfortunately, many teenagers do not seek care, or care is unavailable or delayed for financial or other reasons. Adolescents who receive adequate prenatal care have no significant increase in health risks during the pregnancy. About 4% of teenagers receive no prenatal care or do not initiate care until the third trimester (Neinstein & Farmer, 2002).

Adolescents express many reasons for delayed or inadequate prenatal care, such as a fear of the reaction to news of the pregnancy by parents or significant others (including the baby's father), not recognizing the pregnancy, denial of the pregnancy until the second or third trimester, not understanding the importance of early prenatal care, confusion about available services, lack of transportation, and lack of health insurance or finances. Other difficulties and concerns mentioned by some adolescents are negotiating paperwork, their perception of negative attitudes of community clinic clerical and nursing staff, fear of physicians primarily because of their lack of previous contact with them, and the lack of availability of adolescent-only clinics.

During early pregnancy, adolescents may experience the same conditions that threaten pregnancies in adults. These include ectopic pregnancy and gestational trophoblastic disease (GTD) as a spectrum of disease processes that involve abnormal placental tissue, and threatened, missed, or incomplete abortion (Neinstein & Farmer, 2002). The adolescent may not have been aware that she was pregnant and seek emergency treatment for heavy bleeding, irregular menses, pelvic pain, or abdominal cramping (Emans, Smith, & Laufer, 1998). Bleeding is common in early pregnancy and about half of the pregnancies in adolescents who have severe bleeding end in spontaneous abortion. Some reasons for this include abnormal chromosomal complement, uterine or cervical abnormalities, abnormalities of pelvic structure, maternal systemic illness, or infection (Polaneczky & O'Connor, 1999).

Nutrition

Adolescents are more prone to have an unsatisfactory diet more than individuals in any other age group (Neinstein & Schack, 2002). Two candy bars and a soft drink, or chips and a coke is often their lunch. Poor eating habits, such as missed meals, meals obtained from vending machines or fast food restaurants, and snacks high in sugar with low nutritional value contribute to their nutritional problems (Neinstein & Schack, 2002).

Healthcare professionals should recommend a high-quality well-balanced diet and provide teens with specific concrete examples for how this is accomplished. Cultural and ethnic preferences must be addressed. The pregnant teen, as well as other teens, should be encouraged to eat nutritious, well balanced meals using the Food Guide Pyramid (see Chapter 36) as a guide.

The Food Guide Pyramid is prepared by the U.S. Department of Agriculture and the Department of Health and Human Services (Center for Nutrition Policy and Promotion, 2003). It is available in 30 different languages with cultural and ethnic considerations for requirements.

Findings from the 2003 Youth Risk Behavior Surveillance Survey indicated that 78% of adolescent students nationwide had not eaten the recommended daily requirements of fruits or vegetables during the 7 days preceding the survey and 83% had not ingested the recommended amount of milk (CDC, 2004). Results from the 1999–2002 National Health and Nutrition Examination Survey (NHANES) indicate that an estimated 16% of adolescents are overweight. This is an increase of 5% from the 1988–1994 prevalence of overweight adolescents ages 12 to 19 (CDC, National Center for Health Statistics, 1999–2002).

During pregnancy, daily caloric needs increase from 2,200 to 2,500. Weight gain during pregnancy should range from 25 pounds for an overweight teen to 40 pounds for an underweight teen. If the teen is overweight, her healthcare provider should counsel her about dieting and the school nurse should reinforce these recommendations. In most cases, dieting during pregnancy is not recommended (Neinstein & Farmer, 2002).

Prenatal Vitamin and Mineral Supplementation

Iron deficiency anemia is a common medical disorder of pregnancy, occurring in 15% to 25% of all pregnancies. Iron for the fetus comes from the maternal serum and diet alone does not replace the gestational iron losses (Wenstrom & Malee, 1999). Pregnant adolescents are at particular risk for this condition. Symptoms of iron deficiency during pregnancy can include fatigue, headache, lightheadedness, and exercise intolerance. At delivery blood loss may be poorly tolerated and healing may be compromised (Wenstrom & Malee, 1999). Iron deficiency during pregnancy can put a teen at increased risk for preterm birth and fetal growth restrictions (Cunningham et al., 2001).

The current recommended supplementation for nonanemic women during pregnancy is 30 mg of elemental iron. If the maternal diet is questionable or if the young female is at nutritional risk, a multivitamin is also recommended (Cunningham et al., 2001).

Each year, about 4,000 pregnancies in the United States are affected by neural-tube defects (NTD) such as spina bifida. More than half of these defects could have been prevented with daily intake of 0.4 mg of folic acid throughout the childbearing years (CDC, 2005). In 1996, the U.S. Food and Drug Administration (FDA) established standards for fortifying cereal and grain products, including cereal, bread, rice, and pasta with folic acid in an effort to better supply this important dietary supplement (Tinkle & Sterling, 1997). Natural sources of folate (vitamin B) include dark green leafy vegetables, dried beans, oranges, and orange juice. Hilton (2002) investigated the folic acid intake of 18- to 24-year-old women in a private college and all were found to have an inadequate diet, especially for folic acid. Only 33% reported taking a daily multivitamin.

The school nurse may have an opportunity to observe some of the dietary habits of the pregnant student and to counsel the student about making healthy food choices and about following her healthcare provider's instructions regarding food selection. If a specific diet has been suggested or dietary supplements (i.e., vitamins, iron, folic acid) are prescribed, the nurse should inquire if the student has obtained them, review the reasons for taking them, and encourage the teen to ask questions or help her clarify information she does not understand. The nurse also needs to determine if food is available at the student's home or living arrangement. This is especially important with an economically deprived student in case the nurse needs to assist the teen in obtaining help from school or community resources.

The link between adequate intake of folic acid and the incidence of NTDs, the devastating effects of iron deficiency anemia on the mother and fetus, and the poor dietary choices of many adolescent females make a strong case for school nurse intervention with all adolescent females in an effort to improve birth outcomes for all their pregnancies. The school nurse has the opportunity in most schools to make presentations in the classroom and to suggest or provide resources for health education and/or parenting. In the clinic, the nurse has opportunities for spontaneous or planned teaching about nutrition and health and, in this way, can guide young people in making better choices regarding their nutrition.

Immunizations

The Advisory Committee on Immunization Practice (ACIP) of the CDC gives specific recommendations for vaccines that should be administered, if indicated, and vaccines that are contraindicated during pregnancy (CDC, 2003). Despite state laws requiring immunizations for school attendance in most states, many adolescents are not on schedule with these requirements. Revised schedules for boosters and new vaccines cause previously immunized adolescents to be out of compliance. Current ACIP immunization recommendations and schedules are available online (see Chapter 21), and healthcare providers should access these at frequent intervals to be aware of changes.

Routine vaccines that should be given if the pregnant adolescent is not currently protected are hepatitis B, influenza (inactivated), and tetanus/diphtheria. Live virus vaccines are generally contraindicated during pregnancy because of the theoretical risk of transmission of the vaccine virus to the fetus (CDC, 2003). These live attenuated vaccines include influenza, measles, mumps, rubella, and varicella. Other vaccines are not usually required unless the pregnant teen is traveling to a specific location or there is an outbreak of the disease (i.e., typhoid, rabies, etc.). These are listed in the ACIP online document.

Health and Human Services Departments have vaccine information fact sheets for each vaccine that are written in an easy to read style. These provide information about each disease, who should or should not receive the vaccine, what risks or problems are associated with the vaccine, what to do if there is a reaction, and how to obtain more information about the vaccine.

Substance Use, Misuse, and Abuse

Almost everything taken into the body during pregnancy is passed on to the fetus. Nicotine and other pollutants in cigarettes, alcohol, prescription medications, over-the-counter drugs, illegal drugs, and many chemical products used for cleaning or as weed and insect killers may be dangerous to the mother and to the fetus. Some of the consequences of the use of drugs include miscarriage, low birth weight babies, congenital anomalies, growth retardation, central nervous system abnormalities, and learning difficulties (Neinstein & Farmer, 2002). More information on the effects of substances on the fetus is available from prenatal clinics and health departments.

Alcohol, drugs, and other substances of abuse easily pass from a mother to her baby through the placenta. The effects of maternal smoking on the rate of spontaneous abortion, prenatal mortality, fetal growth, and childhood development make cigarette smoking one of the major hazards of pregnancy (Lee, 1999). In a study of pregnant adolescents with addiction, Bragg (1997) found pre-pregnancy substance abuse to be high, particularly among inner-city youth. Alcohol results in the possible development of fetal alcohol syndrome (see Chapter 35), which causes significant deficiencies in the child's mental development.

The FDA has assigned a pregnancy risk category to each systemically absorbed drug (medication) based on available clinical and preclinical information. The five categories—A, B, C, D, and X—reflect a drug's potential to cause birth defects. Although all drugs are best avoided during pregnancy whenever possible, this rating system permits an assessment of the risk/benefit ratio should a medication be required by a pregnant female. Drugs in category A are generally safe to use during pregnancy; categories B, C, and D carry progressively more risk. Drugs in category X are generally contraindicated (Deglin & Vallerand, 2005).

Herbal preparations are becoming increasingly popular and are easily accessible in health food, grocery, and drug stores. The FDA does not regulate these products for potency and content, nor does it study their claims of health benefit. Because they are advertised as "natural" and "traditional," some adolescents and adults do not consider them to be medications and do not realize they can be harmful to the mother or developing fetus (Lee, 1999). One such example is pennyroyal. Common names of pennyroyal are *squawmint*, *mosquito plant*, and *pudding grass*. The oil has been used by natural health advocates as an abortifacient and as a means to induce delayed menses. Herb teas made from this substance are generally without side effects, but toxicity is possible and there have been reports of adverse events and fatalities following its use (DerMardersoian & Beutler, 2002). Many herbal preparations contain toxic levels of heavy metals and other substances that could be harmful to the fetus (Lee, 1999).

It is important that the healthcare provider monitor correct use of the pregnant adolescent's medications and ensure that the adolescent understands the risk of substance abuse or misuse to herself and her fetus. The school nurse can discuss the proper use of prescribed medications and allow the student to ask questions to clarify her understanding of the purpose of medications. If the adolescent has used substances in the past that could have jeopardized the well being of her child, discussing or reading about possible birth defects can be frightening. She will need reassurance and will also need to understand the dangers and take precautions for the infant's health during the rest of her pregnancy.

Sexually Transmitted Diseases

Unprotected sexual intercourse places teenagers (and adults) at risk for human immunodeficiency virus (HIV) infection and other sexually transmitted diseases (STDs) (see Chapter 42). Compared to older adults, adolescents (10- to 19-year-olds) and young adults (20- to 24-year-olds) are at a higher risk for acquiring STDs because they may be more likely to have multiple (sequential or concurrent) sexual partners, rather than a single long-term relationship, and they may select partners at a higher risk for these diseases. For some STDs, such as *Chlamydia trachomatis* infection, adolescent women may have a physiologically increased susceptibility to infection due to increased cervical ectopy (CDC, Sexually Transmitted Disease Prevention, 2000b). Forty percent of all chlamydia cases reported are among young people ages 15 to 19. In addition, females in that age group have the highest rate of gonorrhea infection. If they are not detected and treated, these STDs and others can cause pelvic inflammatory disease, infertility, and ectopic pregnancy, and increase the risk for HIV transmission (CDC, STDP, 2000a,b).

CDC examined the sexual risk behavior in high school students during 1991–2001. Data from the national Youth Risk Behavior Survey indicated that during this 10-year period, the percentage of U.S. high school students who ever had sexual intercourse and the percentage who had multiple sex partners decreased (CDC, 2002b). The report also showed that among sexually active students from 1991 to 1999, the prevalence of condom use increased. These findings show that overall, fewer students are engaging in risky behaviors that might result in pregnancy and STDs, including HIV infection (CDC, 2002b). The improvements in health outcomes during the past 10 years are attributed to the combined efforts of parents and families, schools, community organizations that serve young people, healthcare providers, religious organizations, the media, and government agencies (CDC, 2002b).

Adolescents often lack knowledge of the symptoms of STDs, and frequently experience barriers to quality STD prevention and treatment services, including lack of insurance and ability to pay, lack of transportation, discomfort with facilities and services designed for adults, and concerns about confidentiality (CDC, 2002). The 1999 Youth Risk Behavior Survey (YRBS) (CDC, STD, 2000a) found that only 42.8% of females and 26.4% of males among high school students who received a routine health examination during the previous year, reported discussing STD or pregnancy prevention with their healthcare provider.

The school nurse is frequently the staff member who can share information with students about the dangers of STDs and how they can protect themselves from these diseases. This may be on a one-to-one basis or in health education or other classes. The nurse may also provide resource materials or invite presenters from local or state Health and Human Service departments, health educators from local universities, or other creditable sources to speak to students. State and local school policies and guidelines vary in what can be taught in the classroom about human growth and development and sexuality. The nurse should always obtain information about school regulations and guidelines and honor the state law and board of education policy before introducing resources or guest presenters. In one-on-one situations, school personnel generally may answer any questions a student may ask.

It is important for school nurses to be knowledgeable and willing to use their expertise and skills to pursue a change in regulations, policies, and guidelines that restrict information that might prevent harm to the students.

Spontaneous Abortion (Miscarriage)

Miscarriage is the most common complication of pregnancy. Approximately 15% of pregnancies end with a spontaneous abortion. It is estimated that two or three times more spontaneous abortions are unrecognized as a pregnancy loss (Scott, DiSaia, Hammond, & Spellacy, 1999). Bleeding, spotting, cramping or low backaches are frequent complaints of pregnant females. Symptoms of miscarriages vary, and the school nurse should refer pregnant students who report any bloody vaginal discharge or uterine bleeding to their healthcare provider or obstetrician for further diagnosis and treatment. If the healthcare provider determines that the cervix is still closed, the usual recommendation is for the pregnant female to remain at home on bed rest until symptoms cease or the condition worsens (Scott et al., 1999). If symptoms persist and the miscarriage proceeds, the healthcare provider may determine the need for medical or surgical intervention.

The school nurse should talk to the teen about physical and mental health needs following a miscarriage or on her return to school. The student may have recommendations from her healthcare provider to rest during the day or be excused from physical education until she receives written permission to resume all activities. Psychological and emotional needs may also need to be resolved and often the school nurse can initiate a conversation to open dialogue about the student's needs or concerns. While some may feel relief at the resolution of the problem, others may have feelings of guilt or ambivalence about the pregnancy loss. Anger, disappointment, and grief are generally present and may be misunderstood or misinterpreted by her friends and family. She may mourn the death of her potential child and question what is wrong with her body that she could not hold a pregnancy. It is important for the student and her partner to be able to express their feelings and resolve their concerns. If mental health counseling is needed, the school nurse can encourage one or both to seek help and she may refer them to a counselor in the school or community.

Hypertensive Disorders

Despite intensive research, how pregnancy increases or aggravates hypertension is not clearly known. "Hypertensive diseases that complicate pregnancy include gestational hypertension (formerly referred to as pregnancy-induced hypertension or transient hypertension), preeclampsia, eclampsia, preeclampsia superimposed on chronic hypertension and chronic hypertension" (Cunningham et al., 2001, p. 568).

An individual is diagnosed with hypertension when his or her blood pressure is 140/90 mm Hg or greater on two measurements taken 6 hours apart. Edema is no longer considered a diagnostic criterion because it occurs in many normal pregnant women. The risk of a hypertensive disorder in teens is due to their primigravida state, not necessarily their age. While the disease occurs most commonly in the last trimester, the adolescent who is late in beginning prenatal care may be seen for the first time in an advanced disease state. Hypertension may progress rapidly from mild to severe, and if untreated, to eclampsia (Cunningham et al., 2001).

In *gestational hypertension,* in addition to a blood pressure of above 140/90 mm Hg for the first time during pregnancy, headaches and epigastric discomfort may occur. However, proteinuria is not present (Cunningham et al., 2001).

In *preeclampsia*, in addition to an elevated blood pressure, proteinuria is present. There may also be persistent headaches, visual disturbances, and persistent epigastric or right upper quadrant pain. As *preeclampsia* continues and becomes more severe, thrombocytopenia is seen. The occurrence of seizures that cannot be attributed to other causes in a woman with *preeclampsia* indicates *eclampsia*. The seizures are grand mal and may start before, during, or after labor (Cunningham et al., 2001).

If the blood pressure measurement prior to pregnancy is not known, readings of 140/90 after 20 weeks of gestation are considered sufficiently elevated for a diagnosis of *preeclampsia*. This elevation must be present at two measurements taken 6 hours apart (Roberts, 1999, p. 833).

The school nurse can schedule the pregnant student for visits to the school nurse's office between the student's appointments with the healthcare provider. On these visits and other nonscheduled visits to the clinic, she needs to take the student's blood pressure and record the results on the student's healthcare record. Should any significant change be noted, she will need to make an immediate referral for the teen to her healthcare provider for care. The nurse will need to impress the importance of medical care to the pregnant teen and her parents or guardians and partner.

Preterm Labor, Preterm Birth, and Low Birth Weight

"Low birth weight" is the term used to define infants who are born too small (usually weighing less than 2,500 grams), and preterm or premature birth are the terms used to define infants who are born at less than 37 weeks' gestation (Cunningham et al., 2002). Preterm labor is defined as cervical changes and uterine contractions occurring between 20 and 37 weeks of pregnancy (American College of Obstetricians and Gynecologists [ACOG] and the American Academy of Pediatrics [AAP], 1997). Preterm labor and births result in approximately 75% of all perinatal mortality, and are second only to congenital anomalies as the leading cause of infant mortality in the United States (March of Dimes Birth Defects Foundation, 1997).

Risk factors for preterm labor and birth include being unmarried, African American, less than 17 years of age, of a low socioeconomic status, or having a decreased education level. It is also more common in those with a history of a previous preterm birth; multiple abortions (miscarriages or elective); anemia; poor nutrition; use or abuse of tobacco, alcohol, or other substances; and having late or no prenatal care (Cunningham et al., 2002). Medical and obstetrical complications include preeclampsia, fetal distress, fetal growth restriction, abruptio placentae, and fetal death (Cunningham et al., 2002).

Low birth weight describes infants weighing less than 2,500 g at birth, very low birth weight refers to infants weighing 1,500 g or less, and extremely low birth weight refers to infants weighing 1,000 g or less (Cunningham et al., 2001). Neonatal mortality rates are directly proportional to the infant's weight at delivery. Cities with large urban populations or with high poverty rates commonly have the highest incidence of low birth weight infants (Cunningham et al., 2001).

In recent years, the term "small for gestational age" has been used to categorize infants whose birth weight is below the 10th percentile for their gestational age. Other terms now used are fetal growth restriction and intrauterine growth restriction (Cunningham et al., 2001). Risk factors for low birth weight (fetal growth restrictions) include the following: constitutionally small mothers; poor maternal weight gain; poor nutritional status; social deprivation associated with lifestyle factors such as smoking, alcohol or other substances of abuse; fetal infections such as rubella, cytomegalovirus, and hepatitis A and B; congenital malformations; chromosomal abnormalities; primary disorders of cartilage and bone (such as osteogenesis imperfecta); maternal ingestion of chemical teratogens; chronic maternal hypoxia; maternal anemia; placental and cord anomalies; and multiple fetuses (Cunningham et al., 2001).

Many of the risk factors for low birth weight infants can be prevented or controlled prior to or during pregnancy. Births to adolescents account for a higher percentage of low birth weight infants and up to 25% of premature infant births in the United States (Davidson, 1998).

PSYCHOSOCIAL DEVELOPMENT OF ADOLESCENTS

Many pregnant teens have not yet reached cognitive or psychosocial maturity (see Chapter 16). The early adolescent (ages 10 to 14) is interested in being with the peer group and more often with a member of the same sex, a "best friend." Family relationships are usually important to them, but often take second place to peer relationships. Early adolescents are still moving in and out of the world of childhood, seeking guidelines and support as they attempt to define a new status and become independent (Radzik, Shere, & Neinstein, 2002). They are preoccupied with self and uncertain about their appearance (Hamburg, 1998). They are beginning to question almost everything and attempting to determine who they are and where they are going. This search for identity is described by Erickson's (1963) psychosocial theory as identity vs. role confusion. The early adolescent may show some degree of self-assurance, test parental and adult authority, have self-doubts, and may be rebellious (Radzik et al., 2002). However, many remain on good terms with their family members.

During middle adolescence (ages 14 to 17), pubertal changes are completed and sexual drives emerge. In many situations, the peer group sets behavior standards. Adolescents in this phase may vacillate between independence and dependence. They want parental support and guidance and they also want and take independent action. Abstract reasoning and introspection begin during this phase as well (Hamburg, 1998).

In late adolescence (> 17 years of age) physical maturation and identity formation should be near completion. Relationships in late adolescence are characterized by reciprocal giving and sharing. Typically, more time is spent in a relationship with one person rather than a peer group. Final independence from parents is almost complete, as is cognitive development (Hamburg, 1998). In late adolescence, positive outcomes include practical, realistic vocational goals leading to emotionally and economically autonomous adulthood (Radzik et al., 2002).

Extending Erikson's theory, Marcia (1966) identified four different styles or processes adolescents may use to establish and maintain their sense of personal identity. These classifications may be used to better understand how young people make career, marriage, and other crucial choices. The levels of the classifications are *achievement, moratorium, foreclosure*, and *diffusion*. Adolescents who demonstrate *identity achievement* have resolved their crisis regarding their identity, made judgments about their personal beliefs and goals, generally have high self-esteem, and accept a high level of responsibility. Individuals who are exploring possible alternatives are in the *moratorium* level. *Foreclosure* refers to the level where the individual takes the views of their parents or others as their own without a period of exploration or experimentation. *Identity diffusion* refers to a state of uncertainty about life choices and a lack of effort to make the choices (Hockenberry et al., 2003; Marcia 1966).

Adolescents in school who demonstrate identity achievement status generally have greater ego strength than the other three status groups. They persevere and perform better in stressful situations or crises (Marcia, 2002). When in the moratorium identity stage, the adolescent's behavior varies, but resembles identity achievers. With a foreclosed identity, there is typically a strong commitment to obedience, strong leadership, and respect for authority (Marcia, 2002).

Opportunities and experiences in the young person's social environment influence his or her identity development. With the more restrictive opportunities of some minority groups or among those living in poverty, foreclosure identity may be more common. Identity diffusion seems more common in minority males than other groups. Two barriers to identity formation among minority youth are conflicting values of the group to those of society and lack of adequate role models (Hockenberry et al., 2003).

All of these processes in psychosocial development may be altered in the pregnant teenager, although many deviations were present before the pregnancy occurred. Decisions made by the pregnant adolescent and her partner have serious consequences for their future. Some drop out of high school; others graduate from high school and continue their education for a chosen career; others get full time jobs. The school nurse has more contact with these students during this time of crisis and may be able to guide the adolescents and their parents, or to recommend appropriate guidance counselors in the school or community, who can assist with deliberations and decisions related to their education and careers.

SEXUAL BEHAVIOR

Physical, hormonal, cognitive, and social changes significantly impact adolescent sexual development (Hockenberry et al., 2003). Adolescents' concerns with their body image and new sexual feelings and practices cause them to compare themselves to peers and role models and to seek peer group approval and acceptance.

As they mature physically, part of their identity formation involves their sexual identity. Sexual feelings become stronger, libido is present in both sexes, and sexual fantasies or dreams are common. Beginning in early adolescence, males typically practice masturbation; the age at which females begin masturbation varies (Hockenberrry et al., 2003).

Close friendships established with same-sex peers in early adolescence may change to relationships with members of the opposite sex during middle adolescence. This usually begins with male and female group activities. Pairing as couples becomes more common as middle adolescence progresses. Relationships generally are not long lasting and deep romantic attachments are seldom formed during this time (Hockenberry et al., 2003).

As the adolescent's need for independence increases, rebellion against parents and their values and beliefs frequently results. Becoming involved in sexual relationships outside of marriage may be a way to demonstrate their independence. Sexual activity is more common in middle adolescence (see Chapter 40), and the relationship between love and sexual expression becomes important. Many view each relationship as real love.

POSTPARTUM DEPRESSION

Varying levels of depression, sometimes referred to as postpartum blues, are experienced by 80% of females (teens and adults) in the first few days and weeks following childbirth. It is likely caused by hormonal fluctuations (Fontaine, 2003). Females typically report feeling miserable, sad, discouraged, anxious, irritable, and sometimes mentally confused; they also cry easily.

If the depression continues and becomes more severe, as exhibited by constant feeling of tiredness, difficulty sleeping, and loss of appetite, a referral for professional counseling may be needed (American Psychiatric Association [APA], 2000). The teen may not be in school at this time, but a school nurse who has developed a relationship with her during her pregnancy may consider calling the teen mother or send a social worker to make a home visit. If signs of severe depression are noted, a referral should be made to a mental health specialist.

DEALING WITH DEATH, LOSS, AND GRIEF

When perinatal deaths occur, the school nurse may be a strong support for the teen. Although the student may not be in school, the school nurse who has developed a trusting relationship with the teen during pregnancy will be in a good position to continue to assist her. The school nurse or social worker should maintain a comprehensive list of resources for referral for adolescents who are grieving and/or depressed before a need arises. Support groups for adolescents may be available in the school and community.

Follow-up visits with adolescents who experience the death of their baby are recommended. The grief experience is a process that stretches over a lengthy period of time and may not proceed in a linear pattern to resolution. The stages in the grief process include denial, anger, bargaining, despair, and acceptance. Each stage may be "revisited" at any time before acceptance occurs (Kubler-Ross, 1969).

The pregnant teen or new mother may experience grief with spontaneous abortion (miscarriage), abortion, infant death related to prematurity, or the loss of the baby after adoption or foster care placement. The grief experience may occur immediately or much later in the life of the teen mother, especially on the anniversary of the child's birth, death, or loss. The school nurse may gently probe during conversation with the adolescent following these experiences. While grief following the death of a baby may be readily observed, the adolescent who experiences loss by adoption or foster care placement may not be able to realize or verbalize their feelings. The school nurse must remember to engage the adolescent in conversation privately and with sensitivity. The nurse needs to use compassionate inquiry to assess for signs and symptoms of grief and/or depression. A referral for professional counseling may be appropriate.

PREGNANT AND PARENTING STUDENTS IN SCHOOL

A successful school program for adolescent pregnant and parenting teens generally has two major components: *the development of an effective, comprehensive program and a staff committed to the program goals*. Initially, those who see the need for the program begin by forming work groups or committees, seeking funding, writing grants, and making proposals. These individuals are ultimately responsible for the initiation, ongoing development and evaluation of the program, or for identifying the persons who can assume these responsibilities. In large school districts, personnel may include the program director of health services (if this individual is not a nurse, a nurse representative should also be selected), counseling services, and/or psychological/social services or other program administrators. A school nurse needs to serve on this team also. In smaller districts it may be personnel in middle management or at a staff level. The success of any program for adolescents and especially those who are pregnant or parenting is also dependent on the second component, the effectiveness of the persons who actually implement the programs by facilitating and guiding this special group of young people toward successful outcomes in education and social and emotional growth (Wolf, 1999).

Pregnant and parenting teens often struggle with the dual challenges of meeting the normative developmental needs of adolescence and the demands associated with pregnancy and becoming a parent. Continuing school during pregnancy and returning to school following the birth of a child are not easy tasks. While still a high school student, the young mother and sometimes the young father must learn to cope with some very adult situations and are expected to make mature decisions regarding the child. Even with the very best of financial, home, and educational situations and opportunities, this is difficult. Teen mothers are not usually in stable family units. Finances are almost always a problem since many teen mothers may have little or no income. School pressures such as mandatory attendance, homework, and some teachers and staff who lack understanding of the student's situation add to the burden.

Unfortunately, many schools do not provide assistance to teens, and may actually discriminate against pregnant and parenting teens (Wolf, 1999). The teens may be placed in alternative programs rather than allowed to return to their original school; they may have excessive unexcused absences following the birth of their infant, or as a result of the infant's illness that may require them to repeat a class; they may be excluded from certain extracurricular activities such as the honor society. These barriers are not in accordance with federal law (Wolf, 1999).

Protecting Their Rights

Title IX of the Education Act of 1972 prohibits discrimination in educational institutions based on gender, and marital, pregnancy, or parenting status (FIGURE 41.5). The teen mother and father have equal rights to an education (Wolf, 1999). The school is required to treat absences due to childbirth the same way it treats absences due to other temporary disabilities (Wolf, 1999). In addition, Title IX makes it clear that pregnant and parenting students must be allowed to choose either to continue to attend their regular school or, if they choose, they may attend an alternative program or school. Alternative schools are required to have instructional programs equal to those of other school educational programs. Female teen parents cannot be required to take parenting education unless male student parents are also required to take the course (Wolf, 1999).

Title IX requires that policies regarding absences and leave of absence are the same for both

ARE YOU A PREGNANT TEEN, OR A TEEN MOTHER, AND STILL IN SCHOOL OR DID YOU LEAVE SCHOOL WHEN YOU BECAME PREGNANT OR AFTER YOUR BABY WAS BORN?

IF YOU ARE A PREGNANT TEEN OR A TEEN MOTHER, YOU HAVE THE RIGHT TO FINISH YOUR EDUCATION.

You have the right to:

- Stay in school and stay in your regular classes while you are pregnant and after your baby is born.
- Participate in all school and extracurricular activities, including sports and honors programs, if you are medically able to do so. Your school may need a letter from your doctor saying that you are medically able to participate in school activities, but only if it requires all other students to see a doctor for health problems.
- Participate in special programs for pregnant students, if one is available, and if you voluntarily choose to do so. No one in your school can force you to go to a special program. No one in your school can force you to take a special class for pregnant and parenting students, either.
- Have excused absences for health problems related to your pregnancy or childbirth.
- Follow your doctor's advice to stay home from school for as long as your doctor says you should.
- Return to your regular classes and activities after your baby is born at the same academic status you had before you left school because of your pregnancy.

Your school may not discriminate against you for being pregnant or for being a mother. This means that your school must treat pregnancy and childbirth the same as other medical conditions. For example:

- If other students who miss school for health reasons receive make-up assignments from their teachers, then you are entitled to receive make-up assignments for the classes that you miss because of pregnancy or childbirth.
- If home instruction is available for students who need to stay home due to a medical condition, then you are entitled to home instruction if your doctor says that you need to stay home from school because of your pregnancy or childbirth.

If you would like help enforcing any of your rights, we may be able to help you. We[1] can provide free legal services to help pregnant teens and teen mothers enforce their rights to stay in school and be treated fairly.

If you need help enforcing your rights, or if you would like more information about your rights, please contact the national Women's Law Center at 202-588-5180 or write to them at 11 DuPont Circle, NW, Suite 800, Washington, DC 20036.

[1]National Women's Law Center.

Figure 41.5 ■ Handout for students, their families, community members, teachers or others who have contact with pregnant teens. National Women's Law Center.

nonpregnant and parenting students. Schools may not require students to be absent for a specific number of days following the birth of the infant. Schools must make the same requirements for making up assignments and for home instruction for pregnant students as for any student who may be absent frequently due to a diagnosed health problem. Students may not be penalized for absences due to childbirth. If the school has a policy regarding the maximum number of days a student may be absent and still pass and this policy is waived for students with medical conditions or temporary disabilities, the policy must also be waived for pregnant and parenting students (Wolf, 1999). In addition, no restrictions can be placed on pregnant or parenting students' participation in extracurricular activities. More information on the interpretation of Title IX and details of the information to be included in drafting a school policy (Figure 41.5) are available from the National Women's Law Center, 11 Dupont Circle NW, Suite 800, Washington, DC 20038.

Providing Programs of Support and Services in the Schools

Some pregnant students will have special needs for their comfort and well being during the school day. Often these can be handled by understanding and helpful school personnel. They may include a need for more frequent restroom use; a need for more fluids and snacks to relieve nausea in early pregnancy; and help with difficulty in climbing stairs, carrying heavy books or book bags, and fitting into a chair/desk in some classrooms. If uniforms are worn by students, an adjustment for the pregnant student should be made. Pregnant students should be encouraged to share these or other problems or concerns with the school nurse, counselor, or other staff as she identifies a problem and needs help in resolving it.

After the birth of the baby, most adolescents will benefit from follow-up and intensive support for several years to achieve success and wellness. It is helpful if the school, community health centers, or pediatric clinics provide programs teaching specific tasks of child care such as infant holding, diapering, feeding, and burping. Helping the students learn about infant stimulation and how to accomplish this is also important. They need to know about normal developmental stages and realistic expectations for their child's abilities at different stages of development. In addition, they may need child care, job training, and information to help them with basic homemaking skills (Stephens, Wolf, & Batten, 1999).

The critical services needed to ensure the best outcomes for teen parents and their children include core services of developmentally appropriate child care; prenatal care and family planning services; preventive health care for infants and young children; and case management that includes assessment, care planning, and coordination of services in the areas of health, nutrition education, parenting, psychosocial development, life skills, and economic self-sufficiency (Stephens et al., 1999). Additional services and supports needed by some young parents and their child include transportation; counseling, including substance abuse counseling and treatment; housing assistance; and economic assistance (Stephens et al., 1999).

Some states and/or individual school districts have comprehensive programs for pregnant teens that provide many or all of these services, especially when personnel from the school district, community, and private and government agencies come together to address the needs of teen parents and their children. Additional information on these program components can be found at Web sites of the Center for Assessment and Policy Development Web site (http://www.capd.org) and the National Organization on Adolescent Pregnancy, Parenting and Prevention (http://www.noappp.org).

School-based programs may struggle with community expectations that the schools meet the needs of parenting students. Resources for educational dollars are continously stretched thin and school-based programs frequently struggle to meet even the basic non-educational needs of this population. Many services and supports necessary for these young families are outside of the school's domain (Stephens et al., 1999). Bringing the school and existing community-based services together in a comprehensive system may be faciliated by the school nurse or other school personnel who encourage systems to come together to develop a coordinated and comprehensive program in efforts to maximize their collobrative efforts and avoid duplication of services. Often schools have no state or local policies or administrative guidelines for pregnant and parenting teen programs. When a school program is supported by funding from grants or from other sources, specific requirements of the grant often determine the services and activities that are to be provided. School policies may limit providing some of the core services recommended and needed by these students. The school nurse needs to be an advocate for these students in the school setting.

FUNDING FOR PREGNANCY AND PARENTING PROGRAMS

To prevent students who are "at risk" from dropping out of school, state and local education agencies may commit additional educational funds to develop alternative instruction methodologies and other innovative educational approaches in regular and alternative schools (Stephens et al., 1999). Several states provide funds to local school districts through formulas based on the number of teen parents served through the schools. Funds may come to the district as a supplement to the average daily attendance (ADA) dollars. The ADA formula may generate additional funding for pregnant students when they are attending school and for a brief period of time following the birth of the infant. Some states require the school to use this money for core services or other programs for pregnant and parenting students, while others do not stipulate a requirement and the money may go to other programs.

State and local public health and social service agencies may also have monies available for use in school programs for teen pregnancy and parenting. Federal welfare reform legislation created the Temporary Assistance to Needy Families (TANF) program to replace an open-ended entitlement program of Aid to Families with Dependent Children (AFDC) program. TANF benefits are provided only to teen parents who are: 1) living under adult supervision, usually with their parents or other adult relatives; 2) younger than 18; and 3) enrolled in and attending an educational program if they have not completed their high school education or the equivalent (Stephens et al., 1999).

Program Personnel and Responsibilities

It is the responsibility of every adult in the school to be sensitive to the feelings and concerns of the adolescent who thinks she is pregnant or who is pregnant. The professional personnel most often employed in public schools who are capable of assisting pregnant and parenting students are the school nurse, social workers, school counselors, and/or school parenting education teachers. Suggested roles these professionals assume, or could assume, are designated in FIGURE 41.6.

The school nurse is often the first person the student confides in regarding her suspected pregnancy. The first step the nurse usually takes is to refer the teen to a healthcare agency or primary care physician. The teenager may also confide in school counselors, school social workers, teachers, or other adults because of an acute need of help, and/or a relationship of trust and respect.

The school nurse will develop an Individual Health Plan (IHP) similar to the one in Figure 41.6 and will assess, monitor, and advise the student who is pregnant. The nurse will ensure that the student is making and keeping appointments with her healthcare provider at required intervals and will schedule visits to the school health room between prenatal or physician visits to monitor the pregnant adolescent's weight, blood pressure, and general health status. This may be kept on a Healthcare Monitoring and Counseling Record for Pregnant

Assisting and Educating the Adolescent Who Is Pregnant

NURSING DIAGNOSIS: Ineffective individual coping Situational crisis (pregnancy) as evidenced by inability to meet age-appropriate role expectations	**NURSING DIAGNOSIS/ KNOWLEDGE DEFICITS:** Signs and symptoms of pregnancy as evidenced by adolescent's health-seeking behavior (or) as evidenced by adolescent's visit to school nurse regarding a diagnosis of pregnancy.
EXPECTED OUTCOME: Adolescent makes decisions regarding the outcomes of the pregnancy.	**EXPECTED OUTCOME:** Adolescent will verbalize understanding of signs and symptoms of pregnancy and will express willingness to seek advice from her primary care-provider or appropriate counselor.
NURSING INTERVENTIONS/ RATIONALES: Encourage discussion of feelings of helplessness and confusion and, refer adolescent to resource clinic/agency or private care-provider who will explore with adolescent alternative ways for handling this issue; provide support and positive feedback to her as new coping strategies are tried in an effort to empower her to deal appropriately with feelings. Discourage displacement of anger regarding this situation crisis onto others and encourage the use of acceptable behaviors.	**NURSING INTERVENTIONS/ RATIONALES:** Provide information regarding pregnancy, nutrition, and rest. Monitor weight, blood pressure. Ensure psychosocial support. Plan to meet academic needs during absence for the delivery.

Individual Health Plan

Figure 41.6 ■ Individual Health Plan.

Students as in Figure 41.7 or a similar record that will help ensure that findings are recorded in a systematic consistent and confidential manner.

Frequently nurses use the student visits to the clinic for planned or incidental teaching. Brief conferences with pregnant students regarding some of the physical changes she may anticipate or be experiencing during her pregnancy, her personal health concerns during pregnancy, the availability of special community health or medical services, her nutrition, healthy lifestyle, the use and misuse of medication, and the upcoming hospital experience are often beneficial to the young teen and may reinforce what she is learning from her parenting classes and from her healthcare provider. It is also important to ensure that she has sufficient psychosocial support.

CONCLUSION

The outcomes of successful school and community programs for pregnant and parenting teens are students who have a healthy pregnancy and a healthy baby, who complete high school, do not have repeat unintended pregnancies, have adequate parenting skills, and provide a healthy start for their children. The support and understanding of school personnel can assist the pregnant teen through this monumental crisis in her life and in her partner's life to

(text continues on page 986)

HEALTHCARE MONITORING AND COUNSELING RECORD FOR PREGNANT STUDENTS

Demographic Data:

Student's Name:			Date:	Home School:
Married: ☐ yes ☐ no	If yes, Husband's Name:			
Address:				Home Phone:
Maternal Grandmother of Baby:				Work Phone:
Address:				
Maternal Grandfather of Baby:				Work Phone:
Address:				
Student's Age:	DOB:	LMP:	EDD:*	Week or Month of Pregnancy:
Current Gravida:	Para:	AB:		
Clinic or Physician:		Phone:		First Appointment:

Routine prenatal healthcare visits are scheduled: Every 4 weeks up to 32 weeks (end of this period) ______
Every 2 weeks up to 36 weeks (end of this period) ______
(Write in pencil)

Then prenatal visits every week until delivery. Record date below for next prenatal appointment and school nurse visit. When the appointment/visit has been kept or changed, record the new date. Student to be seen by school nurse approximately midway between obstetric visits.

Next Prenatal Appointment: ______ *(Write in pencil)* **Next School Nurse Visit:** ______ *(Write in pencil)*

HISTORY

I. Health problem(s) during past 12 months (list and describe management/treatment):

II. Past History (list with date and age):

Hospitalizations (overnight stay, emergency room visit, outpatient, day surgery):

Illness (contagious diseases, childhood diseases, high fever, etc.):

Injuries (accidents, ingestions, head injury):

Medications:

Allergies:

Last HealthCare Visit Before Pregnancy: ______ Name of Provider: ______

Purpose of visit (acute care, routine physical exam): ______

Last Dental Care Visit: Purpose: Provider:

III. Family History:

Biological Father: Age: ____ Health: ______

Maternal Grandparents of Baby:
1. Grandmother - Age: ____ Health: ______
2. Grandfather - Age: ____ Health: ______

Paternal Grandparents of Baby:
1. Grandmother - Age: ____ Health: ______
2. Grandfather - Age: ____ Health: ______

Familial Diseases: (circle) heart disease, stroke, hypertension, diabetes, asthma, allergy, anemia, sickle cell disease or trait, arthritis, cancer (breast, ovarian), epilepsy, cataracts, glaucoma, kidney disease, tuberculosis, mental problems, mental retardation, learning problems, congenital anomalies, other.

Explain: ______

*Expected Date of Delivery

Figure 41.7 ■ Healthcare monitoring and counseling record for pregnant students.

IV. Psychosocial History:

Family Support System (friends, relatives, relationships, interactions):
Household Members:
Self-concept (positive/negative feelings about self):
Housing:
Plans for Future:

Child: Discussion with student date:
Referral for counseling date:
Follow up / Decision about relinquishment or keeping:
Childcare Plans:

Self: Education:
Parenting Classes:
Prenatal Classes:
High School:
Trade School/Alternative School:
College;
Marriage:

V. Past OB History (previous pregnancy if applicable):

Gravida:__________ *(# of pregnancies)* Para:__________ *(# of live babies)* AB:__________

Delivery Date(s): 1.________ Type: (circle) Vaginal C-Section If C-Section, why?________
Maternal Age:________ Length of Pregnancy:________

2.________ Type: (circle) Vaginal C-Section If C-Section, why?________
Maternal Age:________ Length of Pregnancy:________

3.________ Type: (circle) Vaginal C-Section If C-Section, why?________
Maternal Age:________ Length of Pregnancy:________

Habits: (circle) smoking, drinking, drugs, pica, other__________
Explain:__________

High Risks: (circle) infections, bleeding, high blood pressure, anemia, fever, RH factor, trauma, inherited diseases(s), medications, weight gain, chronic disease, hospitalization, other__________
Explain:__________

VI. Review of Systems (includes past and present history of each system): (circle and explain)

General: Changes in weight, appetite, activity level, bowel habits, resistance to disease, other. Birth defects (congenital anomalies)
Skin: Rashes, easy bruising changes in skin color or texture, eczema, impetigo, growths, or tumors
Head: Headache, trauma, infections
Eyes: Vision changes, trauma, infections, cataracts, glaucoma, other
Ears/Nose/Throat: Infections (specify), trauma, epistaxis, allergies, hearing changes, voice changes, canes, speech problems
Neck: Trauma, swollen lymph nodes, limitation of movement
Respiratory: Infections, breathing problems, trauma, wheezing, cough, asthma
Cardiovascular: Murmur, fatigue with exertion, cyanosis
Gastrointestinal: Abdominal pain, nausea, jaundice, vomiting, diarrhea, constipation, ulcer
Genitourinary: Infections, enuresis, encopresis, discharge, rashes, menstruation, sexual development
Musculoskeletal: Trauma, limitation of movement, joint pain or swelling, growths of tumor, curvature of the spine, braces, corrective shoes
Neurological: Birth injury, trauma, seizures (febrile vs. afebrile), staring spells, poor coordination or balance, dizziness, syncope, developmental evaluation
Endocrine: Increased thirst, appetite, urination, diabetes, thyroid problems
Hematologic: Anemia, blood transfusions, blood dyscrasia, sickle cell
Psychosocial: Changes inactivity level, behavior, relationships, punishment, rewards
Nutrition: 24-hour recall including snacks

VII. Post Delivery History (current pregnancy):

Labor and Delivery: Location:__________
Length of Labor (hrs):________ Type of Delivery: (circle) Vaginal C-section
Condition of Mother (list problems):
Condition of Newborn: Birth Wt.________ lbs.________ oz. (breathing, infections, RH factors, jaundice, transfusions, bleeding, congenital anomalies, feeding other)

Postnatal: Home from Hospital: Mother in________ days. Baby in________ days.
Complications:

Neonatal (28 days): Complications:

Return to School:________ Postpartum Check Up:________

Childcare Arrangements:________ Lives with:________

Pre-Pregnant Weight:________ Date:________ Pre-Pregnant BP: ____/____ Date:________

Figure 41.7 ■ *(continued)*

MONITORING–COUNSELING RECORD

To be completed at specific intervals between healthcare provider visits.

DATE	WT.	B.P.	VISITS WITH SCHOOL NURSE – COMMENTS: Inquire specifically about nutrition, headaches, altered vision, abdominal pain, nausea, vomiting, bleeding, vaginal discharge, dysuria. Ask about health, nutrition, classes (i.e., prenatal, parenting, taken by student). The school nurse may review a common health problem or concern at each visit and discuss with student.
		/	
		/	
		/	
		/	
		/	
		/	
		/	
		/	
		/	
		/	
		/	
		/	
		/	
		/	
		/	
		/	
		/	
		/	
		/	
		/	
		/	
		/	
		/	
		/	
		/	
		/	
		/	
		/	
		/	

Figure 41.7 ■ *(continued)*

be successful and to provide a successful life for their family.

References

Alan Guttmacher Institute. (1999a). *Teen sex and pregnancy: Facts in brief*. New York: Author. Retrieved November 23, 2003 from http://agi_usa.org/pubs/fb_teen_sex.html.

Alan Guttmacher Institute. (1999b). *Teenage pregnancy: overall trends and state by state information*. New York: Author. Retrieved November 17, 2003 from http://www.agi_usa.org/pubs/teen_preg_stats.html

Alan Guttmacher Institute. (2002). *Teen pregnancy: Trends and lessons learned*. The Guttmacher Report on Public Policy, 5(1) New York: Author. Retrieved November 21, 2003 from/http://www.agi_usa.org/journals/tgr–archive.html

Alan Guttmacher Institute (2003a). *State policies in brief: Minors rights as parents*. New York. Author. Retrieved November 17, 2003 from http://www.agi_usa.org/pubs/spib.html

Alan Guttmacher Institute. (2003b) *State policies in brief: parental involvement in minors' abortions*. New York: Author. Retrieved November 17, 2003 from http://www.agi–usa.org/pubs/spib.html

American College of Obstetricians and Gynecologists (ACOG) and the American Academy of Pediatrics (AAP). (1997). *Guidelines for perinatal care* (4th ed.). Washington, DC: Author.

American Psychiatric Association (APA). (2000). *Diagnostic and statistical manual of mental disorders (4th ed., text revision)*. Washington, DC: Author.

Barr, L., & Monserrat, C. (2002). *Working with pregnant and parenting teens*. Family Service Division of the Health and Environment Department of New Mexico. Albuquerque, NM.

Bragg, E. (1997). Pregnant adolescents with addictions. *Journal of Obstetric, Gynecologic and Neonatal Nursing, 26*(5), 577–584. Retrieved November 17, 2003 from http://www.cdc.gov/mmwr/preview/mmwrhtml/00056982.htm

Centers for Disease Control and Prevention (CDC), Sexually Transmitted Disease Prevention. (2000a). *Most teens not provided STD or pregnancy prevention counseling during check-ups: Opportunity to educate often overlooked according to CDC study*. Retrieved October 22, 2003 from http://www.cdc.gov/nehstp/dstd/Pree Releases/Teens 2000.htm

Centers for Disease Control and Prevention (CDC), Sexually Transmitted Disease Prevention. (2000b). *Sexually transmitted diseases in adolescents and young adults*. Special Focus Profiles. Retrieved November 22, 2003 from http://www.cdc.gov/std/stats001/2000SFAdol&YAdults.htm

Centers for Disease Control and Prevention (CDC), National Center for Health Statistics. (2002a). *Prevalence of overweight among children and adolescents: United States, 1999–2002*. Retrieved October 18, 2004 from http://www.cdc.gov/nchs/products/pubs/pubd/hestats/overwght99.htm

Centers for Disease Control and Prevention (CDC). (2002b). *Trends in sexual risk behaviors among high school students – United States, 1991–2001*. Morbidity and Mortality Weekly Report, 51(38), 856–859. Retrieved November 21, 2003 from http://www.cdc.gov/mmwr/preview/mmwrhtml/mm5138a2.htm

Centers for Disease Control and Prevention (CDC). (2003). *Guidelines for vaccinating pregnant women: Recommendations of the Advisory Committee on Immunization Practices*. Retrieved October 24, 2003 from http://www.cdc.gov/nip/publications/ preg_guide.html

Centers for Disease Control and Prevention (CDC). (2004). Youth risk behaviors surveillance – United States 2003. *Morbidity and Mortality Weekly Report, 53* (SS–2), 21. Retrieved October 19, 2004 from http://www.cdc.gov.mmwr

Centers for Disease Control and Prevention (CDC). (2005). *Folic acid: PHS recommendations*. Retrieved September 28, 2005 from http://www.cdc.gov/ncbddd/folic acid/health_recomm.htm

Center for Nutrition Policy and Promotion. (2003). *Food guide pyramid images*. United States Department of Agriculture and the Department of Health and Human Services. Retrieved November 22, 3003 from http://www.usda.gov/cnpp/graphics.html

Chandra, A., Abma, J., & Bachrac, C. (1999). *Adoption, adoption seeking and relinquishment for adoption in the United States. Advanced data from vital and health statistics*. No. 306, 1–14. Hyattsville, MD: National Center for Health Statistics. Retrieved November 22, 2003 from http://www.cdc.gov/nchs/data/ad/ad306.pdf

Cohn, D., Gelfman, M., & Schwab, N. (2001). Adolescent issues and rights of minors. In N. Schwab & M. Gelfman (Eds.), *Legal issues in school health services: A resource for school administrators, school attorneys, and school nurse* (pp. 231–260). North Branch, NM: Sunrise River, Press.

Culp, R., Appelbaum, M., Osofsky, J., & Levy, J. (1988). Adolescent and older mothers: Comparisons between prenatal, maternal variables, and newborn interaction measures. *Infant Behavior Development, 58*, 964–975.

Cunningham, F., Gant, N., Leveno, K., Gilstrap, L., Hauth, J., & Wenstrom, K. (2001). *Williams obstetrics* (21st ed.). New York: McGraw-Hill.

Davidson, N. W. (1998). Adolescent pregnancy. In S. Friedman, M. Fisher, S. Schonberg, & E. Alderman (Eds.), *Comprehensive adolescent healthcare* (2nd ed., pp. 1128–1141). St. Louis: C. V. Mosby.

Davies, S., DiClemente, R., Wingood, G., Harrington, K., Crosy, R., & Sionean, C. (2003). Pregnancy desire among disadvantaged AfricanAmerican adolescent females. *American Journal of Health Behavior, 27* (1), 55–62.

Deglin, J. H., & Vallerand, A. H. (2005). *Davis's Drug Guide For Nurses* (9th ed.). Philadelphia: F. A. Davis.

DerMarderosian, A., & Beutler, A. J. (Eds.). (2002). *The review of natural products. Facts and comparison* (3rd ed.). Philadelphia: Lippincott Williams & Wilkins.

Emans, S. J., Smith, V. A. M., & Laufer, M. R. (1998). Teenage pregnancy. In S. J. Emans, M. R. Laufer, & D. P. Goldstein (Eds.), *Pediatric and adolescent gynecology* (pp. 675–713). Philadelphia: Lippincott-Raven.

Erickson, E. (1963). *Childhood and society* (2nd ed., pp. 216–274). New York: W. W. Norton.

Esparza, D., & Esperat, M. (1996). The effects of childhood sexual abuse on minority mothers. *Journal of Obstetric, Gynecologic, and Neonatal Nursing*, 25(4), 321–328.

Fontaine, K. (2003). *Mental health nursing* (5th ed.). Uper Saddle River, NJ: Prentice-Hall.

Get Real About Teen Pregnancy. (2002). *Cultural differences influence teen pregnancy prevention efforts*. News release by California Wellness Foundation. Sacramento, CA. Retrieved November 23, 2003 from http://www.letsgetreal.org/english/nr_Voices_2002.htm

Hamburg, B. A. (1998). Psychosocial development. In S. Friedman, M. Fisher, S. Schonberg, & E. Alderman (Eds.), *Comprehensive adolescent healthcare* (2nd ed., pp. 38–49). St. Louis: C. V. Mosby

Henshaw, S. (1999). *U.S. Teenage pregnancy statistics with comparative statistics for women age 20–24*. New York: Alan Guttmacher Institute.

Hilton, J. (2002). Folic acid intake of young women. *Journal of Obstetric, Gynecologic and Neonatal Nursing, 31*, 172–177.

Hockenbery, M., Wilson, D., Winkelstein, M., & Kline, N. (2003). *Wong's nursing care of infants and children* (7th ed.). St. Louis: C. V. Mosby.

Juszczak, L. (1998). Adolescent parenthood. In S. Freidman, M. Fisher, S. Schonberg & E. Alderman (Eds.), *Comprehensive adolescent healthcare* (2nd ed., pp. 1142–1147). St. Louis: C. V. Mosby

Kirby, D. (1997). *No easy answers: Research findings on programs to reduce teen pregnancy*. Washington, DC: The National Campaign to Prevent Teen Pregnancy.

Kirby, D. (2001). *Emerging answers: Research findings on programs to reduce teen pregnancy*. Washington, DC: The National Campaign to Prevent Teen Pregnancy. Retrieved November 23, 2003 from http://teenpregnancy.org/resources/data/pdf/emeranswersvm.pdf

Kirby, D. (2002). Antecedents of adolescent initiation of sex, contraceptive use and pregnancy. *American Journal of Health Behavior, 26*(6), 473–485.

Klerman, L. (1993). Adolescent pregnancy and parenting: Controversies of the past and lessons for the future. *Journal of Adolescent Health, 14*, 553–561.

Kubler-Ross, E. (1969). *On death and dying*. New York: Macmillan.

Lee, R. G.(1999). Substance abuse. In G. Burrow & T. Duffy (Eds.), *Medical complications during pregnancy* (5th ed, pp. 495–513). Philadelphia: W. B. Saunders.

MacKenzie, R. G., & Kipke, M. D. (1998). Substance use and abuse. In S. Freidman, M. Fisher, S. Schonberg & E. Alderman (Eds.), *Comprehensive adolescent health-care* (2nd ed., pp. 825–848). St. Louis: C. V. Mosby.

Marcia, J. (1966). *Ego identity status: Relationship to change in self esteem, general maladjustment and authoritarianism*. Research paper presented at the European Psychiatric Association convention.

Marcia, J. (2002). Adolescence identity and the Bernardone family. *Identity: An International Journal of Theory and Research, 2*(3),

March of Dimes Birth Defects Foundation. (1997). Statbook. White Plains, New York: Author.

Mazza, C. (2002) Young dads: The effect of a parenting program on urban African American adolescent fathers. *Adolescence, 37*(148), 681–687).

Miller, B., Bayley, B., Christensen, M., Leavitt, S., & Coyl, D. (2003). Adolescent pregnancy and childbearing. In G. Adams and M. Berzonsky, *Blackwell handbook of adolescence* (pp. 415–449). Malden MA: Blackwell Publishing.

Mosher, W., & Bachrach, C. (1996). Understanding U.S. fertility: Continuity and change in the national survey of family growth 1988–1995. *Family Planning Perspectives, 28* (1). Retrieved 10/10/2003 from http://www.guttmacher.org/pubs/journals/280049b.html

National Association of School Nurses (NASN). (1997). *Adolescent parents position statement*. Retrieved 8/16/04 from www.nasn.org

National Association of State Boards of Education (NASBE). (1998). *A call to action: What schools can do to prevent teen pregnancy and promote student achievement*. Proceedings from a National Forum for Representatives of State and Local Boards of Education. Washington, DC: Author.

National Campaign to Prevent Teen Pregnancy. (2001). *Half way there: A prescription for continued progress in preventing teen pregnancy*. Washington, DC: Author.

Neinstein, L. S., & Farmer, M. (2002). Teenage pregnancy. In L.S. Neinstein (Ed.). *Adolescent health care: A practical guide* (pp. 810–833). Philadelphia: Lippincott Williams & Wilkins.

Neinstein, L. S., & Schack, L. E. (2002). Nurtition. In L. S. Neinstein (Ed.). *Adolescent health care: A practical guide* (pp. 170–185). Philadelphia: Lippincott Williams & Wilkins.

Newton, J., Adams, R., & Marcontel, M. (1997). *The new school health handbook* (3rd ed.). Upper Saddle River, NJ: Prentice Hall.

Olds, S., London, M., Ladewig, P., & Davidson, M. (2004). *Maternal–newborn nursing & women's health care*. Upper Saddle River, NJ: Pearson, Prentice-Hall.

Perrin, K., & Dorman, K. (2003). Teen parents and academic success. *Journal of School Nursing, 19*(5), 288–293.

Polaneczky, M., & O'Connor, K. (1999). Pregnancy in the adolescent patient: Screening, diagnosis and initial management. *Pediatric Clinics of North America, 46*(4), 649–668.

Radzik, M., Sherer, S. E., & Neinstein, L. S. (2002). Psychological development in normal adolescents. In L. S. Neinstein (Ed.), *Adolescent healthcare. A practical guide* (pp. 52–58). Philadelphia: Lippincott Williams & Wilkins.

Roberts, J. M. (1999). Pregnancy related hypertension. In R. Creasy & R. Resnik (Eds.), *Maternal–fetal medicine* (pp 833–872). Philadelphia: W. B. Saunders.

Schultz, K. (2001). Constructing failure, narrating success: Rethinking the problem of teen pregnancy. *Teachers College Record, 103*(4), 582–607. Teachers College, Columbia University, New York.

Scott, J., DiSaia, P., Hammond, C., & Spellacy, W. (1999). *Danforth's obstetrics and gynecology*. Philadelphia: Williams & Wilkins.

Stephens, S., Wolf, W., & Batten, S. (1999). *Improving outcomes for teen parents and their young children by strengthening school-based programs: Challenges, solutions and policy implications*. Center for Assessment and Policy Development. Byla Cynwyd, PA. Retrieved 11/23/2003 from https://www.capd.org./home/publications/PDF/policy pdf

Strasburger, V., & Brown, R. (1998). *Adolescent medicine: A practical guide*. Philadelphia: Lippincott-Raven.

Tinkle, M., & Sterling, B. (1997). Neural tube defects: A primary prevention role for nurses. *Journal of Obstetric, Gynecologic and Neonatal Nursing, 26*, 503–511.

U.S. Department of Health and Human Services (2000). *Healthy People 2010: Understanding and improving health* (2nd ed.). Washington, DC: U.S. Government Printing Office.

Ventura, S., Matthews, T., & Curtin, S. (1998). Declines in teenage pregnancy rates, 1991–1997: National and

State patterns. *National Vital Statistics Reports, 47*(12). Hyattsville, MD: National Center for Vital Statistics. Retrieved 11/23/2003 from http://www.cdc.gov.nchs/data/nvsr 47/nus47___12.pdf

Ventura, S., Martin, J., Curtin, S., Matthews, T., & Park, M. (1998). Births: Final data for 1998. *National Vital Statistics Reports, 48*(3) Hyattsville, MD: National Center for Vital Statistics. Retrieved November 23, 2003 from http://www/nber.org/natality/1998/docs/nvsr48/nvs48___12pdf

Ventura, S., Matthews, T., & Hamilton, B. (2001). Births to teenagers in the United States 1940–2000. *National Vital Statistics Reports, 49* (10), Hyattsville, MD, National Center for Health Statistics. Retrieved 8/14/2003 from http://www.cdc.gov/nchs/data/nvsr49/nus49_10.pdf

Ventura, S., Matthews, T., & Hamilton B. (2002). Teenage births in the United States: State trends 1991–2000, an update. *National Vital Statistics Reports, 50*(9). Hyattsville, MD: National Center for Health Statistics. Retrieved November 23, 2003 from http://www.cdc.gov/nchs/data/nvsr/nvsr50/nvsr50_09pdf

Ventura, S., Mosher, W., Curtin, M., Abma, J., & Henshaw, S. (2001). Trends in pregnancy rates for the United States 1976–97: An update. *National Vital Statistics Reports, 49*(4), Hyattsville, MD: Center for Disease Control and Prevention. Retrieved November 22, 2003 from http://www.cdc.gov/nchs/data/nvsr49/nvsr49_04.pdf

Wenstrom, K., & Malee, M. P. (1999). Complications of pregnancy. In J. Scott, P. DiSaia, C. Hammond, & W. Spellacy (Eds.), *Danforth's obstetrics and gynecology* (pp. 327–361). Philadelphia: Lippincott Williams & Wilkins.

Wolf, W. (1999). *Using Title IX to prevent the rights of pregnant and parenting teens*. Center for Assessment and Policy Development. Retrieved February 26, 2003 from http://www.capd.org.home/publications/PDF/policy.pdf

Chapter 42

Sexually Transmitted Diseases

LYNN E. KELLY

Chapter Outline

INTRODUCTION

"STDs are hidden epidemics of enormous health and economic consequences in the United States. They are hidden because many Americans are reluctant to address sexual health issues in an open way and because of the biologic and social characteristics of these diseases" (Institute of Medicine, 1997, p. 43). Although the origin of sexually transmitted diseases (STDs) remains obscure, references to them are found in writings from thousands of years ago. Symptoms consistent with diseases including herpes and syphilis are found in writings about the lives of such famous individuals as Cleopatra and Christopher Columbus (Luger, 1993).

Today, STDs among teenagers and young adults remain a major health problem in the United States. Of all age groups, adolescents are at greatest risk for contracting an STD. It is estimated that 25% of all new cases of HIV infection occur in individuals younger than the age of 20 (Centers for Disease Control and Prevention [CDC], 2000).

Two-thirds of those who contract an STD are 25 years of age or younger (Braverman, 2000). One in four teenagers in the United States contract an STD. Almost 46% of high school students report having ever had sexual intercourse. Only 57.9% of this population reported using a condom during the last sexual intercourse, and 20% of high school seniors have had four or more sexual partners (CDC, 2002a).

Adolescents are also at risk for re-infection because of reluctance to notify partners who would then also be treated (Macke & Maher, 1999). In fact, partner notification by an infected individual occurs in only 30%-60% of the cases (Van De Loar, Termorshuizen, & Van Den Hoek, 1997). It is clear that STDs are a major problem among school-age youth. School nurses should take an active role in providing students with sound knowledge and strategies on the prevention and treatment of STDs.

WHAT IS SEX?

Various reports and studies have amassed a large database on adolescent sexual activity. Almost exclusively, however, these data have focused on vaginal intercourse. This focus has partially been explained by the concern over teenage pregnancy. Adolescent pregnancy rates have been decreasing, but STD rates remain high among this population. It is apparent that adolescents are participating in other forms of sexual activity that do not present the risk for pregnancy, but continue to provide exposure to STDs. These behaviors include oral sex, mutual masturbation, and anal sex (Panchaud, Singh, Feivelson, & Darroch, 2000).

Present-day adolescents are growing up in the age of acquired immunodeficiency syndrome (AIDS). They associate the risk of transmission of the virus that causes AIDS with vaginal intercourse. Unfortunately, STDs can be transmitted during other forms of sexual activity as well. Human immunodeficiency virus (HIV) can be transmitted via rectal sex; human papillomavirus, herpes simplex virus, hepatitis B, gonorrhea, syphilis, and chlamydia can be transmitted during oral sex (Remez, 2000). Girls perceive oral sex to be less risky and preferable to vaginal intercourse because there is no risk of becoming pregnant, believe that they will not contract a disease, and know that they will not lose their virginity using this modality. Some studies have shown that almost half of the adolescents surveyed stated that oral sex did not count as sex (Remez, 2000).

Adolescents and adults may differ in whether a particular activity is sexual, and this may present a challenge when providing adolescents with information related to sexual behaviors. Programs for adolescents where the focus is on pregnancy prevention may unintentionally be promoting sexual behaviors that place members of this group at increased risk for contracting an STD. When stressing abstinence, it is necessary to be specific in defining those behaviors that constitute sexual activity. Adolescents also need to be aware of the risk of contracting an STD from non-intercourse modalities such as in hot tubs.

ADDRESSING THE STD PROBLEM

Numerous governmental and private organizations have committed funds and resources directed at screening for and preventing STDs. Healthy People 2010 (U.S. Department of Health and Human Services [USDHHS], 2000) identifies responsible sexual behavior as one of the priority national health objectives for adolescents. However, adolescents face multiple barriers to adopting safe sexual behaviors as well as accessing services for both the prevention and treatment of STDs.

Practicing safer sex requires a level of thinking and behavior often beyond typical adolescent developmental characteristics. First, the adolescent must admit to him- or herself that the likelihood for sexual intercourse exists. Often this denial of anticipation for sex prevents prior planning and the provision of protection. Next, adolescents must recognize that they are at risk for acquiring an STD. Romantic thoughts about the perceived or fantasized virtues of their partner may limit teenagers' ability to believe that previous sexual experience by the partner may expose them to an infection. Poor communication skills and lack of experience make it difficult for adolescents to discuss touchy subjects such as safer sex practices. Female adolescents often lack the assertiveness to insist that their partner use a condom.

Adolescents face challenges accessing services for prevention of and treatment for STDs. Most communities have free clinics where adolescents can receive STD screening and treatment. However, many teens are unaware of these services or are reluctant to seek out care in a setting that is primarily for adults. In addition, the stigma associated with an STD may make the adolescent feel self-conscious in the health care setting (McEvoy & Coupey, 2002). Adolescents have the legal right to confidential STD diagnosis and treatment (Schwab & Gelfman, 2001). Ensuring that the findings of their test will remain confidential may make the teen more likely to seek treatment.

Among the recommendations made by The Institute of Medicine's Committee on Prevention and Control of Sexually Transmitted Diseases (1997) was that schools play an active role in providing age-appropriate STD-related services focusing on prevention and treatment. School nurses, therefore, should take the leading role in the implementation of programs that provide school-age children and adolescents with information about their developing sexuality, including information related to prevention and treatment of sexually transmitted diseases.

Box 42.1 ▪▪▪

RESOURCES FOR STUDENTS AND FAMILIES

Coalition for Positive Sexuality (http://www.positive.org). Information is presented in Spanish and English. Teens are able to pose questions to experts.

Families Are Talking (http://www.familiesaretalking.org/teen). Sponsored by the Sexuality Information and Education Council of the United States (SIECUS). This site provides extensive information for teens and parents on a wide range of sexuality issues.

Go Ask Alice (http://www.goaskalice.columbia.edu). From Columbia University's program in Health Education. This site provides extensive information on not only sexual health, but also a wide range of health subjects. Teens can search for topics or ask questions.

Iwannaknow (http://www.iwannaknow.org). The American Social Health Association sponsors this site, on which teens can find games that provide information on sexual health services, join a chat room, and search for special topics of interest.

Scarleteen (http://www.scarleteen.com). A site for gay, bisexual, transgender, and questioning youth.

Sex Etc. (http://www.sxetc.org). This site is sponsored by the Network for Family Life Education. There is an online newsletter, advice and information on a wide range of topics, message boards, and information for parents.

Sex Sense (http://www.ppsp.org/tpe.html). Planned Parenthood of Southeastern Pennsylvania sponsors this site that provides advice for teens by other teens.

Teenwire (http://www.teenwire.com). A site with a wide range of pertinent information on sexuality issues, sponsored by Planned Parenthood Federation of America.

Box 42.2 ▪▪▪

RESOURCES FOR SCHOOL NURSES

AIDSinfo (www.aidsinfo.nih.gov). AIDSinfo is a U.S. Department of Health and Human Services project that provides information on HIV/AIDS clinical trials and treatment.

American Social Health Association (http://www.ashastd.org). This is a non-governmental source for accurate information on STDs.

National Center for HIV, STD, and TB Prevention, Division of Sexually Transmitted Diseases (http://www.cdc.gov/nchstp/dstd).

National Vaginitis Association (http://www.vagina/infections.com). Includes a panel of vaginal health experts whose goal is to improve knowledge of the symptoms and treatment of vaginitis.

Sexuality Information and Education Council of the United States (SIECUS) (http://www.siecus.org). SIECUS' mission is to affirm that sexuality is a natural and healthy part of living; to develop, collect, and disseminate information; to promote comprehensive education about sexuality, and to advocate the right of individuals to make responsible sexual choices.

The Alan Guttmacher Institute (http://www.guttmacher.org) is a nonprofit organization whose purpose is to perform sexual and reproductive health research, policy analysis, and education. The organization publishes *Perspectives on Sexual and Reproductive Health*, which is available online.

The Medical Institute for Sexual Health (http://www.medinstitute.org). This organization promotes abstinence until marriage and provides information on sexually transmitted diseases.

National STD Hotline (1-800-227-8922). The hotline is staffed 24 hours, 7 days a week. All calls are private, personal, and confidential.

Teens are comfortable getting information from the Internet and the school nurse can provide students and families with Web sites that have accurate information. Box 42.1 is a list of Web sites that are appropriate for teens. Additional Web sites (Box 42.2) are good resources for school nurses to access science-based information on STDs and other sexual health issues.

STDs can have either a bacterial, viral, or parasitic origin and are contracted by sexual contact that includes vaginal or anal intercourse, as well as oral–genital contact. Twenty-five viral and bacterial infections can be sexually transmitted, producing a wide range of symptoms including genital ulcers, blisters, or papules, discharge from the vagina or penis, dysuria and urinary frequency, itching, burning, and abdominal pain. Symptoms may also include fever, joint swelling and pain, and muscle pain (Braverman, 2000). Some STDs produce no symptoms until years later when serious complications, such as liver or cervical cancer, occur.

CHLAMYDIA

Chlamydia is caused by the bacterium *Chlamydia trachomatis*. In the United States, chlamydia is currently the most commonly reported infectious disease (CDC, 2004a). For females, the highest reported rates of chlamydia are for ages 15 to 19. Rates for males, although significantly lower than female rates, are also highest within this age group. However, with newly developed diagnostic testing, it is anticipated that more males will be identified during screening. Currently, chlamydia is the cause of about one third to one half of all cases of nongonococcal urethritis in men. The high rate among teenage girls is partly attributed to the physiologic characteristics of the immature cervix. The cells that make up the cervix provide easy attachment for particular infectious organisms, especially chlamydia (Vermillion, Holmes, & Soper, 2000). In fact, females, between the ages of 15 and 19 represent 46% of all chlamydia infections (Stoner, 2000). The bacterium lives only on mucous membranes and transmission occurs during oral, anal, and vaginal sexual contact.

It is common for females and especially males infected with chlamydia to have no symptoms. Because of this, all sexually active adolescents and young adults should be screened at least annually (CDC, 2002b). Studies have identified high recurrence rates among females who are becoming reinfected by males who are asymptomatic (Burstein et al., 2001). If symptoms are present, females typically experience burning with urination and a thin, nonpurulent vaginal discharge. Both males and females are at risk for becoming sterile after an infection with chlamydia. Females are at higher risk of becoming sterile after an infection with chlamydia than gonorrhea (Boekeloo et al., 2002). Adolescents infected with chlamydia who are pregnant place their infant at risk for prematurity, pneumonia, and conjunctivitis.

In 2002 the CDC expanded their recommendations for screening for chlamydia (CDC, 2002b). These recommendations include screening annually all sexually active females younger than 20 years of age, as well as women between ages 20 and 24 who are sexually at risk, due to having a new sexual partner or multiple sexual partners. Newly developed screening measures have provided a means for accurate diagnosis. These new diagnostic tools do not require that females undergo a pelvic exam. The nucleic acid amplification tests can be performed on a vaginal swab obtained by the adolescent or on a urine sample. This highly accurate diagnostic test is able to identify chlamydial infection in females who have had previous negative cultures (Kissin et al., 2002). Because of its non-invasive nature, this form of screening can be performed in school based health clinics, health fairs, or even in the adolescent's home (Orr & Fortenberry, 1998). Samples can also be obtained during a pelvic examination. These new non-invasive options for screening may promote increased testing among previously reluctant teens.

Individuals with chlamydia infection often have a concurrent gonococcal infection. Recommended treatment regimens include antibiotics that are sensitive for both infections. Currently the recommended drugs include azithromycin (Zithromax) or doxycycline. Azithromycin often is preferred as only a single dose treatment is required. Side effects experienced with azithromycin are generally rare and typically consist of abdominal pain, diarrhea, and nausea and vomiting (Braverman, 2000). The adolescent is more likely to experience adverse effects when taking the larger single dose regimen. Side effects associated with doxycycline are also rare but potentially more serious, consisting of allergic reactions including hives, rashes, and angioedema. For individuals with allergies to these drugs, erythromycin can be prescribed (CDC, 2002b). Side effects to erythromycin are gastrointestinal in origin and are similar to those associated with azithromycin.

Abstinence from sexual intercourse is necessary until seven days after the completion of the antibiotic course (CDC, 2002b). It is important that both partners complete the treatment to prevent passing the infection back and forth.

Implications for the School Nurse

Chlamydia infections are prevented by consistent condom use. Teens need to be instructed that the infection often produces few symptoms so that a partner may pass the disease on without realizing it. Because the bacteria require contact with mucous membranes, casual contact including sharing food or using the same eating utensils or glass does not transmit the infection (CDC, 2002a). School nurses should be alert for the adolescent girl who complains of dysuria and burning, as irritation of the urethra may produce symptoms similar to those of a urinary tract infection.

Females should be discouraged from self-treatment with over-the-counter medications. Some girls may misinterpret their symptoms as signs of a yeast infection. Wearing cotton panties and gently washing the perineal area with mild soap should be encouraged. Douching should never be done without consulting a physician or advanced practice nurse.

GONORRHEA

Gonorrhea is caused by a bacterium, *Neisseria gonorrhoeae*. After years of a steady decrease in the incidence of gonorrhea, recent rates are increasing, with 335,104 cases reported in 2003 (CDC, 2004b). Some of this increase is attributed to expanded testing and improved screening and reporting procedures. However, the CDC believes the rate of infection has increased, particularly among some populations and in some geographic areas. Highest rates are found among African Americans and teens ages 15 to 19 (Stoner, 2000).

The bacterium requires a warm moist environment and thrives on mucous membranes in the urethra, vagina, rectum, mouth, throat, and eyes. Up to 70% of females may exhibit no symptoms, while 75% of males will experience painful urination and frequency, and a thick yellow or green discharge (Kissin et al., 2002) (Figure 42.1). Symptomatic females experience burning and dysuria and may have a green or yellow discharge. Often this discharge is minimal and may not be noticed. Gonorrhea is the most common bacterium cultured in females with pelvic inflammatory disease (PID) (Faro & Soper, 2001). Bacteria previously found only within the vagina enter the uterus by way of the cervix usually during menstruation, infecting the endometrium and Fallopian tubes. This infectious process often results in scarring, placing the women at risk for sterility and tubal pregnancies.

Males and females contracting rectal gonorrhea after anal sexual intercourse may have bloody stools and a purulent discharge. During delivery, a woman who has gonorrhea can pass the infection on to her infant. Because the organism infects only mucous membranes, newborns are exposed to these membranes in the delivery process; they are at increased risk of contracting eye infections (gonococcal ophthalmia neonatorum), which can result in blindness. In the United States, drops are placed in the eyes of all infants at the time of delivery to prevent a possible gonococcal infection.

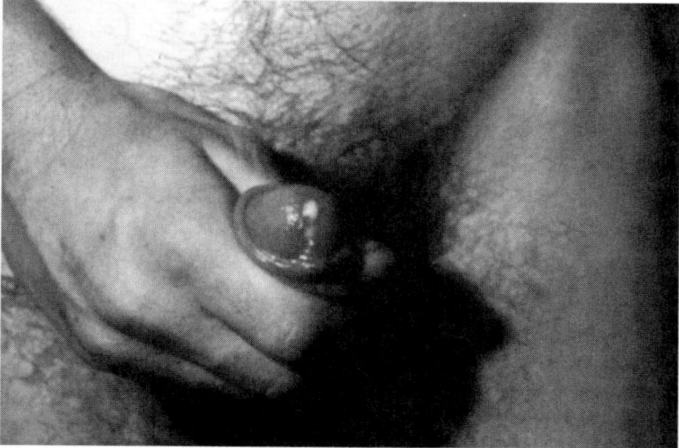

Figure 42.1 ■ Gonococcal urethritis. (*Source*: CDC, Division of STD Prevention.)

In a small number of untreated cases, gonococci invade the bloodstream (disseminated gonococcal infection) (Faro & Soper, 2001). The symptoms include a skin rash consisting of papules and pustules, chills, fever, and swollen painful joints. Early recognition and treatment with antibiotics are necessary to minimize the risk of joint damage resulting from development of arthritis (Sloane, 2002). Gonorrhea is diagnosed by identifying the bacterium by culture. Like chlamydia, gonorrhea can be diagnosed from a urine specimen or cultures obtained from the penis or during a pelvic exam.

At one time, penicillin was highly effective in curing individuals infected with gonorrhea. It became the drug of choice in the 1940s. Starting in the 1980s, however, larger doses were required to destroy the bacteria and cure the infection (CDC, 2002e). More troubling was the identification of some strains resistant to penicillin. In addition, in 2002, the CDC reported identification of ciprofloxacin-resistant strains of the bacteria, first in Hawaii and then spreading to the West Coast (CDC, 2002e). To complicate the treatment further, many individuals infected with gonorrhea also test positive for chlamydia. The *Chlamydia trachomatis* organism is not sensitive to penicillin (Faro & Soper, 2001). Currently the CDC recommends that individuals infected with gonorrhea receive one of the following drugs: ceftriaxone in a single injection, or a single oral dose of ciprofloxacin, ofloxacin, or levofloxacin. In addition, if a chlamydial infection has not been ruled out, the individual should also receive azithromycin or doxycycline (CDC, 2002c).

Implications for the School Nurse

Transmission of gonorrhea requires that the organism come in contact with mucous membranes. Although the bacteria may survive outside of the body for a short period, it is rare to transmit the infection in ways other than intimate sexual contact (King, 2002). Individuals can, however, transmit the infection to their eyes by their hands, resulting in ocular gonorrhea. The infection can cause severe symptoms including swelling, redness, and purulent drainage (Faro & Soper, 2001). Students should be instructed on good hand washing techniques as a means of reducing the risk of transmission to the eyes. Also students should use a separate washcloth and towel for washing the genital area. Although the risk of transmitting the infection from one person to another on personal items is rare, sharing of towels is discouraged.

The discomfort associated with gonorrheal infections, including burning and dysuria, will resolve after antibiotic treatment. Females are discouraged from douching, as this may result in pelvic inflammatory disease (Faro & Soper, 2001). Both males and females should cleanse the genital area with mild soap and water only.

The incidence of pharyngeal gonorrhea has grown because teens are increasingly engaging in oral–genital sex (Faro & Soper, 2001). The student may experience a mild sore throat, but many infections produce no symptoms. It is unlikely that an individual with gonococcal pharyngitis will pass the infection on during kissing (Sloane, 2002).

PELVIC INFLAMMATORY DISEASE

Untreated chlamydia and gonorrheal infections in females can involve the reproductive organs, leading to pelvic inflammatory disease (PID). Yearly, 1 million women of childbearing age develop PID. Teens make up 20% of these cases and are at a much higher risk of acquiring PID than adult women (Faro & Soper, 2001). This is explained by their high rates of infection with chlamydia and gonorrhea, which account for most cases of PID (Braverman, 2000). Scarring within the Fallopian tubes occurs following a single infection. Data show that as many as half of women with PID are not diagnosed early in the infectious process or are inadequately treated (McEvoy & Coupey, 2002).

The adolescent girl with PID typically experiences lower abdominal pain and dysuria. In addition, there may be complaints consistent with flu-like symptoms including malaise, vomiting, and diarrhea. The diagnosis of PID is based on clinical findings outlined by the CDC (2002b), including lower abdominal tenderness, adnexal tenderness (pain in those organs adjacent to the uterus including the ovaries and fallopian tubes), and cervical motion tenderness.

In the past, treatment for adolescents with PID usually required admission to the hospital for intravenous antibiotic therapy. Hospital admission also provided an opportunity to educate the teen and encourage partner notification (Braverman, 2000). However, the current CDC (2002b) recommendations state that most women with PID can be effectively treated on an outpatient basis.

Antibiotics used to treat PID include doxycycline, ceftriaxone, and metronidazole. The adolescent usually receives two different drugs to ensure that both gonorrhea and chlamydia are treated. It is important that adolescents understand that they must abstain from alcohol while taking metronidazole, as it will result in nausea and flushing (Braverman, 2000).

Implications for the School Nurse

PID is a serious complication of an STD. The risk of infertility and ectopic pregnancy are present after a single infection (King, 2002). Other sequelae include chronic pelvic pain, longer and more painful menstrual periods, and pain during sexual intercourse (Faro & Soper, 2001). With the increase use of outpatient treatment, an adolescent girl may return to school before completing the 10 to 14 days of antibiotics. Resolution of symptoms should occur within 96 hours after the initiation of treatment (Faro & Soper, 2001). A student who continues with severe pain and fever after this period of time should be reevaluated immediately. During the acute infection, bed rest in a semi-Fowler's position increases comfort and helps with the drainage of purulent secretions (Faro & Soper, 2001). Some females who have experienced PID will have abdominal pain for up to 6 months after treatment (Faro & Soper, 2001). Nonsteroidal anti-inflammatory drugs (ibuprofen) are effective in relieving pain. Students are instructed to abstain from sexual intercourse until antibiotics are completed, symptoms have resolved, and their partner has completed treatment.

SYPHILIS

Although rates of syphilis are not close to the levels of chlamydia or gonorrhea, recent data indicate an alarming increase in the infection rates to the highest level in 40 years (Sloane, 2002). In 2003 7,177 cases of primary and secondary syphilis were reported, up from 6,862 reported in 2002 (CDC, 2004c). Like chlamydia and gonorrhea, cases of syphilis are required to be reported to public health departments. The highest number of cases is found in the South, encompassing the states of Alabama, Florida, Arkansas, Delaware, District of Columbia, Georgia, Kentucky, Mississippi, North and South Carolina, Tennessee, Maryland, Oklahoma, Texas, Virginia, and West Virginia. The behaviors of men, particularly gay and bisexual men, as well as minorities within the inner cities, are attributed to be most associated with the increase (CDC, 2001a). The high incidence within the inner cities is thought to relate to the concurrent problems of drug abuse and poverty.

Since 1950, laws have required that cases of syphilis be reported to public health departments. Until recently, the ability to contact sexual contacts and educate the public has been thought to be responsible for the decrease in the incidence. However, the number of cases reported has doubled since 1986 (CDC, 2003). The genital ulcers produced by syphilis increase the risk of HIV transmission two to five times. Health officials are concerned that the recent increases in the number of cases of syphilis could also signal an increase in the number of people newly infected with HIV (CDC, 2001b).

Syphilis is caused by a spirochete, *Treponema pallidum*. Individuals can be infected through vaginal, anal, or oral–genital sexual intercourse. The organism enters the body through moist mucosa, or rarely, through a break in the skin. The disease occurs in four stages. The individual remains asymptomatic for a period of time, anywhere from 10 to 90 days after exposure. After this period, the first symptom appears, a lesion at the site of entry of the spirochete. The lesion, a chancre, is firm, painless, and highly infectious (Faro & Soper, 2001). The surface of the chancre breaks down and an ulcer forms. In males, the lesion occurs anywhere on the external genitalia (FIGURE 42.2). In females, it typically is found on the vulva, vagina, or cervix (FIGURE 42.3). With or without treatment, the chancre will heal, leaving no signs of the previous infection.

If the individual has not been appropriately treated, the disease will progress to a second stage, during which the individual will experience symptoms that are consistent with a minor illness, such as the flu. The typical symptoms include headache, low-grade fever, anorexia, and body aches. Also at this time, a maculopapular rash appears over the body, including the palms of the hands and soles of the feet. The rash does not cause pruritus or any discomfort. The rash is also found in the genital area, where it has an appearance similar to genital warts (Faro & Soper, 2001). These genital lesions are highly contagious and the symptoms also resolve without treatment. However, the symptoms are typically concerning to the individual and many infected people are treated during this stage.

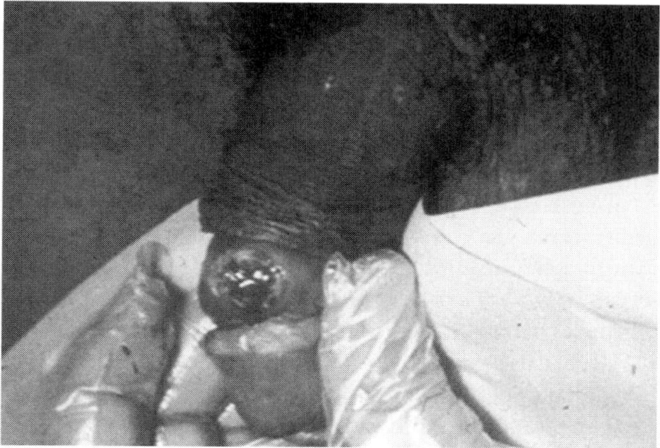

Figure 42.2 ■ Primary syphilis—male. (*Source*: CDC, Division of STD Prevention.)

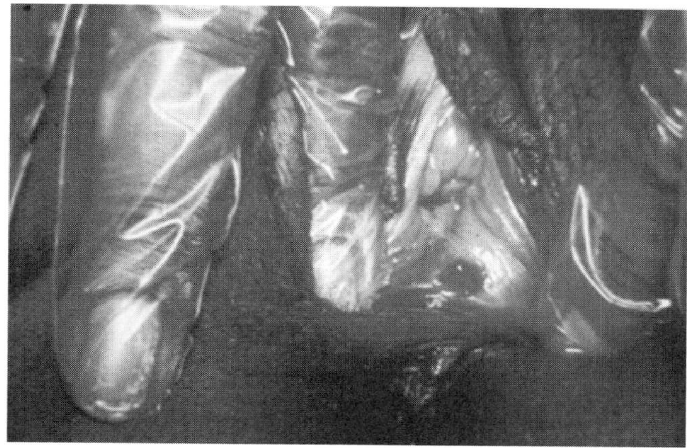

Figure 42.3 ■ Primary syphilis—female. (*Source*: CDC, Division of STD Prevention.)

Treatment of syphilis involves parenteral administration of penicillin G. Treatment options for penicillin-allergic individuals have limited efficacy, but include doxycycline and tetracycline (CDC, 2002b). Without treatment, the disease enters the latent stage, where the individual is free of any symptoms. About two-thirds of those who go untreated remain symptom free for life and are no longer contagious to others. The major exception is the pregnant woman who can pass the spirochete on to the fetus, causing spontaneous abortions, stillbirths, and severe deformities. About one-third of those infected with syphilis will develop symptoms consistent with the tertiary or late stage. Among the manifestations of tertiary syphilis is cardiac involvement including aortic aneurysms and neurosyphilis, which can result in dementia (Rawlins, 2001).

Syphilis is diagnosed by identifying the spirochete, typically in blood using the VDRL (Venereal Disease Research Laboratory) test. This highly cost-effective and accurate test has its limitations. In primary syphilis, 30% of those with the disease will test negative (Sloane, 2002). Certain conditions, including some forms of arthritis, can result in a false-positive result.

Transmission of syphilis occurs during vaginal, anal, or oral sex. All sexual partners are treated if they have had sex within the three months prior to the diagnosis (CDC, 2002b). The infection is transmitted through direct contact with the lesions. It is unlikely that an untreated individual will transmit the infection to another if no lesions are present (Faro & Soper, 2001). Syphilis cannot be transmitted through shared clothing, eating utensils, or in hot tubs (CDC, 2001d).

Implications for the School Nurse

Since the lesions caused by syphilis are painless and resolve with or without treatment, students may not recognize the importance of early diagnosis and treatment. A student who contracts syphilis during oral sex may mistake the lesion for a cold sore. School nurses may need to consider syphilis when evaluating students with oral lesions.

TRICHOMONAS VAGINALIS

Trichomonas vaginalis is a parasitic protozoan that causes one of the most prevalent of STDs in the United States, with 5 million individuals infected annually (CDC, 2001a). It is estimated that this infection makes up almost half of all the curable sexually transmitted infections worldwide. It is often seen concurrently with another STD, particularly gonorrhea. Although almost always transmitted during sexual intercourse, it is slightly possible to acquire the infection from infected water on a washcloth or in a swimming pool (Sloane, 2002).

Trichomonas infections can be asymptomatic for long periods of time. The protozoan survives best in an environment where the pH is less acidic than normally found in the vagina. Therefore, when conditions cause an increase in vaginal pH levels, the organism is likely to multiply and the infection becomes symptomatic. Several factors can alter the vaginal environment, including douching and sexual intercourse (Faro & Soper, 2001). Symptoms in women during an active infection include itching and burning around the vulva and a green, yellow, or gray discharge that may also be frothy. Males who are symptomatic experience symptoms consistent with urethritis, including burning when urinating. A disturbing recent finding is that T. vaginalis infections may promote HIV transmission (Sorvillo, Smith, Kerndt, & Ash, 2001). The pathophysiologic response of the body to the infection can increase HIV shedding (CDC, 2001a). Exposure is increased as the inflammation produced by the infection increases the number of white blood cells, including those carrying HIV. Furthermore, the genital lesions produced by the infection facilitate the entry of the HIV virus. For the individual who is infected with both *T. vaginalis* and HIV, the level of HIV virus within the body fluids is higher, increasing the probability of transmission during sexual intercourse. Diagnosis is made by microscopic examination of vaginal secretions that identify the protozoa.

Treatment for *T. vaginalis* is metronidazole (Flagyl, Metryl, Protostat) orally in a single dose; this has been demonstrated to be 95% effective in curing the infection (Braverman, 2000). Male partners of women infected should also be treated. It is important to warn adolescents not to drink alcohol while taking metronidazole, because they will experience nausea and flushing.

Implications for the School Nurse

Because *T. vaginalis* infection is asymptomatic in many individuals, all sexually active students should be encouraged to discuss STD screening with their primary care provider. Almost all infections are transmitted during sexual intercourse. However, the protozoan has been isolated in urine on toilet seats for up to 45 minutes after deposit, on washcloths 3 hours after contamination, and in hot tubs for 48 hours after last use (Faro & Soper, 2001). Given these data, students should be counseled regarding sharing of personal items and activities where they come in contact with water that may be poorly chlorinated, such as hot tubs and swimming pools (Faro & Soper, 2001).

GENITAL HERPES

One million new cases of genital herpes are diagnosed each year in the United States, with 45 million currently infected (CDC, 2001c). The incidence of genital herpes among teens continues to rise as teens increasingly engage in oral–genital sex. White teens are fives times more likely to be diagnosed with herpes today than in 1970 (Amador & Eyler, 2000). However, HSV is more common in blacks than in whites.

There are eight different types of herpes simplex virus (HSV). Three of these viruses are sexually transmitted; type 1 and type 2 are the most common, with 25% to 40% of genital herpes infections diagnosed being caused by herpes simplex virus type 1 (HSV-1) rather than HSV-2. Type 8 produces Kaposi's sarcoma, which is found in individuals with AIDS. Until recently, each type of the herpes virus was site specific. Type 1 generally produced the typical oral lesion known as the cold sore, while the type 2 virus caused almost all cases of genital herpes. Because of changes in sexual practices, including increased oral–genital sex, both types 1 and 2 can produce lesions found both around the mouth and in the genital area (Thomas, 2001). Herpes is spread by direct skin-to-skin contact or during oral–genital contact with an individual with a fever blister (HSV-1). Genital herpes from HSV-1 is much less likely to produce episodes of recurrence than HSV-2 (Sloane, 2002).

Most individuals experience mild symptoms and the disease may go unrecognized; others, however, experience severe discomfort due to painful blisters found on the genitals or around the rectum (Figure 42.4). The blisters rupture producing ulcers, which will heal in 2 to 4 weeks (Figure 42.5). The initial episode produces the most severe symptoms (Faro & Soper, 2001). As the body produces antibodies to the virus, subsequent attacks usually result in less severe symptoms. HSV remains in the body indefinitely and is incurable. Most individuals experience fewer outbreaks over time. The herpes virus can be isolated from the fluid within ulcers. A more definitive way to determine HSV type is analysis of a small sample of blood for the presence of HSV-1 or HSV-2 antibodies (CDC, 2002b).

Use of nonoxynol-9 (N-9), a spermicidal contraceptive cream, places the person with genital herpes at risk for extension of lesions into the vagina. Even more serious is that this form of spermicide may increase susceptibility to HIV infection (CDC, 2002b). The presence of genital ulcers allows for easy entry of other organisms. Therefore, individuals who are infected with the herpes virus are much more at risk of contracting HIV during intercourse with an HIV-positive person (CDC, 2001d).

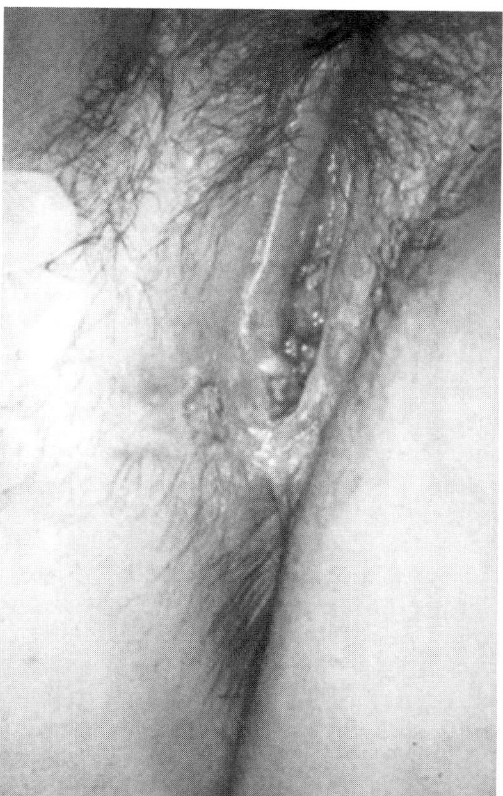

Figure 42.5 ■ Primary herpes—female. (*Source*: CDC, Division of STD Prevention.)

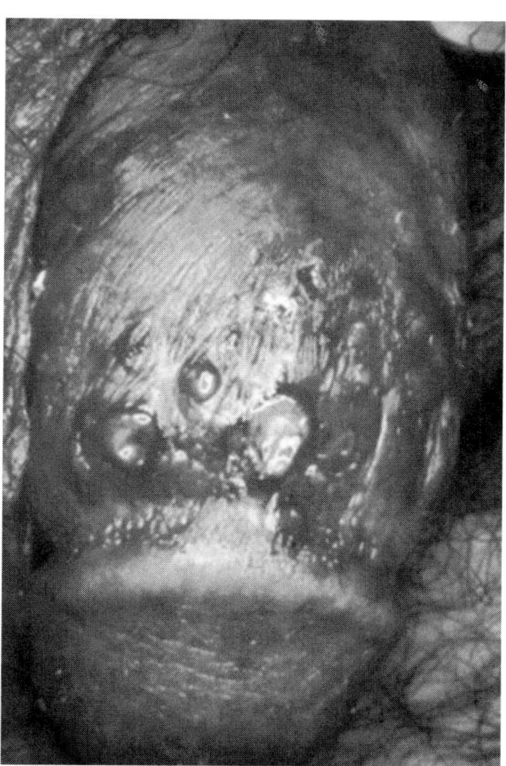

Figure 42.4 ■ Primary herpes—male. (*Source*: CDC, Division of STD Prevention.)

Condoms lubricated with N-9 are no longer recommended by the CDC as a form of STD prevention, as they are more costly, have a shorter shelf life than other condoms, and have been linked to urinary tract infections in females (CDC, 2002b). Although condoms provide significant protection against genital herpes, the male condom does not provide a barrier to all skin-to-skin contact during intercourse.

Currently there is no known cure for herpes. Antiviral drugs, such as acyclovir, help to speed up the healing of the ulcers during outbreaks. Daily suppressive therapy with an antiviral drug may be appropriate for individuals who experience frequent episodes (Romanowski, Marina, & Roberts, 2003).

Implications for the School Nurse

Teenagers need a good understanding of the transmission characteristics of HSV. Many may not be aware that they can acquire the infection from their partner's cold sore during oral–genital sex. It is not possible for the individual with HSV to determine infectious periods, as some individuals continue to shed the virus even when symptom free (Faro & Soper, 2001). Therefore, it is important to use condoms during all sexual contacts.

The herpes virus survives for a short period outside of the body. Items that may come in contact with lesions, such as towels, should not be shared and should be laundered as soon as possible after use. It is unlikely that HSV can be transmitted through sharing of food, community showers, or during sports activities (CDC, 2002b).

Treating the discomfort produced by lesions during outbreaks includes application of lukewarm cloths or sitz baths, keeping the area clean and dry, and wearing loose clothing and cotton underwear. Drying the lesions with a hair dryer on a low setting may reduce the discomfort (Thomas, 2001). Students should be instructed not to break the blisters or apply any ointments unless prescribed by their physician. Use of feminine sprays or douches is also discouraged.

Currently, HSV is a lifelong infection. Factors that have been demonstrated to trigger outbreaks include menstruation, sexual intercourse, fever, and emotional stress (Pereira, Antoni, & Danielson, 2003).

HEPATITIS B AND C

Hepatitis is an inflammation of the liver, either of an acute or chronic nature. There are many causes of hepatitis. Viruses cause the forms of hepatitis that are sexually transmitted.

The hepatitis B virus (HBV) is responsible for 5,000 deaths annually due to chronic liver disease and liver carcinoma. There were 8,064 new cases reported in 2002. Two-thirds of hepatitis B infections are sexually transmitted (CDC, 2004d). The hepatitis B virus can be transmitted in saliva, blood, semen, menstrual blood, and vaginal secretions (Sloane, 2002). The virus enters the body through small openings in the skin or across mucous membranes.

Although a safe and effective vaccine against the virus was developed in 1985, initially only those at high risk for the virus were vaccinated, including healthcare workers, intravenous drug users, and men who had sex with men (MSM). In 1991, hepatitis B immunization became part of the recommended infant schedule. Measures to immunize adolescents began in some states in 1997. However, not all states have this requirement. Adolescents who are not within areas participating in efforts to immunize 13- to 18-year-olds are at risk for contracting the virus. Adolescent males who have sex with other males are at an especially high risk for contracting HBV. Studies have shown that up to 70% of adult MSM have been infected with HBV (MacKellar, Valleroy, & Secura, 2001). MacKellar and colleagues collected data on 3,432 young MSM, ages 15 to 22 years. Only 9% had been immunized against HBV. HBV infection rates ranged from 2% for those age 15 to 17% of those age 22 years.

Hepatitis C (HCV) affects 2.7 million people in the United States and is the most common blood-borne infection in the United States. Almost three million people in the United States suffer from the disease, while 170 million worldwide are affected (CDC, 2004d). Thirty thousand people are newly infected yearly in the United States. Of those who contract the virus, 20% will develop cirrhosis within 20 years. Liver disease due to HCV accounts for 35%-40% of all liver transplants worldwide. While most individuals contract HCV through exposure to infected blood, 20% of those infected contract the disease through sexual contact (CDC, 2004d).

The clinical manifestations are similar for both forms of hepatitis. Some infected individuals will experience no symptoms. When symptoms are present, they typically consist of nausea, vomiting, jaundice, and fatigue.

There are limited treatment options for both hepatitis B and C and the focus is on monitoring and treatment of symptoms. In chronic hepatitis B and C, interferon has been demonstrated to decrease the progression of fibrosis in some individuals. The viruses may produce severe liver damage, leading to cirrhosis and liver failure.

Implications for the School Nurse

The school nurse is reminded of the importance of adhering to the guidelines for standard precautions and good handwashing technique in the prevention and control of hepatitis in the school. Children who have had acute viral hepatitis will need to have their activity monitored and may require periods of rest. Caution should be used when administering any medications to a student who has had hepatitis, as drug selection or dosage may need to be altered due to an impaired ability of the liver to detoxify and excrete them (Hockenberry, Wilson, Winkelstein, & Kline, 2003).

BACTERIAL VAGINOSIS

Bacterial vaginosis (BV) is the most common vaginal infection found in young women. It is caused by an overgrowth of bacteria normally found in the vagina in minimal levels. The organism responsible for most infections is *Gardnerella vaginalis* (Faro & Soper, 2001). When an infection occurs, there is an interruption in the production of lactobacilli. These organisms secrete a substance that works as a disinfectant. The cause of the overgrowth of bacteria is not well understood. Frequent douching may be associated with bacterial growth. It is also unclear as to whether BV is truly a sexually transmitted disease, as females who are not sexually active may also develop BV. However, the infection is found more frequently in women who became sexually active at a young age, report larger numbers of sexual partners, and those who have a current or past STD (Faro & Soper, 2001).

Symptoms include a thin gray-white discharge. There can be very small to large amounts of vaginal discharge. The odor of the discharge is described as similar to "stale fish." This odor is most obvious after intercourse when the vaginal discharge mixes with semen. The same odor can be produced during pelvic examination by placing the vaginal secretions on a slide with a drop of 10% potassium hydroxide (Sloane, 2002). Microscopic examination of vaginal secretions demonstrates the presence of "clue cells," which are epithelial cells covered with bacteria. The vaginal pH in individuals with BV tends to be less acidic than normal, above 4.5 (Sloane, 2002). The CDC (2002b) states that it is unnecessary to treat the male partners of females with BV. Research has not demonstrated a relationship between a female's response to treatment or the likelihood of recurrence and partner treatment. The most effective treatment is metronidazole orally, twice daily, for seven days (Faro & Soper, 2001). Women are encouraged to not use any douches or sprays to deal with the odor and to not douche prior to evaluation.

There is increasing evidence that BV can lead to serious conditions in women, including PID, endometritis, and even cervical cancer. In pregnant women, BV has been linked to preterm birth and postpartum infections (Faro & Soper, 2001). The condition may be missed or misdiagnosed owing to the complex clinical picture.

Implications for the School Nurse

Lack of a clear diagnosis or treatment option may lead the student to self-medicate, which may produce more severe symptoms. School nurses can assist female students in composing a list of questions to ask their healthcare provider that may assist with the diagnosis and treatment of the symptoms.

Secor (2001), in an extensive review of the literature on BV, identified helpful strategies to manage symptoms and prevent recurrences. Students are encouraged to wash their genital area with plain warm water. Applying unscented mineral oil up to twice daily may help with the discomfort. The student should be counseled to avoid douching, using tampons, or wearing tight pants or panty hose. Cotton panties should be consistently worn. Other recommendations are to avoid swimming pools, hot tubs, and the overuse of soaps.

HUMAN PAPILLOMAVIRUS

There are 75 different types of human papillomavirus (HPV); 30 infect the genital tract. Visible lesions may or may not be present. In males, lesions are most commonly found on the tip or shaft of the penis or the scrotum. In females, the lesions may be found on the external genitalia, vagina, cervix, or rectum. Condyloma acuminatum is the most common type of visible lesion; they are raised with an irregular surface resembling a cauliflower (FIGURES 42.6 and 42.7). Four or more of the types of HPV cause cervical cancer.

HPV infections are divided into risk categories, low, intermediate, and high, according to their risk of malignancy (Apgar, 2000). It is estimated that almost 50% of females will have contracted HPV before the age of 25 (Tumolo, 2000). Studies of adolescents with HPV show that up to 90% of the infections will resolve over a period of months (Moscicki, 1999). Because HPV is the most important risk factor for cervical cancer and because there is an increased incidence of abnormal Pap smears in adolescent girls, medical groups, including the American Academy of Pediatrics (AAP), recommend that all

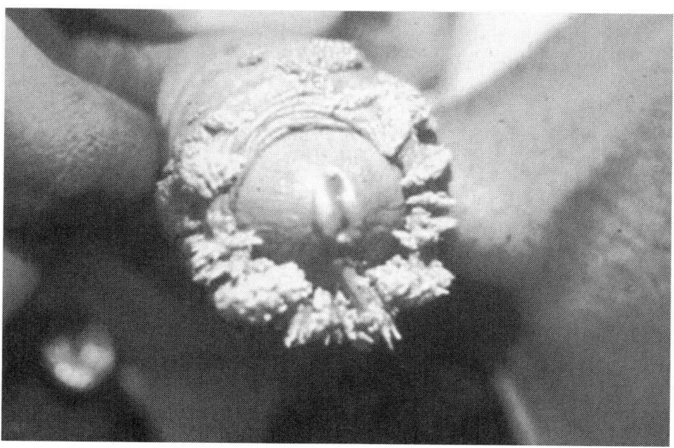

Figure 42.6 ■ Condyloma acuminata—penile. (*Source*: CDC, Division of STD Prevention.)

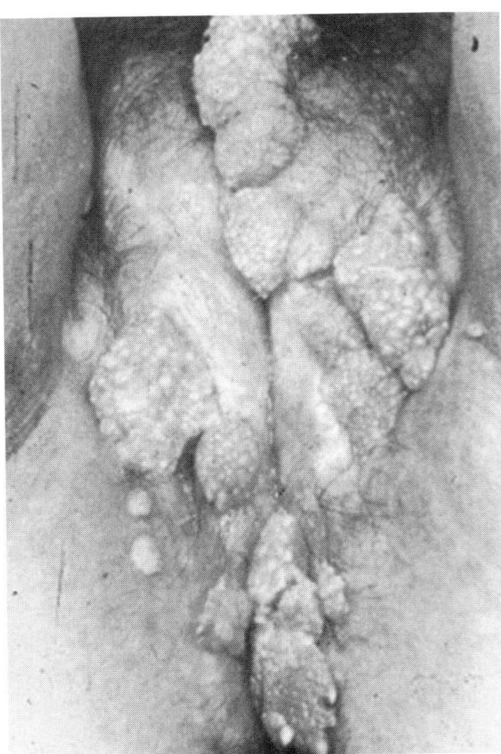

Figure 42.7 ■ Condyloma acuminata—vulva. (*Source*: CDC, Division of STD Prevention.)

sexually active adolescent girls receive a yearly pelvic examination and Pap smear (Brentjens, 2002). Unfortunately, currently only about 15% of sexually active adolescent girls receive Pap smear screening.

Treatment for HPV is dependent on the type of atypical squamous cells found. These cells are graded by the characteristics of the cervical dysplasia. About 15% of women who are infected with high-risk HPV will develop cervical cancer (Apgar, 2000). Currently there exists controversy over the recommended follow-up schedule for abnormal Pap smears. The CDC (2002b) states that the presence of genital warts alone is not an indication to change the frequency of Pap smears. Others recommend that women with low-grade cervical dysplasia undergo a repeat smear in 3 to 6 months (Apgar, 2000). However, follow-up is a concern with adolescents who may not be compliant. When abnormal cells are continually identified, the woman usually undergoes a colposcopy. With magnification, cervical lesions can be visualized and a biopsy of the tissue obtained.

Treatment options for genital warts range from ongoing observation to removal, using various forms of treatment modalities. Currently there is no evidence that removal of the lesions eradicates the virus. The current CDC guidelines (2002b) state that it is acceptable to not initiate any treatment, as many infections will demonstrate spontaneous regression. Patient preference should guide treatment options. Generally those lesions that are visible and produce symptoms are removed. Products are available that can be applied by the individual and include those that enhance the immune response (Imiquimod cream) or prevent cell division (Podofilox gel) (CDC, 2002b). Other treatments are administered by a physician and include cryotherapy, surgical removal, as well as application of other topical agents. Because the virus may not be totally eradicated, recurrences are possible following any of the treatment approaches. Recently a vaccine against HPV16 (most commonly linked to cervical cancer) was tested and found to reduce the incidence of the virus (Koutsky et al., 2002). Further testing is planned before recommendations for expanded use of the vaccine are instituted.

Implications for the School Nurse

Female students who are infected with HPV need to be informed that most types of HPV are not correlated with an increased risk of cervical cancer (CDC, 2002b). However, a thorough evaluation is important to determine the best mode of treatment. Because treatment of cervical warts has not been proven to prevent cervical cancer, the student's preferences should guide treatment (CDC, 2002b). The school nurse can explore and help explain the various approaches to the management of HPV infection.

Sexually active students should continue to use condoms during sexual intercourse. They should be aware, however, that lesions may be located on areas not protected by the condom, including the scrotum, thighs, and perineum.

HIV DISEASE

Beginning in the 1980s, physicians began to see increasing numbers of men infected with unusual diseases (*Pneumocystis carinii* pneumonia and Kaposi's sarcoma) that were usually seen only in individuals whose immune systems were impaired. In 1982 the disease was assigned the name acquired immune deficiency syndrome (AIDS), and in 1984 it was discovered that a virus, human immunodeficiency virus (HIV), caused the disease. Once certain symptoms are present, a diagnosis of AIDS is made; prior to that time, it is referred to as HIV disease.

HIV is in the category of retroviruses. Retroviruses impair cells by reversing cell function in a way that allows the virus to be incorporated into the cell's normal DNA within the nucleus. HIV attacks cells in the body that possess a specific surface molecule, CD4 receptor. These receptors are present on lymphocytes called T-helper lymphocytes. Once the virus invades the lymphocyte, it is no longer able to perform normally. The resultant impairment in immune function places the individual at risk for a number of opportunistic infections (Sloane, 2002). In the United States, sexual contact is the primary etiology for HIV exposure. Adolescents are at great risk for HIV related to unsafe sexual practices. The CDC estimates that in 2003, 3847 individuals between the ages of 13 and 19 years contracted HIV (CDC, 2004e). HIV is most readily transmitted during anal intercourse, as there is a likelihood that some bleeding will occur during this activity. Any lesions on the genital area increase the risk of transmission during vaginal intercourse. There is a very small chance of HIV transmission occurring during oral sex.

An individual infected with HIV initially shows very few signs of the disease. However, some will experience acute retroviral syndrome which occurs a few weeks after acquiring the infection and consists of mild symptoms including fever, rash, and swollen glands (USDHHS, 2002). Other individuals remain asymptomatic for as long as 10 years or longer. After a period of time, the clinical symptoms typical of HIV infection, including lymphadenopathy, weight loss, rashes, fever, ongoing fatigue, night sweats, diarrhea, and respiratory symptoms including cough and dyspnea begin. With the progression of the disease into AIDS, symptoms become more severe as the levels of normal T-helper lymphocytes are reduced and immune system function is impaired. Infections that a healthy immune system is usually able to fend off occur. These "opportunistic infections" are often life threatening and include tuberculosis, herpes simplex, cytomegalovirus, toxoplasmosis, and *Pneumocystis carinii* pneumonia. Malignancies resulting from an impaired immune system, including Kaposi's sarcoma, can occur. Another consequence of the disease is "wasting syndrome," producing chronic diarrhea, fever, and weight loss. Neurological complications can result in AIDS-related dementia (Hockenberry et al., 2003).

Diagnosis of HIV is made by identifying HIV antibodies in the blood. The focus is on prompt diagnosis soon after the HIV infection and well before the onset of AIDS. Starting treatment early in the disease helps to slow down immune system impairment. Until recently, blood samples were sent to laboratories delaying notification of the HIV- positive person for days to weeks. In November 2002 the FDA approved a rapid screening test for HIV. The OraQuick Rapid HIV-1 Antibody Test is able to detect antibodies to HIV from a sample of blood collected by finger-stick. The results are available in about 20 minutes. This provides the opportunity for an individual to receive immediate counseling and follow up (CDC, 2002c). Individuals who have positive findings on the screening test undergo additional blood analysis before the final diagnosis of HIV is made. Testing for HIV is voluntary and requires the individual's permission. While AIDS is a required reportable disease, HIV is not.

Prior to the development of new drug therapies, most people with HIV developed AIDS within eight years after infection (Sloane, 2002). Currently, individuals infected with HIV are started on treatment with a combination of drugs that make up the highly active antiretroviral therapy (HAART). These drugs have produced a dramatic change in the outcome for those infected with HIV. The drugs suppress the ability of the virus to replicate in the body. Zidovudine (AZT) and nucleoside analogs interfere with the enzyme necessary for the replication of HIV (Sloane, 2002). Protease inhibitors, another class of drugs, slow or stop the production of the enzyme protease needed for HIV replication. The decision of when to start treatment is a complex one and is based on the level of HIV present in the blood (viral load) and CD4 T-cell count which is a measure of immune system functioning (USDHHS, 2002).

Implications for the School Nurse

The American Academy of Pediatrics published a position statement on children with HIV in school (AAP, 1999). Included was the recommendation that it was unlikely that children would pass on the virus during normal school activities. Therefore, they recommend that HIV-positive children be permitted to participate in any school activity that they wish to and are physically capable of doing. HIV-positive children should not be barred from any competitive sport.

A common concern of staff is the probability of exposure to blood and body secretions as children experience nose bleeds, falls, and upset stomachs. Sports injuries are another area with a high prevalence of injury and body secretions. These can be addressed by teaching standard precautions to all staff and assuring that staff are implementing them. Staff can keep rubber gloves in their desk drawers. Another common question is the risk of transmission when children bite each other. "Bites with blood exchange among children are thought to be rare" (Dominquez, 2000, p. 211). Should a bite occur, wound management protocols should be in place. If part of the protocol, it might be recommended that both the biter and the victim be tested. Remember that transmission of HBV is considerably higher than for HIV because "HBV is present in higher concentrations in the blood and is more stable in the environment than is HIV" (Dominquez, 2000, p. 213).

HIV quickly dies when exposed to air and is not transmitted in air or water (Sloane, 2002). An infected student who sneezes or coughs in close proximity to another may transmit a cold virus, but not HIV. The concentration of HIV in tears, sweat, urine, and feces is low. These bodily fluids have not been demonstrated to play a role in HIV transmission. There is no need for any special precautions in the cafeteria during meals, as activities such as sharing of food will not transmit the virus. Surfaces contaminated with bodily fluids that contain blood can be disinfected by using a 1:10 diluted solution of household bleach.

The child with HIV is at serious risk for life-threatening infections. The school nurse must be alert to signs of an infection in an HIV-positive child or infectious diseases in the general school population. Stressing good handwashing habits for all children and school personnel will reduce the risk of infectious diseases for all individuals in the school. Contact with pets by the HIV-positive child may produce the risk of certain serious infections such as salmonella. Classroom pets to avoid include all reptiles, chicks, and ducklings (USPHS & IDSA, 2001). The issue of opportunistic infections in HIV-positive students is complex, and the reader is referred to an excellent publication published by the U.S. Public Health Service (USPHS) and Infectious Diseases of America (IDSA) (http://aidsinfo.nih.gov/guidelines/op_infections)

It is known that HIV-positive individuals typically do not develop AIDS for up to 10 years after they are infected. Large numbers of people with AIDS are diagnosed as young adults. Many of these young adults acquired the virus during adolescence. School nurses need to be active in developing programs that provide the school-age population with knowledge and skills that help reduce their risk for acquiring HIV. One program initiated by a school nurse in Smyrna, Delaware involved high school students who developed a media campaign to get the word out to their peers about the risks they take regarding sex and HIV The students developed posters and a television commercial that was aired on local stations.

CONCLUSION

Sexually transmitted diseases are a serious problem among teens. The school nurse may be the person to whom the student comes for information and advice. Recognizing that adolescents face many barriers to services that provide assistance for issues related to sexuality is important as the school nurse is in the ideal position to help teens find the information and services that help to minimize the risk for STDs and provide appropriate treatment. A summary of each STD can be found in TABLE 42.1.

(text continues on page 1009)

Table 42.1 ■
COMMON STDs

DISEASE	ETIOLOGY	MODE OF TRANSMISSION	SYMPTOMS	DIAGNOSIS	TREATMENT	NOTE
Chlamydia	Bacterial: *Chlamydia trachomatis*	Vaginal intercourse Oro–genital sex	Often asymptomatic Females: thin, nonpurulent discharge, dysuria, lower abdominal pain, low back pain, nausea, fever, bleeding between menstrual period, painful intercourse Males: penile discharge, dysuria, burning and itching around opening of urethra, pain and swelling of testicles	Screen all sexually active adolescents yearly. Nucleic amplification test performed on vaginal swab or urine sample	Azithromycin or doxycycline All sexual partners must be treated. Abstain from sexual intercourse for 7 days after treatment.	Often concurrent gonococcal infection present If left untreated: Females: development of pelvic inflammatory disease (PID) and possibly infertility Males: Urethral infection and possibly infertility
Gonorrhea	Bacterial: *Neisseria gonorrhoeae*	Vaginal and anal intercourse Oro–genital sex	Can be asymptomatic, especially in females. Males: dysuria, urinary frequency, thick yellow or green discharge, painful or swollen testicles	Bacteria can be cultured from urine or secretions from the vagina or penis. A Gram stain can be performed in a practitioner's office for quick results.	Ceftriaxone IM, ciprofloxacin PO, or ofloxacin PO, or levofloxacin PO Reinfection is possible after successful treatment if there is sexual contact with an infected person.	If not ruled out, treat also for chlamydia. If left untreated: Females: Can develop PID leading to infertility.

(continued)

Table 42.1 ■ *(Continued)*

DISEASE	ETIOLOGY	MODE OF TRANSMISSION	SYMPTOMS	DIAGNOSIS	TREATMENT	NOTE
			Females: minimal discharge, dysuria, vulvar burning Rectal gonorrhea: purulent rectal discharge, bloody stools, anal itching, painful bowel movements		Drug resistant strains of gonorrhea have been identified.	Males: Can develop epididymitis that can lead to infertility.
Pelvic inflammatory disease (PID)	Untreated chlamydia and/or gonorrheal infections	The mechanism of bacterial ascent to the upper genital tract is unclear.	Produces only mild symptoms in some women. Flulike symptoms: malaise, vomiting, diarrhea, fever Lower abdominal pain, dysuria, foul smelling vaginal discharge, painful intercourse, irregular menstrual bleeding.	Lower abdominal tenderness Adnexal tenderness Cervical motion tenderness Pelvic ultrasound Laparoscopy may be necessary to confirm diagnosis	Typically treated on an outpatient basis Antibiotic regimens vary; most common: single parenteral dose of ceftriaxone, metronidazole, or doxycycline. Treat all partners within 60 days prior to the onset of symptoms. Follow up for outpatient treatment in 72 hours. Surgery may be necessary if an abscess does not resolve.	If untreated, can lead to infertility, ectopic pregnancy, abscess formation, and chronic pelvic pain.

Syphilis	Spirochete — *Treponema pallidum*	Direct contact with lesion during vaginal, oral, or anal intercourse Transmission can occur only when lesions are present.	Asymptomatic 10 to 90 days after exposure Stage 1: firm, round, painless and highly contagious ulcer Stage 2: flu-like symptoms; maculopapular rash over body, especially on palms of hands and soles of feet; rash in genital area resembles genital warts and is highly contagious Stage 3: Can affect any body system including the central nervous system, heart, and lungs.	Isolation of spirochete in fluid from lesion Blood test: Venereal Disease Research Laboratory (VDRL) to identify spirochete	Single IM dose of penicillin G If penicillin allergy—doxycycline or tetracycline orally for 14 days All sexual partners from 3 months prior to the onset of symptoms should be treated.	Syphilitic lesions greatly increase the risk of HIV transmission. All individuals diagnosed with syphilis should be tested for HIV. Having syphilis does not produce immunity. Individuals infected with syphilis and treated successfully are still at risk for acquiring it again during sexual contact with an infected person.
Trichomonas vaginalis	Parasitic protozoan	Vaginal intercourse Small possibility to acquire from infected water on washcloth or in a swimming pool.	Can be asymptomatic for long periods of time. Females—itching and burning around the vulva, foul smelling green or yellow discharge that may be frothy	Microscopic examination of vaginal secretions for presence of the parasitic protozoan Results may take up to 1 week.	Single dose of metronidazole PO Treat all male partners.	Often seen concurrently with another STD, particularly gonorrhea. Infection may promote HIV transmission.

(continued)

Table 42.1 ■ *(Continued)*

DISEASE	ETIOLOGY	MODE OF TRANSMISSION	SYMPTOMS	DIAGNOSIS	TREATMENT	NOTE
			Most males are asymptomatic; those with symptoms experience those consistent with urethritis: discharge from the urethra, urinary urgency, burning during urination.			
Genital herpes	Herpes simplex virus (HSV) (type 1, 2, and 8)	Direct contact during oral, anal or vaginal intercourse The virus can be shed and transmitted to a partner even during symptom-free periods.	Vesicular lesions that rupture are found on the genital area or around the rectum. Lesions usually heal in 2 to 4 weeks. Burning and dysuria Can have psychological effects for some infected individuals.	Visual inspection Isolation of virus within fluid from lesions Serum analysis for HSV-1/HSV-2 antibodies	No known cure for HSV Antiviral drugs may be used during outbreaks or for suppressive therapy.	There are eight types of HSV; three of them are sexually transmitted. Outbreaks average four or five per year. Outbreaks become less severe in time.
Hepatitis B virus (HBV)	Hepatitis B virus	Transmitted in saliva, blood, semen, menstrual blood, and vaginal secretions.	Can be asymptomatic until manifestations of liver damage occur.	Serum analysis for HBV antigens and antibodies	Limited treatment options Focus on monitoring and treating symptoms.	HBV is more infectious than HIV. Hepatitis B vaccine is the best protection.

			Nausea, vomiting, jaundice, abdominal pain, fatigue, anorexia, and joint pain		Interferon may reduce liver fibrosis in some. Can have psychological implications for some infected individuals.	Hepatitis B vaccine is part of the infant vaccine schedule.
Hepatitis C (HCV)	Hepatitis C virus	Exposure to infected blood Sexual contact is a possible mode of transmission, but less likely than exposure to infected blood.	Can be asymptomatic until manifestations of liver damage occur. Nausea, vomiting, jaundice, abdominal pain, fatigue, anorexia, and joint pain.	Serum analysis for HCV antigens and antibodies	Limited treatment options Focus on monitoring and treating symptoms. Interferon may reduce liver fibrosis in some individuals. Can have psychological implications for some infected individuals.	Approximately 60% to 70% of infected individuals will develop chronic disease.
Bacterial vaginosis (BV)	Overgrowth of normal vaginal flora—most commonly *Gardinella* bacteria	Not fully understood—associated with multiple sex partners, douching, lack of vaginal lactobacilli	Thin, gray white vaginal discharge with odor of "stale fish" Burning during urination External vaginal itching	Presence of "clue cells" in secretions Vaginal pH above 4.5 Fishy odor when 10% KOH is added to vaginal secretions on a slide	Metronidazole orally, twice daily for 7 days Avoid consumption of alcohol while taking metronidazole for at least 24 hours after last dose.	Not necessary to routinely treat sexual partners. If untreated, there is the possibility of development of PID. Infected women have an increased susceptibility to other STDs. Recurrence after treatment is possible.

(continued)

Table 42.1 ■ *(Continued)*

DISEASE	ETIOLOGY	MODE OF TRANSMISSION	SYMPTOMS	DIAGNOSIS	TREATMENT	NOTE
Human papillomavirus (HPV)	There are 75 different types of HPV; more than 30 infect the genital tract.	Vaginal and anal intercourse	Can be asymptomatic with flat lesions only visualized using magnification techniques. Papular warts Condyloma acuminata—clusters of soft pink or red cauliflower-like lesions Site of lesions: Females: vulva, labia, anus, vagina, and cervix Male: tip of shaft of penis, scrotum, and anus	Visual examination During routine Pap smear Culdoscopic examination	Yearly pelvic examination Treatment depends on type of atypical cells and patient preference. Options range from observation to removal using various forms of treatment modalities. Many infections will demonstrate spontaneous regression.	HPV infections are divided into low, intermediate, and high categories according to their risk of malignancy. Fifteen percent of women who are infected with HPV will develop cervical cancer. Sexual partners should be encouraged to be evaluated for HPV and other STDs.
HIV disease	Human immunodeficiency virus (HIV)	Exposure to infected blood Sexual intercourse Most readily transmitted during anal intercourse Small chance of transmission during oral–genital intercourse	Some will experience acute retroviral syndrome which occurs a few weeks after acquiring the infection and produces fever, rash, and swollen glands. Typically asymptomatic for period of up to 10 years Onset of symptoms include lymphadenopathy, weight loss, fatigue, night sweats, diarrhea, pneumonia, and other infections.	Presence of HIV antibodies in the blood OraQuick Rapid HIV-1 Antibody Test can provide results in 20 minutes.	Highly active antiretroviral therapy (HAART), which includes Zidovudine (AZT), nucleoside analogs, and protease inhibitors	Students diagnosed with any STD should be counseled to be tested for HIV as early diagnosis and treatment can prevent opportunistic infections and help to minimize the rapid decline of the immune system.

References

Amador, L., & Eyler, A. E. (2000). Diagnosis and treatment of sexually transmitted diseases in adolescence. A practical approach. *Clinics in Family Practice, 2*(4), 5–28.

American Academy of Pediatrics (AAP) Committee on Pediatric AIDS and Committee on Infectious Diseases (1999). Issues related to human immunodeficiency virus transmission in schools, childcare, medical settings, the home and community. *Pediatrics, 104*(2), 318–324.

Apgar, B. S. (2000). Cervical cancer prevention for adolescents. *Clinics in Family Practice, 2*(4), 1–22.

Boekeloo, B. O., Snyder, M. H., Bobbin, G. R., Burstein, G. R., Conley, D., Quinn, T. C., & Zenilman, J. M. (2000). Provider wiliness to screen all sexually active adolescents for chlamydia. *Sexually Transmitted Infections, 78*, 369–373.

Braverman, P. (2000). Sexually transmitted disease in adolescents. *Medical Clinics of North America, 84*, 869–889.

Brentjens, M. (2002). Human papillomavirus: A review. *Dermatologic Clinics, 20*(2), 315–322.

Burstein, G. R., Zenilman, J. M., Gaydos, C. A., Diener-West, M., Howell, M. R., Brathwaite, W., & Quinn, T. C. (2001). Predictors of repeat chlamydia trachomatis infections diagnosed by DNA amplification testing among inner city females. *Sexually Transmitted Infections, 77*, 26–32.

Centers for Disease Control and Prevention (CDC). (2000). *Tracking the hidden epidemics: Trends in STDs in the United States. Atlanta: U.S. Department of Health and Human Services.*

Centers for Disease Control and Prevention (CDC). (2001a). *Trichomonas vaginalis*, HIV, and African-Americans. *Emerging Infectious Diseases, 7*(6), 1–12.

Centers for Disease Control and Prevention (CDC). (2001b). Primary and secondary syphilis among men who have sex with men – New York City. *Morbidity and Mortality Weekly Report, 51*, 853–856.

Centers for Disease Control and Prevention (CDC). (2001c). *Genital herpes*. Division of SexuallyTransmitted Diseases. Atlanta: U.S. Department of Health and Human Services.

Centers for Disease Control and Prevention (CDC). (2001d). *The role of STD detection and treatment in HIV prevention*. Division of Sexually Transmitted Diseases. Atlanta: U.S. Department of Health and Human Services.

Centers for Disease Control and Prevention (CDC). (2001e). *Syphilis elimination: History in the making. Division of Sexually Transmitted Diseases. Atlanta: U.S. Department of Health and Human Services.*

Centers for Disease Control and Prevention (CDC). (2002a). Trends in sexual risk behaviors among high school students – United States – 1991–2001. *Morbidity and Mortality Weekly Report, 51*(38), 856–859.

Centers for Disease Control and Prevention (CDC). (2002b). Sexually transmitted treatment guidelines – 2002. *Morbidity and Mortality Weekly Report, 51*(RR–6), 1–80.

Centers for Disease Control and Prevention (CDC). (2002c). Approval of a new rapid test for HIV antibody. *Morbidity and Mortality Weekly Report, 51*(46), 8–9.

Centers for Disease Control and Prevention (CDC). (2002d). *Sexually transmitted disease surveillance – 2001*. Atlanta: Department of Health and Human Services.

Centers for Disease Control and Prevention (CDC). (2002e). Increases in fluoroquinolone resistant *Neisseria gonorrhoeae*—Hawaii & California, 2001. *Morbidity and Mortality Weekly Report, 51*, 1041–1044.

Centers for Disease Control and Prevention (CDC). (2003). *Recommendations for public health surveillance of syphilis in the United States*. Atlanta: U.S. Department of Health and Human Services.

Centers for Disease Control and Prevention (CDC). (2004a). *Sexually transmitted disease surveillance 2003 supplement, chlamydia prevalence monitoring project*. Atlanta: U.S. Department of Health and Human Services, Centers for Disease Control and Prevention.

Centers for Disease Control and Prevention (CDC). (2004b). *Sexually transmitted disease surveillance 2003 supplement: gonococcal isolate surveillance project annual report – 2003*. Atlanta: U.S. Department of Health and Human Services.

Centers for Disease Control and Prevention (CDC). (2004c). *Sexually transmitted disease surveillance 2003 supplement, syphilis surveillance report*. Atlanta: U.S. Department of Health and Human Services, Center for Disease Control and Prevention.

Centers for Disease Control and Prevention (CDC). (2004d). *Hepatitis surveillance report No. 59*. Atlanta: U.S. Department of Health and Human Services, Centers for Disease Control and Prevention.

Centers for Disease Control and Prevention (CDC). (2004e). *HIV/AIDS surveillance report, 2003* (Vol. 15). Atlanta: U.S. Department of Health and Human Services, Centers for Disease Control and Prevention.

Dominquez, K. (2000). Management of HIV-infected children in the home and institutional settings. *Pediatric Clinics of North America, 47*(1), 203–239

Facente, A. C. (2001). Adolescents and HIV: Knowledge, behaviors, influences and risk perceptions. *The Journal of School Nursing, 17*, 198–203.

Faro, S., & Soper, D.E. (2001). *Infectious diseases in women*. Philadelphia: W. B. Saunders.

Hockenberry, M. J., Wilson, D., Winkelstein, M. L., & Kline, N. E. (2003). *Wong's nursing care of infants and children*. St. Louis: C. V. Mosby.

Institute of Medicine. (1997). *The hidden epidemic: Confronting sexually transmitted diseases*. Washington, DC: National Academy Press.

King, B. M. (2002). *Human sexuality today*. Upper Saddle River, NJ: Prentice-Hall.

Kissin, D. M., Holman, S., Minkoff, H. L., DeMeo, L., McCormack, W. M., & DeHovitz, J. A. (2002). Epidemiology and natural history of ligase chain reaction detected chlamydial and gonococcal infections. *Sexually Transmitted Infections, 78*, 208–209.

Koutsky, L. A., Ault, K. A., Wheeler, C. M., Brown, M. D., Barr, E., Alvarez, F. B., Chiacchierini, L. M., & Jansen, K. U. (2002). A controlled trial of a human papillomavirus type 16 vaccine. *New England Journal of Medicine, 347*(21), 1645–1651.

Luger, A. (1993). The origin of syphilis. *Sexually Transmitted Diseases, 20*, 110–117.

Macke, B. A., & Maher, J. E. (1999). Partner notification in the United States: An evidenced based review. *American Journal of Preventive Medicine, 17*, 230–242.

MacKellar, D. A., Valleroy, L. A., & Secura, G. M. (2001). Two decades after vaccine license: Hepatitis B immunization and infection among young men who have sex with men. *American Journal of Public Health, 91*, 965–971.

McEvoy, M., & Coupey, S. (2002). Sexually transmitted infection: A challenge for nurses working with adolescents. *The Nursing Clinics of North America, 37*, 461–474.

Moscicki, A. B. (1999). Human papillomavirus disease in the adolescent. *Pediatric Clinics of North America, 46*, 783–807.

Orr, D. P., & Fortenberry, J. D. (1998). Screening adolescents for sexually transmitted diseases. Journal of the American Medical Association, 280, 564–565.

Panchaud, C., Singh, S., Feivelson, D., & Darroch, J. E. (2000). Sexually transmitted diseases among adolescents in developed countries. *Family Planning Perspectives, 32*, 24–32.

Pereira, D. B., Antoni, M. H., & Danielson, A. (2003). Stress as a predictor of symptomatic genital herpes virus recurrence in women with human immunodeficiency virus. *Journal of Psychosomatic Research, 54*, 237–244.

Rawlins, S. (2001). Nonviral sexually transmitted infections. *Journal of Obstetric, Gynecologic, and Neonatal Nursing, 30*, 12–17.

Remez, L. (2000). Oral sex among adolescents: Is it sex or is it abstinence? *Family Planning Perspectives, 32*, 298–304.

Romanowski, B., Marina, R. B., & Roberts, J. N. (2003). Patient's preference of valacyclovir one–daily suppressive therapy versus twice–daily episodic therapy for recurrent genital herpes: A randomized study. *Sexually Transmitted Diseases, 30*, 226–231.

Schwab, N. C., & Gelfman, H. B. (2001). *Legal issues in school health services*. North Branch, MN: Sunrise River Press.

Secor, R. M. (2001). Bacterial vaginosis: Common, subtle, and more serious than ever. *Clinician Reviews, 11*(11), 59–68.

Sloane, E. (2002). *Biology of women*. Albany: Delmar.

Sorvillo, F., Smith, L., Kerndt, P., & Ash, L. (2001). *Trichomonas vaginalis*, HIV, and African-Americans. *Emerging Infectious Diseases, 7*, 927–932.

Stoner, B. P. (2000). Comparative epidemiology of heterosexual gonococcal and chlamydial networks. *Sexually Transmitted Diseases, 27*, 215–223.

Thomas, D. J. (2001). Sexually transmitted viral infections: Epidemiology and treatment. *Journal of Obstetric, Gynecologic, and Neonatal Nursing, 30*, 316–322.

Tumolo, J. (2000). Sexually transmitted diseases in adolescents. *Advanced Nursing Practice, 8*(9), 49–52.

U.S. Department of Health and Human Services (USDHHS). (2000). *Healthy People 2010* (2nd ed.). Washington, DC: U.S. Department of Health and Human Services.

U.S. Department of Health and Human Services (USDHHS). (2002). *HIV and its treatment: What you should know*. Washington, DC: HIV/AIDS Treatment Information Service.

U.S. Public Health Service (USPHS) and Infectious Diseases Society of America (IDSA). (2001). *USPHS / IDSA guidelines for the prevention of opportunistic infections in persons infected with human immunodeficiency virus*. CDC: Atlanta: Centers for Disease Control and Prevention.

Van De Loar, M. J., Termorshuizen, F., & Van Den Hoek, A. (1997). Partner referral by patients with gonorrhea and chlamydial infections: Case-finding observations. *Sexually Transmitted Diseases, 24*, 334–342.

Vermillion, S. T., Holmes, M. M., & Soper, D. E. (2000). Adolescents and sexually transmitted diseases. *Obstetrics Gynecology Clinics of North America, 27*(1), 163–179.

PART VIII

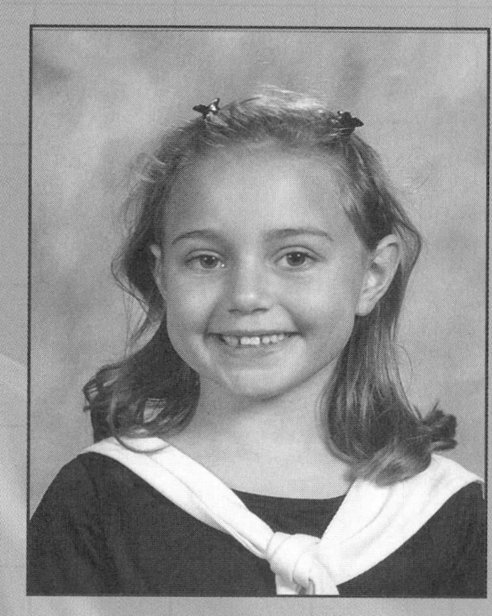

Health Services Management

Chapter 43

Setting Up the School Health Office

BERIT PETERSON ■ LINDA C. WOLFE

Chapter Outline

INTRODUCTION

The school health office is the hub for delivery of health services at school. It houses the health program and the services that are provided by, or under the direction of the school nurse(s). The primary goal is to provide a safe and welcoming environment that efficiently and effectively meets health needs in the school setting. A large number and diversity of services and programs are provided through the school health office, reflecting the health needs of the school community. Clients, including students, their families, school staff, volunteers, and, at times, the surrounding community, seek the services of the school nurse to address their growing physical and emotional healthcare needs, both acute and chronic. "Today's health issues are so complex and diverse that the facilities have had to develop to meet these needs" (Massachusetts Department of Health, 2004, p. 1). Unfortunately, the school nurse's office has not always kept up with these demands (McKibben and DiPaolo, 1997). The ability of the facility to provide privacy, technology, adequate supplies, up-to-date equipment, and storage can create either a gateway or a barrier to prompt and successful interventions.

This chapter assists the school nurse to establish a safe, efficient, and effective setting for the delivery of school nursing services. Within the chapter are recommendations for floor plans, office features, supplies, and equipment. Based on the needs of the school community, the school nurse can customize recommendations and guidelines to each unique school setting. Because little research exists specific to this topic, this chapter presents best practices developed by state agencies and local districts.

The term "school health office" is used in this chapter to describe the room allocated for the delivery of school nursing services. Because not all school health services are provided by a full-time registered nurse, it is important to avoid calling this area "the nurse's office," unless it is in fact always staffed by a registered nurse. Other names frequently used are "health office," "health suite" or "health room," But whichever is chosen, it should be posted, along with the school nurse's name and credentials, where it is easily seen. In addition, signs leading to the school heath office from major entrances are important to students, staff, and visitors alike.

FIRST IMPRESSIONS

The school health office visually represents the health services program and should reflect quality. For most people, the physical appearance of the health office is the first impression of the health services program, reflecting the quality, philosophy, and mission of the provider (Frasca-Beaulieu, 1999). The physical layout, furnishings, equipment, cleanliness, and supplies should be consistent with current standards and recommendations to meet the school community's health needs. Besides being neatly organized, clean, and efficiently laid out, the health office should be a welcoming, caring environment that promotes healthy choices and reflects the professional competence of the school nurse.

Many factors need to be considered when planning a school health office. Before a health office is set up, each school will need to identify its own functions based on a needs assessment, the staffing plan, the school health services' goals, state and national standards, relevant laws, and the responsibilities of the school nurse. All of these affect the health office layout, furniture, and equipment.

FUNCTIONS OF THE SCHOOL HEALTH OFFICE

The two major focuses of the school health office are to prevent illness and disability and to provide early detection and correction of health problems (Butin, 2002). Functions of the school health office are impacted by the number of clients who access services; the health conditions and needs of students and staff, the number and qualifications of health office personnel, the expected role of the school nurse, and the equipment and supplies available. Functions must be identified and individualized by and for each school. The office should be used for health services only (Massachusetts Department of Health, 1995).

The framework for school health services is built on the district's policies and procedures, the mission statement, goals specific to the school, and relevant state or national standards and laws. For instance, if a law or policy mandates vision screening, this impacts the need for adequate space and specialized equipment. If first aid is provided in the health office, then specific equipment and supplies are necessary along with trained personnel. Medication procedures, too, dictate the amount of space, privacy, and locked storage areas that will be needed.

While specific needs are identified for each school community, general functions include the following:

- A private conference space where the nurse, teacher, student, parent, or others concerned with health counseling and guidance can discuss specific health issues of individual students in privacy.
- An isolated area for the care of students who become ill or are suspected of having a communicable disease, until they can be placed under their parents' care or returned to class.
- A service area for provision of first aid and general health care (treatments and medications).
- A space where students' health records are easily accessible, but secure and within the requirement outlined by relevant laws and policies.
- A service area where health assessments are made; vision, hearing, and other screening procedures are carried out; and where immunizations may be provided
- A resource center for health education materials
- A place for those who require a rest period because of specific health needs
- A storage area for health supplies and equipment
- A secured area with locked storage for medication, which meets Board of Pharmacy requirement for securing controlled substances.
- A bathroom meeting Americans with Disabilities Act (ADA) requirements with toilet, ventilation, and a sink with hot and cold running water.

(Adapted from Massachusetts Department of Health, 1995; Minnesota Department of Health, 1996; New Mexico Department of Education, 1999; Virginia Department of Education and Department of Health, 1999.)

ASSESSING THE NEEDS OF THE COMMUNITY

When planning a school health office, it is essential to understand the clientele and their needs specific to the school. As the role of the school nurse has expanded, so have the clientele and their needs. Today's school nurse extends services to students, their families, school staff, volunteers, and the community at large. Given such a large and diverse group, a needs assessment must consider all aspects of health services delivery that is or will be available within the school setting. Such a needs assessment can be a proactive activity to educate the district on the unique needs of a school health office when "building a new structure or renovating one" (McKibben & DiPaolo, 1997, p. 23).

Needs assessments can be done in a formal or informal way depending on the time and resources available. With enough time and resources, surveys can be developed, distributed, collected, and evaluated. With less time and fewer resources, one nurse can collect and analyze data about health needs. An example of the information to be collected and the implications of the data related to planning is provided in TABLE 43.1. Each school nurse then needs to individualize the information and its impact on the local school setting.

(text continues on page 1018)

Table 43.1 ■
HEALTH NEEDS ASSESSMENT

INFORMATION TO BE COLLECTED	IMPLICATIONS FOR PLANNING THE SCHOOL HEALTH OFFICE
Numbers • How many students attend the school? • How many school staff and volunteers are in the school? • What is the average number of clients seen per day?	• The numbers impact the size of the health office, space and furniture needs, supply needs, and number/types of telephones.
Age Groups • What ages/grades are in the school? • What age groups are the staff and volunteers?	• The age, and resulting physical size, of the students impact the size of the furniture, including chairs, cots, and the need for diaper changing space and furniture. • Adolescents and adults need space for privacy. • The physical size of the students influences the size of the supplies that are needed, such as bandages and BP cuffs. • Developmental age of the students influences the room décor; i.e., cartoon characters for elementary ages.
Setting • Is the school in a rural, suburban, or urban setting? • Who are local community and school partners? How do they interact with school health services?	• EMS response times and skill levels may be different in different locales. • Community access to local health care impacts the number of students, staff, and community members for whom the school nurse provides services. • There may be space requirements of community partners for on-site services, such as mental health counseling or dental services. This may affect shared space, furnishings, and equipment.

(continued)

Table 43.1 ■ *(Continued)*

INFORMATION TO BE COLLECTED	IMPLICATIONS FOR PLANNING THE SCHOOL HEALTH OFFICE

Special Needs
• How many students and staff have chronic health conditions?
• What conditions are these?
• What are the unique needs?
• How many students require nursing treatments on a daily or p.r.n. basis?
	• Specific treatment and medication needs require:
	  • Specialized equipment and space for storage of equipment, feedings and medication
	  • Treatment areas for diapering, assessing/monitoring of health conditions, providing treatments (i.e., catheterizations, gastric feedings) and administering medications.
	• Students with disabilities may require assistance with daily living skills.
	• Students using wheelchairs or other assistive equipment need adequate space for moving.

Screenings • What screenings are mandated/provided?	• Younger children require smaller furniture and special vision charts. They are more likely to need typanometer and oto-acoustic emissions equipment available to them. • Early childhood screening programs require space that is available only to the screeners and the children being screened. A waiting and consultation area for parents is essential. • Effective screening tools are needed for each age level (i.e., a Snellen vision wall chart is valid for testing younger children, whereas a Titmus machine may be preferable for older students). • Children with developmental delays need developmentally appropriate screening tools. • Non-English speaking students need effective screening tools to measure health, not language skills.
Illness • What is the average number of students seen and sent home by the school nurse per day for illness?	• The number and trends of past illnesses help identify the size of the isolation and rest areas.
Injury • What is the average number of students seen and sent home by the school nurse per day for injury? • What injury data are available for students in this school?	• The number and types of injuries direct planning for first aid supplies. • Age-specific injury data identify needs for quantities and sizes of supplies, such as dressings and bandages.

(continued)

INFORMATION TO BE COLLECTED	IMPLICATIONS FOR PLANNING THE SCHOOL HEALTH OFFICE
Special Needs • How many students are assessed for special education services?	• Special education assessments require space for student health assessments, treatments, and confidential consultation with parents. A telephone in a private area is important. • Computer and printer availability is needed for writing individual education programs (IEPs), individual healthcare plans (IHPs) and for quick access to complete health records.
Immunizations • Do school personnel administer immunizations?	• Space, furniture, and supplies for immunization administration are needed. • A computer for recording and record review facilitates documentation. • A refrigerator with controlled temperature monitoring is necessary to store vaccines.
Communicable Diseases • Are students in compliance with immunization recommendations? • Are there special considerations relative to communicable disease in the school? • What is the school history of common communicable diseases?	• Space, good lighting, and privacy are needed for personal screenings for communicable disease (i.e., pediculosis). • Isolation is needed when a student with a communicable disease is waiting for a parent to take him/her home.
Off-Site Activities • Will students go on field trips?	• If students participate in school trips, a first aid kit will be needed. • Plans for administration of medication may include a bag for medications, a portable storage container for cold items, and snacks for students with diabetes.
Health Records • What protocols exist for maintaining student/other records? • Are health records computerized or on a hard copy?	• If students' records are electronic, the school nurse needs computer and printer access in the office for daily log input, health records, IEPs, and IHPs. • Computer furniture needs to include an ergonomically correct desk and chair. • Secured storage is essential for paper documents • It is preferable for the school health office to have a fax machine available for confidential communication.
School-Based Health Center (SBHC) • Do students have access to a health clinic within the school? • What is the relationship between the health office and the SBHC? • What are the distinct roles of the SBHC and the school nurse?	• Access to a SBHC may impact on the health office space, equipment and supply needs depending upon the role delineations and the relationship between the health office and the health clinic.

(continued)

Table 43.1 ■ *(Continued)*

INFORMATION TO BE COLLECTED	IMPLICATIONS FOR PLANNING THE SCHOOL HEALTH OFFICE
Medical Advisor • Is there a medical advisor to the school? • What is his or her role and relationship with the school nurse?	• The medical advisor may perform physical exams in the health office, which requires a private space with an exam table, supplies, and equipment.
Communication • How does the school nurse communicate with staff? • Do classrooms have telephones? • Do staff take telephones to recess?	• Consideration should be given to how communication should ideally take place during the day, especially in the event of an emergency. A cell phone, pager or two-way radio may be needed depending upon student needs and the size of the school campus.

Whether planning a new or renovated school health office, the health needs can also be evaluated by obtaining information on other local, regional, or state school health offices that serve a similar population in ages and size. Considerations should be made regarding programs or populations with special health needs that attend the school.

When available, a School Health Advisory Committee can be an important resource to planning (see Chapter 19). The members are usually knowledgeable in areas of health, child development, or the community and recognize both the needs and the assets of the school community. Survey development, distributions, analysis, and subsequent planning are enhanced by the diverse expertise of the members.

In addition to looking at the school as a whole, it is important to look at the unique needs of individual students and staff who require ongoing nursing assessment and anticipated interventions for chronic or acute conditions. Table 43.2 provides several examples and implications.

STAFFING NEEDS

An important consideration in planning a school health office is consideration of who will staff the site. Every student should have access to a full-time registered school nurse all day in each school (National Association of School Nurses [NASN], 2003b), yet this is not a universal practice.

Each school should have an adequate school nurse-to-student ratio. The nationally recommended caseload is 1:750 in the general population. In schools with students who are mainstreamed, the caseload is recommended at 1:225, and in schools with students who are severely chronically ill or developmentally disabled, the caseload should be no more than 1:125. Nursing ratios for medically fragile children need to be based on the individual needs of each child (NASN, 2004a). Depending on the state nurse practice act and the school's health services plan, school nursing services may be augmented by others to whom nursing care is delegated or supervised. Volunteers may also contribute to health services with varying degrees of skills and expertise.

If the current staffing plan does not meet the school's health needs, the school nurse should present his or her concerns to her immediate supervisor with local and national data to support his/her position. Assuming the administration is receptive, it will then be important to plan for the needs of additional staff, such as space, furniture, and equipment. Planning and design assumptions should include an evaluation of future trends to determine proper space allocations (Frasca-Beaulieu, 1999).

Each school needs a staffing plan for times when the scheduled staff person is not able to work. Orientation for substitutes is critical for ensuring seamless delivery of services. An orientation should include some time in the school with the school nurse. The substitute should be aware of the location of the substitute folder, which contains the known daily student health needs, the substitute's responsibilities, the location of necessary documentation and emergency plans, any delegated care, and

Table 43.2 ■
IMPACT OF SPECIAL MEDICAL NEEDS ON SCHOOL HEALTH SERVICES

HEALTH CONDITION/ NEED	EQUIPMENT/ SUPPLY NEEDS	ROOM SET-UP NEEDS	MINIMUM STAFFING NEEDS
Asthma	• Locked medication cabinet • Nebulizer • Peak flow meters with disposable mouth pieces • Stethoscope • Pulse oximeter	• Table • Telephone/other immediate access between nurse and classroom • Electricity	• Full-time access to RN to evaluate for PRN medications
Depression	• Locked medication cabinet • Blood pressure monitoring equipment • Scales	• Private and comfortable space for counseling • Therapeutic environment	• RN with counseling skills
Diabetes	• Glucometer • Refrigerator for snacks and possible medication storage • Locked cabinet for insulin syringes	• Telephone/other immediate access between nurse and classroom	• Full-time access to RN to evaluate for PRN medications
Spina bifida with paraplegia	• Clean area for catheterization • No latex products • Wedges • Skin care products	• Bathroom with wheelchair accessibility	• Scheduled nurse or aide to assist with catheterizations, as allowed by law

so forth. An example of essential information for the substitute folder is outlined in FIGURE 43.1.

THE HEALTH OFFICE

Location

The health office is ideally located near the administrative office. While it should meet the federal requirements for accessibility (Butin, 2002), it should also be located for optimal client use. A location adjacent to other student support services (counseling, psychological, social work, and chemical health) is advised (Minnesota Department of Health & MDCFL, 1996). The office should be convenient and easily accessible to both students and families, but not in a high traffic or noisy area that negates efforts to create a calm and healing environment. Noisy areas include the playground, music room, cafeteria, gymnasium, and rooms with noisy machinery (MDH & MDCFL, 1996). Choosing a room that allows some natural lighting enhances the ability of the nurse in physical assessment.

Facility Design

The health office is planned to optimally support the school nurse in providing safe and efficient care. Considerations should be given to the design in order to create a welcoming milieu and space that models a healthy environment. Optimally, it should be stress reducing, convenient and easily accessible, accommodating, and client-focused (Frasca-Beaulieu, 1999).

School *School Nurse Hours*____________

DAILY SCHEDULE:

Location/description of keys:____________
Voicemail access:____________ **Computer Access:**____________
Break time:____________ **Lunch time:**____________
Role with absentees:____________

CONFIDENTIAL HEALTH CONCERNS

Confidential health list____________
Special Procedures list:____________
Role in delegation of care, if applicable:____________

MEDICATIONS and TREATMENTS:

Medications/treatments list and schedule

GENERAL STUDENT INFORMATION:

School class lists and schedules:____________
Student emergency information:
Student health records location:____________
Class Periods:____________ **Lunch periods:**____________
End of Day Routine:____________

SCHOOL STAFF INFORMATION:

School staff contacts information____________
School nurse contact information for assistance____________

ILLNESS:

Equipment/supplies____________
Communicable disease recording & reporting forms____________
List of students who are exempt from immunizations____________

INJURIES:

First aid guidelines, equipment and supplies:____________
Required Injury/Incident Reports:____________

REFERENCES:

School health manual, protocols and guidelines:
Pediatric reference books:____________

OTHER:

Map of building with fire escape plans:____________
Fire Drill and Crisis Plan, with information on students needing special assistance:____________

Figure 43.1 ■ Health services substitute information.

The physical layout, client control of the environment, noise level, colors, and decorations all influence the overall milieu of the health office. Individuals receiving even short-term treatments can often feel anxious, which is a natural consequence of illness (Frasca-Beaulieu, 1999). Designs can create an aesthetically pleasing, comfortable, emotionally supportive, and stress-reducing space. Designs also support a healthy environment.

Physical Layout

The physical layout of the health office needs to focus on the students and accommodate to their needs. Patient education and service delivery are supported by a well-planned space. Even the philosophy and image of school health services and its future growth are apparent in the design. Variables that affect the design include the amount and location of space allocated for a health office, the budget, the health services staffing, and school resources that may exist in other locations of the school (e.g., counseling, private conference area, screening rooms).

Because of the number of students who will be in the health office at one time, the physical layout should allow the school nurse to visually supervise all areas of the health room as well as provide privacy. Visual supervision is critical in providing a safe and secure environment (Maryland State Department of Education [MSDE], 2002). A desk or other suitable writing surface with a nearby telephone outlet allows the student to speak directly and privately with a parent when needed.

At some time during a school nurse's career, the school nurse may be involved in a renovation project or work with a team creating a new health office. Many hours may be spent planning with a team of nonclinical professionals, such as architects, contractors, designers, and facilities staff. It is important to participate to ensure that patient welfare and clinical efficiencies are considered in the planning and implementation phases. Your role will be that of a liaison and interpreter between your staff or your needs and the project team. This will include:

- Being actively involved in the planning as early as possible, as soon as an architect has been hired
- Keeping a copy of the most current plans
- Keeping your own project meeting notes and being on the mailing list for project meetings and notes
- Involving all staff who have knowledge about the workings of the health office and those who may be working there (Greenberg, 2000)

When designing a school heath office, it may be helpful to examine different floor plans. Guidelines for square footage and floor plans are in TABLE 43.3 and FIGURES 43.2, 43.3, 43.4, 43.5, AND 43.6.

Table 43.3 ■
MINIMUM NET SQUARE FOOT GUIDELINES

ELEMENTARY SCHOOLS			
Function	**Student Enrollment**		
	<300	<600	>600
Waiting	75	75	100
Treatment/medication	100	100	120
Office/consult/exam	150	100–150	100
Exam/isolation	100	100	100–150
Rest area	100	150	200
Toilet room(s)	50–60	50–60	50–100
Storage area	25–30	30–40	40
Total	500–515	555–625	710–785
MIDDLE/HIGH SCHOOLS			
Function	**Student Enrollment**		
	<600	<1,200	>1,200
Waiting	80	100	150
Treatment/medication	100	125	140

(continued)

Table 43.3 ■ *(Continued)*

MIDDLE/HIGH SCHOOLS			
Office/consult/exam	100–150	100–150	100–150
Exam/isolation	90–100	100–125	100–125
Rest areas	200	200	200
Toilet room(s)	50–60	50–100	100
Storage room	30–40	40–50	50
Total	610–680	715–800	840–865

Source: MSDE (2002).

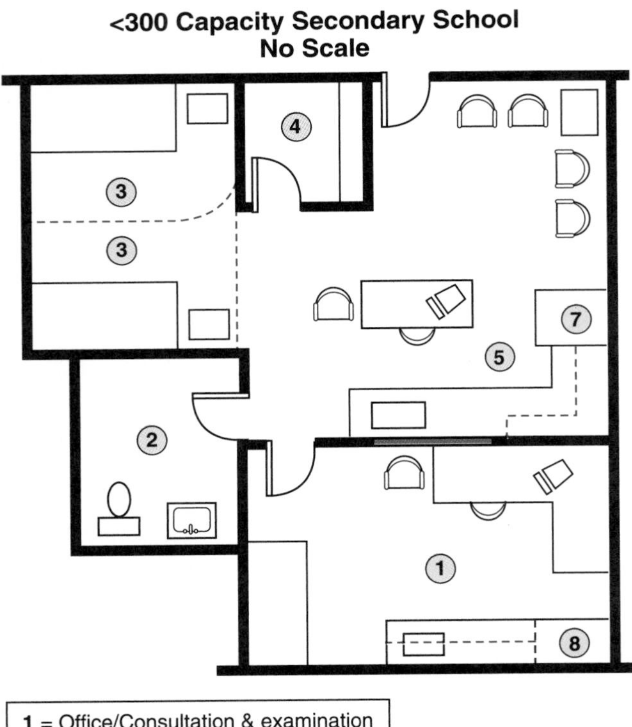

Figure 43.2 ■ Less than 300 capacity elementary school.

Control of the Environment

Pioneering interior designers are embracing psychoneuro-immunology, an emerging field of both art and science, to enhance well-being, creativity, and performance. This approach "combines color, art, interior design, music, and science to produce wellness-enhancing environments. This new scientific method brings more attention to creating wholesome and healthy environments and the holistic approach of healing through appropriate balance of light, color, and space" (Beckwith, 2000, p. 1).

This philosophy believes that tranquil spaces can enhance healing. A decrease in clutter with closed cabinets that hide office paraphernalia can create a sense of order and a calming atmosphere (Beckwith, 2000). Attention to control-related issues enhances nurse–client interactions. A sense of privacy and a feeling of security reduce stress levels (Frasca-Beaulieu, 1999).

Noise Level

Noise levels can induce or reduce stress. "Noise alone is one of the most significantly detrimental environmental factors known to cause physiological changes in the body and affect healing . . . Thoughtful space planning can reduce noise levels" (Frasca-Beaulieu, 1999, p. 69). Positive distractions can help make noises less noticeable. Music is an example of a positive distraction that influences the perception of noise.

Color

Lighting affects color. Effective integration of lighting and color can create spaces that appear to be not only warm, caring, friendly, and supportive but also

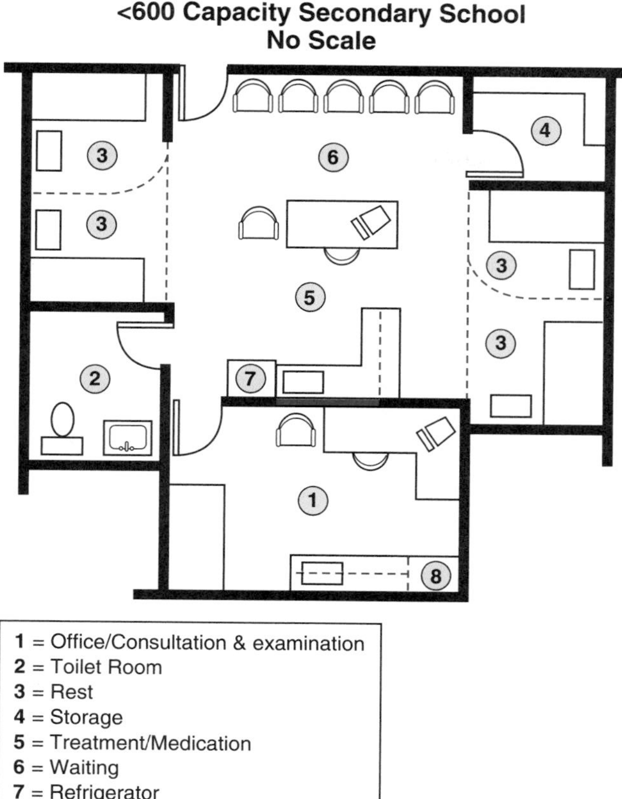

Figure 43.3 ■ Less than 600 capacity elementary School.

dignified and technically proficient. Color can reduce institutional appearance, reinforce the philosophy of the health services, support function, reduce stress, and create a visually interesting, aesthetically pleasing, and stimulating space while creating a supportive, nurturing, and healthy environment. Colors are introduced in furnishings, drapes, and artwork. Sufficient lighting also enhances safety. In addition to natural light, bright and adjustable overhead illumination (2 × 4 fluorescent) is recommended in rest areas, in closets, and over the treatment area (Texas Department of Health [TDH], 2001).

Decoration

Decorative touches enhance the space and create a familiar atmosphere. Warm colors, varied lighting, and furnishings can create a more inviting, homelike, and user-friendly room that is more familiar and relaxing. Different textures minimize the institutional feel, reduce stress, and add interest. Nature scenes can reduce blood pressure and muscle tension (Frasca-Beaulier, 1999). All interior design considerations should appeal to the age group of the students being served.

Healthy and Safe Environment

Cleanliness and serenity are closely linked. Cleanliness is associated with neatness, orderliness, and methodical activity and can give students and staff a higher level of confidence in the health services provided. The design must support a sanitary and safe environment that promotes good health. The ability to clean and sanitize the environment requires consideration when purchasing furnishings and/or planning work areas. "The surface finishes in these areas should be designed for easy cleaning and sanitizing without sacrificing an aesthetically pleasing environment. This would include the treatment of floors, walls, windows, window blinds/

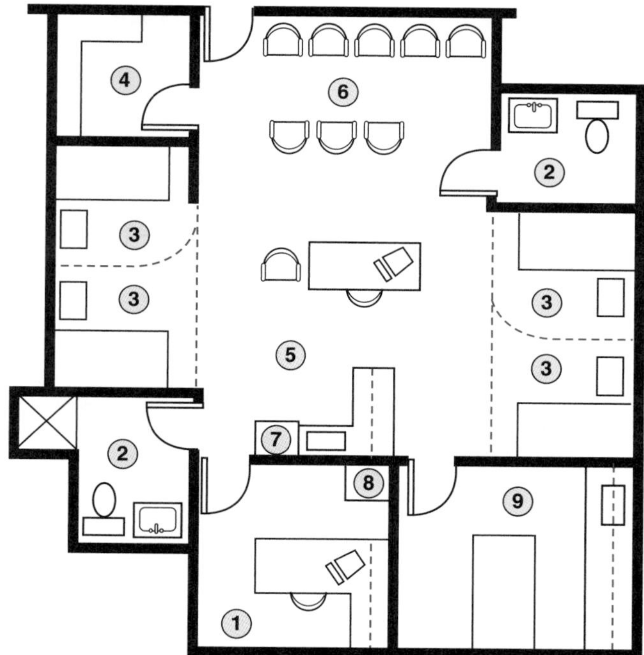

Figure 43.4 ■ Greater than 600 capacity elementary/regional special education school. Less than 1,200 capacity secondary/regional special education school.

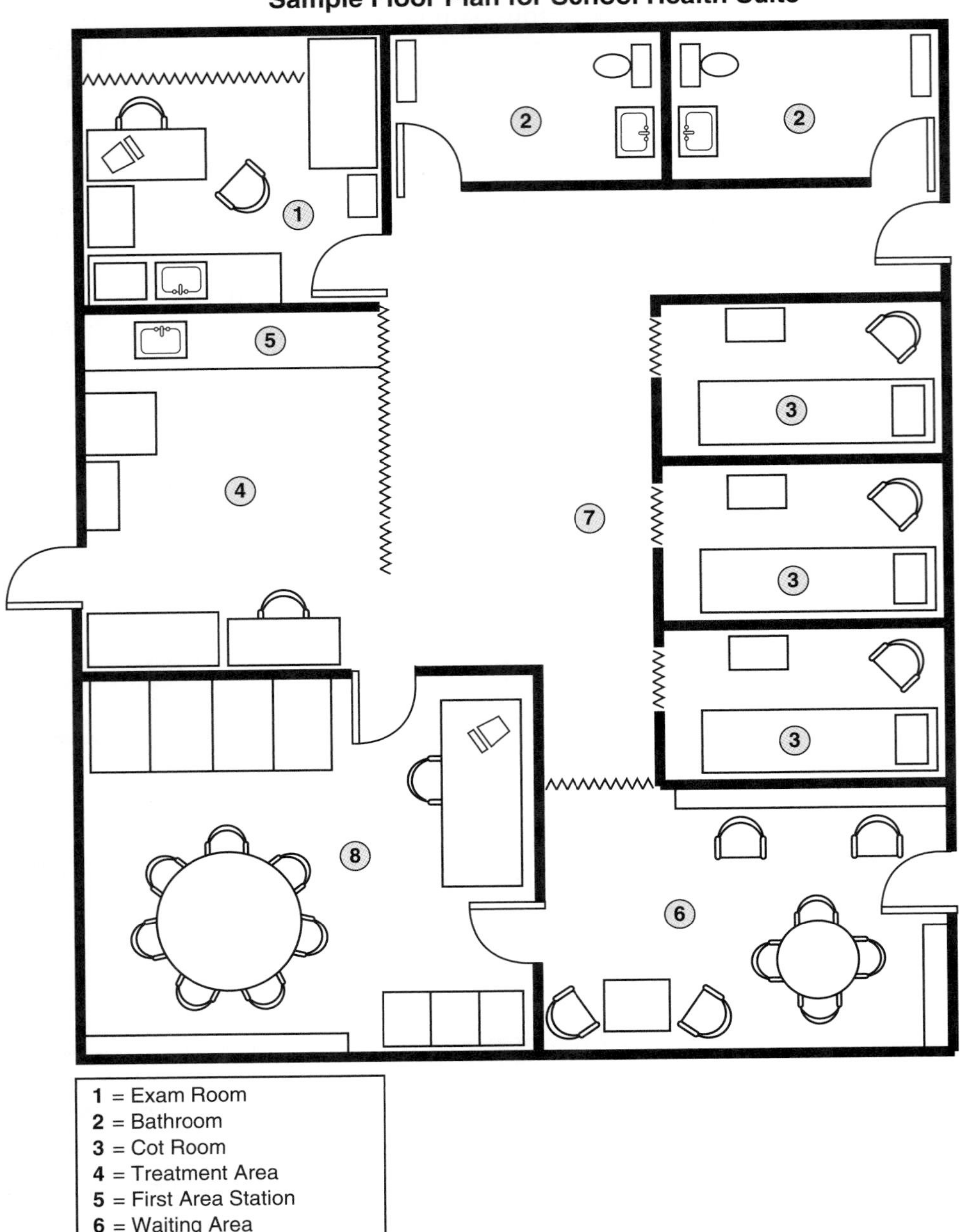

Figure 43.5 ■ Sample floor plan for school health suite.

shades, and counter tops" (MSDE, 2001). It is advised that areas should be reserved for health services purposes only (MDH & MDCFL, 1996). A space with adequate ventilation supports infection control and helps to eliminate foul odors. While aromatherapy is gaining in popularity, it can create strong smells that can trigger asthma and allergic reactions in sensitive people; thus, it should be avoided.

Infection control is a priority in the health office. There is daily risk of communicable disease exposure from one child to another. A rare case in 1981 of a measles outbreak in a pediatrician's office highlights possibilities for a school health office. In this case a symptomatic 12-year-old, with vaccination at 11 $^1/_2$ months, spent one hour in the office. Although most of this time was in a separate examining room, seven other children later presented with secondary cases. Of these, three never saw or were in the same room as the first child. Investigation revealed the exposure came through office airflow (Bloch et al., 1985). While such air-

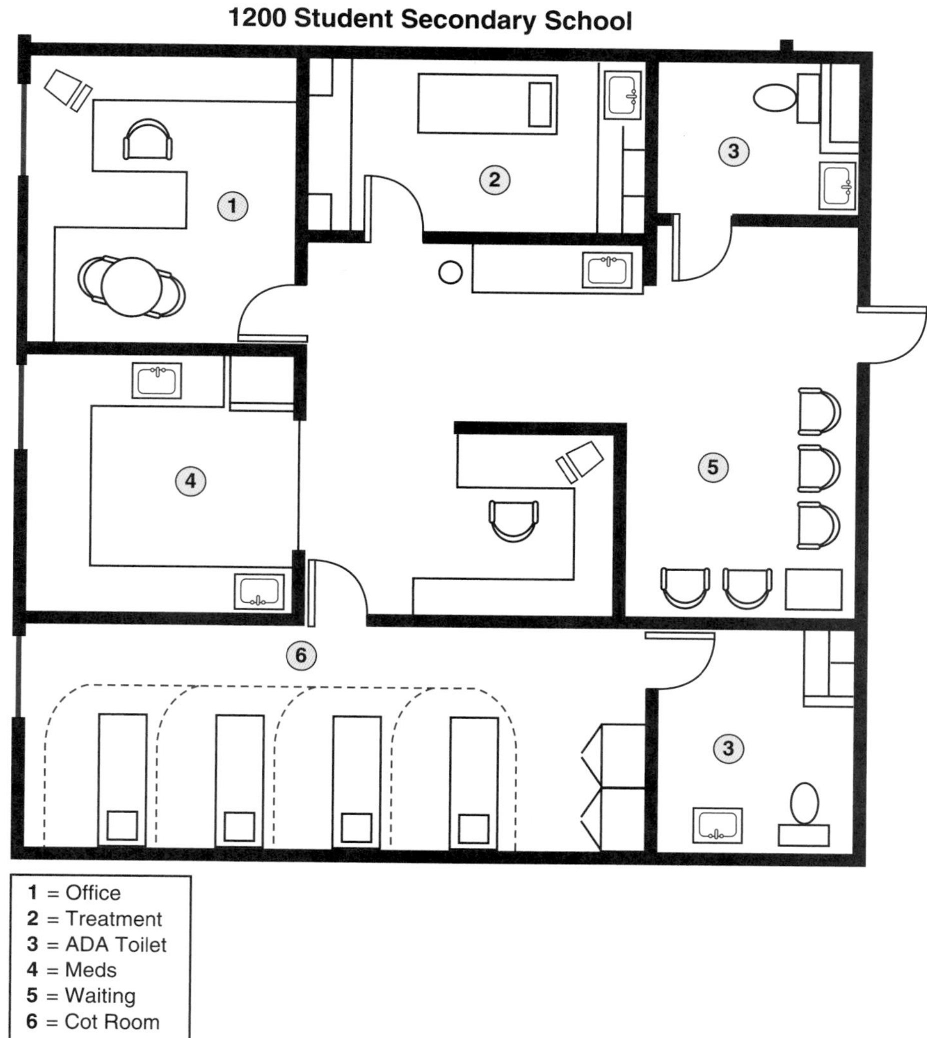

Figure 43.6 ■ 1,200-Student secondary school.

borne transmission is unusual, it illustrates the need for expert architectural designs and for mandatory immunization compliance.

The American Academy of Pediatrics (AAP) recognizes that while infection control in the hospital settings is updated on a regular basis, there are no comprehensive, national guidelines for the practice of infection control in the outpatient setting (AAP, 2000). To meet this void, the AAP released a policy statement, Infection Control in Physicians' Offices, in 2000. Their recommendations are available in FIGURE 43.7. Adequate equipment and supplies are needed to integrate these recommendations into the school setting.

In 1991, the Occupational Safety and Health Administration (OSHA) established rules to protect employees, who may potentially be exposed to blood or other body fluids as a result of their job duties in the healthcare setting (OSHA, 1991). While states may adopt the federal standards as presented or develop their own plan (NASN, 2003a), their guidelines serve as a gold standard for reducing exposure to bloodborne pathogens and planning for safety in the work site. Six OSHA standards apply specifically to physician offices (Guglielmo, 2004) and should be considered in planning for the school health office (TABLE 43.4).

Waiting and Triage Areas

The waiting and triage areas are used for students who are waiting to be seen by the school nurse or waiting to go home after being seen. An adequate number of chairs for seating are needed corresponding to the student enrollment and frequency of use. This area can contribute to health education if wall space allows for educational posters, racks are available for health information and referral materials, bookcases are accessible with age-appropriate read-

Summary of AAP Infection Control Policies

1. All healthcare professionals should wash their hands before and after patient contact. Parents and children should be taught the importance of hand-washing.
2. Standard precautions should be used in dealing with all patients.
3. Contact between infected, contagious children and uninfected children should be minimized. Policies to deal with children who present with infections, such as varicella or measles, should be implemented. Prompt triage of immunocompromised children should be performed routinely.
4. Alcohol is preferred for skin preparation before immunization and routine venipuncture. Skin preparation for incision, suture and collection of blood for culture, requires iodine; solutions of choice are 1% or 2% tincture of iodine or povidone-iodine.
5. Needles and sharps should be handled with great care. Needle disposal units that are impermeable and puncture-proof should be available near the areas used for injection or venipuncture. The containers should not be overfilled and should be kept out of the reach of young children. Policies should be established for removal and incineration or sterilization of contents.
6. Policies for the management of needlestick injuries should also be in place.
7. Standard guidelines for sterilization, disinfection and antisepsis should be followed.
8. Judicious use of antimicrobial agents is essential to limit the spread of drug-resistant bacteria.
9. Outpatient offices and clinics should develop policies and procedures for communication with local and state health authorities regarding reportable diseases and suspected outbreaks.
10. Ongoing educational programs that encompass appropriate aspects of infection control should be implemented, reinforced, and evaluated on a regular basis.

(AAP, 2000)

Figure 43.7 ■ Summary of AAP infection control policies.

Table 43.4 ■
OSHA STANDARDS APPLIED TO THE SCHOOL HEALTH OFFICE

STANDARD	OFFICE DESIGN AND FURNISHINGS	OFFICE SUPPLIES & EQUIPMENT	OTHER
Bloodborne pathogens		• Protective equipment (gloves, face & eye protection, gowns) • Sharps container	• Current (annual) plan with exposure plan • Standard precautions • Plan for Hepatitis B vaccines to indicated staff and record-keeping • Staff training
Hazardous chemical communication (alcohol, disinfectants) (information to staff and others)	• Proper storage	• Manufacturer-supplied material safety & data sheets	• Staff training
Exit routes	• Clearly marked exits	• Posted exit routes	
Electrical	• Electrical capacity for equipment	• Safe use and location of all electrical items	

(continued)

STANDARD	OFFICE DESIGN AND FURNISHINGS	OFFICE SUPPLIES & EQUIPMENT	OTHER
Reporting occupational injuries and illnesses			• Protocols for reporting and documenting
OSHA poster of employee rights		• Poster in easily visible location (available at www.osha.gov/Publications/poster.html)	

Source: Adapted from Guglielmo (2004).

ing materials and a computer with software for health education and/or health games can be easily accessed.

Assessment and Treatment Areas

The assessment and treatment areas require hot and cold running water, a refrigerator with ice-making capability, wall-mounted liquid soap dispenser, access to an electrical outlet, furniture suitable for the age of the student population, a locked medicine cabinet, trash/sharps receptacles, computer access for prompt documentation, and easily accessible cabinet space for supplies. Privacy and close access to a restroom are preferable. The number of beds or cots should correspond to student enrollment and frequency of use.

Counseling Area

Literature supports the link between environmental factors and the patient's health (Peck, 1996). Normalizing the environment through furnishings, sounds, colors, and layout allows students to relax more quickly and find the school health office to be a "safe haven" in the school.

Some students are uncomfortable knowing that others may be aware of their visit to the health office. Ideally, there should be a back entrance for them to enter or exit when they express this concern. The counseling area should ensure privacy of both sight and sound and be easily accessible. A private telephone line as well as an extension telephone are important assets. This area, too, is an ideal site for health education and promotion through availability of health materials.

All students should feel welcome in the school health office. School communities are becoming more and more diverse. The school nurse's choice of health posters and artwork can create an atmosphere of acceptance and respect.

Storage

Locked storage space is essential for equipment, supplies, records, and medication. One security option for locking the health office and medication cabinets is a magnetic card-reader key that tracks whose card unlocks the door and when this occurs. Computerized health records reduce the amount of locked storage space required, but filing cabinets are still necessary. The storage space for supplies can be a large cabinet(s) or a walk-in closet fitted with floor-to-ceiling shelving.

Other

Additional recommendations to optimize the health office include: air conditioning, foot operated soap dispensers and hospital faucets in the lavatory and treatment area, a private lavatory by the assessment area, sound-absorbing ceiling tiles, adjustable door closers to eliminate excess noise, and double-grounded electrical outlets (MDH & MDCFL, 1996). Other suggestions include a wireless computer for moving around in the office and partitions to create new space and privacy.

EQUIPMENT AND SUPPLIES

Equipment

It is helpful to maintain an inventory of equipment and supplies. Recording the dates of purchase and expiration dates expedites efficient tracking. Equipment needs vary with each school. An example of a school health office equipment inventory form is seen in FIGURE 43.8.

The school nurse's planning calendar should include an annual time for restocking and for regular calibration of equipment as recommended by the

Health Office Equipment Inventory

____

____

(School) (Month/Year)

REFERENCE BOOKS: Year

- Control of communicable diseases manual ____
- Medical dictionary ____
- Medication teaching manual ____
- Pharmacological reference ____
- Physical assessment book ____
- School health reference manual ____
- School nursing/pediatric textbook ____
- Other________________ ____
- Other________________ ____

COMPUTER: Model________________ PRINTER________________ FAX________________
AUDIOMETER: Model ________________ Serial #________________ Otoscope________________
VISION TESTING: Stand__________ HOTV Chart__________ Snellen__________ Other Chart__________
Glasses Repair Kit__________ 20 foot Measuring Tape__________ Ophthalmoscope__________
BLOOD PRESSURE: Stethoscope________________ sphygmomanometer________________
Cuffs - Large__________ Adult__________ Child__________
SCOLIOMETER__________ BLOOD GLUCOSE METER__________ REFLEX HAMMER__________
BEDDING: Cots (#)__________ Blankets (#)__________ Soft pillows with vinyl covers (#)__________
LIGHTING: battery pen light (#)__________ magnifying light__________ flashlight__________
PEAK FLOW: Meters (#)__________ Disposable mouth pieces (#)__________ Nebulizer (#)__________
FIRST AID KITS(#) __________ CRUTCHES(#) __________ RING CUTTER __________
WHEELCHAIR with leg lifts:__________ STRETCHER:__________ BACKBOARD__________
SCALES: Upright__________ Portable__________ Stadiometer__________ BMI CALCULATOR__________
BEDSIDE TABLES (#)__________ BASINS (wash/emesis) (#)__________ PORTABLE FAN (#)__________
EXAMINING FLOOR LAMP__________ CLOCK with second hand__________ TIMER__________
REFRIDGERATOR__________ EXAM TABLE__________
COLD PACKS(#): large__________ small__________ INSTANT (#)__________
THERMOMETERS: Electronic__________ Ear__________ Small battery (#)__________
IPECAC (expiration)__________ GLUCOSE GEL (expiration)__________ EYE WASH BOTTLE__________
CPR MASK adult__________ child__________ AIRWAYS__________ AMBU BAG__________
AED__________ DISPOSABLE SUCTION UNIT__________ ELECTRONIC SUCTION UNIT__________
OTHER

____

Figure 43.8 ■ Health office equipment inventory.

manufacturer, the State Department of Health, or the State Department of Education.

Any equipment list needs to be customized to the individual school community. For example, one school may need a Hoyer® lift and another school will require an adjustable table for diapering. Table 43.2 can help the school nurse anticipate needs for specific conditions. Some schools may have additional medication or equipment needs, especially if they have a long emergency medical system (EMS) response time.

Cardiovascular disease remains the most common cause of death in the United States. Sudden, out-of-hospital cardiac arrest claims more than 1,000 lives each day (Caffrey, Willoughby, Pepe, & Becker, 2002). Each year, there are 12 to 20 cases of sudden cardiac death among youth athletes, with another five cases of commotio cordis, which is a blunt, nonpenetrating chest blow causing sudden cardiac arrest (Lovinger, 2002). Most of the cardiac arrests are caused by ventricular fibrillation, which are highly reversible with the rapid application of a defibrillator. An increased long-term survival rate with a good neurological outcome has been demonstrated when patients underwent defibrillation within five to seven minutes (Caffrey et al., 2002).

Recent developments in automated-external-defibrillator (AED) technology have provided a means of increasing prompt defibrillation.

It is hoped that school-based, public access AEDs will strengthen the Chain of Survival in the United States. At least one state has passed legislation that requires the placement of AEDs in every school. A national consensus group, including NASN and Emergency Medical Services for Children, recommends an AED on a list of essential school emergency equipment (Bobo, Hallenbeck, & Robinson, 2003).

Supplies

As with equipment, supply needs differ with each school. Some items may be included depending on recommendations of a medical advisor or state protocols. An ongoing supply list provides an annual record of what exists in the health office and what supplies were used during the school year. This is particularly helpful if there are staffing changes or if other programs and staff use the health office when the school is not in session. A comprehensive list of supplies is included for review and consideration (FIGURE 43.9) when planning a new health office or expanding an existing one. A number of vendors who serve the school health community can be helpful in choosing state-of-the-art supplies and in identifying funding sources.

SPECIAL CONSIDERATIONS

Americans with Disability Act Requirements

The *Americans with Disability Act* (U.S. Department of Justice, 1994) *Accessibility Guidelines* dictate that schools must meet the standards regarding handicap access space and equipment. The *ADA Accessibility Guidelines for Buildings and Facilities* include specific requirements that can be applied to the school health office. Special attention should be given to the most current revisions of law regarding the section labeled *Accessible Elements and Spaces: Scope and Technical Requirements that included Accessible Route, Toilet Stalls, Urinals, Toilet Rooms, and Sinks. Sec.36.304 Removal of Barriers*. It stipulates specific requirements to accommodate individuals with disabilities. Architectural barriers in existing facilities have to be removed, including communication barriers. Examples include:

- Installing ramps;
- Repositioning shelves;
- Rearranging tables, chairs, display racks, and other furniture;
- Repositioning telephones and computers;
- Adding raised marking on room entry, lavatory, and other areas;
- Widening doors or installing hardware for easy widening;
- Installing grab bars in toilet stalls;
- Rearranging toilet partitions to increase maneuvering space;
- Insulating any sink pipes to prevent burns;
- Installing a raised toilet seat;
- Installing a full-length bathroom mirror;
- Repositioning the paper towel dispensers for access; and
- Removing high-pile, low-density carpeting.

(U.S. Department of Justice, 1994)

It is often the school nurse's responsibility to ensure that the accessibility needs of students and staff are identified and that measures are taken within the school to accommodate to these needs. While all of the above recommendations have impact for the entire school building, they also have implications for setting up the school health office.

Record-Keeping Requirements

"One of the most challenging responsibilities of school nurses is managing the many types of student health records, both paper and electronic" (NASN, 2004b). Maintaining confidentiality and ensuring safe storage is often the responsibility of the school nurse. Policies should be developed at the state or local levels to mandate that adequate mechanisms are in place to protect student data. The school health office must provide a means for safe storage, limited access, and simple retrieval of files and easy access to technology that can transmit and receive electronic information. A state of the art computer with printer and fax and a shredder are no longer luxuries, but necessities for the school nurse.

RESOURCES TO ACCESS EQUIPMENT AND SUPPLIES

School health services have been historically covered by the general school budget (Duncan & Igoe, 1998). Funding is now more diverse, and sources may be pieced together from state, nonprofit, and other agencies with targeted outreach goals that can be met in the school setting. Medicaid, private insur-

(text continues on page 1032)

Health Services Supply Order Worksheet

The anticipated yearly needs should be listed in the first column, *"NEEDS for the Year."* The current inventory should be listed in the second column, "MINUS current Inventory." When the current inventory in the second column is subtracted from the yearly needs in the first column, the resulting number should be placed in the third column, *"EQUALS PURCHASE number for the following school year".*

Supplies	**Needs For the Year ____ *(date)***	**Minus Current Inventory**	**Equals Purchase number for following school year _____ *(date)***
Alcohol (bottle -70% Isopropyl)			
Applicators (1000/box)			
Cotton-tip			
Plain			
Bandages/dressings			
Bandages:			
3/8″ Junior (50/box)			
3/4″ Strips (100/box)			
1″ Strips (100/box)			
2″ large strips (100/box)			
Small fingertip (100/box)			
Knuckle (50 box)			
Medium butterfly (100/box)			
Large butterfly (100/box)			
Sheer spot (100/box)			
Elastic wrap:			
2″ (each)			
3″ (each)			
4″ (each)			
Eye pads (box)			
Gauze roll 1″ stretch (box)			
Gauze roll 2″ stretch (box)			
Gauze roll 3″ stretch (box)			
Gauze pad 2×2 indiv. pkg (box)			
Gauze pad 3×3 indiv. pkg (box)			
Gauze pad 4×4 indiv pkg (box)			
Gauze sponges:			
2×2″ Non-sterile (200/bag)			
3×3″ Non-sterile (200/bag)			
4×4″ Non-sterile (200/bag)			
Non-adhering pads:			
2×3″ (100/box)			
3×4″ (100/box)			
Eye pad			
Sanitary pads (individually wrapped)			
Triangle muslin bandage			
Tape			
Cloth 1/2″ (24/box)			
Cloth 1″ (12/box)			
Cloth 2″ (6/box)			
Splints:			
Finger splint (roll)			
Board splint (package of 12)			
Batteries			
Blanket (one/cot)			
Bleach (qt)			
Cotton balls (large bag)			
Cot paper pillow covers			
CPR pocket mask (one per school)			
Cups:			
Paper (1200/case)			
Medication			
100 Plastic			
250 Paper			
Dental floss (each)			
Diabetic supplies			

Figure 43.9 ■ Health services supply order worksheet.

Supplies	Needs For the Year ____ *(date)*	Minus Current Inventory	Equals Purchase number for following school year _____ *(date)*
Glucose test strips			
Control solution			
Lancets			
Glucose meter battery			
Disinfectant			
Disposable diapers			
Emergency medication*			
Eye chart – HOTV/Snellen			
Eye cup			
Eyewash solution			
First aid kit (tool box)			
Fingernail clipper (each)			
Fingernail brush (each)			
Gowns, disposable			
Hazardous labels			
Ice cold pack – small			
Large			
Quick Cold			
Lotion – hand (10 oz)			
Magnifying glass			
Masks			
Medication/Pill envelopes			
Medication spoon (each)			
Office supplies			
Ointments, creams			
Otoscope			
Battery			
Light bulb			
Disposable speculum 3 mm			
Disposable speculum 4 mm			
Disposable speculum 5 mm			
Peak flow meter mouthpieces			
Pen flashlight			
Light battery			
Light bulb			
Pharmaceuticals:			
Antibiotic ointment (tube)			
Antiseptic solution (8 oz)			
Calamine (8 oz)			
Contact lens solution (spray)			
Ipecac (one/school)			
Petroleum jelly (1 oz tube)			
Pillow cover, Vinyl			
Plastic bags:			
Bags – small (box)			
Bags – large (box)			
Zip bags – small (box)			
Zip bags – large (box)			
Red contaminate			
Safety Pins:			
Small (bag)			
Medium (bag)			
Large (bag)			
Scissors:			
Bandage			
Straight (one/school)			
Manicure			
Sharps container			
1 Qt needle storage container			
5 Qt needle storage container			
Slings:			
Triangular bandage			
Soap			

Figure 43.9 ■ *(continued)*

Supplies	Needs For the Year ____ *(date)*	Minus Current Inventory	Equals Purchase number for following school year ____ *(date)*
Standard precautions clean-up kit			
Tape			
Thermometer			
Small digital			
Battery (small digital)			
Covers (small digital)			
Battery (ear)			
Probe covers (ear)			
Battery (large electronic)			
Probe covers (large electronic)			
Tissues			
Tongue blades (box)			
Junior			
Regular			
Towels			
Paper			
Cloth			
Tweezers			
Fine point			
Broad point			
Vaseline			
Wax, dental			
Washcloths			
Miscellaneous items:			
Baking soda			
Salt			
Sugar packets			
Non-latex supplies:			
Bandages:			
Junior (non-latex)			
3/4″ (non-latex)			
1″ (non-latex)			
2″ (non-latex)			
Fingertip – small/medium (non-latex)			
Fingertip – large (non-latex)			
Sheer Spot (non-latex)			
3″ Wrap (non-latex)			
Gloves:			
Small (non-latex)			
Medium (non-latex)			
Large (non-latex)			

(Supply lists are compiled from recommended lists from Departments of Education or Health in Delaware, Maine, Massachusetts, Minnesota, Virginia and Texas. Epinephrine availability is a standard in Delaware and Maine.)

Figure 43.9 ■ *(continued)*

ance, federal block grants, and foundation dollars may cover all or part of the school health services program (Duncan & Igoe, 1998).

School nurses are creative in their approaches to funding equipment and supplies; they often look outside of the school budget. Each state and local jurisdiction allocates funds differently and it is important for the school nurse to understand the options that are available even though he or she may not be directly involved with accessing them. Seeking new funding sources relieves some of the school's financial burden and engages new collaborative partners (see Chapters 19 and 44). These include local foundations, community service organizations, and local clinics and pharmaceutical companies whose missions are to support community health initiatives. School nurse *Wish Lists for Kids* are welcome in parent newsletters, the local paper, the health advisory committee communications, and local health agencies.

CONCLUSION

School nurses are leaders and change agents for the health of children in schools. The school health office facility can facilitate the outreach of health services to the school community. Students have the right to receive quality services within an environment that is safe, efficient, welcoming, and effective.

References

American Academy of Pediatrics (AAP). (2000). Policy Statement: Infection control in physicians' offices. *Pediatrics, 105*(6), 1361– 1369. Retrieved on March 12, 2005 from http://aappolicy.aappublications.org/cgi/content/full/pediatrics;105/6/1361

Beckwith, D. (2000). Influences of color in healthcare: Nature, technology, and culture. *HermanMiller for Healthcare*, pp. 1–5. Retrieved on March 2005 from http://www.hermanmiller.com

Bloch, A. B., Orenstein, W. A., Ewing, W. M., Spain, W. H., Mallison, G. F., Herrmann, K. L., & Hinman, A. R. (1985). Measles outbreak in a pediatric practice: Airborne transmission in an office setting. *Pediatrics, 75*(4), 676–684.

Bobo, N., Hallenbeck, P., & Robinson, J. (2003). Recommended minimal emergency equipment and resources for schools: National consensus group report. *Journal of School Nursing, 19*(3), 150–156.

Butin, D. (July, 2002). School health centers. *National Clearinghouse for Educational Facilities*, 1–4.

Caffrey, S., Willoughby, P., Pepe, P., & Becker, L. (2002). Public use of automated external defibrillators. *New England Journal of Medicine, 347*(16), 1242–1247.

Duncan, P., & Igoe, J. B. (1998). School Health Services. In E. Marx & S. F. Wooley with D. Northrup (Eds.), *Health is academic* (pp. 169–194) New York: Teachers College Press.

Frasca-Beaulieu, K. (1999). Interior design for ambulatory care facilities: How to reduce stress and anxiety in patients and families. *Journal of Ambulatory Care Management, 22* (10), 67–73.

Greenberg, L. (2000). A clinician's guide to construction/renovation project success. *HermanMiller for Healthcare*, pp. 1–6. Retrieved 3/05 from http://www.hermanmiller.com

Guglielmo,W. (July 1, 2004). Your guide to OSHA regulations. *RN*, 2–4.

Lovinger, S. (2002). How useful are automated external defibrillators? *Journal of the American Medical Association, 228*(23), 2952.

Maine School Health Advisory Committee. (2002). *School health manual*. Retrieved on August 21, 2004 from http://www.state.me.us/education/sh/Schoolnurse.htm#FacilitiesandSupplies

Maryland State Department of Education. (2001). *Guidelines for Maryland school-based health centers, 2001–2003*. Retrieved July 14, 2003 from http://www.healthinschools.org/sr/states/MD/ MD–guidelines.asp#up

Maryland State Department of Education. (2002). *School health services: A facility planning and design guide for school systems*, pp. 1–15.

Massachusetts Department of Health. (1995). I. Goodman & A. F. Sheetz (Eds.), *Comprehensive school health manual* (pp. 2–19). Boston, MA: Author.

Massachusetts Department of Health. (2004). *School health facilities*. Draft for School Health Manual. *Comprehensive school health manual*. Boston, MA: Author.

McKibben, C., & DiPaolo, S. (1997). Promoting the construction of an optimal nurse's office facility: one school district's experience. *Journal of School Nursing, 13*(2), 22–29.

Minnesota Department of Health and Minnesota Department of Children, Families and Learning. (1996). *Minnesota school health guide*, 2–14, 2–18, 2–19, Exhibit 2–6–1, 2–7–1 to 2–7–5.

National Association of School Nurses (NASN). (2003a). *Position statement: Regulations on bloodborne pathogens in the school setting*. Retrieved on August 30, 2004 from http://www.nasn.org/positions/pathogens.htm

National Association of School Nurses (NASN). (2003b). *Resolution: Access to a school nurse*. Retrieved on September 7, 2004 from http://www.nasn.org/resources/resolutionaccess.htm

National Association of School Nurses (NASN). (2004a). *Position statement: Caseload assignments*. Retrieved on March 8, 2005 from http://www.nasn.org/positions/2004pscaseload.htm.

National Association of School Nurses (NASN). (2004b). *Position statement: School health records*. Retrieved on September 9, 2004 from http://www.nasn.org/briefs/records.htm

National Association of School Nurses (NASN). (2003b). *Resolution: Access to a school nurse*. Retrieved on September 7, 2004 from http://www.nasn.org/resources/resolutionaccess.htm

New Mexico Department of Education. (1999). New Mexico school health manual. *Health room facility*, p. 1–7. Retrieved on September 5, 2004 from http://www..nmschoolhealthmanual.org/manual/shm_01.pdf.

Occupational Safety and Health Administration (OSHA), Occupational Exposure to Bloodborne Pathogens. 29CFR Part 1910.1030. (1991).

Peck, R. (1996). The office as 'therapy assistant.' *Health Source: Nursing / Academic Edition, 16*(4). Retrieved on September 2, 2004 from ERBSCO Host at http://web3. epnet.com

Texas Department of Health. (2001). Chapter 2, *School nursing practice*. Retrieved on September 9, 2004 from http://www.tdh.state.tx.us/schoolhealth/chap2.pdf.

Texas Department of Health. (2002). *Environmental health considerations for schools*, checklist for school inspections.

U.S. Department of Justice (1994). *Americans with disabilities act standards for accessible design*. Code of federal regulations 28 CFR Part 36 (1994, July1). Retrieved January 10, 2003 from http://www.usdoj.gov/crt/ada/stdspdf.htm

Virginia Department of Education and Virginia Department of Health. (1999). Overview of school health services. In *Virginia school health guidelines* (2nd ed., pp. 127–146). Retrieved September 5, 2004 from http://www.vahealth.org/schoolhealth/chapter3.pdf

Chapter 44

Budgeting and Accessing Funding

LINDA DAVIS ALLDRITT

Chapter Outline

INTRODUCTION

Traditionally, school health services and programs have been funded at the local level through general education funds from the state government. In school districts where student health is seen as related to academic achievement, general fund monies typically have been designated to ensure the presence of professional school health staff, including school nurses and, in some districts, school physicians. Any economic deficit challenges this model of school health funding, especially in states where school nurses are not legislatively mandated. Even in prosperous economic times, school health program managers (i.e., nursing and non-nursing administrators who are responsible for the school health budget) and school nurses must be vigilant in their search for fiscal support to cover base costs or to augment insufficiently funded programs. Consequently, school budgets are increasingly dependent on a variety of funding streams to pay for student health services.

Demonstrating the ability to access funds for school health programs and to successfully receive funds for reimbursable services is one way for school nurses to demonstrate their effectiveness in their role as well as to demonstrate fiscal responsibility. In addition to reviewing potential funding resources and cost recovery programs, this chapter suggests other important elements in finding and maintaining funding. A section of the chapter focuses on methods to acquire funding through proposal writing. Another section covers marketing skills that will advance school health services as funding priorities for school districts and communities. The final section of the chapter covers the essential costs of setting up the school health program, from hiring the staff to furnishing the health office.

FUNDING SOURCES

School health services are commonly supported by several funding streams. This section reviews resources for funds typically available to local education agencies (LEAs) for the provision of school health services. FIGURE 44.1 graphically represents available funding sources.

State Government

The degree of state funding for school health services varies by state. In most states, federal funds are passed through state departments of education or health, and are added to state tax dollars made available to schools. In some states, tax dollars are targeted separately for school health services.

Federal Education and Health Dollars (Categorical Programs)

The federal government provides some funding for school health services. Some of these funds are in the form of entitlements and others must be periodically reauthorized. Federal education dollars from *No Child Left Behind* legislation (previously the *Improving America's Schools Act*, and before that the *Elementary and Secondary Education Act [Public Law 107-110]*) support education system reform, including the removal of obstacles, such as poor health, that impede children's academic success. Within *No Child Left Behind* there are 10 major sections referred to as "Titles," some of which impact on funding.

a. *No Child Left Behind (NCLB), Title I* funds programs for low-income and low-achieving students. This funding is to be used for supplementary educational and related services as identified by a comprehensive needs assessment of the entire school. Funds available through *Title I* are intended to provide opportunities for all children to meet the state's student academic achievement standards, but particularly are intended to address the needs of low-achieving children and could include additional health and social services that are necessary, but not funded by some other source.

b. *No Child Left Behind (NCLB), Title II* provides funds for the training, recruitment, and

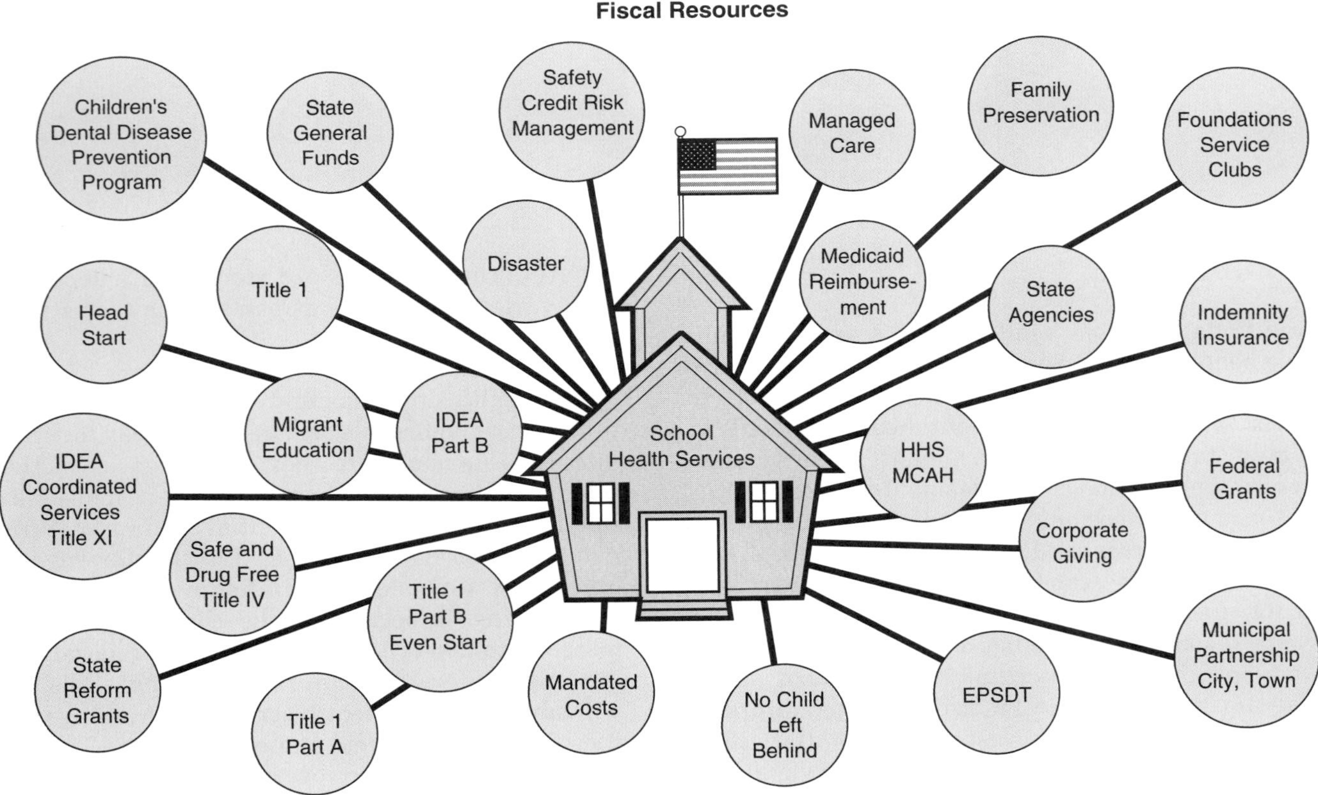

Figure 44.1 ■ School House Fiscal Resources diagram. (Used with permission from Los Angeles County Office of Education/Cathy Bray/January 2004.)

retention of teachers and principals. *Title II* funds may be used for pupil services personnel as long as the local educational agency is meeting its annual measurable objectives as identified in the state plan, and the employment of pupil services personnel aids its schools in effectively recruiting and retaining highly qualified teachers and principals.

c. *No Child Left Behind (NCLB), Title IV* (Safe and Drug Free Schools and Communities) provides funds to school districts to support safe, violence- tobacco-, alcohol- and other drug-free school environments for teaching and learning.

d. *No Child Left Behind (NCLB), Title V* provides funds to states in the form of block grants. A block grant is a fixed amount of money given to states by the federal government to run programs within defined guidelines. In the case of *Title V*, the federal government provides block grants to fund innovative programs to improve student achievement. One of the innovative programs for which states may use *Title V* funds is the hiring and supporting of school nurses.

Other federal laws speak to funding certain initiatives. *Individuals with Disabilities Education Act (IDEA)* is federal legislation that mandates and provides partial funding for health services for children with disabilities (see Chapters 14 and 27). Additional funds for low-income children with disabilities are provided by Medicaid.

Title XIX of the Social Security Act (Medicaid's Early and Periodic, Screening, Diagnostic, and Treatment [EPSDT]) is Medicaid's comprehensive and preventive child health program for low-income children and adolescents ages 0 through 21 years. EPSDT includes periodic health screening, and vision, dental, and hearing services. It requires that any medically necessary health care service listed as part of the federal EPSDT program be provided to an EPSDT recipient even if the service is not available through the state's Medicaid plan to the general Medicaid population. The goals of the EPSDT program are to assure the availability and accessibility of required health care resources and to help Medicaid recipients and their families effectively utilize these resources.

Title V of the Social Security Act (Maternal and Child Health Services Block Grant) provides a lump sum of money to individual states for the funding of health and health-related services to mothers, children and adolescents for the reduction of infant mortality and preventable diseases, and enhances access to necessary health services.

Other Federal and State Programs

Other federal and state agencies make available a variety of competitive funding sources for which schools and districts can apply to implement health programs and services. For instance, the Centers for Disease Control and Prevention (CDC) provide categorical support to state agencies and school districts for programs such as coordinated school health; prevention of Human Immunodeficiency Virus (HIV) and hepatitis B infections; and prevention of childhood obesity and type 2 diabetes. Often, federal and state categorical grants are of multiyear duration, thus allowing grantees time to fully develop their particular programs. LEAs (Local Education Agency) can keep up to date on funding opportunities by subscribing to publications such as the *Federal Register* or accessing online information from government agency Web sites. Special interest and government-sponsored listservs are another source of information about federal and state categorical offerings (TABLE 44.1).

Many states have received large litigation settlements from the tobacco companies that may be available for funding school health services. In November 1998, 46 states settled their lawsuits against the major tobacco companies to recover tobacco-related health care costs. Four states, Minnesota, Mississippi, Florida, and Texas, reached individual settlements earlier in the 1990s. These settlements require the tobacco companies to make annual payments to the states in perpetuity, with total payments over the first 25 years estimated at $246 billion. The multistate settlement, known as the Master Settlement Agreement, also imposed limited restrictions on the marketing of tobacco products. It is estimated that the states will collect $19.5 billion in tobacco-generated revenue from tobacco taxes and the tobacco settlements for 2004 (*Special Reports: State Tobacco Settlement*, 2004, p. 4).

Other Grants and Local Resources

Public and Private Grants

Currently, there are numerous sources of outside funds, both public and private, for school-related programs and projects, including health specific activities; however, many of these resources are narrow categories and typically short-lived. Some of these grants are privately funded, while others are publicly funded. Often these funds are targeted for the development of pilot programs that test the efficacy of a politically sensitive idea or intervention on a specific subset of students, such as family planning for pregnant and parenting teens. Rarely are these type of funds geared toward providing resources for

Table 44.1 ■
SELECTED FEDERAL WEB SITES PROVIDING INFORMATION ON AVAILABLE FUNDS

Early and Periodic Screening, Diagnostic, and Treatment (EPSDT)	http://www.cms.hhs.gov/medicaid/epsdt/default.asp
Federal Register – Main Page	http://www.gpoaccess.gov/fr/index.html
Health Resources and Services Administration (HRSA) – Maternal Child Health Branch	http://mchb.hrsa.gov/grants/default.htm
Medicaid	http://www.cms.hhs.gov/medicaid/
No Child Left Behind	www.ed.gov/policy/elsec/leg/esea02/index.html
U.S. Centers for Disease Control and Prevention	http://www.cdc.gov/funding.htm
U.S. Department of Education – Federal Register Documents	http://www.ed.gov/news/fedregister/index.html

school health services for the general population of students. Consequently, while these funds allow for creativity, the result is a piecemeal approach of short-term, problem- or population-specific funding that is frequently given only once (Allensworth, Lawson, Nicholson, & Wyche, 1997). Even so, schools should not overlook these sources of competitive dollars as they may supplement gaps in the overall school health program.

While both public and private entities accept grant applications, private foundations and public grantors operate somewhat differently. Public grants may be provided directly to the school district or to agencies and organizations that have partnerships with the school district. Private foundations tend to supply smaller amounts of funding than do public funders. Private foundations commonly provide one-time seed money for short-term projects (Bray, 2003). Depending on the foundation, the application process for these private dollars may be quite informal. Public grants tend to be more formal, requiring more detail, more evidence of need, and collaboration with community partners; they typically provide more funds spread over a slightly longer timeframe and include some type of evaluation component.

Local Resources

As school nurses and health services administrators seek funding for their programs, a variety of local resources may be available. Besides funding from the school district itself, other local funding may be available from the county health and social services departments, and other city, county, or regional offices. Fetro (1998) reminded fund seekers that some cities have implemented community-wide children's services initiatives that provide funding for health and human services addressing children's needs. Local service clubs (such as the Elks, Kiwanis, Lions, Shriners, and Soroptomists), local chapters of volunteer health and professional organizations (such as state chapters of the American Lung Association, American Heart Association, American Cancer Society, American Red Cross, Medical Society, and Dental Society), and private healthcare providers may also have funds available to support school programs. In addition to available funds, some organizations and agencies may provide support through adopt-a-school programs that offer resources for use in other areas of the school health program.

Local corporations (such as hospitals, biotech companies, and pharmaceutical firms) may be other sources of funds for schools as those entities have a vested interest in health, particularly in the health of their employees and their families. For instance, Taras (2003) suggested that Local Education Agencies should consider tapping underutilized community resources because hospitals, managed care plans, medical schools, and physician groups are generally interested in preventing student health problems and will often, if asked, donate equipment, such as peak flow meters, and even reimburse school districts for activities such as health education.

RESOURCE MAPPING

As schools and districts work to identify potential funding sources and develop partnerships, it is important that existing resources are recognized and needs for supplemental support determined. Mapping existing funding is basic to a thorough review and allocation or reallocation of assets. Fetro (1998) suggested that prior to looking for new funding to implement additional services, "schools should determine whether (1) the district already receives funds that could support new or expanded initiatives, (2) the district is eligible for such funds, (3) the district makes allocations to schools, and (4) the school is free to pursue additional funding independently" (Fetro, p. 31). Fetro further asserted that "creative thinking, patience, and perseverance are critical" (Fetro, p. 31). TABLE 44-2 provides a sample

Table 44.2 ■
SAMPLE FUNDING/RESOURCE MAP FOR SCHOOL HEALTH SERVICES

	HEALTH SERVICES STAFFING	HEALTH OFFICE EQUIP-MENT	HEALTH SCREEN-INGS	HEALTH ADMINIS-TRATION	EDUCATION/ HEALTH COUN-SELING	OUTREACH/ INSURANCE ENROLL-MENT
NCLB Title I	X		X		X	
NCLB Title II					Staff ed.	
NCLB Title IV	X					
NCLB Title V	X					
Medicaid Billing	X	X	X	X	X	X
Medicaid Adminis-trative Claiming	X	X	X	X	X	X
EPSDT	X		X			
MCH block Grant	X		X			
Tobacco Settlement	X	X	X		X	X
Tobacco tax	X	X	X		X	
State $$	X	X	X	X	X	X
Local $$	X	X	X	X	X	X

funding map. School nurses who understand the funding streams that are available to support school health programs are in an ideal position to assist their school and district in this process.

PROPOSAL WRITING

School districts have numerous opportunities to obtain public and private grants to fund portions of the school health program. Many private foundations offer grants to support research related to specific health problems of the school-age population or to provide health services to targeted student populations. Similar to grant funding from government sources, the funding time period varies and cannot be relied on to provide sustained funding for programs. However, grants do provide funds to meet specific needs and, in some cases, to expand or enhance the school health program. This section focuses on writing and submitting successful grant proposals.

A large amount of information on grant writing is available on the Internet, in libraries, and through nonprofit organizations and for-profit companies. Successful proposal writing entails the synchronization of several activities, including planning, locating funding sources, identifying necessary data, contacting funders, writing and packaging the proposal, submitting the grant proposal to the potential funder, and following up with the funder. The following proposal writing steps may help develop a grant proposal for funding.

Preparatory steps are time consuming. If done well, they tend to simplify the actual writing phase of the grant process. Preparation includes: (1) defining the project and establishing project goals and objectives, (2) identifying appropriate funding sources for the specific project (Table 44.3), (3) accessing the grant proposal guidelines from potential funders, (4) developing a realistic timeline based on the submission deadline, and (5) determining the grant proposal writing team. Once this is done, the team can determine what the staffing and supply needs will be.

Important components of the writing phase of the project include attention to the specific information required by the funder, use of clear, concise, and persuasive language, and a realistic project budget. Grant proposals are commonly composed of the (1) narrative which includes a needs statement, the project goals, objectives and expected outcomes, a work plan, the evaluation method, a timeline for the project, and project staff resumes; (2) project budget showing specific cost estimates; (3) appendix with supplementary attachments, such as support letters, organizational charts, and reference information; and (4) authorizing signatures approving the submission of the proposal. Depending on the funder's requirements, proposals also may include a

Table 44.3 ■
LOCATING FUNDING SOURCES (EXAMPLES)

I. Federal	U.S. Department of Education (http://www.ed.gov/fund/landing.jhtml?src=rt), Health and Human Services (http://www.hrsa.gov/grants/default.htm), Centers for Disease Control (http://www.cdc.gov/funding.htm), and other federal agencies
II. State	State Departments of Education (http://www.cde.ca.gov), Health (http://www.tdh.state.tx.us), Social Services (http://www.dss.state.va.us), and Mental Health (http://www.dhmh.state.md.us), and other state agencies
III. Private corporations and foundations	Examples of companies and foundations at the local, regional, and national levels: Sierra Health Foundation (http://www.sierrahealth.org), The California Endowment (http://www.calendow.org), The Merck Corporation (http://www.merck.com/about/cr/policies_performance/social/philanthropy.html)

Source: Based on Lyon (2003). Reprinted with permission from Los Angeles County Office of Education, Cathy Bray, January 2004.

cover letter, cover sheet, an abstract, a budget narrative, and assurances that any conditions required by the funder will be met.

In addition to developing the content of the proposal, it is imperative to adhere to the technical specifications in the proposal guideline. For instance, the proposal must include only the number of pages allowed and the directions for the format must be followed exactly. Successful proposals are neat, complete and submitted on time (*Basic Elements of Grant Writing, 2003*). Follow directions carefully! Finally, whether or not the proposal is accepted for funding, following-up with the funder will provide valuable information about the proposal's strengths and weaknesses. This information will be of assistance in preparing the next proposal. Box 44.1 provides some tips that successful grant writers have learned through experience. Large districts may have grant writers; medium and small school districts rely on professional staff to write grants in addition to their other duties. As you might imagine, there are many more medium and small school districts than there are large districts that can afford to devote a position within the district structure to a grant writer.

Box 44.1 ■ ■ ■

20 TIPS FROM SUCCESSFUL GRANT WRITERS

1. Do preparation work.
2. Contact the funder.
3. Obtain a Request for Proposal (RFP), application form, or proposal guidelines.
4. Carefully read the guidelines for the grant.
5. Convene a team for brainstorming.
6. Keep in mind that most funders want the same basic information. Do not assume the funder or grant reader knows anything about the subject area.
7. Involve the community through a needs assessment or open forum.
8. Be careful about using acronyms and spell out on first use.
9. Follow grant guidelines exactly.
10. Gather letters of support early/provide templates/hand deliver and collect.
11. Align the project with the purpose and goals of the funding source.
12. Hold regular meetings to keep team members informed and to ensure that the timeline is being followed.
13. Develop a budget that matches the scope of work of the project. Get advice as needed. Do not underestimate or inflate costs.
14. Be flexible about the budget in case the funder wants to negotiate costs.
15. Use a computer and back up with diskettes or CD.
16. Unless expressly prohibited, be repetitive as each section must stand alone.
17. Obtain clerical and editorial support. Proofread the proposal more than once.
18. Adhere to submission date and time.
19. Follow-up with the funder whether or not the grant is funded.

(Corporation for Public Broadcasting, 2003; Davis, 2003; Lyon, 2003).

COST RECOVERY

In challenging economic times, school districts must frequently rely on a combination of local, state, and federal dollars to employ school nurses and other health services staff. Participation in cost recovery programs, which allow the district to recover the costs associated with programs or services, may be a way for districts to ensure long-term sustainability. Several current cost recovery programs are described in this section.

Federal Financial Participation Programs

Federal financial participation (FFP) programs are available to school districts. The funding for these programs comes from the United States Department of Health and Human Services (DHHS) through the state agency for Medicaid. Medicaid is the national public healthcare financing program. Authorized by Title XIX of the Social Security Act, Medicaid is financed by state and federal governments, and administered by the individual states. Medicaid provides health services and long-term care coverage to millions of low-income individuals.

FFP programs require matching funds from the state or local agency. School districts can use state or local education funds as the state match for Medicaid and receive federal funds as reimbursement for providing health-related services to students.

The federal government determines specific guidelines for the administration of these programs. However, states have some flexibility, particularly that of enhancing their existing federal program. When the state uses federal monies to provide a minimal program that offers basic services or an enhanced program that augments the basic program elements with extra services, it must file a plan with the Centers for Medicare and Medicaid Services (CMS). State plans may be amended with federal approval. Implementation of these programs usually requires changes in state laws and regulations.

Early, Periodic, Screening, Diagnosis, and Treatment (EPSDT)

The early and periodic screening, diagnostic and treatment program (EPSDT) is a component of Medicaid and authorized by *Title XIX of the Social Security Act*. EPSDT is a required service under Medicaid for categorically needy children and youth from birth to age 21 years. This federal program is matched and supplemented by state health funds. EPSDT was created to provide comprehensive healthcare services to ensure that health problems are identified and treated in a timely manner, before they become more serious and more costly to treat. Services under EPSDT include scheduled health and dental screening, mental health assessments, immunizations, laboratory tests, counseling, case management, disease and disability prevention education and health promotion. EPSDT examinations may be performed by, or under the supervision of, a certified Medicaid physician, dentist, or other provider, such as a nurse practitioner or physician assistant, qualified under state law to provide primary health care services (Center for Medicare and Medicaid Services, 2002b, pp. 5–11).

If the state is not in a managed care program and if it is allowed for school districts to do so under the state plan, a school district may bill Medicaid under the EPSDT program if the district is a qualified provider and provides the covered services for children. EPSDT billing is based on a fee-for-service system, and providers are obligated by Medicaid to bill third party liable resources. In states with managed care plans, districts may not bill for EPSDT services for students who are enrolled in managed care plans unless the district is under contract with the managed care provider to provide such services.

Local Education Agency (LEA) Billing Option

Congress established the LEA Billing Option in 1989 as a way for schools to recover expenditures for health-related services provided to students enrolled in Medicaid. At the state level, the state Medicaid agency administers the LEA Billing Option, typically in collaboration with the state education agency. Medicaid reimburses qualified providers on a fee-for-service system for assessment, direct services, and interventions to eligible students.

For individual schools or school providers to bill Medicaid, the school's LEA must be enrolled as a provider and the services must (1) be covered under Medicaid, (2) be medically necessary, and (3) be furnished by a qualified practitioner. Federal Medicaid regulations dictate some of the Medicaid provider qualifications, while other provider qualifications are enacted by the state. In instances where states have enacted provider qualifications, the state standards must be applied universally to all applicants. When a school or school district offers a variety of Medicaid-covered services, the school must meet all federal and state provider qualifications related to each provided service. In addition, for schools to receive Medicaid reimbursement, the health services the school provides must be included among those identified in the Medicaid law and included in the state's Medicaid plan, or be offered through EPSDT (Center for Medicare and Medicaid Services, 2002a). Depending on the state plan, school-based Medicaid providers may include school nurses, psychologists, dietitians, licensed clinical social workers, school health aides, and speech, occupational, and physical therapists (Bray, 2003).

Schools and school districts that want to participate in the Medicaid program and receive Medicaid reimbursement must have provider agreements in place between the state Medicaid agency and the healthcare provider who actually furnishes the reimbursable services. Schools and districts may become Medicaid providers, either by qualifying to furnish services directly, or through contracts with independent service providers (Centers for Medicare and Medicaid Services, 2002a).

Billing for Medicaid reimbursement is complex and small and some mid-sized LEAs may require more administrative resources than school districts have available to invest in the process. Claims for services must be processed in a timely fashion, which means that providers must submit all claims within 12 months of the date of service. LEAs must also keep detailed and confidential records of services to students and maintain the records for specified periods in the event of an audit. Consequently, many LEAs hire vendors to assist with the billing activities. Although the vendors can provide guidance through the billing process, LEAs should also avail themselves of the free technical assistance and information offered by their state Medicaid and education agencies (Centers for Medicare and Medicaid Services, 2002a).

Two issues related to Medicaid billing that are particularly problematic for schools and school districts are the concepts of "free care" and "third party liability." With some exceptions, Medicaid does not reimburse for free care, such as health services that are provided to everyone at school without charge. This policy regarding free care may affect the ability of LEAs to bill Medicaid for covered services provided to Medicaid-eligible students unless the LEA bills all students for the services provided or meets one of the exceptions described below. In addition, Medicaid is the payer of last resort; therefore, payment for eligible services must be sought from liable third parties before Medicaid can be billed (Centers for Medicare and Medicaid Services, 2002a).

To allow Medicaid to be billed, LEAs must ensure that the health services they provide do not constitute free care. The following three conditions must be met for Medicaid billing reimbursement to occur. The school or school district:

"(1) Establishes a fee schedule for the services provided (it could be sliding scale to accommodate individuals with low income);

(2) Ascertains whether every individual served by the provider has any third-party benefits, and

(3) Bills the beneficiary and/or any third parties for reimbursable services" (Centers for Medicare and Medicaid Services, 2002a, pp. 44–45).

As mentioned previously, there are two exceptions to the free care rule regarding school health services. The first exception relates to the fact that Medicaid is the primary payer for services provided to children with disabilities. These services are funded under the Individuals with Disabilities Education Act (IDEA) for children with Individual Education Programs (IEP) or Individual Family Service Plans (IFSP), even though the same services may be provided at no cost to children who are not eligible for Medicaid. However, LEAs should bill all liable third parties for provided services (Centers for Medicare and Medicaid Services, 2002a).

The second exception to the free care policy is for services in schools that are supported by *Title V of the Social Security Act* (*Maternal Child Health Services Block Grant*). *Title V* legislation provides funds to states for health and related services for mothers and their children for the reduction of infant mortality, preventable diseases, and access to necessary care. Some LEAs qualify for funding under *Title V* and consequently are able to provide Medicaid-covered services that are exempt from the free care rule and the requirement that Medicaid is to be the payer of last resort, as Medicaid will pay before *Title V* for eligible services (Centers for Medicare and Medicaid Services, 2002a).

Medicaid Administrative Claiming (MAC)

Medicaid reimburses LEAs for administrative activities required for the efficient and appropriate management of the LEA's Medicaid program under Medicaid Administrative Claiming (MAC). For administrative services to be reimbursable under Medicaid, the provider furnishing the services must participate in the Medicaid program and bill Medicaid for the service (Centers for Medicare and Medicaid Services, 2003b). LEAs are reimbursed for carrying out health-related administrative duties and training, including providing information to families through outreach activities; assisting families to enroll their children in the State Children's Health Insurance Program (SCHIP) and Medicaid programs; referring, coordinating, and monitoring covered services; providing translations related to Medicaid services; and promoting interagency coordination and developing related policies and programs.

To be eligible for reimbursement for administrative services, LEAs must complete time surveys, either quarterly or random moment, in which the employees who perform eligible activities record the time they spend in those activities over a specified period. Reimbursement is based on the averages recorded during the survey period. Depending on the state, the funds reimbursed to the LEA under MAC may or may not be restricted. In those states where the funds are not restricted, dollars claimed for administrative services go into the LEA's general fund. Restricted funds are typically required to be reinvested in health and human services programs and activities within the LEA.

The requirements for administrative claiming differ from those regulating the LEA Medicaid Billing program. For instance, provider qualifications and the free care issue do not apply to claims for administrative activities. Under administrative claiming, LEAs may perform certain Medicaid administrative functions without meeting provider requirements. There is no need to keep individual documentation and submit individual claims for provided services. However, LEAs must meet medical service requirements when they provide both health services and administrative claims. In addition, if

LEAs file for reimbursements under both administrative claiming and LEA Medicaid Billing, some activities that may be claimed as administration may not be allowable as separate health services claims when the LEA becomes a Medicaid provider (Centers for Medicare and Medicaid Services, 2002).

Each individual state's plan provides guidance in determining whether an activity qualifies for reimbursement under administrative claiming. If the activity is performed to support the eligibility determination process, or any service covered under the state plan (such as transportation to a medical provider, assistance completing the eligibility application, or marketing via school bus posters and pamphlet distribution), the actions needed to manage such activities may be eligible for reimbursement. Activities unrelated to the Medicaid program, even if performed in the best interest of the student and his or her family, are generally not reimbursable (such as help finding suitable housing or a free food pantry). The activity must be in the approved Medicaid state plan for its related administrative costs to be eligible for reimbursement under the Medicaid program (Centers for Medicare and Medicaid Services, 2002). Depending on the size of the school district and whether or not the district has elected to participate in the federal Medicaid reimburse programs, school nurses should understand how these programs work, so that the nurse can effectively support their district's participation.

Section 1115 of the Social Security Act

The purpose of Section 1115 is to give the U.S. Secretary of Health and Human Services authority to sanction experimental, pilot, or demonstration projects that show promise in advancing Medicaid objectives. Section 1115 Waivers provide funding flexibility and allow states to test the merit of new and innovative ideas. Waivers allow for the provision of health services that would otherwise not be eligible for federal matching funds. Waivers can also expand eligibility for individuals who, without the waiver, would not be eligible for Medicaid. For instance, the savings achieved from the induction of Medicaid eligible individuals into managed care programs can then be used to finance coverage for people previously ineligible for Medicaid. A key factor in the federal decision to accept or decline a waiver is that the pilot cannot be anticipated to cost more than it would have cost without the waiver (Centers for Medicare and Medicaid Services, 2003d).

The manual *Medicaid and School Health: A Technical Assistance Guide* (2002a) provides information on how waivers may be utilized to benefit LEAs. As states have developed waivers and have moved Medicaid beneficiaries into managed care programs, associated services for those who are disabled are frequently not included in the waivers. Consequently, if Medicaid-covered IDEA services are not included in the state waiver, LEAs may provide those services on a fee-for-service basis under an IEP or an IFSP and bill Medicaid directly. However, LEAs cannot bill Medicaid for other services that are being provided under managed care plans in the waiver, such as primary and preventive services provided under EPSDT that are commonly provided in school-based clinics. School nurses should be aware of the status of section 1115 waivers in their state so that the nurse can help school administrators be aware of this potential source of support for school-based health programs.

Transportation

Generally, there is no Medicaid reimbursement for the transportation of Medicaid-eligible students to school, even if Medicaid-covered school-based health services are provided at the school during the regular school day. This is because education is the primary purpose of attending school, while medical services, if provided, are secondary. In addition, schools provide transportation at no cost to all students attending school; therefore, the Medicaid free care policy applies so that Medicaid funds cannot be used for services that are provided free to all others (Centers for Medicare and Medicaid Services, 2002).

However, Medicaid will reimburse (under IDEA) LEAs for transportation to onsite school-based services for students who receive special services, based on their IEP or IFSP. Thus, LEAs may bill Medicaid for transportation to school-based health services for students when both of the following conditions are met (1) The student receives transportation to obtain a Medicaid-covered health care service, *and* (2) both the Medicaid-covered healthcare service and the need for transportation are written in the student's IEP or IFSP.

When the two conditions are met, the LEA is eligible to receive Medicaid reimbursement for transportation to and from the school (Centers for Medicare and Medicaid Services, 2002a). However, Centers for Medicare and Medicaid Services (CMS) Director Richardson (2002) cautioned that the IEP should only include specialized services that a student would not ordinarily receive while attending school. Therefore, when a student with special needs under IDEA rides the regular school bus with non-disabled students, transportation should not be included in the IEP and the cost of the transportation should not be billed to Medicaid. In addition,

LEAs that claim Medicaid reimbursement for transportation services must provide thorough documentation when making such claims.

LEAs may also be reimbursed for transportation if a student receives a Medicaid-covered IDEA intervention service at an off-site facility during the school day. In this situation, transportation costs from the school to the facility and back are reimbursable, but not the transportation from home to school and back on that same day (Centers for Medicare and Medicaid Services, 2002a).

Case Management

Defined by sections 1905(a)(19) and 1915(g)(2) of the Social Security Act, case management includes those activities that help eligible individuals under a state's Medicaid plan to gain access to necessary medical, social, educational, and other services. Case management also involves coordinating services to prevent duplication of services while maximizing the individual's access to needed services. LEA involvement and opportunity for reimbursement from case management activities are dependent on the individual state's Medicaid plan (Golden, 2002).

The school, through daily access to children and youth, can play a major role in case management by identifying students' health problems and facilitating contacts among the family, health services, and social services. Case management activities can assist families in identifying, choosing, and maintaining contact with healthcare providers, making appointments, finding transportation, maintaining records, and providing follow-up to ensure that students receive needed services (Centers for Medicare and Medicaid Services, 2002a).

Several different forms of case management are available and states have the flexibility to provide any or all of the case management type services approved by Medicaid. Medicaid will reimburse schools for the types of case management services that are included in the state plan. The following are examples of case management for which schools may be reimbursed: (1) schools may provide case management as a medical service, such as the coordination of care for specific medical needs identified in EPSDT activities; (2) schools may do case management under Medicaid waivers, such as when school-related health services are exempted from a state's managed care waiver, or (3) schools may provide targeted case management (TCM), such as managing services provided to a targeted group of individuals such as students with disabilities who are served under an IEP or IFSP (Centers for Medicare and Medicaid Services, 2002).

State Children's Health Insurance Program (SCHIP)

At the start of the 21st century, there were almost 11 million uninsured children younger than 19 years of age in the United States. Health insurance coverage is a key factor in determining children's access to and use of health care. Uninsured children are more likely to go without necessary medical care and more likely to get their health care in emergency rooms. Uninsured children are also more likely to be absent from school due to untreated chronic and acute health problems. It is well recognized that high rates of absenteeism from school are associated with school failure. SCHIP provides the opportunity for states to develop effective programs to decrease the number of uninsured children and to improve access for those insured by the program (American Academy of Pediatrics [AAP], Committee on Child Health Financing, 2001); the goal is to improve their health so that they can attend school regularly and succeed academically. Increasing the number of insured children also may have the added benefit for LEAs to increase reimbursement through the programs previously described in this chapter.

Public Law 105-33 (Balanced Budget Act of 1997) established the State Children's Health Insurance Program (SCHIP) as Title XXI of the Social Security Act. This piece of legislation is the largest expansion of children's health care coverage since the inception of Medicaid nearly 40 years ago. While SCHIP does not provide universal insurance coverage for every child, the program does give coverage to uninsured children through age 18. SCHIP is a federal and state partnership, similar to Medicaid. The goal of SCHIP is to extend health insurance coverage to children of working families who are ineligible for Medicaid, but who do not earn enough money to buy private health insurance. SCHIP provides coverage for "targeted low-income children," that is, children living in families whose income is below 200% of the federal poverty level (FPL) or whose family earnings are slightly higher than the state's Medicaid eligibility threshold. With the flexibility allowed by SCHIP, some states have extended the program past the FPL, while other states have expanded insurance coverage to whole families (Centers for Medicare and Medicaid Services, n.d.).

From fiscal years 1998 through 2007, Title XXI will make more than $40 billion available to states to provide health insurance to the eligible children of working parents. Each state receives an annual allotment of these federal funds based on the number of eligible low- income children in the state.

States are required to provide non-federal dollars in matching funds in order to participate in the program (Bray, 2003). Under SCHIP, for expenditures that qualify, the states receive an enhanced federal matching rate, which provides the incentive for state participation in SCHIP. Once awarded, state allotments remain available for expenditure for up to three years (Centers for Medicare and Medicaid Services, n.d).

Under SCHIP, states choose from one of three plans to provide children's health insurance coverage: (1) expansion of the state's Medicaid program; (2) development or expansion of a non-Medicaid health insurance program for children; or (3) a combination of both options. All states have approved SCHIP plans and receive enhanced federal matching reimbursements for SCHIP expenses up to a state SCHIP allocation that varies based on the federal fiscal year. States are allowed to use up to 10% of their total annual SCHIP monies (state and federal) on non-benefit activities, such as: outreach focused on identifying and enrolling children in SCHIP, administrative costs, health services initiatives, and other health assistance for children. Many states have successfully used schools to disseminate SCHIP and Medicaid program information (Centers for Medicare and Medicaid Services, 2003b).

States with separate state programs have great flexibility in providing coverage and are able to direct funding to areas with the most intense needs. In addition, programs that are separate from Medicaid may more easily garner public support, particularly if the state implements cost-sharing (see Box 44.2). There are challenges in developing a

Box 44.2 ■■■

GLOSSARY OF TERMS RELATED TO MEDICAID AND MANAGED CARE

Capitation—A method of payment for health services in which an individual or institutional provider is paid a fixed, per capita amount for each person served without regard to the actual number or nature of services provided to each person.

CMS—The Center for Medicare and Medicaid Services (CMS) is the federal agency responsible for administering Medicare and overseeing the state's administration of Medicaid.

Cost Containment—Terms used to describe efforts to control the growth of medical care costs. Two different strategies are used in the formulation of government policy to contain healthcare costs: regulation and competition.

Cost sharing—Provisions of a health insurance policy that require the insured or otherwise covered individual to pay some portion of his covered medical expenses. Common forms of cost sharing are deductibles, co-insurance and co-payments. For individuals enrolled in SCHIP, states are allowed to impose cost-sharing; however, states may not charge for some services, such as preventive services and immunizations, and states may not impose cost sharing that exceeds 5% of a family's gross or net income.

Encounter—An encounter is a record of a medically related service (or visit) rendered by (a) provider(s) to a beneficiary who is enrolled in the plan during the date of service.

Enrollee—Eligible Medicaid beneficiary who has enrolled in a contracted health plan.

Fee-for-service (FFS)—Method of charging whereby a physician or other practitioner bills for each encounter or service rendered.

Gatekeeper—The term used in referring to the physician who has primary responsibility for the enrollee's medical care and costs. This is the person who authorizes expenditures for external medical services. The term is sometimes used interchangeably with primary care physician or primary care provider.

Health maintenance organization (HMO)—An organized system for providing health care, in which an entity accepts the responsibility to provide or deliver an agreed on set of basic and supplemental health services to a group of enrolled individuals for which that entity is reimbursed through a predetermined, fixed periodic prepayment made by or on behalf of each enrolled person, without regard to the amounts of actual services provided.

Indemnity insurance—Indemnity insurance is the fee for service type of health insurance such as

Blue Cross or Blue Shield. The insured may use providers of their choice. This is the most costly type of health insurance.

Individual Practice Association (IPA)—An association of physicians from various settings that contracts with an HMO to provide health services; the physicians are usually reimbursed on a fee-for-service basis.

Managed care—A health care system that combines the delivery and financing of health care services.

Medicaid—A federally aided, state operated program which provides medical benefits for eligible low income persons in need of health and medical care.

Medically needy—Persons who have sufficient enough income and resources to be ineligible for Temporary Assistance to Needy Families (TANF) or SSI, but not enough to pay for medical care or health insurance. To qualify as medically needy, these individuals must be aged, blind, disabled, or be a pregnant woman.

Primary care —Basic or general health care provided when an individual first makes contact with the medical care system and the provision of care for common illnesses and conditions.

Primary care provider—A person responsible for supervising, coordinating, and providing initial and primary care to patients, particularly those enrolled in a health care plan.

Prospective payment—Any method of paying hospitals or other providers an amount or rate of payment in advance, regardless of the costs of services that will be incurred.

Quality assurance—Activities and programs intended to assure the quality of care in a defined medical setting or program.

Quality of care—The level of excellence with respect to medical services received by enrollees, administered by providers or programs, in terms of technical competence, need, appropriateness, acceptability, humanity, structure, etc.

Supplemental Security Income (SSI)—A federally administered public assistance program for individuals who are aged, blind or disabled and meet income requirements criteria. Such individuals receive a Medicaid card.

(Used with permission from the Los Angeles County Office of Education, Cathy Bray, 2004.)

separate state program. States must implement a separate administration to oversee the new program and this administrative body must coordinate with Medicaid to correctly determine eligibility and enrollment of eligible children. It is also important to clarify that separate state programs do not create an entitlement for children's access to healthcare insurance. If the allotted funds run out, the states with separate programs are not required to continue health care coverage for these low-income children (Bray, 2003).

States are required to develop strategies to prevent families and employers from dropping private health insurance coverage and replacing it with SCHIP. The practice of dropping private insurance in favor of SCHIP is referred to as "crowd out." States can discourage this by restricting the eligibility of families who have or have had access to private insurance, regardless of whether or not they received or could afford to purchase coverage. States may impose waiting periods that require a specified length of time children must be uninsured before being eligible for SCHIP. States are allowed to prohibit employers from dropping or modifying insurance coverage and states may subsidize an employer's cost of expanding health insurance to employees (Bray, 2003).

The American Academy of Pediatrics (AAP) (2001) developed a list a recommendations to reduce barriers and ensure children's access to services. These include the following:

1. States should establish reimbursement rates for Medicaid and SCHIP programs that are comparable to rates offered in private insurance plans and based on the current market rate. Low reimbursement rates and resulting low provider participation could create barriers to access for individuals and families enrolled in Medicaid or SCHIP.
2. States should offer students 12 continuous months of eligibility rather than allowing their eligibility to alternate depending on the parents' eligibility for assistance.
3. States should expand outreach activities that inform working parents that their children may be eligible for federal health programs.

4. States should also expand health coverage to parents as a way to increase the number of children who are enrolled; a study of three states that expanded Medicaid to parents had greater Medicaid participation rates for low-income children than states whose programs did not include parents (Ku & Broaddus, 2000).
5. States should provide access to pediatric medical sub-specialists and surgical specialists as well as reasonable compensation for healthcare providers providing case management when developing ways to care for children with special health care needs.

The impact of the uninsured population on schools is a significant issue for education. As the health professional in the school community, the school nurse must learn to maneuver in the complex system of healthcare eligibility and access.

SCHOOL NURSING AND MEDICAID

Box 44.3 presents a list of potentially reimbursable school nursing services. The list is not intended to be all-inclusive. Implied throughout the list is the importance of quality assurance and documentation of services.

Box 44.3 ■■■

CATEGORIES OF SCHOOL NURSING SERVICES FOR MEDICAID FUNDING

- Case finding is the use of regular health screenings and assessments to identify students with potential health deficits, and includes the making of referrals for care based on the findings. Examples of case finding are:
  1. Nursing assessment of early child development program applicants.
  2. Preschool health appraisals for kindergarten registrants and health appraisal of eligible middle school entrants (EPSDT).
  3. Health assessment of students referred for special education evaluation.
  4. Health history review, developmental assessment, and screening of vision, hearing, dental, posture, blood pressure, and nutrition.
  5. Nursing assessment of new or previously identified health problems from student-initiated, teacher, or staff referral, such as for substance use, child abuse, or pregnancy.
  6. Home visits for health and developmental or environmental assessments.
- *Nursing care procedures* include immunization and medication administration, medically prescribed procedures performed by the nurse, and interventions listed in the Individualized Education or Family Service Plans (IEP or IFSP). Examples of nursing care procedures include:
  1. Administration of immunizations to students who are out of compliance with state immunization law.
  2. Assessment of student medication needs, monitoring compliance, and administration.
  3. Provision of specialized health care services, including but not limited to feeding and nutrition assessment; urinary bladder catheterization; respiratory care; medical support services, such as oxygen administration and shunt monitoring; and the development of protocols including emergency care protocols and health objectives for IEPs or IFSPs.
- *Care coordination* involves outreach, access to care, status monitoring, and follow-up. Examples of care coordination include:
  1. Outreach to identify Medicaid-eligible students.
  2. Follow-up on referrals for evaluation, diagnosis, and treatment, home visits for follow-up and coordination for students with health deficits, monitoring prenatal or family planning, or for arranging transportation for eligible students to medical and dental appointments, and for other necessary care.
- *Health counseling and instruction* entails nursing assessment, preventive health counseling and health education, and anticipatory guidance for diagnosed or possible health problems.
- *Emergency management and care* includes nursing assessment, planning, and intervention for school emergencies, and the follow-up of those emergencies through evaluation and future planning.

(Bray, 2003; National Association of State School Nurse Consultants, 2000)

ADDITIONAL FUNDING SOURCES

Private Insurance Reimbursement

The free care policy of the LEA Medicaid Billing Option requires school districts to bill private insurance carriers (third-party payers) before billing Medicaid, as Medicaid is the payer of last resort in most situations. In some cases, school districts have received reimbursement from these third-party payers. However, most private insurance carriers do not reimburse for health services provided at school. When private insurers reimburse for school health services, generally the rate is somewhat higher than the rate obtained from Medicaid (Bray, 2003). School districts should pursue developing service agreements with private insurance companies and health maintenance organizations (HMO), even though at present, these are insignificant sources of revenue for school districts. As the school health professional, the school nurse can play a pivotal role in developing such service agreements. Taras (2003) cites an agreement one school district has with an HMO whereby the HMO pays the school district every time one of their school-age health plan members receives health education at school.

Managed Care Plan Reimbursement

Managed care combines the delivery and financing of health care services into one health care system. Managed care organizations (MCOs) offer their members a broad spectrum of medical services and specialties. Managed care potentially can provide increased access to preventive and primary care because each member is assigned to a primary healthcare provider who is responsible for coordinating the member's care within the system (Centers for Medicare and Medicaid Services, 2002a).

Efforts by states to enroll Medicaid-eligible individuals in managed care programs have increased as states have faced budget reductions and increased healthcare costs. Managed care allows states to increase health care access, reduce unnecessary care, improve the quality of care, and contain related costs (AAP, Committee on Child Health Financing, 1999).

Managed care plans typically reimburse healthcare providers at a capitated, prepaid premium for providing a set package of health services. In exchange for the premium, the managed care plan accepts the financial liability for provision of the health services package. The managed care plan pays healthcare providers, develops a provider network, and informs providers and plan members about covered services (Centers for Medicare and Medicaid Services, 2002a). While plan providers (physicians and hospitals) may share the risk for the cost of service, capitation also provides guaranteed income and potential to share in profits (Bray, 2003).

The growth of managed care has created complications for LEAs pursuing Medicaid reimbursement for school health services. According to the *Medicaid and School Health: A Technical Assistance Guide*, updated 2002, school providers who operated under the Medicaid fee-for-service practice may find the system very different when a state decides to move its Medicaid beneficiaries into a managed care program. When a state is mandated to move Medicaid beneficiaries into managed care, it does so under a waiver. There are no specific statutory requirements for states to establish relationships between school-based providers and managed care entities. As states apply for waivers related to managed care, the Centers for Medicaid and Medicare Systems (CMS) encourages states to promote collaboration between school districts and managed care plans. Schools should also reach out to the state and managed care organizations to establish relationships to ensure a place at the table when waivers are being developed. The school nurse is the ideal school staff member to act as liaison between the school community and the managed care community as he or she has the skills and knowledge to effectively communicate in both communities. In this way, school health services providers and managed care organizations can ensure that children receive the services they need without duplication.

While managed care providers understand primary care delivery, they are not usually well acquainted with school health programs. Therefore, schools need to work with their state Medicaid agency, as 1915(b) and 1115 waivers are developed and implemented, to create a role for themselves in managed care. Schools should develop agreements or contracts with managed care organizations that describe each organization's responsibility regarding the provision of health services and the receipt of reimbursements. The details of these agreements need to be locally determined, as they will depend on the types of local services that are available from both the LEA and the local managed care providers (Centers for Medicare and Medicaid Services, 2002a). Two examples of school and managed care organization agreements follow.

Oregon

"A 1991 Oregon state law requires prepaid managed care plans to contract with county health departments and other providers of services to children and adolescents. Contracts must cover immunizations, diagnosis and treatment of sexually transmitted diseases, and testing and treatment for communicable diseases. Under this state law, Medicaid managed care plans are required to reimburse school-based health centers for the provision of these services. Plans are also encouraged to contract with school-based health clinics for provision of other health care services, such as maternity case management, well-child care and prenatal care" (Centers for Medicare and Medicaid Services, 2002, p. 31).

Rhode Island

"Under the Rhode Island 1115 waiver, RIte Care, all Medicaid-covered services under an IEP or IFSP under IDEA are considered "out of plan" services and carved out of the waiver. As such, these services are provided in the school settings and billable to Medicaid under the fee-for-service reimbursement methodology. The state has three school-based clinics that provide a wide range of primary and preventive care services. The managed care contract is required to include these three school-based clinics in its network for delivery of RIte Care covered services available at the school-based clinic. The state retains the right to change the number of clinics included in the network during the term of the contract" (Centers for Medicare and Medicaid Services, 2002. pp. 31–32).

MARKETING YOUR PROGRAM

Marketing and public relations are key components in successful efforts in obtaining funding for school health services and programs. While school nurses for many years have spent considerable resources in improving *visibility* through items and activities, such as bumper stickers, logo mugs, and health fairs, marketing goes well beyond such promotional efforts. Synder (as cited in California School Nurses Organization [CSNO], 1999) describes *marketing* as a "set of activities necessary to bring about an 'exchange relationship.' The exchange occurs when someone is willing to give something in exchange for a product or service. The exchange cannot take place unless there are people who want the product or service. These people are the markets."

Synder (as cited in CSNO, 1999) suggested several strategies for school nurses to use to move from promotional activities to marketing a program. For example, the school nurse must:

- Determine which individuals and groups have the desire and means (education and health care dollars) to enter the exchange relationship with school nurses. These groups may include businesses, organizations, community agencies, students, parents, administrators, legislators, and health care system(s).
- Understand the community in which they work, its needs, and its expectations of school nurses. The deliverables that school nurses provide must match with some of the community's expressed needs and expectations.
- Engage in and utilize research to support the relationship of school health services and programs to students' academic success.
- Understand (and communicate that understanding to administrators) how Medicaid and other funding mechanisms work so that revenue is brought into the school district and the nurse is viewed as an invaluable expert who must be maintained on the payroll.
- Establish partnerships with HMOs, school-based and school-linked health centers, after-school programs, and other health-related programs. The personnel and administrators of such programs have the potential to be powerful allies and proponents of school health services once professional relationships are established.

Bogden (2003) argues that the most critical component of marketing the school health policy or program is the enlistment of broad support for its goals and strategies. He further asserts that because education policymaking in the United States tends to be based on local priorities and opinions, it is important to garner support from local constituencies such as healthcare and social service providers, influential community groups, youth-serving community agencies, respected business leaders, and key private-sector employees who may have influence over corporate priorities. An important aspect of marketing is deciding which of the markets is the most important and narrowing the focus based on those determinations. Attempts to engage too many markets at the same time may not have positive outcomes for anyone (Synder [as cited in CSNO, 1999]).

Once the markets are identified, the next steps include determining the most effective way to bring the school health program to the key decision makers, and planning strategies that are likely to gain approval. Bogden (2003) suggests that education decision makers may be more likely to accept a school health program that has a great amount of public support. In addition, he recommends that well-organized public relations campaigns may help to increase school and community awareness of the value of school health programs.

The California School Nurses Organization has several publications that provide a myriad of marketing and public relations strategies and other supports for the school nurse. There are many strategies for communicating the message about the value of school health programs; presenting the school health message in a public forum is a skill every school nurse must nurture. "The image of a school nurse has much to do with the advancement and effectiveness of our programs" (Bays [as cited in CSNO, 1999]). Most images have some basis in reality, and the public's limited and perhaps inaccurate perceptions of the school nurse will be reinforced if members do not consistently present a dynamic and competent picture. The foundation of the school nurse image must be built on each individual nurse's professionalism.

Bays (as cited in CSNO, 1999) made several recommendations to school nurses who are planning presentations:

- To protect school nursing services from being eliminated, it is not enough for school nurses to keep doing the same thing more efficiently; the school nurse must identify the trends and 'meet the future head on.'
- Sharing information with colleagues, teachers, administrators, school board members, potential funders and the general public on a regular basis creates visibility and credibility for school nursing and school health.
- In all areas of the school and community systems, the school nurse must seek occasions to communicate his or her professional image effectively, confidently, and conspicuously.
- All school nurses must work together to ensure that the professional school nurse that the public sees reflects a healthy and positive appearance.

Bogden (2003) suggested that most administrators "dislike surprises and want to know about policy and program initiatives being planned, especially if the matter might come to the school board." Therefore keep the administration informed. Bogden reinforced the need to stay focused on the final goal and not be sidetracked by details. He suggested that compromise should not be considered a defeat, but rather a "partial victory that lays the foundation for future efforts." Success may not come quickly or easily; be patient but persistent. Lastly, effort needs to be sustained after implementation by periodically evaluating the program and taking appropriate action to keep the program on track (Bogden, 2003).

SETTING UP A HEALTH SERVICES PROGRAM

LEAs commonly set aside a portion of their annual budget to address student health care needs. However, the annual budget for school health services varies by state, and in states where there are no state mandates for either specific health services or for school health services personnel, the annual school health care budget may vary greatly from LEA to LEA. It is important for school nurses and school health services administrators to be aware of and involved in (if at all possible) the annual budget development process in their LEA.

To successfully negotiate the annual budget development process that typically occurs several months in advance of the LEA's next fiscal year, school nurses and health services administrators must have a clear picture of core health services that every school should provide and the costs associated with those core services. Not only do schools need to provide urgent care for acute health problems, but schools also need to provide screening for early identification of health problems, treatment of chronic conditions, communicable disease control through immunization monitoring and education, specialized physical healthcare services for students with special needs, record maintenance, health education and health counseling, and referrals to community providers. These core services are costly.

To provide the wide variety of activities identified as core health services, schools must employ qualified and properly educated professionals and other support personnel. Schools also need to provide these individuals with the equipment and supplies needed to render the designated services effectively. There are many models of functioning school health services programs. The following information about personnel and equipment is intended to assist schools in setting up a basic and adequately staffed health services program.

Staff and Salary Suggestions

Physician Consultant

The school physician provides a connection to the medical community and to the district administration. He or she is available for medical consultation on individual students, and is a resource for procedures, programmatic issues, and curriculum (Allensworth et al., 1997). Compensation will depend on the services the school has contracted; some physicians may be willing to donate some consultation time to the school.

Registered Nurse Certified/ Credentialed as a School Nurse

The credentialed school nurse uses specialized clinical knowledge in the decision-making process and a systematic problem solving approach in dealing with school health issues. The credentialed school nurse contributes to the education of students with special healthcare needs through assessment, planning, and providing proper nursing care and evaluating the outcomes. The credentialed school nurse collaborates with school staff, families, students, and care providers to meet the health and educational needs of students. The individual works with members of the community and utilizes knowledge of community health and human services to act as a liaison between the school and the community (Allensworth et al., 1997). The salary of the school nurse should be similar to that of other comparably educated professional support staff, such as school psychologists and school counselors.

Licensed Practical/Vocational Nurse (LPN/LVN)

The LPN/LVN provides specialized nursing care, if allowed by state law, to individual students under the supervision of the school nurse. The salary for the LPN/LVN should be in line with that of similarly titled staff in comparable healthcare facilities.

Unlicensed Assistive Personnel (UAP)/ Health Office Paraprofessional

The trained UAP assists with health office and nursing procedures as permitted by state law. The UAP works under the supervision of the school nurse. The UAP's salary should be comparable to that of other classified staff, such as teacher assistants.

Health Clerk

The health clerk plays an important role within the school health team by maintaining student health records and performing other office tasks. The salary of the health clerk should be similar to that of other school clerical staff. It may be possible to get members of the community to volunteer their services to assist in the health office if allowed by state law and school district policy.

THE SCHOOL HEALTH OFFICE

School health services should be provided in a designated health room or clinic that has appropriate physical facilities for meeting student health needs and adequate equipment and supplies to ensure proper care of students with chronic or acute health problems (see Chapter 43).

Setting Up the Health Office

A budget for office equipment and supplies needed to set up a health office should be established, with ongoing budget provisions for regular maintenance, repair, and replacement of furniture and equipment (Table 44.4). An annual supply budget must be established to replace disposable supplies.

CONCLUSION

The school nurse is intimately involved in budget and funding issues within the school. These may include accessing funding for health-related projects or supplies or accessing reimbursement for services provided. It is also necessary to understand budgetary

Table 44.4 ■ HEALTH OFFICE BUDGET

Essential Equipment and Supplies
Desk(s)/work surface for each staff member housed in the health office. Itinerant staff may share desks, but should have individual space to store job-specific records and supplies.
Chair(s) for each health office staff member housed in the health office. Itinerant staff may share chairs. Chairs need to be available for students who are visiting the health office.
Telephone with direct outside line

(continued)

Essential Equipment and Supplies
Computer, monitor, and printer networked to the building or district data system, if that option is available
School health-related software as needed and/or if computer is not networked
Locking file cabinet(s)
Locking medication cabinet
Locking refrigerator with a separate freezer compartment
Vision screening equipment: • Wall charts and developmentally appropriate materials • Vision tester (optional) • Color vision plates
Hearing screening equipment: • Audiometer • Tympanometer (optional) • Otoscope
Scoliometer
Sphygmomanometer, appropriate cuff sizes, and stethoscope
Beam balanced scale
Cot(s) with washable surface
Stretcher chair
Folding screen (depends on the physical arrangement of the facility)
Examination lamp
Wheelchair
Flashlight
Electronic thermometer
Adequate first aid supplies for the number of students in the building

constraints and how and when to request additional resources. Above all is the need for the school nurse to understand the law in both its restrictions and availability of funds to promote the health of students.

References

Allensworth, D., Lawson, E., Nicholson, L., & Wyche, J. (Eds.) (1997). *Schools and health: Our nation's investment*. Institute of Medicine. Washington, DC: National Academy Press.

American Academy of Pediatrics (AAP), Committee on Child Health Financing, (1999). Medicaid policy statement, *Journal of Pediatrics, 104*, 344–347. Retrieved August 6, 2003 from http://www.aap.org

American Academy of Pediatrics (AAP), Committee on Child Health Financing, (2001). Implementation Principles and Strategies for Title XXI (State Children's Health Insurance Program). *Journal of Pediatrics, 107*, 1214–1220, Retrieved August 6, 2003 from http://www.aap.org

Bogden, J. F. (2003). *How schools work & how to work with schools: A primer for professionals who serve children and youth*. Alexandria, VA: National Association of State Boards of Education.

Bray, C. (Ed.) (2003). *School nurse orientation and review manual*. Downey, CA: Los Angeles County Office of Education.

California School Nurses Organization (CSNO). (1999). *Public relations for school nurses*. Sacramento, CA: Author.

Centers for Medicare and Medicaid Services (2002a). *Medicaid and school health: A technical assistance guide* Retrieved September 12, 2003 from http://www.cms.hhs.gov/medicaid/schools/scbintro.asp

Centers for Medicare and Medicaid Services. (2002b). *State medicaid manual: Part 05 – Early, periodic, screening, diagnosis, and treatment (EPSDT) services*. Retrieved September 12, 2003 from http://www.cms.hhs.gov/manuals/45_smm/sm_05_5_5010_to_5360with_toc.asp

Centers for Medicare and Medicaid Services . (2003a). *Medicaid and EPSDT* Retrieved September 12, 2003 from http://cms.hhs.gov/medicaid/epsdt/default.asp

Centers for Medicare and Medicaid Services. (2003b). *Medicaid school-based administrative claiming guide* Retrieved January 1, 2004 from http://www.cms.hhs.gov/medicaid/schools/macguide.pdf

Centers for Medicare and Medicaid Services. (2003c). *SCHIP Enrollment Reports*. (n.d.). Retrieved November 30, 2003 from http://www.cms.hhs.gov/schip/enrollment

Centers for Medicare & Medicaid Services. (2003d). *1115 Waiver Research and Demonstration Projects*. Retrieved August 3, 2003 from http://www.cms.hhs.gov/medicaid/1115/default.asp

Centers for Medicare and Medicaid Services. (n.d.). *Welcome to the State Children's Health Insurance Program*. (n.d.). Retrieved November 30, 2003 from the http://www.cms.hhs.gov/schip/about–SCHIP.asp

Corporation for Public Broadcasting. (2003). *Basic elements of grant writing*. Retrieved August 5, 2003 from http://www.cpb.org/grants/grantwriting.html

Davis, B. (2003). *Writing a successful grant proposal*. Retrieved August 5, 2003 from http://www.mcf.org/mcf/grant/writing.htm

Elementary and Secondary Education Act (see Public Law 107–110).

Fetro, J. V. (1998). Implementing coordinated school health programs in local schools. In E. Marx & S. F. Wooley (Eds.), *Health is academic: A guide to coordinated school health programs* (pp. 15–42). New York & London: Teacher's College Press.

Golden, O. A. (modified 2002). *Letter to state child welfare and state Medicaid directors, January 19, 2001*. Retrieved September 12, 2003 from http://www.cms.hhs.gov/states/letters/smd119c1.asp

Improving America's Schools Act (see Public Law 107–110).

Individuals with Disabilities Education Act (IDEA) (See Public Law 105–17)

Ku, L. & Broaddus, M. (2000). *The importance of family-based insurance expansions: New research findings about state health reforms*. Retrieved August 15, 2004 from http://www.cbpp.org/9_5_00healthrep.htm

Lyon, J. (2003). Grant writing. In C. Bray (Ed.), *School nurse orientation and review manual* (pp. 21–23). Downey, CA: Los Angeles County Office of Education.

National Association of State School Nurse Consultants. (2000). *Medicaid Reimbursement for School Nursing Services*. Retrieved August 6, 2003 from http://207.28.33.2/swp/tadkins/nassnc/NASSNC_Medicaid.html#DICAID

National Institutes of Health. (n.d.) *Grants & funding opportunities*. (n.d.). Retrieved August 5, 2003 from http://grants1.nih.gov/grants/

No Child Left Behind Act (See Public Law 107–110).

Public Law 105–17; 111 Stat. 37; 20 U.S.C. §§ 1400–1485; (H.R. 5). *Individuals with Disabilities Education Act Amendments of 1997*.

Public Law 107–110; 115 Stat. 1425; 20 USC 6301. *No Child Left Behind Act of 2001*.

Richardson, S. K. (modified 2002). *Letter to state Medicaid directors, May 21, 1999*, Retrieved September 12, 2003 from the Centers for Medicare and Medicaid Services Web site: http://www.cms.hhs.gov/states/letter/smd52199.asp

Special Reports: State Tobacco Settlement. (2004) Retrieved January 11, 2004, from http://tobaccofreekids.org/settlements/

Taras, H. (2003). Maximizing student health resources. Retrieved July 30, 2003, from *The School Administrator Web Edition* site www.aasa.org/publications/sa/2003_01/Cooper_Taras.htm

Title V of the Social Security Act (*Maternal and Child Health Services Block Grant*); (42 U.S.C. 701–710).

Title XIX of the Social Security Act (*Medicaid's Early and periodic, screening, diagnostic, and treatment* [EPSDT]); Section 1905; (42 U.S.C. 1396d)(r).

Chapter 45

Staff Health

SANDRA MCHENRY ■ REBECCA SILVER ■ LINDA C. WOLFE

Chapter Outline

INTRODUCTION

For more than 100 years, school nurses have provided comprehensive care to students. While their primary charge was focused on the illness needs of the student, even the earliest school nurses extended their reach beyond the student and school boundaries. Children cannot be treated successfully in isolation from the family and community, nor can one address illness without consideration of health promotion and wellness. Likewise, a student's health is impacted and interconnected with the health and well-being of the school staff. By striving to maximize the potential of each individual in the school environment, the school nurse's "client" now includes the student, his or her family, the community, and the school staff (Wold, 2001; Wold & Dagg, 2001). This chapter explores the expanded role of the school nurse in promoting the physical, emotional, and social well-being of school staff.

SCHOOL STAFF

Health promotion and disease prevention are important for staff, as individuals, role models, and members of the community. Implementation of employee wellness programs is consistent with the National Association of School Nurses' (NASN) *Scope and Standards of Professional School Nursing Practice* (NASN and the American Nurses Association [ANA], 2001) (see Chapter 4), as well as the Centers for Disease Control and Prevention's (CDC) eight-component Coordinated School Health Model (see Chapter 3). For the purpose of this chapter, several definitions are assumed.

- *School staff* is the diverse group of faculty, administration, and professional/nonprofessional support staff, which includes but is not limited to bus drivers, classroom aides, dietary/cafeteria workers, grounds/custodial/

Table 45.1 ■
SCHOOL STAFF COMPOSITION—UNITED STATES

TOTAL	NUMBER (FTE-FULL TIME EQUIVALENT)	PERCENTAGE
Staff	5,902,916	
Teachers	2,997,741	50.8
Student/other support staff (library support staff, student support services staff, and all other non-administrative support staff, including school nurses)	1,392,677	23.6
Instructional aides	675,038	11.4
Administrative support staff	412,968	7.0
School administrators	160,806	2.7
Guidance counselors	100,052	1.7
School district administrators	63,351	1.1
Librarians	54,349	0.9
Instructional coordinators and supervisors	45,934	0.8

Source: National Center for Educational Statistics (2002).

maintenance staff, secretaries, and therapists, for example, speech, vocational.

- *Staff wellness* is the attainment of an optimal health status for each member.
- *Worksite* is the setting(s) where staff work directly or indirectly with students

The school nurse's ability to identify health needs and risk factors, based on the specific school community, enables him or her to be proactive in providing the prevention, identification, or intervention that will have the most impact. TABLES 45.1 and 45.2 illustrate the diversity of school staff members. BOX 45.1 highlights compelling statistics related to unhealthy adult behavior among school employees in a specific geographic area.

Table 45.2 ■
TEACHER DEMOGRAPHICS (2000–2001)

	MEAN SALARY	MEAN AGE	RACE	GENDER
Teacher	$43,262	43	90% White	21% Men
		(14% <30; 37% >50)	6% Black	79% Women

Source: National Education Association (2003).

Box 45.1 ■■■

WORKPLACE STATISTICS

Statistically, if there are 100 people in your workplace:

1 uses cocaine

7 use marijuana

10 are heavy drinkers (two or more of beer, wine, liquor a day)

60 sit all day to do their work

10 have high blood pressure

25 or more have high blood cholesterol (over 200 mg/dL)

50 don't wear their seat belt regularly

30 smoke

27 have cardiovascular disease

35 are overweight by 20% or more

50 feel under moderate stress

5 have diagnosed diabetes and 5 have undiagnosed diabetes

(Kentucky Association for School Health, 2001)

STAFF WELLNESS

Investment in the health of employees benefits both employees and employers (Partnership for Prevention, 2001). In terms of employee health behavior and health status, research indicates that staff wellness results in improved health behavior and health status, reduced healthcare costs, and lower employee absenteeism as well as higher productivity and morale (Allegrante, 1998). Worksite health programs that are health promotion and disease prevention oriented provide cost savings in a number of areas. Some of the outcomes demonstrate that productivity improves as absenteeism decreases, healthier employees recover from illness sooner, healthy employees have a greater sense of responsibility to come to work, and improved morale results in a more satisfied and committed employee base (DeGroot, 2003; Houghton, 2001). It is believed that attention to employee health in the school setting further leads to a greater commitment of the employee to the school's health program. Thus, with improved staff health, it is postulated that there will be a heightened commitment to student health and increased numbers of healthy role models.

"Staff Wellness" is one of the eight core programs within the CDC's Coordinated School Health Model (see Chapter 3). School-site health promotion for school staff is defined as "assessment, education, and fitness activities for school faculty and staff," which are "designed to maintain and improve the health and well-being of school staff, who serve as role models for students" (McKenzie & Richmond, 1998, p. 4). Essential components include one or more programs targeted at "screening, education and supportive activities to reduce risk-factors, organizational policies that promote a healthful and psychologically supportive work environment, an integrated employee assistance program ..., and employee healthcare, including health insurance, managed care organizations, and access to school health services" ... (Allegrante, 1998, p. 226).

School staff health promotion is specifically identified within *Healthy People 2010* (USDHHS, 2000), which is a comprehensive set of health objectives that establishes targeted goals for the U.S. population for the year 2010. These objectives focus on disease prevention and health promotion. They create a framework from which states, communities, professional organizations, and other agencies can develop local initiatives to improve the health of all Americans. Building on scientific research and expert consultation, two overarching goals of *Healthy People 2010* are:

1. Increase quality and years of healthy life, and
2. Eliminate health disparities.

Twenty-eight focus areas outline 467 specific objectives. As seen in TABLE 45.3, several are specific to worksites, which include the school setting (U.S. Department of Health and Human Services [USDHHS], 2000).

Healthy Workforce 2010 is a document based on the *Healthy People* 2010 objectives. It recognizes the importance of businesses and communities working together to improve the health of Americans through worksite health promotion. "This [*Healthy Workforce 2010*] ambitious effort is guided by *Healthy People 2010* – the prevention agenda for the United States. And it won't succeed without private and public sector employer participation" (Partnership for Prevention, 2001, p. 2). Three reasons are identified by *Healthy Workforce 2010* as rationales for implementation of health promotion within the worksite: improved productivity, lowered healthcare costs, and enhanced corporate image and long-term interests.

As an employer of millions of workers, schools offer an opportune environment to promote wellness

Table 45.3 ■
HEALTHY PEOPLE 2010—WORKSITE OBJECTIVES

FOCUS AREA	OBJECTIVE
7. Educational and community-based programs	7-5 Increase the proportion of worksites that offer a comprehensive employee health promotion program to their employees
	7-6 Increase the proportion of employees who participate in employer-sponsored health promotion activities.
19. Nutrition and overweight	19-16 Increase the proportion of worksites that offer nutrition or weight management classes or counseling.
20. Occupational safety and health	20-9 Increase the proportion of worksites employing 50 or more persons that provide programs to prevent or reduce employee stress
22. Physical activity and fitness	22-13 Increase the proportion of worksites offering employer-sponsored physical activity and fitness programs.
27. Tobacco use	27-10 Increase the proportion of worksites with formal smoking policies that prohibit smoking or limit it to separately ventilated areas.

Source: U.S. Department of Health and Human Services (2000).

for both students and staff. Yet, schools often underestimate the potential impact that worksite health promotion can have on school staff and the school community at large.

> Since the 1980s the Kent Intermediate School District (KISD) in Grand Rapids, Michigan, has been involved in worksite health promotion, with activities ranging from health risk assessments to a healthy heart program to group outings. Dr. George Woons, KISD Superintendent, thinks the health promotion activities have paid off in more ways than one. "Of all the staff development programs, the health improvement programs have done the most to improve employee morale," he asserts. Woons believes part of the reason is that health promotion programs are a great equalizer. School district staff at all levels—cooks and custodians and teachers and superintendents—often have the same health risks. And together we participate in activities to reduce those risks. We're all going through this together to improve health; the morale boost is an extra bonus." (Partnership for Prevention, 2001, p. 10)

THE ROLE OF THE SCHOOL NURSE IN STAFF WELLNESS

The school nurse is uniquely positioned to be an advocate, leader, and provider of both health promotion activities and health services for school staff. Often the school nurse is the primary, or only, health professional employed by a school. As such, his or her expertise and recommendations can help schools to identify needs and institute needed programs.

Health risks within the general community equally affect school employees. Potential health risks among school staff may be easily identified through review of local data relative to such factors as age, gender, race, etc. The school nurse has the knowledge and skills to be a primary advocate, facilitator, and provider for school-site programs and services.

NASN identifies seven core roles of the school nurse (NASN, 2002). All of these link directly or indirectly to staff wellness, staff health, or both. There are references throughout the NASN Issue Brief to the challenging role of working with school staff. Specifically identified activities that relate to staff health include providing care for injury or acute illness, "monitoring chronic health conditions," providing for the "physical and emotional safety of the school community," training staff to respond to emergencies, offering wellness programs, providing programs on health topics, and being a member of the coordinated school health team (NASN, 2002).

Chapter 6 addresses the unique and expanding roles of school nurses. Establishment of a wellness outreach program is congruent with the school nurse's historical public health focus and concern for high-level wellness. Provisions for access to school health services is one area where schools can support staff wellness (Allegrante, 1998). As the primary health resource within a school, the school nurse is often the person who develops and assumes responsibility for staff wellness programs. This enables health initiatives to be provided at little or no cost to the district. Common inexpensive programs include weight management, monitoring hypertension, nutrition education, tobacco cessation, stress management and lifestyles change programs, including walking programs.

SCHOOL NURSE AS SKILLED CLINICIAN

Students and staff recognize the school nurse as a healthcare professional who will assist them in maintaining wellness and coping with health crises. The school nurse may provide individualized health promotion measures for staff through monitoring, which may include blood pressure and weight, and wellness programs. If permissible by state law, the nurse will assess both acute and chronic alterations in the staff's health status and plan appropriate interventions.

The school setting provides a challenging opportunity for independent, autonomous practice. It is vital for the school nurse to maintain a high level of assessment, critical thinking, and decision-making skills to be successful in providing high-quality healthcare services for both students and staff. While school nurses are noted "experts" in pediatrics, their knowledge and skills in adult care may be minimal. Sound practice for adult care is equally essential. Maintaining current resources and referrals for adult physical and mental health is crucial when providing assessment, intervention assistance, or advice to school staff members.

Emergency Care

School districts are responsible for responding to emergencies that occur on school grounds or during school programs. Emergencies will, at times, include school staff. The responsibilities of the nurse, in preparing for school emergencies and in responding to an event, will vary from state to state, district to district, and even school to school. Current knowledge of state practice requirements, district policies, and local job descriptions is needed (Hootman, Schwab, & Gelfman, 2001).

Emergency care of school staff members may be needed anywhere on school grounds. Well-prepared school nurses will have a stocked "Go Bag" to accompany them to emergencies away from the school nurse's office. The Go Bag's contents should suffice for either a student or an adult emergency (see Chapter 10). Careful content planning and maintenance is imperative (Bobo, Hallenbeck, & Robinson, 2003; Grant, 2002). It is prudent to have additional equipment readily available in the health office and have support staff prepared to transport it to an emergency site. In the school setting, the school nurse is one of the first responders.

For school staff emergencies, the school nurse will determine if the employee can be adequately treated by first aid in the school setting or if activation of emergency medical services (EMS) is warranted. Because of the adult status of the employee, there sometimes is negotiation with the employee regarding what the most appropriate next level of medical care should be. In situations where the nurse is in disagreement with the staff member, based on a nursing assessment that warrants further medical intervention, it is prudent to communicate concerns to an administrator.

The school nurse may have authorization to administer lifesaving or over-the-counter (OTC) medications to school staff. Standing Orders for adult emergency medications, such as epinephrine, must be obtained from a provider as permitted through state statute. The practice of providing staff members with over-the-counter (OTC) medications, such as analgesics and antacids, is an accepted practice in many schools. In some instances, OTCs are available for use at the staff member's discretion. In other cases, the school nurse is involved in recommending the appropriate OTC based on presenting symptoms. This practice should be carefully reviewed and based on local statutes, guidelines, and needs. If the school district is willing to accept liability for OTC drug provision for school staff, a policy should be developed and standing orders may be needed.

A staff member who is injured at work will need direct nursing care. In the event the injury resulted from a violent act, the school nurse will need to provide emotional support and reassurance as well as safety. The nurse may be responsible for completing an accident report, notifying the building administrator, and, when warranted, eliciting intervention from the crisis management team or guidance department. The staff member may also be encouraged to seek additional medical or mental health intervention.

Care for Chronic Conditions

School staff members with chronic health conditions are as likely as students with chronic health conditions to request and need more intensive interaction and support from the school nurse. This may come in the form of staff members seeking knowledge regarding their condition or medications from the school nurse. The staff member may also present with requests for medication administration, treatment intervention, or ongoing assessment, and may include daily injections, blood pressure monitoring, or dressing changes. It is not uncommon for a staff member with troubling symptoms or a new diagnosis to seek the professional assistance and advice from the school nurse. The school nurse's acumen in referral arrangements and knowledge of existing systems and resources will be of great value to the school (see discussion of Referrals, below).

Healthy People 2010 proposes several goals for persons with chronic conditions. Healthcare delivery and supervision in the school setting can contribute to their success. TABLE 45.4 illustrates two goals for persons with asthma. Both goals are ones that a school nurse can directly influence by providing an immunization clinic as well as providing interventions to enhance knowledge of the condition and/or compliance with the prescribed regimen.

Because the school nurse's primary responsibility is to provide services to students, individual staff requests and expectations may be a challenge unless reasonable parameters are established. In determining which services will be provided to staff with chronic conditions, the school nurse should collaborate with administration while maintaining staff members' confidentiality. Both the school and the school nurse have duties to provide care, based upon state statutes and staff contracts. In addition, the liability of the school and the school nurse, along with consideration to maintaining quality student services, must be considered.

The establishment of Emergency Care Plans (ECPs) for students is expected practice for the school nurse. The importance of such plans for staff should not be overlooked. The nurse will need to find opportunities to educate school staff about the importance of informed, expedited care in case of an emergency; the purpose and value of having on-site emergency information and an ECP; and the need to share medical concerns with the nurse prior to an emergency. If an employee has informed the school nurse of a healthcare issue (such as diabetes, seizure disorder, cardiac problem, hypertension, asthma, or anaphylactic allergic reaction), he or she should be asked about providing or developing an ECP for the school. The staff member and the nurse may then determine how the information should be maintained and with whom it could be shared. It must be recognized that staff participation in the development of such a healthcare resource is optimal and issues related to confidentiality must be addressed. Should the employee refuse to provide adequate information or resist assistance, the school nurse may need to discuss the concerns with his or her supervisor. The severity of the health problem and the concern for the safety of students or staff are issues that will influence the need to pursue further assistance.

Documentation

Standards of school nursing practice demand quality documentation that gives a complete picture of the client, the nursing care provided, and the

Table 45.4 ■
***HEALTHY PEOPLE 2010*—WORKSITE ASTHMA GOALS**

FOCUS AREA	OBJECTIVE
14. Immunization and infectious disease	14-29 Increase the proportion of adults who are vaccinated annually against influenza and ever vaccinated against pneumococcal disease
24. Respiratory diseases	24-5 Reduce the number of school or workdays missed by persons with asthma due to asthma.

Source: U.S. Department of Health and Human Services (2000).

desired outcomes. Documentation of the health care provided to staff is as important as documentation of that provided to students.

School staff medical records vary by district or state. In addition to nursing notes that may be created by the school nurse, records may include: the employee's medical history; a healthcare professional's complete physical form; the school district's reasonable accommodation for an employee's disability; worker's compensation claims; accident and incident reports; bloodborne pathogen exposure reports; immunization records; sick or long-term disability records; and family or medical leave requests. State or district policy will determine the frequency of routine health examinations and screening, which will affect the number of records maintained on each employee; however, some states/districts do not require any routine health examinations or screenings after employment. Mental health and substance abuse evaluations may also be required if there is concern about the employee's ability to function in the school setting.

Employee health records are generally maintained as a confidential component of the employee's personnel file. This file is often housed in an administrative office of the school or district. Information, such as that found on medical examinations, is regulated under federal laws, specifically the Americans with Disabilities Act (Code of Federal Regulations [CFR], 2003, T.29, Subt. B, Ch. XIV, Pt. 1630). Generally, employee medical information and inquiries kept "shall be collected and maintained on separate forms and in separate medical files and be treated as a confidential medical record" [CFR, Pt. 1630.14 (b) (1)]. However, pertinent information may be shared with supervisors and "first aid and safety personnel may be informed, when appropriate, if the disability might require emergency treatment" [CFR, Pt. 1630.14 (b) (1) (ii)]. This implies that the district may choose to house or share employee health data with the school nurse in instances where the school nurse may be required to render emergency care.

As the need for availability of aspects of an employee's health record varies, some districts are developing policy to address multiple storage sites. In large districts, some employee health information may be kept online, while other components may be kept in personnel department files, the school building, or the nurse administrator's office. It is important to note that a generic employee health record policy is often written and adopted by the state Board of Education. Administrators in the health services department, employee assistance department, and the legal department should then develop guideline and procedures to meet local needs.

The Health Insurance Portability and Accountability Act (HIPAA) privacy laws continue to be clarified related to healthcare record keeping in the school setting. Knowledge of both HIPAA and the Federal Educational Rights and Privacy (FERPA) is essential to the oversight of documentation relative to staff and student data (see Chapter 13). HIPAA guides the activities of documentation related to school staff, while FERPA protects students' health and educational records.

HIPAA was adopted in 1996 to provide standards for facilitating electronic transactions within the healthcare system, as well as to protect the security and confidentiality of health information. It mandates that identifiable health information be protected as it is maintained and transferred. The Department of Health and Human Services (DHHS) provides clarifying statements about the law, while the Office of Civil Rights (OCR) is responsible for enforcement. These agencies may be contacted for clarification and interpretation of the regulations (HIPAA Privacy Rule, 2003). HIPAA is intended to protect privacy and enhance security; it is not meant to stand in the way of treatment or care of clients.

An important aspect of HIPAA regulations is the protection of medical records and individually identifiable health information in any form, including paper, electronic storage and transfer, and oral communication. Paper to paper faxes using fax machines are not subject to HIPAA Transaction Rules, as they are not considered electronic transactions. Faxed authorizations are allowed and electronic signatures are equivalent to written signatures (Bergren, 2003). The establishment of a HIPAA compliant release form is vital if medical records are to be obtained (Box 45.2).

School staff members should be made aware of district regulations related to their personal medical information. They should be cognizant of the school nurse's role in safeguarding incidental disclosure of protected health information, which is heard or seen, or in written form in the health office. This pertains to both students and staff alike. Record keeping of individual employee health data resulting from participation in health promotion programs should ideally be the responsibility of the participating staff member.

Referrals

It is not uncommon for the school nurse to be asked for advice related to employee healthcare plans, available services of local healthcare providers and facilities, and the Employee Referral Program, sometimes called the Employee Assistance Program (EAP). A school nurse's knowledge of these resources

Box 45.2 ■ ■ ■

COMPONENTS OF A HIPAA-COMPLIANT RELEASE OF INFORMATION FORM

- Plain language
- Specific information request (e.g., not "medical records on J. Jones," but rather "medical records from 9/12/03 hospitalization for asthma")
- Specific person disclosing and receiving the information (e.g., not "Highlands Middle School," but rather "L. Smith, RN, Highlands Middle School Nurse")
- Expiration date
- Right to revoke permission in writing
- Purpose of each request
- Signature and date
- An explanation of the potential for the information to be subject to redisclosure by recipient and no longer protected by the Privacy Rule

Taliaferro (2003, p. 1)

and skills in navigating the health system will be beneficial.

Many school employers or unions offer EAPs in the workplace. Programs offered by the EAP strive to meet the needs of employees and their families through identification and confidential treatment of substance abuse and other mental health issues. Frequently, the EAP referral is initiated by the recommendation of a supervisor, but self-referral without the involvement of management occurs as well. Informal referrals may occur when through social interaction and discussion, an employee is encouraged to seek help (Roman & Blum, 2002). This may involve an information dialogue with a supervisor, the school nurse, or a peer. The school nurse may have an opportunity to positively influence an employee's decision to seek assistance from the EAP. In any case, the participation in treatment or counseling must be a decision made by the employee. There are, however, federal regulations that address preemployment drug and alcohol screening, random testing and follow-up testing for school bus drivers (Omnibus Transportation Employee Testing Act, 1991). The school nurse should be aware of district policies regarding the EAP program and school staff testing.

The resources possible for referrals and the specific programs and services offered to enhance health are influenced to some degree by the healthcare insurance plan for the district. In some districts, the negotiated insurance carrier may pay for a specific agency to provide treatment; otherwise, the employee is free to choose from a list of providers who will be reimbursed by the insurance carrier.

AMERICANS WITH DISABILITIES ACT (ADA) AND HIRING PRACTICES

The school nurse may be consulted by administration regarding a facility non-compliance issue with the ADA (ADA, 1990) that involves either students or staff. In large school districts, the nurse may be a member of a committee that reviews ADA requests and recommends resolutions. As hiring practices disallow discrimination on the basis of disability, both new and existing employees may require accommodations under the ADA law (see Chapter 14). This is one of the many ways in which the school nurse addresses the Healthy School Environment, thus supporting the health and safety of all employees.

SCHOOL SITE HEALTH PROMOTION

The CDC defines health promotion for staff as:

> Opportunities for school staff to improve their health status through activities such as health assessments, health education and health-related fitness activities. These opportunities encourage school staff to pursue a healthy lifestyle that contributes to their improved health status, improved morale, and a greater personal commitment to the school's coordinated health program. This personal commitment often translates into greater commitment to the health of students and creates positive role modeling. (CDC, 2001, p. 7)

Staff health promotion can be specific to an individual's unique needs or targeted at all or identified groups of staff.

Healthy People 2010 describes essential components of a comprehensive worksite health promotion program as including:

1. Health education that focuses on skill development and lifestyle behavior change in addition to information dissemination and awareness building, preferably tailored to employees' interests and needs;

2. Supportive social and physical environments, including established norms for healthy behavior and policies that promote health and reduce risk of disease, such as worksite smoking policies, healthy nutrition alternatives in the cafeteria and vending machines, and opportunities for obtaining regular physical activity;
3. Integration of the worksite program into the organization's structure;
4. Related programs, such as employee assistance programs; and
5. Screening programs, preferably linked to medical care delivery to ensure follow-up and appropriate treatment as necessary and to encourage adherence. (USDHHS, 2000)

Partnerships for a Healthy Workforce adds two additional components:

6. A process for supporting individual behavior change with follow-up intervention; and
7. An evaluation and improvement process to help enhance the program's effectiveness and efficiency (Partnership for Prevention, 2001, p. 12).

Individual Health Promotion

Individual health promotion occurs when interventions are directed at the individual employee based on his or her unique needs or condition. Examples would include the school nurse counseling a teacher who is overweight to seek a thorough evaluation by his or her primary healthcare provider or a dietitian; the school nurse teaching a bus driver to monitor his/her asthma using a peak flow meter; or the school nurse sharing resources for a teacher to get free nicotine patches to help with smoking cessation.

Group Health Promotion

Health promotion in a group provides a program or service that is available to more than one person, but may not be relative to all school staff members. Looking at similar examples as the ones used to illustrate individual health promotion, in group health promotion, the school nurse may set up an after-school walking club for staff members who are overweight; provide monthly health lessons to a group of staff members who have asthma; or establish a support group for staff who are trying to quit smoking. Often, the school nurse will not directly lead the health promotion activity, but may organize the formation of a group or schedule experts to work with the group.

Role of the School Nurse in Staff Wellness Programs

Implementation of an effective employee wellness program is a significant endeavor; it is therefore prudent to engage leaders in health promotion from within the school setting (Galemore, 2000). Members may include nursing, health and exercise science, guidance counselors, crisis intervention teams, and substance abuse prevention coordinators. Utilization of these experts enables health initiatives to be provided at a minimal additional cost to the district. Establishment of wellness outreach is congruent with the school nurses' public health focus and concern for high-level wellness.

Common examples of staff health promotion and disease prevention activities include hypertension monitoring, nutrition education, stress management, tobacco cessation, weight management, and lifestyle change programs, including walking groups. Annual surveys may be conducted to determine staff interest in and need for on-site programs. Incentives, such as prizes, recognition, reserved parking, and release time may engender enthusiasm, competition, and commitment (Petch-Levine, Cureton, Canham, & Murray, 2003; Wold, 2001). Record-keeping of individual employee health data resulting from participation in these programs may be the individual participant's responsibility, which alleviates the nurse from maintaining confidential employee health data.

As the individual with the greatest healthcare expertise in the school setting, the school nurse is viewed as an expert resource and a role model. It should be noted that the school nurse may be too busy caring for others to care for him- or herself; thus, the school nurse may not always model a healthy lifestyle in all areas. While school nurses generally eat breakfast, wear seat belts, and avoid alcohol and tobacco, they are often negligent in modeling other health-promoting lifestyle behaviors (Petch-Levine et al., 2003). School nurses are much less likely to get eight hours of sleep, exercise regularly, utilize relaxation strategies, eat lunch, and maintain a healthy weight. Personal reflection regarding the power of role modeling, as well as enhancing one's personal health, should be considered an important component of wellness promotion.

Conceptual Approaches to School Health

The Coordinated School Health Program Model outlines a nine-step process for developing a school-site health promotion program. These include:

1. Initiate the idea.
2. Establish a planning committee.

3. Assess the health needs and priorities of staff.
4. Develop goals and objectives (process, impact, outcome objectives).
5. Design program (include timeline, budget, incentives, identify materials needed, administrative approval).
6. Market the program.
7. Implement the program.
8. Evaluate the program.
9. Modify the program (Allegrante, 1998).

The CDC School Health Policies and Programs Study has specific recommendations for school staff health promotion (CDC, 2001). The *School Health* Program Report Card requires that schools have a faculty and staff health promotion coordinator (FSHP); however state-level summaries reveal that in 2001 only nine states (Arkansas, Delaware, Kansas, Maine, Nevada, New Hampshire, North Carolina, Texas, and Wisconsin) had a state-level FSHP coordinator. Only Mississippi requires each district to have a FSHP coordinator, while Wisconsin reported that each school was required to have one. The *Report Card* requires funding or sponsoring of employee assistance programs and health services for staff, in addition to providing staff health screening and the availability of physical activity facilities or equipment to staff.

CDC also offers a self-assessment and planning guide to promote healthy and safe behaviors within schools. The *School Health Index* assesses the eight core components of the Coordinated School Health program (see Chapter 3). The school team is asked to evaluate the specific areas to determine the degree to which the standard is in place within the school, that is, "fully in place" to "not in place." The team uses the scores to highlight potential areas the school can address (CDC, 2004). The Score Card is highlighted in TABLE 45.5.

Another approach is recommended by the Comprehensive Education Model (CHEM) (Galemore, 2000), which recommends the following steps:

1. Identification of the target population, program developers, and individuals recognized as experts in the area of health promotion
2. Development of outcome goals, which generally relate to indicators of health status, personal lifestyle changes, health education practices, and health promotion resources
3. Determination of personal and environmental health problems through the conduction of a needs assess

Table 45.5 ■

SCHOOL HEALTH INDEX—HEALTH PROMOTION FOR STAFF

	FULLY IN PLACE	PARTIALLY IN PLACE	UNDER DEVELOP-MENT	NOT IN PLACE
Health screening for staff	3	2	1	0
Stress management programs for staff	3	2	1	0
Promote staff participation	3	2	1	0
Training for staff on conflict resolution	3	2	1	0
Training for staff on first aid and CPR	3	2	1	0
Programs for staff on physical activity/fitness	3	2	1	0
Programs for staff on healthy eating/weight management	3	2	1	0
Programs for staff on tobacco-use cessation	3	2	1	0

Source: CDC (2004, Module 7, p. 3).

4. Establishment of a design plan which may include the organizational approach, operational objective, a time-table, resources, activities, a pre-test, program evaluation and budget approval
5. Implementation of the program
6. Evaluation of the program outcomes

Galemore's findings are compelling because her evaluation of this program format assessed not only change in employee health status/behaviors, but also the impact on health insurance claims and sick days. School districts often appreciate receiving these positive outcomes.

Perhaps the easiest way for the school nurse to develop an effective program is to apply the well-known nursing process.

1. Data Collection—Collecting data from school staff can be accomplished through surveys, review of community health data, interviews, personal observations, expert opinions, and so forth. The primary goal is to gain an understanding of the unique strengths and needs of a given population.
2. Assessment—Thorough analysis of the data will identify school needs. Combining this information with knowledge of local existing programs and resources will help to match needs with viable solutions. Assessment will be enhanced with the input of experts, both internal and external to the school setting.
3. Planning and Goal Setting—Goal setting must be reasonable and measurable. Once short-term objectives are identified to support the overall goal, the fundamental process of planning can begin.
4. Implementation—This phase should not be solely the responsibility of the school nurse. Facilitating implementation activities can yield success, as well as directly providing the services.
5. Evaluation—The process must include an evaluation to determine the outcomes of the program related to the established goals, so that changes can be made for the next time the program is offered.

PROMISING PROGRAMS FOR SCHOOLS

Given the large number and variety of potential programs that can be offered or provided to promote staff wellness, it is often difficult to choose the best and most effective one. Choosing programs that promote national goals, such as *Healthy People 2010*, or ones that address specific needs of the local school staff are likely to yield the best outcomes. Materials from the *U. S. Preventive Services Task Force* can be helpful in reviewing preventative services that have demonstrated effectiveness in the work setting (Agency for Healthcare Research and Quality, 2003). Another resource is the National Business Group on Health (National Business Group on Health, 2004), which provides fact sheets, resources, and measures to determine cost effectiveness. *Partnerships for a Healthy Workforce* is another program that provides tools for employers to set goals and implement measures to create and maintain a healthy workforce (Partnership for Prevention, 2004).

Education

Education is the foundation for all programs. Staff members need to perceive the need for and value of programs before they will be motivated to participate. As members of an educational community, they respect the educational process and appreciate quality presentations. However, as adult learners, they respond best when they perceive a need for the information.

Administration often expects the school nurse to present formal programs for school staff on a variety of health issues including Standard Precautions (formerly Universal Precautions) and regulations pertaining to blood borne pathogens, hepatitis and immunizations, and contagious diseases. Providing education is clearly within NASN's Health Education standard that addresses the nurse's role as an educator with students, community, and school staff (Lordi & Bradley, 2000). Chapter 7 details the role of the school nurse as health educator. The frequency of providing this type of information will depend on district/state requirements, staff needs, and nurse capabilities.

Screening/Health Assessment and Measurement

Screenings or health assessments are the most likely programs to be offered by school nurses, often in an informal manner. Common screenings include blood pressure and weight, which are easily provided by the school nurse. For example, the school nurse may offer blood pressure screenings to school staff on the first Monday of each month. Other screenings, such as cholesterol or mammograms, are coordinated with local healthcare providers and can be delivered on-site. This service alleviates use of staff sick leave to get important screenings.

Risk Factor Reduction

Safety and Crisis Response Programs

The overall health of the school community is enhanced when prior planning assures a prepared school staff with a viable response plan to crises of any kind. A prepared school means a safe environment for everyone. Safety and accident prevention programs, frequently offered in schools, include job site safety, first aid, cardiopulmonary resuscitation (CPR), and back injury prevention (James, 2001). Effective training will include return demonstrations of learned skills and periodic drills.

A key area of safety training is preparing staff to respond to emergencies. A New Mexico survey of school nurses revealed that 37% of their schools had activated emergency medical services for an adult emergency (NASN, 2004b). Some staff members are reluctant to perceive themselves as a first responder to a situation requiring healthcare intervention; yet, all school staff should know basic first aid measures so that care can be initiated or a patient safeguarded until the school nurse or EMS arrives on the scene. Teaching the Heimlich maneuver is especially important, if not required, for cafeteria employees and other staff who monitor students during meals. CPR instruction should be available to all staff members. As it becomes more common for schools to keep automatic external defibrillators (AEDs) on the premises, orientation and annual updates will be required on their use. The school nurse can provide the training or arrange for qualified organizations, such as the American Red Cross and the American Heart Association, to train staff. Safety programs require ongoing updates and re-certification to ensure ongoing competency of responders.

Violence

Violence in schools is a concern to all, and numerous programs have been developed to address school safety (Brown, 2002a). The New Jersey State Department of Education began electronic tracking of school violence and vandalism in the 1999–2000 school year. It was found that 48% of the incidents of violence, vandalism, and substance abuse occurred at the high school level. Although 1,810 of the 15,971 incidents of violence were directed at school personnel, there continues to be little attention to the staff as victims (Brown, 2002b). As with student victims, the staff may need medical treatment or mental health counseling to deal with an incident.

Violence prevention should be a priority in all schools (see Chapter 39). Staff members can learn to identify suspicious individuals and/or situations that may result in violence. They can further learn skills to de-escalate conflict situations and to intervene appropriately when confronted with any type of violence.

Group intervention may be necessary when an incident involves multiple staff members or creates generalized anxiety among a given group. The witnesses of violence or harassment may need psychological support and counseling. Anxiety, mounting stress, or post-traumatic stress disorder may occur and interfere with their personal well-being and job performance. The school nurse can intervene by advocating for worksite services and encouraging staff members to participate.

A form of violence to which school staff members are not immune is domestic violence. While domestic violence occurs in the home, it can affect the workplace as well (Partnership for Prevention, 2002). The school nurse can provide a valuable service to communities by making accessible materials and resources for victims of domestic violence and by providing a safe haven for staff members to share personal concerns.

Immunizations

Compared to children, adult immunization rates are much less successful (Poland et al., 2003). While *Healthy People 2010* sets goals for high risk adults (ages 19 to 64) at 60% for annual influenza immunization and for one dose of the pneumococcal vaccine, CDC data from 1999 revealed rates of 31% and 17%, respectively (Pollard et al., 2003). The Advisory Committee on Immunization Practices has highlighted the need to focus on immunizations for adults as well as for children (NASN, 2001). This is especially true because of the close contact between staff and their young students, who are frequently the carriers of contagious diseases; this places staff at high risk for contracting infections. School nurses are well positioned to influence adult compliance through education about the value of adult immunization and facilitation of easy access to immunization clinics.

Stress Reduction

Teaching is a “high stress” occupation (Moriarty, Edmunds, Martin, & Blatchford, 2001). In Sweden, the statistically most stressful position in a workplace environment is that of the comprehensive school teacher (Jacobsson, Pousette, & Thylefors, 2001). Stressors identified in the Swedish study are similar to those present in American schools:

- Perceived work demands, including issues of coordination, excessive paperwork, and time constraints;

- Pupil misbehavior. Large classes, and difficulty meeting individual student needs;
- A loss of empowerment resulting from administrative unilateral decision-making, especially related to curriculum and education initiatives; and
- Negative feedback (Jacobsson et al., 2001).

Educators can use both direct action techniques and palliative techniques to deal with workplace stress (Kyriacou, 2001). Aspects of direct action include having more effective personal organization, obtaining new knowledge/skills, and negotiating for a change in a situation or responsibility. Palliative techniques can be physical or mental and while they do not deal with the source of the stress, they lessen the feeling of stress. The teacher may change the perception of the stressor or engage in physical activities to decrease tension and anxiety and thus develop a renewed sense of control. Houghton (2001) suggested finding allies in the school setting to sustain both health and well-being. By taking a proactive stance, the school nurse may strive to ameliorate staff stress through alleviation of workplace stressors and stress management programming. Many schools address employee stress by offering after-school peer support groups, fitness activities, music therapy, aromatherapy, and Eastern arts (yoga, Tai Chi). Others may offer training in meditation, mediation, or journaling. Schools should consider ways to create places within the school that are quiet, nurturing, and relaxing environments for staff to use for lunch and/or planning periods. If teachers perceive that their physical and emotional needs are being met, they will have additional motivation and energy to better address the needs of their students (James, 2001). The school nurse can be instrumental in convincing the administration to create or support programs in which the nurse may assume the organizational or leadership role.

Fitness

While there does not appear to be a universal definition of "fitness" or "physical fitness," the most common one is defined in a Report of the Surgeon General as: "A set of attributes that people have or achieve relating to their ability to perform physical activity" (President's Council on Physical Fitness and Sports, 2000). Using this general definition, it can be assumed that to be fit, individuals would have the physical ability and stamina to participate in activities of their choosing. Weight, nutritional condition, health status, and level of physical activity are all part of overall fitness.

As with other programs, the school nurse can be instrumental in establishing activities to enhance the overall fitness of the school staff. In addition to strengthening cardiovascular status and enhancing weight management, group fitness activities are a way to improve staff morale and support a sense of community within the staff as a whole. Activities such as walking clubs, running groups, team sports, or aerobic dance classes can be held before or after school and can easily include students and families. Schools are ideal sites for exercise programs as they likely already house equipment for student athletes. In addition, physical education teachers are experts in fitness activities and can be leaders in fitness initiatives.

Organizational Policies and Environmental Changes

The health of the entire school community is affected by both policies and the overall school climate. Policies can facilitate access or create barriers to health programs and services. The school climate, in terms of physical structure and emotional climate, directly impacts on daily health and well-being. The school nurse can be instrumental in assessing these components and facilitating an organizational response to ensure a healthy environment. In some instances, change may come about only with rules to direct programs and mandate sustainability. In other instances, change can occur by convincing decision-makers, from the local custodian who oversees playground equipment to the superintendent who authorizes expenditures for medical equipment, to make decisions that underpin good health.

Environmental Health Promotion

The school environment should exude a positive climate and a healthy/safe environment. School staff are in a position to be able to identify potential health hazards related to school safety, air quality, temperature, mold on the walls, exposed asbestos, noise levels, water quality, food, and/or the spread of communicable disease. When staff members are concerned that an assigned classroom, the school building or a play area is an unhealthy place, the school nurse must be prepared to address their concerns with accurate information or appropriate resources. These concerns should be addressed in a professional way through proper evaluation of the problem and when warranted, a prompt plan of correction. School nurses work closely with state and local public health departments and the Environmental Protection Agency (EPA) to enforce regulations and promote established health practices. The school nurse can provide valuable data to any school investigation by sharing epidemiological data that demonstrate specific building locations where clusters of symptoms have been reported to occur. These environmental concerns of staff are often of immediate interest to them, since they can directly impact on their health.

Indoor Air Quality (IAQ)

Complaints of "sick building syndrome," as it applies to schools, have been used to express the increased concern of school employees regarding the health and safety of the school environment (Hootman et al., 2001; National Education Association, 2001). Since children and adults spend more time indoors than they have in the past, their exposure to indoor pollutants has raised the concern of both nonprofit agencies and the EPA (Epstein, 2001). School nurses recognize the potential for both long and short-term effects for pollutants, especially for those with allergies and altered immunity.

The school environment includes the physical plant (the building and grounds), the occupants (staff, students, parents, visitors), the furnishings (equipment and room materials), and the activities (eating, physical activity, laboratory, cleaning, health care, cooking, industrial shop) (NASN, 2004a). Any school building can have air quality issues. Heating, ventilation, and air conditioning systems in need of maintenance or with insufficient capacity of operation have been identified as fostering the growth of mold and dust mites, which influence the incidence of allergies and asthma (Epstein, 2001). During building renovation, the possibility of exposure to toxic substances such as asbestos, asphalt, and solvent also exists (New Jersey Education Association, 2002). While new school designers focus more on air quality (Sack, 2002), new buildings are not necessarily risk-free.

In addition to issues with the physical building, the underlying ground, or the surrounding community's pollutants, the school staff may inadvertently contribute to poor IAQ. They should be reminded to eliminate or keep in moderation such things as perfumes, potpourri, candles, classroom clutter, dust, and classroom pets. The EPA created an effective school program, *Tools for Schools*, to address IAQ. Released in 1996, the kit is available at no cost to any school. Its comprehensive approach helps staff who are not experts in either health or IAQ to use a team approach to identify and correct problems in the school.

Smoke-Free Schools

Concerns about the effects of second-hand smoke as an asthma trigger, a pollutant, and a cancer-causing agent have provided the impetus to develop non-smoking rules in most schools. The reduction of tobacco use by adults in the workforce is the number one objective of *Partnerships for a Healthy Workforce* (Partnership for Prevention, 2004). The trend during the last decade has been for districts to totally ban smoking on school premises. In the wake of the No Child Left Behind Act of 2001 (P. L. 107-110), the Department of and Health and Human Services announced the reauthorization of the Pro-Children Act of 1994 that prohibits indoor smoking in places utilized to provide educational services to children under the age of 18 (Pro-Children Act, 1994). This is a continuation of the 1994 regulations that ban smoking in facilities that are funded by the federal government, as well as state or local government facilities that receive federal funds, including school districts.

School nurses have been strong advocates for enacting and enforcing these laws; however, when enforcing these laws, school nurses find a new challenge with staff members. Suddenly many are confronted with their smoking habit and have no place to smoke on school grounds. This is an opportune time for school nurses to increase dissemination of literature and resources that offer alternatives to smoking and assist with smoking cessation.

Exposure Control

Staff members may potentially be exposed to a number of agents in the school setting. Three common agents are bloodborne pathogens, hazardous materials, and communicable disease.

Bloodborne Pathogens

Because *bloodborne pathogens,* such as HIV and hepatitis B virus, have such serious sequelae and are prevalent in the school-age population, schools have been examining district policies and procedures and implementing staff education programs. In 1991, the Occupational Safety and Health Administration (OSHA) established rules to protect employees who may potentially be exposed to blood or other body fluids as a result of their job duties in the healthcare setting (OSHA, 1991). These federal standards for healthcare settings were subsequently adapted to the school venue, as evidenced by NASN's 1994 publication, *Occupational Exposure to Bloodborne Pathogens: Implementing OSHA Standards in School* Settings (Bradley, 1994). States may adopt the federal standards as presented or develop their own plan (NASN, 2003). School nurses should be involved with any development, implementation, or evaluation of such a plan.

The concept of *Universal Precautions* changed to *Standard Precautions* and expanded to protect everyone. The practice of *Standard Precautions* by all school employees serves to reduce the risk of communicable disease transmission (Hootman et al., 2001).

The school nurse collaborates with administrators to determine employees at risk for exposure to bloodborne pathogens or other communicable disease as a result of their school assignment. In accordance with OSHA regulations, persons identified as at risk for bloodborne pathogen exposure should receive immediate training and a yearly inservice (Hootman et al., 2001). Based on their job description, some employees will need to have personal protective equipment and/or HBV immunization. Commonly, schools include all employees in annual inservices. Any presentation will ensure that participants understand the critical need for frequent, thorough handwashing. Documentation is an important component of tracking trainings, incidents of exposure, referrals, treatment, and monitoring of activities.

Hazardous Materials

Another potential source of environment exposure is *hazardous materials*, that is, chemicals and/or toxic agents that are in the school building. Cleaning agents, pesticides, building materials, and chemicals in science labs are potentially dangerous items if not handled properly. OSHA maintains standards for storing and handling such material and for informing employees of the presence of these materials in the workplace. The Hazard Communication Standard (HCS) covers all hazardous chemicals in all worksites. "The concept behind HCS is that providing information to employer and employees enables them to take steps to ensure protection in their work places" (OSHA, 2004). Another OSHA safeguard is the Material Safety Data Sheets (MSDS). The sheets contain specific information about the hazards and necessary protective measures to be used with a chemical. Employers "are required to provide access to the labels and the MSDSs, and to train workers" (OSHA, 2004).

While the school nurse is not the safety coordinator, he or she should still be aware of school practices and procedures in order to advocate for and facilitate safe practices. The Materials Safety Data Sheets can be a vital resource for directing first aid responses to chemical exposure. From assessing a student who has ingested soap in the bathroom to determining care for a custodian who splashes a cleaning agent in his eye, the MSDS will outline what level of care and follow-up is needed.

Communicable Disease

Exposure to communicable disease must be addressed in every school setting. Assuring prompt identification and treatment of both students and staff diminishes the spread of any contagion and decreases fear and rumors. Rules governing student exclusion, relative to illness, should be applicable to staff. Staff must recognize that the school is legally authorized to prohibit the attendance of teachers as well as students to prevent the spread of communicable disease (Harrigan, 2002). The school nurse should review the role of the state and local health department in providing guidelines to schools regarding communicable disease detection and control (Hootman et al., 2001).

Education for staff members will set the stage for healthy practices. Essential components should include information regarding the signs and symptoms of common communicable illnesses, modes of transmission, and periods of communicability (Harrigan, 2002). Distribution of materials and resources from the local and state health departments, such as information about influenza immunizations, are helpful for staff.

Student illness (such as Fifth disease, conjunctivitis, meningitis, ringworm, or impetigo) or infestations (such as head lice and scabies) create anxiety for some staff members. Sound explanations, concurrent with treatment of the condition, can help to alleviate some concerns. Staff manuals may also cover these topics to provide general information in a proactive way.

Since September 11, 2001, there has been heightened concern regarding bioterrorism. The school nurse is well positioned to provide a sentinel watch, that is, observe for and recognize unusual symptoms or patterns of illness, and to report unusual symptoms or patterns to a public health authority. The school nurse is also in a place where he/she may likely be the first responder in the event of a biological event (see Chapter 10). The CDC's Web site, www.cdc.gov, provides the most accurate and up-to-date resource for the school nurse in obtaining current information on possible bioterrorism agents, their symptoms, and recommended treatment. This site is also noteworthy for its information on communicable and vaccine-preventable diseases. Response to this and other catastrophic events should be included in the school crisis plan.

Teams

The value of the school nurse serving as a member or leader of a team addressing school health cannot be over emphasized. It is an opportunity that is often overlooked, taken for granted or underestimated; yet, working with a group of professionals offers a promising means of tackling hard issues. The ability to effect change is often dependent upon the work of many, not one. As a member of the coordinated school health team, district ADA team, or community improvement committee, the school nurse can share needed nursing expertise to change policies and initiate programs to enhance the health of the school community.

CONCLUSION

The school nurse plays a pivotal role in the maintenance and promotion of staff health. Through awareness and implementation of local, state, and federal regulations, the journey begins. Through creativity and collaboration, employee wellness programs can be developed that will enhance the school staff's overall health and personal job satisfaction. The expanded role of the school nurse in the health care and health promotion of school staff contributes to the health of the entire school community.

References

Agency for Healthcare Research and Quality. (2003). *U.S. Preventive Services Task Force*. Retrieved August 30, 2004 from http://www.ahcpr.gov/clinic/uspstfix.htm.

Allegrante, J. P. (1998). School–site Health Promotion for Staff. In E. Marx & S. F. Wooley with D. Northrup (Eds.), *Health is academic* (pp. 224–243). New York: Teachers College Press.

Americans with Disabilities Act (ADA) 42 U.S.C. 12101. (1990).

Bergren, M. (2003). National conference on the HIPAA privacy rule. *NASN Newsletter, 18*(4), 20–22.

Bobo, N., Hallenbeck, P., & Robinson, J. (2003). Recommended minimal emergency equipment and resources for schools: National consensus group report. *Journal of School Nursing, 19*(3), 150–156.

Bradley, B. (1994). *Occupational exposure to bloodborne pathogens: Implementing OSHA standards in school settings*. Scarborough, ME: National Association of School Nurses.

Brown, P. M. (2002a). Programs that work. *NJEA Review, 75*(9), 20–25.

Brown, P. M. (2002b). Violence prevention in New Jersey schools. *NJEA Review, 75* (9), 12–18.

Centers for Disease Control and Prevention (CDC). (2001). Coordinated school health programs make a difference. *Chronic Disease Notes & Reports, 14*(1), 6–9. Retrieved July 26, 2004 from http://www.cdc.gov/nccd-php/cdwin2001.pdf.

Centers for Disease Control and Prevention (CDC). (2004). *School health index: A self–assessment & planning guide*. Atlanta: Centers for Disease Control and Prevention.

Code of Federal Regulations Act (CFR). (2003). *Regulations to implement the equal employment provisions of the Americans with Disabilities Act, CFR, Title 29, Subtitle B, Chapter XIV, Point. 1630.* Retrieved October 2, 2005 from http://www.access.gpo.gov/cgi-bin/cfrassenble.cgi?title=200329.

DeGroot, T. (2003). A meta–analysis of the non–monetary effects of employee health management programs. *Health Resource Management, 42*(1), 53–69.

Epstein, B. L. (2001). Childhood asthma and indoor allergens: The classroom may be a culprit. *Journal of School Nursing, 17*(95), 253–257.

Galemore, C. A. (2000). Initiation of a school employee wellness program: Applying the comprehensive health education model. *Journal of School Nursing, 16*(3), 39–46.

Grant, T. W. (2002). Bring your first aid kit: An unannounced mock drill. *Journal of School Nursing, 18*(3), 174–178.

Harrigan, J. F. (2002). *Overview of school health services*. Scarborough, ME: National Association of School Nurses.

HIPAA privacy rule and public health guidance from CDC and the U. S. Department of Health and Human Services. (2003). *Morbidity & Mortality Weekly Report (Suppl.), 52* (17), 1–12.

Hootman, J., Schwab, N. C. & Gelfman M. H. B. (2001). School nursing practice: Clinical performance issues. In N. C. Schwab & M. H. B. Gelfman (Eds.), *Legal issues in school health services* (pp. 167–230). North Branch, MN: Sunrise River Press.

Houghton, P. (2001). Finding allies. *Phi Delta Kappan, 82*(9), 706–711.

Jacobsson, C., Pousette, A. & Thylefors, I. (2001). Managing stress and feelings of mastery among Swedish comprehensive school teachers. *Scandinavian Journal of Educational Research, 45*(1), 37–53.

James, G. (2001). A seven–year follow–up comparing attendees and nonattendees at a statewide school employee wellness conference. *The Journal of School Health, 1* (4), 127–131.

Kentucky Association for School Health (2001), *Statistically if there are 100 people in your workplace:*. Retrieved on August 22, 2004 from http://www.kyschoolhealth.org/Staffhealth.html

Kyriacou, C. (2001). Teacher stress: Directions for future research. *Educational Review, 53*:(1), 27–35.

Lordi, S., & Bradley, B. (2000). *Standards of professional school nursing practice: Applications in the field*. Scarborough, ME: National Association of School Nurses.

McKenzie, F. D., & Richmond, J. B. (1998). Linking Health and Learning: An Overview of Coordinated School Health Program. In E. Marx & S. F. Wooley with D. Northrup (Eds.), *Health is academic* (pp. 1–14). New York: Teachers College Press.

Moriarty, V., Edmonds, S., Martin, C., & Blatchford, P. (2001). Teaching young children: Perceived satisfaction and stress. *Educational Research, 43*(1), 33–46.

National Association of School Nurses (NASN). (2001). *Position statement: Immunizations:*. Retrieved August 27, 2001 from http://www.nasn.org/positions/immunizations.htm.

National Association of School Nurses (NASN). (2002). *Issue brief: School health nurse's role in education, role of the school nurse*. Retrieved January 6, 2003 from http://www.nasn.org/briefs/role.htm.

National Association of School Nurses (NASN). (2003). *Position statement: Regulations on bloodborne pathogens in the school setting*. Retrieved August 30, 2004 from http://www.nasn.org/positions/pathogens.htm.

National Association of School Nurses (NASN). (2004a). *Issue brief: Environmental concerns in the school setting*. Retrieved August 26, 2004 from http://www.nasn.org/briefs/environmental.htm.

National Association of School Nurses (NASN). (2004b). *Joint position statement: The emergency response plan for schools.* Retrieved on August 24, 2004 from http://www.nasn.org/positions/ahajoint.pdf.
National Association of School Nurses (NASN) and the American Nurses Association (ANA). (2001). *Scope and standards of school nursing practice.* Scarborough ME: NASN.
National Business Group on Health. (2004). Retrieved August 27, 2004 from www.wbgh.org.
National Center for Educational Statistics. (2002). *Quick tables & figures, elementary & secondary*. Retrieved July 26, 2004 from http://nces.ed.gov/quicktables/.
National Education Association. (2001). Breaking the mold on air quality. NEA Today, 13–15.
National Education Association. (2003). *Status of the American public school teacher 2000–2001, NEA Research*. Washington, DC: Retrieved July 24, 2004 from http://www.nea.org/edstats/images/status.pdf.
New Jersey Education Association. (2002). Renovation risks. *NJEA Review, 75* (9), 26–27.
Occupational Safety and Health Administration, Occupational Exposure to Bloodborne Pathogens. 29CFR Part 1910.1030. (1991).
Occupational Safety and Health Administration (OHSA). (2004). *Hazard communication in the 21st century workplace, executive summary*. Retrieved August 30, 2004 from http://www.osha.gov/dsg/hazcom/finalmsdsreport.html.
Omnibus Transportation Employee Testing Act. FR Doc. 49 383. (1991).
Partnership for Prevention. (2001). *Healthy workforce 2010*. Retrieved August 21, 2004 from http://www.prevent.org.
Partnership for Prevention. (2002). *Issue brief: Domestic violence and the workplace*. Washington, DC: Author.
Partnership for Prevention. (2004). *Partnerships for a healthy workplace*. Retrieved August 21, 2004 from http://www.prevent.org.
Petch-Levine, D., Cureton, V., Canham, D., & Murray, M. (2003). Health practices of school nurses. *Journal of School Nursing, 19* (5), 273–280.
Poland, G. A, Shefer, A. M., McCauley, M., Webster, P. S., Whitley-Williams, P. N. Peter, G. & National Vaccine Advisory Committee. (2003). Standards for adult immunization practices. *American Journal of Preventive Medicine, 25*(2), 144–150.
President's Council on Physical Fitness and Sports, Research Digest. (March, 2000). Series 3, Number 9. Retrieved August 25, 2004 from http://www.fitness.gov/activity/activity2/digest_mar2000/digest_mar2000.html
Prochildren Act. FR Doc. 94 32136. (1994).
Roman, P. M. & Blum, T. C. (2002). The workplace and alcohol problem prevention. *Journal of Alcohol Research and Health, 26*(1), 49–57.
Sack, J. (2002). EPA pushing improved air quality in schools. *Education Week, 21*(22), 1–2.
School Health Policies & Programs Study (SHPPS). (2001). Atlanta: Centers for Disease Control and Prevention.
Taliaferro, V. (2003). HIPAA and schools [Special supplement]. *School Health Alert*.
U.S. Department of Health and Human Services (USDHHS). (2000). *Healthy People 2010*. Retrieved August 21, 2004 from http://www.healthypeople.gov.
Wold, S. J. (2001). School Health Services: History and Trends. In N. C. Schwab & M. H. B. Gelfman (Eds.), *Legal issues in school health services* (pp. 7–14). North Branch, MN: Sunrise River Press.
Wold, S. J., & Dagg, N. V. (2001). School nursing: A framework for practice. *Journal of School Health, 71*(8), 401–404.

Chapter 46

Staff Management

JAN HOOTMAN

Chapter Outline

INTRODUCTION

Organizational goals for health services can be achieved and quality school nursing services provided only under the direction of and through the services of qualified health professionals, such as school nurses. Successful employee performance is essential to the accomplishments of any organization; availability and effective management of staff resources also contribute to the productivity and well-being of organizations. This chapter describes important issues in managing the school health services staff. Although the chapter is focused on supervisory activities of personnel, it may be used by persons working in lead positions in school health who may monitor the job performance of others. In addition, school nurses should understand the systems in which they work and the management issues in their systems.

School systems are influenced not only by education issues but also by factors from other aspects of the local and global community, for example, legal, business, and health system trends. Subsequently, human resource policies and practices and job performance expectations are ever changing in all work settings. For example, the *aging work force* will continue to increase as the population grows older and will influence the work environment. In addition, the *rate of change* in the world and the workplace is phenomenal, and businesses, including school and health systems, will likely cycle through change even faster for sustainability in the future. This rapid change necessitates staff performance assets such as continuous learning and skill building, improved individual coping mechanisms, and increased job flexibility.

Changing economies and demands for increased quality and efficiency are prompting many organizations, including health and education systems, to *downsize*. For staff to be effective at doing more with less requires organizational support to the work force. This support may include job redesign, retraining, and skillful and sensitive communication as well as empowering workers to have more control over their jobs. Subsequently, staff performance will benefit through facilitating competency in such work activities as delegation, participatory management, and goal setting.

Regardless of the changing work environment, professional performance that provides safe and quality client care is the expectation of all school health and nursing services. School nurses must provide services according to scientifically validated nursing principles and local, state, and national standards for general nursing practice and specialty school nursing practice, as well as legal mandates and professional ethics (Schwab & Gelfman, 2001).

One or more persons in an organization may perform the work of staff management and responsibilities may vary from supervisor, to manager, to human resources director. The goals of staff management are to have the right number and types of people in the right places at the right time to effectively and efficiently complete the tasks to help an organization meet its objectives (DeCenzo & Robbins, 1994). Planning for human resources should be aligned with the strategic plan of an organization. Generally, four activities are necessary in staff management: recruitment, orientation, motivation, and maintenance. This chapter focuses on these activities. However, the responsibilities of a supervisor extend far beyond these management activities and include activities such as budgeting (see Chapter 44), project management, visualizing and projecting the future, and managing legal issues (Chapters 12 to 14).

STAFF RECRUITMENT

The goal of recruitment is to attract qualified and preferably the "best" candidates for a staff or administrative position. Recruitment constraints, such as a nursing shortage, organization policies limiting recruitment to internal promotion, governmental regulations, and salary issues are examples of factors that can challenge the ability to attract applicants. These conditions may call for the recruiter's ingenuity in surmounting such limitations. Recruitment techniques include advertisements, recommendations from current employees, use of employment agency services, and solicitation through educational systems and related health service agencies, such as hospitals, clinics, and public health systems. Some companies recruit via the Internet.

Creating an Applicant Pool

Advertisements are one way to communicate a job vacancy. Advertisements can be posted within the hiring organization or externally to the general labor market via professional journals or newspapers. The higher the position, the more specialized the skills, or the shorter the supply in the labor force, the more widely dispersed the advertisement may need to be. A job advertisement generally contains information about:

- Job duties to be performed
- Qualifications required, including work experience and minimum educational preparation or certification or other qualifications required or desirable
- Application process (for example, phone for an interview, send in a resume, or e-mail the application)
- Application deadline

When seeking employment or seeking to fill job positions, employment agencies may be helpful in job location and recruitment efforts. An agency may advertise the position, screen candidates against the employer's criteria, and provide guarantees for a time to the employer should the applicant not perform satisfactorily. All states provide a public employment service. A private employment agency must charge for its services. The fee can be absorbed by the employer, the employee, or split between the two.

Educational institutions are excellent sites for recruitment. Colleges and universities were previously considered to graduate only young and inexperienced workers; now they are a resource for experienced workers who have returned to school to upgrade skills or pursue new educational and career opportunities. Some school districts also employ BSN-RNs without experience and provide an orientation and on-the-job preceptor opportunities. Professional organizations, including labor unions and state and national nursing organizations, generally distribute job opportunities to their members. Other healthcare systems, such as hospitals and community health, may be resources for staff looking to make a change into school nursing.

Another recruitment option, and perhaps more viable for school nursing, is the use of independent contractors. This technique has cost saving features because a company does not have to consider this person an employee who is entitled to the benefits of regular staff. The independent contractor will need to have the skills and nursing competencies necessary to perform the job. Consult with the business office and legal counsel for assistance in the language and content of the work agreement for an independent worker. Be aware that a consultant who is required to comply with instructions about when, where, and how work is to be done is ordinarily deemed an employee (Gagliardi & Johnston, 2002).

JOB APPLICATION AND INTERVIEW PROCESS

Primarily, state and federal laws direct the types of information employers can use for employment decisions. The current guidelines can generally be found through the state and federal departments of labor (the federal Web address is http://www.dol.gov/). Court decisions and agency policies and guidelines also influence recruitment and hiring decisions. These may be confusing and often change. Avoid any recruitment techniques that have the intent or effect of excluding on the basis of race, color, national origin, sexual preference, religion, age, pregnancy status, or disability. The employer has the right to ask if the applicant meets the legal age requirements for work in your city or state. Check the state's guidelines and obtain legal counsel if there is no human resources department to provide guidance through the recruitment, interview, and hiring activities to fill health service staff or administrative positions. See FIGURE 46-1 for federal laws that prohibit job discrimination questions. All requests for information must be related to the duties of the job in question and all applicants for the job should be asked the same questions to ensure fairness. The job application questions can help you determine whether the applicant has the minimum experience and education required for the position.

Job Description

All candidates should have access to the job description before the interview meeting. A job description is a concise list of the expected work and responsibilities as well as the knowledge, skills, and abilities required of the person filling the position. A job description does not usually dictate how to do the work. The description indicates the person to whom the worker will report and with whom the employee will interact. Action verbs (i.e., assesses, provides, and manages) give clear description of the work activity to be performed. There is no standard job description for the school nurse, for roles and responsibilities vary based on multiple factors including population size and characteristics, local expectations of the role, and state regulations regarding scope of nursing practice. Even job title will vary depending on the scope of the position, for example, "staff nurse," which generally implies direct student care, to "consultant," which often implies more responsibility with case management and less direct nursing care in the health room. See FIGURES 46.2A and B for examples of school nurse job descriptions.

Other job descriptions for school health services include school nurse supervisors or administrators (FIGURE 46.3) and unlicensed assistive personnel (UAP) (FIGURE 46.4). A variety of titles identify persons assigned to assist the registered nurse in

(text continues on page 1080)

FEDERAL LAWS THAT PROHIBIT JOB DISCRIMINATION* QUESTIONS

- *Title VII of the Civil Rights Act of 1964 (Title VII)* prohibits employment discrimination based on race, color, religion, sex, or national origin (http://www.eeoc.gov/laws/vii.html).
- *The Equal Pay Act of 1963 (EPA)* protects men and women who perform substantially equal work in the same establishment from sex-based wage discrimination (http://www.eeoc.gov/laws/epa.html).
- *The Age Discrimination in Employment Act of 1967 (ADEA)* protects individuals who are 40 years of age and older (http://www.eeoc.gov/laws/adea.html).
- *Title I and Title V of the Americans with Disabilities Act of 1990 (ADA)* prohibits employment discrimination against qualified individuals with disabilities in the private sector and in state and local governments (http://www.eeoc.gov/laws/ada.html).
- *Sections 501 and 505 of the Rehabilitation Act of 1973* prohibits discrimination against qualified individuals with disabilities who work in the federal government (http://www.eeoc.gov/laws/rehab.html).
- The Civil Rights Act of 1991 provides monetary damages in cases of intentional employment discrimination (http://www.eeoc.gov/laws/cra91.html).

Figure 46.1 ■ Federal laws that prohibit job discrimination questions *The U.S. Equal Employment Opportunity Commission (EEOC) enforces all these laws.
(*Source:* U.S. Equal Employment Opportunity Commission, 2002.)

> "The job description will serve as the most important local standard of care against which a school nurse's performance will be measured in a civil action to determine if the school nurse met the standard of a reasonable, prudent school nurse" (Schwab & Gelfman, 2001, p. 145).

SAMPLE SCHOOL NURSE JOB DESCRIPTION

Based upon sample from and used with permission of Edina Public Schools, Minnesota
Qualifications and job duties vary with local expectations, staffing pattern, and legal regulations

Organizational Relationship: Reports and is administratively accountable to the Coordinator of Health Services and to the building principal in matters of school building administration and provision of heath services in the building.

Qualifications:

1) Baccalaureate degree in nursing
2) Licensed as a registered nurse in accordance with the MN Board of Nursing
3) Licensed as a school nurse, in accordance with the MN Department of Children, Families, & Learning
4) Previous experience as a Licensed School Nurse or Public Health Nurse preferred

Primary Objectives:

1) To strengthen and facilitate the educational process by modifying or removing health-related barriers to learning
2) To promote optimal levels of well-being in students and staff

Major Areas of Responsibilities:

I. Recommend school district policies and philosophy related to the Health Services Program
- Participate in developing, implementing, and evaluating school health program goals, objectives, and procedures
- Participate in planning programs that eliminate or minimize student health concerns that may interfere with learning

II. Assess and evaluate the health and developmental status of school children
- Assist in developing, implementing, and evaluating procedures and programs to assess the health and developmental status of students
- Identify student health needs through health assessment and communicate with parents and staff

III. Promote and maintain health and well-being of students, families, and school personnel by teaching and counseling
- Participate on the child study team: assists in the identification of students with health conditions and disabilities, interprets health factors pertinent to the student's disability and develops, implements, and evaluates the health component of the individual educational plan (IEP)
- Assist students and parents in identifying and utilizing available and appropriate community health resources

IV. Implement an individual plan for the care of students with chronic health conditions and disabilities and students needing treatments or medications
- Develop individualized health plans (IHP) with specific goals, objectives, and interventions based on student health needs
- Supervise health assistants/paraprofessionals in assigned buildings
- Administer medications and treatments to students per physician order and parent authorization

V. Prevent communicable disease
- Monitor immunization status and provide appropriate immunizations
- Screen for contagious diseases and provide referral and treatment information
- Work with local health agency to track reportable communicable diseases

VI. Develop and maintain a system of first aid, recommend school safety measures, and promote a healthful school environment
- Participate in developing and maintaining a system for providing first aid and emergency care
- Participate in identifying and reporting current or potential environmental health and safety hazards for students and staff

VII. Provide health education
- Provide consultation and assistance to teachers in their planning, implementation, and evaluation of health education units
- Provide health counseling to students to assist them in making decisions regarding their health and health behaviors
- Provide in-service education opportunities for school staff on health-related issues

VIII. Assume responsibility for continuing education and own professional development
- Complete yearly goal setting for professional growth
- Participate in self evaluation of performance and continuing education activity

IX. Collect data and maintain records within professional and legal boundaries and school guidelines
- Initiate, maintain, and annually reviews student health records
- Maintain daily, monthly, and yearly statistical information regarding health status of students and staff and utilization of school health service programs

Figure 46.2 ■ Sample school nurse job description.

SAMPLE JOB SCHOOL NURSE DESCRIPTION

Based on a sample from and used with permission of Willamette Education Service District, Salem, Oregon

Qualifications and job duties vary with local expectations, staffing pattern, and legal regulations

JOB TITLE: Nurse Consultant

REPORTS TO: Direct Supervisor

SUMMARY: To provide evaluation, assessment, consultation, or direct services to children with health needs in educational settings, as well as train staff and delegate nursing tasks as appropriate; to provide school health services at district request and direction; to provide general training (CPR, First Aid, Blood-Borne Pathogens) as requested.

ESSENTIAL DUTIES AND RESPONSIBILITIES (including performance standards.) Other duties may be assigned.

1. PLANNING AND PREPARATION

1.1. Develops expectations and goals appropriate for position and responsibilities, based upon identified needs.
1.2. Designs a process and identifies and organizes resources for achieving expectations and goals.

Specific Indicators of Standard Attainment:

a) Plans, develops, and follows a weekly schedule based upon IFSP/IEP service needs and caseload. Demonstrates flexibility in adjusting schedule to meet emergency needs.
b) Plans, organizes, and schedules appropriate meetings.
c) Displays knowledge of, or is able to research, etiology, characteristics and prognosis of relevant medical conditions.
d) Displays knowledge of normal developmental sequences and learning patterns in the areas of sensory, motor, psychosocial and cognitive development and can use this knowledge in the development of Health Management Plans.
e) Displays knowledge of health issues and safety needs of children.
f) Displays knowledge of laws, regulations and current professional practice standards affecting nursing services, especially in educational settings.
g) Orders supplies as needed and effectively plans distribution of equipment and materials.
h) Provides assistance and/or recommendations to families and school districts regarding selection, ordering, and funding of appropriate equipment and materials. Nurse effectively evaluates factors related to safety, availability, and cost when choosing equipment or intervention options.

2. IMPLEMENTATION AND MANAGEMENT

2.1. Carries out plans and uses strategies and resources, adapting as needed to achieve desired goals.

Specific Indicators of Standard Attainment:

a) Uses and manages time effectively.
b) Effectively manages, evaluates, and modifies needed school health programs and Health Management Plans.
c) Provides service coordination to parents and children, including referral to other agencies for health care issues, as needed. Functions as a student advocate when appropriate.
d) Completes required paperwork in specified time and manner. Manages and maintains accurate records. Completes Medicaid forms as needed.
e) Creates an environment and provides instruction that engages staff and students and enhances learning.
f) Communicates expectations and monitors and reinforces staff and student behavior positively to facilitate learning, using effective behavior management skills and teaching practices.
g) Evaluates the quality and effectiveness of her practice and stresses quality improvement through the development of improved policies and procedures or practice guidelines.

3. ASSESSMENT AND THE USE OF ASSESSMENT INFORMATION

3.1. Selects or develops methods of collecting information, and uses these methods appropriately.
3.2. Interprets, analyzes, and acts upon information to make decisions, guide improvement, and report results.

Specific Indicators of Standard Attainment:

a) Uses assessment data to establish appropriate Health Management Plans, training goals and objectives or school services.
b) Provides constructive, timely feedback to students and staff to enhance learning.
c) Develops, selects, and uses appropriate assessment tools, and interprets results effectively.
d) Writes necessary assessment summaries and recommendations in a clear, informative and timely manner.
e) Monitors, evaluates and modifies student and staff performance using observation and data.

4. COMMUNICATION

4.1. Conveys information and ideas in modes, forms and in a style that is appropriate to audience, purpose, and context.
4.2. Listens and responds respectfully to information and ideas conveyed by others

Figure 46.2 ■ *(continued)*

Specific Indicators of Standard Attainment:

a) Participates knowledgeably and collaboratively on IFSP/IEP/504 teams.
b) Employs appropriate counseling and crisis intervention strategies as needed.
c) Participates collaboratively on a team to develop an integrated IFSP/IEP. Writes goals which are appropriate and measurable, reflecting students' health needs, preferences and expected outcomes.
d) Provides effective and collaborative consultation. Provides inservice training (including First Aid, CPR, Blood-Borne Pathogen/Standard Precautions, and Medication Administration Training) and follow-up to children, school staff, and parents. Promotes public awareness of relevant health issues.
e) Maintains confidentiality.
f) Communicates clearly and effectively with students/children, parents, colleagues and other service providers with consideration for culture and background; is sensitive to listener's level of understanding when using medical terminology.
g) Offers/volunteers assistance when appropriate.

5. LEADERSHIP AND PROFESSIONAL SERVICE AND CONDUCT

5.1. Envisions future needs and opportunities appropriate for position and program.
5.2. Acts on the basis of professional principles and generally accepted norms of professional behavior.
5.3. Contributes to the advancement of the profession and the agency as a whole.

Specific Indicators of Standard Attainment

a) Demonstrates an awareness of individual professional strengths and limitations and sets and meets appropriate performance goals.
b) Fosters effective inter- and intra-agency collaboration.
c) Participates in continuing education essential for provision of services appropriate to current nursing practice standards.
d) Contributes to a positive, supportive, and healthy work environment by:
    - understanding and tolerating differences in points of view
    - demonstrating a positive attitude
    - working effectively to resolve conflicts
    - listening and responding respectfully to information and ideas conveyed by others
    - responding calmly and effectively to crisis situations
    - actively participating in staff and planning meetings
    - interacting with and contributing to the professional development of peers and colleagues
e) Adheres to a code of professional ethics as identified by agency, professional organization, or licensing commission (ANA and NASN).
f) Supervises staff to whom nursing tasks have been delegated.
g) Envisions future needs and opportunities appropriate for position and program.
h) Contributes to the advancement of the profession and the agency as a whole.

SUPERVISORY RESPONSIBILITIES: None except as may be needed to monitor delegated healthcare tasks.

QUALIFICATION REQUIREMENTS: To perform this job successfully, an individual must be able to perform each essential duty satisfactorily. The requirements listed are representative of the knowledge, skill, and/or ability required. Reasonable accommodations may be made to enable individuals with disabilities to perform the essential functions. This position requires the employee to have reliable transportation.

EDUCATION AND/OR EXPERIENCE: Graduate of an approved college or university program.

CERTIFICATES/LICENSES: Current valid Oregon Nursing license. Current CPR and First Aid teaching certification for infants, children, and adults.

OTHER SKILLS AND ABILITIES: Ability to participate as an active and supportive member of an educational or therapy team.

PHYSICAL DEMANDS: The physical demands described here are representative of those that must be met by an employee to successfully perform the essential functions of this job. Reasonable accommodations may be made to enable individuals with disabilities to perform the essential functions. While performing the duties of this job, the employee is regularly required to sit and communicate or hear. The employee frequently is required to use hands to finger, handle, or feel objects, tools, or controls. The employee is occasionally required to stand and reach with hands and arms.
The employee must frequently lift and/or move up to 10 pounds and occasionally lift and/or move up to 50 pounds.

WORK ENVIRONMENT: The work environment characteristics described here are representative of those an employee encounters while performing the essential functions of this job. Reasonable accommodations may be made to enable individuals with disabilities to perform the essential functions.
While performing the duties of this job, the employee works with standard office and/or instructional equipment or personal mobility equipment (wheelchairs) with moving mechanical parts.
The noise level in the work environment is usually low to moderate.
This job is itinerant. Nurses serve children in their educational environment which may include homes, preschools, and classrooms.

EMPLOYEE: "I have read this job description and agree with its contents."

Employee:____________________ Date:__________
Direct Supervisor:____________________ Date:__________

Figure 46.2 ■ *(continued)*

SAMPLE JOB DESCRIPTION FOR SCHOOL NURSE ADMINISTRATOR

Based on a sample from and used with permission of Multnomah Education Service District, Portland, Oregon
Qualifications and job duties vary with local expectations, staffing pattern, and legal regulations

JOB TITLE:	Supervisor, School Health Services
FUNDAMENTAL ASSIGNMENT:	To supervise staff in the planning and implementation of direct healthcare to students in Multnomah Country public schools.
SUPERVISED BY:	Director, School Health Services
REPORTS TO:	Same
SUPERVISORY RESPONSIBILITY:	Responsible for the supervision, coordination and evaluation of assigned personnel and activities of various programs in the Department of School Health Services.
MAJOR DUTIES AND RESPONSIBILITIES:	1. Supervise and evaluate department staff and make recommendations to the director regarding their continued employment. 2. Assist in the development, implementation, and evaluation of practice and procedures appropriate to specific health professions license requirements. 3. Observe and evaluate the nursing practice of regular, temporary and substitute staff and provide follow-up including consultation, recommendations and/or demonstrations of nursing technique as required. 4. Provide orientation and inservice for staff, substitutes, and student nurses. 5. Make recommendations to the director regarding personnel matters relating to the department. 6. Conduct interviews for new regular, substitute and temporary staff and make recommendations to director for hiring. 7. Assist staff assigned to other SHS supervisors in the absence of that supervisor. 8. Coordinate health services such as clinics and health screenings with community health care providers. 9. Consult and collaborate with parents, teachers, school administrators and community health or social service agencies to address student health problems and plan health services. 10. Participate as assigned by director in interdisciplinary/interagency collaborative efforts to enhance health programs/services to the school community. 11. Supervise and coordinate activities of volunteers and temporary employees within department as assigned by the director. 12. Collaborate with university faculty to provide clinical/practicum experience for baccalaureate and graduate students in appropriate health professions. 13. Communicate the agency and department mission and values to staff, local district personnel, parents, students and community agencies. 14. Collaborate with other ESD departments, school personnel, community providers (agencies), and constituent districts to develop, implement, direct and evaluate community-based services that address the mission of MESD and SHS. 15. Contribute to a positive and productive work environment. 16. Perform other job-related duties as assigned by director.
LIMITS OF AUTHORITY:	This position is subject to board policies, administrative rules and procedures, department regulations and applicable state and federal statutes. This position carries specific administrative authority to effect the responsibilities in this job description. All commitments outside of authorized programs and services are subject to prior approval by the supervisor of this position.
QUALIFICATIONS:	1. Required: a. Valid Oregon license to practice as a registered nurse. b. Minimum of 3 years experience within the last 7 years in school nursing. (Two years of community health nursing experience may be substituted for up to 1 year of school health experience.) c. Demonstrated leadership skills which reflect a variety of problem-solving strategies. d. Demonstrated skill in organization of ideas and resources. e. Demonstrated effective human relation skills that include ability to listen to and accept differing opinions, ability to manage and resolve conflict and ability to respond tactfully. f. Demonstrated flexibility and adaptation to change. g. Demonstrated effective written and verbal communication skills. h. Bachelor's degree in nursing, management or other health-related field, or 3 years experience in MESD Department of School Health Services as a school nurse.

Figure 46.3 ■ Sample job description for school nurse administrator.

JOB DESCRIPTION FOR SCHOOL HEALTH ASSISTANT

Sample based upon Job Description from and used with permission of Reading School District, Pennsylvania

QUALIFICATIONS:

1. High school diploma or its equivalent
2. Valid CPR and First Aid certification
3. Certified nursing assistant preferred
4. Experience working with children

REPORTS TO: School nurse

JOB GOAL: To assist the school nurse in the smooth and efficient operation of the school health service in order to realize that services maximize a positive impact on the educational environment.

PERFORMANCE RESPONSIBILITIES:

1. Help maintain the health room under the direction of the school nurse
2. Maintain records and perform clerical work
3. Have a working knowledge of Health Services to interpret to others as necessary
4. Attend regularly scheduled meetings
5. Keep First Aid and CPR certification current
6. Keep all matters pertaining to school health with strictest confidentiality
7. Maintain effective health room schedule
8. Make telephone calls and send appointments to parents
9. Is available for any temporary reassignment
10. Contacts parents to pick up or notifies parents of a sick or injured child
11. Assists with immunization program and kindergarten registration
12. Completes height, weight, vision and hearing screenings and refers to school nurse per direction
13. Administers medications per medication policy
14. Performs all other work-related duties as assigned by school nurse or principal

Figure 46.4 ■ Job description for school health assistant.

the delivery of health services (i.e., certified nursing assistants, paraprofessionals, and in schools even administrators and faculty). These persons are considered to be UAPs. The official definition is one who is "trained to function in an assistive role to the registered professional nurse in the provision of care activities as delegated by and under the supervision of the registered professional nurse" (American Nurses Association [ANA], 1994, p. 2). In some school districts, the school administrator may be the legally responsible person for choosing the UAP. But the nurse must be involved in the decision making to affirm that the UAP demonstrates competence and a willingness to accept responsibility for the assignment (NASN, 2004).

Job description information can help applicants consider whether they seriously want to be considered for the position, and it may help unqualified or marginally qualified applicants to withdraw from the selection process. Schwab and Gelfman (2001, p. 146) caution that "It is inadvisable for licensed nurses to work in positions with job descriptions that do not require and support their licensed responsibilities to clients." It is the position of the National Association of School Nurses (NASN) that every school-age child deserves a school nurse who is minimally a graduate of a baccalaureate degree program from an accredited college or university and licensed by that state as a registered nurse. In addition, NASN supports state certification, where required, and promotes national certification of school nurses through the National Board for Certification of School Nurses (NBCSN) (NASN, 2002a, 2002b) (see Chapter 5).

Job application forms give the opportunity to collect a job-performance synopsis of the candidates' skills and accomplishments. Based on the job description, some of the applicants may be eliminated in the initial application screening because of experience or education that is inadequate for the position. Questions should be stated in ways to encourage the sharing of information versus writing evasive answers. *Have you ever been dismissed or asked to resign from a position? If yes, please explain the circumstances*. In addition, the application process affords an opportunity for applicants to demonstrate their ability to follow directions, an essential job competency. An application should require a signature from the applicant attesting to the truthfulness of the information provided and giving permission to check references.

It should be recommended that at least one of the references should be from a current employer. However, if a current employee knows the candidate, the employee's recommendation would be most respected. Knowing their integrity and credibility is at risk otherwise, current employees will generally use critical judgment in making referrals. In addition, the applicant will often get a very detailed and accurate job description from a current employee as compared to the information obtained from printed descriptions or from an employment agency. The applicant thus has a clearer description of the available position to determine if the job is truly of interest.

When reviewing applications, remember that these documents are generally written as the best work of the applicant. Check for:

- A comparison of the candidate's qualifications against the established criteria (e.g., is the education appropriate for the job to be done?)
- Neatness and overall appearance of the document. (Poor penmanship will likely continue in job documentation and report writing.)
- General construction for organization, logic, grammar, and spelling. (Typographical errors can reflect a careless applicant and poor grammar portrays weak communication skills.)
- Work history and primary job responsibilities. (Are there unexplainable gaps in the work history? Is there evidence of frequent moving?) Be sure to probe for information about the gaps and moves. Such behaviors may indicate risks for lack of commitment to an organization and/or competency challenges.

Medical Examination/Drug and Alcohol Screening

Employers can require a medical examination only after a job offer has been made. Employers may not inquire about any physical or mental conditions or impairments that affect an applicant's ability to perform the job, or ask if an applicant needs a reasonable accommodation to do the job. Even if the applicant has an obvious disability, the Americans with Disabilities Act (ADA) prohibits questions about the nature and extent of the disability. Employers may evaluate whether an applicant is qualified for the job by asking:

- If the applicant has the ability to perform the specific job functions that are described. For example, an employer may state the physical requirements of a job (such as the ability to lift a certain amount of weight or the ability to do cardiopulmonary resuscitation on the floor), and ask if an applicant can satisfy these requirements.
- Applicants to describe or demonstrate how they would perform job tasks.

Once a conditional job offer is made, the employer may ask disability-related questions and require medical examinations as long as this is done for all entering employees in that job category. If the employer rejects the applicant after a disability-related question or medical examination, investigators will closely scrutinize whether the rejection was based on the results of that question or examination. If the question or examination screens out an individual because of a disability, the employer must demonstrate that the reason for the rejection is job-related and consistent with business (EEOC NOTICE Number 915.002, 10/10/95). The health-care provider may disclose only the conclusions about the employee's ability to work with or without restrictions. Medical data must be kept in a separate file, available only to those with a "need to know" (NOLO Law Centers, 2002a).

Employers can generally require job applicants to submit to drug testing; there are restrictions on the right to drug test current employees. The ADA prohibits discrimination based on past drug and alcohol problems. It is, however, appropriate to check that drug use is not recurring. Illegal use of drugs means the use of one or more drugs, the possession or distribution of which is unlawful under the Controlled Substances Act. It does not include use of controlled substances pursuant to a valid prescription, or other uses that are authorized by the Controlled Substances Act or other federal law. Alcohol is not a "controlled substance," but alcoholism is a disability (ADA, 1990). Questions asking whether an applicant has participated in an alcohol rehabilitation program are forbidden (EEOC NOTICE, 1995). Again, guidance from the human resources department or legal counsel is appropriate. An employer can refuse to hire someone with a history of alcoholism or illegal drug use if it can be shown that the person poses a direct threat to health or safety. This means that the employer can demonstrate that there is a high probability that the person will return to the illegal drug use or alcohol abuse, resulting in substantial harm to the person or others. Harm infers that something cannot be reduced or eliminated through what the ADA deems a "reasonable accommodation," such as changing the employee's job duties to eliminate working with triggers to the addictive behavior (ADA, 1990).

Reference Checks

It is prudent practice to do background and reference checks to verify information provided in the application and interview processes. Information regarding educational experience, degrees and licensure (including any encumbrances/practice limitations), and employment history should be verified. The legal doctrine of "respondeat superior" means the employer can be held liable for the wrongful acts of employees who act within the scope of their employment (Employers, Beware of Negligent Hiring and Retention, 2000). Court decisions have held employers negligent when failing to select competent and safe employees and third parties were injured (Outlaw, 1998). Such cases include *Evan F. v. Hughson United Methodist Church* (1992) 8 Cal.App.4th 823, 843 and *Chevron USA, Inc. v. Superior Court* (1997) 4 Cal. App.4th544. The accountability for liability extends as well to independent contractors. Reserve reference-check action for your final candidates. The application should state that all information will be verified and all references checked. Put in writing that any information will be kept confidential and communicated only to those individuals who are directly involved in the hiring process. Explain clearly to candidates what information will be checked and how you will gather the information. This allows candidates to remove themselves if there is something they want to keep private. If a candidate refuses to consent to a reasonable request for information, you may legally determine not to hire the person on that basis (NOLO Law Centers, 2002a). Employers may implement immediate dismissal if they find any application information was falsified.

There is no formula for determining the exact number of references to check. Some personnel departments have a set requirement. A minimum number would be two references in order to compare information. Sources include:

- Former bosses or supervisors
- Peers
- Subordinates (if in management) or customers (if the job involved customer contact).

Other sources include school of nursing faculty for new graduates or RNs in graduate study. Persons who provide the references should not be related to the candidate. Refer to FIGURE 46.5 for samples of reference questions.

Because many organizations are concerned about being sued for defamation or violating an employee's right to privacy, it is often difficult to get more than a verification of employment in reference checks. The consent statement should include the ability to contact former employers, waiving any legal action against them for responding truthfully to reference inquiries, and authorize the types of information that may be specifically released. Applicants generally identify only references who will speak favorably about job performance. To obtain job performance information, ask candidates to supply copies of performance evaluations received from previous employers. Reference checks can be done for a fee by a professional agency. In addition to reference checks, persons working in school systems will need to complete a criminal records check.

SAMPLE QUESTIONS FOR REFERENCE CHECKS

Regarding Candidate/Reference Relationship:
- *What were your position and responsibilities when you supervised the applicant?*
- *How long have you worked with the candidate?*

Regarding the Circumstances and Facts in Previous Work Settings:
- *What were the dates of the applicant's employment?*
- *What was the candidate's position? Primary Responsibilities and Duties?*
- *What was the applicant's reason for leaving?*
- *Was the applicant terminated or did she or he leave under less than desirable circumstances?*

Regarding Previous Job Performance:
- *Compared to other employees in the same classification, how did this applicant perform?*
- *How would you rate the applicant's contribution to your agency?*
- *Was the applicant's attendance "excellent," "satisfactory," or "poor"?*
- *Please comment on the applicant's dependability?*
- *What are the applicant's strengths?*
- *In what areas should the candidate improve to increase future success?*

Regarding Personal Trait Characteristics:
- *How did this person accept supervisory direction?*
- *What are her/his communication skills like?*
- *Would you rehire this applicant? Why?* Or *Based on the last annual evaluation, would this employee be eligible for rehire in your district?*

Figure 46.5 ■ Sample questions for reference checks.

State laws vary on the extent of an applicant's criminal history information that can be obtained and used in making hiring decisions. Seek guidance from the human resources and legal counsel staff. An employer may use information in the public record from a Workers' Compensation Appeal only if the injury in question might interfere with the ability to perform required duties (Workers' Compensation and the ADA, 2002). It is prudent to check the driving record of applicants whose job will require large amounts of driving as well as any encumbrances against professional licenses. These are not confidential records and can be released without the licensee's consent (NOLO Law Centers, 2002a). Document all information received.

Job Interview

Resumes and application forms are valuable tools but they do not tell about an applicant's interpersonal skills and often focus on a few key job duties rather than describing in depth candidates' responsibilities and capabilities. Thus, an interview is a universal employee selection tool. The interviewer has dual roles: to represent the organization and to evaluate the candidate. As an agent of your organization, your actions and information will influence applicants' impressions about the organization. The primary purpose of the interview is to determine how well the person will perform on the job, not how well he or she performed during the interview. If the interviewer should identify in the interview process that this is not the best candidate for the position, it is still important to treat all persons respectfully and answer their questions. They, in turn, can influence others about your organization based upon their perspectives of the interaction and what information they received about the organization.

Proper staff selection is the goal of all hiring activities. Costs to an organization for hiring an incompetent employee include:

- Low staff morale
- Inadequacy of the new employee
- Needing increased assistance by co-workers, thus decreasing their productivity
- Recruitment and screening of applicants
- Legal fees

The ratio of staff turnover costs to average salary can exceed 15% (Rosenberg, 2000). Subsequently, interview systems should be developed and conducted to attain proper staff selection. See Figure 46.6 for a sample framework in developing and completing an interview. Interviews are generally done by two or more persons who have authority to make hiring recommendations. A team helps increase objectivity by having several persons listen to the information. Often, the interviewers will be from different job classifications in order to have a holistic interview process.

INTERVIEW AND SELECTION PROCESS

1. Screen out unqualified candidates (those lacking minimum qualifications).
2. Be on time for the interview to show respect for the candidate.
3. Structure the interview process through a designated time frame and standardized questions. (Clarify the maximum length of the interview but not necessarily the ending time.)
4. Select a quiet location where interruptions will not occur.
5. Set the tone of the interview.
   a. Be punctual and welcoming. Greet and escort the applicant to and from the interview area.
   b. Make introductions and initiate through social dialogue and transition questions, a relaxed exchange of information, e.g., *How did you come to be interested in this position/this organization?*
   c. Explain the interview process (time allotted, taking of notes, what you will share about the job, ask questions of them, allow them to ask questions of you).
6. Provide realistic information about the job.
   a. Give a job description and job expectations.
   b. Describe hours, special policies or procedures, working conditions.
7. Conduct the interview.
   a. Limit your talk to about 25% of the time to get the information you need. Use silence appropriately to prompt the applicant to elaborate or continue discussion.
   b. Allow the candidate adequate time to consider the question and form an answer.
   c. Do not interrupt the candidate; re-clarify and restate questions, as needed, to help the candidate's understanding.
   d. Avoid anticipating answers and poor listening.
   e. Maintain eye contact. Observe the candidate's body posture, eye contact, voice, and so on to provide cues about his or her reactions and feelings.
   f. Avoid approval or disapproval of candidate's statements. Use positive reinforcement such as *"uh-huh," "that's interesting,"* and nodding your head to affirm your interest and desire to hear more.
   g. Make notes unobtrusively to assist later information recall. Complete necessary documentation immediately after the interview for clear memory recall at a later time.
   h. Ask only job-related questions.
   i. Ask open-ended, objective, meaningful questions to obtain more information. (Begin with what, why, how, describe, tell me about. *What do you find the most challenging part of the school nurse's job? Describe two job accomplishments of which you are most proud.)* Ask pertinent follow-up questions. Use reflective responses to get more information from candidates who have volunteered information that raises questions for you.
   j. Maintain control of the process. (Redirect if candidates focus on irrelevant subject; direct them back to a topic, etc. For candidates who will not talk or are vague, use soft, non-threatening questions and several questions to better coach the candidate in how to more fully respond to a question. *Tell me about your recent position. What aspects do you really enjoy? With whom do you work?* For persons who talk too much, try more specific questions. *"Tell me about three incidents when you needed to call for emergency care."*

Figure 46.6 ■ Interview and selection process.

INTERVIEW AND SELECTION PROCESS

8. Provide an opportunity for the candidate to ask questions.
9. Close the interview.
   a. Review next steps with specific time line.
   b. Thank candidates for their time.
10. Evaluate using a scoring process based on predetermined criteria that may include:
    a. Work experience, education, training
    b. Cognitive skills and capacity for continuous learning
    c. Motivation and interest for the job
    d. Ability to perform the job
    e. Needs of the department/organization
    f. Reference verification

    See also Figure 46-7 for characteristics of exemplary school nursing practice.
11. Use multiple, trained interviewers to increase the validity of the interviewing process and promote buy-in of selection and promotion decisions.

Figure 46.6 ■ *(continued)*

The application and interview information is used to help analyze the likelihood of a good match between the organizational culture, job requirements, physical environment, and the skills and traits of the job applicants. Prior to posing the interview questions, it is essential to create a milieu where the candidate feels comfortable in talking. All candidates have some level of anxiety. The interviewer's task is to reduce the candidate's anxiety level so that sharing information is more comfortable and delivered more natural.

While there is no set number of questions to pose, you will want to pose a sufficient quantity of questions to give you the depth of information needed for an adequate assessment about the candidate's skill level. Today's work world leaves new hires with little time to learn the job and with high expectations to produce results immediately. Do not be limited by seeking the performance traits of the incumbent worker. Identify "nice-to-have" traits versus mandatory traits. Cognitive ability and the capacity to learn are essential traits. Since transformation within organizations is a continuous action in the current work environment, applicants must be able to continuously learn and change behaviors and thinking. Since humans make mistakes, interviewers should inquire about performance mistakes and what candidates learned from them and subsequently used in later job situations or decision-making.

Motivation level has a significant influence on job performance and is another vital trait to predict successful performance. Without self-motivation, employees require an external source, often the "boss." High performers are self-motivated (Quinn, 2002). Influencing employees' motivation and subsequently job productivity are their:

- Perceived locus of control (assume personal ownership and responsibility for action),
- Initiative and persistence (degree to which action is self started and maintained toward reaching a goal), and
- Interests and desires (performing tasks that do not appeal to them enhances no one's motivation.)

It is important to assess these critical qualities. Pulcini, Couillard, Harrigan, and Mole (2002) identify that little is known about the components of exemplary school nursing practice. Their study identified personal and professional characteristics needed for exemplary school nursing practice (FIGURE 46.7). Remember that the behavior demon-

OVERARCHING CHARACTERISTICS OF EXEMPLARY SCHOOL NURSING PRACTICE

I. Mastery of the Science of Child Health Nursing: Is a professional expert, is knowledgeable, handles emergencies well, is a source of information, knows limits, pursues continuing professional education (seeks continuing education, professional standards used in job)

II. Mastery of the Art of Child Health Nursing: Is honest and trusted, has a caring attitude, has a rapport with students, sees the uniqueness of each child, is a child advocate, is committed to the total well-being of the child, is child focused, provides continuity of care, is family focused, is able to see the child's perspective

III. Effective in School and Community Systems: Is flexible, encourages teamwork, is effective at educating administrators, works toward autonomy within the school system, maintains focus on health in an educational environment

IV. Excellence of Communication Skills: Listens, follows up, has a positive attitude, maintains confidentiality

V. Leadership Qualities: Is a problem solver, exudes confidence, is empowered, is able to prioritize.

Reprinted with permission from *Journal of School Nursing*
Pulcini, J., Couillard, M., Harrigan, J., & Mole, D. (2002). Personal and professional characteristics of exemplary school nurses. *Journal of School Nursing, 18* (1), 33–40.

Figure 46.7 ■ Overarching characteristics of exemplary school nursing practice.

Box 46.1 ■■■

IMPORTANT EMPLOYEE CHARACTERISTICS

- Attendance patterns
- Capacity for flexibility, change, ambiguity, and chaos
- Commitment to the organization and profession
- Competencies for and interest in doing the work
- Communication assets/weaknesses
- Cooperation/collegiality
- Critical thinking skills/problem solving ability
- Grooming
- Integrity
- Interests and goals
- Involvement in continuous learning (must be quick to learn and a perpetual learner)
- Locus of control
- Maturity
- Motivation (intrinsic versus extrinsic focus)
- Patience, tolerance, persistence
- Professional goals
- Reliability
- Respect for authority, organizational values
- Self management
- Work experience

strated in the interview may be the best you will ever see in this person. Qualities found by most employers to be important characteristics in employees are listed in Box 46.1.

To objectively obtain information about qualities and skills, use a blend of behavioral questions (75%) and dilemma situations (25%) (Rosenberg, 2000). Just as in taking a health history from a client, the job interview questions should encourage information sharing from job candidates. Behavioral questions help relay the past patterns of the candidate's actions. Such questions may start with "*What has been your experience with ....*" or, "*Tell me about a situation when....*" Listen for a description of the situation, the candidate's action, and an outcome or end result from that action to identify the candidate's ability to achieve objectives, produce results, think logically and perceptively as well as process information. Dilemma questions often start with "*What if....*" It is appropriate to use current situations from your organization for these questions. Listen for the candidate's ability to transpose his or her skills into your work environment. Avoid too many questions with a "yes" or "no" response. See Figure 46.8 for some suggested interview questions.

As well as listening for content, observe for candidates' behaviors. Tense persons have rigid shoulders and clenched or fidgeting hands. Adjust the warm-up time until the applicant shows evidence of relaxing (more normal posture, relaxed hands, etc.).

POSITIVE BEHAVIOR SIGNALS

- Answers questions fully
- Open, eager, and approachable

BEHAVIOR SIGNALS SUGGESTING CAUTION

- Changes subject quickly rather than answering question
- Excessive talker
- Becomes defensive
- Abrupt, ill-mannered
- Speaks negatively about former employers or coworkers

POSSIBLE INTERVIEW QUESTIONS

Intended as behavioral questions unless marked (D) for dilemma question.

To Assess Job Skills:

- Describe your most recent job duties and responsibilities. How would those prepare you for this position?
- Describe how you have used the skills of ___ in your past work situations?
- Provide several clinical scenarios and have the candidate describe his or her projected action. (D)
- In your most recent performance evaluation, in what three areas were you rated the highest? In what two areas were you rated the lowest?

To Assess Collegiality, Ability to Work Independently:

- In the past how have you ensured that staff/work colleagues trust and respect you?
- Describe a conflict situation you experienced in your job? What did you do to resolve it?
- You are assigned to work with several paraprofessionals. You observe that neither expresses much enthusiasm for her work; both have frequent absenteeism, and one is reported to you by the principal as being rude to students and staff. You determine that poor motivation is a driving factor. What would you do? (D)
- What are the advantages and disadvantages of working independently in the school setting?
- Among the supervisors and principals with whom you have worked, which do you admire the most and why?

To Assess Goals and Expectations:

- What is important to you in your work setting?
- What are your career goals for the next 2-5 years? What steps have you taken towards these goals.
- What have you been doing to increase your knowledge and skills?
- Why are you interested in changing job positions?
- What benefits are important to you?

To Assess Interests:

- What did you like most about your previous job? What did you enjoy the least?
- What do you like most about nursing (school nursing)? What do you enjoy the least?
- What do you identify as your strengths? Your weaknesses? How do you compensate for those weaknesses?
- What would be the ideal model of school nursing in which you would like to work? (D)
- Of your past jobs, which was your favorite and why? Which was your least favorite and why?

To Assess Locus of Control:

- Tell me about a situation where you managed successfully unwanted changes thrust upon you by your organization.
- Tell me about a time when your were unable to meet a project's deadline. What were the obstacles you encountered? How did you try to overcome them?
- Share about a situation where you were given a project without any guidelines or structure other than a due date. How did you go about the project?
- You have been asked by your supervisor to participate in a special pilot mental health project. You have a special interest in doing more with mental health. However, you are feeling overloaded this year with an additional school in your assignment, new immunization requirements for 20% of your students, and some exacerbating personal health issues for you. What action will you take? (D)

Figure 46.8 ■ Possible interview questions.

Complete evaluations promptly after the interview while your memory is most clear. Remember that good candidates offer evidence of their talents. In addition, analyze the candidates' personality fit with the institution and the job position. Studies have supported that performance improves when there is a suitable job match between an individual's personality strengths and the requirements of a job (Atencio, Cohen, & Gorenberg, 2003; Blohowiak, 1998). Every candidate is part task-oriented, part affiliation-oriented, and part power-oriented. However, candidates may have a predominant need and it behooves interviewers to look for behavioral indicators that an employee may need much supervisory redirection to fit with the job description and/or the work culture. A comparison (Rosenberg, 2000) of historical problem areas for the three orientations include:

TASK ORIENTED	AFFILIATION ORIENTED	POWER ORIENTED
Problems with human relations.	Friendly interaction takes precedence over productivity	Not working up to their potential.
Profuse paperwork	Passive–aggressive behavior	Always pushes for more and wants the highly visible assignments.

TASK ORIENTED	AFFILIATION ORIENTED	POWER ORIENTED
Being right and consequently argumentative with others	Difficulty in coping with change	Publicizes and blows activities out of proportion.
Taking responsibility for their mistakes	Lacking in good organizational and time management skills	Overwhelming concern about status and reputation

A matrix or scoring form will assist interviewers to objectively validate selection of candidates to whom a job is to be offered. For the matrix, determine the essential criteria, which includes skills as well as personal traits. Refer to FIGURE 46.9 for a format that can be used in ranking the candidates and determining final selections. Verify conclusions by comparing them to the preceding reference information.

Job Offer

Make the job offer to one candidate. This applicant may want to counter-negotiate your offer. Be prepared with your limits of negotiation. Once an offer has been accepted, it is best protocol to notify all other applicants as soon as possible that they were not chosen. It is prudent to put your job offer into a formal letter and to include the following elements:

1. Starting date of employment
2. Official job title to be given employee
3. An attached contract or statements that
   a. Retain the right to terminate employment for any reason or no reason.
   b. Represent the complete terms and conditions of employment.
   c. List the benefits associated with employment (including salary).
   d. State the agency's/school district's policy on discrimination and sexual harassment.

SCHOOL NURSE INTERVIEW SCORING SHEET

Based on a Sample from and Used with Permission of Highline School District, Everett, Washington

Select questions pertinent to the job description for which the candidate is interviewing

Applicant's Name__________

Interviewer__________

Interview Date__________

Score each question from 1 (low) to 10 (high)

______ 1. Please describe your nursing experience, particularly with children (birth through 21 years).

______ 2. The state immunization law now requires entering kindergarten students to have proof of hepatitis A vaccine. There has been no previous requirement for this vaccine for school children. What factors do nurses need to include in planning for ensuring compliance with this law?

______ 3. You are the school nurse at an elementary school with a program for developmentally disabled students. A teacher calls on the intercom and asks you to come & check an 8-year-old girl who has been having a seizure for 6 minutes. Describe your planning and actions.

______ 4. In this district, we usually do student health screenings for hearing, vision and spinal screening on a school health screening day. What factors would you consider in setting up a school health screening day?

______ 5. A kindergarten student comes to the health room crying loudly and holding his right wrist with his left hand. The teacher follows him in and states no one saw what happened. When you ask the boy what happened, he cries louder and shrinks away from you. What are some ways you might assess the student?

______ 6. Describe possible ways of meeting the needs of students who come to school without breakfast.

______ 7. What are some possible ways of meeting the needs of students who do not have health insurance?

______ 8. You are dealing with a student emergency at one of your schools when your other school calls and requests that you come immediately to help with an emergency. What would you do?

______ 9. In planning for potential natural disasters, what steps would you take to meet the needs of students with health problems such as seizures, diabetes, ADHD, tube feedings, and so forth?

______ 10. A deaf high school student comes to see you in the health room and hands you a note saying she doesn't feel well. You do not know sign language. How would you assess her problem?

______ 11. Describe your experiences in jobs requiring self-direction, organization and/or management.

______ 12. If we asked your present or past supervisor, what would he or she say are your strengths as a nurse? (0–5), your challenges as a nurse? (0–5)

______ 13. What are your professional goals?

______ Total Score Recommend for hire: Yes ☐ No ☐

Figure 46.9 ■ School nurse interview scoring sheet.

4. A mechanism for a signature by you (or the designated human resource contact) and the candidate indicating acceptance and agreement of the conditions set forth in the letter and contract. (Rosenberg, 2000)

NEW EMPLOYEE ORIENTATION

Orientation Goals

A well planned and delivered orientation is crucial to helping new employees establish firm foundations for effective relationships with the organization and other work colleagues as well as for the specific performance of the assigned job. New members to any group generally have some level of anxiety due to uncertainty about expectations and processes, being accepted, and succeeding. A new worker often feels a lack of identification with the organization, colleagues, and regulations. Anxiety can heighten employees' motivation to learn quickly the values and norms of their new role, but orientation must provide the special attention to soon reduce the tension. Otherwise, new employees' motivation will be dulled by an inability to be ready to learn owing to their high anxiety level. An effective orientation will, at minimum:

- Foster an understanding of the organizational culture, its values and its diversity,
- Help new employees understand their role and fit within the organization,
- Reduce employees' anxiety and assist the development of positive working relationships,
- Assist new employees to successfully adjust to the new job, and subsequently reduce startup costs (Quicker learning gets employees more rapidly to higher performance.),
- Reduce employee turnover, and
- Save time for supervisor and co-workers.

(A Quick Guide to Employee Orientation, 2002)

Brown (2002) says the most important principle to convey during orientation is commitment to continuous improvement and continual learning. This directs new employees to be comfortable in seeking data, problem solving, and making decisions. These information management and critical thinking skills are crucial in business today, including the business of school nursing. Orientation should address the uniqueness of school nurses who are providing health care in an education system and having education laws impact the delivery of health services.

Orientation Process

Orientation activities may be presented by a variety of persons within an organization or primarily by one individual, such as an immediate supervisor, human resource or professional development staff, or a lead staff member. Content should include everything employees need to know about an organization and assigned job tasks that will make them knowledgeable and productive employees. See FIGURE 46.10 for general orientation and program process and content ideas. During orientation, provide in writing to all new employees the standards of conduct for the organization. It is wise at this time to have the nurse review and acknowledge basic school nurse competencies required for the position and his/her knowledge, understanding, or experience in each job assignment area. This is then used as a basis for planning further staff development and orientation on an individual basis by continuing education staff or a nurse teacher or preceptor. It is prudent to have employees sign an acknowledgment that they are aware of and have read pertinent Board of Education or Board of Public Health policies and standards of conduct. In addition, a signature to verify the employee's agreement to follow these rules should be required. The acknowledgment may include a statement that failure to follow these guidelines can lead to discipline, including termination.

The complexity and large scope of practice for a school nurse position makes it imperative that adequate clinical practice training (job data) be provided to each school nurse. To help augment an organization's training, check on the availability of a state or school nurse organization-sponsored orientation program that is specific to school nursing. NASN publishes a school nurse orientation manual (Zaiger, 2001). Many individual districts, schools of nursing and state school nursing organizations provide a school nurse orientation program. Reference materials may be obtained from local and state resources as well as from the National Association of School Nurses (http://www.nasn.org). At minimum, all school nurses should have immediate access to the state nurse practice act and the scope and standards of school nursing practice (NASN & ANA, 2005).

Ideally, the chief executive officer (i.e., the superintendent or alternatively the department chair or school principal) is involved in the orientation's welcoming activity. This affords new employees an interaction with the administration and provides an opportunity for administration to share with new employees the organization's mission and goals while telling about the organizational culture. This welcoming approach helps to build the new

CONTENT AND ACTIVITIES FOR NEW EMPLOYEE ORIENTATION

Not All Inclusive

Prior to orientation:

- Distribute an announcement to current staff about new employees
- Send a welcoming letter to the new staff with content about
  - ✓ Job description
  - ✓ Affirmation of first work day
  - ✓ Time and location to report
  - ✓ Suggested attire
  - ✓ Required/recommended readings and form completion
  - ✓ Orientation schedule and activity description, including meal information

Within Orientation:

- Welcoming greetings and general introductions
- General organization information—e.g., history, mission, values, goals, funding streams, organizational structure, internal and external relationships, products and services provided, policies and procedures, employee services, introduction to organization's policies and procedures
- Complete necessary documentation—e.g., for insurance and health benefits, citizenship verification, RN licensure/certification verification
- Business details—e.g., work hours, time cards, vacation/sick, leave policies, key distribution, reimbursement for travel/other expenses, credit card use, dress code, parking arrangements, malpractice coverage
- Review of job description, expectations, and performance evaluations
- Equipment use—e.g., phones, office machines, special assessment equipment
- Computer training and support—policies and procedures, including confidentiality and privacy; assessment of knowledge and comfort with hardware and software
- Tour of work location(s)
- Introduction to key persons
- Safety and security, injuries on the job
- Employee's position—responsibilities, duties, expected level of performance
- Program evaluation process—timelines, data collection tools, employee's role (e.g., reports)
- New or updated skills/procedures required in the position

SCHOOL NURSING CLINICAL ORIENTATION CONTENT

- Professional Issues—e.g., professional preparation, education team, school nursing practice, legal issues, professional organizations, data collection
- Practice Issues—e.g., medication, immunizations, communicable disease, documentation, age of legal consent, informed consent, transporting students, confidentiality, delegation, and specific clinical conditions, i.e., diabetes, asthma, allergies, reproductive and mental health issues, and drug and alcohol situations
- Managing emergencies; crisis preparation
- Resources—e.g., local providers; access to care for medically indigent or emergent conditions; parent, school and community groups; consultation resources
- Screening programs—e.g., hearing, vision, spinal screening, pediculosis
- Child protection laws, reporting processes, documentation, interview technique
- Special health care and special education management—Individual Education Program (IEP), Individual Family Service Plan (IFSP) and 504 plans
- Health education, wellness promotion—guidelines for class presentations
- Working with paraprofessionals and other professionals in the school community—e.g., training, supervising
- Supplies and accessing equipment

Figure 46.10 ■ Content and activities for new employee orientation.

employee's relationship with the organization and interest for the orientation.

Orientation should also strive to decrease the anxiety inherent in new employees. While trying to create a comfortable environment for orientation, consider the pace of delivering information. No one can absorb everything at once. Too much information too quickly can be overwhelming and cause greater anxiety and self-doubt regarding one's ability to meet performance expectations adequately. Introduce new employees to people they need to know in a controlled way. Space out introductions just like information. Orientation should begin with the most important information. The length of an effective orientation will vary depending upon the quantity and complexity of the content as well as the experience and skill of the new employee. It may work best to extend orientation over weeks and months depending upon the frequency, timing, and complexity of job tasks. For example, it may be best to break certain procedures (such as immunization management) into multiple training sessions that approximate the implementation time of the associated processes.

Partnering a new employee with a more experienced person is an effective way to reinforce the orientation process and to provide ongoing support. Be sure the experienced person wants to "buddy" and has the appropriate job skills and especially interpersonal and communication skills. A good "buddy" or "mentor" is a resource and a source of accurate organizational knowledge, provides a positive perspective, is a skilled listener, dialogues well, and is effective at building relationships. Refer to Chapter 7 on the educator role for considerations in developing the format of the orientation session(s).

Mentoring, Role Modeling, and Coaching Employees

Supervisors can teach through their role modeling. Supervisors more effectively teach by showing "how" rather than "giving orders." Supervisors can help staff keep looking for opportunities to learn new skills and subsequently expand capabilities. Encourage staff to ask "what" and "why." Nudge employees to inquire as to *What can we learn from that? What do we need to do to improve?* Encourage employees to be problem solvers. *What help do you need from me at this time? What would you like to do with this problem?* To be a positive example, supervisors must consistently meet and demonstrate the standards of the organization and profession. Likewise, supervisors' behavior influences staff's behavior and attitudes. Supervisors who welcome change and show personal drive develop similar qualities in others.

Coaching is the art of improving the performance of others (Ali et al., 2001). Coaching can be spontaneous or formally planned. Be ready to adapt your coaching style to the reason for the coaching. Coaching can build staff skills, move a project's progress, solve problems, enhance careers, overcome conflicts, re-motivate staff, and afford brainstorming. Sometimes staff need clear direction and definite answers, such as for skill building. Other times, staff wants to develop their own solutions with the coach's support. Coaching should be:

- Specific,
- Helpful (not an outlet for the supervisor's feelings; own your observations through "I" statements),
- Timely (in close proximity to a situation),
- Focused on work behavior rather than personality (describe the actions seen in job performance and effects seen on the job) (Academic Human Resources, 2002).

EMPLOYEE MOTIVATION

The fact that employees have job skill ability is not an assurance of their satisfactory job performance. Motivation is a critical component of job performance. People work to satisfy their needs and wants. There are multiple motivation and needs theories about job motivation. Maslow's hierarchy of needs is probably the best known. None can solely explain job motivation. Nelson (1996) says people will do their jobs for what they are paid, but it will do little to get them to do their best job. Their extra effort is more a function of how they are treated.

Internal and Intrinsic Motivation

Previous commentary in the job interview section regarding internal or intrinsic motivation suggests that these are significant influential employee performance factors. Intrinsic rewards include satisfaction that is self-initiated, such as a feeling of accomplishment from or pride in one's work. External motivators are incentives such as rewards, job perks, promotions, money, and discipline coming from outside the employee. Money is seldom the top employee motivator. The strength of financial motivation varies with life circumstances. However, employees who just want more money will never be satisfied; their expectations rise with each salary increase (Nelson, 1996). External motivation stops its effectiveness when there is nothing to sustain it. This inconsistency negatively influences employees' productivity. Waiting for another external motivator to "jump start" productivity reduces accomplishments. Persons who are internally motivated have greater ability to put themselves into motion and subsequently to achieve more.

Motivation and Individual Variables

Motivation is a complex process because individuals are unique in their needs and wants. Research shows that needs are neither instinctive nor fixed for individuals (Bowey, 2002). Supervisors will need to assess and be sensitive to individuals' differing and changing priorities. Neuhauser (2002) reminds that if people are all treated the same way, they begin to feel like robots. Research suggests that professionals value challenge, autonomy, and opportunities to use their skills. Workers in minimum wage jobs place high priority on security, earnings, benefits, and working conditions (Ali et al., 2001). People are motivated to do what they like doing. Subsequently, it will be helpful to know employees' values and then to correlate assignments accordingly. Using measured continuous change in small, tolerable increments can also stimulate staff to learn and try new approaches. Consider generation differences in finding motivation strategies. For example, seasoned nurses may value more meaningful work where they can match values and the

GENERATION	MATURES (VETERANS, TRADITIONALISTS) Born 1922–1943	BABY BOOMERS Born 1944–1960	GENERATION XERS Born 1961–1980	GENERATION YERS (MILLENIALS) Born after 1981
MOTIVATORS AND REWARDS	• Knowing work is valued by employer • Quantify how their work drives profit and affects the bottom line • Take time for personal touch; hand write a note rather than e-mail • Let staff chat and socialize between assigned tasks • Honor their hard work with symbolic records of achievement	• Pay attention to Boomer's contributions and recognize without being reminded • Give lots of public recognition • Give a chance to prove themselves and their worth • Give perks with status • Assist them in gaining name recognition through the company; get them quoted in a publication • Ask for their input • Get their consensus • Reward their work ethic and long hours	• Invest in training and development to give employees a sense of career growth • Pass along praise from clients to help them feel satisfied and productive • Give lots of projects with as much freedom and control as possible • Give constant contructive feedback • Give time to pursue outside interests and allow to have fun at work • Invest in the latest computer technology; they see it as an investment in their work • Be conscious of perks "up the ladder." Xers do not crave status symbols, but resent others getting very visible, expensive recognition.	• Create a collegial environment • Do not micro-manage • Recognize the need for autonomy • Learn about their personal goals and show how they mesh with the company's goals • Make all opportunities equal • Forget traditional gender roles • Be sensitive to the potential for conflict with Xers • Open avenues for education and skill-building • Establish mentor programs • Provide opportunities for team work, but be certain team leaders are strong • Emphasize impact can have on agency
FEEDBACK PREFERENCE	• No news is good news	• Once a year with documentation	• Instantaneous feedback	• Whenever I want it at the push of a button
(Generational Stereotypes, 2002; Hicks & Hicks 1999; How veterans, baby boomers, generation Xers and generation nexters can all get along in the workplace, 2002; Lancaster & Stillman, 2001; and Northwest AHEC, Nursing Regional Workforce Planning Group, 2000.)				

Figure 46.11 ■ Comparisons of the diversity among workers' generations.

ability to practice nursing. Younger nurses may need more emphasis on career movement and compensation. Refer to FIGURE 46.11 for comparisons of generation differences.

ORGANIZATIONAL CLIMATE AND MOTIVATION

The organizational climate influences employee motivation (Snow, 2002). Initial research (Litwin & Stringer, 1968) and ongoing study (Hay, 1995) found six key dimensions of culture that consistently affect performance.

- Flexibility—The feeling employees have about constraints in the workplace (unnecessary rules, procedures, policies, and practices that interfere with accomplishment and the acceptance of new ideas).
- Responsibility—The feeling that employees have appropriate authority delegated to them to do their jobs.
- Standards—The emphasis that employees feel management puts on improving performance and doing one's best, including the degree to which employees perceive that challenging but attainable goals are set for the organization and employees.
- Rewards—The degree to which employees feel they are recognized and rewarded for good work and that recognition is directly and differentially related to levels of performance. Plan retention strategies, such as job sculpting, for the top performers. These are an organization's most valuable financial and professional assets.
- Clarity—The feeling that all know what is expected of them and understand how the expectations relate to the larger goals and objectives of the organization.

- Team Commitment—Staff feel proud to belong to the organization and subsequently provide extra effort when needed.

Abrashoff (2002) adds communication as a significant cultural dimension affecting employee performance. Communication includes praise, sharing ideas, and explaining goals. Change is rampant today in all aspects of life. Change frightens many workers. Workers' "fears thrive in silence. The antidote is to keep talking" (Abrashoff, 2002, p. 54). Explain decisions honestly. The work climate can and should be periodically measured through direct observation of employee performance by trained observers, interviewing key staff by trained assessors and by paper and pencil survey.

MANAGERS' MOTIVATION PRINCIPLES

Managers find the following principles to be critical in establishing successful individual motivation systems:

- Involvement—Participating in decision making is respectful of and motivates people. Staff should be involved in the development of new systems and consulted about problems they foresee. Persons closest to a problem generally have the best solutions. Ask staff for their ideas. This affords staff commitment and a sense of ownership. Give staff responsibility and authority. These demonstrate to staff a sense of trust and respect. Ensure sufficient communication pathways to encourage staff's being informed, asking questions, and sharing information and ideas. (Examples include involving the school nurse in quality oversight and process improvement groups; allowing the school nurse the authority to implement schedule changes that will facilitate increased utilization of professional nursing services.)
- Remove demotivators—Staff will be distracted without the right quality, quantity, and accessibility of supplies, equipment, space, tools, etc. Likewise, inconsistent supervisory and school district practices, confusing information, and unclear expectations are not well tolerated in the work environment. People do not like working inefficiently, having no control over the pace of their work, or being continually under pressure (Ali et al., 2002). Good employee support (i.e., providing positive feedback on performance), clear communication, and consistency in practices (i.e., following the district's policies and procedures) need to be available from the supervisor. Provide appropriate training at the teachable moment; for example, model conflict management in a crisis event with an angry parent. Include teaching "people skills", such as relationship building and active listening, for use in all components of the work and especially for interacting, problems solving, and decision making. All staff should have at least part of their jobs be of high interest to them (Nelson, 1996). This might be accomplished by unusual approaches such as having someone attend a meeting for you or read and summarize a journal article on a topic of special interest to him or her. Build confidence by welcoming input, encouraging ability, and reducing fear through open communication. Ensure trust by keeping commitments, communicating honestly, and avoiding gossiping.
- Equity—Performance standards should be fair and comparable for all staff doing the same job in the same organization. Be willing to do whatever you ask of others.
- Reinforcement—People learn faster from successes than failures (Byham & Cox, 1988). Procedures should be in place to give reinforcement, encouragement, guidance, and feedback. The reinforcements must be of interest to the employee. Ask employees what most motivates them, such as autonomy, continuing education and/or leadership opportunities. You can do this routinely with all new employees and recheck periodically with all employees. You may want to use a formal survey but can obtain the same information from their narrative description in writing or shared verbally with you.

Give encouragement and praise to staff. Never assume your staff knows their work is appreciated just because they do not hear you complain. Catch people doing the right things and acknowledge their positive actions. Find a variety of ways to acknowledge and appreciate staff's work such as saying thanks, giving recognition at a board meeting, and sharing accomplishments with all staff promotions. Nelson (1996) says praise should be done as soon, as sincere, as specific, as personal, as positive, and as proactive as possible.

Listen actively ("aggressively," as Abrashoff [2002] says) to staff. This includes avoiding interruption while speaking, asking questions and paraphrasing to ensure understanding, asking open questions, reading body language, looking at the whole meaning of what is being said, being respectful, and giving undivided attention. Implement staff's viable suggestions. Celebrate staff and organization successes (Ali et al., 2001; Manning & Brugh, 2001). Rewards can include providing paid conference registrations, leadership of special projects, and recognition, such as in newsletters, personal notes, and formal presentations to the school board.

INDIVIDUAL MOTIVATORS

Ask people if they have enough responsibility. Ask staff what motivates them or what would be an enticing award for them. Staff can grow through delegation; it can stretch their abilities. Delegate to encourage staff's ownership in the work. Delegation is discussed in more detail later in this chapter. Of primary importance is the maintenance of employee self-esteem and the supervisor's ability to support employees' sense of self-respect and dignity. Neuhauser (2002) advises that people will like working for a healthcare organization and choose to stay because they are respected and feel pride in their work. Abrashoff (2002) reinforces the importance of relaying respect and individual dignity and identifying the lack of such treatment to staff as the primary reasons for lack of reenlistment or job turnover. Although Neuhauser's and Abrashoff's findings are specific to healthcare organizations, their principals appear applicable to school nurses who have a unique healthcare role as an employee of an education system. Beside needs and drives, adult workers have expectations of their employers and supervisory staff. Often workers' expectations are not overtly expressed (see Box 46.2).

Box 46.2 ■■■

KNOWLEDGABLE, EXPERIENCED, EXPERT EMPLOYERS

- Clear and fair policies, procedures, and employment practices
- Business integrity
- Personal respect
- Clear job descriptions
- Two-way communication (especially to be listened to)
- Effective management and supervision
- Positive discipline
- Opportunities for personal growth
- Ability to make an impact on the organization
- Appropriate rewards, especially more personal responsibility

(Abrashoff, 2002; Bellios, 1997)

Employer Caring and Employee Motivation

Nurses are masters at caring. Caring should not be reserved only for nurses' clients. Employees connect and commit themselves to an employer when there is individual respect and care, when they can use satisfying skills and when they find meaning in a work community. Five processes are said to be essential to caring for another person:

- *Maintaining belief*—Conveying that there is personal meaning to be found in the current situation. It includes a commitment to stay with them and to convey hope and optimism.
- *Knowing*—Striving to understand another's situation, seeking information, and establishing a partnership.
- *Being with*—Being present and actively listening to another person while conveying that what happens truly matters to you. Talk to staff regularly and create safe places for dialogue. The relationship the worker has with the supervisor determines 50% of work-life satisfaction. (Neuhauser, 2002).
- *Doing for*—Performing for others what they would do for themselves if it were possible. It includes setting up opportunities for people to solve problems and perform well.
- *Enabling*—Making it possible for others to practice self care. It involves informing, coaching, assisting and supporting another person (Henry & Henry, 2002).

Caring provides support to employees. It demonstrates a willingness to be a partner with staff in providing the agencies' services and products. Caring can be a motivational tool.

PERFORMANCE EVALUATION

Responsibilities and Goals for Employee Evaluation

Organizations have a responsibility to ensure that individual clinicians have access to appropriate supervision and support in the exercise of their job responsibilities (Winstanley, 2000). Several nursing researchers have shown that clinical supervision can lead to improvements in personal growth (Paunonen, 1991), increased satisfaction with nursing care and work (Butterworth, 1994; Hallberg, Hansson, & Axelsson, 1994) and decreased tedium and burnout (Berg, Hansson, & Hallberg, 1994). Feedback to employees about their performance is a motivation tool as well as a quality assurance device for employers.

Tustin, Canham, Berridge, Braden, and Starke (2002) say the "final goal of nursing evaluation should be to promote excellence in nursing practice, and ultimately, excellence in the programs and services provided by the professional nurse" (p. 229). Performance evaluation is a professional responsibility intended to enhance one's professional growth and competencies. If employees are performing well, they deserve recognition. If their performance needs improvement, they need to know the specifics and to form a plan for improvement. In addition, an effective performance review system gives direction and facilitates agreement on expected contributions, identifies educational needs, and is a mechanism for gathering ideas for change.

In addition to employers' liability for hiring incompetent or potentially unsafe employees, employers are just as liable for retention of unsatisfactory employees. Subsequently, organizations are accountable for monitoring employee competency. Thus, if an employee is found to be unfit after being hired, and corrective action is not taken, the employer is liable for negligent retention (Smith Publishers, 2000).

Assessment of employee performance should take place routinely, with formal assessments usually varying from every 6 months to every 2 years. Performance evaluation is a supervisory responsibility and cannot be delegated to another staff person. Some employees need more attention than do others, depending on factors such as their length of employment, their level of competency, and the complexity of their assignment. Competence assessments and performance evaluations are different supervisory actions. A competence assessment evaluates whether an individual has the knowledge, education, skills, experience, and proficiency to perform assigned responsibilities. A performance evaluation assesses how well persons actually perform their responsibilities. Competence must be assessed before conducting a performance evaluation (Herringer, 2002).

The Evaluation Process

All performance evaluations should be conducted using established agency or school district policies and guidelines, as well as the employee's job description and pre-established performance goals. The ways of measuring and collecting information should be suitable for the purpose of evaluation and the instruments used should also report adequate validity and reliability testing. Competence assessment cannot be undertaken adequately until the measurement instruments are known to have these properties. Several groups (The National Association of School Nurses, The National Consortium of School Nurse Educators, and the Southern Regional Education Board [Poster & Marcontel, 1999]) have developed curriculum and competency guidelines for school nurses (see Chapter 11).

Evaluations must be objective and job related. Court cases [for example *Brito v. Zia Co.* (1978) and *Watson v. Ft. Worth Bank & Trust Co.* (1988)] have clearly stated that evaluations are legally questionable on job-relatedness grounds, especially if adverse impact against federally protected classes of employees is seen in terms of the average appraisal ratings that are given. Evaluations must be based on facts, specific behaviors, and direct observations that are compared to agency policies and procedures, legal mandates, professional practice standards, and established performance benchmarks. These approaches assist employers to meet Equal Employment Opportunity (EEO) Program Evaluations and Compliance Reviews (2002) regulations for bias-free evaluations. Evaluation criteria will vary based on the practice settings, whether rural and urban environments, single-campus and multiple-campus assignments, alternative programs, and diversity of population, and will vary with the years of school nursing experience. Examples of evaluation documents can be found in FIGURES 46.12A, B, and C.

It is important to keep documentation of all formal evaluations as required by the local school district or parish. Such data support the legal needs of an organization (i.e., the tracking of an employee's performance, or validating grounds for termination or promotion). Refer to the human resources guidelines, legal advisement, and state educational records archivist to determine the length of record retention. A variety of evaluation approaches may be used, such as multiple raters (more than one person scores employees) and peer evaluations (conducted by co-workers doing the same job). Generally, both positive and negative outcomes are associated with the various evaluation approaches. Determine what provides the best data for the organization and employees' needs to encourage professional performance and to meet the agency or school district's employee evaluation guidelines.

"Since only nurses can accurately evaluate the clinical, technical, and judgment aspects of nursing practice, it is important to have nurse supervisors evaluate these aspects of school nurse performance....

(text continues on page 1099)

SCHOOL NURSE EVALUATION

Based on sample from and used with permission of Edina Public Schools, Minnesota

Nurse____________________ Date____________

Assignment____________________ Years in District____________

I. Recommends school district policies and philosophy related to the Health Services program.
- Participates in developing, implementing, and evaluating school health program **goals, objectives, and procedures.**
- Participates in **planning programs** that eliminate or minimize student health concerns that may interfere with learning.

Does not meet expectation *Needs improvement* *Meets expectation* *Exceeds expectations*
Supporting comments:

II. Assesses and evaluates the health and developmental status of school children.
- Assists in **developing, implementing, and evaluating procedures** and programs to **assess the health and developmental status of students.**
- Identifies student health needs through **health assessment.**

Does not meet expectation *Needs improvement* *Meets expectation* *Exceeds expectations*
Supporting comments:

III. Promotes and maintains health and well-being of students, families, and school personnel by teaching and counseling.
- Participates on the child study team: assists in the identification of students with disabilities, interprets health factors pertinent to the student's disability and develops, implements, and evaluates the health component of the individual educational plan (IEP).
- Assists students and parents in identifying and utilizing available and appropriate **community health resources.**

Does not meet expectation *Needs improvement* *Meets expectation* *Exceeds expectations*
Supporting comments:

IV. Implements an individual plan for the care of students with handicaps, students needing treatments or medications.
- Develops individualized health plans (IHP) with specific goals, objectives, and interventions based on student health needs.
- **Supervises health aides/paraprofessionals** in assigned buildings.
- Administers **medications** and treatments to students per physician order and parent authorization..

Does not meet expectation *Needs improvement* *Meets expectation* *Exceeds expectations*
Supporting comments:

V. Develops and maintains a system of first aid, recommends school safety measures, and promotes a healthful school.
- Participates in developing and maintaining a system for providing **first aid and emergency care.**
- Participates in identifying and reporting **environmental health and safety hazards** (current and potential) for students and staff.

Does not meet expectation *Needs improvement* *Meets expectation* *Exceeds expectations*
Supporting comments:

VI. Is active in health education.
- Provides consultation and assistance to teachers in their planning, implementation, and evaluation of **health education** units.
- Provides **health counseling** to students to assist them in making decisions regarding their health and health behaviors.
- Provides **inservice education** opportunities for school staff on health-related issues.

Does not meet expectation *Needs improvement* *Meets expectation* *Exceeds expectations*
Supporting comments:

VII. Assumes responsibility for continuing personal education and professional development.
- Initiates, and completes **professional development goals.**
- Seeks **independent learning opportunities** to build new skills.

Does not meet expectation *Needs improvement* *Meets expectation* *Exceeds expectations*
Supporting comments:

VIII. Collects data and maintains records.
- Initiates, maintains, and annually reviews **student health records** (pupil health record, emergency card, immunization record, and reports of physical examinations).
- Maintains daily, monthly, and yearly **statistical information** regarding health status of students and staff and utilization of school health services programs.

Does not meet expectation *Needs improvement* *Meets expectation* *Exceeds expectations*
Supporting comments:

____________________ ______
Supervisor Signature *Date*

Nurse Comments:

____________________ ______
Nurse Signature *Date*

Figure 46.12 ■ School nurse evaluation.

SAMPLE EVALUATION FORM

Based on Sample Form and Used with Permission of Willamette Education Service District; Salem, Oregon

PERFORMANCE STANDARDS REVIEW FORM

Name: ______________________ **Date:** ______________________

Position: Nurse **Program:** WESD Health/Sensory-Nursing

Shaded areas show a common core of standards intended to apply across departments and roles. **"Indicators of Standards Attainment"** show specific expectations for particular positions; indicators will vary depending on one's responsibilities. The sample indicators below are intended to apply to many, but certainly not all, specialist positions.

Performance Standards	Standards Attainment Scale: Does not meet standard: below essential job requirements	Standards Attainment Scale: Meets standard: appropriate, effective, proficient
1. PLANNING AND PREPARATION 1.1. Develops expectations and goals appropriate for position and responsibilities, based upon identified needs. 1.2. Designs a process and identifies and organizes resources for achieving expectations and goals.		✓
Specific Indicators of Standard Attainment: a) Plans, develops, and follows a weekly schedule based upon IFSP/IEP service needs for assigned caseload. Demonstrates flexibility in adjusting schedule to meet emergency needs. b) Plans, organizes, and schedules appropriate meetings. c) Displays knowledge of, or is able to research, etiology, characteristics and prognosis of relevant medical conditions. d) Displays knowledge of normal developmental sequences and learning patterns in the areas of sensory, motor, psychosocial and cognitive development and can use this knowledge in the development of Health Management Plans. e) Displays knowledge of health issues and safety needs of children. f) Displays knowledge of laws, regulations and current professional practice standards affecting Nursing services, especially in educational settings. g) Orders supplies as needed and effectively plans distribution of equipment and materials. h) Provides assistance and/or recommendations to families and school districts regarding selection, ordering, and funding of appropriate equipment and materials. Nurse effectively evaluates factors related to safety, availability, and cost when choosing equipment or intervention options.	Comments	

Performance Standards	Standards Attainment Scale: Does not meet standard: below essential job requirements	Standards Attainment Scale: Meets standard: appropriate, effective, proficient
2. IMPLEMENTATION AND MANAGEMENT 2.1. Carries out plans and uses strategies and resources, adapting as needed to achieve desired goals.		✓
Specific Indicators of Standard Attainment: a) Uses and manages time effectively. b) Effectively manages, evaluates, and modifies needed school health programs and Health Management Plans. c) Provides service coordination to parents and children, including referral to other agencies for healthcare issues, as needed. Functions as a student advocate when appropriate. d) Completes required paperwork in specified time and manner. Manages and maintains accurate records. Completes Medicaid forms as needed. e) Creates an environment and provides instruction which engages staff and students and enhances learning. f) Communicates expectations and monitors and reinforces staff and student behavior positively to facilitate learning, using effective behavior management skills and teaching practices. g) Evaluates the quality and effectiveness of her practice and stresses quality improvement through the development of improved policies and procedures or practice guidelines.	Comments	

Figure 46.12 ■ *(continued)*

Performance Standards

Standards Attainment Scale

	Does not meet standard: below essential job requirements	Meets standard: appropriate, effective, proficient
3. ASSESSMENT AND THE USE OF ASSESSMENT INFORMATION 3.1. Selects or develops methods of collecting information, and uses these methods appropriately. 3.2. Interprets, analyzes, and acts upon information to make decisions, guide improvement, and report results.		✓
Specific Indicators of Standard Attainment: a) Uses assessment data to establish appropriate Health Management Plans, training goals and objectives or school services. b) Provides constructive, timely feedback to students and staff to enhance learning. c) Develops, selects, and uses appropriate assessment tools, and interprets results effectively. d) Writes necessary assessment summaries and recommendations in a clear, informative and timely manner. e) Monitors, evaluates and modifies student and staff performance using observation and data.	Comments	

Performance Standards

Standards Attainment Scale

	Does not meet standard: below essential job requirements	Meets standard: appropriate, effective, proficient
4. COMMUNICATION 4.1. Conveys information and ideas in modes, forms and in a style that is appropriate to audience, purpose, and context. 4.2. Listens and responds respectfully to information and ideas conveyed by others.		✓
Specific Indicators of Standard Attainment: a) Participates knowledgeably and collaboratively on IFSP/IEP/504 teams. b) Employs appropriate counseling and crisis intervention strategies as needed. c) Participates collaboratively on a team to develop an integrated IFSP/IEP. Writes goals which are appropriate and measurable, reflecting students' health needs, preferences and expected outcomes. d) Provides effective and collaborative consultation. Provides inservice training (including First Aid, CPR, Blood-Borne Pathogen/Standard Precautions, and Medication Administration Training) and follow-up to children, school staff, and parents. Promotes public awareness of relevant health issues. e) Maintains confidentiality. f) Communicates clearly and effectively with students/children, parents, colleagues and other service providers with consideration for culture and background; is sensitive to listener's level of understanding when using medical terminology. g) Offers/volunteers assistance when appropriate.	Comments	

Performance Standards

Standards Attainment Scale

	Does not meet standard: below essential job requirements	Meets standard: appropriate, effective, proficient
5. LEADERSHIP AND PROFESSIONAL SERVICE AND CONDUCT 5.1. Envisions future needs and opportunities appropriate for position and program. 5.2. Acts on the basis of professional principles and generally accepted norms of professional behavior. 5.3. Contributes to the advancement of the profession and the agency as a whole.		✓
Specific Indicators of Standard Attainment a) Demonstrates an awareness of individual professional strengths and limitations and sets and meets appropriate performance goals.	Comments	

Figure 46.12 ■ *(continued)*

b) Fosters effective inter- and intra-agency collaboration. c) Participates in continuing education essential for provision of services appropriate to current nursing practice standards. d) Contributes to a positive, supportive, and healthy work environment by: • Understanding and tolerating differences in points of view • Demonstrating a positive attitude • Working effectively to resolve conflicts • Listening and responding respectfully to information and ideas conveyed by others. • Responding calmly and effectively to crisis situations • Actively participating in staff and planning meetings • Interacting with and contributing to the professional development of peers and colleagues. e) Adheres to a code of professional ethics as identified by agency, professional organization, or licensing commission (ANA and NASN). f) Supervises staff to whom nursing tasks have been delegated. g) Envisions future needs and opportunities appropriate for position and program. h) Contributes to the advancement of the profession and the agency as a whole.	

SAMPLE EVALUATION FORM

Sample from 1 of 9 standards from the Evaluation document from Lubbock Independent School District, Lubbock, Texas

Standard III: Education - The school nurse acquires and maintains current knowledge and competency in school nursing practice.			
MEASUREMENT CRITERIA: a) The school nurse acquires knowledge and skills appropriate to the specialty practice of school nursing on a regular and ongoing basis. b) The school nurse consistently participates in continuing education activities related to current clinical knowledge and professional issues. c) The school nurse seeks experience to maintain current clinical skills and competence.			
EVALUATION CRITERIA			
Exceeds Expectations	*Proficient*	*Below Expectations*	*Unsatisfactory*
1. The school nurse shares with colleagues new knowledge, research and innovative practices through continuing education programs related to professional setting. 2. The school nurse shares with colleagues new knowledge, research and innovative practices through a variety of professional resources. 3. The school nurse assists colleagues in the implementation of new knowledge, research and innovative practices. 4. The school nurse develops and provides professional experiences to promote clinical and relaxed competence of colleagues.	1. The school nurse attends continuing education programs offering new knowledge, research and innovative practice related to professional setting. 2. The school nurse seeks new knowledge regarding research and innovative practices through a variety of professional resources. 3. The school nurse implements new knowledge, research and new practices in the professional setting. 4. The school nurse seeks clinical experiences to promote professional competency.	1. The school nurse occasionally attends continuing education programs offering new knowledge, research and innovative practices related to professional setting. 2. The school nurse occasionally seeks new knowledge regarding research and innovative practices obtained through a variety of professional resources. 3. The school nurse occasionally implements new knowledge, research and new practices in the professional setting. 4. The school nurse seeks clinical experiences to promote professional competency.	1. The school nurse rarely attends continuing education programs offering new knowledge, research and innovative practice related to professional setting. 2. The school nurse rarely seeks new knowledge regarding research and innovative practices obtained through a variety of professional resources. 3. The school nurse rarely implements new knowledge, research and new practices in the professional setting. 4. The school nurse seeks clinical experiences to promote professional competency.

Figure 46.12 ■ *(continued)*

Otherwise, non-nurse evaluators determining the appropriateness of a nurse's clinical decisions and actions might be considered practicing nursing without a license" (Bourne in Schwab & Gelfman, 2001, p. 146). It is the position of NASN that it is essential to provide supervision and evaluation of school nurses by school nurses knowledgeable in school nursing practice, supervision, and administration, and that evaluations should be based upon standards of professional school nursing practice (NASN, 2003). Refer to Chapter 11 on measuring school nurse efficacy.

In preparation for the evaluation, employees may be asked to complete a self-appraisal, using the same evaluation form to be used by the supervisor or perhaps focusing on his or her strengths and weaknesses. This is not only good evaluation practice but also part of school nursing standards of practice (NASN & ANA, 2005). The self-evaluation may be discussed with the employee during the staff meeting. It is beneficial to provide employees with a copy of their evaluation prior to the actual meeting to allow the employee to be prepared with questions and as a means of avoiding surprise. There should be no surprises in a formal evaluation. Employees should be aware as soon as possible about any concerns regarding their job performance. Surprise information can negatively impact their ability to listen, have clear dialogue, and be receptive to problem solving. Provide privacy for an appraisal discussion.

As the evaluation meeting begins, review the purpose and the accomplishments for the meeting. Review past performance and the quantity and quality of the work since the last review. Include a discussion of how tools and training have affected job performance and how these can be used in the future for the growth of job performance. Also include a comparison of the employee's perceptions (received prior to the evaluation meeting) with your observations. At the conclusion of the meeting, determine mutual understanding of the appraisal and future goals. Both the employee and the supervisor should sign the evaluation and goal forms affirming there has been an exchange of information on the content. The documents should be retained within the personnel file and in accordance with agencies or school policies on file retention.

Be consistent in your approach with all employees' evaluation. Rating scales may rank employees as "meets standards/expectations," and "does not meet standards/expectations." Other weighting systems are used but generally are found to be less satisfactory as supervisors tend to over rank employees to ensure salary advancement or avoid demerits in merit systems (Toropov, 2001). When working within a merit and competency system, remember that a comparison of evaluation scoring can be the determining factor in position reductions or promotions. Supervisory commentary should be included in all formal evaluations to validate the documented scoring. Avoid general statements that do not provide validation of an accurate assessment or do not describe how the employee is not meeting expectations. For example, the commentaries "*an excellent nurse*" and "*a poor performer*" are general statements. Rather, describe observed behaviors, just as one does in documenting client care so that others can draw conclusions from the written data.

Evaluations should include the employees' strengths and weaknesses in order to improve weak performance and encourage higher motivation in strong areas. Be cautious of the "halo" effect (high competence in one area overshines all other performance areas) or its opposite (poor performance in one area overshadows all other areas). Always ask employees to identify how improvement can be achieved. A supervisor's goal is to help employees find their own solutions to weak and unacceptable behaviors. Record employees' perspective of their performance, including concerns, suggestions, and requests for support.

Set performance goals with the employees, working together to create a plan of action to help in deficient areas. Goals should:

- Have meaningful results;
- Be attainable (a little stretch promotes professional growth);
- Be readily understood;
- Be measurable in quality, quantity, time, and cost; and
- Be aligned with the program or organizational goals.

Determine a follow-up time. Record the actions to which you both have agreed and the target dates for completion. Professional performance is a goal for all school nurses, new and long term. Professionalism implies expert knowledge, credibility, critical thinking, sound decision making, innovation, continuous learning, and respect for legal and ethical frameworks. A supervisor's help to staff in their goal accomplishment will vary from person to person. Seasoned school nurses may need more autonomy; help them plan ways that their experience can help others. For new staff, encourage easier goals and check more frequently with staff and give them feedback more often. "Performance evaluation requires on-site observation of performance and skills, record review, and discussion of student care and assigned responsibilities" (Schwab & Gelfman, 2001, p. 133). Depending on your job responsibilities and number of assigned staff, you will need to identify ways to effectively provide the oversight and evaluation that will support staff's performance. Although on-site observation is the best mechanism for evaluating employee performance, it may be necessary to utilize audits, written reports, and electronic and phone communication as alternative means for collecting performance information.

Although no research currently exists to determine appropriate ratios for nurse and nurse supervisor ratios, it would be important for the supervisor to establish the maximum ratio possible for managing staff supervision and all other job responsibilities. Then one can use this information in negotiation with school district administrative staff and/or the district's school board and request policy and procedural development for ongoing reference in staffing considerations.

EMPLOYEE DISCIPLINE

General Discipline Principles

Regardless of efforts at employee selection, orientation, coaching, or job design, there will be problem employees (DeCenzo & Robbins, 1994). Some employees will require extrinsic disciplinary action. To avoid litigation, it is prudent to have agency or school district policies about performance concerns, the discipline process, and behaviors for which an employee can be terminated immediately (e.g., theft and endangering students or employees). Each year employees should be reminded that the policies are in print and/or online. The object of discipline is to correct undesirable behaviors. It is a basic fact that the more quickly the discipline follows the offense, the more likely it is that the employee will associate the discipline with the offense rather than the supervisor.

In most instances advance warning is given in writing prior to initiating formal disciplinary action. Exception is when danger to students or staff is anticipated, such as with drug/alcohol abuse.

- Be consistent with all disciplinary action.
- Direct the discipline at the behavior and not the individual employee.
- Be specific, positive, and constructive in your feedback.
- Set boundaries when initiating a discipline meeting.
- Allow time to listen and to give responses to the employee.
- Avoid reacting to defensive behaviors.
- Explain the consequences of the employee's failure to demonstrate performance improvement (Academic Human Resources, 2002).

The nature of the performance problem will influence the disciplinary action. Refer to Box 46.3 for factors that can influence the disciplinary decision.

Disciplinary Actions

Counseling, discipline (e.g., warnings, suspension, plans of assistance) and termination must be handled appropriately. Generally, disciplinary intervention is progressive through these preceding steps. Closely follow the agency's or school policies and procedures for these actions and obtain guidance through the entire proceedings from human resources staff and legal counsel to assure a fair and legal implementation process. Although discipline is often regarded as punitive, the intent is to change behaviors in order to have a satisfactory job performance. Subsequently, some organizations are reframing the historical terminology associated with discipline and moving toward "positive discipline," "oral reminder," "written reminder," and "decision-making leave" (DeCenzo & Robbins, 1994). Although it may seem to some as merely a selection of different semantics, the philosophical intent is to demonstrate more caring and concern for the employee.

Box 46.3 ■ ■ ■

FACTORS THAT INFLUENCE DISCIPLINARY DECISIONS

- Seriousness of the problem
- Duration of the problem
- Frequency and nature of the problem.
- Extenuating factors (for example personal health problems, recent death of a close family member).
- Degree of the organization's formalized training and performance guidelines regarding the behavior of concern.
- History of the organization's discipline practices. (There should be consistency in responses to substandard performance.)
- Administrative and legal backing. (DeCenzo & Robbins, 1994)

Performance Counseling

The intent of counseling is to empower the employee through effective guidance to have more control over his or her work and behavioral changes affecting performance. The supervisor still retains responsibility for monitoring outcomes and intervening with discipline and termination for unsatisfactory performance that is not amenable to coaching and other strategies. Corrective counseling should occur in a quiet and closed office. If possible, schedule the meeting early in the day and early in the week. Generally, persons are less tired and stressed at these times. Be sure all facts are precisely accurate and you have recent, clear examples of deficient behavior to cite in your dialogue. A planned agenda for the meeting will help you deliver the necessary information more effectively and assist you to cover all the important information.

Anticipate emotional reactions, more so if health or personal issues are involved. Allow the person a few minutes to regain composure. It is important to listen, not talk, and to hear the feelings (i.e., fear, resentment, and frustration). Avoid arguing or trying to convince someone when he or she is angry. Do not get angry yourself. Do not stop an employee who wishes to leave the room; resume the discussion later. Be clear in describing the problem and describing expected behavioral changes. Maintain your focus on the behavior in question, not on the person.

State and demonstrate your faith that the employee can change and that you want him or her to remain on your team. Give the employee an opportunity to explain the situation and to make suggestions for how to improve; avoid being drawn into excuses. Assure the employee of your assistance in making improvements, but clarify that the final responsibility for change lies with the employee. Employees' personal problems are private until job performance begins to be impacted. If the employee identifies that substance abuse or other personal problems are the cause for the behavior problem, refer the employee to appropriate counseling, healthcare providers, or the agency's employee assistance program. Even if qualified, supervisors should not provide the health counseling an employee may need. Dual roles create a conflict of interest and confusion for the employee. Document actions, verbal responses, and the employee's attitude.

Verbal Warning

Inform the employee about the substandard behavior or the rule violation, the evidence of the violation, and the difficulties the behavior causes. (*All staff are to be in their schools by 8 a.m. unless a schedule change is approved by the supervisor. Your principal reports you consistently arrive around 9 a.m. You were not available for my phone call at 8:15 a.m. on the past three mornings. The school is complaining about the poor quality of service they are receiving; the principal shared that you missed two important staff meetings for children with serious health conditions.*) Allow the employee to respond. Ask as many questions as you need to understand the situation from the employee's perspective.

Determine if there are justifications for the employee's behavior and whether the employee has an adequate solution. Determine what specific actions must be done and by when and communicate this to the employee. The objective is for performance at an acceptable behavioral level. Describe the consequence of the continued behavior. The time period for correction should be the shortest time reasonable for correction. It should be immediately for attitude and attendance (Ali et al., 2001). Affirm that the employee understands the supervisor's plan for follow up and the consequences if the problem reoccurs.

Advise the employee that a *verbal warning* or *oral reminder* is being given. Document this action as a memo of understanding to the employee and retain a copy in the supervisor's file. The employee should receive a copy of all written communication issued as part of the disciplinary process. The employee is asked to sign the original document indicating by signature that he or she has read the warning, received a copy, and had the opportunity to discuss the contents. Should an employee refuse to sign any document, make such a note on the original document. This document is generally not retained in the permanent human resource file. The supervisor should plan for follow up and share the projected action plan with the employee.

Written Warning

The written warning is the same as for the verbal warning. This is known as the first step of a disciplinary process because the documentation becomes part of the employee's official personnel file. The employee is advised at the end of the dialogue that a written warning is being issued. The documentation states the problem, any rule or standard violation, any acknowledgment by the employee, behavioral corrections to be made by the employee, and the consequences of recurrent deviant behavior. A copy is filed in the official personnel file and is given to the employee. Again, a plan for follow-up by the supervisor is essential.

Job Suspension

The use of this action varies from agency to agency. A suspension with or without pay usually occurs only if the prior warning actions have been implemented without the desired outcome. Suspension without prior verbal or written warning generally occurs only for a serious infraction—for example, theft or being on the job under the influence of alcohol or illegal chemicals. The purposes of suspension generally include the need to complete an investigation or to convince the employee of the serious nature of the performance deficiency and the necessity to accept responsibility for changing performance behaviors.

Plan of Assistance (Improvement Plan)

The use of this action also varies from district to district. This process is used as a formal and last step to providing direction and support to an employee with substandard job performance. The content conveys:

- How the inadequate performance was determined,
- The expectations of and actions to be taken by the employee,
- The assistance to be offered by the supervisor and agency, when performance will be evaluated in the future, and
- Notice that termination will occur for unsuccessful completion of the plan.

Have legal counsel review all plans before implementation.

Job Termination

Employees may depart from an organization voluntarily (resignation) or involuntarily (firing for poor performance or just cause, layoff due to lack of work or loss of job position). Follow company policies exactly for termination proceedings. To avoid accusations of discrimination and violation of termination protocol, consider firing only if:

- You have given the employee clear information regarding performance expectations (via the job description);
- The employee has been given and verifies reading the policy handbook;
- You warned the employee in successive and dated memos that clearly describe the deteriorating job performance even after employer assistance; and
- There is clear observation of continuing performance problems (Parting Ways, 2001).

Not all of these preceding actions may be necessary if the employee is in a probationary time with the organization. However, proceed cautiously and with support of legal counsel and human resources. Have legal counsel review all letters of termination for use of proper language. Yet, move quickly once there is a firm decision for termination. Otherwise, it becomes easy to procrastinate and the employee (if he or she becomes aware) may hold this against you in legal proceedings. Have ready before your meeting with the employee a letter of termination to the employee. This reiterates the observed behaviors, your actions, and the subsequent consequence that must now be enacted according to your organization's policies.

Meet with the employee in a private area. It is often good practice to have another supervisory or personnel department staff person in the environment when the information is given to the employee about termination. This provides another available person to help with the listening to and dialogue with the employee as well as serving as a witness. The presence of two persons may decrease the risk for violence. The tone of delivery should be cordial and empathetic. It is appropriate to acknowledge the positive contributions but keep this sharing short so the individual does not misinterpret the information. In this meeting, little new information is necessary about the performance concerns. The employee gets the majority of the talking time. Offer words of confidence for the future career of the employee. Have ready for the employee the final pay due and information about available benefits and legal rights, for example, COBRA (health insurance) rights. The terminating agency will be responsible for unemployment compensation.

Obtain all passwords from the employee and advise appropriate offices of the need to close all electronic device access. Obtain immediately the organization's supplies, including all keys and any credit cards issued. As appropriate, facilitate the employee's collection of all personal items and accompany the employee off campus.

CONFLICT MANAGEMENT

General Considerations

A more common performance challenge involving supervisory intervention is the issue of conflict management. Differences amongst people and subsequently conflict is part of life and working relationships. Confrontation is the key intervention to prevent conflict's escalation to destructive proportions (Mayer, 1990). However, conflict is associated with negative emotions and situations (e.g., antagonism and uncomfortable relationships). Consequently, humans often tend to avoid confrontation. Conflicts are often caused by communication failures, especially in listening. The need to be right, a strong drive in all humans, is generally a primary contributor to any conflict. Conflicts are invariably the result of many compiling minor issues and incidents, rather than one single situation. Mind reading the motives of others is a source of many destructive conflicts, for example,, perceiving that someone is ignoring you and thus is upset with you, when, in actuality, the person may actually be distracted by personal issues. Supervisors may find themselves involved in a conflict with an employee, may need to act as a mediator or facilitator in conflict resolution between employees, or may need to coach an employee through appropriate action regarding a conflict with co-workers or clients.

Conflict Management Skills and Steps

It is important to remain calm, listen carefully (listen 80% of the time, talk 20%) and be kindly assertive (Ali et al., 2002). Sometimes listening is all that is needed to defuse emotions and calm persons to allow them to think differently or more clearly. In addition, conflict resolution skills include direct, assertive communication, describing behaviors and emotions rather than personalities, and checking perceptions. Helping persons to understand that caring more about the relationship rather than about being right is helpful in conflict resolution. Caring includes having concern about what the other person has to say. Effective listening, as nurses know well, requires patience and persistence in overcoming listening barriers. Examples of listening barriers include allowing personal biases to interfere with hearing the message, responding before hearing the other's viewpoint, having to be right or having the last word, and mentally rehearsing responses rather than paying full attention to the sender.

One-on-one meetings with involved persons are often the most efficient way to intervene with conflict. Use an open body language, for example open arms and chin up. Avoid prolonged eye contact in a confrontational situation. This is generally perceived as threatening behavior. One's words, actions and body language must be in alignment, sending a positive and consistent message. If the timing, location or environment is wrong for successful conflict resolution, listen closely and show interest, but at the first reasonable opportunity, identify that a more suitable time or location needs to be arranged. Steps to use in working through conflict include:

- Outline the situation as you see it.
- Listen to the other person's view.
- Gain agreement that a problem exists.
- Use questioning to identify ways of resolving the problem.
- Negotiate a resolution to the dispute. Agree on an action plan.

Harassment

Schwab and Gelfman (2001) define harassment as offensive activities of sufficient intensity and persistence that they interfere with an individual's work or learning. Harassment can be any form of behavior that offends or intimidates, such as:

- Written material
- Verbal comments, intrusive questions, jokes
- Gestures
- Ignoring, isolating, or segregating a person or group
- Staring or leering
- Sexual or physical contact
- Intrusive questions about sexual activity
- Sexual assault (Gringberg, 2002)

Employers, including schools, have an obligation to maintain a workplace free from harassment. Work organizations must create written policy that addresses harassment and a hostile work environment and consistently follow the policy. The policy should define "harassment" and "aggression" and state that neither is tolerated. This information should be written into the employee handbook and be included in new employee orientation. Training should be conducted to raise awareness of harassment and aggression, clarify misconceptions about the behaviors, explain the manager's responsibilities for providing a safe and supportive work environment and share the organization's specific policy (American College of Healthcare Executives, 2002). A procedure should accompany policy that specifies the reporting process, investigation, and standards for corrective action.

Any time an employee expresses a feeling of harassment or the supervisor perceives harassment is occurring or that a hostile work environment is evident, immediately stop the behavior and investigate. Some guidelines to follow in the investigation include:

- Keep an open mind for conclusions until the investigation is complete.
- Be respectful of the complainer. Often

employees feel vulnerable and afraid when making the complaint.

- Document your investigation. It will protect you should there be questions about your action and your approach.
- Consult with legal counsel.
- Take appropriate action against the wrongdoer. Action may vary from warning or counseling to termination for more serious situations, such as threats and stalking. Take action quickly, document it, and notify the accuser that action has been taken (NOLO, 2002b).

Title IX of the 1972 Education Amendments requires schools to adopt and publish grievance procedures to investigate and resolve sexual harassment complaints. Schools must have policies against harassment. The school is also liable for hostile environment harassment, which is permitting harassment to continue once notice of the behavior is made. School nurses must be familiar with this school policy and take prompt action once a report of such behaviors is made (Cohn, Gelfman, & Schwab, 2001).

PROFESSIONAL BURNOUT

Although little, if any, research has been done in school nursing on worker burnout, the issue should be of concern because of its increasing incidence and its related cost to all work organizations. School nurses are not likely to be exempt. The U.S. National Institute for Occupational Safety and Health (NIOSH) reports job stress (a key factor in burnout) as a growing occupational safety and health problem (NIOSH, 1999). There is a high incidence of this syndrome among all healthcare providers and especially nurses (Happel, Martin, & Pinikahana, 2003). Job costs include not only the direct care to the employee incurring the physical and mental ailments but also to the employer for stress-related expenses (e.g., increased employee absenteeism, decreased productivity, increased health insurance premiums, increased injuries, job turnover expenses, or legal fees).

Worker burnout results in physical, psychological, and emotional exhaustion and eventually alienation from work. Burnout is complex, multidimensional and a byproduct of both personal and organizational variables. Burnt out employees are often those who care; they are many times the "superstars" (Moore, 2002). Burnout occurs when workers experience increasing amounts of negative stress that, in due course, harmfully affects well-being and productivity.

Stress itself is a neutral event. The employee interprets the stress as either being positive or negative. With positive stress, employees are motivated to put in the extra time and effort to do their best work; they feel a strong sense of accomplishment when their work is done. Employees who interpret the stress as negative can feel overwhelmed, be irritable, and start to worry. These employees generally put the same amount of work into a project, but at the conclusion of projects, they will feel drained and not energized for the next project. Put enough of these negative events together and employees can become very vulnerable for burnout. Burned out workers perceive their efforts as being futile toward any successful accomplishments. Subsequently, they appear absent-minded, apathetic, and unproductive.

Influencing Factors in Professional Burnout

Job conditions can lead to stress and stress, likewise, is positively or negatively influenced by individual and situational conditions including a:

- Balance between work and personal life,
- Support network (of friends and co-workers), and
- Relaxed and positive outlook.

Job conditions that may lead to negative stress include:

- The design of tasks (heavy workload, infrequent breaks, long work hours, hectic pace, routine tasks with little inherent meaning, little sense of control)
- Management style (lack of worker involvement in decision making, poor managerial communication, insufficient reward, unfairness, lack of recognition)
- Interpersonal relationships (poor social connections, including lack of support from coworkers and supervisors)
- Work roles (conflicting or uncertain job expectations, value conflict)
- Career concerns (job insecurity, lack of growth or advancement opportunity, rapid changes for which workers are unprepared)
- Environmental conditions (crowding, noise, ergonomic issues, etc.)

Mehrabian (2001) said that burnout could occur in three major ways:

1. The worker performs the same routine and work daily for years. Repetitious, boring, and uninteresting work is associated with

feelings of stagnation, helplessness, and depression.

2. A person in the same job for some time identifies no avenues or opportunities for job advancement. In addition, the work being done has become routine, highly predictable, and unexciting. This combination tends to create feelings of hopelessness and stagnation.
3. The third kind of burnout occurs when the worker is overwhelmed daily with complex and varied tasks, being continuously required to respond to a variety of urgent, demanding, and changing circumstances. Nurses are prime candidates for this kind of burnout. Persons juggling family and work are also more vulnerable.

Workplace Intervention Strategies for Professional Burnout

No generalizations can be made for all workers about precipitating factors of job stress. However, supervisors will be prudent to review all data to see what interventions might be made in the work environment to minimize vulnerability to job stress and subsequently job burnout. Prevention strategies can include:

- *Increase the frequency of connections with staff*. Relationships are crucial to the development of trust and effective working partnerships. Facilitate connections with other work colleagues and allow for some social interaction in the course of work to develop a sense of community. Establish work schedules that are compatible with responsibilities outside of the job. Afford two-way communication. Reduce uncertainty about career status.
- *Diminish intensity in assignment responsibilities*. Ensure the workload is compatible with workers' capabilities and resources. Facilitate and encourage delegation as appropriate. Change job descriptions when work responsibilities are unrealistic. As possible, give momentary respite and support related to assigned work.
- *Be attuned to employees' motivators and stressors*. Align, as possible, job assignments with interests and strengths. Thomas and Morris (2002) report that job satisfaction is a significant predictor of burnout in nurses. Delegate to staff special projects in which they hold special interest. Buckingham and Clifton (2001) remind supervisors of the uniqueness of each employee and the importance of focusing on employee strengths as the basis of performance success and reward for each employee. Give staff opportunities to participate in decisions affecting their job and in problem solving in order to afford a sense of personal control. Create job diversity. Provide comprehensive orientation programs to clarify job responsibilities and explain the culture of the organization. Facilitate access to educational opportunities that upgrade job skills and enhance self-confidence.
- *Create a work culture that promotes employee health, one that emphasizes personal balance along with hard work*. Provide choices as possible. Provide adequate support and timelines for the quantity of work being requested. Give clear and nonconflicting direction. Acknowledge and reward employee contributions. As possible, give prestige to job roles. Buckingham and Clifton (2001) share that the more prestige an organization offers to job positions, the healthier are the employees. Provide resources for employees to access personal stress management measures. Design an employee survey to measure perceptions of job conditions; collect and analyze data. Plan appropriate interventions such as organizational redesign or securing employee assistance programs, and evaluate.
- *Model self-care and stress management*. Use positive words in difficult situations rather than say "I can't," and "This is too hard." Share personal techniques of breaking jobs into small manageable components to make job accomplishment possible in an apparent overwhelming task. Model self-care through daily exercise. Diversify and become involved in new, enjoyable tasks. Show how you tap into your creativity and seek control by looking for solutions for issues that have frustrated or stressed you. Tell others what you enjoy about your work.
- *Identify early warning signs*. Irritability, overreaction in situations, reports of feeling overwhelmed, or having minor health ailments may be examples indicative of feeling stressed.
- *Dialogue with and counsel employees in whom you have observed warning signs*. Dialogue between supervisor and employee may help staff to stop denying symptoms, seek professional help, and begin self-care measures, such as setting limits, changing circumstances in a relationship or situation,

and reprioritizing activities. Share school/school district and community helping resources and encourage and support effective self-management strategies. Be aware that clinical depression can mimic the symptoms of burnout; refer accordingly.

A supervisor can never alleviate all stress, but can minimize stress and support employees through stressful times and nurture effective coping skills.

DELEGATION

Supervisory Task Delegation

Delegation is a way for supervisors to teach (new skills and expertise), support (instill confidence and self-reliance), and improve morale (afford participation in decisions and projects) and motivation (build commitment and engagement in the work; encourage creativity and initiative) in employees. The primary purpose of supervisor delegation is employee growth, but it can release time for the supervisor to do other managerial work and provides the opportunity to mentor new leaders in an organization (Simmons, 2000; Tyme, 2000). Some parameters to help selection of supervisor tasks to delegate include:

- All necessary information is available to the employee.
- The parameters of the work are clear.
- The task does not involve managerial responsibilities (i.e. hiring, performance appraisal, disciplinary action, promotion).

The principles of nursing task delegation apply to supervisory delegation, that is, adequate training and ongoing monitoring of performance.

Nursing Task Delegation

Although not all school nurses are in a supervisory position, many school nurses will likely encounter the issue of delegation in their practice setting. With the increasing incidence of chronic health conditions (i.e., diabetes and asthma), complex medical conditions, and correlating health technology, more students are in need of ongoing health management and nursing procedures during the school day. Federal laws (Section 504 of the Rehabilitation Act of 1973, the Americans with Disabilities Act of 1990, and the Individuals with Disabilities Education Act [IDEA] of 1990) require that school health services be provided as a related service to all eligible students. Some school districts cannot meet this mandate without delegation by school nurses.

Delegation has been defined as "the transfer of responsibility for the performance of an activity to another, with the former retaining accountability for the outcome" (ANA, 1994, p. 11). State nurse practice acts and their associated rules and regulations define the guidelines and standards regulating delegation of nursing tasks. Some states and territories restrict the procedures that can be delegated; others do not allow delegation at all. (NASN, 2002b) Delegation of nursing care is a complex legal and clinical issue in any setting, especially in schools due to the unique situation of providing healthcare in an academic system. School nurses must know and understand their state's regulations as well as the school nurse specialty standards of practice for delegating nursing care in the school setting. A number of organizations (i.e., NASN, ANA, the National Association of State School Nurse Consultants, and the National Council of State Boards of Nursing) have published position statements and guidelines on the issue of delegation. These guidelines and standards are in place to ensure the health and safety of clients.

The school nurse may need supervisory interpretation and guidance related to delegation and in following the critical processes meticulously. Pohlman (2001) advises that litigation involving school nurses is often about the issue of delegation. It is critical that school nurses communicate to schools the intent of delegation, the parameters for safe delegation, and the process to ensure student safety. Parents and school staff can be confused about why tasks done at home are held to a different standard in schools. The school nurse must be ready to describe that the need for such regulatory practices is to protect the health and safety of students during the school day. The school nurse must be involved in development of district policy that addresses the delegation of care in the school setting.

Nursing Delegation Process

Only a registered nurse can delegate nursing care. The school nurse is responsible for using professional nursing judgment to determine the appropriate level of care needed for each student, including whether or not tasks can be delegated. Once the school nurse, in accordance with the state's nurse practice act and by assessment of the unique characteristics of the individual student needing nursing services, determines that a task can be delegated, an appropriate delegatee must be chosen (NASN, 2002b). Although states vary in their approach, registered nurses (RNs) may delegate to a Licensed Practical Nurse (LPN), also known as Licensed Vocational Nurse (LVN), or unlicensed assistive personnel (UAP) (i.e., school staff) certain tasks within the scope of RN practice. The nurse remains accountable for the actions of the delegatee designated by the delegation process. By definition, a delegated nursing service requires that the professional nurse train and supervise the delegatee and evaluate the health outcome of the student needing the procedure(s). The training must be documented. The documentation must reflect that the delegate understands what needs to be done and demonstrates proficiency in performing the delegated task. Ongoing and regular evaluation by the registered nurse is required in accordance with state, district, and/or school policy. Supervision is generally categorized as "on-site," that is physically present and/or being immediately available. This may limit the potential for delegation when a nurse has a part time or a multi-school assignment (Pohlman, 2001). The National Council of State Boards of Nursing (1995) identified five "rights" that nurses must use (see FIGURE 46.13) as guidelines for delegation:

- Right task
- Right circumstances
- Right person
- Right direction/communication
- Right supervision/evaluation

Unlicensed Assistive Personnel (UAP)

While school administrators have responsibility for student safety, they cannot legally decide the level of special healthcare needed by a student. The

All decisions related to delegation of nursing activities must be based upon the fundamental principle of public protection. Licensed nurses have ultimate accountability for the management and provision of nursing care, including all delegation decisions. However, seldom is a single nurse accountable for all aspects of the delegation decision-making process, its implementation, supervision, and evaluation.

The Five Rights of Delegation, identified in *Delegation: Concepts and Decision-making Process* (NCSBN, 1995) can be used as a mental checklist to assist nurses from multiple roles to clarify the critical elements of the decision-making process. Nursing service administrators (all levels of executive/management nurses) and staff nurses each have accountability in ensuring that the delegation process is implemented safely and effectively to produce positive health outcomes.

Nursing service administrators (NSA) and staff nurses must work together collaboratively and cooperatively to protect the public and maintain the integrity of the nursing care delivery system. The following principles delineate accountability for nurses at all levels from NSA to staff nurses.

Right Task

Nursing Service Administrator (NSA)	Staff Nurse
▪ Appropriate activities for consideration in delegation decisions are identified in UAP job descriptions/role delineation.	▪ Appropriate delegation activities are identified for specific client(s).
▪ Organizational policies, procedures and standards describe expectations of and limits to activities.	▪ Appropriate activities are identified for specific UAP.

Generally, appropriate activities for consideration in delegation decision-making include those:
1. Which frequently reoccur in the daily care of a client or group of clients.
2. Which do not require the UAP to exercise nursing judgment.
3. Which do not require complex and/or multi-dimensional application of the nursing process.
4. For which the results are predictable and the potential risk is minimal.
5. Which utilize a standard and unchanging procedure.

Right Circumstances

Nursing Service Administrator (NSA)	Staff Nurse
▪ Assess the health status of the client community, analyze the data and identify collective nursing care needs, priorities, and necessary resources.	▪ Assess health status of individual client(s), analyze the data and identify client specific goals and nursing care needs.
▪ Provide appropriate staffing and skill mix, identify clear-lines of authority and reporting, and provide sufficient equipment and supplies to meet the collective nursing care needs.	▪ Match the complexity of the activity with the UAP competency and with the level of supervision available.
▪ Provide appropriate preparation in management techniques to deliver and delegate care.	▪ Provide for appropriate monitoring and guiding for the combination of client, activity and personnel.

(Continued)

Figure 46.13 ■ The five delegation rights.

Right Person

Nursing Service Administrator (NSA)	Staff Nurse
■ Establish organizational standards consistent with applicable law and rules which identify educational and training requirements and competency measurements of nurses and UAP.	■ Instruct and/or assess, verify and identify the UAP's competency on an individual and client specific basis.
■ Incorporate competence standards into institutional policies; assess nurse and UAP performance; perform evaluations based upon standards; and take steps to remedy failure to meet standards, including reporting nurses who fail to meet standards to board of nursing.	■ Implement own professional development activities based on assessed needs; assess UAP performance; perform evaluations of UAP based upon standards; and take steps to remedy failure to meet standards.

Right Direction/Communication

Nursing Service Administrator (NSA)	Staff Nurse
■ Communicate acceptable activities, UAP competencies and qualifications, and the supervision plan through a description of a nursing service delivery model, standards of care, role descriptions, and policies/procedures.	■ Communicate delegation decision on a client specific and UAP-specific basis. The detail and method (oral and/or written) vary with the specific circumstances.
	■ Situation specific communication includes: ◆ Specific data to be collected and method and timelines for reporting, ◆ Specific activities to be performed and any client specific instruction and limitation, and ◆ The expected results or potential complications, and timelines for communicating such information.

Right Supervision/Evaluation

Supervision may be provided by the delegating licensed nurse or by other licensed nurses designated by nursing service administrators or the delegating nurse. The supervising nurse must know the expected method of supervision (direct or indirect), the competencies and qualifications of UAP, the nature of the activities which have been delegated, and the stability/predictability of client condition.

Nursing Service Administrator	Staff Nurse
■ Ensure adequate human resources, including sufficient time, to provide for sufficient supervision to assure that nursing care is adequate and meets the needs of the client.	■ Supervise performance of specific nursing activities or assign supervision to other licensed nurses.
■ Identify the licensed nurses responsible to provide supervision by position, title and role delineation.	■ Provide directions and clear expectations of how the activity is to be performed: ◆ Monitor performance ◆ Obtain and provide feedback ◆ Intervene if necessary ◆ Ensure proper documentation
■ Evaluate outcomes of client community and use information to develop quality assurance and to contribute to risk management plans.	■ Evaluate the entire delegation process: ◆ Evaluate the client ◆ Evaluate the performance of the activity

THE FIVE DELEGATION RIGHTS

Reproduced from the NCSBN Web site (www.ncsbn.org) and used with permission from the National Council of State Boards of Nursing (NCSBN), Chicago, IL, copyright 1995.

Figure 46.13 ■ *(continued)*

registered nurse is responsible for determining if delegation is appropriate, even if ordered by a physician, unless the physician or other healthcare professional assumes responsibility for the training and supervision of the unlicensed assistive personnel (UAP) (National Association of State School Nurse Consultants, 2000). The determination to delegate must be made case by case, for each student's health condition, responses and needs are different as are the available school community resources. FIGURE 46.14 contrasts appropriate and inappropriate delegation.

It is preferable when delegating to use someone with health training. If such persons are not

Appropriate Delegation Activities	Inappropriate Delegation Activities
Asks UAP to follow specific directions when assisting the student with a *prn* medication. **Clear direction without modifications must be given to the UAP.**	Tells UAP to use her judgment about when to report to her that the student with diabetes is not feeling well. **Assessment may not be delegated to a UAP.**
Determines the nursing diagnoses for the student newly entering with a gastrostomy tube and develops a care plan that she reviews with the IEP team and delegates the feeding to the UAP. **Nursing diagnoses may be identified and care plans may be developed only by the professional nurse.**	Requests UAP to develop a seizure procedure for the new student since she has cared for so many students; the nurse will review it after it is written. **The care plan may be developed only after a nursing assessment and the nurse must identify procedures needed and provide appropriate training.**
Identifies the goals for a student's IHP and shares with the IEP team for a student newly eligible for special education services after incurring a head injury 6 months ago on the football field. **After assessment and identification of nursing diagnoses, the nurse identifies appropriate student goals and implements them advising the team as appropriate and documenting in the IEP as legally required for special health needs affecting learning.**	Asks UAP to evaluate the student's breath sounds and report whether the lungs sound better and to implement the prn nebulizer treatments if necessary. **The professional nurse is solely responsible for assessment; this may not be delegated nor may nursing interventions that require nursing knowledge, judgment and skill.**
You clarify that you cannot delegate the injection of epinephrine to a certified nursing assistant parent volunteer going on an overnight experience with Jill who is known to be allergic to bees and peanuts. You request that you or a substitute professional nurse accompany the class. **Delegation may be done only when the task is one that is repeated frequently, has a predictable outcome, and does not involve ongoing assessment.**	Acquiesces to principal's selection of a classroom aide for the caregiver of a child needing feeding monitoring due to risk for choking. This aide has been unable to accurately demonstrate CPR and Heimlich techniques. Your principal warned you that she does not believe this is a delegated activity. **It is the professional nurse who has final accountability for the selection of unlicensed staff when delegation is needed in the school setting. Unsafe delegation requires action by the school nurse, even if it means job resignation.**

Figure 46.14 ■ Comparison of appropriate and inappropriate delegation.

obtainable, the selected UAP (Unlicensed Assistive Personnel) must be willing to perform the task following the nurse's training. The school nurse must define and supervise the education, training, and utilization of the UAP. The UAP's training and competency evaluation must occur on an individual student specific basis. For example, training for blood sugar testing must be different for each student—based upon the individual medical orders and a student's usual responses to his or her health condition. Training cannot be generically applied by the UAP to all students needing help with glucose testing. The school nurse must provide clear, succinct directions, including the objectives of the task as well as the limits and expectations for the UAP. Communication includes the school nurse's verbal as well as written direction with verification of the UAP's understanding by accurate return demonstration of the procedure. The UAP must understand the school nurse's responsibility for the quality of care provided by the UAP and the process to be used for supervision. A memorandum of understanding (FIGURE 46.15) and skills check-off list are tools to document these requirements. The school nurse must monitor and evaluate performance. According to state regulations, school policy, and the competency of the UAP, the school nurse will determine the type and frequency of UAP supervision.

Just as for employee evaluation, UAP evaluation should be based on objective criteria, including direct observation, reports, and conferences. Mutually determine with the school principal his or her level of involvement in the evaluation process. In addition, school nurses must be informed about the associated legalities of delegation (i.e., scope of practice of licensed practical nurses, the use of volunteers and delegation, and relation of Good Samaritan laws in job performance). School nurses and supervisors must have access to current and appropriate in-depth resources on this topic in order to practice legally and safely as well as provide appropriate direction to school administrators.

CONCLUSION

Recruitment and retention of quality employees is a challenge, but it is an important issue related to the future of school nursing. Employee recruitment and retention is primarily about the work culture (i.e.,

Sample of Memorandum of Understanding Regarding the Specifications of Delegation
Based on Sample from and Used with Permission of Department of School Health Services, Multnomah Education Service District, Portland, Oregon

DELEGATION AND SUPERVISION OF NURSING TASKS*

Student________________ DOB__________ School________________

Delegable nursing tasks/specialized training regarding:________________________

*Delegation of nursing tasks to unlicensed persons is done in accordance with OAR 851-047-0000. Appropriateness of delegation of a nursing task is determined by a registered nurse. The training of the unlicensed person(s) is done by a registered nurse. The training is student specific and is not transferable to another student or staff person.

As designated caregiver for the above procedures, I do understand that:

- The information for this student is confidential and cannot be discussed with anyone other than those designated and directly responsible for the student's care.
- This intervention is for this student's needs only and is not transferable to other individuals without specific re-training by the school/special needs nurse.
- All delegated caregivers must be supervised at least every 60 to 120 days as to competency in the performance of the above noted procedures. This procedure is good for one calender year from this date, or until a change in the student's status necessitates a procedural change. This student will be periodically reassessed for his/her continued need for this named intervention.

My training did include:

- Reason for task
- Written and verbal direction for doing procedure.
- Demonstration and practice of technique.
- Directions for emergency situations, adverse reactions, risks.

I am willing and able to perform the listed procedures.

____________	____________	____________
Delegated Caregiver Signature/Date	Delegated Caregiver Signature/Date	Delegated Caregiver Signature/Date
RN Signature/Date	RN Signature/Date	RN Signature/Date

Figure 46.15 ■ Sample of Memorandum of Understanding Regarding the Specifications of Delegation. (Based on sample from and used with Permission of Department of School Health Services, Multnomah Education Service District, Portland, Oregon.)

fairness, respect, and responsibility). "Healthcare is known for attracting people who are kind, caring human beings. The trick is to use those traits on each other" (Neuhauser, 2002, p. 477). Creating a positive climate creates a direct link to productivity, job satisfaction, retention, and commitment of employees (Snow, 2002).

Fairness is not sameness, but rather looking at each situation and making decisions based on need and what best serves the entire organization. Each employee is entitled to technically and interpersonally competent supervision. Supervisors and lead staff must also be continuous learners and able to accept and implement change as well as utilize, mentor, and encourage the diversity of the future workforce. Each staff member wants a feeling of connection with and respect from administration.

It is unethical to allocate resources disproportionately, for example, providing less coaching and counseling to the poor or average employee facing performance problems as compared to the "super stars." Ethical supervisors find ways to develop retention plans for the top performers but do not excuse all employees from accountability. Accepting the role of supervisor means responsibility for being the organization's agent, that is, the representative of an organization's core values to their employees. Likewise, supervisor responsibility includes representing to the organization the needs, interests, and well being of the employees. Being effective in a supervisory role is critical to both organizational and individual employee successes.

References

Abrashoff, D. (2002). *It's your ship. Management techniques from the best damn ship in the navy*. New York: Warner Books.

Academic Human Resources and Personnel Services Office. (2002). *Performance review training*. Retrieved December 11, 2003 from http://webster.uihr.uiuc.edu/ahr/PDF%20Forms/PerformanceAppraisal.pdf.

Ali, M., Boulden, G., Brake, T., Bruce, A., Eaton, J. Holden, R., Johnson, R., Langdon, K., Osborne, C., Renshaw, B., Seymour, J. Shervington, M., & Tee, R. (2002). *Successful manager's handbook*. New York: DK Publishing.

Ali, M., Brookson, S., Bruce, A., Eaton, J., Heller, R., Johnson, R., Langdon, K., & Sleight, S. (2001). *Essential managers manual: Managing for excellence*. New York: DK Publishing.

American College of Healthcare Executives. (2002). *Preventing and addressing harassment and aggression in the workplace*. Retrieved December 14, 2003 from http://www.ache.org/policy/harass.cfm

American Nurses Association (ANA). (1994). *Position statement: Registered professional nurses & unlicensed assistive personnel*. Washington, DC: Author.

Americans with Disabilities Act (ADA), Title II. (1990). *Technical assistance manual*. Retrieved December 11, 2003 from http://www.usdoj.gov/crt/ada/taman2.html

A quick guide to employee orientation—Help for managers & HR. (2002). Retrieved December 11, 2003 from http://www.work911.com/articles/orient.htm

Atencio, B., Cohen, J., & Gorenberg, B. (2003) Nurse retention: Is it worth it? *Nursing Economics, 21*(6), 262–268.

Bellios, C. (1997). *Understanding employee drives and motivations*. Retrieved December 11, 2003 from http://www.easytraining.com/motivation.htm.

Berg A., Hansson U., & Hallberg I. (1994). Nurses' creativity, tedium and burnout during one year of clinical supervision and implementation of individually planned nursing care. *Journal of Advanced Nursing, 20*, 742–749.

Blohowiak, D. (1998). *Your people are your product*. Worcester, MA: Chandler House Press.

Bowey, A. (2002). *Motivation at work*. Retrieved December 16, 2003 from http://www.enclopedia.netnz.com/gainsharing/Motivation.html

Brown, J. (2002). *Employee orientation, Keeping new employees on board*. Retrieved December 16, 2003 from http://www.humanlinks.com/manres/articles/employee_orientation.htm

Buckingham, M., & Clifton, D. (2001). *Now, discover your strengths*. New York: The Free Press.

Butterworth, T. (1994). Preparing to take on clinical supervision. *Nursing Standard, 8* (52), 32–34.

Byham, W., & Cox, J. (1988) *Zapp! The lightning of empowerment*. New York: Fawcett Columbine.

Cohn, S., Gelfman, M., & Schwab, N. (2001). Adolescent issues and rights of minors. In N. Schwab and M. Gelman (Eds.), *Legal issues in school health services*. North Branch, MN: Sunrise River Press.

DeCenzo, D., & Robbins, S. (1994). *Human resource management*. Englewood Cliffs, NJ: Prentice-Hall.

EEOC NOTICE Number 915.002, 10/10/95 Retrieved December 16, 2003 from http://www.eeoc.gov/docs/preemp.html

Employers, beware of negligent hiring and retention. (2000). Retrieved December 16, 2003 from http://www. hrhero.com/topics/hire/hire-negligence.shtml

Equal Employment Opportunity Program Evaluations and Compliance Reviews. (2002). Retrieved December 16, 2003 from http://www.aphis.usda.gov/oa/%20crec%20web%20team/crecinside/

Gagliardi, V., & Johnston, T. (2002). *Legal considerations when a board hires a consultant*. Retrieved December 23, 2003 from http://www.pbnlaw.com/PressRoom/legal_consider.shtml

Generational Stereotypes. (2002). Retrieved December 16, 2003 from http://www.boomercafe.com/randstad.htm

Gringberg, D. (2002). *Sexual harassment*. Your workplace newsletter XVIII. Retrieved December 14, 2003 from www.westaff.com/yourworkplace/ywissue18_full.htm

Hallberg, I. R., Hansson, U. W., & Axelsson, K. (1994). Satisfaction with nursing care and work during a year of clinical supervision and individualized care. *Journal of Nursing Management, 1*, 297–307.

Happell, B., Martin, T., & Pinikahana, J. (2003). Burnout and job satisfaction: A comparative study of psychiatric nurses from forensic and a mainstream mental health service. *International Journal of Mental Health Nursing, 12*(1), 39–47.

Hay, M. (1995). *The organizational climate dimensions*. Boston: McBer and Company.

Henry, J., & Henry, L. (January-February, 2002). Leading with soul/Retaining employees. *The Physician Executive, Journal of Medical Management*, 50–53.

Herringer, J. (2002). Once isn't enough when measuring staff competence. *Nursing Management, 33* (2), 22.

Hicks, R., & Hicks, K. (1999). *Boomers, Xers and other strangers: Understanding the generational differences that divide us*. Wheaton: Tyndale House Publishers.

How veterans, baby boomers, generation Xers and generation nexters can all get along in the workplace. (2002). Retrieved December 23, 2003 from http://www.committment.com/getalong.html

Lancaster, L., & Stillman, D. (2001). *When generations collide: Who they are. Why they clash. How to solve the generational puzzle at work*. Retrieved December 16. 2003 http://www.powerhomebiz.com/News/generations.htm

Litwin, G., & Stringer, R. (1968). *Motivation and organizational climate*. Boston: Harvard University Press.

Manning, P., & Brugh, J. (2001). *Recruiting and retaining employees for dummies*. New York: Hungry Minds.

Mayer, R. (1990). *Conflict management: The courage to confront*. Columbus, OH: Battelle Press.

Mehrabian, A. (2001). *Understanding and overcoming work burnout*. Retrieved December 16, 2003 from http://www.kaaj.com/psych/burnout.html

Moore, T. (2002). Job burnout. Retrieved December 16, 2003 from http://www.buildingbetterhealth.com/topic/burnout;$sessionid$JGrSMCYAABFPOCTYA

National Association of School Nurses. (2002a). *Position statement: Education, licensure, and certification of school nurses*. Scarborough, ME: Author.

National Association of School Nurses (NASN). (2002b). *Position statement: Delegation*. Retrieved December 14, 2003 from http://www.nasn.org/positions/delegation.htm

National Association of School Nurses (NASN). (2003). *Position statement: School nurse supervision / evaluation*. Scarborough, ME: Author

National Association of School Nurses (NASN). (2004). *Guidelines for delegating care in the school setting*. Scarborough, ME: Author.

National Association of School Nurses (NASN) & the American Nurses Association (ANA). (2005). *School Nursing: Scope and standards of school nursing practice*. Silver Spring, MD: Nursebooks.org. American Nurses Association.

National Association of State School Nurse Consultants (NASSNC). (2000). Retrieved December 23, 2003 from http://lserver.aea14.k12.ia.us/swp/tadkins/nassnc/NASSNC_del-unlic.html#DELEGATION

National Council of the State Boards of Nursing (NCSBN). (1995). *Position paper: Delegation concepts and decision-making process*. Retrieved December 16, 2003 from http://www.ncsbn.org/public/regulation/delegation_documents_delegati.htm

Nelson, B. (1996). *Motivating today's employees*. San Diego, CA: Nelson Motivation Inc.
Neuhauser, P. (2002). Building a high-retention culture in healthcare: Fifteen ways to get good people to stay. *Journal of Nursing Administration, 32*(9), 470–478.
NOLO Law Centers. (2002a). *Background checks on job applicants and employees*. Retrieved November 9, 2003 from http://www.nolo.com/lawcenter/ency/
NOLO Law Centers. (2002b).
NOLO Law Centers (2002c). *Guidelines for handling discrimination and harassment complaints*. Retrieved December 14, 2003 from http://www.lawsguide.com/mylawyer/guideview.asp?layer=3&article=191
Northwest AHEC, Nursing Regional Workforce Planning Group. (2000). *Generating effective teamwork across the generations: Educational modules for healthcare managers*. Retrieved December 16, 2003 from the World Wide Web: http://www.northwestahec.wfubmc.edu/brochures/genera~1.ppt
Outlaw, W. (1998). *Smart staffing*. Chicago: Dearborn Financial Publishing.
Parting ways: Effective termination techniques. (2001). Retrieved December 12, 2002 from http://www.onlinewbc.gov/Docs/manage/terminations.html
Paunonen M. (1991). Changes initiated by a nursing supervision programme: An analysis based on log-linear models. *Journal of Advanced Nursing, 16*, 982–986.
Pohlman, K. (2001). Legal framework and financial accountability for school nursing practice. In N. Schwab & M. Gelfman (Eds.), *Legal issues in school health services: A resource for school nurses, administrators, and attorneys*. North Branch, MN: Sunrise River Press.
Poster, E., & Marcontel, M. (1999). School nursing role and competence. *Journal of School Nursing, 15* (2), 24–42.
Pulcini, J., Couillard, M., Harrigan, J., & Mole, D. (2002). Personal and professional characteristics of exemplary school nurses. *Journal of School Nursing, 18*(1), 33–40.
Quinn, C. (2002). *Don't hire anyone without me*. Franklin Lakes, NJ.: Career Press.
Rosenberg, D. (2000). *Hiring the best person for every job*. New York: John Wiley & Sons..
Schwab, N., & Gelfman, M. (Eds.) (2001). *Legal issues in school health services*. North Branch, MN: Sunrise River Press.
Simmons, K. (2000). *How to cure "delegation deficiency."* Retrieved December 14, 2003 from http://www.centeronline.org/knowledge/article.cfm?ID=938
Smith, M. L. Publishers. (2000). Excerpt from *West Virginia Employment Law Letter*. Retrieved December 16, 2003 from http://www.hrhero.com/topics/hire/hire-negligence.shtml
Snow, J. (2002). Enhancing work climate to improve performance and retain valued employees. *Journal of Nursing Administration, 32* (7/8), 393397.
Thomas, K., & Morris, R. (2002). Job satisfaction among nurses: A predictor of burnout levels. *Journal of Nursing Administration, 32* (12), 648–654.
Toropov, B. (2001). *Manager's portfolio of model performance evaluations*. Upper Saddle River, NJ: Prentice-Hall.
Tustin, J., Canham, G., Berridge, J, Braden, D., & Starke, T. (2002). Professional development and appraisal system for school nurses. *Journal of School Nursing, 18*(4), 229–236.
Tyme, J. (2000). Delegation trains everyone. Retrieved December 14, 2003 from http://www.ideasandtraining.com/DelegationTrains.html
U.S. Equal Employment Opportunity Commission. (2002). *Federal laws prohibiting job discrimination questions and answers*. Retrieved December 16, 2003 from http://www.eeoc.gov/facts/qanda.html
U.S. National Institute for Occupational Safety and Health (NIOSH). (1999). Retrieved December 16, 2003 from http://www.cdc.gov/niosh/about.html
Winstanley J. (2000). Manchester Clinical Supervision Scale. *Nursing Standard, 14*(19), 31–32.
Workers' Compensation and the ADA. (2002). Retrieved December 16, 2003 from http://www.elinfonet.com/fedarticles/5/37
Zaiger, D. (2001). *School nursing practice: An orientation manual* (2nd ed.) Scarborough, ME: NASN Press.

Court Cases and Legal Decisions

Brito v. Zia Co., 478 F.2d 1200, 1204 (10th Cir.) (1978). Retrieved December 16, 2003 from http://www.usdoj.gov/eoir/OcahoMain/publisheddecisions/Looseleaf/Volume8/1041.pdf
Chevron USA, Inc. v. Superior Court. (1997). 4 Cal. App.4th544,549. Retrieved December 16, 2003 from http://www.tlpj.org/briefs/107-Ting.htm
Evan F. v. Hughson United Methodist Church (1992) 8 Cal.App.4th 823, 843. Retrieved December 16, 2003 from http://www.employmentlawnews.com/negligent.htm
Watson v. Ft. Worth Bank & Trust Co. (1988). 487 US 977, 987, 108 Sup.Ct. 2777, 2785. Retrieved December 23, 2003 from http://billslater.com/uop/Course_work/LAW_529_WFS_Case_Analysis_%20Watson_v_Fort_Worth_Bank_&_Trust.htm

Chapter 47

Dealing with Controversy in the Practice of School Nursing

MARILYN MARCONTEL-SHATTUCK ■ ELIZABETH K. GREGORY

Chapter Outline

INTRODUCTION

Controversy implies at least two different opinions. Some controversies involve interpreting the law; others involve ethical decision-making; still others are just differences of opinion. In the school setting, the outcomes of this process should be in the best interest of the student, the school, and the family.

The goal of school health services is to assist students to obtain, maintain, or improve their health in order that they may be able to take full advantage of their educational opportunities and attain their educational objectives. Along the way, this goal presents multiple issues. The issues presented in this chapter do not easily fit into the preceding chapters. Many schools have dealt with these issues and the content stated here is only a starting point for further exploration.

The school nurse needs to be open to new ideas, knowledgeable, a lifetime learner, and a catalyst for consensus building. Doing things the way they have "always" been done ("Tradition" as the song from *Fiddler on the Roof* goes) means "we will continue to do something one way because we have always done it that way." While some policies or habits do not always need to be changed, the ability to see, plan, and consider all sides of a situation will allow for personal growth and consistently positive outcomes.

The school nurse is an advocate for students and their families. At the same time, the school nurse is part of the professional education team. The nurse who is employed by a school district is expected to support the mission of the district, to follow the laws and policies, and to generally assist all students to reach their full potential. Decisions must be based on facts and logical thinking, not left to chance. However, when policy is not addressing student needs or when school staff needs to address sensitive issues, the school nurse is in an ideal position to lead the process and discussion. The school nurse needs to be knowledgeable and proactive. The ethical code of conduct for professional nursing as well as the principles of ethical decision-making will assist the school nurse when making decisions.

ETHICAL DECISION-MAKING

Being ethical does not mean responding based on feelings or religious beliefs, or abiding by laws or norms. Ethics are standards of right and wrong that prescribe what humans ought to do; they are a set of values, such as honesty and loyalty. Ethics may be called a set of obligations, like being of benefit to others or being fair (Velasquez, Andre, Shanks, & Meyer, 2003). Ethics are the standards by which we live. "Taking care" of every student in the same way may be considered "fair," but it will not be in the best interest of each individual. "Sharing" confidential information about a student, such as about a teen who is a hepatitis B carrier, may be detrimental to the student and affect the teachers' perception of the teen; in addition, it is not ethical. Ethics requires thinking and decision-making. In this situation, ensuring that all the teachers understand standard precautions for bloodborne pathogens and have the protective supplies they might need is sufficient. The law prevents disclosure of healthcare information to non-healthcare providers (i.e., teachers and administrators) without parental permission unless an individual's health or safety would be at risk (see Chapter 13).

Ethics is a systematic, critical reflection of obligations to a client. Ethical decision-making is a rational process for determining the most morally desirable course of action in view of conflicting value choices. Bioethics reflects issues related to healthcare actions. If all parties agree, then no ethical issue exists. To be a true issue, there has to be a realistic choice between at least two possible equivalent courses of action.

The two primary approaches to ethical decision-making are deontological and utilitarian. In the deontological approach, acts are considered to be intrinsically right or wrong independent of their consequences or circumstances. Decisions are based on formal rules of conduct and principles that are absolute in all decisions; there is no gray zone. An example would be that *any* untruth is a lie and deserves the same punishment regardless of the reason or circumstances.

The utilitarian approach attempts to maximize good for the greatest number of individuals affected (Aiken, 2004). No action in and of itself is considered to be right or wrong; rather, it is the intent that decides. The decision is for the good of humanity. Public health laws are based on this approach, in which the end (or protection against disease for most individuals) justifies the means (such as mandated immunizations or clean water standards). In using the above example on lying, a person who "lies" in order not to hurt someone else's feelings might not be punished as severely as someone who lies to absolve responsibility for an act.

Inherent in all ethical decisions are the principles of autonomy, nonmaleficence, beneficence, justice, and veracity (Aiken, 2004). Autonomy refers to the individuals' right to self-determination; that they are free to make decisions for themselves. This principle becomes cloudy when discussing minors, as it becomes the responsibility of the parent to make "reasonable" decisions in the "best interest of the child." However, autonomy is not an absolute right; the student who intends to harm himself or others does not have the right to do so and the school nurse is mandated to seek assistance to stop that process. Autonomy promotes the nursing principle that each individual is unique.

Nonmaleficence is the obligation to make decisions that "do no harm" and beneficence is one's duty to balance the possible benefits against the possible harms of an action. Justice is the principle that all people are equal but that resource allocation is based on need and availability. The final principle is veracity or truthfulness; school personnel must not intentionally deceive a family or student.

Each issue requires the nurse to not only collect pertinent physiological and psychosocial data, but also to assess the relevant values and preferences held by the parents. Decisions are often more palatable to all parties when they incorporate the values of the involved parties. Because of their strong communication skills, school nurses are often in an ideal position to be the liaison with the family.

The *Code of Ethics for Nurses* (American Nurses Association [ANA], 2001) states that nurses must assume responsibility and judgment for their actions. It espouses many of the above ethical principles. Other healthcare professionals adhere to many of the same core beliefs. In school systems, legal guidelines and public policy steer change and decision-making; the background for a decision can therefore be documented to a parent. However, parents need to know that they can dispute administrative decisions.

As part of a school decision-making team, the school nurse should consider and share the following:

1. What benefits and what harms will each course of action produce, and which alternative will lead to the best overall consequences?
2. What moral rights do the affected parties have, and which course of action best respects those rights?
3. Which course of action treats everyone the same, except where there is a morally justifiable reason not to, and does not show favoritism or discrimination?
4. Which course of action advances the common good?
5. Which course of action develops moral virtues (Velasquez, Andre, Shanks, & Meyer, 2004, p. 3)?

The objectives for school health services may conflict with an administrative or school board objective to maintain a balanced budget; but each is trying to further the students' educational goals as they see them. Parents generally want their children to thrive in the educational setting. Their goals may be in conflict with the nurse's goal for the students' special health needs. Consensus is essential for the student's benefit.

DEALING WITH ANGRY PARENTS

Scenario: *When Ann Jackson, the school nurse in a large elementary school, returned to the office after lunch, she had several messages on her answering machine: The first one started with a question, "Ms. Jackson, did you find other children in my daughter's class who had head lice? I happen to know that Marsha got them at your school because other parents have told me their kids got them there, too. Why can't y'all get rid of the kids who are bringing lice to school and leave us alone?" As she continued and left a call back number, the tone of her voice became louder and more demanding.*

Another angry message from a parent was as follows: "Ms. Jackson, the teacher told us that we had to get another shot for Lucinda before she comes back to school. I took her to the clinic Friday and they told me she had all the shots she needed. Now, you say I have to go back to get this other one. I can't take off work again, and the clinic doesn't give her a shot unless I am there." The parent left a phone number so Ann could call her back.

Ann sat at her desk, took a deep breath, and picked up the phone. Two angry parents in one hour were unusual—but the calls were not unlike other calls from frustrated parents.

Definitions

Aggression refers to action, such as attacking a person or a group. It can be a verbal or physical attack.

Anger is a result of a feeling of lack of control over self, the environment, circumstances, or a perception of being treated unfairly (Wegger, 2004). Anger is feeling mad in response to frustration or injury and is an emotional state that varies in intensity from mild irritation to intense fury and rage. Generally it is a normal, healthy emotion. When anger is out of control and a person becomes destructive, it may lead to more serious problems.

Anger management is a way to reduce emotional feelings and the physiological arousal that anger causes. One can not get rid of, or avoid, the things or the people that cause the anger, nor can they change them, but they can learn to control their reactions (American Psychological Association [APA], 2004).

Frustration is the feeling we get when we do not get what we want, or when something interferes with our goals. This may lead to anger.

Hostility is described as a more constant state of anger, antagonism, or unfriendliness.

Issues

1. Parents generally want what is best for their children and follow rules and requirements. However, they consider their child and their time as top priorities. The school nurse may be caught between school district policy, state laws, health department requirements, and parental desire.
2. Frustration with the "system" and erroneous information may lead to anger at the messenger (the nurse). This may come from school

personnel, parents, or students. The school nurse must learn to deal with anger from others and ways to control stressful encounters.

Policy and Management

School nurses rarely work with parents who do not want the best for their child. Parents may not know what their child needs or how to obtain good health care, but it is important to most parents to do the best they can for their child. Even when parents are receptive to the school nurse's suggestions and advice, they may be frustrated by school or health department policies. Frequently these laws and guidelines are the cause of friction with parents.

The more the school nurse is able to reduce the level of anger in a parent, the more likely the parent will receive the information that is needed in order to understand a policy or requirement and, ultimately obtain the proper health care for the child.

One of the most important skills in dealing with anger is the skill of being an effective listener. To help parents or others who become angry it is important to exhibit traits of effective listeners:

- Be attentive (give a nod of the head, make eye contact without challenging).
- Be genuinely interested in the other person's needs or problems.
- Allow the other person to express himself without reacting judgmentally.
- Resist getting drawn into the anger.
- Discuss what needs to be accomplished cooperatively to resolve the conflict (Luhn, 1992).

When interacting with an angry parent, some appropriate nurse responses are to:

- Encourage the parent to express his/her concerns and feelings.
- Ask the parent questions to clarify your understanding.
- Try to negotiate when possible.
- Give the reason for the policy, law, or requirement.
- Encourage alternative solutions (if there are any).
- Restate the rules, guidelines, laws or requirement if the parent seems confused.
- Encourage participation.
- Take the opportunity or initiative to resolve the problem, if you can.
- Be as empathic and understanding as possible.

When the nurse and the parent cannot resolve their differences, it is time to end the meeting and suggest an appointment with the principal, nursing supervisor, or the next level as in a grievance. Parents have the right to "due process" and school districts have those guidelines in place. Another reason for ending discussion would occur if the parent's anger or frustration escalates to being abusive or threatening.

What if the school nurse gets angry? Try to remember it is normal for adults to get angry and important to recognize feelings of anger; however, it is not appropriate, nor will it resolve the current situation for the school nurse to demonstrate anger. As a school professional, it is important to learn and practice positive ways to deal with frustrating situations. Remember that a positive outcome for the client (the student) is the nurse's concern.

DEALING WITH NONCOMPLIANT PARENTS

Scenario: *John came to the school health office for the second time that week. The school nurse knew why he was there. It was fourth period; time for his daily medicine and the teacher always sent him after the second bell rang. For the first four months this year, John's mother had brought his medication to the school like they had discussed. This was a surprise to the nurse because last year she was on the phone weekly to remind the mother to bring it. She knew by memory every excuse the mother used about why she hadn't brought the medicine. Last year the nurse even had to ask the principal to talk to the mother in order to get her to bring the medicine. When the nurse gave John the next to last pill in the bottle this week, she reminded him to tell his mother he needed a refill and she gave him a note to take home and give her. She hoped he was in the health office now to tell her his mom was on her way to school with of his medicine refill. This year she had done better, at least up to now.*

Definition

The nursing diagnosis of noncompliance is the extent to which a person's and/or caregiver's behavior coincides or fails to coincide with a health-promoting or therapeutic plan agreed upon by the person (and/or family, and/or community) and healthcare professional (North American Nursing Diagnosis Association [NANDA], 1999).

Issues

1. Parents who request that medications and treatments be given at school and who do not provide the medications or equipment

necessary may cause further discomfort or illness to their children.

2. Parents who are noncompliant in obtaining immunizations or in providing appropriate treatment of infections or infestations may be a threat to the health and safety of their own child and to other children.
3. School nurses have a role in assisting parents to understand the child's illness and the need to comply with instructions of the healthcare provider.

Policy and Management

The majority of parents want the best for their children, especially when it comes to healthcare. They are cooperative and concerned and appreciate the assistance the nurse and other school personnel provide for students. Unfortunately, there are a few parents who are noncompliant.

Reasons for noncompliance vary, but frequently are one (or more) of the following:

- Concerns about the child's discomfort (as experienced in immunizations)
- The parent's misunderstanding and uncertainty of the need (as with medications prescribed); poor understanding of the seriousness of the illness
- Poor communication about the diagnosis and treatment required (such as with directions for the use of a pediculicide for treatment of head lice)
- Inadequate information and understanding of illness in general or of the child's specific illness or condition
- Frustration with the length of treatment
- Fear of side effects
- Cultural or religious differences (may cause parent or student to refuse treatment or use alternative therapies or faith healers)
- Lack of resources, including finances, time to get the medication or treatment, or no access to a phone or to transportation
- Negative media publicity or information from the Internet or other sources that confuse or misguide the parent and may cause the parent to stop medication or treatment (Adapted from the International Confederation of Childhood Cancer Organizations [ICCCO], 1999)

Whatever the reason for noncompliance, it is best to do everything possible to identify and eliminate deterrents to compliance and enhance factors that will encourage it. This will take some time and effort, but seeing a change in parent behavior and in the health of students are always positive.

Whenever possible, prevention of this problem is in the best interest of the student. Some ways to prevent this problem are through better and more nurse–parent communication by telephone, e-mail or personal counseling, and by putting information or instructions in writing. Using simple instructions in the language of the parent is also necessary. Indications that would sometimes predict a tendency toward noncompliance (i.e., warning signs of parent or family dysfunction, noncomprehension or low socioeconomic status) may allow the nurse to deal with the issues in a different way and cause fewer problems later. Discussing parent noncompliance with the healthcare provider may also be appropriate.

Extreme parental noncompliance where the parent refuses to consider the child's best interest may represent a form of child abuse or neglect (Menahem & Halasz, 2002). If the school nurse suspects that a student's health is threatened by lack of medical treatment, a referral to Child Protective Services or the police is required (Hootman, Schwab, Gelfman, Gregory & Pohlman, 2001). Additional information on child abuse is found in Chapter 39.

SELF-MEDICATION AT SCHOOL

Scenario: *Stuart, age 15, was diagnosed with asthma at age five. His asthma is controlled with medication and careful monitoring by his mother and the asthma specialist. Stuart takes Singular, Rhinocort aqua, and Advair daily, carries a Maxair inhaler as a rescue medication, and has allergy injections once or twice a month. Stuart is currently in the tenth grade. He has a physician's order and a written request from his parents to carry his Maxair inhaler. The school nurse, who is not in the school every day, keeps Stuart's Epi-Pen should he need it. Stuart is a conscientious student and has been carrying his rescue inhaler since third grade. He uses his inhaler prior to orchestra (he plays the flute) and physical education classes (Soccer team). He rarely misses school since he has been in good control of his asthma for years.*

Definition

Self-medication is defined as the ability of and legal authority of a student to carry a prescribed medication on his person in the school setting and to use that medication as prescribed by a healthcare provider without the intervention of an adult.

Issues

Students with chronic conditions who require medication on demand, commonly students with asthma, diabetes, seizure disorders, and severe allergic conditions, need to have their medications *immediately* to control symptoms. In the school setting, students who should have medications on hand but need to obtain these medications in the school health office may skip a dose if they do not want to be late for Physical Education or recess. When students are forced to go to the school health office to get their medicine or check their blood glucose level, they may choose not to go. This may put their health in jeopardy.

Policy and Management

The following questions will help guide the options available to deal with issues related to self-medication at school.

1. *Do school board policies and state laws about self-medication already exist?*

   State government regulates education, medical practice, and nursing practice; therefore there is no national "plan" for medication administration in schools (Schwab, Gelfman, & Cohen, 2001). The practices and customs in one state do not necessarily hold true in another. Thirty-eight states allow students to carry medication for asthma (Jones & Wheeler, 2004).

   If state law does not address students' self-administering medications, has the school district prepared its own policy? Many districts have policies that do not permit students to carry medications at school or at school events (Schwab et al., 2001). There are three federal statutes that may require public schools to permit students to carry emergency medications under certain conditions: The Individuals with Disabilities Education Act, Section 504 of the Rehabilitation Act of 1973, and the Americans with Disabilities Act (Jones & Wheeler, 2004) (Chapter 14). It is against these laws to deny a student the right to maintain health and prevent untoward outcomes; however, the request for permission to carry medications must come from the parents and be included in a student's Individualized Education Program or their 504 Accommodation Plan.
2. *Will a particular student be responsible for self-medication?*

Self-management is important for controlling many chronic conditions. Children and adolescents will vary in their ability to assume management of their condition. The desired outcome for interventions is independent self-care. Factors include their knowledge and beliefs about their condition, the need to be normal, feelings of invulnerability or vulnerability to health problems, and credibility with adults (Velsor-Friedrich, Vlasses, Moberley, & Coover, 2004).

Self-administration of medication by students with chronic health problems is appropriate only if there is a written school board policy to address the practice (Schwab et al., 2001). "Policy should address when and under what circumstance self-administration is permitted and the decision making process" (Schwab et al., 2001, p.218). Even if six-year olds check their own blood glucose levels at home and administer their insulin, does this automatically make it appropriate in the school setting? If so, what location will best suit the student? How much observation should the parent expect? However, before plans are developed, written permission from the healthcare prescriber and from the parents requesting self-administration of medication by the student is required.

As an example, students with asthma need to understand their triggers, management strategies to treat symptoms and/or prevent an attack, what their medications are for, and the proper use of rescue inhalers before they can manage medications on their own (Gregory, 2000). Findings of four high school focus groups for students with asthma were: wanting to be normal; the unpredictability of the disease; credibility of a teen with asthma; and self-management issues (Velsor-Friedrich et al., 2004). Students in the focus groups from the same school did not know anyone else had asthma. One student said, "Like you don't really bring it up" (Velsor-Friedrich et al., 2004, p. 144). Students voiced feelings of powerlessness around second hand smoke or teachers who really do not "cut them any slack" if their asthma is bothering them. One student said, "... so I swam and I could not breathe underwater ... I know I am not going to pass ..." (Velsor-Friedrich et al., 2004, p. 145).

Questions that must be addressed are as follows: How likely are students to "lend" their friends their inhaler, even though the friend does not have a diagnosis of asthma? Is a student with an inhaler at jeopardy for another student swiping the inhaler and throwing it away or depressing the valve to empty the can? How well does the student keep a record of doses used, since the manufacturers recommend going by doses dispensed, rather than shaking the canister to see if it is empty or not (*Allergy & Asthma Today*, 2004).

3. *Does the student understand the principles of treatment and the signs of stress caused by the chronic condition? What is the role of the school nurse?*

   The school nurse should be involved in determining the competency of the student to assess symptoms related to his or her chronic condition and take appropriate steps (Schwab et al., 2001). This includes, but is not limited to:

   - Welcoming students and discussing how they are and what they are currently doing.
   - Assessing the student's knowledge of signs and symptoms and skills in carrying out the action plan. Is remedial action necessary?
   - Observing the students' ability to get an accurate peak flow reading; manage their nebulizer or inhaler; accurately use the blood glucose monitor; or use an Epi-Pen. Determine that the student can decide on an insulin dose and measure the insulin accurately. Does the student know how to determine if the inhaler is nearly empty?
   - Encouraging students with chronic conditions to tell friends and teachers about their diagnosis and what they might need to do it the student started acting 'different.'
   - Making a realistic plan to assist the student to avoid triggers (Velsor-Friedrich et al., 2004).
   - Preparing an Individualized Healthcare Plan (IHP) and an Emergency Action Plan (EAP) that non-medical individuals in the school can understand (see Chapter 9).
   - Communicating with teachers and coaches to provide information on management challenges they may encounter. Do they understand the EAP? Are they supportive of students with chronic conditions? Do they have the necessary supplies to assist the student?
   - Identifying school employees who need to know about a student's condition and EAP. Protocol sheets should be used for training and signed by the nurse who provides the instruction and the participants.
   - Assessing family dynamics, knowledge, and issues, since every student is a part of a family. Does the student have a usual source of health care? Can the student and family access health care? Does the treatment plan seem logical and follow current protocols? How well do the parents understand their child's chronic condition? What barriers to well-managed care do they face? How can the school nurse assist to remove barriers?

The nurse should provide a listening ear to the student with a chronic condition who might need medications or other assistance. The school nurse should emphasize that while having a chronic illness is "different" and can make life more difficult, preventing complications is a goal to better health.

National Association of School Nurses (NASN) Position Statements

The NASN has issued a number of position statements regarding emergency medications and self-medication and treatment in the school setting. Because it is recognized that easy access and prompt intervention with epinephrine is vital to saving lives of those having severe allergic or asthmatic reactions, it is the position of the NASN (1999, 2000b) that school nurses supervise the management and treatment of life-threatening allergies and asthma, but that the self-managed administration of epinephrine should be evaluated on a case-by-case basis by the school nurse, the parent, the healthcare provider, and the student. Medication and emergency policies in school districts must be developed with the safety of all students and staff in mind.

Because medical studies show that management of near normal glucose levels will prevent and slow the development of diabetes complications, NASN (2001) supports the self-management of diabetes, while considering the individual status of each student. "Each student with diabetes is unique in regard to his or her disease process, developmental and intellectual abilities, and required level of assistance with blood sugar monitoring. Academic productivity may be impaired if a student with diabetes is unable to monitor blood sugar levels promptly on an "as needed" basis in the least restrictive educational setting."

The American Academy of Pediatrics (AAP) supports the NASN positions. They state that if the healthcare provider believes the student is qualified for self-administration, the student should be allowed to do so. They reinforce that school districts should have policies in place that allow this practice "in some cases on the basis of a student's level of responsibility and the drug in question" (AAP, 2004, p. 17). AAP (2003) suggests that parents provide written notification "acknowledging that the school bears no responsibility for ensuring the medication is taken" (p. 699).

STUDENTS WITH SPECIAL NEEDS (MEDICATIONS AND/OR SPECIALIZED TREATMENT) ON FIELD TRIPS

Scenario: *Miranda, age 11, is wheelchair bound. Miranda requires medication every four hours because of a seizure disorder and gastrostomy tube feedings every four hours, because of problems with her esophagus. Miranda has a full-time attendant at school to help her with her needs and she must lie down for 20 minutes once a day for a change in position. Miranda enjoys her friends and her classes at school. She is on grade level and uses a laptop to complete assignments. All fifth graders are going to the museum in a week. The personal attendant notified the school nurse and is requesting assistance to prepare for Miranda's trip. The class trip is scheduled for 5 hours. Miranda will need supplies for a tube feeding, medications, and a mat for a rest in a supine position.*

Issues

Students scheduled to participate on a field trip need to receive their scheduled medications or have specialized procedures as ordered. The school nurse is responsible for developing an Emergency Healthcare Plan and training staff who will accompany students on field trip.

Policy and Management

"All students are entitled to participate in the educational program even if special accommodations are needed to meet their special health needs" (NASN, 2000c). Students cannot be denied the opportunity to participate in a field trip if the field trip is part of the student's educational goals. If a student requires a medication or a specialized procedure during the school day and the class is on a school-sponsored field trip, that medication or procedure must be provided. Careful preparation on the part of the school nurse for a student's daily needs will make planning for a special event or substitute nurse easy to accomplish.

The process to be followed related to medications, treatments, and field trips is dependent on state and local mandates. State school board policy and state board of nursing requirements, as well as local district policy, must be in place and will define appropriateness of allowing school personnel to be trained to administer daily medications to students if a registered nurse is not present. State regulations may require a registered nurse to accompany every field trip when students require medication or specialized procedures (Fibison, 2001).

Students must be provided the same level of nursing or healthcare at any school function. Parents can be asked if they will accompany their child on a field trip, but parents cannot be required to attend (Hootman et al., 2001). For example, a student cannot be denied the opportunity to go on a field trip just because he must have an intramuscular medication during the day. However, a registered nurse may have to accompany the student, if the parent is not available.

The school nurse should receive a list of students participating in a field trip and prepare medications and materials for their specialized treatments. A review of the steps for medication administration or the specialized procedure may be in order. Include a written copy of the steps to follow. It is important for the individual giving the medication to a student to write down the time and any untoward results and return that information to the school nurse. "During field trips individual student medications should be individually packaged by a pharmacy in 'travel packs' (one dose per package) or sent in their original container. Original containers can include small, properly labeled containers from a pharmacy filled only with the number of doses needed on the field trip" (Hootman et al., 2001, p. 223).

Emergency medications, such as epinephrine, albuterol inhalers, glucogon, and diazepam suppositories (for seizures), may also need to be placed in an emergency bag and clearly marked (AAP, 2004). At least one adult chaperone must be trained to administer these medications. "Overnight trips require a physician's order for medications not usually taken during the school day" (AAP, 2004, p. 18).

School nurses need to ensure that school personnel are prepared and knowledgeable about their students' specialized physical healthcare needs since these individuals are often primary caregivers and first responders in an emergency (Heller & Tumlin, 2004). Staff must be able to demonstrate to the school nurse that they know how to perform the skill. Emergency healthcare plans need to be expanded to include specific action plans for common problems on and off campus. Emergency care plans should also provide school personnel with possible problems that might occur and the plan for immediate action. These may be related to safety issues, as with a student with a seizure disorder or steps to take should a gastrostomy tube come out.

Requests for providing specialized procedures, as with medication administration, require an order from a healthcare professional and a parental request. Students may also be taught, if appropriate, to participate in their healthcare procedures. When a student's goal is to participate and maybe become independent with healthcare procedures, that goal should be in that student's IEP and IHP (Heller & Tumlin, 2004).

DRUG TESTING OF ATHLETES

Scenario: *Jim had a game coming up Friday night. The coach promised him on Thursday that he would be in the starting lineup and would play the entire game if he continued to play as well as he had all week. He wasn't sure what he was doing that was different, but he knew he was playing better ball than he ever had before. He truly felt like a part of the team. Jim got to the locker room early on Friday afternoon. His teammate, Larry was already there. It was too soon to change clothes, so they walked out to the field. When they passed the water fountain, Larry took an envelope out of his pocket and took a pill. Jim asked him what it was. Larry grinned and said "It's what makes me the fastest guy on the team. One of these white crosses before a game and I'm all over the field." Jim knew it was amphetamine. He had tried some his freshman year and he remembered the good feeling it gave him. During his sophomore year the school started testing athletes for drugs and he quit taking it because playing meant a lot to him. Now his senior year he was finally playing well. Larry held the envelope out and said, "Want one? Go on, they aren't heavy ones. Sometimes I even take two." Jim thought about it. They might have a drug screen thing coming up, but by Monday surely he'd be clear. He reached for the envelope; after all, this was his big night.*

Definitions

Ergogenic aids are various substances used, usually by athletes, in an attempt to enhance performance or add weight to qualify for certain weight categories of competition (see Chapter 40). Some types of ergogenic aids and substances in each type are:

- Medications, such as over-the-counter decongestants, antihistamines, laxatives, antidiarrheal agents, and weight loss medications
- Performance-enhancing drugs such as stimulants (amphetamines, cocaine, caffeine), muscle and strength aids (anabolic steroids), pain relievers (narcotic analgesics), and dietary supplements (androstenedione, dehydroepiandrosterone, and creatine)

Some of these substances are legal and helpful when used appropriately under the direction of a healthcare provider (Hergenroeder & Neinstein, 2002). Others are illegal and it is against the law to possess them.

Psychoactive drugs are drugs that have an impact on thinking, mood, or behavior. The term usually describes the effects of drugs or toxins. Some psychoactive drugs have performance-enhancing side effects, but often decrease performance because of cardiovascular effects and impaired judgment. Drugs in this category are alpha-adrenergic agents, caffeine, nicotine, alcohol, marijuana, cocaine, benzodiazepines, narcotics, and amphetamines (Schwenk, 1997).

Toxicological screening is the testing used to identify traces of drugs and/or alcohol in the blood or urine.

Issues

1. Does a student have a right to privacy and protection from unreasonable search? What is the degree of control and supervision a school may exert over school-age children and youth?
2. Are resources in place to assist the student who "fails" the test, but has no health insurance or sufficient parental income or interest to seek help?
3. Drug screening has limitations: (a) the cost to the school to perform the tests; (b) drug tests do not test for all possible substances used by students to enhance performance; and (c) drugs vary in the amount of time they are in the body prior to excretion (see Chapter 24).

History and Background

Identifying drugs and alcohol in the urine or blood was initially used to determine possible intoxification in a patient with acute medical or psychiatric symptoms. This toxicological screening was expanded over the years to help psychiatrists and other physicians confirm a diagnosis of substance abuse and to determine if medicines were taken as prescribed. Urine and blood tests have been used in more recent years by business, government, courts and schools in an effort to identify drug abuse or drug abuse problems of employees, persons under arrest, and students (American Academy of Child and Adolescent Psychiatry [AACAP], 1990).

In 1995 the U.S. Supreme Court held that random drug screening for athletes did not violate the U.S. Constitution and was permissible (Cohn, Gelfman, & Schwab, 2001). In 2002, the U.S. Supreme Court upheld the legality of a drug testing program for students participating in competitive, extracurricular activities (National Drug Control Policy Office [NDCPO], 2002). In these rulings, the Court only interprets the Federal law. Schools are also subject to state laws that often provide more protection of students' privacy rights. These laws vary from state to state, and some states are in the process of changing their previous state laws. Legal advice is recommended for schools considering drug testing of students.

A recent large-scale national study on student drug testing found no difference in rates of drug use between schools that have drug testing programs and those that do not. This study was based on data collected from 1998 to 2001 on 76,000 students nationwide. The study found that drug testing did not have an impact on illicit drug use among students, including athletes (Yamaguehi, Johnson, & Malley, 2003).

Policy and Management

Some school districts have developed a student drug testing policy. Some of these are available online and could be used as models for schools that choose to develop a student drug testing policy. Representatives from the athletic staff, athletes, school health services, health education staff, physicians, and parents should be involved in policy discussion and development. The following five components should be included in the written policy and guidelines:

1. The purpose of the drug prevention program, the methods of collection, and consequences should be detailed.
2. An educational component must be written and implemented.
3. Testing must be defined and preferably be random.
4. Guidelines for disciplining students with positive test results must be written, approved by the school board, published, and announced to the students.
5. Evaluation of a treatment plan for drug users must be planned, implemented, and ongoing (Hergenroeder & Neinstein, 2002).

The American College Health Association (1999) has written comprehensive guidelines for drug education and testing of student athletes. These guidelines stress the importance of evaluation and counseling for those who test positive or those who identify themselves as needing assistance; these are important components of every program. In addition, confidential counseling without risk of sanctions should also be available to students who want to discuss their drug abuse problems. The guidelines for the collection, testing, education, discipline, and evaluation programs will need to be clearly written and shared with all stakeholders. As with all policy, legal assistance will be needed to ensure that state and federal laws are followed if the school chooses to test.

Some of the alternatives to drug testing suggested in *Making Sense of Drug Testing* (Gunga, Cox, Rosenbaum, & Appel, 2003) are:

- Engage students in after school programs.
- Incorporate reality based drug education into the school curriculum.
- Provide counseling for students/staff who request help for drug abuse.
- Allow students to be assessed and treated by a healthcare professional.
- Encourage parents to be better informed.
- Cultivate trust and respect among students and adults.

TRUANCY AND ABSENTEEISM

Scenario 1: *John and Sally got "busted" after skipping their afternoon classes so they could sit in John's car and drink beer. The officer who arrested them took them to a juvenile center. Both sets of parents were called to pick them up since this was a "first" arrest for truancy and drugs. They were released to their parents and given a date to appear in court. John and Sally were told to be in school all day, every day, and their parents were told to call school officials to check on their attendance in each class.*

Scenario 2: *Bill walked in the front door of his school at 7:30 A.M. He walked down the hall and out the back door. His mother had been bringing him 45 minutes early each morning for a week to serve out a detention for cutting class. Last night he had decided enough was enough. No more detention hall. He was going to skip the whole day today. He knew he could be expelled, but detention was worse. It was like a prison where the teacher never spoke or smiled.*

Scenario 3: *Sara was sick again on Tuesday. She hadn't felt like going to school Monday and the week before she missed three days. School just wasn't fun. She had so much homework to do and her grades were awful. Her mother didn't really care whether she went to school or not. Sara thought her mom enjoyed the time they spent together when she was at home. Her mother didn't finish the ninth grade and she seemed to do as well as the women in the neighborhood who did finish school. Maybe her mom would just let her quit. At least she was going to stay home today.*

Definition and Extent of the Problem

Generally truancy is defined as any unexcused absence from school. Each day, hundreds of thousands of young people are absent from school; many are absent without an excuse and deemed truant. Although national data are not available (in part because no uniform definition of truancy exists), many large cities report staggering rates of truancy and chronic absenteeism (Baker, Sigmon, & Nugent, 2001). Truancy has been labeled as one of the top 10 educational problems in this country's schools, negatively affecting the future of young people (Dekalb, 1999).

It is no longer considered unusual to find young elementary students with a significant truancy problem. Many large city elementary schools report students missing numerous days of school each year. When children are truant at younger ages, problems usually have as much to do with parent issues as with the student.

An adolescent or younger student who is truant or drops out of school makes a conscious decision to miss school. One of the most common causes of this is school failure. High-risk social behaviors (gang involvement, violence, running away, sexual promiscuity, and excessive drug and alcohol use) are often seen in connection with truancy and in students dropping out (Schubiner, Robin, & Neinstein, 2002).

Some absences for illness may be part of truancy. Students who state illness as a reason for missing school may be reflecting somatic complaints. These somatic complaints do not have to be associated with a psychiatric disorder, but for those who do, anxiety and depression are common (Houck & Perri, 2002). The students in the above study stated they were absent because of pain or fatigue, but they did not routinely seek healthcare professionals for health complaints.

Absenteeism is common in the student with a chronic medical condition. Those with severe asthma, cystic fibrosis, diabetes mellitus, sickle cell anemia, juvenile rheumatoid arthritis, epilepsy, congenital heart disease, or other disorders may have had absences due to their symptomatology and those absences may cause them to have academic problems. In addition, the side effects of the medication(s) these students take may also impair their cognitive function (Schubiner et al., 2002).

Issues

1. Because behavior problems leading to truancy are often followed by more serious behavior problems, truancy has been linked to delinquent and criminal activity (burglary, auto theft, vandalism), substance abuse, and gang activity, in young people.
2. Adults who were frequently truant in school are more likely to have poorer physical and mental health, lower paying jobs, increased chance of living in poverty, and more reliance on welfare support, and have children who exhibit problem behaviors and an increased likelihood of incarceration (Baker et al., 2001).
3. School nurses are not often included in the student assistance teams in the schools, especially related to truant students.

Types and Reasons for Truancy

Baker et al. (2001) grouped the numerous reasons for truancy into four general categories: family, school, economics, and student. The family category includes a lack of guidance or parental supervision, parental drug or alcohol abuse, lack of awareness of attendance laws, and differing views about education. In the school category, the highest numbers of truant students are usually from inner city schools and poverty in these areas is cited as a cause. In addition, the attitude of teachers, students, and administrators, inconsistent attendance policies, and lack of meaningful consequences are cited as causes. Economic issues sometimes require students to work; more often these students are from a single-parent home or are parenting teens who lack child care (Baker et al., 2001). Student factors include drug and alcohol abuse, misunderstanding or ignorance of attendance laws, physical and emotional ill health, lack of school-engaged friends, and lack of proficiency in English. Low academic achievement and weak basic skills are other major reasons for truancy.

Policy and Management

Intervening early in the school year with those students who are absent for vague complaints may provide that feeling of connectedness to the school community that may increase attendance (Houck & Perri, 2002). School nurses need to be a part of the school team that evaluates students with unexcused absences in order to provide available health history information or to assess the students' health history and physical condition and, if appropriate, refer the student for medical, psychological or psychiatric evaluation.

To successfully help students stay in school, the issue of truancy must be a priority of school personnel and the community. An important step to be taken is to determine a definition and policy for truancy. The National Association of Secondary School Principals (cited by Dekalb, 1999) has suggested that creating effective attendance policies requires following these guidelines:

- The policies should be strong. Schools that invest thought and effort into solving the problem make the most headway.
- Participation in the formulation of the attendance policies should be broadly based.
- Attendance expectations, as well as consequences of good and poor attendance, should be specified in writing.
- Policies should be well publicized.
- Policies should be consistently enforced at every level: by teachers, counselors, and the principal.
- Every absence should be followed up by a telephone call or a letter.

Numerous examples of state and local policies and guidelines are on the Internet under "truancy." An exploratory look at some these may be helpful for those who are developing policies and interested in creative and successful methods to eliminate absenteeism.

SCHOOL REFUSAL

Scenario: *Juan and his family moved from Mexico to the United States two years ago. He is the youngest of six children and lives with his parents and three siblings. The other siblings are still living in Mexico. Juan entered the third grade and did well. He is now in the fifth grade. He did not return to school after the December holidays this year due to illness. In February, at the request of the principal, the school nurse visited Juan and his mother in their home. The mother told the nurse that when she mentioned school, Juan would cry and become physically sick, often to the point of vomiting. The mother had taken him to the doctor, and the doctor was unable to find anything physically wrong with him. The doctor told Juan and his mother that he should be in school; however, he continues to cry, scream, complain of stomachaches, and vomits when she tries to take him to school. She said she wants Juan to be in school, but is not willing to "force" him to go.*

Definition

School phobia, school avoidance, and school refusal are terms used to describe the signs of anxiety in children who have a persistent, abnormal and irrational fear of going to school. Approximately 1% to 5% of school-age children experience school refusal at some time and to some degree. The condition is more common in children 5 to 6 and 10 to 11 years of age, but may occur at any age. It occurs in boys and girls from all socioeconomic levels (Fremont, 2003).

Refusal to go to school often starts after a time when the child was at home for a summer vacation or a holiday break. Sometimes it is after a brief illness. These are times when the child has become closer to the parent. It may also come after a stressful occurrence at home or at school, such as the death of a relative or pet, a bullying or embarrassing incident at school, a move to another neighborhood, or a change in schools (AACAP, 1998).

The student may complain of not feeling well just before time for school. The "illness" soon goes away but reappears the next morning at school time. Some children just refuse to leave the house (AACAP, 1998).

Issues

1. Absenteeism is a huge problem in schools. Many school nurses are actively involved in school attendance issues, and are often the ones who identify a student with school refusal (Karasik, 2003). Identifying the absent student and the cause of the absence may be the responsibility of the school nurse.
2. Students who do not attend school are sometimes dropped from the school enrollment records without the school identifying the cause of the absence.
3. Students with school refusal often have other behavioral problems. Dysfunctional family interactions are frequently seen in families of children with school refusal (Fremont, 2003).

History and Background

The term "school phobia" was used in the 1930s to describe the child who was anxious or fearful about school attendance. Professionals criticized the use of the word "phobia" because the behaviors involved did not meet the criteria for true phobias. Researchers prefer to use the terms "school avoidance syndrome" or "school refusal" (Paige, 1998). Some students fear school-related activities, such as the behavior of other children toward them, examinations, or riding the bus. Some children may be anxious about being separated from their caregiver or have other issues surrounding home or family. If it is caused by a fear of another child or of a teacher, of taking a test or of parent separation, it may be more easily resolved than when the cause is less obvious or more severe (see Chapter 34).

The child may enjoy receiving additional attention from caregivers, may have more fun at home than at school by being able to watch TV and play games and may enjoy the home routine more than school pressures. School avoidance or refusal is not a formal psychiatric diagnosis. A student with school refusal may exhibit emotional distress and some 30% to 50% may show an associated psychiatric disorder, such as anxiety or depression (Houck & Perri, 2002).

Truancy is distinguished from this group by antisocial and delinquent behaviors. In addition, a truant student is not anxious about school, and is not with parents or caregivers when out of school (see issue on Truancy and Absenteeism, above).

Policy and Management

As with many issues involving health and healthcare, school refusal is not generally included in school board policy. Guidelines developed by personnel in departments such as health services, psychological services, social services, and counseling should ensure that efforts are made to assist the parents and students with support and counseling, and provide information to faculty and staff concerning assisting students with this problem. Professionals in these disciplines may also need to work with the student, the family, and administration to deal appropriately with student absences as the issue is being resolved.

Treatment for school refusal depends on the cause. In some instances, helping a parent understand how to deal firmly with the child will be sufficient. Many times a child's family reinforces the school refusal symptoms. More involved cases may require the help of a psychologist or psychiatrist. Some students require medication, depending on severity and underlying problems, which could be family dysfunction or clinical phobia (Schubiner et al., 2002).

Children with an unreasonable fear of school may throw tantrums, have panic attacks, cry, display shyness, irritability, or unhappiness, make demands for parental attention, feel unsafe in a room by themselves, display clinging behavior, or have difficulty going to sleep (AACAP, 1998).

A variety of somatic complaints and symptoms may occur in students with school refusal. These include dizziness, diaphoresis, headaches, palpitations, abdominal pain, nausea, vomiting, diarrhea, and back and joint pain (Fremont, 2003). The parent who understands that there may be times when the child is truly ill will need to know what symptoms to look for when the child complains of illness before taking the child to school. Basically, these would include fever over 100°F, vomiting more than one time, frequent cough, frequent diarrhea, widespread rash, earache, or toothache. It may require a trip to the doctor to determine wellness or illness, but the parent can then take their child to school for the rest of the day.

In an effort to prevent school refusal, the school nurse and other school staff involved with the student need to encourage parents to assist or allow their children to become independent. This process starts in early childhood and continues throughout childhood. The school nurse can provide a site for support to assist the student to return to the classroom. For children who are very fearful, extra help may be needed for longer periods of time. If the child is extremely upset and needs to be forced to attend school, if there is a great deal of family stress, or if the refusal is becoming habitual, the family should ask for help from the school psychologist, school counselor or other mental health provider (Paige, 1998).

GENDER IDENTITY AND SEXUAL ORIENTATION: LESBIAN, GAY, BISEXUAL, TRANSGENDER, AND QUESTIONING YOUTH (LGBTQ*)

Scenario: *Terry and Pat are inseparable. While they do not have classes together, they travel to and from school together and both are members of the drama club and tennis team. The school nurse has heard students talk about the pair's closeness in terms that make the nurse wonder about health and safety issues with any same-sex relationship. Since Pat sees*

*LGBTQ is used in the current literature (Benton, 2003; NASN, 2003).

the nurse at least weekly because of asthma, the nurse decides to set out some pamphlets on lesbian and gay relationships and support group hotlines. Meanwhile the nurse should review current literature in this developmental area and review an effective communication manual in order to plan some leading questions to begin discussion.

Definitions

Lesbian—females who partner only with females

Gay—males who partner only with males (*also homosexual*)

Bisexual—a person who partners with both males and females

Transgender—"an umbrella term describing a number of distinct gender positions and identities including: transsexual, transvestite, transgeneralist, androgyne, intersex, hermaphrodite, and the states of cross-gender, cross living, and cross-dressing" (Bakker & Cavender, 2003. p. 66).

Questioning youth—"Youth who desire or engage in same-sex behavior. Questioning is often used as a shorthand term for this diverse group of young people who do not identify as being lesbian, gay, or bisexual" (NASN, 2003, p. 1).

Homophobia—an irrational fear of, aversion to, and prejudice against individuals perceived to be other than hetersexual (Rutgers University School Health Services (RUHS), 2004).

Heterosexism—the institutionalizing of heterosexuality as the norm (RUHS, 2004). It "resembles racism or sexism and denies, ignores, denigrates, or stigmatizes nonheterosexual forms of emotional and affectional expression, sexual behavior or community" (Center for Substance Abuse Treatment, 2003, p. xiv).

Heterosexuality—"erotic, romantic, and affectional attraction to people of the opposite sex" (Bakker & Cavender, 2003, p. 66)

Sexual orientation—an individual's pattern of physical and emotional attraction to and arousal by other persons. This is not synonymous with sexual activity (Frankowski, 2004) and falls within a continuum of opposite sex attraction to same-sex attraction.

Gender identity—the sense of oneself as a male or female

Gender role—outward expression of maleness or femaleness as viewed by a particular culture

Issues

1. School-age children and youth who are LGBTQ may experience developmental difficulties.
2. Students who are LGBTQ have unique health and safety concerns.
3. The role of the school nurse with students who are LGBTQ must be specific enough to meet their multiple needs and must not be affected by the school nurse's personal feelings of variations of sexual preferences.

Problems

Developmental Difficulties of Being LGBTQ in School-Age Children and Youth

Developing a sexual identity is part of growth and development and is one component of a person's identity. Homosexuality is considered to be a *normal* variation of human sexual and emotional expression and is *not* a form of mental illness or defective development (Center for Substance Abuse Treatment [CSAT], 2003). In most cases, one's sexual orientation is not a choice and is due to a combination of genetic, hormonal, and environmental influences (Frankowski & Committee on Adolescence, 2004).

While sexual identity is usually identified as a developmental task of adolescents, (sexual attraction often coincides with gonadarche [age 12 for females and 14 for males]), sexual attraction often begins in elementary school (Harrison, 2003). From the age of 10 on, students are developing and dealing with their sexuality. While initial awareness of feelings for someone of the same sex may have occurred at age 10, the first experience with someone of the same sex often occurs between ages 13 and 15, allowing most teens to identify their sexual preference by age 16 (CSAT, 2003).

Adolescents, as well as younger students, may be confused or concerned about their sexuality and/or gender identification issues. Experimentation is part of this process, yet some students may misperceive behaviors and thoughts as a permanent and telling characteristic of one's sexual identity. The number of students who consider themselves to be LGBTQ ranges from 1% to 10%, with more males than females. Up to 25% of 12-year-olds are uncertain about their sexual orientation; by age 18, only 5% are still uncertain (Frankowski & Committee on Adolescence, 2004). Students with disabilities may also be among the LGBTQ group (Benton, 2003).

Youth who are LGBTQ are at higher risk of being rejected by friends, dropping out of school, and being kicked out of their homes (Frankowski & Committee on Adolescence, 2004). They may feel there is no one in whom they can trust. They may become homeless and may resort to prostitution to support themselves, thus putting themselves at greater physical risk as well as risk from psychosocial deficits due to a lack of love, trust, and security.

LGBTQ youth represent mainstream and diverse cultural and minority groups "for whom identity concerns may be particularly salient during adolescence" (APA, 2002, p. 19). Questions about sexual identity may arise from feelings of being "different" because of attractions to their own sex, experimentation, or concern when they do not share an attraction for the opposite sex that their friends profess. Confusion about sexual orientation may lead adolescents to deny their feelings, seek out the opposite sex, or isolate themselves.

Unique Health and Safety Concerns for LGBTQ Youth

To cope with the confusion, loneliness, and social ostracism, many LGBTQ students turn to drugs and alcohol. Coping difficulties may be exacerbated by anti-gay violence in the school. Students with gender issues are at a higher risk for beatings or personal injury because of stigma or prejudice. This may occur in the form of physical or verbal abuse, bullying, or harassment. The more stereotypically gay a student is, especially for youth of color, the more chance there is of victimization (CSAT, 2003). CDC (1999) reported increased fears among these students of physical attack at school. These attacks often lead to truancy, more for an attempt to be safe rather than avoidance of school.

LGBTQ may be at higher risk for health problems than their peers depending on their lifestyle. "Non-heterosexual youth are more likely to have had sexual intercourse, to have had more partners, and to have experienced sexual intercourse against their will, putting them at increased risk of STDs including HIV infection" (Frankowski & Committee on Adolescence, 2004, p. 1829). Sexually active males who have sex with males account for 34% of all new AIDS cases among 13- to 24-year-olds in the United States (CDC, 2000). Girls with lesbian feelings are at higher risk of teen pregnancy, sexually transmitted diseases (STDs), and human immunodeficiency virus (HIV) infection because they feel pressured to experiment or hide their true feelings and have unprotected sex (Bakker & Cavender, 2003; Benton, 2003).

Homosexual and bisexual youth are at higher risk for depression and are two to seven times more likely to attempt suicide than their non-LGBTQ peers (Frankowski & Committee on Adolescence, 2004). The suicidal thinking may have more to do with stress, violence, family problems, lack of support, and other problems (Bakker & Cavender, 2003). These issues may also put them at risk for low self-esteem, altered body image, and eating disorders. Their social isolation decreases their ability to develop dating skills. Their need to keep their sexuality a secret interferes with their ability to find positive role models (Harrison, 2003).

Policy and Management

All students are equally deserving of respect and fair treatment and have the right to a school environment that is safe and supportive. The stress brought about by discrimination and stigmatization of LGBTQ youth leads to increased health and safety risks. Because of this, NASN (2003) issued a statement that reads:

> It is the position of the National Association of School Nurses that all students, regardless of sexual orientation, gender expression, and gender identity are entitled to equal opportunities in the educational system. The school nurse needs to be aware of students who are lesbian, gay, bisexual, transgender and questioning; sensitive to their needs; knowledgeable about the health needs of this group of students; and effective in interventions to reduce risk factors. The school nurse should be actively involved in fostering a safe environment, demonstrating an understanding of the issues and modeling respect for diversity.

Perhaps first on the agenda for students who are LGBTQ is to provide the safety and acceptance for them to disclose their preferences or questions. The adolescent tends to tell a trusted friend first, and if family members know, the mother is told before the father (Savin-Williams, 1998). Students who disclose to the school nurse want someone they trust to listen. At the same time, when students disclose sexual explorations, the professional should not assume that the student is developing a LGBTQ identity (APA, 2002). When they choose to disclose to the school nurse or other school professional, their feelings should be kept in confidence. There is no reason for this information to be shared unless the student is depressed or suicidal. Students may not be sure of their feelings or may be seeking your reaction. They want acceptance.

It is essential for the school to provide each student with a safe environment. This ensures an environment free of violence and harassment, free of judgment, and confidential for their sharing of real or perceived health and developmental issues. Students do *not* want to hear that they are too young to be sure (APA, 2002). They do *not* want to hear that this is a phase they will outgrow, nor do they want to hear your religious views.

The school nurse, often the trusted confidant for students with a variety of concerns, should provide a compassionate, listening ear for adolescents with concerns about their sexuality and provide much needed health education. Identifying students who may consider themselves LGBTQ is not as important as having these students being able to identify the school nurse as safe and approachable (Benton, 2003).

Disclosure to family is more successful if the family is cohesive and there are positive family dynamics and acceptance of those who are different. Students who have low self-esteem, have poor relationships with their family members, and are abused or rejected in the home are less likely to disclose their sexual preference (Harrison, 2003). It may be helpful for students to role-play the disclosure process with the school nurse before going to their parents. This role-play should include how they might handle the hostility or disappointment they might receive. The school nurse might also offer to be with the student when he or she tells the parents. The student needs to understand that parents might need time to grieve for themselves.

The role of the school nurse with students who are LGBTQ must be specific enough to meet their multiple needs and must not be affected by the school nurse's perceptions of variations of sexual preferences. Benton (2003) reported on data from Sawyer's (2001) study of school nurses' attitudes and practices in addressing LGB adolescent physical and mental health in schools. While 48% of school nurses surveyed stated nurses should counsel students about their sexual orientation, only 23% actually did. While 84% of the same nurses believed nurses should counsel LGBTQ students to practice safer sex, only 32% provided that counsel. If needed, the school nurse should confer with the school counselor or district psychologist for educational literature for themselves and their students for discussion with them. Being nonjudgmental is essential. Use gender-neutral language, such as "partner" rather than "boyfriend" or "girlfriend."

LGBTQ youth must develop interpersonal skills that allow them to meet interested others while they are developing a sense of who they are (self-esteem) and a personal identity (Bakker & Cavender, 2003). They need accurate sexuality information regarding sexually transmitted diseases and how they are transmitted by some sexual practices and what measures might be taken to prevent these. If this form of sex education is not allowed in the school, the school nurse can have an information sheet with available community resources to provide assistance. It certainly needs to be reinforced that "most homosexual adolescents develop into productive healthy adults" (Harrison, 2003, p. 110).

The school nurse needs to assess:

- What resources are available in the community?
- What policies are in place to prevent discrimination and harassment to students who are LGBTQ? Are they followed?
- Are there safety issues in the school related to sexual orientation?
- Do the parents or a trusted friend know? (Does the student have a support system?)
- Do the parents accept their child's sexual orientation? Parents may need referral to a support group.
- Has sexual activity been initiated and, if so, is protection used? Does the student need to be screened for STDs?
- Is the student depressed? If so, has the student considered suicide (see Chapter 34)?

Two intervention practices *strongly discouraged* by multiple healthcare and educational groups include "reparative therapy" that attempts to convert someone who is homosexual to heterosexual by eliminating their desire for members of their own gender, and "transformational ministry" that uses religion to eliminate homosexual desires. Since homosexuality is not a mental disorder and is not listed in the *Diagnostic and Statistical Manual of Mental Disorders*, it does not need correction. Nor should one religious belief be imposed on others. Health and mental health organizations, as well as multiple education groups "do not support efforts to change young people's sexual orientation through "reparative therapy" and have raised serious concerns about its potential to do harm" (Just the Facts About Sexual Orientation, 2000). Laws that prohibit discrimination and separation of church and state also apply here.

DO NOT RESUSCITATE ORDERS IN SCHOOLS

Scenario: *Rita, a 10-year-old student in a special class for students with learning difficulties and physical handicaps, has been enrolled at J. R. Lewis Elementary School for three years. Rita has not been able to move her body since birth, but can follow movement and sound by moving her head. She recognizes her mother's voice and can track light. When unhappy, she cries. Her mother provides excellent care and Rita does not have any reddened skin areas on her body. Rita has a seizure disorder involving involuntary arm movements. The seizures seem to be triggered by atmospheric changes. She experiences episodes of difficulty in breathing, which have worsened in the past few weeks. She is sleeping more than usual. Rita has had repeated upper respiratory infections and pneumonia twice in the past three months. She does not have bladder control and is catheterized every three hours. In the past six months, Rita has been treated four times for bladder infections.*

Rita's doctor discussed her deteriorating condition with her parents last week. He also signed a Do Not Resuscitate Order at the family's request and he advised them to contact Family Hospice for assistance. They are working with that agency, and the outreach nurse has counseled the parents and will continue assisting them.

The school nurse is scheduling a meeting with the parents, the Family Hospice nurse, the school counselor, principal, teacher and herself to discuss and plan how the school and school personnel can work with this family and continue to provide care and support for Rita when she is at school.

Definitions

Do Not Resuscitate (DNR) order—A physician's order for a patient indicating that no basic or advanced cardiac life support efforts will be initiated in the event of cardiac and/or respiratory arrest. The physician's order or directive is addressed to emergency medical responders indicating the predetermined request by the patient or guardian or surrogate to withhold cardiopulmonary resuscitation (CPR) and other end-of-life resuscitative treatments once breathing and/or heartbeat have ceased. It is a directive that allows the patient to be able to die without emergency intervention. Positioning for comfort and all other needed care (i.e., administration of oxygen, suctioning, use of the Heimlich maneuver for choking, and control of bleeding or pain) are continued.

Advanced cardiac life support (ACLS)—This term refers to attempts at restoration of spontaneous circulation using basic CPR plus advanced airway management, endotracheal intubation, mechanical ventilation, defibrillation, and intravenous medications.

Basic life support (BLS)—BLS is the phase of emergency care that includes recognition of cardiac and/or respiratory arrest, access to the EMS system, and basic CPR. Basic CPR is the attempt to restore spontaneous circulation using the techniques of chest compressions and pulmonary ventilation.

Issues

1. School personnel are rarely asked not to consider providing all care they can for a student. Even when a child's condition is irreversible, complying with a DNR order is emotionally painful for everyone concerned. Parents of healthy children and many school personnel find it unacceptable for a child to die at school (AAP, Committee on School Health and Committee on Bioethics, 2000).
2. Parents and students have rights.
3. In some instances, parents of medically fragile, chronically ill, and terminally ill students do not wish CPR to be initiated in the case of respiratory or cardiac arrest. The school district may be petitioned to honor a DNR order (NASN, 2000a).
4. A DNR order could be misinterpreted by untrained staff and therefore mishandled.

History and Background

An increasing number of students with life-threatening medical problems are enrolled in the nation's school. School personnel including nurses are routinely dealing with challenges unique to the care of this population. School officials may receive requests from some of these families and their physicians to limit resuscitative efforts in the case of respiratory or cardiac arrest of the child.

When a medical condition is too far advanced to expect recovery and death is imminent, the family may ask the physician for a Do Not Resuscitate (DNR) order. The purpose for the DNR order is to provide the dying child supportive and compassionate care without prolonging the process or discomforts of dying (Wold, 2001). When families choose to do this, there is a possibility the child will die while in school. The ethical, moral, and legal issues involved cause school officials to deal with issues with which most have never dealt.

Policy and Management

In the 1970s when Public Law 94-142 (The Education for All Handicapped Children's Act) was passed, school personnel were not sure medically fragile children would be able to attend public schools. Gradually, procedures and facilities were developed to accommodate these students. As more state laws allow for DNR in schools and more families request this for their child, it appears that this issue, too, will be resolved. Nevertheless, "DNR orders for children should be considered rare and extraordinary measures intended strictly to benefit the child. Such unusual directives should only be used when death is inevitable in light of a terminal medical condition" (Costante, 2001, p. 423).

The American Academy of Pediatrics (2000) recommends that pediatricians:

- Assist to develop plans and procedures that respect the rights and interests of a dying child.
- Meet with parents and school officials—nurses, teachers, administrators—and emergency medical services personnel, to develop plans for in-school medical interventions.
- Help parents and schools understand a child's condition.
- Review the plans for in-school care at least every 6 months.
- Review the plan with the board of education and its legal counsel. Work with school systems and parent/teacher organizations to develop age-appropriate education programs about death and dying.
- Be available to assist teachers and parents when a child dies at school.

School personnel and district administration will need to discuss and plan in order to make complex decisions regarding a DNR request. "As a basic requisite any school having a student with a DNR order should have a full time professional nurse to manage the student's care and implement the medical directives" (Costante, 2001, p. 432).

Each child with a DNR order should have an IHP and an EAP developed by the professional school nurse with involvement from the parents, administrators, physicians, teachers and the student when appropriate (Constante, 2001; NASN, 2000a). Developing a DNR policy in a public school requires the identification of local, state, and federal laws related to DNR orders and care of medically fragile students; assessment of practices currently associated with care of these students; establishment of community and administrative support, and the guidelines and support services necessary for individuals who will care for this student if the student dies at school.

HEALTH INSURANCE FOR CHILDREN

Scenario: *Joanne, who is 10 years old, was diagnosed with asthma when she was 7. Her symptoms are moderate but tend to worsen in the presence of dust, mold, cigarette smoke and cold weather. Since her diagnosis, her mother has made continuous efforts to keep their apartment free from allergens. Joanne has used several medications to control her asthma and she sees her primary care provider on a scheduled basis and as needed with acute problems. Joanne lives with her mother and a younger brother. The mother has worked for the same employer for 15 years, and Joanne and her brother have been covered under her health insurance plan at work since birth. Her employer recently told her that a cost-cutting measure necessary for the company would eliminate insurance coverage for her and her children. The mother's options are CHIP, Medicaid, private health insurance, or community clinics.*

Definitions

Community clinics—Hospitals and religious groups may finance a freestanding clinic for walk-in type healthcare (URI, chronic health problems) but are not usually equipped for fractures or emergencies. Payment is on a sliding scale fee-for-service basis.

Medicaid program—Title XIX of the Social Security Act was established in 1965. It is also known as Medicaid. The program is a joint-funded federal-state program. Medicaid provides medical assistance to certain families and individuals with low incomes. These are primarily the aged, poor, blind, disabled, and families with dependent children (Behrman, 2003).

Privately purchased health insurance—A fee-based service of some insurance companies. this insurance is usually costly and may have high deductibles, especially for parents with young children or those with chronic conditions.

State Children's Health Insurance Program (SCHIP)—The Balanced Budget Act of 1997 was responsible for Title XXI of the Social Security Act. This is called the State Children's Health Insurance Program (SCHIP). It allows each of the states to establish their own programs, to expand their Medicaid program, or to use a combination of these programs to provide health insurance for low-income children. States are allowed a great deal of flexibility in the design and operations of SCHIP, and receive an enhanced match rate for services provided to eligible children (Behrman, 2003). Availability is based on income.

Issues

Health insurance should be available and affordable for all children.

1. Existing programs can provide insurance for most children.
2. Program funding needs improvement.
3. Outreach, enrollment, and retention of clients are critical for program success.
4. School nurses can be leaders and collaborate with other community members to expand outreach efforts.

History and Background

Medical insurance was first offered in 1847 by a commercial insurance company. The purpose was to defray financial loss from disability after accidents or from specific communicable diseases, such as smallpox and scarlet fever (Stanhope & Lancaster, 2000).

Ensuring healthcare for children in poverty has developed over several decades. Maternal and child health programs started in the Depression era and evolved into entitlement programs for low income children (Mann, Rowland, & Garfield, 2003).

Public health insurance coverage for children has evolved into an important national priority. This began in 1965 with the creation of Medicaid and continued with the State Children's Health Insurance Program (SCHIP) in 1997. Filling the gap between Medicaid and employment-based coverage, SCHIP focuses on the uninsured children of working, low-income families. According to census data of 2001, 16.5 million children (23% of all children nationwide) were covered by Medicaid or SCHIP; and about 8.5 million children (12% of all children nationwide) were uninsured (Bennett & Shields, 2003).

As of September 30, 1999, each of the states and territories had an approved plan in place (Centers for Medicare and Medicaid Services [CMMS], 2004). When designing state programs, there are three options. The state can either:

- Use SCHIP funds to expand Medicaid eligibility to children who previously did not qualify for the program;
- Design a separate children's health insurance program entirely separate from Medicaid; or
- Combine both the Medicaid and separate program options.

Since 1997, significant progress has been made in reducing the number of uninsured children; however, funding problems and state budget short falls are threatening these programs. Despite the success of Medicaid and SCHIP, there are high uninsurance rates among low-income children due to a weak economy, rising healthcare costs, and funding shortfalls (Behrman, 2003). It is clear that the federal and state governments and local community resources will need to continue to work together to ensure that these public health programs are ongoing.

Policy and Management

The majority of low-income children who still lack health coverage are eligible for either Medicaid or SCHIP. There are several barriers to enrollment. Many parents are still unaware that programs exist or that their children are eligible. If the children are successfully enrolled, they may lose coverage when the parents do not comply with enrollment requirements.

Schools and school nurses are vital links to identifying uninsured children and to encouraging enrollment into Medicaid and SCHIP (NASN, 2002). They are involved in outreach programs and collaborate with state and local organizations to expand outreach activities to assist eligible families obtain healthcare coverage. Successful outreach programs in schools may include:

1. Identifying students who do not have health insurance and mailing a letter or making personal contact to inform parents and enroll students in the SCHIP program.
2. Ensuring that Free and Reduced Lunch forms include health insurance eligibility and consent to share information.
3. Providing Medicaid and SCHIP information on Back to School night (or other meetings with parents), in all appropriate languages.
4. Linking SCHIP information with school registration forms.
5. Writing articles for the school and district newsletters to inform parents of SCHIP.
6. Including SCHIP information with athletic physical and school athletic insurance information.

7. Including SCHIP information in report card mailings.
8. Having the school-based health center serve as an application center for SCHIP.
9. Collaborating with community groups to provide financial incentives to enroll uninsured children (Council of Chief State School Officers, 2001 cited in NASN, 2002).

In 2004, the National Education Association (NEA) and the Children's Health Insurance (CHI) encouraged teachers, school administrators, counselors and school nurses to join a national effort to connect children with affordable healthcare coverage. They provide free Back to School Action Kits with suggestions and materials for school program emphasis (NEA-CHI 2004). This program or other similar programs of these organizations will assist in enrolling all eligible students into programs providing healthcare coverage.

FEDERAL SCHOOL NUTRITION PROGRAMS AND ISSUES RELATED TO VENDING MACHINES

Scenario: *A school board member, the school nurse, and the physical education department chair are asked to represent their school district at a state education agency meeting that introduces ideas and concrete suggestions for implementing a wellness program for students and staff. Materials include plans for nutrition education and school lunch reform. The school nurse and the PE teacher have already implemented some steps to motivate students and staff on their campuses and the school board member, a dietician, has been questioning the quality of the school lunch program for several years. At the conference they strategize with some parents, teachers, school nurses, and food service personnel. The debate involves understanding how the Federal food commodity system works to defray expenses for the district as well as the value of the vending machine profits for each school campus.*

Issues

1. Does district administration, including the school board, support national and local concerns on the quality of school meals?
2. Do administrators utilize federal reports of the effects of hunger and/or inadequate diets on health and learning?
3. Do administrators utilize health reports related to the epidemic of childhood obesity and the link to food in the school?
4. What is the "big picture" for the food services budget? What percent of the food service budget depends on the federal commodities program?
5. Do district food service menus reflect the tenets of nutrition curriculums?
6. How much revenue from vending machines or other moneymaking ventures (popcorn sales, carnivals, etc.) is used to subsidize education dollars for basics and for enrichment?
7. What alternative money-generating projects that do not involve non-nutritive foods are readily available?

Policy and Management

It is difficult to change ingrained lifestyle patterns, yet it is known that good nutrition among school-age children and adolescents results in increased cognitive development, increased attention span, higher test scores, better attendance, and fewer behavior problems in school (AAP, 2004). Yet, the food companies that buy ads for distribution through the various media, constantly sent their message to buy foods that are often non-nutritious, fat laden or sugar filled items. School districts need to partner with families and the healthcare community to wean staff, parents, and their "couch potato" children off chips, pizza, sodas, and so forth and increase their exercise.

The latest published Youth Risk Behavior Surveillance - 2003 (Centers for Disease Control and Prevention [CDC], 2004, p. 1) reported that 78% of teenagers do not eat the recommended five fruits and vegetables/day; 33.4% report insufficient amounts of physical activity; and 13.5% are overweight for height. What will the health and knowledge of these children be as they become adults and parents themselves? How much responsibility do schools have for sound nutritional and health information? Integrating information about healthy nutrition throughout school activities and modeling sound nutrition via a coordinated school health program approach are means of correcting this problem.

Under laws promulgated by the Department of Agriculture, surplus agricultural commodities are distributed to schools. Initially this program addressed the problem of childhood hunger via the National School Lunch Program. In 1966, the program was expanded to include a school breakfast program. "Students from families with incomes at or below 130% of the poverty level receive meals free, while those between 130% and 185% of the poverty level pay a reduced price" (AAP, 2004, p. 154). Schools are reimbursed based on the number of full price, reduced price, and free meals they serve.

Food service staff for the school district usually develop school menus based on the commodities available from the USDA as well as nutrition guidelines for age. Because the commodities do not supply all required nutrients, the district must purchase the other foods. Schools may contract with food service vendors to provide all or part of the food-related services. Some school administrators have entered into corporate sponsorships with commercial food companies for guaranteed external funds. These come with a cost, as schools must guarantee that their foods and beverages will be the only ones served. This may include setting up vending machines, advertising on book covers, and hanging posters in the school and at school events (AAP, 2004).

One example of a state taking action is the Texas Department of Agriculture (TDA) guidelines that limit fat content and portion size and prohibit fast food chains from being on a public school campus during the school day. The TDA goal was written with community input, including PTAs and PTOs; their goals are to provide healthier food for students (Zuniga, 2004).

There is a mounting drive to eliminate or curtail student access to vending machine drinks and snacks. Vending machine profits may be prized moneymakers for a school or district or a pet PTA/PTO project; therefore it is important to find out why vending machines or outside food vendors are in the school before beginning a campaign to modify or abolish them. According to an industry statistic, an estimated 20,000 schools have vending machines in their corridors, common areas, and gymnasiums. Yet, federal and state governments heavily regulate where and how vending machines can be used. Federal laws prohibit the sale of foods that have "little nutritional value" in competition with the school lunch program (School Vending Machines Generate Funds, 2004). State laws are often stricter. California has banned vending machines from elementary and middle schools (Chang, 2004).

The National Secondary School Principals' Association recommends that "the importance of providing healthy choices to students, faculty, and school visitors should be paramount for school officials in discussions with beverage companies" (Engein, 2004, p. 1). Schools should provide alternatives to soda and candy. This report for principals provides important guidelines when contracting with vending machine companies. However, the National Soft Drink Association says parents and local school districts, not states, should determine what children eat and drink in school. The trade group says soft drink companies already offer a variety of drinks to students including bottled water, juice and sports drinks (Chang, 2004).

In a Center for Science in the Public Interest survey (School Vending Machines "Dispensing Junk," 2004) of schools in Illinois, with 13,650 drink vending machines, 70% stocked sodas, juice drinks with less than 50% juice, iced tea, or sports drinks. Some 12% of the available drinks were water and 5% were milk, but only whole or 2% milk. Vending machines with snack foods had candy (42%), chips (25%) and sweet baked goods (13%).

Augenblick and Silverstein (2003), national cost consultants for school districts, use formulas to project district financial costs. Some items considered include the enrollment and adjustments associated with the proportion of students in special education programs, students eligible for free/reduced-price lunch, and limited-English proficient (LEP) students. Then there are textbooks, salaries, maintenance, etc. Expenses are high.

What food commodities does the school plan rely on for their food budget? How much whole milk and yellow cheese is provided at no cost? These and other federal commodities save school districts a lot of money. For success, it is important to work within the system.

The school nurse, along with others interested in improving nutritional intake in the school setting, should be prepared and garner support before approaching administrators with a plan to eliminate or introduce healthful food goals. The resources at the end of this chapter provide information on plans already prepared by the CDC. You will be more successful if you can include an administrator, parents, food service personnel, and the district dietician, if one is available, in your plan.

In addition, be prepared with simple, no cost strategies for incorporating exercise activities into classroom drills. Look at what is available in your community; seek out proactive, supportive people for nutrition reform or monitoring, if your community has a sound nutrition program. Written school board policies for dietary modifications in food services may already exist but may have been ignored. If vending machines must stay in the school, determine where they should be and what should be sold in them. In addition to vending machines, discourage fund-raising efforts that involve selling candy; multiple alternatives now exist to sell wrapping paper and other gifts instead.

Ask about the amount of money vending machines bring into the school monthly. Perhaps parents or community businesses would subsidize that amount? Find out where the profit from vending machines or popcorn sales goes. Understand the school's financial plan and school or district goals. Revenue is usually accounted for to the penny; understand the expenses before you propose modifications. There is daily media attention to the growing size of Americans, yet people continue to eat and not exercise. Encourage no cost exercise programs. Publish the nutritional plan and how it meets nutrition standards. School staff need to be good role models regarding their choices for meals and snacks. School personnel, whether administrators, teachers, bus drivers, or school nurses, also may not "walk their talk." It is best to lead by example. A school team committed to making a difference in the health of their students will be discussing food choices and participating in physical exercise daily.

Materials for teaching about informed choices and exercise programs can be started with minimal expense. Check with local voluntary organizations, county extension agencies, registered dieticians at local hospitals, and state education agencies for current, reliable information.

THE ENVIRONMENT: CONDITIONS AND AIR QUALITY INSIDE AND OUTSIDE THE SCHOOL

Scenario 1: *A school district called the health department when 15 students in one school were sent home with abdominal complaints and flu-like symptoms. For the most part the students were feeling well when they arrived at school. The health department epidemiological division sent personnel to the school within the hour. Air and surface residue in air ducts and in the cafeteria were collected and a thorough history was collected via phone on each student. As more students and a few staff appeared in the school health office with similar complaints, the health deparment asked parents for permission to draw students' blood and collect urine samples as well. The school was closed the next day and more illnesses were reported. Everyone recovered quickly, the building air ducts were cleaned even though no organisms were ever identified. In all 45 students and staff missed an average of three days from school.*

Scenario 2: *Smith Elementary School is located within 2 miles of several chemical processing plants. Last week everyone in the community heard the sirens give one continuous blast that lasted for 10 minutes. The school went into lockdown mode which included turning off the ventilation system and moving everyone to the inside classrooms. The principal anticipated a call from the factory risk manager announcing that this was a drill, but no call came. Parents began arriving at school, some on foot, to pick up their children. Parents have been notified that in the event of a lockdown for any reason, no one would leave the building and no one could enter. Community members were allowed to enter the gymnasium by an unlocked, outer door, but could not enter the building.*

Issues

- What is the school nurse's role in monitoring air and water quality on campuses?
- Are action plans (or school crisis plans) in place for sudden multiple illnesses in the school? (See Chapter 10.)
- How does air and water quality impact on students with special needs?

Problems

"A school environment is the complex interaction of the physical plant (the building and grounds), the occupants (staff, students, parents, visitors), the furnishings (equipment and room materials), and activities (eating, physical activity, lab work, cleaning, healthcare, cooking, and industrial shop). Schools provide specialty areas that include art, music, classrooms, cafeteria, science, swimming pool, industrial shop, consumer science, office, health office, gymnasiums, sports fields, grounds, playgrounds, bus areas, and parking lots, as well as heating/cooling ventilation areas and storage and custodial spaces" (NASN, 2004).

The quality of air and water can be affected by bacteria and toxins that can cause health problems. Some exposures that result in adverse health effects for children depend on the agent, dose, age of the student, the length of exposure, the route of exposure, individual sensitivities, and the student's health status. Exposures of most concern involve those causing neurotoxic effects. Because so many mineral, chemical, and biological contaminants are now recognized to impact on human health, it is even more important to manage the school environments to eliminate potential toxins and allergens.

Monitoring Outside Air Quality

States have established ambient air monitoring sites, which collect and report detailed data for volatile organic compounds, nitrogen oxides, ozone, and meteorological parameters. This is in response to the 1990 Clean Air Act Amendments, in which the U.S. Environmental Protection Agency (EPA) requires more extensive monitoring of ozone and its precursors in areas with persistently high ozone levels (mostly large metropolitan areas). States and the EPA are collecting data to better understand the underlying causes of ozone and air quality pollution, to devise effective remedies and to measure environmental improvement (U.S. Environmental Protection Agency, 2004). There are 10 regional data collection and education areas covering all 50 states (http://www.epa.gov/ttn/ atw/nata/index.html).

The last step of the EPA's national-scale assessment is to characterize the quantitative estimates of risk posed by 32 common air toxins identified by the EPA's Integrated Urban Air Toxics Strategy. The 33rd air toxin in this assessment, diesel particulate matter, is reported separately in a more qualitative manner. These air toxins were chosen because they pose the greatest potential risks to public health in urban areas (U.S. Environmental Protection Agency [U.S. EPA], 2004). Investigation is exploring the risk of both cancer and noncancer effects from inhalation of these air toxics nationwide, in both urban and rural areas.

Federal regulation of environmental toxins in schools began with the passage of the Asbestos Hazard Emergency Response Act (AHERA) in 1986 (U.S. EPA, 2003). Ozone alert readings are sometimes reported with the weather in areas with chronic ozone problems. Ozone alerts can occur for miles around centers of manufacturing. Local health departments have Web sites so school personnel receive instant alerts when air quality is in question. Ozone alerts have caused schools to cancel field trips and restrict physical education and recess to indoor activities.

Suburban and rural areas have their own air quality problems, if large-scale animal feeding farms, usually for chickens, beef and pigs, are located near where people live. Sewage holding ponds permeate the air with noxious odors for nearby residents. In addition the refuse can seep into the ground water causing local pollution of water. Additional issues can include management of water contamination by reduction of infectious organisms, mercury, and polychlorinated biphenyls (PCBs).

Monitoring Air Quality Inside a School

"The building, its occupants, and their activities, as well as equipment and supplies, must be maintained and controlled in a way that uses existing knowledge and practices to promote the health of the inhabitants" (NASN, 2004, p. 1). The school nurse should be acquainted with the facilities coordinator and ask when and how the school plant is inspected. It is important to know who to call before a problem arises related to the air and water quality within the school. For example, outbreaks of Legionnaires' disease still occur in office buildings, cruise ships, and schools. The first report of the illness was in the 1980s when an American Legion group was meeting at a hotel (Legionnaires' disease on rise in hospitals, nursing homes, 2004). Many people became ill with flu-like symptoms (hence the name of these water-borne bacterial (*Legionella*) or fungal (*Aspergillus*) organisms that grow and contaminate water faucets and air conditioning systems.

Remembering that the school environment is part of the coordinated school health effort (Chapter 3), the nurse is concerned with preventing adverse health reactions for students exposed to physical, chemical, and biological toxins occurring in the school environment. This includes prevention of asthma aggravation by exposure to particulates, such as tobacco smoke, dust mites, and cockroach parts. The school nurse is also concerned with exposures that could disturb the learning capacity (lead) or could be implicated in acute illness and allergy (mold) (U.S. Department of Labor [USDL, 2003), chronic illness (asbestos), or cancer (radon, tobacco smoke, ultraviolet light exposure) (NASN, 2004). Ventilation systems in homes or schools can harbor bacteria, molds, viruses, and other toxins (Rosenfeld, 2004). Mold can result from leaking air conditioning units, excessive humidity, leaking roofs, damp carpets, and areas that have a great deal of water, such as bathrooms, kitchens, and shower/ changing areas for physical education.

NASN prepared an Issue Brief on the School Health Nursing Services Role in Healthcare: Environmental Concerns In The School Setting (2004). It covers a wide range of environmental concerns including asbestos, radon, ultraviolet light, lead, mercury, tobacco smoke, carbon monoxide, particulate matter, solvents and volatile organic compounds (VOCs), pesticides (organophosphates, carbamates, organochlorines), noise, molds, animal dander, fur saliva, and feathers, and cockroach parts.

Some environmental toxins that may impair the health of children and/or occur as school exposures are listed below:

- **Asbestos**

  Source: Disturbed or deteriorating asbestos-containing building materials (insulation, ceilings, floor tiles)

  Effects: Lung cancer, mesothelioma, asbestosis
- **Radon**

  Source: Radioactive decay of radium in the earth core

  Effects: Cancer
- **Ultraviolet light**

  Source: Outdoor sun exposure

  Effects: Skin erythema, sunburn, melanoma, nonmelanoma skin cancer

- **Lead**

  Source: Deteriorating paint, dust, soil, water (via solder absorption)

  Effects: Decreased cognitive ability, attention dysfunction, aggression; deterred grow pattern, headaches, loss of appetitive, decreased activity, vomiting, convulsions

- **Mercury**

  Source: Industrial discharges in water, equipment containing mercury (thermometers, sphygmomanometers, thermal switches)

  Effects:

  1. Inhalation of elemental mercury vapor: necrotizing bronchitis and pneumonitis, central nervous system effects (tremor, insomnia, forgetfulness, loss of appetite, emotional lability, memory impairment)
  2. Consumption of organic mercury in food (fish and food treated with mercury): central nervous system effects include weakness, visual and hearing impairment, tremor, muscle spasticity, paresthesias, ataxia, coma, death

- **Environmental tobacco smoke**

  Source: Tobacco smoke environments

  Effects: Respiratory tract illness, middle ear effusions, asthma and asthma exacerbation, cancer

- **Carbon monoxide**

  Source: Combustion of fuel in furnace boilers and vehicles (e.g., idling vehicles in school parking lots near air intake)

  Effects: Headache, dizziness, fatigue, drowsiness, nausea, vomiting, loss of consciousness

- **Particulate matter**

  Source: Outdoor air pollution

  Effects: Asthma aggravation, respiratory irritation

- **Solvents and volatile organic compounds (VOCs)**

  Source: Formaldehyde, construction materials, acetone, paint solvents, machine degreasers, acetone, benzene

  Effects: Mucocutaneous irritation, respiratory effects, rhinitis, nasal congestion, rash, pruritus, headache, nausea, vomiting

- **Pesticides (organophosphates, carbamates, organochlorines)**

  Source: Agriculture, pest management, lice treatment

  Effects: Neurological impairment including behavioral disturbances, impaired coordination, depressed cognition, coma, fatigue, irritability, depression, tremor

- **Noise**

  Source: Multiple

  Effects: Noise-induced hearing loss, psychological effects

- **Molds**

  Source: Ubiquitous in the environment. Some species are known to produce adverse health effects.

  Effects: Eye, nose, throat irritation; allergic or toxic reaction; asthma aggravation

- **Animal dander, fur saliva, and feathers**

  Source: Pets

  Effects: Allergic reactions for susceptible persons, asthma aggravation

- **Cockroach parts**

  Source: Roach infestations are common in numerous areas including housing, other buildings, and outside areas

  Effects: Allergic reactions for susceptible persons, asthma aggravation

  (NASN, 2004)

Policy and Management

The school nurse should be a major player on the school crisis team or action team. These teams are part of the safe and secure school initiatives and they may go by many names. Planning for school emergencies requires the cooperative effort of all the school staff to provide for the safety of everyone in the building. A school-wide action plan (or school crisis plan [Chapter 10]) must be in place. Plans to move students to a safe place must be developed and known to all staff for incidents such as noxious odors in the school or the lock-down of the building if noxious odors are being emitted from a nearby petrochemical plant.

Planning and preparedness are required for school health services personnel. Everyone will be counting on the nurse for counsel and reassurances. In this age of cellular phones, perhaps the school would be able to provide this for the nurse's use. Parents should know in advance of an emergency that their school takes their responsibility for their child seriously and plans are in place. The school nurse's role is to plan and prepare some type of portable means for moving IHPs and EAPs, medications, treatment materials, first aid supplies, and emergency information cards for students and staff. If everyone is relocated off site, the nurse may plan to have fragile students located near the first aid setup. IHPs, 504 plans, and emergency action plans should be developed for students with health needs, including allergies and sensitivities to environmental agents. The NASN Issue Brief contains many interventions.

The school nurse is the health expert in the school building and can provide scientifically sound information about environmental issues and exposures. The maintenance department is responsible for cleaning the building, maintaining the heating, cooling, and ventilation systems, and doing building repairs. The school nurse can be of assistance by serving on committees or serving as a consultant regarding these activities as they may impact on safe environmental practices. The Occupational Health and Safety Administration (OSHA) (U.S. Department of Labor, 2004) has many regulations that impact on the safety of school workers, especially those relating to occupational exposure to environmental toxins. The school nurse can assist in implementing safety standards and in making the standards understandable and applicable to the school setting (NASN, 2004).

NASN (2004) recommends the following interventions for the school nurse related to environmental health:

- Develop IHPs, emergency plans, or 504 plans to address individual student sensitivities and health needs.
- Develop IHPs, emergency plans, or 504 plans for persons with health impairments from toxin exposure.
- Develop a school committee to implement the EPA's *Tools for Schools IAQ Management* program.
- Be aware of asbestos compliance activities (AHERA) in your school and district.
- Promote use of an Integrated Pest Management system for insect control in the school.
- Support environmental toxin exposure risk and management education programs for staff and children.
- Follow hazardous waste management (EPA) policies in your school and district.
- Participate in educational opportunities about environmental toxins, their health impact, reduction, and exposure prevention.
- Participate in OSHA-required Workplace Safety Teams to develop policies and practices that reduce hazard exposure.
- Be familiar with OSHA-required Material Safety Data Sheets, their content, and where to obtain them in your school.
- Become familiar with resources on promoting reduction of toxic exposures in children.
- Participate in community programs to protect children from environmental toxic exposure.
- Promote school and district policy development for management of potential hazards and activities in schools that advance safe environmental management.
- Support and enforce smoke-free school environments. Support students and staff who are interested in addressing environmental issues.
- Be aware of immediate care actions and first aid for persons exposed to chemical spills, toxin inhalation, or other toxin exposure.
- Assist in development of school and district Emergency Response Plans for chemical or toxin exposures.

TELEMEDICINE—TELEHEALTH

Scenario: *John, age 8, has had asthma for 6 years. John lives in a rural farming area that is 140 miles from the nearest medical facility, a hospital with 150 beds, five physicians and a nurse practitioner. John's parents work on a farm 30 miles from the school. The school district where John is enrolled has a telemedicine unit managed on site by two registered school nurses. The district also employs two clinic assistants. The district received a grant to help finance the telemedicine unit, so there is no cost for parents to use this service at this time. The network is connected to a room at the area hospital and to a medical center 200 miles from the community. Now consults and treatments are paid for through the grant and every student is eligible. The school nurse monitors John's peak flow tests and medications and has called for a consult because John has been in the yellow zone for two days and is coughing frequently. His temperature is normal, but peak flows are not. His throat and tympanic membrane are reddened. The nurse faxed the peak flow report and medication administration (home and school) forms after making the appointment. The physician examines John's ears when the nurse inserts an otoscope with the camera attached. John answers the physician's questions. A diagnosis of an acute upper respiratory infection is made and antibiotics are recommended. An order will be sent to the local pharmacy for the parents to pick up and suggestions for follow up care will be with the prescription for the parents. John must continue to see the school nurse for peak flow testing and a follow up appointment is set for one week.*

Definitions

E-health is the broad category of health merged with electronics or technology in some manner (American Telemedicine Association, 2004). Telemedicine and telehealth are actually subsets of e-health.

Telemedicine or telehealth is a subset of e-health. It is the delivery of actual patient health care over a videoconferencing or telecommunications system.

Telehealth is more specific and encompasses evaluations and education via technology.

Telepharmacy is the same system between a pharmacy and the local site where the pharmacist uses a video-conference session to oversee the dispensing of prepackaged medications to patients while they are at the telemedicine clinic. The client can interact with the pharmacist as well (Telepharmacy Goes Online, 2003).

Issues

What are the legal and practice parameters for telemedicine?

What about confidentiality of the telemedicine examination?

Policy and Management

Every state has at least one telemedicine contact. These sites are available on-line or can be found by calling the state health department for information. Telemedicine should use the same standards of care found in more traditional forms of medicine. The healthcare provider-patient relationship and interaction is a two-way communication; the process should be similar to the patient having the healthcare practitioner in the same room (Texas Tech University, 2004).

There are federal grants, such as from the National Institutes of Health, and foundation grants for start up costs and on-going expenses (see references for national associations). Training is provided for a fee at several locations. For example, The Texas Tech Center for Telemedicine (Lubbock, TX) offers a course called Telemedicine 101 (Texas Tech University, 2004). This 8-hour course provides a broad overview of telemedicine in a small group setting. Participants are able to discuss their organization's telemedicine needs and determine which applications are appropriate. A hands-on practicum is provided to familiarize participants with the technology. This Center and others will also customize trainings, provide ongoing continuing education, and collaborate on-site.

Most telemedicine occurs over specialized videoconferencing equipment with special medical peripheral equipment called Consult Carts and Teledoc Carts (Texas Tech University, 2004). Carts can include EKG equipment, an electronic stethoscope, and special exam cameras attached to the system, such as an otoscope. The physician, nurse practitioner, or physician's assistant at the base and the patient at the remote site communicate via special high-speed telephone lines or satellite. The system is completely interactive, meaning that both parties can talk back and forth, carrying on a live, interactive conversation as if they were in the same room face-to-face. Computer based telemedicine systems also allow for digital images to be stored and sent to a physician at a later time (Texas Tech University, 2004).

Telemedicine is the same as going to the healthcare practitioner's office. Most physicians agree that any limitations created by the separation of healthcare practitioner and patient are more than outweighed by the benefits of providing the distant patient with more immediate access to quality healthcare. A physician can see and hear almost anything over the system that they would see or hear in their office in the presence of the patient. However, the physician cannot touch or feel the patient. The remote provider, in many cases a nurse, who is with the patient touches and feels the patient at the direction of the physician.

The same reasonable and customary standards of confidentiality applied to patients and their records are continued with telemedicine examinations. Providers must adhere to strict patient confidentiality measures and comply with the requirements for the Health Insurance Portability and Accountability Act (HIPAA) (see Chapter 13).

Laws and rules pertaining to the practice of medicine will also apply to telemedicine. The key is to not let the technology alter the manner in which the physician practices. The healthcare provider is advised to not take chances or make assumptions because of the technology. Rather, the healthcare provider needs to refer the patient for an in-person visit as needed. Healthcare providers must be licensed to practice medicine in every state in which they practice, so state boarders must be observed for site locations.

The American Nurses Association (ANA) has participated in the national dialogue on telemedicine/telehealth since 1996. ANA's position provides guidance for all professional nurses.

> ANA strongly believes that the strength and promise of telehealth lie in providing increased access to healthcare services by augmenting existing services, not in replacing them. Telehealth technologies should not be used to replace needed access to in-person healthcare services. The potential for abuse of these technologies by providing "cheaper" substitutes for in-person care needed in homes, communities, schools, nursing homes, hospitals, and other settings requires the development and enforcement of standards that ensure these technologies will be used appropriately. (ANA, 1997, p. 2)

School nurses have been on the forefront of telemedicine. The process allows students to receive an evaluation by a healthcare professional without the student having to leave school; fundamental to its effectiveness, however, is the presence of a licensed professional on both ends of the transmission to assure accurate input and subsequent directed intervention (the registered nurse/school nurse) and the other to provide diagnosis and prescriptive interventions. While School-based Health Centers could provide the same services, difficulty keeping them funded has resulted in this technology-driven approach.

Young and Ireson (2003) examined the effectiveness of a telehealth program in an elementary school. Of the 3461 visits to the school nurses, 150 telehealth referrals were made. The most common diagnoses were otitis media, pharyngitis, dermatitis, and upper respiratory infections. Providers, school nurses, students, and families were very satisfied with the system and it saved families from $101 to $224 per encounter. The service was also able to provide telepsychiatric evaluations.

It is the position of the National Association of School Nurses that technology has the potential to greatly enhance the services provided by the school nurse, but not to replace in-person healthcare provided by the registered professional school nurse (NASN, 2002). Therefore, the issues of telehealth in the school setting must be thoroughly evaluated, and school nurses practicing in this new environment must partner with regulatory and professional agencies to develop and use standards for safe and effective practice.

CONCLUSION

Each of the issues addressed in this chapter requires investigation, consensus, and discussion after all players consider their personal views and the needs of the student for a specific situation. The school nurse must be a member of the decision-making team when issues affect the health and safety of students in his or her care. A review of the ethical decision-making processes will help the school nurse as well as all others involved seek the best ethical decision.

Resources

American Nurses Association (ANA). (1997). ANA policy series: *Telehealth–Issues for nursing.* Washington, DC: Author.

American Telemedicine Association—http://www.atmeda.org/Q&A; video clip, information.

Center for Disease Control and Prevention (2004). Retrieved on September 11, 2004 from http://www.cdc.gov/nccdphp/dnpa/npa–proj.htm.

Links from this site:
- 5-A-Day for Better Health
- ACES: Active Community Environments Initiative
- BAM! Body and Mind™
- IMMPaCt, International Micronutrient Malnutrition Prevention and Control Program
- KidsWalk–to–School
- National Bone Health Campaign
- Obesity and Overweight State Programs
- Well–Integrated Screening and Evaluation for Women Across the Nation (WISEWOMAN)

The Youth Media Campaign, *VERB™*

Fairchild, B. & Hayward, N. (1998). *Now that you know: A parents' guide to understanding their gay and lesbian children* (3rd ed.). New York: A Harvest Book, Harcourt, Brace & Company.

Health Issues for LGBTQ *Students: What you should know and how you can help*. Welcome/Mission. Health Centers. Services. Departments. Immunizations. Insurance. Health Information. Ask The Staff. Forms. Student Involvement. Links/Resources www.health.rutgers.edu/sexual_health/lgbtq.asp.

Kissen, R. (2002). *Getting ready for Benjamin: Preparing teachers for sexual diversity in the classroom*. Lanham, MD: Rowman & Littlefield Publishers.

Outland, O. (2000). *Coming out: A handbook for men*. Los Angeles: Alyson Publications.

PFLAG (Parents, Families and Friends of Lesbians and Gays) offers support groups, educational outreach, and more to families and friends of gay, lesbian, intersexual, and transgender family members (202–467–8180 and www.pflag.org).

Savin-Williams, R. (2001). *Mom, dad, I'm gay: How families negotiate coming out*. Washington, DC: American Psychological Association.

Telemedicine Information Exchange—http://tie.telemed.org/

Telehealth Network— http://telehealth.net/

Texas Tech University Health Sciences Center—http://www.ttuhsc.edu/telemedicine.

Young, T., & Ireson, C. (2003). Effectiveness of school-based telehealth care in urban and rural elementary schools. *Pediatrics, 112*(5), 1088–1094.

Posters

Safe Zone Poster: National Youth Advocacy Coalition—Bridges Project (www.nyacyouth.org).

This Is A Safe Place To Talk About ... Poster. Wildflower Resource Network (wrnetwork@aol.com).

For lead in drinking water, look at http://www.epa.gov/superfund/programs/lead/health.htm.

For ozone information and to check quality of air locally, look on http://www.epa.gov/epahome/ozone.htm.

For more on lung safety and enrichment activities, look at the American Lung Association Web site at http://www.lungusa.org.

References

Aiken, T. (2004). *Legal, ethical, and political issues in nursing*. Philadelphia: F. A. Davis.

Allergy & Asthma Today. (Summer 2004). Publication of the Allergy & Asthma Network Mothers of Asthmatics.

American Academy of Child and Adolescent Psychiatry (AACAP). (1990). *Drug and alcohol screening, policy statement*. Retrieved August 12, 2004 from http://www.aacap.org/publications/policy/ps21.htm

American Academy of Child and Adolescent Psychiatry (AACAP). (1998). *Children who won't go to school*. Facts for families, Number 7: Retrieved August 4, 2004 from http://www.aacap.org/publications/factsfam/noschool.htm

American Academy of Pediatrics (AAP), Committee on School Health and Committee on Bioethics. (2000). Do not resuscitate orders in schools. *Pediatrics, 105* (4), 878–879.

American Academy of Pediatrics (AAP). (2003). Guidelines for the Administration of Medication in School. *Pediatrics, 112* (3), 697–699.

American Academy of Pediatrics (AAP). (2004). *School health policy and practice*. Elk Grove Village, IL: Author.

American College Health Association (ACHA). (1999). *Drug education / testing of student athletes*. Retrieved August 8, 2004 from/http://acha.orginfo-resourcesguidelines.cfm

American Nurses Association (ANA). (2001). *Code of ethics for nurses*. Washington, DC: American Nurses Publishing.

American Psychological Association (APA). (2002). *Developing adolescents: A reference for professionals*. Washington, DC: APA.

American Psychological Association (APA). (2004). *Controlling anger before it controls you*. Retrieved August 4, 2004 from http://www.helping.apa.org/daily/anger.html.

American Telemedicine Association (ATA). (2004). Retrieved January 10, 2004 from http://www.atmeda.org/

Augenblick, J., & Silverstein, J. (2003). *An estimation of the total cost of implementing the results of the school finance adequacy study*. Retrieved August 12, 2004 from www.msbanet.org/pdf/PhaseIIReport.pdf

Baker, M., Sigmon, J., & Nugent, M. (2001). *Truancy reduction: Keeping students in school*. Washington, DC, U.S. Department of Justice, Office of Justice Programs, Office of Juvenile Justice and Delinquency Prevention.

Bakker, L. J., & Cavender, A. (2003). Promoting culturally competent care for gay youth. *Journal of School Nursing, 19*(2), 65–72.

Behrman, R. (Ed.). (2003). Health insurance for children. Statement of purpose; Glossary of terms. *The Future of Children, 13*(1), 246248. Retrieved August 12, 2004 from http://www.futureofchildren.org

Bennett, C., & Shields, M., (Eds.). (2003). *Health insurance for children: Issues and ideas. A guide for policy makers and the press*. Retrieved August 12, 2004 from http://www.futureofchildren.org

Benton, J. (2003). Making schools safer and healthier for lesbian, gay, bisexual, and questioning students. *Journal of School Nursing, 19*(5), 251–259.

Centers for Disease Control and Prevention (CDC). (1999). *Young people at risk: HIV / AIDS among America's youth*. Atlanta: Author.

Centers for Disease Control and Prevention (CDC). (2000). *HIV among African Americans*. Atlanta: Author.

Center for Disease Control and Prevention (CDC). (2004). *Youth risk behavior surveillance–United States, 2003. Morbidity & Mortality Weekly Report, 53* (SS-2). Retrieved September 11, 2004 from http://www.cdc.gov/HealthyYouth/YRBS.

Centers for Medicare and Medicaid Services (CMMS). (2004). *State children's health insurance program*. Retrieved August 12, 2004 from/http://www.cms.hhs.gov/schip/about-SCHIP.asp

Center for Substance Abuse Treatment. (CSAT). (2003). *A provider's introduction to substance abuse treatment for lesbian, gay, bisexual, and transgender individuals*. Rockville, MD: U.S. Department of Health and Human Services.

Chang, A. (2004). *Schools across U.S. target vending machines in obesity controversy: States target school vending machines in battle against childhood obesity*. Organic Consumers Association. Retrieved on September 11, 2004 from http://www.organicconsumers.org/school/obesity031904.cfm.

Cohn, D., Gelfman, M., & Schwab, N. (2001). Adolescent issue and rights of minors. In N. Schwab & M. Gelfman (Eds.), *Legal issues in school health services: A resource for school administrators, school attorneys and school nurses* (pp. 248–250). North Branch, MN: Sunrise River Press.

Costante, C. (2001). Do Not Resuscitate in the School Setting: Determining the Policy and Procedures. In N. Schwab & M. Gelfman (Eds.), *Legal issues in school health services: A resource for school administrators, school attorneys and school nurses* (pp. 419–437). North Branch, NM: Sunrise River Press.

Dekalb, J. (1999). Student truancy. ERIC Digest, Number 125. ERIC Clearinghouse on Educational Management. Retrieved August 23, 2004 from http://www.ericfacility.net/ericdigests/ed 429334.html

Engein, J. (2004). *Business partnerships: NASSP guidelines for school-beverage partnerships*. Retrieved September 12, 2004 from http://www.nassp.org/schoolimprove/school_beverage_partnerships.cfm.

Environmental Protection Agency. (2004). *Enhanced ozone monitoring (PAMS)*. Retrieved October 2, 2005 from http://www.epa.gov/oar/oaqps/pams/.

Fibison, W. J. (2001). Future direction in school health care: The genetic revolution. In Schwab, N. C. & Gelfman, M. H. B. (Eds.), *Legal issues in school health* (pp. 483–488). North Branch, MN: Sunrise River Press.

Frankowski, B. and the Committee on Adolescence. (2004). Sexual orientation and adolescents. *Pediatrics, 113*(6), 1827–1832.

Fremont, W. (2003). School refusal in children and adolescents. *American Family Physician, 68*(4), 1555–1560.

Gregory, E. K. (2000). Empowering students on medication for asthma to be active participants in their care: An exploratory study. *Journal of School Nursing, 16*(1),20–27.

Gunga, F., Cox, A., Rosenbaum, M., & Appel, J. (2003). *Making sense of student drug testing: Why educators are saying no*. Retrieved August 3, 2004, from http// www.drugtestingfails.org/pdf/drug_testing_booklet.pdf

Harrison, T. (2003). Adolescent homosexuality and concerns regarding disclosure. *Journal of School Health, 73*(3), 107–112.

Heller, K. W., & Tumlin, J. (2004). Using expanded individualized educational care plans to assist teachers of students with complex health care needs. *Journal of School Nursing, 20* (3), 150–160.

Hergenroeder, A. C., & Neinstein, L. S. (2002). Guidelines in sports medicine. In Neinstein, L. S. (Ed.), *Adolescent health care: A practical guide* (4th ed., pp. 280–428). Philadelphia: Lippincott, Williams, & Wilkins.

Hootman, J., Schwab, N. C., Gelfman, M. H. B., Gregory, E. K., & Pohlman, K. J. (2001). School nursing practice: Clinical performance. In Schwab, N. C. & Gelfman, M. H. B. (Eds.), *Legal issues in school health* (pp. 167–229). North Branch, MN: Sunrise River Press.

Houck, G. L., & Perri, C. (2002). A support group for absentee middle school students. *Journal of School Nursing, 18*(4), 201–205.

International Confederation of Childhood Cancer Organizations. (1999). *Guidelines for refusal, noncompliance, and abandonment of treatment in children and adolescents with cancer*. Working Committee on Psychosocial Issues in Pediatric Oncology. Retrieved August 8, 2004 from http://www.icccpo.org/articles/ psychosocial/guidelines_refusal.html

Jones, S., & Wheeler, L. (2004). Asthma inhalers in schools: Rights of students with asthma to a free appropriate education. *American Journal of Public Health, 94*(7), 1102–1108.

Karasik, L. (2003). Reducing school refusal: The school nurse role. Poster session presented at the annual meeting of the National Association of School Nurses, Cincinnati, Ohio.

Legionnaires' disease on rise in hospitals, nursing homes. (2004). *Nurse Week, 11*(17), 7.

Luhn, R. (1992). *Managing your anger. Menlo Park, CA: Crisp Publications.*

Mann, C., Rowland, D., & Garfield, R. (2003). Historical overview of children's health care coverage. *The Future of Children, 13*(1), 31–53. Retrieved August 12, 2004 from http://www.futureofchildren.org

Menahem, S., & Halasz, G. (2000). Parental noncompliance—a paediatric dilemma. A medical and psychodynamic perspective. *Child Care Health and Development, 26*(1), 61–72.

National Association of School Nurses (NASN). (1999). *Position statement: The use of asthma inhalers in the school setting*. Retrieved January 2005 from http:// www.nasn.org/positions/inhalers.htm.

National Association of School Nurses (NASN). (2000a). *Position statement: Do not resuscitate*. Scarborough, ME: NASN.

National Association of School Nurses (NASN). (2000b). *Position statement: Epinephrine use in life-threatening emergencies*. Retrieved 2004 from http://www.nasn.org

National Association of School Nurses (NASN). (2000c). *Position statement: Out-of-school educational field trips and camps*. Scarborough, ME: Author

National Association of School Nurses (NASN). (2001). *Position statement: Blood sugar monitoring in the school setting*. Retrieved 2004 from http://www.nasn.org/ positions

National Association of School Nurses (NASN). (2002a). Position statement: *Soft drinks and candy in the school setting*. Scarborough, ME: Author.

National Association of School Nurses (NASN). (2002b). *State children's health insurance program issue brief*. Retrieved/August/14,/2004 from at http:// www. nasn.org/briefs/schip.htm

National Association of School Nurses (NASN). (2002c). *Position statement: Use of telehealth in the practice of school nursing*. Accessed January 2005 from http:// www.nasn.org

National Association of School Nurses (NASN). (2003). *Issue brief: Sexual orientation and gender identity / expression*. Scarborough, ME: NASN. Retrieved April 6, 2004 from http://nasn.org/positions/orientation.htm.

Nationgal Association of School Nurses (NASN). (2004). *Issue brief: School health nursing services role in health care: Environmental concerns in the school setting*. Scarborough, ME: National Association of School Nurses.

National Drug Control Policy Office. (2002). *What you need to know about drug testing in schools*. Retrieved August 8, 2004 from http://whitehousedrugpolicy.gov

National Education Association (NEA), Health Information Network, and Children's Health Insurance. (2004). *Back to school – Get involved!* Retrieved August 20,2004 from http://www.Neahin.org/programs/ childhealth/backtoschool.htm

North American Nursing Diagnosis Association (NANDA). (1999). *Nursing diagnoses, definitions and classifications 1999–2000*. Philadelphia: Author

Paige, L. (1998). *School phobia, school avoidance and school refusal: A handout for parents. Communique, National Association of School Psychologists.* Retrieved August 12, 2004 from http://www.ldonline.org/ ld_indepth/ parenting/naspschool_avoidance.html

Rosenfeld, I. (2004). Second opinion. *Parade* (August 8, 2004), p. 18. *Rutgers University School Health Services Web Page*. (2004). Retrieved July 22, 2004 from http://www. health.rutgers.edu/sexual_health/ lgbtq.asp

Savin-Williams, R. C. (1998). The disclosure to families of same-sex attractions by lesbian, gay, and bisexual youth. *Journal of Research on Adolescence, 8*, 49–68.

School Vending Machines Generate Funds – and Controversy. (2004). *School Nurse*. Retrieved September 11, 2004 from http://www.schoolnurse.com/ med_info/vendingmech.html

School Vending Machines "Dispensing Junk." (2004). *Center for science in the public interest newsroom*. Retrieved on September 11, 2004 from http:// cspinet.org/new/pdf/dispensing_junk.pdf

Schubiner, H., Robin, A. L., & Neinstein, L. S. (2002). School problems and ADHD. In Neinstein, L. S. (Ed.), *Adolescent health care: A practical guide* (pp. 1454–1476). Philadelphia: Lippincott Williams & Wilkins.

Schwab, N. C., Gelfman, M. H. B., & Cohen, S. D. (2001). Fundamentals of U.S. Law. In N. C. Schwab and M. H. B. Gelfman (Eds.), *Legal issues in school health service* (pp. 55–79). North Branch, MN: Sunrise River Press.

Schwenk, T. (1997). Psychoactive drugs and athletic performance. *The Physician and Sports Medicine, 25*(1), 32–40.

Stanhope, M., & Lancaster, J. (2000). *Community & public health nursing* (6th ed.). St. Louis: C. V. Mosby.

Telepharmacy goes on line. (2003). *Telemedicine Report, 5*(1), 1. Retrieved on March 4, 2004 from http://www.ttuhsc.edu/telemedicine.

Texas Tech University. (2004). Retrieved January 10, 2004 from Telemedicine Technology at http://www.ttuhsc.edu/telemedicine.

U.S. Department of Labor, Occupational Safety and Health Administration (OSHA). (2003, October 10). *A brief guide to mold in the workplace*. Retrieved January 10, 2004, from http://www.osha.gov/dts/shib/shib101003.html

U.S. Department of Labor, Occupational Safety and Health Administration (OSHA). (2004). *Safety and health topics: Hazard communication*. Retrieved January 10, 2004, from http://www.osha.gov/SLTC/hazardcommunications/index.html

U.S. Environmental Protection Agency (EPA). (2003). *Asbestos in schools*. Retrieved January 10, 2004, from http://www.epa.gov/asbestos/asbestos_in_schools.htm

Velasquez, M., Andre, C., Shanks, T., S.J., & Meyer, M. J. (2003). *Thinking ethically: A framework for moral decision making*. Markkula Center for Applied Ethics. Retrieved on August 14, 2004 from htttp://www.scu.edu/ethics/practicing/decision.html

Velsor–Friedrich, B., Vlasses, F., Moberley, J., & Coover, L. (2004). Talking with teens about asthma management. *Journal of School Nursing, 20*, 140–148.

Wegger, G. (2004). *What to do when a kid gets mad! Exploring anger through a child's eye*. Presentation at the National Association of School Nurses 36th Annual Conference, Seattle, WA.

Wold, S. (2001). School Health Services: History and Trends. In N. Schwab & M., Gelfman (Eds.), *Legal issues in school health services: A resource for school administrators, school attorneys and school nurses* (pp. 7–54). North Branch, NM: Sunrise River Press.

Yamaguchi, R., Johnson, L., & O'Malley, P. (2003). Relationship between student illicit drug use and school drug testing policies. *Journal of School Health, 73* (4), 159—164.

Zuniga, J. A. (2004). Vendors, PTOs worried as schools banish fast food. *Houston Chronicle*, July 30, 2004, p. A8.

Index

Page numbers followed by b denote boxed material; those followed by c denote charts; those followed by f denote figures; those followed by t denote tables.

D

J

K

L

M

N

O

P

W

X